Mary Katharine Pokman
Meredith N.C. 353

S0-AGV-353

Medical-Surgical
Nursing

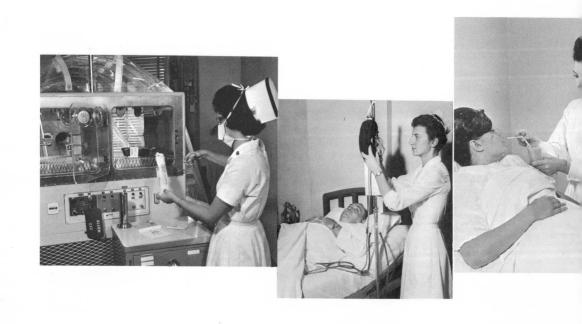

Medical-Surgical Nursing

KATHLEEN NEWTON SHAFER

JANET R. SAWYER

AUDREY M. McCLUSKEY

EDNA LIFGREN BECK

FOURTH EDITION

With 236 figures

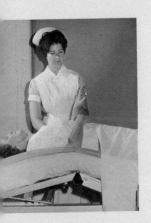

Saint Louis

The C. V. Mosby Company

1967

KATHLEEN NEWTON SHAFER, R.N., M.A.

*Formerly Associate Professor in Out-Patient Nursing,
Cornell University–New York Hospital School of Nursing, New
York, N. Y.; formerly Assistant Consultant in Orthopedic
Nursing, National League for Nursing Education; formerly
Instructor in Medical Nursing and Instructor in Surgical
Nursing, Cornell University–New York Hospital School of
Nursing, New York, N. Y.*

JANET R. SAWYER, R.N., A.M.

*Instructor, School of Education, Department of Nurse
Education, New York University, New York, N. Y.; formerly
Instructor in Surgical Nursing, Cornell University–New York
Hospital School of Nursing, New York, N. Y.; formerly
Instructor in Surgical Nursing, Hartford Hospital,
Hartford, Conn.*

AUDREY M. McCLUSKEY, R.N., M.A., Sc.M.Hyg.

*Director, Nursing Advisory Service of National League
for Nursing and National Tuberculosis Association;
formerly Supervisor, Hamden Public Health and Visiting
Nurse Association, Inc., Hamden, Conn.; formerly Associate
Professor in Nursing, Cornell University–New York Hospital
School of Nursing, New York, N. Y.; formerly Coordinator
of Nursing Instruction in Chronic Illness and Rehabilitation
and Instructor in Medical Nursing, Cornell University–New
York Hospital School of Nursing, New York, N. Y.*

EDNA LIFGREN BECK, R.N., M.A.

*Formerly Associate Director of Nursing Education, Muhlenberg
Hospital School of Nursing, Plainfield, N. J.; formerly
Assistant Professor in Fundamentals of Nursing and Instructor
in Surgical Nursing, Cornell University–New York Hospital
School of Nursing, New York, N. Y.; formerly Clinical
Instructor in Surgical Nursing, Roosevelt Hospital School of
Nursing, New York, N. Y.*

FOURTH EDITION
Copyright © 1967 by
THE C. V. MOSBY COMPANY

*All rights reserved.
No part of this book may be reproduced in any manner
without written permission of the publisher.
Previous editions copyrighted 1958, 1961, 1964
Printed in the United States of America
Library of Congress Catalog Card Number 67-13896
Distributed in Great Britain by Henry Kimpton, London*

*The illustration of a nurse passing sterile equipment through a
porthole in an isolator is courtesy National Institutes of
Health, Bethesda, Md.*

Preface

In this fourth edition of *Medical-Surgical
Nursing*, chapters have been altered substantially, and new material has been added to
bring the book up-to-date with current concepts in the health care of people and with
new developments in medical treatment and
related nursing care.

Each year the hospital becomes more and
more an integral part of the community as
demands upon it increase both for hospitalization and for short-term care in emergency
units and outpatient departments. Although
the importance of prevention has long been
recognized, the concept of prevention has
enlarged. Prevention may mean primary prevention of illness, prevention of progression
of disease, prevention of complications of
disease, or prevention of limitations in living
if handicaps do occur. The concept of the
patient's family as an integral force in his
progress during illness and of the need for
their involvement in any plans for his continuing care is now fully recognized. These
concepts are of vital importance to nurses
both during their school years and as professional practitioners. Therefore, changes in
the arrangement of chapters and emphasis
upon the presentation of material have been
made with them in mind.

With the conviction that the best learning takes place during the actual care of patients in the clinical situation, particular effort has been made in this edition to incorporate the principles of physiology and the other sciences as they relate to care of sick people of all age levels. As in previous editions, the emphasis is upon the whole patient and upon the patient as an individual regardless of his age level or his particular location during phases of treatment.

We acknowledge with gratitude the assistance of Mrs. Betty Pritchard Scott, R.N., in revising the section on nursing in accidents and emergencies in Chapter 13. We wish to thank Miss Margaret R. Bennell and Mrs. William H. McCarthy, Jr., librarians at the Muhlenberg Hospital in Plainfield, N. J., for their unfailing helpfulness; we appreciate the cooperation of Miss Shirley Baty who prepared the medical illustrations.

Kathleen Newton Shafer
Janet R. Sawyer
Audrey M. McCluskey
Edna Lifgren Beck

Contents

Contents

Section 2   **Nursing related to specific medical and surgical care**

Trends and problems influencing patient care

1

The patient and the nurse—
understanding,
interaction, and intervention

Study questions

1 Keep a record for a week of each patient for whom you care. Include the patient's age, his nationality, his place of birth, the language spoken in his home, his education, his place in his family, and his religion. Consider whether or not any of these influenced the nursing care you gave.
2 How has knowledge of the patient's background, as listed above, influenced your teaching of a patient during his preparation for leaving the hospital?
3 What are some of the ways in which anxiety may be expressed? List some questions that patients and members of their families have asked you that indicate anxiety.

Understanding of self and others and the use of self in interaction with others toward a therapeutic goal (the maintenance and restoration of health in people) is basic to all nursing care. In this chapter we can only highlight a few concepts that affect relationships with people. The nurse should deepen her understanding by reading and discussing the many articles and books devoted entirely to such topics as mental health, cultural patterns, emotional responses to illness, and interpersonal relationships.

Nurse-patient interaction begins when the nurse and the patient first encounter each other, but this interaction may be colored by past experiences and preconceptions. The nurse learns to take certain nursing action spontaneously yet appropriately. However, through definitive assessment of the patient's emotional, social, cultural, and physical needs, the nurse learns to take planned, purposeful action to help the patient toward the therapeutic goal. With careful analysis, interpretation, validation, and evaluation of her own and the patient's responses, ideally, the nurse proceeds step by step with the patient toward both short-term and long-term goals of care. There is almost limitless reading material on these aspects of patient care. The starred readings at the end of this chapter are only suggestive.

3

Understanding and interaction

The concept of patient

"The patient is a person" and "patients are people" are phrases used frequently in the nurse's teaching. Often these or similar phrases serve to remind the nurse that the patient, whoever he may be, is a human being with hopes and desires, likes and dislikes, strengths and weaknesses. The patient may be a man or a woman, a boy or a girl, an infant or an elderly person. *Who* he is and *his place* are important. They are of paramount importance to him and they should be a most important consideration in his care.

Being a patient places the person in a unique setting. The number of places where patient care is offered today are numerous and differ greatly. The person who becomes a patient is often described as "one who is under the care of a physician or in a hospital." Patients receive care also in the physician's office, the outpatient service of a hospital, in their own homes, in nursing homes, and in other institutions. Regardless of where care is given, each experience has special meaning to the patient. Perhaps for most people, institutional care has the greatest significance. The fact that the person is away from his home, family, friends, and usual way of life, even though for only a short time, and is faced with threat of disease or illness and unpleasant experiences, may tax his resources in understanding and in adaptation.

The individual who becomes a patient in a hospital takes on a different status and is surrounded by circumstances quite unlike his usual ones. His total environment becomes quite different from the familiar. He is requested, upon admission, to wear clothing he normally wears for sleep. His living quarters become only a room or cubicle with little other than a place to rest. He may have private bathing or toilet facilities, but most likely he will share a community-type room. A public lounge may be available to him and his family, or there may be only a bench in the corridor. His family, perhaps some friends, hospital personnel, and fellow patients complete the group of people who will be his close associates during his hospitalization. The latter two groups of people are determined for him by circumstances and by others rather than by his choice.

A patient in the hospital is the recipient of suggestion, direction, explanation, and treatment. He is observed, tested, exposed to situations over which he may have little or no control, given a variety of medications and treatments, and he may have an operation. As he recovers from illness or completes a diagnostic survey, he usually is given a final checkup, and then he may be declared well enough to resume life at home or he may go to another institution for further care. On the other hand, the hospitalization may be his last life experience.

The patient's response to illness may be quite different from his response to hospitalization. Illness outside a hospital may be accepted and the patient may experience physical and emotional discomfort with little outward expression. With hospitalization, his response to illness may be intensified, or else his reaction may be one of relief with a lessening of his reaction to illness. The significance of the hospital or hospital care to each patient needs careful consideration. Hospital surroundings, atmosphere, and ways of doing things are very familiar to personnel and to some patients. Most patients, however, are not familiar with them and need help to adjust to the experience.

The patient's concept of the nurse

The nurse should be aware that each patient has a mental image of the nurse and that wide variations exist. The same factors influencing his behavioral responses to illness and care will influence his concept and expectations of the nurse.

The image the patient has of the nurse may speed or delay his acceptance of her and of what she helps him to do. For example, his mental image of the nurse may be that of a woman in a white uniform, cap, shoes, and stockings. When a public health nurse comes to his home to continue his care and he is confronted with a nurse in a different colored uniform and accessories, it is not uncommon for him to ask if she *is* a nurse or whether she is the same as the "other" nurses.

The patient's concept of the nurse frequently is based upon the general public's idea, particularly if the patient has had no previous contact with nurses. The nurse is commonly held in a position of respect by the public. She is often thought of as a person who is good, immaculately groomed, efficient, and kind. She is thought of as one who "does for the sick." When the nurse attempts to teach the patient to do things for himself, as he will need to do in readjustment to daily living, he may feel that she is trying to get out of doing her work or that she does not appreciate the fact that he is not well. Unfortunately, in the past much of the "caring" in nurse-patient relationships has been conveyed through doing *for* the patient rather than *with* the patient.

The public frequently turns to nurses for answers to questions regarding health, but the nurse is seldom considered a teacher. When the nurse attempts to teach the patient and family about measures to prevent illness and to maintain health, she may elicit little interest from them. Thus, if continuing nursing care consists primarily of health supervision in the home, the patient and his family may feel that the nurse is not needed. If she must give some treatment, assist with some physical exercises, or carry out some other function that gives concrete evidence of "doing," then her contribution may be recognized by them. When nurses make arrangements for patient care, particularly in the change from care in the hospital to care in the home, these factors should be borne in mind.

Some patients may have had traumatic experiences that lead them to distrust and reject the nurse. Others may have listened to harrowing experiences of their friends and assume that their association with nurses will not be pleasant. The nurse should try to help the patient correct this distortion by encouraging him to relate to her as an individual.

Psychologic factors may affect the patient's response to the nurse. When any person becomes ill and dependent upon others, he regresses to some extent. Just having to be in a hospital and having to abide by the regulations places the patient in a dependent position. Some patients unconsciously respond to the nurse as they did to their mothers during childhood. This may be demonstrated by docile obedience, eagerness for approval, playing childish tricks to see if they can "get away with anything," or by a number of other ways. Their behavioral expressions will depend upon what they learned as appropriate responses. Others may identify the nurse with a domineering mother from whom they may be seeking emancipation or with an unwanted mother-in-law. They may respond with stubborn and contradictory behavior that the nurse must try to understand.

The patient may have come from a cultural background in which women are considered inferior to men, one in which women unquestionably wait upon men. For example, a man who had recently come to this country antagonized all the members of a nursing staff by ordering them about and by refusing to help himself at all. His convalescence was being delayed by his firm conviction that the women about him, the nurses, must "do for him" on all occasions. Only when an alert nurse noticed that he ordered his wife about during visiting hours and that she accepted this in a satisfied fashion did the nurses realize the meaning of his behavior. In this particular instance the situation was remedied by working through the doctor, whose opinions, suggestions, and judgments were accepted readily by the patient as those of the nurses were not. There was no need for resentment on the part of the nurses. There was need only for an understanding of the patient and for appropriate action with this in mind.

Interpretation of all we see is based on our own experiences and learning. Therefore, it is not strange that the nurse is seen in a different light by each person she encounters. Accepting this, she needs to work toward responding to each patient individually, respecting his differences and placing her emphasis on common elements. In this way she will give the most effective care.

The nurse's concept of the patient

The nurse-patient relationship is a term commonly used to identify the complex interaction between the patient and the nurse. Every nurse needs to understand this relationship, for upon it will rest her success in helping the patient and in achieving personal satisfaction.

Each one of us is uniquely different from any other individual. The nurse needs to be aware of her own biases and prejudices and

5

work toward meeting each person with an open mind. To be successful in working with patients as individuals, the nurse needs to accept each as he is without attaching conditions to the acceptance. The patient then does not need to be burdened with trying to earn the nurse's approval, and it also is easier for the nurse to work with the patient and his family with genuine sincerity, sensitivity, and understanding. The nurse who attempts to convey outwardly one response when inwardly she is responding in another way only confuses the patient, and relationships remain superficial.

The nurse may encounter many situations that require acceptance of things that cannot be changed. She cares for patients with incurable illnesses that may result in immediate death or that may become chronic and result in eventual death. Some patients may require disfiguring surgery. Some may have deformities or communicable diseases with attendant social stigma. The nurse needs to develop the ability to accept things that cannot be changed and to respect the opinions of others in the determination of what can be or should be changed within reasonable limits.

The nurse needs to learn to distinguish between her own goals and standards of value and conduct and those of her patient. Discovery of what situations mean to the patient is one of the first steps nurses can take to truly help the patient. Every nurse should realize that although she attempts to anticipate what the patient may need, the patient may be the best interpreter of what he needs and wants, if only someone will listen. Much can be learned about the patient through observation, collection of information by other health personnel, talking to the patient's family, and talking to other nurses who take part in his care. However, the best source of information may be the patient, and he should be given every opportunity to express his own feelings about situations. If the meaning of observed patient behavior is not clear, the nurse should not make assumptions. Verifying the meaning with the patient brings the concern into the open, and together the patient and the nurse learn the meaning.

There will be situations that the nurse finds difficult to understand and that she cannot accept. She herself may need help and should seek help from persons who are prepared to help her understand herself. Through this kind of discussion she then may give care to patients with greater awareness of the meaning of her own behavior and the behavior of the patient.

There can be no set rules or techniques to determine the nurse's responses to patients. Each response is made according to the individual and the situation. The following suggestions may help as guidelines:

1. Be yourself, for nothing else draws more genuine response from others.

2. Let others respond in their own way rather than trying to make them respond the way you would.

3. Reflect upon situations that are unsatisfactory or frustrating and ask yourself the following questions: Why do these situations exist? What did the patient do and say, and what did you do and say? Did you really understand what it meant to him, or were you interpreting by your values?

4. Continue to grow intellectually, emotionally, and socially by developing broad interests both within and outside nursing.

Emotional and cultural responses to illness

In general, the patient's behavior is influenced by his previous knowledge and experience, his cultural background, his emotional makeup, and alterations in his physiologic functioning. These influences are so closely tied to each other that it is often very difficult to sift out a single reason for his behavior. However, the nurse should bear in mind that whatever the patient's behavior may be, it has a very definite meaning. It may be relatively simple or very complex. The patient may not be able to verbalize the reason for his behavior, or if he does, his interpretation may be quite different from the nurse's interpretation.

To understand his behavior, the patient's age needs to be considered along with other factors. A child will react according to his stage of emotional and physical development as well as according to the factors already listed. A discussion of the stages of growth and development cannot be included here, but every nurse should remember that the child's reactions are different from those of the adult and are in keeping with behavioral patterns expected at particular stages of development.

The physically and chronologically adult patient, however, is often expected to face his problems in an adult fashion, when in actuality his behavior may illustrate that the level of emotional maturation he has attained makes this impossible under the circumstances.

Anxiety and *fear* are part of the natural reaction of every normal human being when threats to his health appear. Anxiety has been defined as a feeling of uncertainty and helplessness in the face of danger. It is caused to some extent by the nature of the human organism but can be intensified by lack of knowledge, by lack of trust, and by social, cultural, and economic forces bearing directly upon the affected individual. Fear of cancer, for instance, is becoming almost universal in our society. This fear can be transferred from one person to another in such a way that it has been defined as one of the most common "communicable diseases" of man. It is imperative that the nurse have some understanding of the anxieties and fears of her patients.

Illness may be a new experience for the patient. He may be uncertain of what it will mean for him. He may be uncertain of the reactions expected of him by others and of how others will react to him. His anxiety may be very much oriented toward his present situation. He may be fearful of the many activities that directly affect him and that occur around him, such as diagnostic procedures and treatments. His own incidental observations of other patients in the hospital may cause concern.

Illness often separates the patient from those he loves and those who perhaps know him best and can comfort him most. Even a short hospitalization may seem very long to the patient and his family, who are accustomed to daily support of each other. Being denied this accustomed source of warmth and security increases the patient's anxiety and fear. Small children, who cannot always be given a satisfactory explanation of what may be done to them, often suffer greatly from anxiety.

The loss of financial security and the economic effects of illness may cause the patient and his family to feel threatened. This may be particularly true of the man who is head of a household. One response may be anger and hostility. If this response occurs, the patient needs acceptance of his behavior and a good listener. By listening, the nurse may help the patient to release tensions. Sometimes the social worker can help him to resolve some of his problems. In the hospital it is she who knows the most about such community resources as financial aid, housekeeping services, child-placement facilities, nursing homes, and job-placement agencies.

The signs of anxiety, fear, and tension are variable. An indifference to his symptoms and to the tests being made may mean that the patient has not accepted the possibility that anything may be wrong. He may not be able to face reality and still maintain stability and integrity of his personality. The patient who is noisy and demanding, perhaps declaring that he is not worried, is one who, if closely observed, may reveal what he dares not verbalize. The patient who "forgets" the clinic appointment at which he is to learn the results of a test is probably fearful of these results. Other patients manifest their anxiety, consciously or unconsciously, by repeatedly asking the same question, making many complaints, or being preoccupied with bodily functions. Still others struggle with their fears alone, leaving the nurse unaware of their problems. Insomnia, anorexia, frequent urination, irritability, lack of ability to listen or to concentrate, and detachment are often signs of anxiety. Sometimes marked physical signs, such as perspiring hands, increased pulse and respiratory rates, and dilated pupils, denote anxiety and fear. Perhaps the best way a nurse can estimate her helpfulness to the anxious patient is by his progress. If he becomes more tense, she should seek expert assistance.

Cultural background is related so closely to emotional response that it must always be considered in determining the basis for the patient's behavior. This evaluation may be difficult to make and may necessitate careful observation and study. It is important, however, that the nurse try to identify whether the patient's response is a cultural or an emotional one because her response will, in turn, depend upon this knowledge.

Certain diseases may have implications

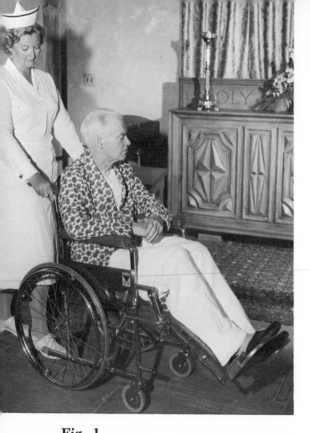

Fig. 1

Many patients derive great comfort from a few moments of silent prayer in the chapel.

that are not culturally acceptable to the patient or his family. In some societies it is a disgrace to become ill at all. Diseases such as epilepsy and mental illness may be carefully guarded secrets within families. Some diseases, such as venereal disease, may be associated with uncleanliness or immorality.

Various parts of the body may have significant meaning in certain cultures. Some patients may refuse to permit amputation of a limb because physical fitness and the "body beautiful" are valued highly. The modern woman in the United States may have an almost intolerable emotional reaction to a mastectomy because of the emphasis placed upon women's breasts in our culture.

Anxiety may be caused by the patient's inability to participate in his usual religious experiences. It is important for the patient to retain religious medals and perform religious rites (Fig. 1). If this is not possible, an interpretation of the reasons by a religious

adviser is usually helpful in decreasing anxiety.

During illness the patient may be denied certain foods considered necessary in his culture. This may produce anxiety. For example, after two weeks in the respirator, one young patient became anxious over his first meal because the food was not sanctioned by his church law. His family and religious leader had to be called to reassure him before he would eat. Some people believe that one should fast when ill. Imagine the anxiety and uncertainty produced when a nourishing diet is served and these patients are told by the doctors and nurses that they must eat.

The patient may be censured for displaying behavior acceptable in his own cultural group. For instance, in one culture "the picture of health contains a normal amount of disease." For this reason, early medical care or a program of prevention may meet resistance. In another culture the family usually prefers to care for the patient at home, but if hospitalization is necessary, many relatives and friends cluster around lest the patient feel rejected in his time of need. In still another culture it is proper to go to bed with much moaning and groaning if one is ill, so that the relatives may fulfill their rightful role of beneficence. Hospital personnel frequently consider these patients "problems" rather than recognizing that such behavior is culturally determined and trying to work out acceptable adjustments. Explanation to the patient and his family of hospital policies, such as visiting hours and isolation requirements, may prevent undue anxiety in both the patient and his relatives.

Nursing intervention

Appraisal of the patient

The nurse's general understanding of the patient and the interaction that takes place between patient and nurse form the basis for planning nursing care. Information from the patient and family supplies more of the framework from which she can begin to plan nursing care. As the nurse learns more about the patient, she is able to identify his potential. She helps the patient to maintain and use his capacities, and especially to find ways of achieving what is most important to him. There may be times when the patient is unable to recognize the strengths he has, but through understanding and building trust the nurse can help the patient to become more aware of his capabilities.

Plans for patient care need to be kept flexible and within practical limits for the patient and his family. Written plans help to keep all nurses informed of what the patient is capable of doing and of the goal he is trying to reach. Keeping plans simple yet up-to-date and pertinent reduces the number of times the patient has to inform the staff about his capabilities and helps to provide a consistent approach toward his nursing care.

The following "Patient Information Guide for the Nurse" is a sample of the kind of information that can be collected by the watchful nurse for her use as well as for the use of other professional persons giving patient care. Although traditionally the physician records the history of the patient over a period of time, the nurse learns many details about the patient's habits, behavior, complaints, and discomforts as well as his reactions and progress during treatment. By using a guide to identify what the patient has to use and what he lacks, the nurse is better prepared to help him proceed toward recovery.

PATIENT INFORMATION GUIDE FOR THE NURSE

I Physical, emotional, and social observations
  A Physical
    1 General appearance
      a Body build, weight, height, posture, gait
      b General day-to-day appearance
      c Changes in appearance
      d Appearance before illness
    2 Symptoms and signs
      a Temperature
      b Pulse
      c Respiration
      d Blood pressure
      e Color
      f Specific complaints such as pain, nausea, fatigue, dyspnea
      g Usual pattern of specific complaints; e.g., in cardiac patient, time and nature of chest pain over a period of days, in relation to activity
      h Intake and output
      i Other physical symptoms and signs that occur in relation to self-care (see II, Self-care activities)

    3 Previous state of health
      a Number of admissions—present hospital and others
      b Contact with other health agencies—public health nursing family service
  B Emotional and social
    1 Behavior
      a Adjustment—to illness, roommates, staff, therapy
      b Previous behavior—collection of observations made by patient and by family and/or friends
      c Usual day-to-day behavior—interest, occupation, general frame of mind or spirits
      d Changes in behavior—circumstances at time of change and before and after change
      e Family relationships—at home, reaction to visitors if in hospital, reaction to lack of visitors, family interest, family members who seem to help
    2 Social activities
      a Usual way patient likes to spend time
      b Amount of free time available and how used
      c Friends or lack of friends
      d Activities at home or outside home or both
    3 Family
      a Nationality
      b Birthplace
      c Religion
      d Place in family—mother, father
      e Siblings
      f Children
      g Language spoken in home
    4 Mental ability and education
      a Vocabulary
      b Ability to understand explanations
      c Ability to carry out functions in relation to care needed
      d Ability to repeat actions, such as giving self-medication after a demonstration
      e Ability to retain knowledge to be used another time
      f Ability to make suggestions regarding own care
      g Amount of schooling
      h Kind of schooling
      i I.Q.—if psychologic testing has been done
    5 Household
      a Importance to patient
      b Importance to family
      c Patient satisfied or dissatisfied
      d Location of home
      e Physical setup of home
    6 Finances
      a Kind of work patient has done

b Kind of work patient is doing

c Income of patient and family

d Attitude toward job—satisfaction, dissatisfaction

e Use of income—values of individual in relation to finances

f Use of public assistance or private funds—acceptance of, reaction to

g Effect of finances on health habits, purchase of prescribed medications, follow-through on prescribed diagnostic tests

II Self-care activities

(Include factors such as patient's interest in doing, specifically how the activity is done, progression in doing activities)

A Personal hygiene

1 Bathing

a By patient, nurse, member of family, or combination

b Usual method—bed, tub, shower

c Frequency

2 Nails

Care of, by patient, nurse, member of family, or combination

3 Hair

a Shampoo by patient, nurse, member of family, or combination

b Where shampooed and type of equipment used or needed

c Usual method

4 Shaving

a By patient, nurse, member of family, barber, or combination

b Usual method and equipment used

c Frequency

B Grooming and appearance

1 General appearance

a Neat

b Untidy

c Interest in

2 Use of cosmetics

a Used by self or with help

b Interest in

3 Combing hair

a By self, nurse, member of family, or combination

b Special device necessary

4 Dressing

a By self, nurse, member of family, or combination

b Special devices used

c Difficulties involved, need for practice

C Eating

1 Type of food

a Regular

b Special diet

2 Appetite

3 Likes and dislikes

4 Accomplished by self, nurse, member of family, or combination

5 Special devices or setup necessary

D Elimination

1 Continent

2 Incontinent

3 Constipation

4 Amount of urinary output

5 Habit

6 Need for special training schedule and management—bladder and bowel

7 Facility used

a Bedpan

b Commode

c Toilet

d Special equipment

E Activity

1 Bed activities

Ability to turn, lift, pull, balance, attain sitting position

2 Special devices for bed activity

a Bars

b Trapeze

c Others

3 Ability to go from bed to chair, from bed to wheelchair, from wheelchair to chair

4 Ability to return to bed

5 Ability to stand

6 Walking and stair climbing

7 Use of any devices in standing and walking

8 Tolerance for activity

9 Amount of activity advised in comparison to that carried out

10 Activity on ward and activity off ward

11 Ability to move about in house and how

12 Ability to go outside house and how

13 Ability in managing transportation

F Rest

1 Usual habit

2 Habit on hospital unit

3 Habit since illness

4 Prescribed amount in comparison to amount taken

5 Problems of maintaining or securing rest —when and how helped

III Special teachings for future

(Need for special teaching may be in relation to any of above activities)

A Special diet—selection, purchase, and preparation of food

B Administering medication

1 Purchasing and obtaining medication and necessary equipment

2 Method

C Household activities

1 Easier ways of managing

2 Relocation of articles in home

3 Scheduling activities

D Care of other members of family by patient

E Care of patient by other members of family

F Provision for follow-up of patient and reevaluation

Maintaining the patient

Physical capacities. Although the nurse may begin with recognizing the patient's emotional strengths and weaknesses, at the same time she should be assessing carefully his physical strengths and weaknesses. The patient should be kept as active as possible within the limitations set by his diagnosis and the physician's prescribed regimen. The nurse should be particularly attentive to the maintenance of activity in the case of patients who are confined to bed or who have severely restricted activity. Patients who have partial restriction of activity and are left without encouragement to move may readily develop limitations in motion or contractures.

Patients confined to bed or allowed only limited activity will have problems of body mechanics. Helping the patient to keep as active as possible within his limitations and to keep good bodily alignment may enable him to resume usual activities sooner. The nurse should have a thorough understanding of joint motion and either should help the patient go through the full range of motion or should move each joint through its range of motion once or twice daily, or as often as necessary to preserve the ability to move freely. The daily bath and assistance with self-care activities provide excellent opportunities for helping to preserve mobility. The nurse should know the ranges of motion in a systematic fashion and should familiarize herself with their terminology (Figs. 2 to 4). As she helps the patient to preserve motion, she should teach the importance of these activities to both patient and family.

If a patient has lost an extremity (amputation) or has loss of function (paralysis), careful attention given to bed posture, changes in position, and follow-through on exercise programs will help prevent development of additional disability. Many patients who require extended periods of bed rest can be helped to maintain muscle tone by use of a footboard, foot exercises, quadriceps setting, self-care within the limits permitted, correct position, and frequent turning unless contraindicated. Specific methods of prevention can be checked with the doctor if there is doubt.

Most patients are placed on progressive activity programs as their condition permits. As new activities are to be done, the nurse should give a clear explanation of the nature of the activity, what she will do to help, and what the patient must do. Preparation of the patient prior to changes in activity will help to pave the way for better acceptance of the change and will help allay the patient's apprehension. For example, the patient who has pain on moving in bed and has been on bed rest for weeks may become apprehensive and fearful when approached with the idea of being moved out of bed. The nurse can do much to allay fears and apprehension by knowing exactly how the patient can be moved—and with the least effort on his part. The nurse with a confident but understanding manner can make a new procedure much less traumatic for the patient than can the competent, technically skilled nurse who lacks understanding.

The nurse can and should contribute suggestions for working out activity problems with her patients. One way of finding a method for a particular body motion is for the nurse actually to assume that she has the same limitation as the patient and proceed from there. For example, if the patient has weak upper and lower extremities, it may be difficult for him to assume a sitting position in bed. Experimenting for herself, the nurse will find that, starting from a back-lying position, she must first place the palms of her hands close to her hips. Then, by pushing on her elbows, she can raise her head and shoulders from the bed. By sliding one elbow back and then the other until both elbows are under the shoulders, she will be in a position in which she is supported but in which the hands are not free. By pushing on the right hand and extending the right elbow, then pushing on the left hand and extending the left elbow, she will find herself approaching a sitting position but not yet in a balanced position. By moving first one hand forward and then the other, she can gradually assume a balanced sitting position. Whereas this may be an easy procedure for the nurse who is strong and not hindered by weakness, it may be painstaking and slow for the patient who has weak extremities. However, through a step-by-step demonstration the nurse can teach the patient exactly how he can achieve a sitting position in bed. Since almost all rehabilitation is a slow process, it is important not only to have an ultimate goal but

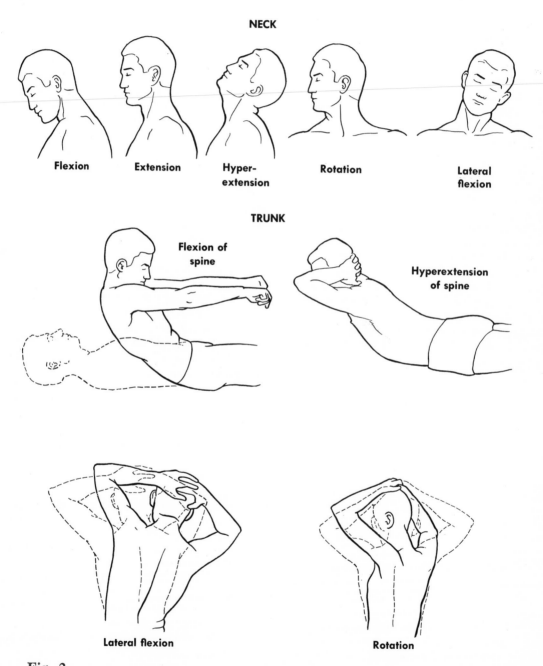

NECK

Flexion Extension Hyper-extension Rotation Lateral flexion

TRUNK

Flexion of spine

Hyperextension of spine

Lateral flexion

Rotation

Fig. 2

Illustrating range of joint motion for the neck and trunk.

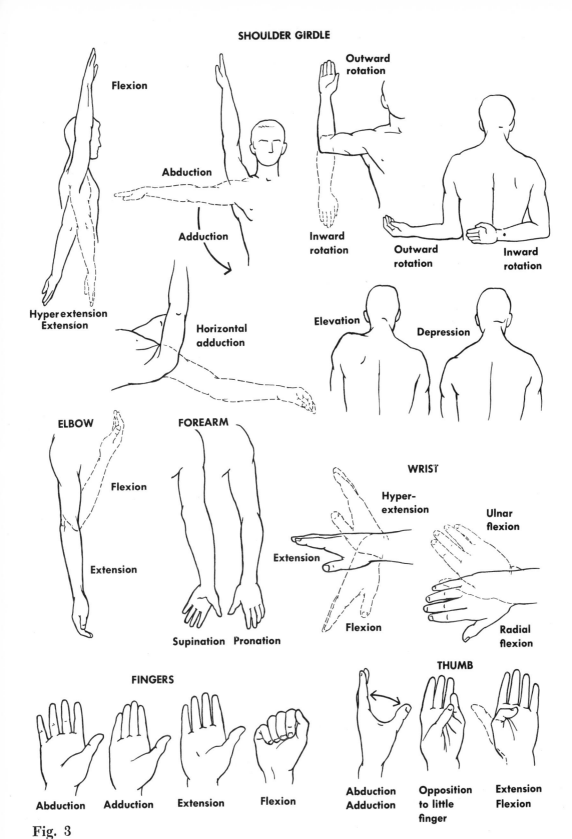

Fig. 3

Illustrating range of joint motion for the shoulder and shoulder girdle, elbow, wrist, forearm, and hand.

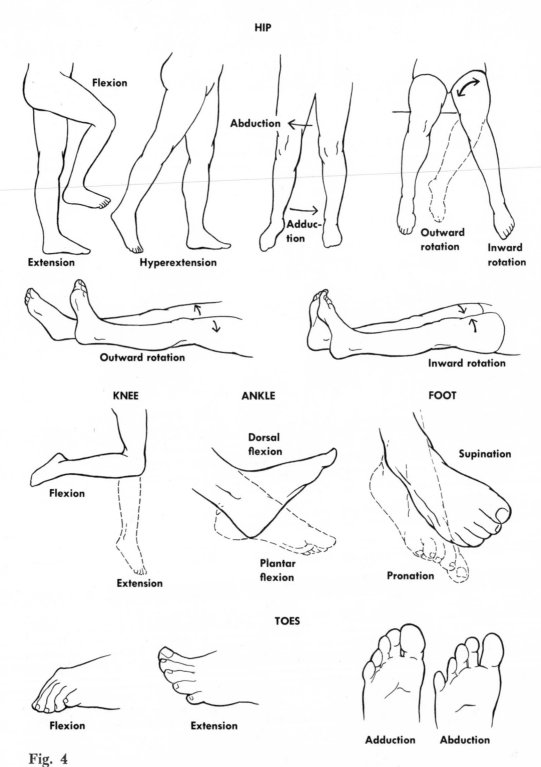

Fig. 4

Illustrating range of joint motion for the hip, knee, ankle, foot, and toes.

also to set intermediate goals that may be obtained in a shorter time. Unless patients experience some success, discouragement usually develops.

The nurse can be a source of encouragement to the patient in finding new ways to manage necessary self-care. However, nurses can learn much about techniques from their patients. Faced with a problem that he knew had to be lived with for the rest of his life, many a patient, as well as doctors, nurses, and therapists, has been spurred to develop easier ways of managing daily needs as well as meeting occupational needs. Extension handles for combs, toothbrushes, and eating utensils are simple to construct and make it possible for many patients to be self-sufficient. If given a picture or sample drawing with explanations of what is needed, members of the family can often help make self-help devices for the patient. In this day of small gadgets, one can find numerous useful articles already on the market. However, patient and family may need help in recognizing the needs for such aids, in learning where to find them, and in learning how to use them effectively.

Careful nursing attention to prevention of decubiti, incontinence, and malnutrition also helps speed the patient's return to his usual activities. Nursing care contributing to prevention of these problems is discussed in detail in subsequent chapters.

Emotional capacities. Although the patient may have serious physical limitations, he may be able emotionally to accept them and either compensate for them or through sheer inner strength manage his own daily care and his life despite them. Discussion of understanding the patient's emotional responses to illness or threat to health was included earlier in this chapter. The nurse cannot possibly know all the factors contributing to anxiety or their particular application for each patient. However, she can do much to help the patient rally the emotional strength necessary to continue with a prescribed medical program.

Nursing action in prevention and release of anxiety

Orienting the newly admitted patient and his family to the hospital routine tends

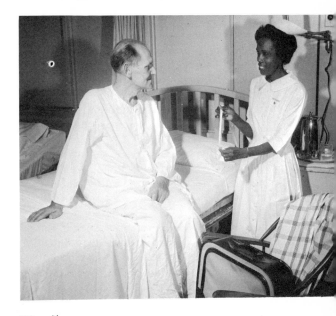

Fig. 5

Admitting a patient provides the nurse with the opportunity to allay some of his fears and anxieties by thorough explanation of environment and of expected procedures.

to minimize anxiety (Fig. 5). Each new experience should be explained to the patient and, if possible, related to familiar experiences. It is helpful to inform the patient how he may call the nurse, when he will see his doctor, the hours the religious adviser is available, and how he may contact his family. In addition, the family should be told how to obtain information concerning the patient, when they may visit, and any immediate plans for the patient.

If a patient is to have a treatment or test, he must be given some idea of what will be done, the preparation involved, and the reasons why the procedure is necessary. To remove the water pitcher and inform a patient that he cannot have any more water until after his x-ray examination can leave him with many anxious thoughts: "What x-ray examination?" "I wonder when it is?" "What will it be like?" "It must be something special if I can't have any water." Lack of knowledge as a cause of anxiety reflects the nurse's lack of consideration for the patient's rights as an individual.

Explanations should be given in the patient's own terms at appropriate times and repeated as necessary. If the patient is very anxious, he may need repeated explanation, since extreme anxiety reduces intellectual function. Detailed explanations should not be given to a patient who is very anxious, under sedation, has a high temperature, or is in severe pain because he will not remember them. Repetition is often required for older persons and children because they may have a short memory span.

Time spent in giving explanations to relatives is not wasted. Not only does it relieve their anxieties, which may be transmitted to the patient, but it also saves having to untangle misinformation. Often the family is helpful in interpreting necessary instructions to the patient in such a manner that he understands and accepts them.

In most instances a large part of the nurse's work is to encourage the patient to express his anxieties, to help him see the universality of fear in his situation, and to help him seek outlets for his fears and tensions and to allay them whenever possible. The nurse should provide opportunities for the patient to talk, but she should not probe. There is a difference between prying into a patient's thoughts and beliefs and eliciting information that will aid in the understanding of his behavior. Without seeming unduly curious, one can usually find some topic of personal interest to the patient that will provide an opening. A picture on the bedside table may create such an opening. Then, if the nurse will listen with sincere interest and without making judgments about the patient, she may begin to gain insight into the patient as a person. And more important, he may begin to speak about his fears.

As soon as the patient begins to talk about his feelings, the nurse should proceed with conversation, taking her cues from what the patient offers. The nurse who feels inadequate herself may cut off the conversation. For instance, if a patient says, "You know, I don't think I'll ever get to see my little boy again," a common response is "Oh, don't say that, certainly you will; you're going to be all right." The patient may very well not be all right. Would it not be better to respond, "What makes you feel this way?"

Such a response helps the patient explore the subject and leaves opportunity for the patient to answer and to examine this fear himself. It also gives the nurse a chance to find out what the patient fears. The nurse who is willing to listen to patients, to be guided by their reactions, and to work with them rather than to make decisions for them will give them needed emotional support. Solving patients' problems for them, even if it were possible, is not the aim of nursing. Indeed, it would tend to make patients less healthy psychologically.

The nurse is prepared only to help the patient look at those problems that he himself is able to bring into awareness. Underlying problems should be handled by people trained in psychotherapy. A nurse needs to be able to recognize normal anxiety reactions and to report exaggerated reactions that may indicate the need for psychiatric referral. Stuttering and blocking of words may indicate increasing tension. Depression and sadness are normal reactions to illness and particularly to surgery, but feelings of guilt and worthlessness should make the nurse aware of the possibility of suicide. Apathy may indicate that the patient has given up not only fear but also hope. Fortunately, most normal and abnormal anxiety is self-limiting and improves with a cheerful and encouraging attitude on the part of the staff, renewed activity for the patient, and a chance to talk. Independence should be allowed and encouraged as soon as possible, since for most people nothing is so demoralizing as complete dependence upon others. Independence cannot be forced, however, because it results from changes within the patient himself. This motivation may sometimes be initiated by first allowing the patient to be dependent. The desired goal is interdependence—the result of collaboration of the health team and the patient to help the patient regain and maintain normal health.

The nurse has a responsibility to her patient for maintaining channels of communication with others who may be better prepared to meet his needs. The patient should feel free to communicate with others, such as the doctor, his family, spiritual advisers, and social workers. At times the nurse may need to be a "go-between" because some patients are unsure as to whether their questions are appropriate. When accompanying the doctor, a statement by the nurse, such as, "Mr. Jones asked about how long he would be hospitalized, and I believe you have some other questions, don't you, Mr. Jones?" may provide the necessary opening.

Providing for the patient's return home

Throughout the patient's illness, the nurse must be aware that he is a member of a family and of a community to which he will return. This fact must be considered in planning for home care, or there will be anxiety, which is often the problem confronting the patient who is said to have "hospitalitis." It is important for the nurse to ascertain with whom the family authority lies, since such a person is usually the one who should be brought into planning. She also needs to gain insight into reactions to such things as disability, infectious diseases, and care of the aged, which may be culturally determined. A patient may find it difficult for others to accept him. In such a case the nurse should try to prepare him for this adjustment.

The aged patient is not always readily taken back into the home of his children. In some cultures the older person rarely has this problem, since he is highly respected as the head of the family. In others it may be expected that the aged person who is widowed will go to a home for the aged when he is no longer able to live by himself. Awareness of any such possibilities should make the nurse alert to early planning with the patient and his family for his discharge, whether it be for convalescent, rehabilitative, chronic, or terminal care. Here again, the plans must stem from the patient and his family.

Planning is also necessary in carrying out any patient-teaching program. The nurse's goal is to help the patient and his family toward self-sufficiency and independence. She suggests needed materials, routines, and techniques. The patient, with his family, should be encouraged to work out the details, such as the equipment available, the best time of day, the best place, and the easiest technique. They must plan, for example, how a special diet can be worked in with the family meals. The nurse should be available to give guidance as needed. In teaching patients, the following suggestions may be helpful:

1. Explain to the patient the desired results, suggesting possible means to these ends.
2. Explore with the patient and his family the possibilities of carrying out instructions. Listen carefully for factors that might interfere with carrying out instructions and try to make adjustments that will make the treatment acceptable and practical to the patient and his family.
3. Have the patient practice the procedure as it is to be carried out in the home.
4. Provide some channel for assistance if the patient should meet with difficulty.

As she gives physical care to her patient, the nurse should always be using her abilities to provide for comprehensive care. Not every problem will be solved during one patient contact. Some may never be solved or at least not in the manner that seems, in the nurse's judgment, to be for the best interest of the patient.

In this chapter great stress has been placed on the nurse's understanding of human behavior, her acceptance of different patterns of living, and her skill in working with people. Most important is the emotional overtone in the "way" things are done, conveying to the patient inherent warmth, responsiveness, sensitivity, and understanding. Good nurse-patient relationships develop from *genuine feelings* and *appropriate techniques.*

References and selected readings*

1 Anxiety recognition and intervention, programmed instruction, Am. J. Nursing 66:129-152, Sept. 1965.
2 *Ashbrook, James B.: Not by bread alone, Am. J. Nursing 55:164-168, Feb. 1955.
3 *Bird, Brian: Psychological aspects of preoperative and postoperative care, Am. J. Nursing 55:685-687, June 1955.
4 *Brown, Esther Lucile: Newer dimensions in patient care, New York, Russell Sage Foundation. 1961, part 1: The use of the physical and social environment of the general hospital for therapeutic purposes. 1962, part 2: Improving staff motivation and competence in the general hospital. 1964, part 3: Patients as people.
5 *Clemence, Sister Madeleine: Existentialism: a philosophy of commitment, Am. J. Nursing 66:500-505, March 1966.

*References preceded by an asterisk are particularly well suited for student reading.

6 *Connolly, Mary Grace: What acceptance means to patients, Am. J. Nursing 60:1754-1757, Dec. 1960.

7 *Dicks, Russell L.: Who is my patient? New York, 1943, The Macmillan Co.

8 *Eldred, Stanley H.: Improving nurse-patient communication, Am. J. Nursing 60:1600-1602, Nov. 1960.

9 Elms, Roslyn R., and Diers, Donna K.: The patient comes to the hospital, Nursing Forum 3:88-96, 1963.

10 Erickson, Florence: When 6- to 12-year olds are ill, Nursing Outlook 65:48-50, July 1965.

11 *Greenhill, Maurice H.: Interviewing with a purpose, Am. J. Nursing 56:1259-1262, Oct. 1956.

12 *Gregg, Dorothy E.: Anxiety—a factor in nursing care, Am. J. Nursing 52:1363-1365, Nov. 1952.

13 *Gregg, Dorothy: Reassurance, Am. J. Nursing 55:171-174, Feb. 1955.

14 Hayes, Wayland J., and Gazaway, Rena: Human relations in nursing, Philadelphia, 1964, W. B. Saunders Co.

15 *Henderson, Virginia: The nature of nursing, Am. J. Nursing 64:62-68, Aug. 1964.

16 *Ingles, Thelma: Understanding the nurse-patient relationship, Nursing Outlook 9:698-700, Nov. 1961.

17 *Jourard, Sidney M.: How well do you know your patients? Am. J. Nursing 59:1568-1571, Nov. 1959.

18 Kachelski, M. Audrey: The nurse-patient relationship, Am. J. Nursing 61:76-81, May 1961.

19 Kelly, Mary M.: Exercises for bedfast patients, Am. J. Nursing 66:2209-2213, Oct. 1966.

20 King, Joan M.: Denial, Am. J. Nursing 66:1010-1014, May 1966.

21 Koos, Earl L.: The sociology of the patient, New York, 1959, McGraw-Hill Book Co.

22 *Macgregor, Frances M. Cooke: Social science in nursing—applications for the improvement of patient care, New York, 1960, Russell Sage Foundation.

23 *Mahaffy, Perry R., Jr.: Admission interviews with parents, Am. J. Nursing 66:506-508, March 1966.

24 McCain, R. Faye: Nursing by assessment—not intuition, Am. J. Nursing 65:82-84, April 1965.

25 *Nayer, Dorothy D.: Skin grafts—the patient, Am. J. Nursing 64:98-101, Nov. 1964.

26 *Neylan, Margaret Prowse: Anxiety, Am. J. Nursing 62:110-111, May 1962.

27 *Neylan, Margaret Prowse: The depressed patient, Am. J. Nursing 61:77-78, July 1961.

28 *Orlando, Ida Jean: The dynamic nurse-patient relationship, New York, 1961, G. P. Putnam's Sons.

29 Peplau, Hildegarde E.: Talking with patients, Am. J. Nursing 60:964-966, July 1960.

30 Perry, George S.: Families of America, New York, 1949, Whittlesey House, McGraw-Hill Book Co.

31 *Prange, Arthur J., Jr., and Martin, Harry W.: Aids to understanding patients, Am. J. Nursing 62:98-100, July 1962.

32 Saunders, Lyle: Cultural difference and medical care, New York, 1954, Russell Sage Foundation.

33 *Skipper, James K., and Leonard, Robert C., editors: Social interaction and patient care, Philadelphia, 1965, J. B. Lippincott Co.

34 Sorensen, Gladys: Dependency—a factor in nursing care, Am. J. Nursing 66:1762-1763, Aug. 1966.

35 Stevens, Leonard F.: What makes a ward climate therapeutic? Am. J. Nursing 61:95-96, March 1961.

36 Tarnower, William: Psychological needs of the hospitalized patient, Nursing Outlook 65:28-30, July 1965.

37 *Taylor, Carol D.: The hospital patient's social dilemma, Am. J. Nursing 66:96-99, Oct. 1965.

38 Travelbee, Joyce: What do we mean by rapport? Am. J. Nursing 63:70-72, Feb. 1963.

39 Travelbee, Joyce: What's wrong with sympathy? Am. J. Nursing 64:68-71, Jan. 1964.

40 Willie, Charles V.: Patient and nurse: members of a group, Nursing Outlook 57:585-587, Oct. 1957.

41 Wu, Ruth: Explaining treatments to young children, Am. J. Nursing 66:71-73, July 1965.

2

Age—a factor in nursing care of patients

Study questions

1 Review the normal schedule for physical development in children. What are the developmental tasks of each age group?
2 Review the conspicuous physical differences between a young adult and a very old person.
3 From what you have read in newspapers and current magazines, what would you select as major problems of old people in our society?
4 From what you have learned in fundamentals of nursing, what are some practical measures you can take to prevent accidents involving elderly patients in the hospital environment and in their own homes?
5 Review the eating patterns of an elderly person of your acquaintance; compare their food intake with your understanding of an adequate diet.
6 Review the care of dentures in your texts on fundamentals of nursing.
7 What services are available in your community for infants and children? What ones are available for the elderly?

Diseases and disorders requiring medical or surgical treatment afflict persons of all ages, from newborn infants to octogenarians. The age of the patient influences his nursing needs and must always be considered in giving care to him. Each person, regardless of his age, and whether he is sick or well, has needs related to his physical and emotional welfare. These include being fed, clothed, and housed, being safe and comfortable both physically and spiritually, and being important to others. It is not possible nor appropriate to discuss each aspect fully in this book. The student should refer to the many excellent books and periodicals related specifically to the various age groups for additional information. Some are listed in the suggested readings at the end of the chapter.

In the United States two age groups in the population have received a great deal of society's attention—the children and the elderly. The number of elderly people in the United States has increased steadily over the past fifty years. Approximately 9.3% of the population (about 17.5 million persons) is 65 years of age or over.[38] By 1970 it is estimated the number will reach or surpass 22 million.[3] At present those persons 75 years of age or over are increasing proportionately faster than the total age group who are over 65. The increased numbers of elderly have come about primarily through the decrease in infant mortality, the prevention and control of communicable disease during childhood, and improvements in medical care in general. At the present time, however, the largest percentage increase in the population of the United States is among those 5 to 18 years of age.[38]

Society's youth. Concern first was aroused about infants and children during the latter half of the nineteenth century. There were extremely high morbidity (illness) and mortality (death) rates among this group. The problem was especially serious among the children of the poor and of immigrants living in urban communities. Children often were housed in crowded and unsanitary tenements, played in the streets, and were utilized and exploited by developing industries as their labor force. In addition to being overworked and subjected to disease and accidents, most children received little schooling. Contaminated water and food also caused much illness. In response to public sympathy for these children, the Children's Aid Society of New York was founded in 1853. Shortly thereafter, children's hospitals and clinics began to be established. Interest in child care *(pediatrics)* has continued since this time. In 1909 the first national effort to conserve children's health was started by the President, who called a White House Conference on Children and Youth. Since then, this group, with nationwide representation from all professional and social groups (both public and private) interested in child care, has convened every ten years to discuss the problems of youth. As a result of the first conference, The United States Children's Bureau (then under the Department of Labor) was formed. This bureau is an excellent source of literature for parents, and it is active in working with the states to help them provide improved services for children and their families.

Stemming from the aroused interest of society in children, much social legislation improving the welfare of children has been enacted. The education of children is now compulsory in most states, and child-labor laws now prohibit hiring children in industries producing goods sent across state lines. Most states have laws limiting child labor within their boundaries.

Through the international activities of the Children's Bureau and through such organizations within the United Nations as the World Health Organization, UNICEF, and UNESCO, as well as the Peace Corps and voluntary groups such as churches, assistance is being given to developing countries throughout the world to improve child care. The Fourteenth General Assembly of the United Nations in 1959 approved the Declaration of the Rights of the Child, which is based on the idea that mankind everywhere owes children the best it can give.[22]

In the United States many services are available to children free of cost. Almost every community has free well-baby clinics and immunization programs. Public schools usually provide free yearly health examinations for children. Financial assistance is available in every state in the country for medical care of crippled children and the blind. The nurse should become familiar with the services available in her community so that she may guide parents to seek help as needed.

Despite all the efforts, there are still many serious problems related to the youth of our society. Physical abuse of infants and young children by adults, especially young ones, seems to be increasing. The injuries sustained by an abused child are known as the "battered-child syndrome." In addition, many children are neglected. The physician is now required by law to report any case of abuse that comes to his attention. Appropriate community agencies then provide for the protection of the child. The abuse and neglect of infants many times is related to the problems of teen-agers and young adults.

Teen-age marriages and pregnancies (often of unmarried mothers) have become exceedingly common. Many, though not all, of these parents are emotionally immature and unprepared to accept the responsibilities of marriage and parenthood. As a result of increased promiscuity, the incidence of venereal diseases, even in young teen-agers, is increasing at an alarming rate (p. 526). Drug addiction among young teen-agers has increased (p. 136). Many of our youth have serious emotional problems, and general lack of respect for law and order is widespread. As a consequence, homicide and suicide, as well as crime in general, have also increased. Accidents among young people have increased because many now own their own cars and motorbikes and they pass many otherwise unoccupied hours driving about the streets.

Society did not foresee these problems and is poorly equipped to handle them. Facilities for giving adequate help to youths frequently are unavailable. Once again, legislation is being drafted in an attempt to prevent some of the problems. For instance, tight federal controls are being placed on habit-forming drugs, and federal legislation relative to driving safely is being enacted. Many communities are instituting free mental hygiene clinics and treatment facilities for young drug addicts. Unfortunately, professional staff to man them is in exceedingly short supply.

Community-sponsored activities to help the young fill their free time also are springing up. The federal government has urged communities to provide jobs for youths, especially during the summer months, and it has even provided antipoverty funds to assist communities in this endeavor. A great deal of government attention is also being given to the school dropout in an attempt to prepare youths for obtaining work as adults, as well as to help them develop interests with which to fill the many hours of leisure time that even working members of society have today.

The elderly person in our society. Unfortunately, social adjustments adequate to meet the challenges presented by the increasing number of elderly persons were not made over the years. It was not until 1950 that much social planning for the elderly was instituted. Meanwhile, the plight of many elderly people had become almost insufferable. Many, typical of their age group, had one or more chronic illnesses, and most had been replaced on the work force by younger people. Consequently, the problems of this group often were overwhelming. As the number of elderly people was increasing, the patterns of living were changing. No longer were homes large enough to accommodate aging relatives. In fact, society seemed to have begun to frown upon elderly parents' living with their children. This arrangement, therefore, even if possible, frequently was distasteful to both the elderly and their chil-

dren. The provision of living facilities for this group of persons, many of whom needed some nursing care or homemaking assistance, and many of whom could barely afford even the basic essentials of life, became a tremendous challenge. Formerly, the elderly person could continue to work as long as he wished, and many, now being forced to retire, had been accustomed to working long hours in their earlier years. Consequently, many of the elderly had not prepared for retirement. Not only did they have little money, but they frequently had no interests or hobbies with which to fill their new-found leisure time.

In 1950 the first National Conference on Aging was held in Washington. Following this, the Committee on Aging and Geriatrics (the care of the elderly) was formed within the federal government. In the same year the National Social Welfare Assembly, a voluntary organization, formed a Committee on Aging. This committee became an independent organzation, the National Council on Aging,* in 1961. This group has concerned itself with matters affecting the aged, such as standards for sheltered care, employment of the aged, and retirement regulations. It is a valuable source for literature relating to the elderly. In 1956 a Federal Council on Aging was created to coordinate efforts in behalf of the elderly in the various departments of government and to broaden the range of federal activities. In the same year, the Center for Aging Research in the National Institutes of Health was established. Recently, an Office of Aging was created within the Department of Health, Education, and Welfare. This office publishes a monthly newsletter, *Aging.*

Many state and local committees have been formed and have a broad area of interest. In several states, joint legislative committees have been formed to guide lawmaking bodies in passing legislation concerning the welfare of older people. Many church and other local groups have set up special committees to study what their contribution can be to housing, recreation, and other community planning for the aging. Most county medical societies now have geriatric

---

*Headquarters, 315 Park Ave. South, New York, N.Y. 10010.

sections, as does the American Nurses' Association. There are two national scientific societies devoted exclusively to the aging and the aged, the Gerontological Society, Inc., and the American Geriatrics Society.[24]

As a result of society's interest in the elderly, the majority of them now have a small income from one or more sources, such as voluntary insurance plans, state and federal government plans, and individual savings. The average income per family unit, however, is still substantially below that of families the heads of which are 45 to 65 years of age, and the elderly, as a group, have a lower standard of living. Persons whose income is largely from pensions, which do not increase or decrease with the cost of living, have the greatest difficulty.

It is impossible to determine exactly how many receive benefits, since sources overlap. However, in March, 1963, about 10 million persons 62 years of age and over received income from Old-Age, Survivors, and Disability Insurance (Social Security) and 4,645,-000 wives and other dependents of retired and deceased workers also received income from this source.[38] In 1962 the average monthly income of a retired single man worker from Social Security benefits was $81.70; that of a single retired woman worker was $62.40; that of the retired worker and aged wife was $127.10; and that of the aged widow was $65.40.

Unfortunately, it is still very difficult for the person over 65, even if he is physically able and anxious to work, to find employment. Gradually, however, society is learning that gainful employment seems to be essential for many people to be happy. It cannot be replaced by provision for economic security. There is presently a genuine effort to encourage job development and employment for the elderly.[24]

There has also been a great deal of concern about suitable housing for the elderly. Many aged persons live in private homes that are too large, in poor neighborhoods, in isolated rural areas, in the top floor of walk-up tenements, and in housing that is otherwise unsuitable. They may live in these dwellings for financial reasons or because they may wish to remain in familiar surroundings. Many still live with children, and disturbing problems have occurred from crowding, economic pressures, and dissimilarity in cultural backgrounds of various members of the family. Some elderly persons live with distant relatives or friends, only visiting their children, and sometimes they are happier than those who live with sons and daughters.

Progress has been made recently in setting aside a portion of low-cost housing for elderly persons. These facilities are located on ground floors of buildings with special heating and safety features, such as electric instead of gas stoves, good lighting, and doorways without sills to minimize the danger to the person with locomotor disability from stumbling and falling.

At first there was a movement to provide communal homes (homes for the aged) and building developments exclusively for the aged. Soon, however, it was learned that a variety of housing facilities was needed. What one older person prefers, another may not. Although homes for the aged and group housing planned specifically for the aged are good for those who fear to be alone and who need the security and protection of group living, they are not the answer for everyone. Many wish to live where they may associate with all ages (Fig. 16), and indeed this is preferable.

Every effort should be made to enable the aged person to live in his own home and in his customary setting if he so wishes. This is sometimes made possible by providing such services as housekeeping for the frail and visiting nursing for the ailing. Sometimes arrangements for bringing one hot meal each day to the home may be all that is necessary to enable a feeble elderly couple to carry on together. Others can maintain a home if provision can be made for assistance with some relatively simple tasks such as grocery shopping. Provision for a telephone and for daily visits by a neighbor is frequently all that is necessary. Making prior arrangements to enter a home for the aged whenever the need arises has made it possible for many elderly persons to continue on their own with less apprehension.

In an effort to help the elderly use their free time in a satisfying manner and to help them maintain social contacts, despite the death of a husband or wife and lifelong friends, many community and voluntary agencies have organized clubs for the elderly. Here they can make new friends (Fig. 6) and participate in activities suitable to their physical stamina (Fig. 7).

Visitors, either voluntary or employed, are provided by some community agencies to go into the homes of elderly shut-ins solely for socialization. They are also being used for lonely hospitalized patients. Often an elderly person can be used to give this service, thus providing him with a useful occupation.

Compared to other age groups, the geriatric age group requires medical, nursing, and other professional services, as well as drugs and appliances, more often, in larger amounts, and for longer periods. They also have more frequent and longer hospital admissions.[36] Previously (as at present), the implications of illness were more important for the aged person than was the illness or disability itself. He often could not afford to be ill, and he was frequently uncertain who would care for him during illness. General hospitals often were reluctant to admit him, and he often found himself in a poorly equipped hospital for the chronically ill or in a poorly staffed nursing home. He frequently put off medical care, delayed the purchase of medications, and refused treatments or home nursing care because he felt

he could not afford them. Recently, with the passage of federal legislation to amend the Social Security Act (Title 18, "Medicare," and Title 19, Medical Assistance), a great step forward has been made to alleviate this problem. Hospital care and nursing home care, for a limited period at least, are now assured by the federal government for all persons over 65 years of age. For three dollars a month, medical insurance to assist in paying for a doctor's services and other medical items can be obtained. The legislation also includes specific requirements that an institution must fulfill to qualify for Medicare and Medical Assistance funds. This legislation has brought about improvements in many facilities.

The adult in our society. Nonelderly adults in the United States are usually considered to be those persons between 21 and 65 years of age. This group makes up the majority of the work force and the homemakers. By far the greatest number are married and have

Fig. 6

Adjustment is difficult when death of a spouse brings loss of the companionship developed over many years. (Courtesy New York League for the Hard of Hearing, New York, N. Y.)

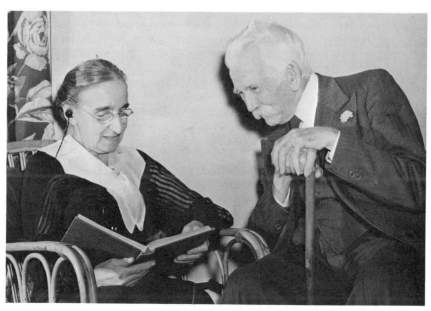

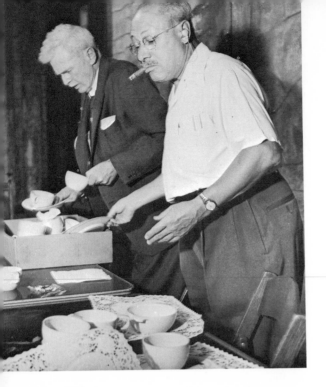

Fig. 7

Community recreational programs fill in many
empty hours. (Courtesy New York League
for the Hard of Hearing, New York, N. Y.)

children, but there is also a sizable number
of single people in this age group.

Most of the community planning and organization is done by the adult age group
and, consequently, health teaching related
to community needs usually is directed toward them. The younger members of this
group often need to be taught about child
rearing and homemaking, and they usually
are receptive to such teaching.

It is at this age that people should begin
to prepare physically, psychologically, and
economically for retirement and their later
years. Maintenance of good health practices
related to diet, exercise, and rest may help
to prevent their suffering from many of the
chronic ills of the aged. Yearly medical examinations, even though they feel well, may
help to assure that early symptoms of disease are recognized and treatment instituted
before conditions become acute or chronic.

Adults should be taught the early signs of
cancer, since it frequently occurs in the later
adult years. Certainly they need to maintain immunizations (p. 299). People in this
age group, especially those having jobs in

industry and construction, are frequently involved in accidents. Accident prevention
programs, the institution of safety devices,
and the supervision of their use are important for this group. Teaching working people and homemakers how to prevent stasis
of blood in the legs may prevent them from
developing peripheral vascular disease (p.
364). Teaching this age group to avoid obesity is certainly essential (p. 121) and may
help to prevent serious chronic diseases such
as diabetes and arteriosclerosis in later
years. Avoidance of the use of tobacco also
is essential teaching and may prevent diseases such as cancer of the lung, emphysema, and peripheral vascular disease.

In our society today, people undergo great
stresses, both on the job and in life in general. We live in a highly competitive and
fast-moving society. The adult is especially
affected by the competition, as it may influence his ability to maintain a job and a
home for his family. The resulting stress may
contribute to such diseases as duodenal ulcers, coronary heart disease, and hypertension. Therefore, it is extremely important
to teach adults how to relax. Physical activities and diversional recreation of all kinds
are essential because they help to reduce
tensions. Some of these activities, especially
in the later adult years, should be ones that
can be continued into retirement.

Labor unions have done more for the welfare of the adult group than any other
agency in our society. They have been concerned with wages and working conditions
and have instituted pension and insurance
plans for many working groups. Insurance
companies have also directed their efforts
toward adults, urging them to participate
in voluntary insurance plans and providing
them with a great deal of literature concerning health practices. Industry, of course,
focuses a great deal of attention on the adult
consumer. Laborsaving devices planned for
adults have often been useful. "Do-it-yourself" materials have also been useful in helping many fill their leisure hours, although
they have also resulted in an increased number of accidents among persons in this age
group.

Recently, some businesses have begun to
help the adult prepare psychologically for
retirement. Programs have been instituted

to gradually reduce the working year. It is hoped that this reduction will help people adjust more readily to retirement.

Age as a factor in development and in illness

The nurse whose patient is an infant, child, or adolescent should remember that he is growing physically and developing physically, mentally, and emotionally. Therefore, she not only has a responsibility to provide for his clinical nursing needs, but she should try to see that his growth and development progresses as well as possible under the circumstances of illness. The nurse also may need to help parents understand and provide for their children's present and future needs.

To give effective care to patients in this age group, the nurse should know the usual stages of growth and development and the special attention needed by each group for maintaining normal development. The emphasis the nurse should place on the various aspects in giving care will vary, depending upon the age of the child, how long he is ill, whether he must be hospitalized, and the nature of his illness. For example, in caring for a 6-month-old infant with diarrhea, she would be immediately concerned with replacing the fluid loss. In a 16-year-old, on the other hand, fluid loss might not be of great concern unless the diarrhea continued unabated for a number of hours or unless the patient was already debilitated by another illness. If the child is chronically ill, providing educational toys for him, allowing him to play with others, and making provision for him to continue his schooling may be very important in his care. For the child with a short-term illness, such provision is not essential. If a child is of preschool age, any illness, whether acute or chronic, that separates him from his mother may affect him emotionally. Special attention, therefore, needs to be given to ways of providing love and security for children in this age group.

The infant (birth to 2 years of age)

Care of the infant. Infants have all the basic needs of the person of any age and they may be afflicted with similar ailments.

However, the ways in which their needs are expressed, their ability to cope with them even when well, and their response to illness are quite different. In caring for an infant a cardinal rule to remember is: *Babies are not little adults, physically, physiologically, or emotionally.*

Physical and physiologic characteristics of infants. An infant's physical development is incomplete, and therefore his metabolism is extremely active. His need for calories, fluids, and all the nutrients is proportionately greater than that of persons in any other age group. His reserves of fat, glycogen, and extracellular water are so limited that he cannot withstand loss of fluid or the omission of food or fluids for more than a few hours without developing signs of acidosis (p. 101) and dehydration (p. 96). If dehydration occurs, the baby will go rapidly into shock from subsequent loss of blood volume. Unless immediate treatment is given, death will soon follow. Parents should know of the need to seek immediate medical attention for any baby who has fever, diarrhea, or vomiting or who fails to take several consecutive feedings. Because of the ease with which they become dehydrated, infants seldom are given cathartics or enemas. Any order for a cathartic or enema should be carefully verified with the doctor, and after it is given the infant should be observed closely for signs of dehydration.

Because his metabolism is so active, the infant generates large amounts of heat. He also loses proportionately larger amounts of fluid than do physically larger persons in dissipating the same amount of heat and therefore becomes quickly dehydrated by fever. The infant also is quickly chilled because his vascular dilation and constriction are poorly controlled, preventing body heat from being retained efficiently. This poor control is probably related to the incomplete development of the nervous system in infants.

Because the nervous system of an infant is incompletely developed at birth, he is not able to do such things as focus his eyes, use his hands to grasp objects, and localize pain. Even after physical development of the nervous system is complete, physical and emotional responses, except for reflex ones, which are part of the body's defense system, must be learned by repetitive practice. Those that produce satisfying results for the person usually are retained. They may or may not be appropriate according to the standards of society. However, responses that are unacceptable to others usually are not satisfying. It is in this way that the family and the community mold behavior according to social and cultural patterns. The child who is given no opportunity to practice physical and emotional responses will not develop normally even if he has no physical or physiologic limitations.

If physical development is incomplete for some reason or if there is a malfunction of some physiologic process, the child may not be able to develop normally in every aspect. For example, the mechanism for seeing or hearing may be incomplete, and as a result the baby will be blind or deaf. A muscle in his leg may be congenitally absent, making it impossible for him to learn to walk. Failure of the anterior lobe of the pituitary gland to secrete the growth hormone may cause him to be a dwarf; oversecretion may cause him to grow excessively. His brain may fail to develop normally for various reasons, making him mentally retarded and, in turn, possibly preventing his learning such activities as walking and talking.

During the first year or two of life the infant's endocrine functions are sluggish. His fluid and electrolyte balance is easily upset and he has little resistance to infection or stresses of any kind. Therefore, babies respond quickly and critically to illness. They may be apparently well one moment and an hour later seriously ill. The younger the child the more pronounced is this response.

Young babies, especially ill ones, are very prone to infections and often die as a result of them. They are more likely than are older children to have generalized systemic involvement even from such seemingly minor conditions as a cut or a cold. Therefore, the nurse and others caring for a sick infant should wear an isolation gown to protect the infant against organisms carried on the clothing. Some authorities advise that a mask be worn, and some feel that sterile masks and gowns should be used. No one with an upper respiratory infection or any staphylococcal infection should care for a baby. Be-

fore giving care to an infant, it is essential to carefully wash one's hands. The baby's room should be kept clean and dust free, and it should be comfortably warm but well ventilated. All treatments should be carried out with the utmost gentleness to prevent traumatizing tissues, and strict surgical aseptic techniques should always be used whenever the treatment involves an opening on the skin or entry into any body cavity.

The infant tolerates respiratory embarrassment very poorly. Special precautions should always be taken to prevent the infant's accidentally suffocating. The importance of these measures should be stressed to parents. No soft pillows, filmy plastic, blankets, or other material that might smother a baby should be in contact with or anywhere near his face. Pins or any small objects that he might put into his mouth and accidentally swallow must never be left within reach.

Any infant who is "croupy," has a dusky color, shows sternal retraction on respiration, or has irregular respirations (Cheyne-Stokes) needs immediate medical attention. The nurse caring for a sick baby should always know how to give mouth-to-mouth resuscitation (p. 241). Teaching parents to do this might at some time save the life of their child. Parents should also be taught the signs of respiratory embarrassment in an infant and be alerted to the need to seek immediate medical attention should they occur.

A baby with any respiratory embarrassment, no matter how slight, may be given oxygen to make each inspiration more effective and to reduce the work of the heart as it attempts to transport adequate oxygen to all parts of the body. This is usually given by a small oxygen tent or a head tent (Burgess box). Steam tents (croup tents) may be needed to provide humidity to loosen mucous secretions. (Pediatric nursing texts should be consulted for detailed discussions of these procedures.) Mucus in the nose and throat may need to be removed with suction (p. 191). A temporary tracheotomy sometimes must be done (p. 598). All these procedures may be very upsetting for the child's parents. The considerate nurse will find time to explain to them the reason they are necessary and arrange for them to talk with the doctor about the child's condition. If oxygen is being used only prophylactically, the parents should be told this fact.

Anticipating the infant's physical needs. Not only is the infant unable to take care of himself in any way, but he is unable to express his needs except by crying. Therefore, others must anticipate them. The nurse who cares for an ill baby must observe his appearance and behavior closely and frequently for signs and symptoms of abnormality. Parents also should be taught to recognize these signs and symptoms so that they will know when to get medical attention for their baby.

A restless, irritable infant may be manifesting pain which he has no other way of expressing. Since pain is difficult to evaluate and localize in babies, any symptoms suggesting it should be reported in detail to the doctor.

Failure of the infant to eat properly may be a sign of any one of many serious disorders and should always be discussed with the doctor. Apathy to food and loss of appetite may signify an incipient infection. It may have many other causes. Failure to gain weight in spite of taking food is always a serious sign. Unusual fussiness between feedings is often indicative of ill health. A satisfied and healthy baby usually sleeps soon after his feeding and awakens prior to the next one. Persistent vomiting, as contrasted with the normal occasional regurgitation that occurs in many well infants, nearly always is a serious sign and may be the first evidence of infection anywhere in the body or of other disease.

Changes in the character and timing of stools may indicate serious gastrointestinal disease. When an infant is sick, the color and amount of each stool should be noted and recorded. The time of each stool also should be recorded. The color, odor, and amount of urine and the frequency of urination should be recorded (p. 102). Any

Fig. 8

The social worker is visiting while the grandmother helps care for the infant. Note that the grandmother is standing so as to protect the child from rolling out of the bed accidentally. (Courtesy Today's Health, American Medical Association, Chicago, Ill.; photograph by Dorothy Reed.)

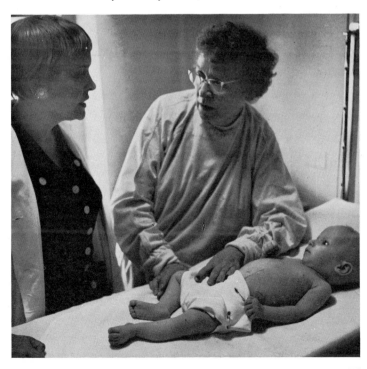

significant changes in the stool or urine from normal should be brought to the doctor's attention at once.

Caring for the infant's needs. Attention must be given to the infant's *general hygiene.* Each day the infant's entire body should be thoroughly inspected. This is usually done during the bath. The eyes, ears, and nostrils should be inspected for discharges and cleaned as necessary. The skin and scalp should be observed for any lesions. Rashes on the back of the head, the buttocks, and perineum are rather common. They can be minimized by keeping the baby clean and dry (Fig. 8). If the baby has any urinary tract infection, special care needs to be taken because the urine is likely to be more acid or alkaline than normal.

If the baby is hospitalized or sick at home for a long period, plans should be made for him to be in the outside air and sun at intervals. Care should be taken not to chill the baby or to overexpose him to the sun.

The infant must be given *food* and *fluids.* If the ill infant can tolerate food and fluid by mouth, he usually is given his regular formula. Otherwise, food and fluids are given parenterally. Occasionally, a baby will have to be gavaged (fed through a nasogastric tube) (p. 107).

Well babies, beginning soon after birth, usually receive prescribed formulas equivalent to 2½ ounces and 50 calories per pound of body weight a day.[22] Formulas may be supplemented by orange juice and vitamins A and D. Solids in the form of the yolks of hard-boiled eggs and strained baby foods are usually started at least by the third or fourth month. They should be fed to the baby before he is given his bottle. When the infant begins to get teeth and learns to chew, he is usually advanced to minced or chopped foods (junior foods). Most children go to an "adult diet" some time between the eighteenth and twenty-fourth month.[22] When a baby no longer takes a formula, his diet should include the basic four food groups (p. 114).

Often a sick infant will need extra fluids, and the doctor should specify the amount and type of fluid. Plans must be made to space this extra fluid between feedings. Medications are usually given by medicine dropper or spoon. Any baby, but especially

an ill one, should be held for his bottles and medications to prevent aspiration. Holding him may also improve his appetite because most infants are used to being fed in this way at home.

If the baby is hospitalized over a period of many months, the nurse should consult the doctor about increasing his diet. There usually is no reason why a hospitalized infant's diet should not progress with his age in the same way it would normally. New foods should be started one at a time. If an infant rejects a food, a substitution should be made and the food tried again later. To help the child to learn to chew, the nurse may give him crackers or dry toast. Chopped food should never be given before he has learned to chew.

Before the baby is discharged from the hospital, the nurse should be sure that the mother knows the formula or food he is receiving and how to prepare it. Nurses from the nursery for newborn infants may be called upon to teach formula preparation, or sometimes the nutritionist or dietitian will teach it. The visiting nurse can be asked to go into the home to give the mother additional help as necessary.

Attention needs to be given to the baby's *physical development.* Not all babies develop at the same rate, and the sick baby may be expected to be somewhat retarded in his development. As the infant develops, he soon should begin to look about him. At around 4 months of age he usually begins to clutch at large objects, although he may be 8 months old or more before he can hold small objects. Around 5 months of age he begins to roll over and by 8 months of age he may be able to crawl. Babies vary greatly in the time they learn to walk and speak. The average age for walking is 12 months. Many children can say several words by this age too.[22] (See pediatric nursing texts for further details.)

The nurse caring for an infant should know the usual schedule of development. She should be alert for any indications of abnormality in the development of infant patients and bring these to the physician's attention. She also should provide care that will in no way impede development. If the infant is ill for a long time, either at home or in the hospital, she should see that provisions are made whenever possible for normal development to continue.

Provisions should be made for the baby to have as much normal movement as possible. A firm mattress helps the sick baby who has poor muscle tone to move about more easily. If possible, the baby should be turned on his abdomen for about an hour twice a day. He may also be propped to either side for periods of time. When any part of the infant's body must be restrained, it is desirable for the restraint to be released for five or ten minutes every two to four hours day and night. This allows the infant to move the part freely at intervals. However, no restraint should be removed without first consulting the doctor.

Equipment appropriate for the infant's stage of development should be provided. Bright rattles or mobiles strung over the crib provide exercise in eye movements. When the baby begins to clutch with his hands, a rattle or some similar toy should be provided. If the baby is beginning to crawl and pull himself up, it is often permissible to put him in a playpen or some other safe area where he can move about more freely than in a crib.

Special attention should be paid to the *safety* of a baby. A baby, no matter how young, should never be left alone with the crib side down or in any other place where he might fall (Fig. 8). Even young babies are usually quite active with their arms and legs and can accidentally propel themselves over the edge of a bed or table. When the baby begins to move about more actively, a harness restraint often is used to secure him even in the crib. The harness slips over the shoulders and chest, fastens in the back, and is tied to the lower bar at the head of the crib with a square knot that holds securely but is easily untied. Preferably, the harness should be made like a vest, and its ties should be short enough to prevent the infant from becoming entangled in them and choking. Any body restraint used for an infant or small child must be approved by the medical staff of the hospital and must be ordered specifically by the doctor for each patient.

Occasionally it may be necessary to use restraining measures to prevent a baby from moving about during a procedure, to prevent him from pulling on catheters or dressings, or to keep him from scratching an itchy rash. Usually, holding the baby's arms and legs firmly at the ankles and wrists provides sufficient restraint for a procedure, but sometimes it may be necessary to place him in a blanket restraint ("mummy" him) (Fig. 9). To prevent the baby from pulling at dressings and tubes or scratching himself, elbow splints usually are effective. They prevent bending of the elbow but allow movement of the arm as a whole. (See Fig. 10.) Since the baby is as agile with his feet as with his hands, a splint may need to be placed behind the knee. Special care must be taken to ensure that any splints are well padded and do not press into soft tissues, lest ulceration of the tissue occur. At other times it may be necessary to apply wrist or ankle restraints. These restraints should be well padded and should allow for maintenance of correct body alignment and slight movement of the part. For a tiny baby a long gown that fastens snugly in the back and can be tied below the feet may suffice to keep dressings and catheters out of reach. A gown with mittens also may give adequate restraint. No restraint should impede circulation to the part and, if permitted, it should be removed periodically (see above).

It is normal and necessary for a baby to be fondled and loved. "Mothering" is essential for his *psychologic development*. The plan for care, therefore, should include time for cuddling the infant of any age, and some time should be taken each day to play with him. If a rocking chair is kept at the bedside, the infant can be held comfortably, talked to, and stroked while he is being bathed, dressed, and fed, and even while he is being given certain treatments. Some babies may have restrictions of movements and cannot be held. The resourceful nurse, however, will still find ways of providing loving care. Even a baby who cannot be held can be talked to and stroked. Wheeling his crib back and forth in a rocking motion often is comforting to a baby too. The baby who has apparatus such as catheters attached usually can be held safely provided that the persons caring for him are properly instructed in the necessary precautions.

The nurse can provide some of the "cuddling" needed by the infant patient as she

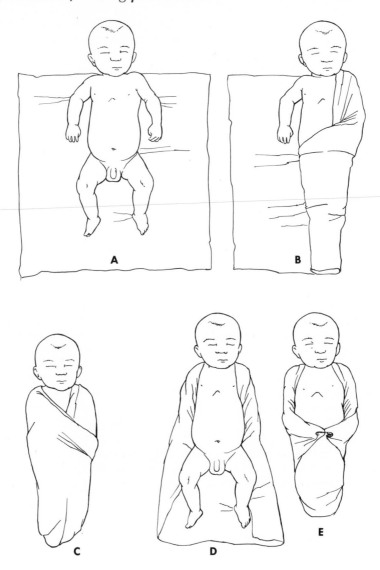

Fig. 9

Mummying an infant. **A,** Place infant on sheet or blanket to be used. **B,** Wrap one side of sheet snugly around and under baby so that the arm is at his side and legs are together. **C,** Bring other side of sheet across body, securing the other arm. Pin the sheet securely at the side and bottom. **D** and **E,** A modification that can be used for treatments requiring that the chest and/or abdomen be uncovered.

gives him care, but her attention must of necessity be divided among many patients. Therefore, she seldom is able to give a baby the necessary amount of attention. Since this is a period of life when the mother and baby are normally together, it is preferable that whenever possible the mother provide the "mothering." It is probably not essential for the welfare of a young infant that the mother be present twenty-four hours a day. However, as he approaches the age of 2 years, it becomes more important. (See discussion later in this chapter.) If the mother cannot be with her baby, another family member,

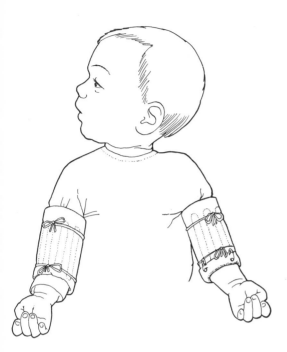

Fig. 10

Elbow splints prevent infant from disturbing dressings or scratching, yet permit free movement of the shoulders and arms.

such as a grandmother, a teen-age sister, or the father, may wish to assist with the care (Fig. 8). Sometimes a volunteer or paid worker may be assigned as "mother" for the infant who must be hospitalized for a long time and whose family is not present.

The infant's *spiritual needs* must not be neglected. The religious or denominational affiliation of the infant's family should be ascertained, and the nurse should be meticulous in assuring that appropriate observances are carried out. She should always ask whether the baby has been baptized, and if not, whether the family wishes him to be. The family also should be consulted about their desire to have a priest, minister, or rabbi informed should the baby become critically ill. In discussing the infant's progress with the family members, the nurse should give assurance that their desires in these matters have been complied with.

The infant's family. The baby who is hospitalized usually belongs to a family who

will be interested in the course of his illness and his general development. Arrangements should be made for the family to speak with the doctor about the infant's medical progress and about plans for his continued treatment. The nurse can tell the family about any new symptoms displayed by the infant, signs of physical or psychologic improvement, and advances in normal development. She can also explain to the family the procedures that the infant is undergoing.

If a family member is assisting in the nursing care of a hospitalized infant, the nurse is still responsible for the care. She should specifically define that care for which the family member will be responsible and plan to teach her about the care and assist her with it as necessary. It is always best to assist the family member at least the first time she gives the care. When the nurse feels that her assistance is no longer needed, she should still plan to observe the care periodically, and she should let the family member know that she is always available to give assistance or to answer questions. The nurse usually gives the infant his medications and treatments, but if he will need continued treatment at home, the family member who will give it should have the opportunity to learn and practice the procedures involved under the guidance of the nurse. Often a baby whose mother has been allowed to assist with his care in the hospital will be able to be discharged from the hospital sooner than otherwise because the family is less fearful and is prepared to provide continuing nursing care in the home.

Home care. It is usually advisable to arrange for a visiting nurse to make a home visit to any baby who has been hospitalized, and she is often asked to give the parents help when a child is receiving his medical care at home. If the baby has been hospitalized, an early referral should be made so that the nurse may visit the home before the baby's return to help the family make the necessary preparations. It may be helpful for the visiting nurse, before doing this, to visit the baby in the hospital. In writing the referral, information concerning nutrition, development, medications, details of dressings, and other treatments should be included so that the nurse in the home can give continuing follow-up care.

31

Trends and problems influencing patient care

The young child

The term young child applies to children in two age groups: those 2 to 5 years of age (preschool children) and those in elementary school. Although both groups are growing and developing rapidly, they differ somewhat physically, physiologically, and psychologically. Children in both groups grow rapidly for a time, slow down, and then have another spurt of growth. Their appetite may parallel the growth pattern. Physiologic controls, especially of fluids and electrolyte balance and temperature, are still not fully developed in the preschooler, although they are somewhat more effective than those of an infant. By about the age of 7 years, physiologic controls appear to be fully developed.

The preschool child is still learning basic muscle coordination and basic speech, is developing the basic behavior patterns necessary for socialization, and is exploring his environment. He does not express himself with complete facility yet and often has not learned to cooperate with spoken instructions. The schoolchild, on the other hand, usually can express himself well, can follow instructions, and has learned to cooperate with others. He often can be reasoned with effectively.

Children in both age groups need love and affection. To be happy, they also need discipline. Knowing the acceptable limits seems to give security to persons of every age.

The ill child. Children, especially those under the age of 5, tolerate any systemic upset, such as may occur with infection, tissue trauma, or anesthesia, poorly. Their ability to withstand fluid and electrolyte loss is still poor, and they still may readily respond with fever. Therefore, extensive bowel preparations for diagnostic procedures or surgery are rarely given, and doctors rarely withhold food or fluids for long. The usual plan when food or fluids must be withheld is described on p. 94. If more than one enema is given to a child under 7 years of age, or if food and fluids are withheld for more than two to four hours, he should be observed closely for signs of dehydration, and the doctor must be notified at once if they appear.

There is rarely any reason why children who are not seriously ill or who do not have a fever cannot be dressed during the day. Most hospitals provide suits and dresses as well as underclothes and nightclothes. Children who are hospitalized should be encouraged to continue activities they have learned to do for themselves at home, such as dressing themselves, washing, and going to the toilet. Bathrooms with low fixtures usually are available, or a sturdy step stool can be used. The nurse should ask the mother what her child does for himself and make as few radical changes from the home routine as possible. The child responds best to as much normality as possible. If the child must be kept in bed, the nurse should be sure he understands about the use of the bedpans, bed bathing, and eating from trays.

Many children in the younger age groups are finicky eaters, and feeding the hospitalized child may present special problems. Most children eat better if given small servings and if they are not constantly coaxed. They usually eat better at a table with others, and making mealtime a "party" occasion is often helpful. Snacks between meals may supplement inadequate meals. Food likes and dislikes should be ascertained from the mother.

The older child may have a voracious appetite, especially if he is growing rapidly and is very active. He should be given foods high in protein and foods that are simple carbohydrates. Starches and fats sometimes should be avoided because overweight may become a problem. The mother should be told about diet requirements because they also apply to the child's diet at home.

Play should be provided for children unless they are acutely ill. A variety of amusements should be available, especially for young children. Even when well, the attention span of children is short, and sick children may tire of an activity even more readily. Preschool children often enjoy crayoning, finger painting, and make-believe activities (Fig. 11). The school-age child may be interested in reading, listening to records, observing and caring for birds or fish, making such objects as model planes or jewelry, painting, or taking part in competitive activities. Playing with others usually is possible even for the bedridden child, but care should be taken that the child does not overexert himself or become overtired. Educational play activity and play with others are

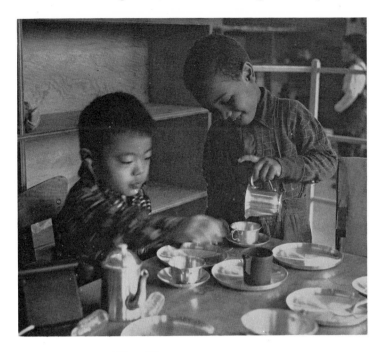

Fig. 11

Make-believe play activities amuse many preschool children. These two little boys are playing house. (Jan E. Ott from Monkmeyer Press Photo Service; from Sawyer, Janet R.: Nursing care of patients with urologic diseases, St. Louis, 1963, The C. V. Mosby Co.)

especially important for the child who has a prolonged illness, so that continued mental and social development is assured.

If a child of school age is hospitalized or is sick at home for a long period of time (usually over two weeks), most boards of education provide visiting teachers. Parents need to be reminded of this service. Continuing with his schoolwork not only provides diversion for the child but also assures him of "keeping up" in school.

Every ill child, whether in the hospital or at home, should receive some special attention from adults. This attention is needed especially by the bedridden child. The form of the attention needed varies with the child. Most children, even those of school age, need to be held and hugged occasionally; others respond better to interest in their activity or just quiet talking. Almost all children like to have stories read to them, and quiet play activities such as games are usually enjoyed. Helping the mother or nurse with such small tasks as picking up toys or cleaning the table may provide the desired attention. A very ill child of any age may want little more than the comfort of a parent's presence, but it is very important to him.

When a child requires treatments or medication, the nurse must adapt the procedures to the age of the child and to his response. Before a procedure is performed, it should be described to the child of any age and his part in it explained. With preschool children, painless but strange procedures can often be accomplished most easily by using play techniques. For example, a rocking-horse seat may be provided for the child while a roentgenogram of the lungs is taken. A similar arrangement can be made for holding a potty for the collection of urine specimens. The resourceful nurse can devise many techniques of this type. The school-age child usually follows instructions well and is surprisingly cooperative if explanations of procedures are given to him. Often he can assist with his tests. For example, he may watch the clock for the time to collect specimens. The capacity to cooperate will, of course, vary from child to child and depends upon the extent of his development.

If the procedure will be uncomfortable, a parent or a nurse who is well liked by the child should be present to comfort and firmly hold him as necessary. The child of any age should be told truthfully what type of sensation he may expect, and it usually is advisable to tell him when he is about to be hurt. Restraining techniques such as "mummying" (Fig. 9) occasionally must be used for the safety of a preschool child who is overactive, but usually just talking to the child and holding him firmly is all that is needed. School-age children who have been properly instructed rarely need restraining. Appropriate praise, comfort, and attention should be given to the child of any age at the completion of a painful procedure.

Giving oral medication to children often requires an individualized technique that should be recorded on the child's nursing care plan. It is helpful to ask the mother about methods she has found successful with her child. Some children will swallow pills disguised with food, and others will take them dissolved in small amounts of fruit juices, but care should be taken not to develop a food dislike by its use with medications. Children's medications often come in both liquid and pill form and usually are flavored. The child may accept one form better than the other. Usually, children accept medicine better when they are among other children who are also receiving it. Therefore, it may be helpful to offer medications to children in a group situation. Special care must be taken, if this method is used, not to give drugs to the wrong child. Medication should *never* be given to any child before his identification band is carefully checked.

Medications should not be forced upon a child. If difficulty is encountered in getting a child to take a medication, the nurse should wait a few minutes and then try a new approach. There usually is some approach that is effective, but if not, the doctor should be consulted.

Special needs of the hospitalized child. If hospitalization is necessary, the child of any age should be prepared for the experience by his parents. The nurse in the doctor's office or clinic should be sure the par-

ents know how to prepare him. They should tell the child truthfully about the hospital and why he must go there. He should not be frightened about the experience, but neither should he be led to expect the experience to be completely pleasant. He should be told about the high beds, bedpans, urinals, bed baths, eating in bed, the attire of nurses and doctors, and the play facilities in a matter-of-fact and reassuring way. If possible, the preparation for hospitalization should be done gradually. Well-written storybooks concerning hospitalization are available in bookstores and may be helpful in introducing the topic. One available book is *Going to the Hospital.** (See Fig. 12.)

Children, especially those between 2 and 5 years of age (preschool age), tend to form attachments to inanimate objects, such as well-loved toys or blankets. Such an object, whatever it may be, gives the child comfort and security. Even a sick child of school age may want to bring some favorite object to the hospital. He should be allowed to do so, and no one should worry if it is old or ragged. The object is the child's link with home, and he should be free to take it with him wherever he goes, even to treatment rooms and to the operating room.

It is important, too, for parents to allow children of any age, prior to their departure for the hospital, to help prepare for their return home. This tells the child he is expected home again. Often the child can pack a bag with clothes that he will wear when he is discharged from the hospital, or he may help prepare the room where he will stay while he is recuperating.

Hospitalization and separation from the mother has been found to be especially upsetting for the child between 2 and 4 years of age. He has a tendency to regress to earlier behavior patterns while in the hospital, on his return home, or at both times. This regression may take many forms. Some children return to earlier behavior of bed-wetting or soiling their clothes; others may have bad dreams and cry during sleep. Some refuse to eat; others revert to baby talk and whining or stop talking altogether. The

---

*Prepared by the Child Development Center, 1953, Children's Hospital of East Bay, Oakland, California.

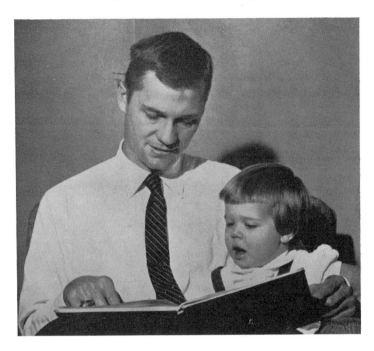

Fig. 12

A child's father can help in preparation of the child for hospitalization. This one is reading to his daughter a book about going to the hospital. (Bloom from Monkmeyer Press Photo Service; from Sawyer, Janet R.: Nursing care of patients with urologic diseases, St. Louis, 1963, The C. V. Mosby Co.)

child may be "too good" or he may be unusually naughty. Temper tantrums and clinging to the mother are common. If the child has to be separated from his mother, the regression may be more noticeable and last much longer. Consequently, doctors now seldom hospitalize children in this age group unless it is absolutely necessary. Whenever possible, the child is cared for in his home, in an outpatient department, or in the doctor's office.

If the child must be hospitalized, many doctors advise the mother to "room in" with the child during the entire hospital stay. Many hospitals have lounging chairs or cots placed at the child's bedside; some of the cots slide under youth beds. The mother's comfort should be considered, and the thoughtful nurse will be sure that she knows the location of rest rooms, dressing and eating facilities, and a telephone booth. The mother should be informed about hospital regulations by which she is expected to abide. For example, it may be customary for her to leave the room during certain treatments or she may be forbidden in other children's rooms or in workrooms of the unit. Often, if the mother stays at the hospital with her child, plans must be made for the care of the rest of the family. The social service department of the hospital or of a public health agency may be helpful in this regard. It is certainly not always possible or practical for a mother to stay with her child constantly, especially if the hospitalization is to be for more than a few days. If she cannot stay, she should not be made to feel that she is a poor mother.

When the mother does not stay with the hospitalized preschool child, he should be cared for by as few nurses as possible. This procedure seems to add to his security. A substitute mother (p. 31) may also be used. Frequent and regular visits from the parents are helpful, even though the child often ignores them during the visit and cries bitterly after they leave. This behavior may be very upsetting to parents, and the nurse should prepare them to expect it. They should be helped to realize that it is a completely normal response and that no amount of reasoning with him will change his reaction. He is angry at his parents because he thinks he has been deserted. They should be cautioned not to add distrust to anger by failing to visit at appointed times or by deceiving him in any way. For instance, they should tell the child when they are leaving and not slip away without telling him they are leaving. If frequent visits cannot be made, children seem to enjoy receiving some daily memento, such as a brightly colored greeting card or a note from the family. Nurses should allow the child to keep the card with him and should be willing to read and reread it for him. Telephone conversations between the older child and his parents also seem to give comfort.

Hospitalization apparently is not too psychologically traumatic for the schoolchild, especially if he has been adequately prepared for it. Unless the child is acutely ill or will be having an operation, he rarely needs the constant attendance of his mother. However, his parents should be urged to visit him regularly or, if frequent visits are not possible, to keep in regular contact with him by telephone or letter.

The parents will want to know about their child's activities, behavior, and progress in the hospital. Although no child should be discussed with his parents when he is present, the nurse is responsible for keeping parents informed and for giving them necessary explanations. Plans also should be made to teach the mother any procedures she will need to know when the child returns home. The parents should be told to expect that a young child on return home may exhibit some form of regressive behavior. He can be managed best by giving him extra "mothering" and resuming former expectations for behavior at once. Arrangements should be made for parents to discuss the medical aspects of the child's care with the doctor.

The teen-ager

The early adolescent (12 to 16 years) is neither a child nor an adult, and he may alternately respond and wish to be treated as either a child or an adult. Adequate handling of this group offers a real challenge. One must feel one's way and alter the approach accordingly.

Many boys and girls in their early teens are physically awkward and ill coordinated because their growth during this period progresses in uneven stages. The young teenager should not be expected to handle any tasks that would put him in the embarrassing position of "falling over" his hands and feet. Great tact is needed to avoid being obvious about avoiding such a situation. He also may drop and spill things but should not be reprimanded.

The teen-ager, especially the young one who is growing rapidly, consumes large amounts of food. Girls between 13 and 15 and boys between 16 and 19 years of age need more calories than at any other time during their life cycle. Teen-agers often need double or even triple servings of food at meals and nourishing snacks between meals. Good food habits should be stressed to ensure an adequate nutritional intake as well as a "filling" one (p. 114). Teen-agers often tend to maintain a hamburger-and-coke diet. Teen-age girls, especially, often omit breakfast.

Young teen-agers of both sexes are likely to be subject to disorders involving the skin. Acne vulgaris is a common condition at this age. It is related to the hormonal changes of puberty. Although it cannot be prevented, the symptoms can be minimized and complications prevented by attention to skin care and to diet (p. 781). This condition is very upsetting to most teen-agers, and they usually are willing to follow suggestions for care.

Teen-age girls often spend much time languishing and primping. They are flattered by attention by men but also enjoy "woman-to-woman" talk. Teen-age boys often try to get a "rise" from young women by acting like a "man-about-town." At other times they may seem quite rude, failing to respond to people who are talking to them or responding curtly. If these reactions are handled matter-of-factly or ignored, they will usually pass.

Teen-agers, especially older ones, are often confronted by ambivalence, and they may become quite confused and worried.

They feel a need to be the same as others in their group and yet they are beginning to become individuals. They may be the size of an adult and have the sexual drive of an adult but still be emotionally immature. Society, however, may expect them to behave as an adult. Teen-agers are inherently idealistic, yet the realities of the world are constantly being revealed to them. They have a great amount of energy and enthusiasm. These qualities are all too frequently rejected by adults, probably because the realization that their own years of life are passing makes them uncomfortable.

Teen-agers need to talk about their problems and feelings. The teen-age boy often likes to talk with an older adult, either a man or woman. The teen-age girl may confide in a young woman. Both boys and girls may find it easier to talk with someone other than a family member. Priests, ministers, rabbis, club leaders, nurses and doctors, and friends of parents may be useful in this role. The teen-ager should be allowed to express his feelings freely and should be helped to explore them. Sometimes professional help may be needed.

The ill teen-ager. When teen-agers, especially the older ones, require hospitalization, they are often assigned to the adult service. They are usually considered adults as far as physical aspects of preparation for diagnostic tests and therapy are concerned. However, their psychologic needs must be met quite differently from those of an adult.

It is most important that the teen-ager's relative maturity be acknowledged by the nurse. She should talk to him as an adult. He is likely to be flattered by this and usually responds well. The teen-ager is usually interested in his disease even though he may appear very blasé and even disinterested. Unless the nurse makes a deliberate effort, this attitude may cause her to be negligent about exploring the true reaction

Fig. 13

Teen-agers usually are interested in learning. Here, one is watching a male nurse prepare a drug for injection before he answers the boy's questions. (Lew Merrim from Monkmeyer Press Photo Service; from Sawyer, Janet R.: Nursing care of patients with urologic diseases, St. Louis, 1963, The C. V. Mosby Co.)

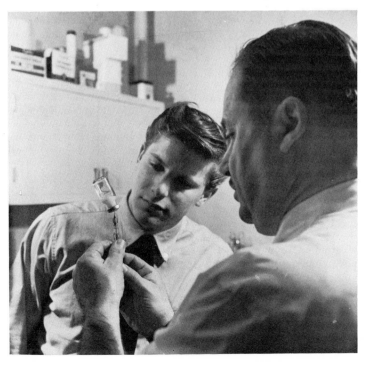

of the patient to his condition and even about explaining procedures to him. Actually, the teen-ager usually is eager for health teaching and is likely to accept it well. He often enjoys discussions of a scientific nature. (See Fig. 13.)

The nurse should realize that the teen-ager has fears. She should anticipate these and by her manner let him know that she does not think less of him for showing them. Teen-agers worry most about being different from others in their age group. They worry about their condition, and, surprisingly, many also worry about death, although they rarely mention it. The comfort and consultation of a priest, minister, or rabbi may therefore be desirable. An adolescent boy may become panicky about the effect of disease on his sexual and reproductive capacity. The nurse, becoming aware of his fear, should refer the problem to the doctor, who can give the best reassurance. Girls often worry about having a vaginal examination. The nurse can help reduce their fears greatly by explaining procedures they must undergo factually, telling them who is likely to be present during examinations, anticipating for them questions that may be asked by the doctor or others, and seeing that they are kept informed about the probable course of their treatment.

Adolescents, both boys and girls, are likely to be quite modest. Their privacy should be ensured, and any personal teaching or supervision, such as that involving physical examination, is more acceptable to them from a nurse of the same sex. If a male nurse is not available, the doctor will often give special attention to supervision of a boy. If a female nurse must attend to situations of this kind, an adolescent boy is much more at ease with a mature nurse than with a nursing student or a recent graduate who is near his own age. When the teen-age girl is hospitalized, on admission she should be given the necessary supplies and instructions for caring for her menses. In this way she may be saved from great embarrassment. She also should be told that her illness may cause her menstrual period to be skipped or to be premature. If a menstrual irregularity occurs without the girl being aware of the possibility, she may be quite concerned, yet not mention it.

Appropriate diversional activities should be provided for teen-age patients, who usually find the days very long. Most of them enjoy watching television, and many like to read and do things with their hands. If they can be out of bed, they may enjoy participating in useful activities about the house or hospital unit. Young friends should be encouraged to visit them, and if they have a hobby, they may be encouraged to work on it. If the duration of the illness is longer than two weeks, plans should be made with the school to continue schoolwork unless contraindicated.

The teen-ager should participate in plans for his convalescence since continuing progress will depend on his cooperation. If he has had a serious illness, he should be helped to assess his health situation realistically and to set short-term and long-term goals for himself accordingly. Sometimes his fondest dreams for the future must be given up. Such an occurrence can be so devastating that he may need to be referred to a psychiatrist.

The adult

By about the age of 22 years, physical growth is complete. Behavior patterns are firmly entrenched and the personality is molded. There is also some evidence that mental faculties may decline gradually after the age of 22, although the adult is perhaps better able than a younger person to use his knowledge effectively.

Adulthood is often referred to as the time of maturity. However, the nurse must understand that a particular patient may not necessarily have attained what would normally be considered "mature adult behavior." Emotional maturity varies from person to person, as do intellectual ability and physical characteristics. In addition, an adult who appears reasonably mature under usual circumstances, may, when under severe stress, exhibit behavior more typical of a child. He may, for example, demand undivided attention or even have a temper tantrum.

Too often the adult patient is considered to be a person who, without outside assistance, can always handle all his problems except his medical one. Actually, the adult often is confronted with the most acute socioeconomic and psychologic problems of any patient, primarily because he is likely to have a spouse, children, or aging parents who depend upon him for support. Regardless of the level of maturity he has attained, these problems may seem almost insurmountable to him, and indeed they may be. Perhaps it is the complexity of the problems that makes nurses reticent about discussing them with patients. Nevertheless, the patient cannot settle down to the business of getting well if his mind is filled with anxieties. Therefore, finding out what may trouble the patient and obtaining suitable help for him as necessary should be one of the primary objectives in giving nursing care to the adult.

The adult patient's major concern often is not about himself. He may be the breadwinner of a family. How is the family being supported during his illness? How is he going to pay the medical bills? The patient may be a mother with a family of small children. Who will care for the children? If she is hospitalized, she often is concerned about how her family is getting along at home. The patient may have no family. Who will look in on him if he is ill at home? If he had an emergency admission to the hospital, who will take care of his unfinished business? Who will care for him during convalescence? These are only a few of the pressing problems frequently facing the adult patient. Some problems of hospitalized patients may be alleviated by providing the use of a telephone or by arranging an unscheduled visit with a family member, friend, or business associate. Help needed by the patient may be available through social work services in the hospital or through public health agencies. It is helpful if assistance in family care can be arranged prior to the patient's being hospitalized. The nurse in a doctor's office or clinic should be alert for patients who need this type of help.

The adult patient is often expected "to act like an adult." He may not feel free to show his emotions, believing that crying is for children. He may not feel free to express his fears or even to respond to pain by groaning or moaning. In consequence, he may unconsciously show his tension in even less desirable ways. He may be demanding, irritable, or perhaps depressed. The nurse should let the patient know she appreciates his concerns and knows he must feel upset. She should also remember that each person may respond differently to similar situations, since response depends upon how a person has learned to handle stress in the developmental years.

All too often the adult patient is given no instruction. This seems to be especially true if he is able to afford private medical care. For some reason, financial affluence and education have come to imply that the patient needs no health teaching or explanations. The nurse should always be sure that the patient knows how to obtain the medical and nursing care he needs and that he knows how to give any self-care that may be necessary. The level at which teaching is done should be determined by the patient's ability to learn and by his interest.

The adult patient quite commonly has been taking medication or following a special diet for a condition other than the one for which he is currently being treated. The nurse should remind the patient that he must tell the doctor about any other treatment he is receiving. He should be told not to take medications other than those prescribed for his current condition without first consulting the doctor. This applies also to drugs that he may be taking without a prescription, such as aspirin and antihistamines. The medications may contain similar ingredients and cause an overdose, or they may be antagonistic drugs or drugs that in combination produce untoward effects.

Occasionally a lactating mother is admitted to the hospital. Arrangements need to be made within a few hours to pump her breasts at regular intervals or to dry up the milk supply. Otherwise, the breasts will become painfully engorged. Nurses on the obstetric service may be consulted for assistance with the procedure. The nurse should always ascertain whether arrangements have been made for the care and feeding of the baby. A visiting nurse may need to be asked to visit the home at once.

Adults who are ill need diversion as much as patients in any other age group. Many relish the opportunity to just relax and read or watch television or listen to the radio. Others are happier keeping actively busy. They may like some occupational therapy (Fig. 14), or they may prefer to do useful activi-

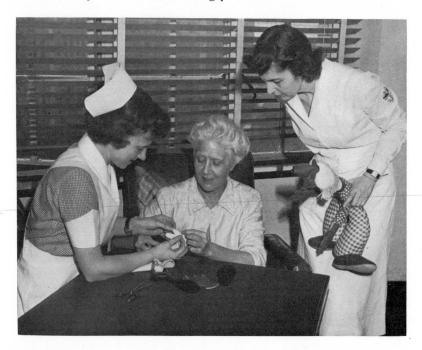

Fig. 14

Adult patients also need diversion. (From Newton, Kathleen, and Anderson, Helen C.: Geriatric nursing, ed. 4, St. Louis, 1966, The C. V. Mosby Co.)

ties about the hospital unit or for their own homes. Diversional activities should be determined by the patient's interest and his physical limitations. Sometimes it may be possible and desirable for adults to carry on their business from their bedside. Adults are more likely than any other age group to need their social and business contacts restricted at times during illness. Since adults are likely to be active in the community, they may have many visitors. These visits sometimes are more tiring than diversional for the ill patient. It is preferable that the nurse or family member explain the situation to the visitors and ask their cooperation.

The elderly person

Although 65 years of age is usually considered the beginning of late maturity or old age, tremendous individual variation exists. Age is really physiologic and not chrono-

logic. Some people may be old at 45 years of age, while others are not old at 80. Persons under 75 are usually considered to be the "young old," and persons 75 years of age and over are the "old old" or "really old." The problems and needs of these two groups may be quite different. The "old old" usually have more physical changes typical of aging and far more social problems, such as loss of friends and loss of independence, than the "young old." The reverse, of course, may be true.

The characteristics of aging. Aging is a normal process in which certain *anatomical and physiologic changes* take place. The speed with which it occurs varies, and depends on hereditary factors and the stresses of life. Tissues become somewhat desiccated (dried out), and cells divide (reproduce) more slowly. Therefore, healing takes place more slowly, and the body's response to infection is less rapid and, apparently, less effective. Tissues gradually lose their elasticity, leading to a decreased speed of muscle response and decreased strength. Loss of tissue elasticity also causes increased rigidity of such body structures as the rib cage. This rigidity, in turn, may cause decreased lung expansion and predisposes the aged person

40

to lung congestion. Bones become rarefied in the aging process and fractures occur easily. This is true particularly of the neck of the femur and the vertebral bodies.

The elasticity of the blood vessels also lessens, causing circulatory changes. The elderly person does not tolerate radical changes in position, such as lowering of the head for postural drainage or elevation of the feet above heart level. Vessels in the head may become engorged, and there is inadequate circulation to the lower extremities. With prolonged standing, blood may accumulate in the lower extremities so that not enough is provided for the brain. Dizziness and accidents may follow.

There is gradual degeneration and atrophy of the nervous system in old age, leading to lessened nerve acuity and impaired sensation. The older person's gag reflex may be less acute than that of a younger person, and, therefore, aspiration of mucus or other foreign material, such as food, may occur easily. He may be unaware of burning himself or of pressure on soft tissues. Mental deterioration, known as senility, may also occur. However, not all old people whose mental processes appear slow and muddled are senile. An inadequate blood supply to the brain may cause this condition. Bed rest causes the elderly person's circulation to slow up, and consequently, many elderly people become confused when they must stay in bed. This is noticeable in some even after several hours of sleep. Loss of interest in life may also make an elderly person appear dull mentally.

The liver, heart, kidneys, and other vital organs of many elderly people may be working hard to maintain normal function with little margin of safety. Any additional burden may be enough to tip the balance unfavorably unless particular care is given. The physiologic controls of fluid and electrolyte balance and temperature also are less efficient in the aged. Faintness and shock may follow relatively short periods without food and fluid because of fluid and electrolyte imbalances. Therefore, the elderly person should receive medical attention for even apparently slight indispositions.

The basic *psychologic needs* of the elderly are no different from those of adults. In one survey[16] elderly persons were asked what they considered essential for their happiness. They mentioned good health, a place to live, enough money to live comfortably, recognition by others, participation with others, and opportunity for a variety of experiences. However, the elderly typically have greater difficulty obtaining their desires than do younger adults. Both their desires and the difficulties that must be overcome to obtain them should be considered in planning the nursing care of elderly people. The primary objective in caring for the elderly person is to help him make the adjustments necessary to make life worth living. Each patient has different limitations and frustrations, and each will react to them differently. In general, the elderly person will react essentially as he has reacted to other stresses throughout his life.

The elderly person who is ill. Most diseases from which the aged suffer are chronic, and many patients have several chronic ailments. Some of these ailments are not particularly troublesome. Most have developed slowly and usually take time to alleviate or cure. Heart disease, cancer, renal disease, vascular disease such as cerebrovascular accident, chronic lung disease such as emphysema, and accidents are the most common problems that bring older patients to the hospital. Other chronic ailments such as arthritis, skin disorders, and mild neuromuscular conditions are very common but are usually cared for while the patient is ambulatory. The most prevalent acute illnesses of later life are acute respiratory conditions such as pneumonia and pulmonary edema.

When the elderly person becomes ill, he is particularly apprehensive and worried, probably because his security is more profoundly affected by illness than that of younger persons. He often fears helplessness and physical dependence upon others. The elderly patient may face many adjustments that make it difficult and sometimes impossible for his basic emotional needs to be met. In addition to illness and the depleted physical energy almost always accompanying it, he may have no family and few friends, or his spouse may be ill too. He often has an inadequate income and housing problems. Even before his illness, he may have been depressed because of feeling unwanted and useless.

Illness may break down the barriers to overt aggression that have been built up over a long period of time, and the aged patient may appear irritable out of all proportion to his circumstances. He may use his illness as an occasion for revolt and aggression against years of neglect to his self-esteem and to almost overwhelming economic and emotional problems. The trivial event precipitating the irritability during illness may be purely incidental. Others who have been quite active with the onset of illness may develop lethargy to a far greater extent than one would anticipate. They may seem to give up all hope or desire to live.

Similiarities between childhood and old age should not be assumed, because they are not valid. Even in the matter of helplessness there is no similarity. The child is in ascendance; he is developing new power daily and marking up achievements over his environment. The aged person's helplessness is infinitely more frustrating because it is increasing rather than decreasing.

Providing for the elderly patient's nursing needs. The goal of geriatric medical and nursing care is to keep the patient well for his age. This includes living with chronic ailments and continuing degenerative changes. The nurse who herself sees aging as a normal, inevitable process, one requiring adjustments in living patterns but not a withdrawal from life, is best prepared to work with the aging patient. Her philosophy of aging should be one of ever-changing life that eventually will end in death, not one of approaching death.

Necessary nursing care depends upon the physiologic and anatomic changes that have taken place, the disease from which the patient is suffering, and his own emotional makeup and apparent adjustment to his particular situation. In planning nursing care for elderly patients, the nurse should consider each patient's physical, social, economic, and psychologic capacities and limitations. The older patient frequently talks at length about his family and the past to the nurse who is willing to listen. His conversation may give clues of interests that should be encouraged and of problems that are confronting him. The nurse should eval-uate these clues and make plans to help the patient maintain as much independence as possible despite his limitations. Sometimes, plans must first focus on ways of encouraging the elderly patient to regain an interest in living.

When giving nursing care to elderly patients, it is necessary to take special care *to build up and protect their sense of worth and their feelings of adequacy.* Remembering the names of patients and calling them by name, instead of using such terms as "grandma" or "grandpa," helps. Giving clear explanations to the patient may spare him the embarrassment of mistakes caused by misunderstanding. Since many elderly patients are deaf, special care must be taken to be sure the patient has heard the explanation. The best method to use to ensure that he hears and understands should be recorded on his nursing care plan. The nurse should always face an elderly patient when speaking and speak distinctly so that he can lip-read inconspicuously if necessary. If hearing is better in one ear than the other, she should talk into the good ear. If the patient uses a hearing aid, she should be sure that it is working properly. Written instructions are helpful for some elderly patients. The nurse should also be thoughtful about repeating instruction because the memory span decreases with age.

Placing equipment conveniently so that assistance need not be requested also makes the elderly patient feel more adequate. Self-help devices may help him maintain some degree of independence. For example, an overbed trapeze or side rails on the bed may allow him to pull himself about in bed. Handrails along hallways and in the bathroom or a walkerette (Fig. 228) may make it possible for him to walk alone. Sturdy chairs with arms and wooden seats make it easier for many elderly patients to get into and out of chairs themselves. Low beds also allow them to be more independent. If the patient uses a cane, glasses, hearing aid, or dentures, these devices should be readily available. Showers or bathtubs equipped with handrails and with nonskid strips may make it possible for some patients to bathe independently.

Many adjustments can be made to help the patient who is confined to a wheelchair retain some measure of independence. If the patient is able to transfer himself to the toilet, having a bathroom fixed in such a way that this maneuver is possible may be desirable. Some patients, especially if they have urinary frequency or incontinence, appreciate their wheelchair or chair being fixed as a commode (p. 159). Removal of door sills may make it possible for an elderly patient confined to a wheelchair to move about the house. Elderly patients are often unable to propel their chair manually. They may, however, be able to use a motorized wheelchair.

Elderly patients often need help with such personal care as arranging the hair, applying cosmetics, shaving, and dressing. This help, if necessary, should be given regularly, and special care should be taken to assure that it is given before the patient goes about his daily activities. Personal appearance is important to everyone's morale.

Many elderly patients can give most or all necessary *physical care* to themselves. Some may need encouragement to do so; others resent not being allowed to care for themselves. The nurse or the family member caring for them, however, must be patient and give them adequate time. The older patient often is exceptionally slow in the morning and, in fact, geriatricians (doctors who specialize in the care of the elderly) instruct their patients to take twice the usual time to shave, to dress slowly, and to avoid hurry of any kind, particularly in the morning hours. Since the elderly patient may tire easily, the nurse should be sure that he is physically able to give his own care.

If the patient is in a general hospital, a slow pace is often hard to assume. For example, many diagnostic procedures must be carried out in the morning, and breakfast must usually be served with that of other patients. However, many hospital routines can be adjusted for the elderly patient. For instance, he may prefer to bathe and shave in the afternoon or early evening. He then will only need minimal personal care during the morning hours and will feel less rushed. The nursing care plan for physical care of each elderly patient should include what self-care he gives, what assistance he needs, the method used, and the schedule the patient follows. Most elderly patients

object to change, and therefore it is important to maintain routines as much as possible. The patient should participate in planning the schedule, since whenever possible it should parallel his pattern of care at home.

Since *physical deterioration* occurs in the aging process, elderly people, especially the "old old," need to use somewhat different hygienic practices than an adult uses to maintain an optimum physical condition. The *skin* of an elderly person is usually thin, delicate, and sensitive to pressure and trauma. The loss of subcutaneous fat and the hardening of the tiny arterioles near the surface cause the skin to be wrinkled, sagging, and sallow. Sweat glands atrophy and the excretory function of the skin is lessened, making the skin dry and flaky and sometimes causing it to itch. Color changes occur in the skin with aging, and seborrheic keratoses, which are lesions resembling darkened, greasy warts, are common (Fig. 175). These lesions are nonmalignant but should be inspected frequently for signs of any irritation or change.

Because the skin is likely to be very dry, daily bathing may be contraindicated for the elderly. Usually, one or two baths a week are sufficient, although the patient who is incontinent needs local sponging at frequent intervals and perhaps more frequent baths. Mild superfatted soaps or detergent solutions should be used because regular soaps can be irritating. After bathing, or more frequently if the skin is very dry, lanolin or some other emollient cream should be applied lightly. Alcohol is drying and should not be used. Bony prominences should be gently massaged.

If the patient is confined to bed, an alternating positive and negative pressure mattress may be extremely helpful in maintaining the skin in good condition. The patient should change position frequently, and bony prominences and weight-bearing areas should be massaged at least every two hours. Chamois or sheepskin pads placed under bony prominences seem to be extremely effective in relieving pressure and in preventing irritation of the skin.

Because of dryness, poor circulation, and low resistance to infection, the skin of elderly persons readily becomes infected. Special care should be taken to prevent fungus infections, such as epidermophytosis (athlete's foot) (p. 779). Elderly persons often need assistance in drying their feet after bathing and in cutting and caring for their toenails. Nails are often hard and scaly; soaking the feet in warm water or applying oil to the nails for a day or two prior to cutting softens them and makes cutting easier and safer. A podiatrist should be asked to care for very hard nails.

As the tissues age and circulation becomes sluggish, the *hair* becomes thin, dry, and colorless. Massage of the scalp and daily brushing with a soft-bristled brush help to preserve its beauty. Lanolin cream in small amounts may be used for massage, and oil treatments may be given before shampoos. Frequent shampooing should be avoided. Every two to four weeks is sufficient for most aged patients, although some people who have washed their hair more frequently throughout their lives may wish to continue to do so. A mild soap dissolved in water or a shampoo with a nonalcoholic base should be used. The older person should not experiment with new shampoos because many preparations contain alcohol and other agents that may have a drying effect.

The distribution and quality of hair change with age. Hair in the axillary and pubic areas becomes finer and scanty, whereas that of the eyebrows becomes coarse and bristly. To many women, hair on the face is a most annoying feature of growing old. If the patient is ill for a long time and is unable to care for herself, the nurse may have to assist in the removal of superfluous hair on the face. Shaving or using a pumice stone, followed by the application of cream to prevent drying, usually suffices. Plucking stray hairs from the face is often necessary. Hairs should not be plucked from moles but may be snipped close to the surface of the skin with small scissors. Stray hairs on the face may be made less conspicuous by bleaching them daily with a weak solution of hydrogen peroxide and ammonia if this can be done without irritating the skin.

Changes occur in the *eyes* with aging. There is a decrease in the conjunctival secretions, and sometimes the lower lid drops (ectropion), causing the moistening fluid of the eye to be lost. Therefore, irritation of the conjunctivas and tearing are common complaints of the aged. Smoke also may be more irritating to their eyes than to those of younger persons.

An accumulation of secretions at the inner canthus of the eye may be present, particularly upon awakening, and may be uncomfortable and unsightly. A sterile cotton sponge moistened with boric acid solution or physiologic solution of sodium chloride can be used to cleanse the eyes. Care must be taken not to press upon the eyeballs or to irritate any exposed conjunctiva.

The lens of the eye loses its ability to accommodate effectively as aging progresses. Most people over 60 years of age need glasses, at least for reading. Care of glasses, making certain that they are not lost or broken, is important in the nursing care of the elderly. Glasses should be kept clean. Smudged glasses rather than failing vision may be the cause of difficulty in seeing. The patient should have his glasses available at all times since confusion and inability to deal with situations in an adequate fashion may result if they become misplaced.

The eyes of older people also accommodate more slowly to changes in light. Bright lights or sunlight may be almost unbearable to some elderly people, and they will want the window shades pulled and the room lights dim. The nurse should arrange lights so that there is no glare. Many elderly persons see very poorly in the dark, and therefore night-lights should always be used to prevent accidents when getting up during the night.

Cataracts, failing vision, and actual blindness are common in the aged. See p. 843 for the care of the patient with visual impairment.

The elderly person should be urged to give special attention to the care of his *mouth* and *teeth*. Free hydrochloric acid in the stomach may be decreased, predisposing to poor oral health as well as to impaired digestion. The gums become less elastic and less vascular. They may recede from the remaining teeth, exposing areas of a tooth not covered with enamel. These areas are sensitive to injury from brushes and coarse dentifrices. Many elderly persons have decayed, broken, or missing teeth. This leads them to avoid foods that are difficult to eat but that may be necessary for health. The effect of mouth health upon nutrition is very real; surprising improvement in appetite has followed correction of unhealthy conditions in the mouth.

Approximately 80% of women and 70% of men have lost their teeth by the time they are 70 years of age and therefore wear dentures. Consequently, care of dentures and prevention of their loss are part of the general nursing care of most elderly patients. Patients may be encouraged by their dentists to keep dentures in place while they sleep as well as when they are awake, since this helps to preserve the normal contours of the face. Dentures should be cleansed following each meal. Because dental plates may be conductors of heat, and since the mouths of aged patients are often not too sensitive to excessive heat, they should be urged not to consume very hot food or fluids.

The feet and legs usually show the results of limitation in peripheral circulation before any other body part. Therefore, it is important for the aging person to *exercise the feet and legs regularly,* to avoid constriction or stasis of the circulation to their lower extremities, and to avoid injury and infections of their feet and legs. Precautions similar to those described for the patient who has peripheral vascular disease (p. 364) should be taken by all elderly people.

As the muscles become less active in age, slumped posture may result. The abdomen may sag, the spine becomes rounded, and the chest and shoulders droop forward. Lessened elasticity of tissue tends to make these changes fixed. Attention to preventive posture is, therefore, essential. Although corrective postural exercises and general exercise must be prescribed carefully by a physician, teaching good posture and encouraging deep breathing are part of the daily nursing care of all elderly patients. Any improvement in posture will enable the elderly patient to use his diminishing resources to better advantage. Good body alignment adds to the comfort of the patient confined to bed, as well as decreasing the need for corrective exercises later. A firm mattress is usually preferable and helps to make the use of pillows more effective. If greater stability is

needed, a fracture board can be placed under the mattress. Bedcovers should be light and warm and should be tucked loosely, giving sufficient room for the patient to move about in bed. A block or board placed at the foot of the bed helps to keep covers off the toes and provides something firm against which the patient may press his feet and thereby get some exercise. A pillow placed lengthwise under the head and shoulders helps to bring the chest forward, thereby permitting good chest expansion. Pillows placed under the arms support the muscles of the shoulder girdle and provide comfort for the patient who must have the head of the bed raised for long periods of time.

Unless there is some particular contraindication, exercises for the arms and legs, exercises to keep abdominal and gluteal muscles in good tone, and exercises to strengthen the extensor muscles of the spine should be performed several times each day by every bed patient. These exercises should be taught to the patient by the nurse, and they should be supervised daily by the nurse or the family member caring for the patient. The regular performance of exercises will help to prevent the loss of muscle tone that occurs in all bed patients, regardless of age, unless activity is continued.

The elderly person should wear the *clothing* that is comfortable for him. He often feels cold and may wear woolen clothing even when it seems very warm to others. The hospitalized patient often wishes to wear socks, woolen underwear, a bed jacket, a cap, or other items of clothing to which he is accustomed. Some provision must be made for the care of this clothing. Sometimes members of the family are glad to care for special clothing that the patient needs.

Elderly women often appreciate assistance with altering their clothes. They may be unable to afford new ones, but they often are interested in remaining stylish. Wearing a well-fitted brassiere and corset not only improves the elderly woman's appearance but the support given to sagging tissues may make her more comfortable.

The elderly person should be encouraged to wear firm, well-fitted shoes with good support to prevent damage to the arches of the feet since the muscles are often weak.

Hospitalized patients should have their shoes and should wear them when they are up. If an elderly person wears slippers, they should also fit well and be firm, since the person is less likely to slip or stumble and fall.

Fresh air is especially necessary for the elderly person because, with his diminished chest expansion, poorly oxygenated air may not provide him with a sufficient blood level of oxygen. The aged, however, may be susceptible to drafts not even noticed by younger persons, and consequently they dislike open windows.

Protective adipose tissue under the skin disappears with age, and the volume of circulating blood, particularly to the small outer arteries, may be diminished, thus affecting the ability to withstand chilling without discomfort. Decreased activity also lessens circulatory function, resulting in lowering of skin temperature and susceptibility to chilling. Many elderly people suffer from mild arthritis and fibrositis, which produce vague muscle and joint pains, and these conditions are aggravated by chilling. Measures to provide fresh air but to avoid drafts and chilling are essential. Sometimes windows can be opened wide in adjoining rooms, or perhaps a screen can be placed in front of an open window to prevent drafts and extra covers given to the patient to keep him warm.

Rest is essential for the aged. However, confusion, decubitus ulcers, lung congestion, and general deterioration may result from prolonged bed rest. Circulation to the brain, as well as to the body in general, is markedly slowed during long periods of inactivity, and therefore rest should be alternated with activity. It is undesirable for an elderly patient to be confined to bed, and even acutely ill elderly people are often gotten up in a chair for most of the day. They may even be encouraged to walk. When the patient is being cared for by his family, the nurse should try to impress upon them the great importance of some activity, since they may be oversolicitous of the patient or it may seem to require too much effort.

Elderly people usually *sleep* lightly and intermittently, with frequent waking. At home the aged person may get out of bed, read, wander about the house, and even prepare something to eat at odd hours. Actually this activity is probably good, since it prevents excessive slowing of circulation. After long periods of sleep, many elderly patients are confused. Some wakefulness, therefore, can be expected in the elderly patient who is hospitalized. If the patient is allowed out of bed, it probably is best for him to get up as he would at home. However, a low bed, night-lights, and adequate supervision should be employed to avoid accidents, and the nurse should be sure that the patient is not constantly wakeful. Elderly patients, similar to all others, may be unable to sleep. They are rarely given sedation, however, since many become excited rather than sedated by it.

The time-tested aids, such as a warm drink, a back massage, and quiet surroundings, may help to get the night of sleep off to a good start. Interesting activities to keep patients awake during the day may result in better sleep at night. Most important, however, are the patient's peace of mind and feeling of well-being, which may be achieved by giving individual attention to the elderly patient, making him feel at home and secure. A kind word and a wish for a good night of sleep or an unobstrusive inquiry into some mentioned fear or uncertainty for which reassurance can be given may alleviate worries and will do much to help the patient sleep (Fig. 15).

Noise should be avoided during the hours of sleep because it is particularly disturbing to the elderly ill person, especially if he has a hearing loss. Partial deafness may set the person "on edge," and alert him to catch every sound. Even those persons with inability to hear conversation may be disturbed by the sound of a distant radio, shrill voices, or rattling equipment.

Many elderly people are undernourished, and for this reason a great deal of emphasis is placed on *nutrition* for the aged. Other than acute and chronic illness, possible causes of malnutrition in the elderly are limited financial resources, psychologic factors such as boredom and lack of companionship in eating, edentia, lifelong faulty eating patterns, fads and notions regarding certain foods, lack of energy to prepare foods, and lack of sufficient knowledge of the essentials of a well-balanced diet. Many elderly persons, particularly those living alone, subsist on a diet high in carbohydrates and low in vitamins, minerals, and protein. Often they think that because they are elderly they do not need much food. A diet composed largely of tea and toast may seem sufficient. The nutritional intake needed by the elderly and ways of improving the appetite are described on p. 118.

The nurse should instruct the patient and those responsible for his care in the essentials of a well-balanced diet. Dietary patterns should not be changed too quickly, and it is useless to attempt to change many established food patterns. Simply prepared and easily digested foods are best, and meals should be distributed throughout the day. Usually elderly persons do not tolerate too much fried food. Large amounts of roughage should be avoided, but bulk is necessary. Fluid intake is important, yet many do not drink much water. Tea, coffee, and other beverages are usually preferred. Drinks prepared with dry skimmed milk supply essential protein and are useful in helping to meet the protein and calcium needs of older patients without supplying too many calories.

Some elderly persons are obese even though they may be undernourished. Excess weight burdens the heart, liver, kidneys, and musculoskeletal system and should be avoided. Weight reduction for the aged person, however, should be gradual and must be supervised by a physician. Sudden loss of weight is poorly tolerated by many elderly persons whose vascular system has become adjusted to the excess weight. Sudden weight reduction may lead to serious consequences, including confusion associated with lowered blood pressure, exhaustion, and vasomotor collapse.

Elderly patients may worry about their *bowel function*. They tend to forget that less food and less activity will result in reduced bowel function. Any marked change in bowel habits, however, and any unusual reactions to normal doses of laxatives should be reported, since malignancies of the large bowel and diverticulitis are fairly common among this age group.

Regularity in going to the toilet is important, since it provides stimulus to evacuate the bowel. Motor activity of the intestinal

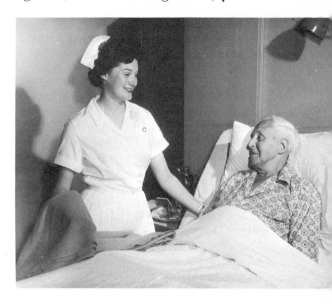

Fig. 15

A kind word, a wish for a good night of sleep, and attention to physical comfort are often as effective as drugs in helping the patient sleep.

musculature may be decreased with age, and supportive structures in the intestinal walls become weakened. Sense perception is less acute, so that the signal for bowel elimination may be missed. Constipation may occur and in turn lead to impactions. The very elderly and somewhat confused patient should be reminded to go to the bathroom following meals.

Daily attention must be given to elimination, and sometimes small enemas may be needed every two or three days. Many doctors now order laxative rectal suppositories such as bisacodyl (Dulcolax). Small daily doses of a mild laxative may be ordered. The mild bulk laxatives, such as psyllium seed and agar-agar combined with mineral oil, are usually preferred to the saline cathartics, which may cause dehydration. If the patient is constipated, it may be necessary occasionally to insert a gloved finger into the rectum to be certain impaction has not occurred.

Frequency of *micturition* is common in old age and becomes a problem during illness. The ability of the kidneys to concentrate urine during sleeping hours usually decreases slowly with age. In addition, decreased muscle tone in the bladder with resultant impairment of emptying capacity may result in residual urine in the bladder and subsequent mild infection. One of the first signs of diminishing or failing kidney function is frequency of micturition during the night. Frequency and slight burning on urination are symptoms of mild bladder infection.

Elderly women have relaxation of perineal structures, which may also interfere with complete emptying of the bladder and predispose to bladder infection. Some elderly patients have decreased sensation and do not realize when the bladder must be emptied. Periodic dribbling of urine suggests that the bladder is not being emptied. The nurse should observe the very elderly patient for distention of the bladder and report its presence to the doctor.

Unless there is a definite contraindication to high fluid intake, the elderly patient should be urged to take sufficient fluids to dilute urine and decrease its irritating properties. Fluids may be limited in the evening if nocturia is troublesome and is interfering with sleep. If the patient is quite feeble, it is well to suggest that a urinal or bedpan be used during the night.

Involutional changes in the lining of the vagina lead to lessened resistance to invasion of organisms. Mild infections with troublesome discharge are not unusual in elderly women. This condition should be reported to the doctor. Frequent local bathing may be helpful in allaying itching.

Almost all elderly men have hypertrophy of the prostate, which makes urination difficult. The nurse must report, or must urge her patient to report, such complaints to his doctor because specific treatment is often necessary and can be safely administered even when the patient is far advanced in years.

Incontinence of urine and/or feces has been found to be over three times more prevalent among the hospitalized or institutionalized aged, but about 10% of the aged being cared for at home also have this problem. It is twice as common among women as men.[36] Care of the patient with incontinence is described on p. 148.

An important part of nursing care for the elderly is helping to meet their *emotional needs*. Elderly patients are often lonely, and individual attention should be given to them. They often appreciate just talking with others. If possible, the nurse should plan time to visit with them herself. Volunteers may also be used to visit the elderly. Some patients appreciate visits with a clergyman.

When visiting with elderly patients, one should remember that, although they commonly talk about events and activities in their own past, they usually are interested in the activities of young people and of the world about them (Fig. 16). These interests often must be satisfied for them through the eyes and ears of others. If the patient is unable to see well enough to read, he may be interested in being read to by others.

Provision should be made for the patient who requires long hospitalization to maintain his family contacts. A grandfather or grandmother often wishes to see a grandchild, and a visit should be arranged, if possible. Sometimes, plans can be made for the patient to make a short visit outside the hospital. This is especially important if a wife or husband is physically unable to visit the patient. Arranging for telephone conversations with family members also is desirable.

If the elderly patient likes to read, reading materials should be provided. If he is unable to see to read, talking books, available through public libraries, may be appreciated. Television and radio also provide desirable diversion. Elderly people often are interested in doing useful tasks.

There are many tasks in which even the elderly person who is ill may be able to participate. Women may enjoy mending or knitting. If they are at home, they may be able to help with dishes or meal preparation. Men may be interested in repairing toys or making useful gadgets for the house. Many elderly persons enjoy painting. The older person may be quite slow in all his activities, and great care must be taken not to show impatience, which may discourage further participation.

Elderly patients are usually aware of death as an imminent possibility and often make surprisingly frequent and casual mention of death. The nurse should not avoid this issue. If the nurse senses that the patient is genuinely concerned about death, she may make a tactful inquiry as to whether he would like to see a clergyman, a family member, or the doctor, or perhaps to arrange to transact some unfinished business. The nurse must always be responsive to such requests, since they frequently are more important for the patient's peace of mind than his medical treatment.

Special precautions related to diagnosis and treatment Elderly persons usually tolerate *drugs* poorly and may have bizarre reactions to them. If the renal or hepatic function is impaired, drugs may be excreted more slowly than normal and cumulative effects may appear. Because of poor circulation, elderly persons are more likely than young patients to have a delayed effect from drugs. The nurse should carefully check for untoward reactions and report them to the doctor. Narcotics and sedatives are tolerated especially poorly, and small doses usually are prescribed. If the patient is emaciated or of very advanced years, the use of full adult doses of drugs should be questioned.

Many elderly patients must administer drugs to themselves. The nurse should carefully determine their ability to do so, and should report to the physician if the practice does not seem to be safe, so that other plans can be made. In planning self-administration of drugs with the elderly patient, it is frequently helpful to determine the easiest time for him to remember to take medication. This time is usually tied in with some incident of daily living, such as arising or taking meals. The use of a medication check sheet is helpful in reminding some patients. Plans may also include placement of the medication, so that seeing it will be a reminder. Special care needs to be taken, however, to put it where it will not accidentally be taken in place of another drug or where other family members, such as small children, may take it.

Elderly patients who are undergoing *diagnostic tests* requiring withholding of meals or the use of enemas or cathartics should be attended unless they are in their beds because they often become quite weak and dizzy. No elderly patient should ever be left unattended on a treatment table, and he should be helped on and off the table. Since he often is quite dizzy, it is advisable for him to arise slowly and sit on the edge of

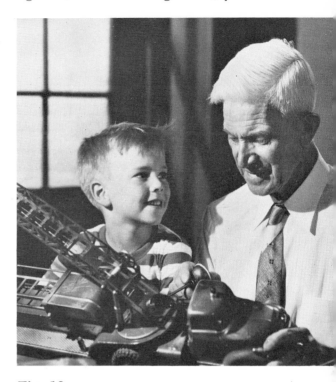

Fig. 16

Older people often enjoy association with youngsters. (© 1958, Parke, Davis & Co.)

the table for a few moments before standing. The dizziness is caused by the slow compensation of inelastic blood vessels. Older patients with cardiovascular disease may also be orthopneic and cannot tolerate lying flat for examinations.

Because of the rapidity with which they develop decubitus ulcers, elderly patients who must lie on x-ray, treatment, or operating room tables for lengthy periods of time need pads placed under the normal curves of their backs and a pad of material such as sponge rubber placed under bony prominences. Skin over bony prominences should be rubbed occasionally to improve the circulation to the area. On return to the unit the patient's skin should always be checked for pressure areas, and if any signs of pressure are evident, these areas should be massaged frequently until the tissue appears normal in color. If possible, the patient should be kept off these areas until signs of pressure disappear.

If the patient is placed in lithotomy position, care must be taken to place both legs in the stirrups at the same time to prevent undue pull on unresilient muscles. Care must also be taken to prevent hyperextension and hyperflexion of the joints since many elderly patients have arthritis.

References and selected readings*

1 Amend, Edith L.: A parent education program in a children's hospital, Nursing Outlook 14:53-56, April 1966.

2 *Austin, Catherine L.: The basic six needs of the aging, Nursing Outlook 7:138-141, March 1959.

3 Bortz, Edward L.: Healthy added years. In 1961 Britannica book of the year, Chicago, 1961, Encyclopaedia Britannica, Inc.

4 *Bozian, Marguerite W.: Nursing in a geriatric day center, Am. J. Nursing 64:93-95, April 1964.

5 *Bruce, Sylvia J.: What mothers of 6- to-10-year olds want to know, Nursing Outlook 12:40-43, Sept. 1964.

6 *Carney, Robert G.: The aging skin, Am. J. Nursing 63:110-112, June 1963.

7 *Cholcher, Mary, and Burtis, Mary: Teens together, Am. J. Nursing 64:104-105, July 1964.

8 *Dahlin, Bernice: Rehabilitation: fact or figure of speech? Nursing Outlook 12:34-37, Nov. 1964.

9 *Dittman, Laura L.: A child's sense of trust, Am. J. Nursing 66:91-93, Jan. 1966.

10 *Drummond, Eleanor E.: Impact of a father's illness, Am. J. Nursing 64:89-91, Aug. 1964.

11 *Erickson, Florence: When 6- to 12-year olds are ill, Nursing Outlook 13:48-50, July 1965.

12 Erikson, E. H.: Youth and the life cycle, Children 7:43-49, March-April 1960.

13 Folsom, Marion B.: Goals of a national health program for meeting health needs, Ann. Am. Acad. Polit. & Social Sc. 337:11-19, Sept. 1961.

14 *Goldfarb, Alvin I.: Responsibilities to our aged, Am. J. Nursing 64:78-82, Nov. 1964.

15 Hammar, S. L., and Eddy, Jo Ann K.: Nursing care of the adolescent, New York, 1966, Springer Publishing Co., Inc.

16 Havighurst, Robert J., and others: Psychology of aging, Bethesda Conference, Pub. Health Rep. 70:837-856, Sept. 1955.

17 *Henley, Barbara M.: Helping the elderly find community services, Am. J. Nursing 63:89-92, April 1963.

18 *Hevey, Lena A.: Vision and aging, Nursing Outlook 12:61-63, June 1964.

19 *Hulicka, Irene M.: Fostering self-respect in aged patients, Am. J. Nursing 64:84-89, March 1964.

20 *Linden, Maurice E.: The emotional problems of aging, Nursing Outlook 12:47-50, Nov. 1964.

21 *Mahaffy, Perry R., Jr.: Admission interviews with patients, Am. J. Nursing 66:506-508, March 1966.

22 Marlow, Dorothy R., and Sellew, Gladys: Textbook of pediatric nursing, Philadelphia, 1965, W. B. Saunders Co.

23 Nelson, W. E., editor: Textbook of pediatrics, ed. 8, Philadelphia, 1964, W. B. Saunders Co.

24 *Newton, Kathleen, and Anderson, Helen C.: Geriatric nursing, ed. 4, St. Louis, 1966, The C. V. Mosby Co.

25 *Outland, Carol Ann Wehr: A child is hospitalized, Am. J. Nursing 64:135-136, June 1964.

26 *Peszczynski, Mieczyslaw: Why old people fall, Am. J. Nursing 65:86-88, May 1965.

27 Piper, Geraldine M., and Smith, Emily M.: Geriatric nutrition, Nursing Outlook 12:51-53, Nov. 1964.

28 *Render, Helena W.: My old age, Nursing Outlook 12:31-33, Nov. 1964.

29 Riccitelli, M. L.: The management of osteoporosis in the aged and infirm, J. Am. Geriatrics Soc. 10:498-504, June 1962.

30 Rodstein, Manuel: The aging process and disease, Nursing Outlook 12:43-46, Nov. 1964.

31 *Schreiber, Frederick C.: Dental care for long-term patients, Am. J. Nursing 64:84-86, Feb. 1964.

32 *Schwartz, Doris: Medication errors made by aged patients, Am. J. Nursing 62:51-53, Aug. 1962.

33 Schwartz, Doris: The elderly ambulatory patient: nursing and psychosocial needs, New York, 1964, The Macmillan Co.

34 Smith, Emily M.: Nursing services for the aged in housing projects and day centers, Am. J. Nursing 65:72-74, Dec. 1965.

35 Smith, Margo: Ego support for the child patient, Am. J. Nursing 63:90-95, Oct. 1963.

36 *Soller, Genevieve R.: The aging patient, Am. J. Nursing 62:114-117, Nov. 1962.

37 Stafford, Nova Harris: Bowel hygiene of aged patients, Am. J. Nursing 63:102-103, Sept. 1963.

38 Statistical abstracts of the United States, 1965, 86th annual edition, Washington, D. C., 1962, U. S. Bureau of the Census.

39 Stieglitz, Edward J., editor: Geriatric medicine, ed. 3, Philadelphia, 1954, J. B. Lippincott Co.

40 Stone, L. J., and Church, Joseph: Childhood and adolescence, New York, 1957, Random House, Inc.

41 The nation and its older people—report of the White House Conference on Aging, 1961, Washington, D. C., 1961, U. S. Government Printing Office.

42 *Toys at work, Am. J. Nursing 65:68-71, Dec. 1965.

43 Wheatley, George M., and Hallock, Grace: Health observation of school children, ed. 3, New York, 1965, Blakiston Division, McGraw-Hill Book Co.

44 *Wu, Ruth: Explaining treatments to young children, Am. J. Nursing 65:71-73, July 1965.

*References preceded by an asterisk are particularly well suited for student reading.

3

Maintaining the body's defenses against harmful factors in the external environment

Study questions

1 What is a normal white blood count? Distinguish between the various types of white blood cells. What is the normal proportion of each? What are the main functions of the polymorphonuclear leukocytes?

2 In disease, what is the significance of a leukocytosis? Of a leukopenia? Study the laboratory findings of a patient who is or has been acutely ill; compare repeated white blood count reports. What treatments or circumstances appear to have contributed to these changes?

3 What is the therapeutic action of aspirin? What untoward symptoms does it have? When is it contraindicated?

4 Review the procedure for an alcohol sponge bath; a sterile dressing; a blood transfusion.

5 Where are the sympathetic and parasympathetic nervous systems located in relation to the central nervous system, and how are they linked to it? What functions are controlled by the autonomic nervous system?

6 Describe the appearance and actions of a frightened person. Describe your own physical and emotional state when you have been frightened or anxious.

7 Distinguish between epinephrine and norepinephrine. Where in the body are these hormones produced? What is the effect of each? Review the commonly used drugs containing these hormones.

8 How is oxygen transported in the blood? What is the reflex mechanism that comes into action when the blood oxygen level is low?

9 What is the normal oxygen concentration of the air? What is the normal atmospheric pressure? As the atmospheric pressure decreases, what happens to the oxygen availability? Review the physical laws relating to the pressure of gases (Dalton's law, Boyle's law, and the law of solubility of gases).

10 What nutrients are essential for life? Which ones are stored by the body? What essential body functions require expenditure of water?

Since the turn of the century great strides have been made in the prevention and treatment of disease and disability. This progress has been made possible by application of the results of epidemiologic investigations. *Epidemiology* is the study of the patterns of health and disease in man. The factors that influence the occurrence and distribution of health, disease, defects, disabilities, and deaths among groups are sought and analyzed. Attempts are made to discover which population groups and which individuals in the group are affected, what the causative agent is, and under what environmental circumstances the disease or disability becomes prevalent. Although epidemiology started as the study of infectious disease, epidemiologists are now studying many noninfectious conditions, such as cancer, heart disease, air pollution, and accidents. With increased knowledge about the causative agents of disease, how they act on the host (person afflicted), and how the host responds (body reaction), much medical treatment has changed from palliative to curative. Increased knowledge of the effect of environment on the host, as well as on biologic agents that attack the host, has

51

made possible the discovery and institution of many preventive and control measures.

Since it usually is easier and more economical to prevent a disease or disability than to cure or correct it, the nurse should become familiar with current epidemiologic knowledge about the cause and prevention of disease and disability, apply it to her nursing practice and her life, and teach it to others. She also should be constantly alert for new developments in this field of rapidly expanding knowledge, and she herself, in the course of practicing her profession, may see relationships (agent-host-environment) that deserve study.

Disease or disability may be caused by *external* or *internal* agents. The external agents may be classified as *biologic* (living matter such as bacteria, viruses, fungi, worms, or insects), *chemical* (poisons), *nutritional* (excesses or deficiencies in diet), *mechanical* (surgery, accidents), or *physical* (exposure to excess heat, cold, or radiation). The internal agents may be classified as *genetic* (anomalies or hormonal, metabolic, or glandular deficiencies), *physiologic* (structural changes due to aging or the body's response to other disease processes), or *psychologic* (structural or physiologic changes due to psychosomatic response). As the nurse studies each disease process, she should try to classify the causative agents.

Much preventive nursing care is concerned with maintenance of the body's defenses against harmful factors in the external environment. The body has built-in mechanisms to protect it from the constantly changing and frequently hazardous external environment. Although some of the defenses are structural parts of the body, many are adaptive processes. To exist, all living matter must constantly adapt to its environment, which consists not only of inanimate matter (air, water, soil, cars, houses) but of living matter (people, other animals, insects, plants, microorganisms). This adaptation is a purposeful adjustment and is necessary to maintain the integrity of the organism. The remainder of this chapter will deal with the body's defense mechanisms against environmental factors that attack it physically, what happens when they fail, and the treatment then instituted to modify them or to supplement them. Chapter 6 deals with the psycho-

logic defense system. Maintenance of the internal environment in a homeostatic state also involves body defense against changes in its equilibrium. These changes usually are brought about originally by factors in the external environment. This aspect will be discussed in the following chapter.

External defenses

Skin. The skin is the first line of defense against injury and disease. If the skin is not broken and its glands secrete normally, pathogenic bacteria cannot enter the body through it. Skin also protects the delicate tissues of the body from injury by such external forces as heat, cold, and trauma.

The normal acid secretion of the skin (pH 5.5) tends to inhibit the growth of disease-producing microorganisms (pathogens). Bacteria that are normally present on the skin (resident bacteria) are usually nonpathogenic. Staphylococci are the exception. Of the transient organisms, only the bacilli causing anthrax and tularemia are able to live or multiply in the acid flora of the skin.

Resident bacteria, including staphylococci, however, are present on the skin in great numbers. They penetrate the hair follicles and the glands of the skin, and perspiration continuously brings them to the surface. Scrubbing with soap and water removes only the surface bacteria. The skin, therefore, can never be considered sterile (free from all organisms). For this reason, in addition to thoroughly scrubbing the hands, sterile gloves are worn or sterile instruments are used to prevent contamination during surgical aseptic procedures.

Thorough hand washing, by its mechanical action, is effective in decreasing the number of bacteria on the skin. Shaving the hair to which bacteria cling also tends to reduce their numbers. The use of bacteriostatic soaps containing hexachlorophene such as pHisoHex and of disinfectants such as alcohol, benzalkonium chloride, and povidone-iodine (Betadine) to cleanse the skin prevents rapid multiplication of bacteria remaining on the skin. These agents are all effective supplements to the body's defenses because a few pathogens, gaining entrance to the body, are more likely to be destroyed by the body's internal defenses than are large numbers of them.

Sensory receptors (touch, pain, pressure, heat, and cold) are located in the skin. These receptors are protective mechanisms against injury because they warn the person against continued contact with dangerous external forces. The responses to the sensations, however, are learned, and their effectiveness depends on mental maturation and consciousness. They are ineffectual in infants and young children and in the unconscious patient. For this defense mechanism to operate, neural pathways along which the sensations are carried to the spinal column and the brain must be functioning. Consequently, persons with diseased or absent nerve pathways will not be protected. The acuity of these sensations also decreases with aging. In the absence of fully functioning sense receptors in the skin, compensatory measures to avoid contact with dangerous external forces must be taken by the person or by others for him.

Melanin (skin pigment) screens out some of the burning rays of the sun and thus acts as a protective agent. However, since people have varying amounts of melanin in the skin, it is not a universally protective mechanism and it needs to be supplemented as necessary with the use of protective lotions and with the use of caution in exposure to sunshine.

Mucous membranes. Mucous membranes protect the eyes and line all parts of the body that have external openings. If intact, the mucous membranes, like the skin, are impervious to bacteria. They also contain some sensory receptors. In addition, their secretions may deter the growth of bacteria, and the cilia along the membranes of the nose and respiratory tract tend to sweep bacteria and other foreign material out of the body. Mucous membranes also are highly vascular, so that internal defenses are readily available to destroy bacteria gaining entrance through them. The danger of bacterial invasion through the mucous membranes is greatest when they are dry and the person is chilled, because dryness causes cracking and chilling causes the superficial blood vessels to constrict.

The eyes. The eyes, including the conjunctivas, are protected from the entrance of bacteria and particles of dirt by the lids and eyelashes. Foreign material that gains entrance tends to be washed out by the tears. The blinking reflex also protects the eyes against damage by shutting out foreign material and bright light. In the absence of these protective devices, special care must be instituted to protect the eyes (p. 165).

Nose, mouth, throat, and respiratory system. The nose and mouth normally contain many pathogens such as streptococci and pneumococci. Usually these organisms are not harmful since most pathogens that enter through the mouth are washed back into the throat by saliva, swallowed, and destroyed by the gastric secretions. Bacteria and other foreign material that are inhaled into the nose are usually blocked by the cilia in the anterior nasal passages. If they succeed in passing through this barrier, the mucous secretions of the nose move the bacteria into the nasopharynx, where they are swallowed and destroyed by gastric secretions. Pathogenic organisms are unlikely to gain entrance to the body through the nose, mouth, or throat unless there is a break in the mucous membrane. Although mouthwashes, gargles, and irrigations with antiseptic solutions decrease the numbers of organisms in the mouth and throat slightly for a limited time, their effectiveness is very minimal.

Occasionally bacteria and other minute particles of foreign material from the nose and throat are aspirated into the lungs instead of being swallowed. If this happens, the movement of the cilia and mucous secretions normally propels them forward into the pharynx, where they are expectorated or swallowed. The cough reflex prevents aspiration of large particles of foreign material into the lungs. The patient must be conscious for this mechanism to be effective. It also is less effective in the very young, the very old, and the debilitated. In these circumstances, special care must be taken.

The greatest threat of pathogens in the nose, mouth, throat, and respiratory system is the spread of the organisms of one person to others who are susceptible owing to such factors as age, wounds, or debility. To prevent the spread of bacteria from the nose and throat, people are taught to cover the nose and mouth when sneezing or coughing and to blow the nose and expectorate into disposable handkerchiefs. A dry mask worn over the nose and mouth helps to decrease the spread of bacteria to others. Acceptable types of masks are described on p. 303. Masks are worn during surgical aseptic procedures and while caring for burned patients to decrease the possibility of introducing organisms from the nose and throat into the wounds. A damp mask incubates bacteria and increases their numbers and their spread. When there is known respiratory disease, a mask worn by the patient may prevent spread of infectious organisms to others.

Where the gastric acidity is low, special precautions need to be taken to avoid introducing organisms through the nose and mouth because they may not be destroyed in the stomach. Since infants have a low gastric acidity, bottles and nipples used for feeding them and equipment used to prepare their formulas are sterilized. Hands should be washed thoroughly before feeding or handling a baby. Sometimes masks are worn by persons caring for an infant to prevent pathogens from their nose and throat from passing to him. This latter precaution is not necessary for the mother or family members to take unless they have an upper respiratory infection. The baby has antibodies that were passed to him from his mother through the placenta. They usually protect him against organisms normally found in the nose and throat of persons in his family. Because of these antigens, unless the mother has a communicable disease, breast feeding probably exposes the infant to fewer organisms to which he has no resistance than other means of feeding him. Special precautions to avoid ingestion of large numbers of organisms by mouth should also be observed by adults who for any reason have low gastric acidity.

The gastrointestinal tract, urinary tract, and vagina. If pathogens get through the stomach into the upper gastrointestinal tract, many of them are destroyed by the proteolytic enzymes or the alkaline bile. However, pathogens such as typhoid and paratyphoid bacilli, the virus that causes infectious hepatitis, and *Entamoeba histolytica,* which causes amebic dysentery, enter through the mouth and are unaffected by the gastric or intestinal secretions. In fact, they set up in-

fection in the bowel and use it as their portal of exit from the body. The bowel is the natural habitat of some pathogens, such as *Escherichia coli* and *Bacillus welchii.* Although these organisms do not produce disease in the bowel, they may be transported in the feces to areas of the body that are favorable for their growth and multiplication and set up infection there. *Bacillus welchii,* the causative agent of gas gangrene, produces disease only when it reaches sites with little oxygen, such as deep wounds. *Escherichia coli* frequently causes infections of the urethra and bladder in women, and it may cause vaginal infections. Therefore, after a bowel movement the anus should be cleansed away from the vagina and urethra.

Some pathogens also are normally present in the anterior urethra and some may leave the body through the kidneys. Unless they are very virulent, are massive in numbers, or are left in an obstructed kidney, ureter, or bladder, however, they rarely cause difficulty. The mucous lining of the urinary tract prevents their invasion of tissue, and normal urine flow from the upper urinary tracts and normal voiding washes them out. Trauma such as may occur in catheterization may, however, predispose to infection by these organisms, especially if the patient is not emptying his bladder completely when he voids. Practices that reduce the danger of infection from catheterization are described on p. 151.

Vaginal secretions contain acid, which usually destroys most pathogens entering the vagina. The spirochete and the gonococcus are notable exceptions. Vaginal secretions, however, are not present before puberty and they decrease in amount after the menopause. Young girls and older women, therefore, should be especially careful not to introduce organisms into the vagina (p. 497). Frequent use of vaginal douches tends to wash away the protective secretions.

If the hands are not washed after using the toilet, bacteria that exist in or pass through the bowel, urethra, or vagina may be transmitted via eating utensils or food to others. All employees of food establishments are required to have laboratory examinations of the stools before employment to determine whether they are carrying infectious organisms in the intestinal tract. The employer is responsible for providing approved toilet and hand-washing facilities and for insisting upon their proper use. All eating and drinking facilities and meat-handling establishments are inspected regularly by a health department sanitarian in an attempt to decrease the spread of infectious diseases by inadequate methods of cleansing utensils and other poor practices. The practice of hand washing after handling excreta, of course, also applies to the nurse. She should teach this practice to patients and provide them with the opportunity to carry it out during hospitalization.

Sheltered areas. All parts of the body with no openings to the outside are considered "sheltered areas" and are normally free of any organisms. Internal defenses seem to be less effective in these parts. Therefore, extreme caution needs to be used to prevent the introduction into or growth of organisms in areas such as the bloodstream, the spinal canal, the peritoneal cavity, and the bones.

Internal defenses against invasion by pathogens

When the external defenses fail to prevent the injury of body tissues or their invasion by biologic agents, the internal defense mechanisms come into action. Pathogens may enter the body to cause primary disease or they may enter in the wake of other conditions. Staphylococci and streptococci frequently invade cells already damaged by other organisms, disease, or injury. *Bacillus welchii* and the tetanus bacilli always enter through traumatized tissues. Regardless of whether the invasion by pathogenic organisms is a primary or secondary condition, the body's defensive response is the same.

Histamine response and phagocytosis

Whenever cells are damaged by any kind of agent, they release histamine into the surrounding intracellular fluid. This is a proteinlike substance and is picked up by the blood. Its release causes a local tissue reaction called *inflammation.* This reaction is an attempt by the body to localize the effects of the injury and to overcome any invading bacteria at the initial site. It is the first line of internal defense against infection.

Blood flow to the site of the injured cells is accelerated, and surrounding capillaries dilate. Because of the increased permeability of the capillaries, which is produced by the histamine, blood cells and serum escape into the tissues, causing the part to become red, hot, and swollen. If an extensive number of cells are damaged, the part may also be painful because of the pressure of the increased intracellular fluid on nerve endings. The swelling may produce loss of function in the part. Redness, swelling, heat, and pain are the cardinal signs of inflammation.

The increased blood flow brings with it polymorphonuclear leukocytes (neutrophils) that histamine has also mobilized. These leukocytes ingest the bacteria and dead tissue cells (phagocytosis) at the site of the tissue damage. They then are carried away through the blood and lymph streams and broken down into elements that the kidneys excrete. The inflammatory process subsides as the leukocytes remove the debris and as the blood, serum, and lymph are reabsorbed into the blood vessels and lymphatics.

If the bacteria fail to be contained locally and are picked up by the lymph stream, which drains all tissues of the body, they will be carried to the nearest lymph node. These nodes are located along the course of all lymph channels, and here, too, bacteria can be ingested and destroyed. If the bacteria are strong enough to resist the action in the lymph nodes, leukocytes are brought in by the bloodstream to attack and engulf the bacteria in the node. The node then becomes swollen and tender because of the accumulation of phagocytes, bacteria, and destroyed lymphoid tissue. This is known as *lymphadenitis.*

If the bacteria are picked up by or introduced into the bloodstream, there are large phagocytic cells called *tissue macrophages* that are located along the course of the blood vessels, in the spleen, liver, lungs, bone marrow, and adrenal glands, and that function similarly to lymph nodes and will engulf and digest these blood-borne organisms as well as any dead cells or other foreign particles that pass through the bloodstream.

Some pathogens that gain entrance to the body resist being engulfed by phagocytes by giving off substances that repel or destroy them. This characteristic of the organism is

55

known as its *virulence.* The number of invading organisms also may be too great for the phagocytes to handle, or the internal defenses of the host may be functioning poorly; that is, the host is *susceptible.* For example, the ability of phagocytes to ingest offending organisms is lessened in any disease that causes a decreased number of white blood cells (leukopenia) or an increased number of immature cells such as occurs in leukemia. In shock, less blood is available and the process is impeded. The numbers of organisms, their virulence, and the susceptibility of the host to invasion by them are known as the *infectivity potential.* If any or all of these conditions are favorable, the organisms have an opportunity to grow at the site of entry or to be transported through the bloodstream to the tissues and organs of their choice, such as muscles, nerves, and lungs) and there to thrive and multiply. In this process, which is called *infection,* cells are damaged by the organisms living on them or by an inflammatory response (autoimmune reaction) to the toxin (poisonous soluble protein) given off by the pathogen and carried by the blood and lymph to organs and tissues especially sensitive to it. Hemolytic streptococci may cause tissue damage in the latter manner, causing such complications as rheumatic fever and glomerular nephritis. Tissues of the heart are damaged by the toxin produced by the bacteria that cause diphtheria.

The systemic reaction caused by the absorption of toxins in the bloodstream is called *toxemia.* If bacteria are present and are growing and producing toxins in the bloodstream, the infection is called *septicemia.* The presence of bacteria in the bloodstream is called *bacteremia.* Pus in the bloodstream is known as *pyemia.* Bacteria circulating in the bloodstream may lodge at points distant to the original site of infection and cause a *secondary infection.* This is the process by which infections such as bacterial endocarditis and pyelonephritis usually occur.

Symptoms of disease or infection caused by biologic agents do not appear until enough cells have been damaged to cause a generalized histamine response—that is, one that produces some systemic reaction. The period between entry of the pathogens into the body and the appearance of symptoms is called the *incubation period.* Pathogens that localize at the site of entry have short incubation periods, while those that must be transported for a distance from the portal of entry to the site of tissue invasion usually have longer incubation periods.

A generalized histamine response causes a rise in body temperature that is believed to stimulate an increased production of white blood cells. A rise in temperature, therefore, is considered an important body response to infection, and infection without an accompanying fever may suggest a poor prognosis. With infection there also is an increased *blood sedimentation rate;* that is, when anticoagulant is added to the blood in the laboratory, the red blood cells settle to the bottom of a test tube more rapidly than normal. (In one method of determination commonly used, the normal for men is 0 to 9 mm. per hour; for women, 0 to 20 mm. per hour.) This increase in the sedimentation rate is believed to be caused by an increase in fibrinogen (a blood protein essential to the healing process). The sedimentation rate is elevated during the acute inflammatory stage of infection. Its elevation, therefore, is an indication that body defense mechanism for the repair of damaged tissue is operating. Because the sedimentation rate gradually returns to normal as tissues heal, it also is used to determine when physical activity can be resumed safely following an acute infection.

Other signs and symptoms vary according to the portal of entry and the specific tissues finally invaded by the pathogen. The symptoms produced depend on where the histamine is released. Often symptoms appear in two stages. The symptoms related to tissues at the portal of entry appear and then subside, only to be followed several days later by symptoms produced by damage of cells in the specific tissues invaded. Localized invasion of skin or soft tissues produces symptoms of local inflammation (p. 55). Invasion of the respiratory tract produces symptoms of a cold, with increased mucous secretions and congestion. Invasion of the gastrointestinal tract produces nausea, vomiting, and diarrhea. Invasion of the central nervous system produces severe headache and stiff neck. Invasion of muscle may cause muscle pain, weakness, or spasms. Organisms producing toxins frequently cause rashes, high fever, and chills. Symptoms of general malaise, anorexia, dull headache, and generalized aching usually occur when there is widespread tissue involvement, as in viral infections such as influenza.

The histamine response varies with age. It is less active in infants, young children, and elderly people, and it is at its peak during young adulthood. Therefore, young children and the elderly are more prone to generalized disease because they are less able to combat injuries and infections locally. Because histamine response is at its peak in young and middle-aged adults, they frequently have more severe symptoms if they contract a generalized infection than do young children and elderly people. However, because of the active response to the initial exposure, they also are less prone to develop generalized infections.

Antigen-antibody response

Pathogens and their toxins are foreign proteins, and the body has a mechanism for dealing with any foreign protein (antigen) that invades it. This mechanism is a very effective second line of defense against pathogenic organisms.

As the cells of the body come into contact with sufficient amounts of any specific foreign protein, they become *sensitized* to it and produce a chemical substance that tends to reject the protein by repelling or damaging it in some way. The chemical substances that are formed in response to pathogens are called *antibodies;* those formed in response to toxins are called *antitoxins.* The antibody or antitoxin for each type of pathogen is specific. The antibodies enable the phagocytes to engulf organisms. The antibody may cause the organisms to stick together in clumps (agglutinate) or to break up (lyse), or it may coat the organisms or prevent their reproduction. The antitoxin neutralizes the toxin released by the pathogen. The process is known as the *antigen-antibody response,* and it is by this mechanism that infecting organisms finally are overcome by the body.

Antibodies and antitoxins are thought to be formed due to a change in the molecular configuration of the amino acids in certain body cells (tissue cells or blood cells), and they are formed in response to a specific foreign protein.[8] The molecular configuration of the amino acids in the cell may be temporarily or permanently changed, and the resulting resistance to the specific pathogen is known as *active immunity.* Antibodies and antitoxins remain in the blood for varying periods of time, and as long as they are present they provide protection for the person against a repeated attack from the specific organism. When the antibodies form in response to disease, the process is called *natural active acquired immunity.* If the molecular structure, or the pattern of the cells, remains permanently changed, the patient remains immune. This condition is called *permanent active immunity.* Not all organisms produce a permanent change in the cellular pattern. An example of one that does not is the virus of the "common cold." Even when a permanent change in molecular structure does occur in the cell, periodic contact with small numbers of the organism seems to be needed to maintain continued effectiveness of antibodies. A permanent immunity against diseases that cause antibody production and appear endemically (some of the population having the disease every few years) is usually maintained in this manner. Immunity acquired for common childhood diseases is an example.

Methods have been developed to artificially inject certain pathogens or their toxins into the body so as to stimulate active antibody production without disease. This is called *artificially acquired active immunity.* It is used to enhance the body defenses against disease-producing organisms. The use of this method is discussed on p. 298.

The young child seems to be best equipped to acquire natural active immunity. He is old enough to withstand infection, and the level of his histamine response, although high enough to stimulate the internal defenses against infection, is also low enough so that symptoms are rarely severe. Consequently, it is considered a good practice to begin to expose the preschool child to the usual environment in which he will live. He should not be intentionally exposed to known disease, but isolation of the child in his home environs should be avoided. Artificially immunizing the child against diseases that might cause serious complications, as well as seeing that he receives natural acquired immunity, is recommended (p. 299).

Studies[9] show that people who have grown up in crowded and unhygienic conditions seem to be less prone to attack by many of the more common infecting organisms than are those whose living conditions have been better. For example, draftees to the armed services who have lived in rural areas are more prone to develop influenzal diseases soon after induction than are their city compatriots. Before the advent of vaccine against poliomyelitis, many children living under slum conditions were less susceptible to the virus that causes poliomyelitis than were rural or suburban children living in more hygienic surroundings.

Natural active immunity sometimes is inherited and does not require actual contact by the body with a pathogen. This is known as *inherited immunity* and is thought to be genetically determined. It probably accounts for the resistance of certain species, races, or individuals to specific diseases. In the study of many diseases, absence of this resistance factor is of more concern than its presence. For example, its absence apparently influences the increased susceptibility or tendency of certain families to such diseases as tuberculosis. Susceptibility to such noninfectious diseases as cancer, coronary artery disease, and diabetes mellitus apparently is inherited also.

In *passive immunity,* antibodies against specific pathogens are present in the bloodstream, but the person has not produced them himself. Therefore, their effectiveness is *temporary.* In infants this kind of immunity is accomplished by a natural mechanism. Antibodies pass through the placental membrane into the infant's bloodstream prior to birth and protect the infant from many of the common infections and communicable diseases (provided that the mother has an active immunity to them) up to the age of approximately 6 months. Other types of passive immunity are acquired by injecting human or other animal serum containing antibodies against specific pathogens into the bloodstream of a person who has been exposed to the disease. This is an emergency measure to supplement the body's defense mechanism, and the effects are temporary. The use of passive immunization is discussed further on p. 299.

The healing process

No healing will occur until infection has subsided and pus and dead tissue have been removed. Pus is a local accumulation of dead phagocytes, dead bacteria, and dead tissue. The bacteria most commonly causing this reaction are the staphylococcus, streptococcus, and *Pseudomonas aeruginosa (pyocyanea).* A collection of pus that is localized by a zone of inflamed tissue is called an *abscess* (Fig. 17). An inflammation in which pus spreads in sheets into the surrounding cellular tissue is called *cellulitis;* whereas an inflammation in which pus collects in a preexisting cavity such as the pleura or gallbladder is called *empyema.* When infection forms an abscess within the body, develops a suppurating channel, and ruptures onto the surface or into a body cavity, it is called a *sinus.* If the infection forms a tubelike passage from an epithelium-lined organ or normal body cavity to the surface or to another organ or cavity, it is called a *fistula* (Fig. 17).

After the infected area is clean, new cells are produced to fill in the space left by the injury. They may be the normal structural cells or they may be fibrotic tissue cells, known as *scar tissue.* If they are fibrotic cells, they will not function as formerly but only serve to fill in the injured area. Some body cells readily regenerate; for instance, after the bowel has healed, it is almost impossible to find the injured area. The respiratory tract also regenerates its tissues readily. Liver tissue regenerates less easily, and some nerve cells are always replaced with fibrous tissue. If a large amount of tissue is destroyed, structural cells may not be replaced, regardless of the type of tissue.

When little scar tissue is produced, the process is called *healing by first intention.* This type of healing usually occurs in a clean, incised wound that is sutured. The edges of the injured tissue are glued together by shreds of fibrin, a thin layer of blood clot, and a crust of dry, protective plasma. Within three days, fibroblasts multiply and grow across the gap while leukocytes, blood, and lymph continue to remove the debris. Collagen fibrils are then formed

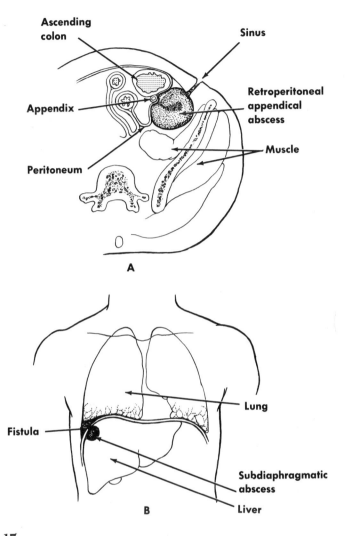

Fig. 17

A, An appendical abscess with a sinus that has developed through the abdominal wall. **B,** A subdiaphragmatic abscess that has developed a fistula opening into the pleural cavity.

to replace the fibrin, and the injured area is quickly filled with granulation tissue composed of new capillaries, fibroblasts, and collagen fibers. Meanwhile, cells typical of the tissue bridge the gap from each side of the wound. As the fibrous connective tissue increases in amount, shrinkage of this tissue occurs and the scar increases in strength. The rapidity with which healing occurs is influenced by the maintenance of a good blood supply, adequate lymph drainage, a

high-protein diet, and a continuous supply of vitamin C.

When there is excessive loss of tissue and the skin edges cannot be brought together, healing by granulation must occur. This process is called *healing by second intention*. It is similar to healing by first intention, but it takes longer because a large area must be filled with granulation tissue. The scar from healing by second intention is usually large and appears uneven. If it involves skin or any other tissue that normally contains nerve endings, it will be numb. As the healing progresses and the scar tissue shrinks, contraction of surrounding tissue may occur and lead to malfunction and deformity.

Some people, especially Negroes, are prone to excessive scar formation. Such tissue formation, known as a *keloid,* is hard and shiny in appearance and may enlarge to a surprising degree. It may cause disfigurement or undergo malignant degeneration, and for this reason is usually excised surgically. Serous membranes sometimes become adherent during inflammatory and healing processes, and as the inflammation subsides, fibrous tissue forms, holding the membranes together. This fibrous tissue is called an *adhesion.* Adhesions may occur in the pleura, the pericardium, about the pelvic organs, and in many other parts of the body. They often occur in and about the intestinal tract, where they may cause an obstruction.

Instead of healing, there may be necrosis, or death of the tissue. Bacteria, both pathogens and nonpathogens, often invade the necrotic tissue and cause putrefaction (decomposition), which is called *gangrene.* The body defenses are useless in preventing or curing gangrene because no blood can get to the area. Gangrenous tissue must be completely removed before healing can occur.

Principles basic to invasion by pathogens

The nurse needs to understand the principles that make invasion of human beings by pathogens possible. The following principles are basic to the prevention of both local and generalized infections and to their spread. They underlie medical asepsis (isolation and reverse precautions) and surgical asepsis.

1. The greater the number of microorganisms (both pathogenic and nonpathogenic), the greater the possibility of infection.

2. By genetic mutation a microorganism can change from a nonpathogen to a pathogen, or a pathogenic organism may become more viable or more virulent. (Since microorganisms multiply at an exceedingly rapid rate, mutations frequently occur.)

3. Desirable conditions for growth (available food supply, warmth, moisture, and an appropriate supply of oxygen and light) increase the number of pathogens.

4. The number of susceptible hosts and the passage of time tend to increase the virulence of organisms because their numbers increase.

5. The more virulent the pathogen, the more serious the disease is likely to be.

6. Resistance of a host to a pathogen usually increases with contact with it, because antibodies against it are produced.

7. A pathogen with which the host is unfamiliar is likely to produce disease.

8. A host with lowered body defenses against infectious organisms is more likely to contract infection.

Surgical asepsis. The purpose of surgical asepsis is to prevent as many organisms as possible from entering body areas that are usually shielded from the external environment during procedures that necessitate perforation or incision through the skin or mucous membranes. All materials that are used in these procedures are sterilized (made free of all organisms), and the patient is protected from other possible sources of pathogens. Before touching sterile materials, hands should be scrubbed, and then the materials should be handled only with sterile gloves or a sterile instrument (p. 202). If there is a large wound or an opening into a body cavity, those in contact with the patient should wear sterile gowns. Caps and masks must be worn by everyone (including the patient) in the room since the hair, nose, and throat are sources of airborne pathogens. Shoe covers also may be used. Excessive talking and movement in the area should be curtailed since this increases spread of airborne pathogens, and the environment should be kept scrupulously clean. Operating rooms may be fumigated periodically with bacteriostatic sprays such as 2% peracetic acid solution, and ultraviolet lights may be used to destroy organisms. Recently some operative procedures, notably organ and tissue transplants, in which any antibody response due to infection may increase the possibility of the body's rejecting the transplanted tissue (foreign protein), have been performed through a plastic "bubble" in which the patient is encased and by which he is isolated from the environment. The skin in the area to be incised usually is shaved and then scrubbed and disinfected (p. 177). The surrounding area then is draped with sterile material. For a perforation such as a venipuncture, scrubbing the area with disinfecting solution is sufficient. To counteract any organisms that may be introduced, antibiotics may be prescribed to be given just prior to an operation and just after it, and they sometimes are introduced into the operative site.

The isolated patient. Medical asepsis (isolation of a patient) has one of two purposes —either to prevent spread of a pathogen from the infected patient to others, or to protect the susceptible patient from pathogens carried by others or present in the environment. The principles basic to preventing spread of a pathogen from an infected patient are discussed on p. 301.

Reverse precautions are used to protect the highly susceptible patient from pathogens. The patient is placed in a single room that should be thoroughly cleaned and aired prior to his admission. It often is fumigated with a bacteriostatic spray and left to air for twenty-four hours. This process may be repeated at one- or two-week intervals, but the repetition means moving the patient from room to room. Anyone entering the room wears a face mask, and sometimes the hair is covered. The door to the room usually is kept closed, and traffic in and out of the room is kept at a minimum. No one with a known infection of any kind (local or generalized) should be allowed in the room. Anyone giving direct care to the patient should wash her hands thoroughly first and wear a freshly laundered (sometimes sterile) gown. If possible, the patient is not transported to other areas of the hospital, but should this be necessary, he usually is asked to wear a face mask, and any open wounds are covered with a sealed dressing. His room should be kept free from dust. How-

Fig. 18

The patient may be placed in an isolator (Life Island), or plastic tent, to completely shield him from the environment. (Courtesy Walter Reed Army Institute of Research; reprinted, with permission, from Ginsberg, Miriam K., and LaConte, Maria L.: Am. J. Nursing 64:88-90, Sept. 1964.)

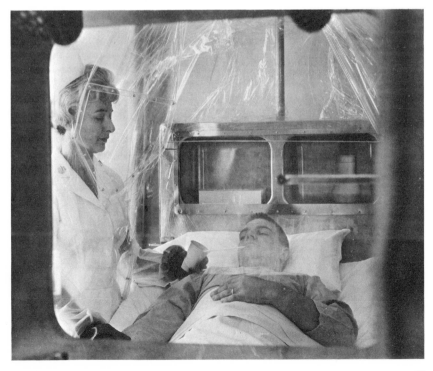

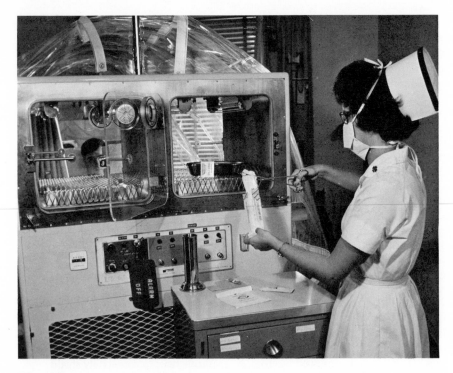

Fig. 19

Only sterile materials are used in the isolator. Here the nurse is passing sterile equipment through a porthole. (Courtesy National Institutes of Health, Bethesda, Md.; reprinted, with permission, from Seidler, Florence M.: Am. J. Nursing **65**:108-111, June 1965.)

ever, only damp dusting and mopping or vacuuming should be permitted.

Sometimes even stricter precautions are desired, and the patient may be placed in an *isolator* (Life Island)— a plastic tent that completely shields him from the environment (Fig. 18). The inside of the tent is rendered nearly microbe-free, and the patient is bathed and his hair shampooed with soap containing hexachlorophene, such as pHisoHex, before he is placed in it. Only sterile materials are used in the tent, and they are passed through portholes (Fig. 19). Even the food is sterilized. The nursing and medical personnel work through gauntlets that protect the patient from their hands. This procedure is completely described in a recent periodical.[42]

Anyone who is medically isolated is socially isolated also. The nurse must be sure the patient and his family and friends understand why the isolation is necessary, and she should make special plans to minimize the social isolation. See the discussion of ways to overcome this problem on p. 284. Unless special care is taken, the patient of any age may have personality changes. The younger child fails to develop at a normal rate, whereas the older child may revert to earlier patterns of social behavior that often persist after he returns home. Adolescent and adult patients sometimes become paranoiac and may even have hallucinations or become delirious. (See p. 127 for the care of the patient with these problems.)

If the patient is isolated from his physical environment for any length of time, he must be reintroduced to it carefully. He should be warned to avoid contact with persons who have known infectious disease and to notify his doctor if he develops any infection. Probably it is best if he does not have to be around school-age children, because they frequently are carriers of pathogens.

Care of the patient with an inflammation

Inflammatory reactions in many parts of the body respond to the administration of hormones produced by the adrenal cortex *(corticosteroids)*. These hormones appear to act as buffer substances between the irritant and the body cells. By this means they lessen the symptoms of inflammatory processes throughout the body, and even though not in any sense curative, they permit tissues aggravated by inflammation to repair more promptly. Consequently, the corticosteroids are used extensively in treating inflammatory conditions that are not self-limiting. Local inflammations often respond well to treatment with heat.

Application of heat. Heat, applied locally, increases vasodilation in an inflamed area and thus augments the natural defense mechanism. Dry heat in the form of heat lamps or diathermy may be ordered, or moist heat in the form of hot compresses or soaks may be used. Many doctors prefer massive warm, moist packs because they insulate the part, preventing loss of body heat from the physiologically dilated vessels. Warm packs, however, may cause reflex vasoconstriction and decrease, instead of increase, the blood supply to the affected part. Hot applications are used rarely and with great caution for infants because their tender skin is easily burned. The temperature of the solution used for soaks should not be over 37.8° C. (100° F.). If moist compresses are used for long intervals on an extensive area, such as an extremity in an infant or small child, the body temperature should be checked at least every two hours, because a large percentage of the body area is exposed to extra heat and deprived of dissipation of heat. If the temperature rises, the compresses should be discontinued and the doctor notified. Sterile procedures are not necessary unless there is an open lesion. These procedures are described in texts on fundamentals of nursing.

The corticosteroids. The corticosteroids may be administered systemically or topically and sometimes are injected into involved joints or into specific lesions. The adrenocortical hormone itself, adrenocorticotropic hormone (the anterior pituitary hormone that stimulates adrenocortical hormone production), or a derivative of either hormone may be used. The adrenocortical hormones used to treat inflammatory processes include cortisone, hydrocortisone, hydrocortamate (an ointment), and their many derivatives, such as prednisone, prednisolone, pregnenolone, fludrocortisone (an ointment). The adrenocorticotropic hormones in current use include corticotropin (ACTH) and dexamethasone. Because knowledge about the corticosteroids is increasing rapidly, new preparations are constantly becoming available to supplement or replace older ones. Indeed, changes may occur before the publication of this book. The nurse should keep continuously informed about the latest developments by reading current literature from drug companies and by regular perusal of medical, nursing, and other scientific periodicals.

Because corticosteroids affect a wide variety of body functions (p. 756), their therapeutic uses are numerous, but their effect also makes them potentially dangerous. They should be used only with the utmost care and discretion. Any nurse may care for patients who are being treated with corticosteroids, and therefore all nurses should be well informed about these drugs.

The nurse working with a patient receiving corticosteroids should know the functions of the body that are controlled by these hormones and be prepared to recognize and deal with untoward reactions and to prevent the disastrous effects of rapid withdrawal of the drugs. The preparation used may have the total effect of the adrenocortical hormones or it may have only a partial effect. Deoxycorticosterone (DOCA) is a mineralocorticoid primarily affecting the fluid and electrolyte (sodium and potassium) balance. Cortisone and hydrocortisone preparations are glucocorticoids exerting effects on glucose metabolism, electrolyte balance, lymphoid tissue, eosinophils, and fibroblasts, and producing anti-inflammatory and anti-stress effects. Adrenocortical extract or corticotropin preparations produce full adrenocortical hormone effects—that is, the effects of deoxycorticosterone and cortisone plus gonadal hormone effects. The adrenogenic hormone, secreted by the adrenal cortex as well as by the testicles (testosterone), stimulates protein anabolism and has masculiniz-

63

ing effects. The estrogenic hormone, secreted by the adrenal cortex as well as by the ovary, exerts its effects on tissues reflecting secondary sex characteristics. Corticosteroids applied topically do not produce systemic effects unless they are used in large amounts in areas where they can be absorbed easily.

The nurse should watch all patients on corticosteroid therapy for side effects and untoward reactions, and she should report the early signs at once. If a patient is being cared for at home, he and/or his family should be taught to watch for the signs. Many of the side effects of this therapy, while unsightly and annoying, do not contraindicate therapy unless more severe untoward reactions occur. Some patients find they become quite "jittery" and may have difficulty sleeping; others feel euphoric. Usually these effects are self-limiting, but some patients may develop psychic reactions. Therefore, personality changes should be recorded carefully and reported. Some patients become very depressed. The typical "moon face" so often described in patients who are on corticosteroid therapy often changes the person's appearance noticeably. Since this change in appearance is related to fluid and electrolyte changes, it forewarns of the need for careful measurement of the serum sodium and potassium levels, but it rarely necessitates stopping treatment. Hirsutism in women and engorgement of mammary tissue in men are common but not serious side effects of adrenocortical extract, or ACTH.

To avoid his undue concern, any patient receiving systemic treatment with corticosteroids should be forewarned that at first he may feel nervous and overalert and may have difficulty sleeping. If this condition continues beyond three or four days or becomes worse, he should contact his doctor. The patient on long-term therapy needs to be told about the "moon face," the hirsutism, and mammary gland changes. The patient often needs help in making an emotional adjustment to changes in physical appearance. He should be observed carefully for any signs of withdrawal from personal contacts or other personality changes that suggest difficulty. A woman who is at the climacteric and receiving ACTH should be told that the

hormone may cause menstrual bleeding. Any change in the menses should be reported.

Serious untoward effects that require immediate attention may result from long-term treatment with corticosteroids. They can follow the use of either cortisone or ACTH. The patient may develop a hypokalemia (low potassium content of the blood) and a hypernatremia (excessive amount of sodium in the blood). Muscle weakness, cardiac arrhythmias, hypertension, edema (dependent and pulmonary), and neurologic symptoms suggest these conditions. He may develop diabetes mellitus due to interference with the body's use of insulin. (See p. 742 for the symptoms.) He also may show signs of tissue wasting due to increased protein catabolism. Wounds may fail to heal well, and old healed lesions, such as peptic ulcer craters and the Ghon tubercle of tuberculosis, may break down. New peptic ulcers may develop. (See p. 651 for the symptoms.) Eosinopenia and lymphopenia may develop. Because of these side effects, corticosteroids are rarely given for a long period to patients with histories of healed peptic ulcer, tuberculosis, heart failure, hypertension, cardiac arrhythmias or blood dyscrasias. They are not used after surgery or for traumatic injury unless the patient has been on the drug previously and must be maintained on it postoperatively. If the nurse is aware of any circumstances that make the use of these drugs dangerous for the patient, she should be sure that the doctor is so informed.

Today many people take drugs prescribed by various specialists, and the doctor ordering the most recent drug may not be aware of other drugs being taken. Before the patient starts taking corticosteroids, the nurse should find out what other drugs he is taking and have him discuss them with his doctor. She also should instruct the patient to inform any other doctor who may be prescribing for him that he is taking corticosteroids. Adrenergic drugs, such as amphetamine, and psychic stimulants are definitely contraindicated because they increase the possibility of hypertension and manic states. Tranquilizers also may be undesirable due to their psychic effects. Corticosteroids may counteract the effects of hypotensive drugs, and the two types of drugs should not be taken simultaneously without medical advice. Patients who are receiving estrogens or androgens may need the dosage of these drugs adjusted.

Because corticosteroids depress the inflammatory process and the production of lymphocytes, the body's first line of defense against invading pathogens, the patient on corticosteroid therapy must be carefully protected against infection. Frequently during hospitalization reverse isolation techniques are used. The patient should be told that reverse isolation protects him from exposure to others who may be carrying infectious organisms and why this protection is important. He should be advised that when he returns home he should minimize his exposure to crowds and his contact with persons who have colds and other infectious disorders. He also should avoid chilling and fatigue. If he sustains even slight cuts or injuries or develops any sign of infection, he should contact his doctor at once. If infection does occur, antibiotics may be used. Several of the antibiotics, however, are contraindicated, owing to the side effects they may cause. For example, chloramphenicol (Chloromycetin) sometimes causes agranulocytosis (a depression of white blood cells), and monilial infections may result from chlortetracycline (Aureomycin). These side effects may produce serious consequences in a patient on corticosteroids, because the hormone makes him very susceptible to infections.

When adrenocorticosteroids are being taken, sodium tends to be retained and to increase the retention of water in the body. Salt intake, therefore, is almost always restricted. The nurse should ask the doctor about the patient who does not have an order for a low sodium diet. Even if the patient is not to be on a special diet, she should suggest that he avoid salty foods and use less salt than usual in food preparation. A diet high in potassium also may be ordered, and additional potassium may be given. The hospitalized patient on corticosteroids usually is on recorded intake and output. Daily weight and blood pressure may be taken, and usually a urinalysis is done at least once a week.

Systemic administration of adrenocorticosteroids suppresses the secretion of ACTH by the pituitary gland. Sudden withdrawal of the drug or a marked decrease in dosage may cause an acute adrenocortical hormone deficiency owing to the failure of the inactivated pituitary hormone to take over effectively at once. This may precipitate addisonian crisis, which, if not treated immediately, can cause death from hypotension and vasomotor collapse. This condition and its medical and nursing treatment is described fully on p. 759. Hypoglycemia also may develop (p. 756). Adrenocortical hormones usually are discontinued gradually. The drug should not be discontinued for diagnostic tests without specific orders from the doctor.

Every patient receiving systemic adrenocorticosteroids on an ambulatory basis should be warned of the serious consequences of omitting the drug and the need to take it at the prescribed intervals. The patient and his family should know the symptoms that may occur if hormones are inadequate, and they should understand the need to seek immediate medical attention if these symptoms occur. The patient should carry an identification card giving his name and address, the drug he is taking, the name and address of his physician, and instructions as to what should be done in event of sudden injury or unconsciousness.

Errors in giving corticosteroids to hospitalized patients and cancellation of orders when patients are transferred from one unit to another or when diagnostic tests or operations are scheduled can lead to serious consequences. Since one of the signs of adrenocortical deficiency is low blood pressure, it is apparent that this deficiency may affect adversely the postoperative course of a patient whose blood pressure may also be lowered by the operation.

Corticosteroids rarely are given to infants and young children. If they are, special precautions should be taken. The infant and young child are likely to tolerate these medications poorly and should be watched carefully for untoward reactions. The younger the child is, the shorter the time he can tolerate an untoward reaction. Therefore, any signs of reaction should be noted promptly and treatment instituted at once.

Care of the patient with generalized infection

A generalized infection is one that causes widespread tissue sensitization and, therefore, a generalized histamine response. The patient usually has an elevation of temperature, accompanied by a hot, dry skin, coated tongue, rapid pulse, general malaise, anorexia, and chills. Profuse diaphoresis may occur. In severe infections with high fever, delirium also may develop. (See p. 128 for care of the delirious patient.) Because the central nervous system is less fully developed and less stable than in adulthood, convulsions are not uncommon in infants and young children who have an infection with a high fever. (See p. 871 for care of the patient who has convulsions.)

Symptoms of generalized infection are seen in many disorders. Symptomatic treatment, however, is similar regardless of the cause and will be discussed here. Care of specific infections with their specific symptoms are discussed in the appropriate chapters in Section II of this book.

Care of the patient with fever. Although fever is an essential part of the defense mechanism, most doctors advise that a patient with a temperature over 38° C. (100.4° F.) stay in bed, since his respiratory and pulse rates are increased. Usually he is permitted to get up to go to the bathroom. Because headache and irritability often accompany severe systemic infection with a high fever, the room should be kept quiet and glaring lights dimmed. The patient should be encouraged to sleep. A warm sponge bath, a back rub, and a smooth bed may help to induce sleep. Frequent baths may be needed since more body wastes may be excreted through increased perspiration. To prevent drying of the mucous membranes of the mouth and nose, the patient should be provided with a vegetable oil with which to lubricate the anterior nasal passages and his lips. He should also be encouraged to brush his teeth several times a day and be urged to take a generous amount of fluids.

In an infection with an accompanying fever, toxins are often excreted through the kidneys, more fluid than usual is lost by evaporation from the skin and by the rapid respiration, and more fluids are needed for accelerated metabolic processes. The adult patient, therefore, usually is urged to take 2,500 to 3,000 ml. of fluid a day. Infants and children should be given smaller amounts. See p. 105 for a detailed discussion of

limitations and precautions to be observed in administering fluids to children and to certain adults. In addition to water, fluids high in calories and containing vitamin C, protein, salt, and potassium, if not contraindicated by the disease, should be taken by the patient, because they help to supply the body's metabolic and electrolyte needs. Solid foods usually are not palatable to the patient with a fever, but may be eaten if desired.

Since kidney damage can occur, the nurse should determine whether or not the urine excreted is normal in appearance and adequate in amount. Often there is an order to measure it. If, despite forcing fluids, the urine becomes concentrated or less than 1,000 ml. are voided daily by an adult, less than 500 ml. by a child, or less than 300 ml. by an infant, the doctor should be notified.

Sudden rises (spikes) in temperature are not unusual in infants and young children who have acute infections because their temperature control mechanism is labile. They do not, however, tolerate fever well. Infants and young children are easily dehydrated because their body surface is proportionately greater than that of an adult. Consequently, they rapidly develop fluid and electrolyte imbalance.

Temperatures that are considered too high to be permitted to continue without heart or other tissue damage (usually over 40° C. [104° F.] in an older child or adult and over 39° C. [102° F.] in an infant or young child) and prolonged elevations that tend to debilitate the patient by increasing his metabolic needs may be lowered to safer levels by the administration of acetylsalicylic acid by mouth or rectum and sponge baths with tepid water or alcohol (half alcohol and half water) (Fig. 20). Ice bags are sometimes applied to the head, groin, and axillas. Care should be taken not to initiate shivering by the excessive use of cold applications. (For details of the procedure, see fundamentals of nursing texts.)

If chills accompany a fever, the patient should be lightly covered to prevent further dissipation of surface heat until the fever can be lowered. Shivering is the body's physiologic response to excessive loss of heat from its surface and acts to raise the body temperature. The mechanism comes into play regardless of fever. The use of warm covering only serves to raise the temperature higher and to produce excessive sweating, which can cause a serious loss of sodium and water in the infant and small child.

A high fever increases metabolism, which, in turn, increases the work load and subsequently the rate of the pulse. It also causes nitrogen wastage and weight loss and increases loss of fluid and sodium through perspiration. For these reasons, hypothermia may be used to treat serious generalized infections, especially in patients who tolerate high fever poorly, such as infants, debilitated patients, and patients who have cardiac or renal disease. Hypothermia decreases the body's metabolic needs. The lowered body temperature also inhibits multiplication of the infecting organism, making it easier for the body's defenses and the prescribed treatment to control the infection producing the fever. (See p. 188 for the nursing care of a patient being treated with hypothermia.)

After a high fever the patient usually stays in bed until his temperature has been normal for twenty-four hours. After a high or prolonged fever most adults feel weak, perspire on physical exertion, and become tired easily. For several days (or even weeks after a prolonged fever) the patient of any age should have extra rest and should eat foods high in protein and calories. Children and young adults usually recover much more rapidly than elderly persons, even when the infection has been severe. During recovery, the patient of any age needs visitors and quiet activities such as reading to help pass the time.

Treatment of local symptoms. Nausea and vomiting often accompany a generalized infection. If they occur, food and fluids should be withheld for a time. Dimenhydrinate (Dramamine), an antihistaminic drug, sometimes can be tolerated and gives relief. If the fever is very high and/or the fluid loss from vomiting is large, fluids may be given parenterally. Infants need fluid replacement much sooner than adults do. Carbonated beverages, tea, broth, and soda crackers or dry toast are usually retained best as nausea subsides.

Symptoms of a "cold" also frequently accompany generalized infections. The doc-

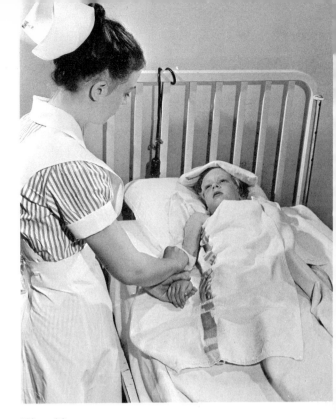

Fig. 20

Elevated temperatures may be lowered to safer levels by sponging the patient with alcohol solution.

tor often prescribes an antihistaminic drug to relieve these symptoms. Otherwise they are treated similarly to those of the common cold (p. 539). Muscle aches and pains, which often occur with an elevation of temperature, are usually relieved by giving aspirin. Rashes that itch may also occur and present a difficult nursing problem. (See p. 769 for the treatment and nursing care.) Antihistaminic drugs sometimes give relief.

Care of the patient with local infections following injury

Wounds. The nurse may be called upon to care for persons with wounds sustained through injury. Therefore, she needs to recognize the seriousness of various types of wounds, know what emergency care to give, and when to advise the patient to seek medical attention.

All wounds sustained accidentally may be infected. If they do not bleed, bleeding should be encouraged to help wash away bacteria. They should be washed well with running water, soap and water, or an antiseptic such as hydrogen peroxide, which bubbles up and helps to debride the wound. Excessive bleeding should be controlled. For minor wounds caused by bites or by dirty or rusty material, the person should seek medical attention. The wound may need to be incised surgically and drained. If there is any danger of its being infected with *Clostridium tetani,* tetanus toxoid or antitoxin is given (p. 69). Medical attention also should be sought for large or deep wounds because sutures may be needed to prevent unsightly scarring. If any appendage, such as a fingertip, has been amputated, the patient and the amputated part should be brought to the doctor at once, since he may be able to suture it in place, and union may occur.

An *incised wound* is one caused by a sharp, cutting object such as a knife, glass, or razor blade. Several layers of tissue are cut and the wound gapes apart. A *laceration* is similar to an incised wound except that it has jagged, rough edges. It may be caused by such things as animal bites, wire, or machinery. Both of these wounds usually bleed profusely, and bleeding may have to be controlled by pressure over the wound or at pressure points (p. 244).

A *puncture wound* is caused by a sharp, pointed, narrow object such as a nail, pin, bullet, or splinter of wood. As the tissues are penetrated by the object, pathogenic organisms may be introduced. Since the skin quickly seals over, the wound rarely bleeds enough to wash organisms out. Bacteria, such as *Clostridium tetani,* that thrive without air may infect these wounds. Because anaerobic bacterial infections are extremely serious, a doctor should be consulted if the puncture was made by a dirty object. Puncture wounds received from objects such as contaminated needles used for any parenteral treatment also should be reported to a doctor. Viral hepatitis may be contracted from this type of injury. Gamma globulin may be given as prophylaxis. Any puncture wound should be made to bleed, and it should be watched carefully for signs of developing infection.

A *stab wound* is caused by a sharp, cutting, pointed instrument such as a knife. Deep tissues are usually penetrated, and the instrument may be plunged into a body cavity or into an organ. In the case of a stab wound of the chest, the instrument should never be removed unless a "sealing" dressing such as petroleum jelly gauze is available for immediate application. Otherwise, air may be drawn into the pleural cavity, breaking the normal vacuum and causing a *pneumothorax* (collapse of the lung) (pp. 574 and 582). All stab wounds require medical attention since they are deep and should be well debrided. If the injury has been on the trunk, the patient should be examined carefully and observed to determine whether an organ has been perforated.

A wound caused by a blunt instrument that breaks the skin and bruises the surrounding tissues is known as a *contusion.* There is hemorrhage into the tissue with a resultant *hematoma* (swelling caused by leakage of blood into the tissues). The immediate application of ice to the area and elevation of the injured part may reduce swelling due to bleeding of superficial tissues.

Complications from contaminated wounds. If the tissue around any wound becomes swollen, reddened, or painful, medical attention should be sought at once because these signs indicate infection. Wounds are most often infected by staphylococci. Both the pathogenic strain (*Staphylococcus aureus A*) and the nonpathogenic strain (*Staphylococcus aureus B*) are found normally in the nose, throat, hair follicles, and sweat glands of man. Most people have a high tolerance for these microorganisms, but the very old, the very young, and those with metabolic disease, acute infections, wounds, or abrasions are very susceptible to them. Although staphylococci are responsible for most suppurative infections of the skin, streptococci and enteric organisms also may infect wounds. Open wounds that are exposed frequently to the air may become infected with the airborne bacteria *Pseudomonas aeruginosa.* Their presence may be detected by the appearance of a blue-green watery discharge.

Staphylococcal infections. The incidence of serious staphylococcal infections in hospitals is increasing and poses one of the most difficult aspects of caring for hospitalized patients today. In recent years staphylococcal organisms have become increasingly resistant to antibiotic drugs, and pathogenic strains have become more virulent. Staphylococci can be isolated from patients and from staff members as well as from dust, hospital equipment such as blankets, pillows and mattresses, and the air. Many authorities feel that the best hope of controlling staphylococcal infection lies in strictest attention to good aseptic techniques. Stress is being placed on cleanliness. Hospital housekeeping is being examined for adequacy and for control of dust. The nurse is primarily responsible for teaching other staff members and supervising good aseptic technique in matters such as washing hands and in the care and handling of linen and all other hospital equipment that may be active in the transfer of infectious organisms. In current practice, patients with active infection are isolated, and strict medical asepsis is observed. All or most hospital personnel may be required to have nose and throat cultures. Those who are carriers of staphylococci usually are treated with antibiotics and are not permitted to be in contact with susceptible patients while they have a positive culture.

If, when the staphylococci are implanted in susceptible tissues, body defenses do not overcome them quickly, they produce coagulase and toxins that destroy cells and phagocytes and cause a dense, hard, fibrinous wall to surround the infected area. This wall protects staphylococci from the body defenses, allowing the bacteria to multiply and extend the infection. Necrosis of tissue develops, and the subsequent degeneration and liquefaction of cells results in abscess formation. If the infection is allowed to progress without adequate treatment, necrosis of soft tissues may occur, underlying bone may become infected, the lymph nodes may become involved, and generalized bacteremia may occur and cause death.

Local infections caused by pathogenic staphylococci usually are treated by hot soaks, incision and drainage of the abscess, and antistaphylococcal drugs. Surgical incision of the abscess is necessary because the drugs are less effective in the presence of pus.

Tetanus. Tetanus, or lockjaw, is an infectious disease caused by the gram-positive, anerobic, spore-forming bacteria *Clostridium tetani*, which are normal inhabitants of the intestinal tracts of men and other animals and can survive for years in soil and dirt. They enter the bloodstream of human beings through wounds and travel to the central nervous system.[3] They produce a powerful toxin that acts at the myoneural junction, causing prolonged muscular contractions. The symptoms of tetanus appear from four days to four weeks after the introduction of the bacteria into a wound. The patient first notices stiffness of the jaws and then develops difficulty in opening his mouth. He complains of rigidity of the facial and sternocleidomastoid muscles. They become hypertonic and cause stiffness of the neck and spasm of the facial muscles, which produces the characteristic sardonic smile (*risus sardonicus*). The abdominal and lumbar muscles also become rigid, and opisthotonos (arching of the back) occurs. Painful muscle spasms may occur upon the slightest stimulation (a draft, jarring the bed, or touching the bedclothes).

Even with rigorous treatment, about 25% of patients with tetanus die. Prophylaxis is the only sure treatment (p. 299). Once tetanus has developed, treatment is directed toward neutralizing the toxin with large intravenous doses of tetanus antitoxin. If the person has ever received horse serum, a possible allergic response is avoided by giving human tetanus immune globulin. All patients receiving serum therapy should be watched carefully for anaphylactic shock (p. 77). The area around the wound is infiltrated with tetanus antitoxin, and then it is widely excised and debrided, flooded with zinc peroxide, and left open. Recently the hyperbaric oxygen chamber has been used to flood the tissues with oxygen.

Prevention of muscle spasms limits the spread of the toxin. Therefore, the patient should be kept in a warm, quiet, darkened room removed from external stimuli. If bedclothes or pajamas cause spasm, they should not be used, and the patient should not be disturbed during the acute stage of tetanus for routine nursing measures such as bathing and bed making. The muscle spasms also may be controlled by giving thiopental sodium (Pentothal) intravenously, curare or curare-like synthetic drugs parenterally, or chloral hydrate or paraldehyde by rectum.

The patient should be protected from injuring himself during muscles spasms by padded side rails on the bed and a padded headboard. If possible, a mouth gag should be inserted between the back teeth to prevent biting of the tongue. No attempt should be made to pry the jaws apart, however.

A temporary tracheostomy may be necessary to prevent respiratory difficulty due to laryngeal spasm. The fluid and caloric intake must be maintained to prevent electrolyte imbalance. It may be necessary to give nourishment intravenously because of dysphagia, but a diet high in calories and fluids sometimes is tolerated without ill effects. A nasal catheter may be used for feeding if it does not cause spasm of the throat muscles. Antibiotics may be given in massive doses to combat concomitant infection.

The nurse must observe the patient at least every half hour, and it may be necessary for him to be attended at all times. He should be observed for signs of respiratory distress, and the type and length of all the muscle spasms should be recorded. Death may occur as a result of spasm of the respiratory muscles, following exhaustion from repeated and prolonged spasm of all the body musculature, or from no apparent cause. Any change in his condition should be reported to the physician.

Gas gangrene. Gas gangrene is a much feared wound infection that usually occurs following traumatic wounds in which there is damage to muscles. It is caused by *Clostridium welchii,* which is found in the intestinal tract of human beings and domestic animals. These bacteria are able to survive for indefinite periods of time in dust, dirt, and woolen clothing.

Gas gangrene is characterized by the onset of pain and swelling in the infected area within seventy-two hours after the introduction of the Welch's bacilli. The patient becomes prostrated with extreme weakness and exhaustion and is very pale. The pulse and respirations become rapid, and the blood pressure falls. The temperature may be only slightly elevated. The infected area is extremely tender, and there may be gas bubbles within the wound and under the skin. A thin, brownish, odorous, watery discharge comes from the wound. This drainage contains large numbers of the bacteria. The involved area is swollen, brick red, and necrotic. The surrounding area may be blanched at first and later a mottled purple.

Because not all wounds containing gas bubbles are infected with gas gangrene, the diagnosis can be made only by culture of wound discharge.

The treatment of gas gangrene consists of radical excision of the infected area, packing of the wound with zinc peroxide dressings, and administration of large doses of antibiotics. Gas gangrene antiserum also is available. Gas gangrene can be spread to others and, therefore, precautions must be taken. The patient should be isolated, his soiled dressings burned, and any instruments used for wound care washed and sterilized immediately after use. Sterilization should be with steam under pressure for twenty minutes. If this procedure is impossible, fractional sterilization should be used. Soiled linen also should be autoclaved or fractionally sterilized before it is sent to the laundry. While the wound is draining, everyone in personal contact with the patient or his belonging should wear gloves and a protective gown. If no protective clothing is worn, care must be taken not to contaminate clothing, and dressings should be handled only with instruments. Whether or not gloves are used, the hands should be scrubbed well with soap and water after caring for the patient or for his belongings. Anyone with hangnails or open wounds on the hands should not care for a patient with gas gangrene. Gas gangrene, fortunately, is less prevalent and less serious since the advent of antibiotic therapy. However, an occasional patient may still develop the disease. Usually the patient is quite alert and requires constant supportive nursing care to keep him comfortable and as free from pain and apprehension as possible.

Wound irrigation and packing. The nurse is often asked to irrigate or pack infected or gaping wounds. It is important that these wounds heal from the bottom since, if the skin and superficial layers of tissue heal first, a collection of pus may form in the unhealed space. When irrigating deep wounds or sinus tracts, a catheter usually is placed as deep into the wound as possible. Then, with an Asepto syringe, the irrigating fluid is instilled until the returns are clear (Fig. 21). The doctor should be consulted as to the direction in which the catheter should be inserted and the depth to which it should go. This information should be recorded on the nursing care plan. In irrigating fistulas

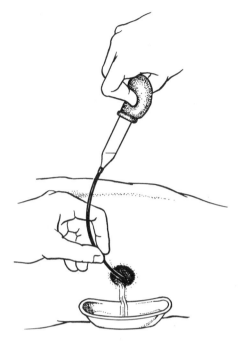

Fig. 21

A catheter and Asepto syringe are often used to irrigate an infected wound that may have a deep abscess or a sinus tract to the exterior.

the fluid instilled in one opening should return from the other. The patient should turn so that all the irrigating solution drains back, or the solution should be aspirated from the wound with an Asepto syringe, since fluid that is left in a deep wound becomes a culture medium for bacterial growth.

If the wound is to be packed, the packing also should be placed into the bottom of the wound cavity to prevent surface healing. Packs should be kept moist. If they become dry, they should be moistened with normal saline solution before being removed to prevent damage to the newly formed granulation tissue. This tissue will ooze readily, and it should be handled gently. The doctor often trims it with scissors to stimulate further healing. The patient feels no pain from this procedure since there are no nerve endings in the new tissue.

Diluted sodium hypochlorite solution, 0.5% (modified Dakin's solution), often is used to irrigate or pack infected wounds. It is a pow-

erful germicide and deodorant, and dissolves necrotic tissue, preparing the area for granulation. It usually is not used if there are catgut sutures, since it may dissolve them. Dakin's solution is irritating to normal skin, and a protective ointment should be applied before it is used. Since Dakin's solution is unstable, it should be made freshly every forty-eight hours. Hydrogen peroxide solution also is ordered for the irrigation of infected wounds and is the solution most often used for home care. It acts as a cleansing agent, removing organic debris, but its bactericidal action is limited in the presence of blood or pus.

Povidone-iodine (Betadine) in 0.5% dilutions, an antiseptic, also may be used. Wounds infected with *Pseudomonas aeruginosa* are treated with irrigations and packs of acetic acid, 0.25 to 1%. Antibiotic solutions and solutions containing proteolytic enzymes, such as *streptokinase* and *trypsin*, which digest the necrotic tissue, may be instilled into the wound. No special care of the skin is needed when using hydrogen peroxide, povidone-iodine, acetic acid, or antibiotic solutions. If solutions containing enzymes are used, however, care should be taken to keep them off the skin, where they will cause irritation. If, in caring for the wound, the nurse notices any increased inflammation or any increased suppuration or necrosis, she should record this change and notify the doctor.

Common local infections

Patients often ask the nurse for advice on minor infections involving the superficial tissues. Therefore, she must be able to recognize the most common infections and know when medical attention is indicated. She also should teach measures for preventing these infections.

Infections of the hand. Infections of the hand occur frequently because the hands are functionally involved in most activities and thus are likely to be injured or exposed to infection. These injuries and infections usually are painful, and rest is essential to healing. Therefore, although the patient rarely is hospitalized, he may be partially incapacitated.

An infection involving the soft tissues around and underneath the nail is called a *paronychia* (Fig. 22). It usually results from

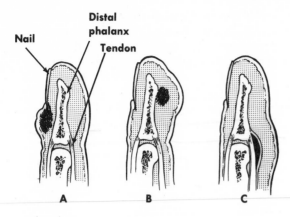

Nail
Distal phalanx
Tendon

Fig. 22

Common infections of the finger. **A**, Paronychia. **B**, Felon. **C**, Tendon sheath infection.

the infection of a hangnail. The involved finger is very painful, and the patient complains of a continuous throbbing sensation in it. The pain is relieved immediately by lifting the soft tissues away from the nail with a scalpel and draining the pus. The patient then may be given an antibiotic and instructed to soak his finger in warm, sterile saline solution for fifteen to twenty minutes several times a day and to refrain from using his hand.

An infection that involves the soft tissue of the fingertip is called a *felon*. It often is caused when staphylococci are introduced into the finger by a pinprick and sometimes can be prevented by making pinpricks bleed. In the early stages the infection responds to warm soaks, and sometimes an antibiotic is given. If it is allowed to progress untreated, the swelling may cause obstruction of the arterial blood supply to the soft tissues of the finger, and necrosis of the tissue and underlying bone may occur. The infected area will then have to be surgically incised and drained and the necrotic tissue excised. A pricked finger should be watched carefully, and if swelling or pain develops, medical treatment should be obtained.

Infection of the tendon sheath, particularly on the palmar surface, often follows puncture wounds of the fingers or hand. Streptococci are most often the infecting organisms.

The hand becomes red and swollen along the tendon, and movement is very painful. This kind of infection usually responds to early treatment with antibiotics and hot soaks, but surgical incision and drainage may be necessary. Untreated infections of the tendon sheath lead to destruction of the tendon with resulting finger and hand deformities. If the tendon has been damaged, a tendon graft to correct deformities may be necessary after healing has occurred.

Lymphangitis and lymphadenitis. Lymphangitis is an inflammation of the lymphatic vessels. It is usually of streptococcal origin and is a sequela of infections of the feet, legs, hands, or arms. The first symptom to appear is a red, tender streak under the skin of the leg or forearm, indicating the spread of the infection to the lymphatic vessels. The lymph nodes above the infection (in the knee, groin, elbow, or axilla) become swollen and tender as the infectious organisms invade them. This condition is known as lymphadenitis. If the infection continues uncontrolled and bacteria reach the bloodstream, septicemia, with fever, chills, malaise, and increase in the pulse rate, may develop. Infections of the lymph channels are treated by drainage of the original infection, antibiotics, hot wet dressings, and elevation of the affected extremity.

Furuncles and carbuncles. Furuncles (boils) and carbuncles (multiples boils) are common local infections. They are discussed on p. 780.

Ulcerations. An ulcer is a superficial loss of skin due to the death of cells. It may be caused by infection, second-degree burns, or inadequate blood supply and nutrients to the part. Debilitated persons are prone to develop decubitus ulcers from prolonged pressure over bony prominences. Ulcers of the lower legs and feet are rather common in persons with poor arterial or venous circulation in the lower extremities. If the ulcer does not become secondarily infected, it will heal by second intention. Because of their location, however, ulcers of the skin usually become infected with staphylococci, streptococci, or enteric bacteria and require extensive treatment with antibiotics both systemically and locally.

Warm saline soaks usually are prescribed to cleanse the ulcer and stimulate granula-

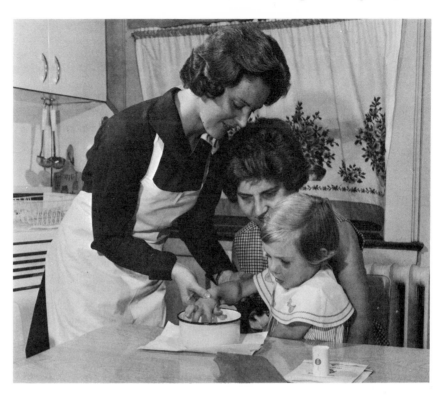

Fig. 23

The nurse in the patient's home is teaching the mother how to carry out the prescribed procedure of hot soaks for her child's infected finger.

tion. If the ulcer is infected, irrigations and packings similar to those described on p. 70 may be ordered. Pressure on the part should be relieved and circulation to it stimulated. Patients with large ulcers on the trunk may be placed in CircOlectric beds or on Stryker frames and turned from the abdomen to the back at one- to two-hour intervals. Patients with ulcers on the legs or feet may be placed on CircOlectric beds and the bed tilted up or down at regular intervals. An oscillating bed may also be used. There may be an order to keep the part elevated, with intermittent exercise prescribed. Alternating air-pressure mattresses should be used. Padding bony prominences with lamb's wool also reduces pressure. If the ulcer does not heal, as often occurs in arteriosclerotic diseases, a skin graft may be necessary to close the wound.

An ulcer of the skin usually is easier to prevent than to cure. The measures discussed above for relief of pressure over bony prominences and for improvement of circulation should be used prophylactically for debilitated patients, patients who must be confined to bed for long periods, and patients with any disease that tends to impair circulation.

Home care of local infections

Many patients with local infections are not hospitalized. Therefore, the nurse will often be asked to instruct patients in applying hot dressings, soaking the hands or feet, providing rest for the part by splinting, or elevating with a sling or pillows (Fig. 23).

Sterile normal saline solution is most often used for hot dressings and soaks to open wounds. The patient can make this solution in the home by adding 8 ml. (2 tsp.) of table salt to each quart of water and boiling the solution for ten minutes. The solution must be allowed to cool until it can be used without danger of causing a burn. Magnesium sulfate (Epsom salt) may be ordered. It should be prepared according to the doctor's orders.

If hot wet dressings are to be applied, the area covered by the dressing should be lubricated with petroleum jelly to prevent burns. Sterile dressings are placed in the solution and wrung out with forceps, eyebrow tweezers, or two sticks. These instruments should be boiled before the initial use. They can then be stored in a sterilized jar containing 70% alcohol or benzalkonium chloride or be boiled before each use. If sterile dressings are not available, the dressing material can be boiled with the solution. Unsterile hot dressings can be prepared by immersing a bath towel in hot water and wringing it out. Heat will be maintained for longer periods if the wet dressing is covered with a piece of plastic and flannel. A hot-water bottle may also be placed over the dressing to maintain the heat. The length of time hot dressings are to be kept in place will be determined by the doctor, but twenty minutes to half an hour, four times a day, is the usual time.

If hot soaks are being used, a basin large enough to immerse the part completely should be obtained. If an open wound is being soaked, the basin and solution should be sterile. Sterilization can be accomplished by filling the basin to the brim with the solution and boiling it. After it has cooled sufficiently for the soak, the excess solution can be poured off. Soaking is usually ordered for fifteen to twenty minutes, three or four times a day. Soaks are often done with the dressing left in place. However, outside layers of the dressing should be removed. The wound usually is redressed after the soak.

Rest for a finger is often accomplished by wrapping it in a bulky dressing. This prevents bending of the joints. A *splint* may sometimes be made by placing a tongue blade under the finger before applying the dressing. If the wound is on the fingertip, a splint of this type is helpful in preventing accidental trauma. Unless contraindicated, the joints should be moved each time the dressing is removed to prevent stiffening.

Slings are frequently used to provide elevation and rest for an infected finger or hand. A scarf or a triangle of muslin will serve as a sling. The sling should be applied so that the hand is supported with only the tip of the little finger showing, and it should be tied so that the hand is elevated above the elbow. In order to prevent pressure sores, care must be taken to avoid knotting the sling over the spinous processes. To prevent "frozen" joints, a sling should be removed several times a day and the joints put through their range of motion. The sling should be removed at bedtime and the part elevated on a pillow.

Elevation of arms or legs on pillows should be done according to the principles of good body mechanics, making sure that the part is in proper body alignment and is supported along the entire length of the limb. Care should be taken that drainage of the vessels is not impeded but rather is enhanced by the position.

If the infection involves the leg or foot, the patient may not be able to be up and about to care for himself, and a family member may need to be taught to prepare the dressings or soaks. However, if no such assistance is available, the patient may be admitted to the hospital. The nurse should discuss plans for home care with the patient and consult the doctor if home nursing care seems inadvisable.

Internal defenses against other foreign proteins

The body's mechanism for dealing with foreign proteins (the antigen-antibody response, p. 57) is not reserved only for pathogenic organisms. It also comes into action against other foreign substances such as pollens, food, animal serum, and dander, as well as a variety of other material such as house dust, cosmetics, synthetic products, and drugs. Some people also develop allergic response (hypersensitivity) to bacteria.

Allergy

Antigenic substances that produce hypersensitivity are known as *allergens,* and the hypersensitivity is called an allergy. The tendency to develop a hypersensitivity seems to run in families and is believed to be inherited genetically. However, any person exposed frequently enough and intensely enough to a substance that stimulates an an-

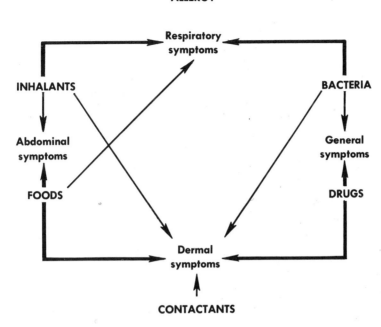

Fig. 24

Illustrating the causes of allergic responses and their relative severity.
(Courtesy Dr. Paul F. deGara, New York, N. Y.)

tigen-antibody response in the body can become allergic to that substance. Any person can be allergic to anything; there are as many possibilities as there are individuals. Susceptible people only develop allergic responses more readily and to more substances. Allergens may be inhaled, ingested, or injected, or they may produce a reaction upon contact with the skin.

When a person who has a tendency to become allergic first comes into contact with the specific allergen to which he is sensitive, antibodies are formed. When this allergen is again introduced into the body, the antibodies combine with it, liberating histamine, and reactions such as sneezing, tearing of the eyes, watery discharge from the nose, wheezy breathing (asthma), skin eruptions, and urticaria may occur. Nausea, vomiting and diarrhea may also be allergic reactions. (See Fig. 24.) Infants and children often are prone to eczema and gastrointestinal symptoms. As they grow older, respiratory symptoms frequently develop. The response tends to be increased with each encounter, and frequently allergies to other substances ensue.

Epinephrine (Adrenalin) and antihistaminic drugs such as tripelennamine (Pyribenzamine), diphenhydramine (Benadryl), and chlorpheniramine (Chlor-Trimeton) may provide temporary symptomatic relief. Antihistamines have a tendency to produce drowsiness, and epinephrine may cause nervousness. Persons who must drive motor vehicles or work around machinery should schedule their doses of these drugs so that they are not understimulated or overstimulated during times when alertness is essential. If drowsiness is a serious problem, they should consult the doctor who prescribed the drug.

It usually is possible to determine the specific allergens to which a person is hypersensitive by taking a detailed history and then testing for sensitivity. *Skin tests* are often used to determine whether a person has a sensitivity to certain substances in his external environment. Several methods of testing are used. Small amounts of extracts of various allergenic substances to which the patient is suspected to have a sensitivity may be injected intradermally at spaced intervals, usually on the outer surface of the upper arm, on the forearm, or in the scapular region. The extract also may be placed on the skin and the skin scratched lightly (*scratch test*). These two methods are used most often to test for sensitivity to pollen, feathers, dander, and dust. They also may be used to test for sensitivity to foods, but the results are often inaccurate. When clothing or other material is the suspected allergen, a small piece of it may be put against the skin under an airtight patch for forty-eight to seventy-two hours (*patch test*). Sensitivity to soaps and other cleaning agents such as detergents often is tested in this way. An infant may be tested indirectly by injecting his blood serum at spaced intervals under the skin of a nonallergic person, and twenty-four hours later injecting the extract of the suspected allergenic substance at these sites. Tests for allergenic substances usually are done in series; for example, pollens from trees are tested first, then pollens from grasses, and so on. Positive reactions are indicated by the appearance of *wheals* or a pronounced redness. Occasionally one drop of a test extract is instilled into the eye to test for sensitivity (*conjunctival test*). Redness of the conjunctiva and tearing will appear within five to fifteen minutes in an allergic person.

A person with a food allergy usually is asked to keep a food diary for at least a week. On the basis of this diary, suspect foods such as milk, wheat products, and eggs may be removed from the diet (*elimination diet*) until symptoms subside and then added one at a time in an attempt to isolate the offending foods. Babies on this diet often must be given a special nonmilk formula made of products such as soybeans or barley. The mothers need instructions in preparing this formula. A similar elimination process may be used for allergy to other substances such as cosmetics or fabrics.

Some hospitals now have nonallergenic rooms, which may be used to remove a highly allergic person from his usual environment and thus facilitate the search for the substances to which he is sensitive. They also may be used for treatment. When the symptoms have subsided, various articles used at home may be introduced one at a time. Only a limited number of staff members are allowed to enter the room, and they may be requested to avoid the use of cosmetics and to wear a special gown.

The nurse may be helpful to the allergic patient during the period of testing by encouraging him to continue the program, which often takes weeks and months. By suggesting common allergenic substances to him, the nurse may help the patient give the doctor a more complete history. She is often called upon to help the patient plan for elimination testing.

As soon as the offending allergens have been determined, an attempt is made to slowly desensitize the patient by the injection of tiny but increasingly larger doses of the allergen at regular intervals (usually one to four weeks) over a long period of time. This treatment may take years, or it may have to be continued indefinitely. It is about 80% effective in hay fever but less effective in asthma and dermatitis.[1]

Patients who cannot be desensitized and those in the process of desensitization need help in planning to avoid allergens to which they are sensitive. If the patient is sensitive to a certain food, he should be instructed to eliminate this food from his diet. He may need help in the selection of substitute foods so that nutritional deficiency does not develop. When he has been desensitized to a particular food, he may resume eating the food, but only small amounts should be taken at first. If any symptoms develop, the food should be stopped and the doctor notified.

When the patient is sensitive to such substances as dust, mold, spores, animal dander, feathers, insecticides, glues, or lint from fabrics, he and his family must decide the best way to avoid them. The nurse may help with suggestions and by explaining the problem to other family members who may need to cooperate. Dust, feathers, and animal dander often must be eliminated since they frequently are troublesome even to patients whose primary allergy is to other substances. Daily damp dusting lessens the amount of dust in the air. If pillows containing feathers cannot be removed, they can be covered with plastic. New homes sometimes must be found for pets, although it usually is some time before the patient consents to this measure.

Specific care of the patient with asthma is discussed on p. 558, and care for the patient with allergic dermatitis is discussed on p. 783.

Anaphylactic shock

The patient may be so sensitive to an allergen that its subcutaneous injection will cause an acute, severe allergic reaction known as anaphylactic shock. The initial symptoms of anaphylactic shock are edema and itching about the site of the injection, apprehension, and sneezing. These mild reactions are rapidly followed, sometimes in a matter of seconds or minutes, by edema of the face, hands, and other parts of the body, wheezing respirations, cyanosis and dyspnea, dilation of the pupils, rapid weak pulse, and falling blood pressure. Death may follow in a few minutes. The respiratory and circulatory symptoms are caused by constriction of smooth muscle by histamine.

Parenteral injections of penicillin are the most frequent cause of anaphylactic shock. Animal serum used in the preparation of antitoxins and extracts of allergenic substances used for testing or desensitization of an allergic patient also frequently cause it. Sudden death resulting from a bee sting is due to anaphylactic shock. Contrast media containing iodide, such as those used for intravenous pyelograms and angiograms, may produce this serious allergic response. Persons also have been known to develop anaphylactic reactions to acetylsalicylic acid as it is absorbed into the bloodstream. Therefore, this drug may not be as innocuous as many people believe.

Since people with a history of allergies are more likely to develop anaphylactic reactions to drugs than are those without such a history, all patients should be questioned about allergies and sensitivity to drugs before drugs are initiated. If there is any positive history, the doctor should be consulted before a new drug is started, and if it is given, the patient should be watched closely for allergic response. In hospitals it is now common practice to have the fact that the patient is sensitive to certain substances posted conspicuously on the outside of his chart where it cannot be overlooked by anyone responsible for the care of the patient.

People who are known to have received a specific type of animal serum and who must receive antiserum should be given another type if it is available in order to lessen the possibility of an allergic response. However, before *any* serum, such as horse, bovine, or rabbit serum, is injected into the body, the person should be tested for sensitivity to it. A small amount of serum (0.1 to 0.2 ml.) is injected just under the skin of the forearm (intradermally). A similar amount of saline solution is injected under the skin of the other forearm as a control. The appearance within five to fifteen minutes of a reddened, itching wheal or hive about the site of the serum injection constitutes a reaction. Conjunctival tests also may be used (p. 76). If the patient has a reaction, the doctor must be consulted before the serum is given. If it is essential and no other type is available, very small doses may be given at intervals.

Any time animal sera, allergenic extracts, or contrast media containing iodide are given, epinephrine hydrochloride (Adrenalin) 1:1,000, an antihistamine such as tripelennamine (Pyribenzamine) or diphenhydramine (Benadryl), aminophylline, and levarterenol (Levophed) should be available, and the patient should be kept under surveillance for at least twenty minutes. Any reaction that occurs within a few minutes forewarns of an impending emergency. At the first sign of untoward symptoms (redness and itching about the injection site, itching of the eyes, nasal symptoms, or tightness in the chest) the doctor should be notified. He usually prescribes antihistamine by mouth to counteract a slight reaction. In case of a more severe one, the antihistamine is given parenterally, a tourniquet is applied above the injection site, and Adrenalin is injected into the site. Additional Adrenalin may be given at intervals until the reaction subsides or tachycardia develops. Aminophylline may have to be given to relax the bronchial spasm and levarterenol to raise the blood pressure. Sometimes, to counteract shock, the patient's lower limbs are elevated, oxygen may be given by positive pressure mask, and an infusion is started. If there is tracheal edema, an emergency tracheostomy may have to be done.

Transfusion reactions

Blood from another person is in itself a foreign protein. It may contain allergens to which the patient is sensitive, antibodies, and pathogens. Consequently, blood is a dangerous therapeutic agent that must be used only with the greatest care.

If the blood contains allergens to which the patient is sensitive, he may have an allergic response. Urticaria usually is the first symptom. It may be followed by dyspnea and cyanosis. If any of these symptoms appear, the blood should be discontinued at once, but the vein should be kept open with the physiologic saline solution until the doctor has been contacted for further orders. Sometimes, if the blood is absolutely essential and the reaction is not severe, an antihistaminic drug is given and the transfusion continued. Epinephrine hydrochloride (Adrenalin) 1:1,000 will cause prompt disappearance of the symptoms. Diphenhydramine (Benadryl) and tripelennamine (Pyribenzamine) also may be ordered to relieve an allergic reaction.

The most serious reaction to a blood transfusion (with the exception of anaphylactic shock) is caused by giving the patient incompatible blood—that is, blood with which antibodies in the recipient's blood react.[7] When this is done, the donor's blood is agglutinated and dissolved (lysis) by the recipient's serum, and the product of this hemolysis is circulated throughout the bloodstream.

After he receives about 50 ml. of incompatible blood, the patient usually complains of fullness in the head, severe pain in the back, and a sensation of constriction in the chest. Nausea and vomiting may occur, and the patient's pulse usually becomes rapid and his blood pressure drops. If the transfusion is discontinued at this point, these symptoms will disappear, but a few hours later the urine becomes red (port-wine urine) and the urinary output is diminished. The urine contains red blood cells and albumin. This reaction is thought to be due to the release of a toxic substance from the hemolyzed blood that causes a temporary vascular spasm in the kidneys, resulting in renal damage and blockage of the renal tubules by the hemoglobin precipitated out in the acid urine (hemoglobinuria). If the patient receives more than 100 ml. of the incompatible blood, irreversible shock with complete renal failure may occur, and death may follow. This renal failure is similar to the renal damage that sometimes results from poisons and highly toxic drugs (p. 429).

At the first sign of a reaction, the blood transfusion should be discontinued and the doctor notified. Epinephrine hydrochloride (Adrenalin) 1:1,000 is given at once, and the urine is rapidly alkalized by an intravenous injection of sterile 1/6 molar sodium lactate solution. This procedure reduces the precipitation of hemoglobin in the kidneys.

As blood cells disintegrate (lyze), large amounts of potassium are released into the bloodstream, and if the renal function is impaired, hyperkalemia (excessive amount of potassium in the blood) will develop (p. 100). If this condition occurs, the patient may be treated with an artificial kidney machine (p. 434).

Pyrogenic reactions can occur with the administration of any intravenous fluid, including blood. Pyrogens are toxic products of bacterial growth, and if tubing, needles, and solutions such as sodium citrate are improperly processed, pyrogens may be present despite sterilization that has killed any viable bacteria. The symptoms of a pyrogenic reaction differ little from early symptoms of reaction to incompatible blood. They include fever, headache, nausea and vomiting, weakness, and lumbar pain. However, they subside shortly and require no definitive treatment.

The most common pathogens transmitted to other persons through blood are the viruses causing infectious hepatitis (both serum and infectious). (See p. 706 for the symptoms and treatment.) This transmission is difficult to prevent because many people appear to be carriers. Blood from a donor known to have had infectious hepatitis is never used. It has been suggested that all patients receiving blood transfusions should be given gamma globulin prophylactically. However, the amounts needed are prohibitive, and, consequently, it is used at this time only for patients who would be poor risks if they did develop hepatitis. Other

78

pathogens, such as gram-negative coliform bacilli, diphtheroids, and staphylococci, can be introduced into the body with blood, and the resulting bacteremia may cause death.

Precautions in administering blood. Before blood is given to the patient, a sample of his blood is drawn for typing and cross-matching. His blood is then matched with the blood of possible donors to see if there is compatibility between the patient's serum and a donor's red cells. If they are compatible, the red blood cells do not clump together or agglutinate when the serum of the donor and the red cells of the recipient are mixed, and vice versa. The blood also is tested for the Rh factor. Approximately 85% of the population are Rh positive, which means that their blood contains agglutinins that will sensitize and later cause agglutination of the red cells of those persons (15% of the population) who are Rh negative (do not have these agglutinins).[45] Several other tests are now done to determine the presence of unusual antibodies, many of which seem to be racial or geographic in origin.[7] With more sensitive testing, blood is less likely to produce untoward reactions, but it becomes increasingly difficult to find appropriate donors. A central clearinghouse for blood, the American Association of Blood Banks,* has been organized to help locate donors with unusual factors in the blood. The donor's blood also is tested for syphilis, and if the test is positive, the blood is not used.

The administration of the blood transfusion is the responsibility of the physician, but the nurse gathers the equipment and prepares the patient. (For the procedure see a fundamentals of nursing text.) The blood should not be obtained from the blood bank until the doctor is ready to start the transfusion, and only one bottle at a time should be brought to the unit. Refrigeration on the unit usually is not suitable for storage of blood, and without adequate refrigeration the blood cells may release potassium that may be detrimental when given to some patients (p. 100). Just before the transfusion is started, the label should be checked against the accompanying card by both the

nurse and the doctor for name and type and for Rh and other factors. If the doctor is assured that the blood is intended for the patient, he starts the transfusion.

If possible, the patient should be attended constantly by a nurse until the first 100 ml. of blood has been received, since any serious reactions usually occur by this time. If he cannot be given special attention, the nurse should check the flow of the blood frequently and observe the patient for signs of any reaction. An infant, young child, or acutely ill person should be attended constantly by someone on the nursing team throughout the procedure. A child's attention can often be distracted from the procedure by reading to him. When the adult patient is not attended constantly, his call bell must be placed within reach of his free hand, and he should be advised to call the nurse if he experiences any unusual sensation such as chilliness, dizziness, or any aches or pains.

Rejection of tissue and organ transplants

One of the most serious problems surgeons face in trying to transplant any tissue from one person to another is failure of the grafted tissue "to take" (become a contiguous part of the body of the recipient). It is felt that the antigen-antibody response is responsible for this failure. Tissue from another person is a foreign protein, and the body proceeds to destroy it. Attempts are made to desensitize the recipient to the donor's tissue before surgery, and total body irradiation is sometimes done before surgery in an attempt to minimize the response. The operation usually is done with the patient inside "the bubble," and he is kept in an isolator (p. 62) preoperatively and postoperatively in an attempt to prevent infection, which may stimulate increased antibody activity.

The body's defenses against stress in the environment

The body has a self-preserving mechanism that automatically and immediately comes into action in times of stress or danger. The stress can be physical, as in injury or disease, or psychologic, as in fear, anger, or frustration. Although stress often arises

---

*Located at the Chelsea Navy Hospital in Massachusetts.

from changes in the external environment that threaten survival, it also may result from changes in the internal environment of the body. This mechanism is called the alarm reaction, or *general adaptation syndrome*. It often is said to prepare the person for "fight or flight," but the response may be that of immobility. The mechanism suppresses functions that are nonessential for life and augments those which facilitate overcoming or escaping the stressful situation. An adequate blood supply to the brain and heart is maintained, that to the skeletal muscles is increased, and provision is made to maintain the body's water, electrolyte, and temperature balance and to supply extra energy. To achieve this state, the nerve endings of the sympathetic nervous system are stimulated to produce a chemical called norepinephrine and the adrenal medullas are stimulated to secrete norepinephrine and epinephrine. This reaction is known as the *sympathoadrenal response.*

Norepinephrine acts as a vasoconstrictor (increases the peripheral resistance to blood flow) and, consequently, causes an elevation in blood pressure. *Epinephrine* stimulates the central nervous system, causes increased cardiac output, dilates the bronchioles of the lungs, which aids in gaseous exchange (the exchange of oxygen for carbon dioxide), and enhances metabolic activity so that more energy is available. Perspiration is increased, allowing for dissipation of excess body heat. Gastrointestinal peristalsis is decreased, and the blood vessels in the kidneys constrict. The pupils dilate, making distance vision and vision in the dark more acute. Clotting of the blood is enhanced. There is some evidence that epinephrine causes the spleen to contract and discharge blood into the general circulation. In addition, it stimulates the production of ACTH by the anterior pituitary gland, which, in turn, causes an outpouring of adrenocorticosteroid hormones. The action of these hormones provides emergency fuel by stimulating the release of glycogen from the liver and muscles, and it helps maintain the fluid and chemical balance that usually is upset by the initial stress response. Later these hormones help to provide the body with materials for repair of any damage incurred.

The protective mechanism used in re-

sponse to stress is called into action frequently in everyday life, but the response usually is minimal and too short-lived to produce symptoms. In times of severe stress or danger, however, the person appears pale, his skin is cool and moist, his pupils are dilated, his muscles are tense, and he is keenly alert. His pulse is full and rapid, his systolic blood pressure is elevated, and his respirations are deep but usually show little increase in rate. The person having a pronounced reaction to stress may have abdominal distention, and he usually becomes nauseated. After the immediate threat has been removed, he may vomit or have diarrhea. If the stress is not severe enough to cause vasoconstriction of the renal vessels, the person usually has a full bladder and a desire to void as soon as the stress is relieved. If the stress continues as it does after severe trauma or during serious illness, the urine may be concentrated and the output reduced.

If moderate to severe responses to stress occur frequently, permanent damage to the body may result. For example, constant exposure to emotional stress is thought to be the cause of gastric ulcers and of coronary heart disease and hypertension in some people. It also appears to play a part in the response of some people to allergenic substances.

The body's response to stress may be detrimental to a patient with heart disease, generalized arteriosclerosis, or aneurysms, because he may be unable to tolerate the increased stress on the cardiac muscle or blood vessel walls. The epinephrine output accompanying the alarm response may cause the patient with diabetes mellitus to go into insulin shock (p. 753), because epinephrine (as well as insulin) facilitates the metabolism of glucose, and the insulin in the blood may not be used. Later, however, when the adrenocortical hormones come into action and release glycogen from the liver, and when the epinephrine response is lessened, the patient may have an elevated blood glucose level unless extra insulin is administered. Patients with inadequate adrenocortical hormones and those with a diseased liver often withstand stress poorly because necessary energy supplies may not be available, and the homeostatic regulation of body fluid and electrolytes is inadequate. Under all these circumstances the nurse may need to help the patient and his family plan their life so as to avoid unnecessary stress. Some special precautions are discussed in the chapters dealing with each disease condition.

Recently, it has been learned that persons do not tolerate stress equally well at all times of the day. For example, the adrenocorticosteroid output seems to be lessened during the night hours. Probably urine specimens will be tested for 17-ketosteroids more frequently in the future because this test done on specimens voided at various hours may give clues as to when an individual should withstand stress best. It is quite likely that in the near future, operations and stress-producing treatments will be scheduled with the individual's optimum period for withstanding stress in mind, so that shock, which is caused by poor accommodation to stress, can be minimized.

The intensity of the response to physical stress seems to be related to the extent of the injury or the severity of the illness. For example, the more tissue removed in an operation, the greater the stress response will be. The sudden appearance or an increase in symptoms of stress and their failure to respond to treatment may be the first sign that the patient's condition is getting worse. Unless measures are instituted to relieve the primary condition causing the stress, the body's mechanism for dealing with it may soon be overtaxed. Transitory signs and symptoms of stress, such as a temporary rise in the systolic blood pressure and the pulse rate and periodic deep breathing, probably signify an increase in emotional stress or that the patient is overexerting physically.

The original stress may be so damaging to the body that it is impossible for the defense mechanism to be effective. Examples of extreme stress situations are arterial bleeding, pressure on the hypothalamus, overwhelming infection, and blockage of a major branch of the coronary artery. In these situations, unless the primary condition can be controlled promptly, death will occur.

Nursing care

Every nurse should understand the body's mechanism for handling stress. Otherwise,

nursing actions may impede rather than complement and supplement the defense mechanism. She should remember that the purpose of the initial response to stress is to help the person escape the stress-producing situation or mobilize all his defenses to resist it. Severe and continuing stress, however, may overtax the body's mechanism for self-preservation.

Physical activity reduces the sympathoadrenal response. Therefore, although physical activity may be useful in reducing anxiety states, it is contraindicated in severe stress caused by trauma or illness because it will impede maintenance of body functions essential for life. Thus, a patient showing signs and symptoms of severe stress usually is kept in bed and sometimes is given sedation. Although he should be kept warm, he should never be too warm, because overheating causes vasodilation, counteracting arteriolar constriction, which assures an adequate blood supply for the vital organs.

Although the patient may be able to cope with one stress-producing situation, his body may not be able to adapt to further stress. Therefore, it always is extremely important to prevent additional physical or emotional stress. Special care needs to be taken to prevent further trauma or superimposed infection. Anxiety and fear both produce stress reactions, and special care should be taken to alleviate them in any patient who has suffered a serious injury, is undergoing surgery, or is seriously ill. Extraordinary thoughtfulness may be required since the patient is likely to be very alert. Anxiety-producing conversations with the patient or in his vicinity should be avoided, and noise, bright lights, and movement should be kept at a minimum. Pain should be alleviated because it increases the stress reaction.

Even a minor stress reaction causes annoying symptoms, which the nurse should attempt to relieve. The backache, general muscle tension, and headache that commonly accompany illness are often symptoms of stress. Comfort measures such as back rubs, frequent position changes, and maintenance of proper body alignment and support help to relax the muscles. After a severe stress reaction, food and fluids should be withheld until nausea subsides and gastrointestinal activity returns to normal.

The body's defenses against inadequate food, water, and oxygen supplies

The body, even under normal circumstances of health, has a very limited ability to withstand inadequate replacement of nutrients, water, and oxygen from the environment. Some oxygen in the external environment must always be available, and a complete absence of water can be tolerated by an adult only for several days. A baby or child can tolerate it for no more than one day because he has less fluid reserve in the body and uses more than an adult. A well-nourished young adult can exist without food for several weeks if necessary, but he will develop electrolyte imbalances. The baby and young child must have daily replacement of nourishment because their needs are great and their reserves minimal. Elderly people need a constant supply of nutrients because they may have limited circulation, which makes the distribution of nutrients to cells inefficient. In addition, vital organs such as the heart and kidneys may be functioning near maximum capacity and be poorly able to withstand inadequate cellular nutrition and the resultant additional strain caused by the electrolyte imbalance. Elderly persons tolerate starvation no better than children but for different reasons.

Food and water

If adequate food is not available, the body burns its own tissues to supply its energy needs. It cannot do this for any length of time, however, without the development of fluid and electrolyte imbalances. Many vitamins and minerals essential for continuance of body processes that help to maintain the homeostatic state are not stored in the body and must be supplied daily in food.

To maintain its energy requirements without adequate food, the body first burns its glycogen stores. Fats are then oxidized, and finally body proteins are mobilized and burned for energy. Burning of body fats produces ketones, and as proteins are burned, nitrogen and potassium accumulate in the blood. If lack of food is associated with an inadequate fluid intake, these end products of metabolism may be retained by the body and electrolyte imbalances rapidly ensue. Symptoms of metabolic acidosis (p. 101) appear, the blood urea nitrogen (p. 421) rises, and symptoms of hyperkalemia (p. 100) develop. Lack of an adequate food and water supply is a stress situation, and the resultant outpouring of adrenocortical hormones causes sodium to be retained to help maintain the blood volume by holding water in the bloodstream. Hypernatremia (p. 99) can result from this retention of sodium. Despite adequate intake of water, electrolyte imbalances will occur eventually because of inadequate mineral replacements.

To maintain essential body functions, an adult uses at least 1,700 ml. of water a day, an infant about 300 ml., and a child about 500 ml. Water produced from the burning of tissues (oxidation) and water pulled from the interstitial spaces can be used to maintain the body's needs for a short time. The kidneys, too, will conserve water as much as possible. However, since only 150 ml. a day is produced by oxidation (proportionately less in infants and children despite their higher metabolic rate), the available supply is rapidly depleted and the patient becomes seriously dehydrated (p. 96). This sequence of events may be speeded up by illness.

Although it is possible to live for short periods without food and fluid, the results are likely to be very serious for the person who is ill. Therefore, seeing that food and fluid intake is maintained is of primary importance in caring for any patient. The nurse should remember that lack of adequate food and water is a stress situation. In stress, energy requirements increase, which quickly compounds the problems.

Oxygen

Although the body must always have a supply of oxygen, it normally can make some adjustments to decreased amounts of available oxygen. For example, people who live at high elevations, where less oxygen is available to the body, gradually develop an increased number of red blood cells. This compensatory mechanism provides for greater oxygen transport in the blood, and although each blood cell may carry less oxygen than normally, the increased number of carriers may provide for adequate oxygenation of tissues.

Since travel has become so rapid and so widespread, it is important to teach the public the implications of this adjustment, which normally is slow. Because extreme or unusual exercise or stressful situations always require extra oxygen supplies, care should be taken to avoid these situations for several days after arriving in a place where the altitude is higher than that to which a person is accustomed. In high altitudes the atmospheric pressure is low, and at low atmospheric pressures less oxygen diffuses across the alveoli into the blood, while carbon dioxide diffuses more rapidly than usual from the blood, causing respiratory alkalosis. This reaction is an application of Dalton's law of gases. If precautions are not taken until the body has had an opportunity to compensate by increasing the number of red blood cells, the tissues may not receive enough oxygen. Men whose work takes them to places where the altitude is high are likely to have serious difficulty if they contract respiratory illness. They also need to avoid strenuous physical activity for several days after arrival.

Because of the dangers accompanying atmospheric pressure changes, most planes now have pressurized cabins as well as additional oxygen supplies. It is unwise for anyone who would be susceptible to the development of problems due to a low concentration of oxygen to fly in a plane without these protections. Elderly persons and those persons who have circulatory or respiratory diseases often tolerate atmospheric pressure changes poorly. They should be advised to consult their physician before planning a trip that entails going to mountainous regions or flying.

A precipitous change from an area of high pressure to one of low pressure can cause rupture of the alveoli because of the expansion of the gases in them. This is an application of Boyle's law. This type of pressure change also causes a decrease in the solubility of the nitrogen in the blood, causing the nitrogen to form bubbles that obstruct blood flow. This is an application of the law of the solubility of gases. The latter condition is commonly known as "the bends" (*decompression sickness* or *caisson disease*)

and may be a problem for pilots, divers, and others who work underwater for long periods of time. Unless pressurized cabins or tanks are used, descent from planes or ascent from diving should be gradual enough to allow time for accommodation to pressure changes. Informing the public about this reaction has become important because many people today engage in flying and diving for recreation.

When extra oxygen is needed, respirations increase in rate and may become gasping, allowing more air to be inspired. This response is bought about by the low oxygen level in the blood with increased carbon dioxide and the stimulating effect of carbon dioxide on the respiratory center. The bronchioles in the lungs also dilate to enhance the gaseous exchange unless disease prevents dilation. This dilation is a stress response that helps to assure an adequate supply of oxygen for the vital organs. Therefore, the person suffering from an inadequate supply of oxygen should be protected from any additional physical exertion or emotional stress that might overtax and consequently decrease the body's stress response. Additional stress also increases the need for oxygen.

If the body is unable to accommodate to an inadequate oxygen supply in the external environment, or if, even though oxygen is available, the blood is unable to carry adequate amounts of it because of a low hemoglobin level (anemia) pure oxygen may be administered. Usually, adequate amounts can be provided by an oxygen tent, face mask, or nasal catheter. Occasionally, oxygen must be administered under positive pressure, and hyperbaric oxygen chambers also may be used.

The body's defenses against temperature changes in the external environment

Life cannot exist unless the temperature of the body is maintained within a relatively narrow range. For normal body function, this temperature is about 37° C. (98.6° F.). The external environment, however, often is much colder or warmer than this temperature, and since heat tends to radiate from a warm area to a cooler one, the body must constantly adjust so as to release or retain heat.

When the environment is hot, the body temperature begins to rise. The blood vessels in the skin then dilate so that heat can be released. The person perspires, and as the moisture evaporates, the air enveloping the skin is cooled so that body heat can radiate to the environment. Respirations also increase and this process, too, releases heat as well as moisture. Usually the person who is too warm instinctively stays somewhat inactive, thus avoiding the burning of additional body fuel with the production of heat.

When the external environment is cold, the superficial blood vessels constrict so that the body radiates less heat. If too much heat is still being lost, shivering occurs. Shivering is a form of muscle contraction that causes additional body fuel to be burned.[27] In the same way, exercise also helps to warm the body.

Even the normal person may be unable to compensate for extremely high or extremely low environmental temperatures. If he cannot compensate, heat exhaustion, sunstroke, or freezing may occur (p. 253). All people should be warned against unnecessary exposure to these extremes.

It is important, in giving nursing care to patients, to avoid measures that counteract the natural defenses for heat control. For example, providing too much warmth for a patient who has a fever, yet feels chilly, may cause the temperature to rise farther. However, if he is not protected enough to prevent shivering, the temperature also will be increased. Sudden warming of a person whose body temperature has been markedly lowered may actually cause it to drop further because, unless the environment is very warm, the heat is lost through the dilated vessels.

Nursing measures may be taken to help the body regulate its temperature. Giving the patient with a fever a sponge bath may help dissipate body heat by increasing evaporation from the skin surface. Giving aspirin also helps to dissipate heat. The physiologic action of aspirin that causes this dissipation is not fully understood, but perspiration usually is increased. Patients who have poor arteriolar constrictive mechanisms, such as the elderly, persons with arteriosclerotic disease, and persons whose symphathetic nervous system is blocked by drugs, surgery, or injury, have a tendency to lose body heat. It is important for them to be protected against the cold by the use of light, yet warm clothing and bed coverings. Patients with disease of the hypothalamus or medulla, those who have just been treated with hypothermia or hyperthermia, and infants, whose nervous system still is not fully developed, need to have their body temperatures carefully checked at frequent intervals, because their body mechanisms for temperature control may be ineffective. The temperature control mechanisms are especially ineffective when there is a wide swing in environmental temperature or if a person has a disease that is causing fever. Therefore, the temperature of the external environment should be carefully controlled when giving care in these situations, and treatment to reduce fever needs to be instituted promptly.

References and selected readings*

1 Allergy and hypersensitivity, a programed review for physicians, ed. 2, New York, 1964, Charles Pfizer & Co., Inc.

2 *Bardsley, Christine, and others: Pressure sores, Am. J. Nursing 64:82-84, May 1964.

3 Beeson, Paul B., and McDermott, Walsh: Cecil-Loeb textbook of medicine, ed. 11, Philadelphia, 1963, W. B. Saunders Co.

4 Benson, Margaret E.: Handwashing—an important part of medical asepsis, Am. J. Nursing 57:1136-1139, Sept. 1957.

5 Bergersen, Betty S., and Krug, Elsie E.: Pharmacology in nursing, ed. 10, St. Louis, 1966, The C. V. Mosby Co.

6 *Bruton, Mary R.: When tetanus struck, Am. J. Nursing 65:107-110, Oct. 1965.

7 *Buchanan-Davidson, Dorothy J.: A drop of blood, Am. J. Nursing 65:103-107, July 1965.

8 Burnett, F. M.: The integrity of the body, New York, 1966, Atheneum Publishers.

9 Burnet, Sir Macfarlane: The natural history of infectious disease, ed 2, London, 1960, Cambridge University Press.

10 Caswell, H. Taylor: Staphylococcal infections among hospital personnel, Am. J. Nursing 58:822-823, June 1958.

11 *Cirksena, William J.: Tetanus, Am. J. Nursing 62:65-69, April 1962.

*References preceded by an asterisk are particularly well suited for student reading.

12 Colbeck, J. C.: Control of infections in hospitals, Chicago, 1962, American Hospital Association, monograph series no. 12.

13 Engler, H. S., and others: Cancer arising in scars of old burns and in chronic osteomyelitis, ulcers, and drainage sites, Surgery 55:654-664, May 1964.

14 Finland, M., and others: Occurrence of serious bacterial infections since introduction of antibacterial agents, J.A.M.A. 170:2188-2197, Aug. 29, 1959.

15 *Frohman, I. Phillips: The adrenocorticosteroids, Am. J. Nursing 64:120-123, Nov. 1964.

16 Fuerst, Elinor V., and Wolff, LuVerne: Fundamentals of nursing, ed. 3, Philadelphia, 1964, J. B. Lippincott Co.

17 *Ginsberg, Miriam K., and LaConte, Maria L.: Reverse isolation, Am. J. Nursing 64:88-90, Sept. 1964.

18 Goth, Andres: Medical pharmacology, ed. 3, St. Louis, 1966, The C. V. Mosby Co.

19 Ham, Arthur W.: Histology, ed. 5, Philadelphia, 1965, J. B. Lippincott Co.

20 Hare, R., and Ridley, M.: Studies on the transmission of Staphylococcus aureus, Brit. M. J. 1:69-73, Jan. 11, 1958.

21 Harkins, Henry N., and others: Surgery—principles and practice, ed. 2, Philadelphia, 1961, J. B. Lippincott Co.

22 *Hershey, Nathan: Infection control, Am. J. Nursing 65:103-104, Nov. 1965.

23 *Hill, Edward J., and Blacha, Lillian T.: Treatment and nursing care of hand injuries, Am. J. Nursing 63:85-91, Aug. 1963.

24 *Johnson, Kenneth J.: Allergen injections, Am. J. Nursing 65:121-122, July 1965.

25 Kline, Patricia A.: Isolating patients with staphylococcal infections, Am. J. Nursing 65:102-104, Jan. 1965.

26 Leavell, Hugh Rodman, and Clark, E. Gurney: Preventive medicine for the doctor in his community, New York, 1965, Blakiston Division, McGraw-Hill Book Co.

27 MacBride, Cyril M.: Signs and symptoms: applied pathologic physiology and clinical interpretation, ed. 4, Philadelphia, 1964, J. B. Lippincott Co.

28 Marlow, Dorothy R.: Textbook of pediatric nursing, ed. 2, Philadelphia, 1965, W. B. Saunders Co.

29 McCallum, Helen P.: The nurse and the isolator, Nurs. Clin. North America 1:587-596, Dec. 1966.

30 Miller, Joseph M.: The proteolytic enzymes, Am. J. Nursing 58:1410-1412, Oct. 1958.

31 *Nahmias, Andre J.: Infections associated with hospitals, Nursing Outlook 13:450-453, June 1963.

32 Nichols, Leola F.: When staph comes home to roost, Am. J. Nursing 63:75-78, April 1963.

33 *Nichols, T., and others: Diurnal variations in suppression of adrenal function by glucocorticoids, J. Clin. Endocrinol. 25:343-349, March 1965.

34 Ordman, L. J., and Gillman, T.: Studies in the healing of cutaneous wounds, Arch. Surg. 93:857-928, Dec. 1966.

35 Pratt, Mary K., Walsh, Helen, and Hazelhurst, Robert C.: A VNA combats staph infection, Nursing Outlook 8:310-313, June 1960.

36 Ravenholt, O. H.: Eliminating blankets as an infection source, Hospitals 32:75-80, June 16, 1958.

37 Riley, Richard L.: Air-borne infections, Am. J. Nursing 60:1246-1248, Sept. 1960.

38 Rockwell, Virginia Tyler: Surgical hand scrubbing, Am. J. Nursing 63:75-81, June 1963.

39 *Rogers, Fred B., editor: Studies in epidemiology, New York, 1965, G. P. Putnam's Sons.

40 *Roueché, Berton: The incurable wound, Boston, 1954, Little, Brown & Co.

41 Sawdust bed therapy, Am. J. Nursing 49:654, Oct. 1949.

42 *Seidler, Florence M.: Adapting nursing procedures for reverse isolation, Am. J. Nursing 65:108-111, June 1965.

43 *Selye, Hans: The stress of life, New York, 1956, McGraw-Hill Book Co.

44 *Shaffer, Joseph H., and Sweet, Lawrence C.: Allergic reaction to drugs, Am. J. Nursing 65:100-103, Oct. 1965.

45 Smith, Alice Lorraine: Carter's microbiology and pathology, ed. 8, St. Louis, 1964, The C. V. Mosby Co.

46 *Some psychological effects of medical and surgical advances, Frontiers of Hospital Psychiatry 3:1-2, 8, June 15, 1966 (Roche Laboratories, Division of Hoffman-LaRoche, Inc., Nutley, N. J.).

47 *Stare, Frederick J.: Good nutrition from food, not pills, Am. J. Nursing 65:86-89, Feb. 1965.

48 Stone, H. H., and others: Verdoglobinuria: an ominous sign of pseudomonas septicemia in burns, Ann. Surg. 159:991-995, June 1964.

49 The use of blood, North Chicago, Ill., 1961, Abbott Laboratories.

50 U. S. Department of Health, Education, and Welfare: Staphylococcal disease: selected materials on nursing aspects, Atlanta, 1960, Communicable Disease Center, U. S. Public Health Service.

51 *Using a Stryker frame, Am. J. Nursing 64:100-101, Feb. 1964.

52 Vesley, Donald, and Brask, Marion: Environmental implications in the control of hospital-acquired infections, Nursing Outlook 9:742-745, Dec. 1961.

53 Wheeler, Margaret, and Volk, Wesley A.: Basic microbiology, Philadelphia, 1964, J. B. Lippincott Co.

54 Whipple, Dorothy V.: Dynamics of development: euthenic pediatrics, New York, 1966, Blakiston Division, McGraw-Hill Book Co.

4

Maintaining the body in a homeostatic state

Study questions

1 What is oxidation? What is catabolism? What is the action of a catalyst? What are some common catalysts in the body?

2 What is the normal blood hemoglobin level? Check the hemoglobin level of the patients on your unit who have oxygen deficits and relate it to their diagnosis.

3 List several body processes, other than anabolism, requiring expenditure of energy. What is the caloric value of a gram of carbohydrate; fat; protein? How many calories do 1,000 ml. of 5% glucose in water provide?

4 Review Chapter 2 to determine how the caloric needs of young children, adolescents, adults, and elderly people differ.

5 What is a complete protein? Name several. Plan an adequate diet without using complete proteins.

6 Review the process of diffusion. How does it differ from osmosis? What happens when a 5% solution of salt is placed in a container in which it is separated by a semipermeable membrane from a 1% solution of salt? What would happen if a solution of sugar or protein, such as gelatin, was separated by a semipermeable membrane from water?

7 What happens to the extra salt and water you consume when ham is served for dinner?

8 Review these procedures: hypodermoclysis, venoclysis, blood transfusion, nasogastric intubation, Murphy drip. What are the special details for the nurse to remember when these procedures are ordered?

9 If you (or a close friend or member of your family) have recently had severe diarrhea, vomiting, or elevation of temperature, what symptoms did you observe that might indicate change in fluid or electrolyte balance?

We live in two environments—an external one of heat and cold, noise, dirt, and physical force and a much more constant internal one of fluid, electrolyte, and temperature balance. The human machinery, carefully steered by the hormones and the central nervous system, is constantly adapting to changes in body requirements and to variations in the availability of essential elements. Upon this adaptive quality rests our ability to survive. Oxygen, energy, and an intact anatomical structure are essential for the operation of the adaptive machinery. The nurse must know how essential body functioning is maintained if she is to help people maintain health and to give supportive nursing care when disease or injury upsets the body's ability to maintain its checks and balances.

Maintaining respiration

Oxygen is essential for the body's metabolic process, oxidation-reduction reaction (catabolism). This reaction releases the energy required for life. For oxygen to be used by the body, it must reach the bloodstream. It does so through the process of respiration.

External respiration, by which air is exchanged between the external environment and the lungs, is a mechanical process steered primarily by the medullary center in the brain. A rise in the carbon dioxide or the hydrogen ion levels in the blood stimulates this center, which in turn sends stimuli to the diaphragm and intercostal muscles and causes them to contract, expanding the chest cavity so that air enters to fill the potential vacuum. Stretching of the lung tissues causes an inhibitory stimulus to be sent to the medulla, stopping the inspiration. Expiration, or the discharge of air from the lungs, is largely a passive process. Any disease that inhibits expansion of the chest or the lungs, including the bronchioles and alveoli, and thus prevents the inflow of air or that decreases the elastic recoil of the lungs, essential for expiration, may lead to an oxygen deficit.

When the levels of carbon dioxide and hydrogen ions in the blood are low *(alkalosis)*, respirations are slow and shallow. As the levels rise *(acidosis)*, respirations become deep and rapid unless the levels become high enough to depress instead of stimulate the medullary centers *(carbon dioxide narcosis)*. If the medullary centers are depressed, chemoreceptors in the carotid bodies that are sensitive to low oxygen tension in the blood stimulate respiration.

It is important for the nurse to realize that respiration in a patient who has medullary damage or in a patient with serious acidosis may be sustained only by the chemoreceptors in the carotid bodies. Respirations under these circumstances usually are *Cheyne-Stokes* in character; that is, the patient may take several breaths, fail to breathe for a few seconds, then breathe again. If oxygen in high concentrations is given at this time, the only stimulus to breathe may be removed. Respirations may need to be mechanically sustained until the body mechanism is reinstated, and every nurse should know how to do the procedure (p. 241). (Mechanical respirators for long-term use are discussed on p. 853.)

When the oxygen reaches the lung, it must diffuse through the alveoli into the blood, where it is picked up by the hemoglobin and transported to cells throughout the body. This process is called *internal respiration*. Failure of the exchange of adequate oxygen and carbon dioxide at this level leads to low oxygen tension in the blood and acid-base imbalance. The failure usually is caused by low atmospheric pressure, anemia, or diseased alveoli.

Maintaining the energy supply and intact body tissues

The energy supply

All body functions require energy, and physiologic oxidation-reduction reactions (the burning of foodstuffs and/or body tissues) are the only source of this energy. Energy production is so vital that, if nutrients are unavailable from other sources, the body has a protective mechanism by which it can burn its own tissues.

Oxygen and carbohydrates, fats or proteins, and usually enzymes (biologic catalysts) are essential ingredients for producing energy. Enzymes are special proteins built under genetic control, and some work only when specific minerals and vitamins (coenzymes) are available. Thus, for adequate energy production all nutrients must be available. This fact demonstrates the great importance of good nutrition.

The healthy adult man of average size who lives in a moderate climate needs 1,500 calories a day just to maintain the basic functions essential to life (those functions that go on even while the person is at rest). However, basic caloric needs vary with age, sex, body size, climate (p. 115), and body temperature (see the discussion of fever, p. 66, and of hypothermia, p. 188). Extra calories are required to sustain additional activity.

The body always meets its energy requirements before nutrients are used for any other purpose. In fact, they cannot be used without energy. Extra caloric intake, therefore, is essential to prevent the burning of body tissues in any situation in which extra energy is being used, whether in normal life or in illness.

Whenever food cannot be ingested, digested, assimilated, and metabolized by the body normally, some body tissues must be burned. For example, patients with untreated or uncontrolled diabetes mellitus (a condition in which carbohydrates are not metabolized effectively) burn excessive amounts of fat for energy. Because they

87

often are unable to dispose of the acid end products of fat metabolism, acidosis (p. 101) may develop. People who are starving also develop this problem as soon as the body's carbohydrate stores are depleted and body fat must be used.

The normal body stores much of its fat intake in the liver as glycogen to be used as needed. The remainder is stored as adipose tissue, which can be metabolized if necessary. Whenever fats cannot be assimilated or stored, such as in some diseases of the liver, additional glucose should be given so that the body proteins are not burned for energy. The burning of body proteins is undesirable because the cells of the body contain most of its protein. Burning body proteins and fats for energy causes weight loss.

Some body proteins are almost always used for energy under conditions of severe stress. When there is extensive tissue damage, however, this metabolic process seems to be accelerated and usually continues for seven to ten days despite adequate intake of food. This acceleration is thought to be due to the action of the adrenocortical hormones. The burning of body proteins often causes serious chemical imbalances in the body because large amounts of nitrogen and potassium are lost in the urine. Potassium and solutions containing amino acids often are given intravenously to patients after operations, burns, or injuries that have resulted in extensive tissue damage. This measure may be contraindicated, however, if coexistent renal damage causes the nitrogen and potassium to be retained in the blood.

It is not possible to meet even the basic energy requirements of a person by the intravenous route. If the nutrient is too concentrated, it will have a diuretic effect and be lost through the kidneys, and the amount of fluid needed to give enough of the nutrient in appropriate dilution is prohibitive. In addition, intravenous feedings often are needed in stress situations, and the increased adrenocortical secretions at this time tend to hold water and sodium in the body, making the danger of overloading the circulation even greater than normal. Stress also tends to increase the energy needs. Thus, it is important to begin to feed the patient by the alimentary route (either by mouth or

through nasogastric intubation) as soon as possible. If a person is expected to be unable to eat for several days, such as after certain operations, special care will be taken beforehand to improve his general nutrition.

Tissue building and repair

The metabolic process by which proteins are synthesized by the body is called *anabolism*. All body cells are basically protein, and anabolism makes possible the development of new cells for tissue growth and replacement. It is also by this process that blood is replaced and that enzymes and hormones are produced. Anabolism, however, cannot take place until after the body's energy requirements are met.

Since catabolism of protein is unavoidable in conditions of severe stress, such as serious infectious disease or extensive tissue damage, patients with these conditions must be provided with the complete proteins essential for synthesis of body protein as soon as possible. The amino acids that are given intravenously are not complete proteins. Therefore, they are only useful to supplement other food or to be burned as energy to conserve body proteins. A nutritious diet should be given as soon as the patient is able to tolerate it. The diet needs to be relatively high in calories (2,000 to 3,000 calories a day) despite the limited physical activity of the patient since extra energy is being expended because of the increased metabolism, resulting at first from the stress and later from tissue repair. The diet should also be high in protein. If the patient is at home or is returning home after an illness, he should be instructed to continue this diet until he regains his normal weight. Caloric and protein intake should then be reduced to normal.

The pituitary gland, adrenals, and thyroid and parathyroid glands all effect metabolic processes in various ways. A disturbance of the function of any one of these glands may cause a disruption in anabolic processes.

Maintaining the circulation of blood

To maintain life, nutrients and oxygen must be transported throughout the body to cells and the waste products of metabolism must be removed from each cell. This process is accomplished by the circulatory system. Maintenance of this system, therefore, is essential to life.

Shock

When oxygen and nutrients become unavailable to vital cells in the body, shock occurs. Shock is a failure of the capillary circulation, resulting in failure of cellular metabolism and a resultant loss of the energy essential for all life processes.[25] It may be caused by a variety of unrelated conditions, such as severe infection, toxemia, anaphylaxis, severe dehydration, hyperinsulinism, severe physical or psychic trauma, massive hemorrhage, or loss of blood plasma such as occurs in burns. Severe cardiac disease also causes shock because the heart is unable to pump sufficient blood through the body. Shock is classified as *hematogenic* (secondary to blood loss), *neurogenic* (secondary to vasodilation and reflex inhibition of the heart), *cardiogenic* (secondary to cardiac failure or to mechanical interference with heart function), or *vasogenic* (secondary to vasodilation by humoral substances such as histamine).

In *hematogenic shock* there is a decrease in the total blood volume. This decrease may result from the loss of large quantities of whole blood or plasma directly from a blood vessel, from a traumatized area, or from the leakage of large quantities of plasma from the blood vessels into other body tissues or spaces. This leakage may be caused by fractures or soft tissue injuries. Some authorities believe that shock in the latter instances may be vasogenic in nature. They feel that a histamine-like substance is released at the site of the injury and circulated through the bloodstream, causing increased permeability of the capillaries, through which the plasma escapes.

In *vasogenic shock*, vasodilation by drugs, such as histamine and alcohol, or histamine released in the body in response to foreign proteins or toxins from infectious organisms causes leakage of plasma into the tissues. Anaphylactic shock, discussed on p. 77, is a type of vasogenic shock.

Cardiogenic shock is caused by failure of the heart to pump an adequate amount of blood into the general circulation. This failure may be due to failure of the venous return, failure of the heart muscle itself, or failure of the blood to be discharged properly from the left ventricle because of valvular malfunction. Cardiac tamponade (compression) also may cause it.

Neurogenic shock is a fleeting type caused by spinal anesthesia, operations and drugs that inhibit the sympathetic nervous system, and psychic trauma such as fear, worry, and emotional tension. Fainting is the commonest form. Symptoms are caused by sudden vasodilation of the peripheral blood vessels into which much of the circulating blood rushes. There is no actual loss of blood volume. Vasodilation caused by psychic trauma is considered an important contributory factor in other types of shock.

Very young patients, elderly patients, and patients with cardiovascular diseases and metabolic disorders such as diabetes are more likely to develop shock following trauma, disease, or surgery than is a young, healthy adult. A patient who is receiving cortisone therapy or who has had it discontinued recently may have a rapid onset of shock because the adrenal glands may be unable to compensate by secreting additional hormones as they normally would. These patients may be given cortisone intravenously.

To prevent the occurrence of shock following elective surgery, the patient is prepared preoperatively so that he is in the best physical and emotional state possible. Typing and crossmatching of blood are done before surgery so that if blood is needed to combat shock, it will be available. An infusion usually is started in the operating room so that if the patient needs blood, it can be given easily.

In shock, regardless of the cause, the systolic blood pressure drops below 100 mm. Hg, the pulse increases in rate and becomes weak and thready, the patient becomes extremely weak, and the skin is pale, cold, and covered with perspiration. As shock progresses, the respirations become rapid and shallow and the temperature becomes subnormal. The patient may be apprehensive and restless or he may become apathetic, indifferent, and finally unconscious. Symptoms of neurogenic shock appear rapidly, but those of other types of shock do not appear until the condition is well established. It is only by careful observation of the vital signs and of the general physical appearance of the patient that shock may be recognized and treated early. Restlessness, apprehension, coldness, and pallor may be the first noticeable symptoms. The blood pressure and pulse usually are within relatively normal limits in the early stages.

When there has been loss of fluid from the circulating blood, the venous return to the heart is slowed and the cardiac output, therefore, is decreased. A compensatory vasoconstriction due to the excretion of epinephrine and norepinephrine maintains the blood pressure at a normal level for a short period of time. However, as fluid losses increase, the vasoconstriction becomes ineffectual and the blood pressure drops markedly, decreasing the blood supply to vital body tissues. This decrease leads to tissue anoxia *(ischemia)*, and if it is allowed to persist, the shock becomes irreversible. The liver, kidneys, and nervous tissues tolerate a lack of oxygen and nutrients for only a very short time before permanent tissue damage occurs. If the systolic pressure remains below 50 mm. Hg for long, the patient usually dies.

Treatment of shock. The treatment of shock is based on its cause. The symptoms of neurogenic shock readily disappear when the patient is placed in a recumbent position. One of the best ways to treat shock caused by fluid loss is to replace the fluid. If the loss is due to internal or external loss of blood or plasma, whole blood usually is given. Plasma or plasma substitutes such as albumin, dextran, or normal saline solution are sometimes used to maintain the blood volume until whole blood can be obtained. The blood is given in sufficient quantities as fast as is safe to restore the systolic pressure to at least 80 mm. Hg. Oxygen may be given by mask to increase the oxygen available to the blood. If the shock is due to electrolyte imbalance, appropriate fluids and electrolytes are given either intravenously or orally to restore the normal balance. When shock is caused by vasodilation by substances within the body, vasoconstricting drugs such as phenylephrine (Neo-Synephrine), levarterenol bitartrate (Levophed), or metaraminol bitartrate (Armine bitartrate) may be given, but they are not used until blood

volume has been restored. When shock is due to cardiac insufficiency, digitalis usually is administered. If the heart has stopped, cardiac massage is started at once, and epinephrine hydrochloride (Adrenalin) 1:1,000 may be given directly into the heart muscle (p. 336).

Nursing care of patients in shock. The patient in shock should be kept quiet and warm, but he should have only enough covering to maintain his body temperature. If he perspires, he is too warmly covered and the peripheral blood vessels have become dilated, dissipating the available blood to the surface vessels. Any movement of the patient in shock is contraindicated. All physical care, except for essentials such as using the bedpan and comfort measures such as washing the face and hands, should be omitted until the blood pressure stabilizes. In the past, the patient was often placed in the Trendelenburg position (a head-low position) to increase the flow of blood to the brain. However, this position has been found to inhibit cardiac output, and many doctors now prefer that the lower extremities be elevated at a 45-degree angle from the hip, with the knees straight and the head on a level with or slightly higher than the chest. This position promotes increased venous return from the legs without interfering with the cardiac output. Neither position should be used without a doctor's order, however, since elevation of the foot of the bed may increase bleeding in some instances, and it may cause the visceral organs to press against the diaphragm, thus inhibiting respiration. The patient should be kept flat until medical orders are received.

Measures to prevent further stress should be instituted at once. The patient's questions should be answered and all procedures explained in an attempt to decrease his anxiety. Barbiturates may be prescribed for their sedative effect. Relief of pain also decreases shock, and morphine sulfate is often ordered for this purpose. Usually it is given by the doctor intravenously since subcutaneous injections may be too slowly absorbed because of decreased circulation to the tissues. Repeated injections of any drug given subcutaneously during shock may cause symptoms of overdosage on the return of normal circulation. If the patient is receiving such drugs as levarterenol bitartrate (Levophed) by infusion, the nurse must take his blood pressure every five to ten minutes so that the rate of flow of the drug can be adjusted according to the rise and fall of blood pressure. The pressure should be kept within normal limits. The site of injection should be watched for signs of infiltration because the drug can cause tissue necrosis.

Hemorrhage

Hemorrhage is the loss of a large amount of blood from the bloodstream due to rupture or injury of a blood vessel, slipping of a ligature from a blood vessel postoperatively, erosion of a vessel by a drainage tube, tumor, or infection, or some interference with the clotting mechanism of the blood, such as occurs in hemophilia. The patient may lose small amounts of blood over a long period of time, or he may lose a large amount of blood in a short period of time. The bleeding may be arterial (bright red and spurting), venous (continuous flow of dark red blood), or capillary (oozing). The blood may be expelled from any body orifice from an incision, or from the site of an injury, or it may collect under the subcutaneous tissues as a tumor mass (*hematoma*) or in a body cavity such as the peritoneal cavity.

Symptoms of massive hemorrhage, both internal and external, are apprehension, restlessness, thirst, pallor, a cold, moist skin, drop in blood pressure, increased pulse rate, subnormal temperature, and rapid respirations. As hemorrhage continues, the lips and conjunctivas become pale and the patient may complain of spots before the eyes, ringing in the ears, and extreme weakness. If the hemorrhage is not controlled, unconsciousness and finally death will occur.

Treatment and nursing care of hemorrhage. The treatment of hemorrhage is to stop the flow of blood if possible and to replace the lost blood. When bleeding occurs, the vessel walls contract, narrowing the lumina of the vessels, and a clot forms over the end of the bleeding vessel. Clotting usually occurs much earlier in the child and very young person than in older patients because the blood vessels of children and young persons are more elastic. In arterial bleeding the clotting phenomenon is not possible until there has been enough blood loss to decrease the pressure of the blood circulating through the bleeding vessel. However, pressure against the artery proximal to the bleeding point decreases the flow of blood through it and permits clotting to take place. Elevation of the part also may decrease arterial bleeding. *Direct pressure* at the site of the bleeding also decreases the blood flow and encourages clotting. This method is frequently used in superficial wounds, and a gelatin sponge (Gelfoam) also may be applied to help form a clot. The principle of direct pressure may also be used to control hemorrhage from esophageal varices. An esophageal balloon is inserted and then inflated until it compresses the bleeding vessels. In a similar way bleeding from the prostate gland, such as may occur following prostatectomy, is controlled by direct pressure. A Foley catheter is inserted and the balloon inflated to compress bleeding vessels.

Cold applications are often used to control bleeding into tissues or into body cavities, since the cold causes the small vessels to contract. In uterine hemorrhage, an ice bag may be applied to the abdomen over the uterus. In gastric hemorrhage, it may be placed over the epigastric region, or a gastric tube with a balloon through which iced alcohol circulates may be passed into the stomach. In hemorrhage from the lung, an ice bag usually is applied over the sternum.

Very *hot applications* cause reflex vasoconstriction and control bleeding temporarily. This method is often used during an operation in which there is considerable vascular oozing. To control the bleeding permanently, large vessels usually have to be ligated, and smaller ones may be electrically cauterized. A ruptured organ such as the spleen may have to be removed to control bleeding. Removal of the spleen also may be necessary to control bleeding due to a blood dyscrasia such as idiopathic thrombocytopenic purpura.

When the bleeding is caused by a prothrombin deficiency, such as occurs in liver diseases in which hepatic ducts are obstructed or in biliary duct obstruction, *vitamin K* is given parenterally. Vitamin K is helpful in controlling hemorrhage following overdoses of bishydroxycoumarin (Dicumarol).

If possible the blood loss should be measured so that the doctor can prescribe replacement more accurately. Dressings saturated with blood can be weighed, and blood in vomitus, both that which is bright red and that which is coffee-ground color, should be measured. Whenever possible, tarry stools and bright blood discharged from the rectum should be measured. If this is not feasible, the blood loss should be estimated. The doctor often will want to see evidence of bleeding, such as bloody stools, vaginal clots, bloody vomitus, and hematuria.

Blood replacement usually is started before complete hemostasis has been accomplished, since the restoration of blood volume is imperative in preventing the occurrence of irreversible shock. Blood plasma or a plasma expander may be given until whole blood is available. Whole blood may be given until the systolic pressure is between 85 and 100 mm. Hg, and it may be necessary to administer from 2,500 to 3,500 ml. of whole blood before this reading is reached. The speed at which blood is given during this time depends upon the patient's condition. If the blood pressure is very low, the blood may be given very rapidly and may even be pumped in under pressure by the doctor. (See p. 78 for additional information about transfusions.)

The patient is usually very apprehensive because of the hemorrhage and because of the emergency measures that follow it. Every attempt should be made to keep him quiet, reassured, and comfortable. He should never, under any circumstances, be left alone while a hemorrhage is occurring. Barbiturates and morphine sulfate are often ordered as sedatives. Evidences of bleeding should be removed from the bedside, and stained linen and clothing should be replaced. Noise and excitement should be kept to a minimum, and all treatments and procedures, such as frequent blood pressure readings, transfusion, the use of unusual positions, and, if necessary, restriction of food and fluids, should be explained to the patient and his family. The patient with a massive hemorrhage usually is given nothing to eat or drink until the hemorrhage is controlled, since he may have to be taken to the operating room. Food and fluid also are often withheld when the bleeding is from the gastrointestinal tract.

Maintaining the fluid, electrolyte, and temperature balance

For normal body functioning, the internal environment of the body must be relatively stable. A certain amount of fluid, distributed in a specific way, is essential, and the fluid must contain specific quantities of certain chemical compounds. Larger or smaller quantities of fluid or chemicals than normal, changes in their distribution, or the presence of chemicals not usually found in the fluids may interfere with essential body processes and may even lead to death. The temperature of the internal environment also must be kept within specified limits.

Body fluid component

The internal environment is made up of intracellular and extracellular fluids. A fluid medium is essential for all body processes. In the normal adult with average body fat, approximately two-thirds of the body weight is fluid.[13] In the infant, however, three-fourths or more of the total weight is fluid.[13] The fluid is contained within three compartments that are separated by semipermeable membranes. In the adult, roughly two-thirds of the fluid is within the cells (intracellular), whereas the remainder is divided between the interstitial fluid that surrounds all living cells and allows for diffusion of nutrients, electrolytes, water, hormones, oxygen and waste products (three-twelfths of the total) and the fluid within the blood vessels (intravascular) (one-twelfth of the total). In the infant, almost half of the fluid is extracellular (Fig. 25), with more fluid between the cells (including bones and cartilage) and less in the circulating blood.

Since fat is essentially free of water, the body type of the person must be considered in estimating his body fluid component.[13] Thus, about 100 pounds (50 liters) of a lean adult weighing 150 pounds are fluid.

Normal exchange of body fluids. Body fluid is constantly being lost and, for normal processes to continue, must be replaced. With an average daily intake of food and liquids, the healthy body easily maintains compartmental balance.

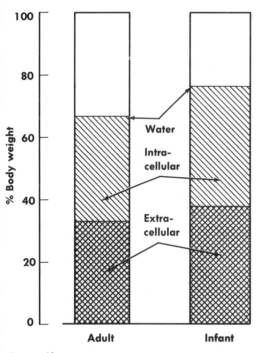

Fig. 25

In the infant, almost half of the total body fluid is extracellular. As the child grows, however, the proportions gradually approximate adult levels.

Loss. Fluid normally leaves the body through the kidneys, lungs, and skin, with very small amounts being lost through the gastrointestinal tract and negligible amounts being lost in saliva and tears. Two vital processes demand continual expenditure of water—the removal of body heat by vaporization of water and the excretion of urea and other metabolic wastes. The volume of water used in these processes varies greatly with external influences. It has been estimated, however, that even with no food or fluid intake an adult of average build loses at least 800 ml. of water daily through the skin and lungs, and he excretes about 900 ml. of water daily through the kidneys. This *compulsory fluid loss* is essential for maintaining normal body processes. The average adult, taking a normal amount of food and fluids, actually loses larger amounts. (See Table 1.)

The daily loss of fluids in babies and growing children is proportionately greater than that of an adult. Their extremely active metabolism generates large amounts of heat that must be dissipated. The baby loses large amounts of fluid through the skin because the skin surface is larger proportionately than that of an adult. In addition, the

Table 1

Normal fluid intake and loss in an adult eating 2,500 calories per day (approximate figures)*

Intake		Output	
Route	Amount of gain (ml.)	Route	Amount of loss (ml.)
Water in food	1,100	Skin and lungs	1,000
Water from oxidation	300	Bowel	100
Water as liquid	1,200	Kidneys	1,500
Total	2,600	Total	2,600

*Adapted from Fluids and electrolytes, North Chicago, Ill., 1957, Abbott Laboratories.

Note that the intake of water in solid food is almost equa to that taken as liquid. Two-thirds as much water is lost from the skin and lungs as from the kidneys. This is significant in the care of patients with severe burns, who have lessened ability to perspire and who have poor pulmonary function.

kidneys of infants do not conserve water as effectively as the kidneys of adults. In the older child and adult, if the body needs water, the pituitary antidiuretic hormone promotes its reabsorption from the renal tubules, and fluid ingested in excess of need is eliminated through the kidneys. This latter mechanism is not fully developed in infants.

Approximately 120 ml. of fluid, which is essentially an ultrafiltrate of plasma (plasma minus the protein content), are filtered through the glomeruli every minute. Normally, however, only 1 ml. per minute is excreted as urine. The remainder returns to the bloodstream. The baby's urinary output is similar to that of an adult, or one-half of intake. His total water "turnover," however, is much larger in that he takes in and excretes proportionately much more water.[20]

Replacement. The body receives water from ingested food and fluids and through metabolism of both foodstuffs and body tissues. Solid foods such as meat and vegetables contain 60 to 90% water. Metabolic processes release about 12 ml. of water for each 100 calories of fat, carbohydrate, or protein oxidized.[13] Table 1 shows the approximate daily intake for an average adult. Note that the normal daily replacement of water equals the normal daily loss. Easily measurable intake (liquid) and easily measurable output (urine) are also approximately equal. These figures, therefore, serve as guides for determining normal fluid balance and emphasize the great need for recording intake and output accurately.

The baby's reserves of extracellular fluid are much more limited than are those of older children and adults. Since his daily turnover of water is more than half of his extracellular fluid volume, it is essential that his fluid losses be replaced at once. He cannot live even as long as an adult without fluids.

Body electrolyte component

All body fluids contain chemical compounds. Chemical compounds in solution may be classified as electrolytes or nonelectrolytes. Electrolytes generally may be thought of as breaking up into separate electrically charged particles known as *ions.* Sodium chloride in solution exists as posi-

tively charged sodium ions, Na$^+$, and negatively charged chloride ions, Cl$^-$. Positively charged ions are called *cations.* Negatively charged ions are called *anions.* Proteins are special types of charged molecules. They have a charge that is dependent upon the pH of the body fluids. At normal plasma pH (7.4) the proteins exist with a net negative charge. (See Table 2.) Nonelectrolytes such as urea, dextrose, and creatinine remain molecularly intact and are essentially uncharged.

Electrolytes account for most of the osmotic pressure of the body fluids, are important in the maintenance of acid-base balance, and help to control body water volume. The three fluid compartments contain similar electrolytes, but the concentration of the various electrolytes in each compartment varies markedly. (See Table 2.)

Differences in individual ion concentrations occur in various fluids. For instance, the gastric secretion is acid; hence the concentration of hydrogen ions is high. Pancreatic secretion, on the other hand, is more alkaline than plasma and contains a high concentration of bicarbonate. Gastric, pancreatic and intestinal juices, and bile all contain high concentrations of sodium ions.[13]

In health the ratio of cations to anions in each of the body fluids and the concentration of the various ions in these fluids is relatively constant. Knowing the common electrolytes found in various body fluids is helpful for nurses in planning to prevent depletion of necessary substances and in noting early signs of imbalance.

Normal exchange of electrolytes. Electrolytes move more readily between interstitial (surrounding the cells) and intravascular (within the blood vessels) fluids than between intracellular and interstitial fluids. Therefore, normally most of the electrolyte exchange occurs between interstitial and intravascular fluids.

Loss. Electrolyte loss is mainly through the kidneys, with smaller losses through the skin and lungs and relatively minimal losses through the bowel. The kidneys selectively excrete electrolytes, retaining those needed for normal body fluid composition. Hormonal influences affect the kidneys' selective function. For example, the adrenocortical hormones favor sodium reabsorption and the

Table 2

Normal electrolyte content of body fluids and normal daily loss of ions in urine*

Electrolytes (anions and cations)	Maintenance levels of fluid compartments			Daily loss in urine (mEq./L.)
	Intravascular (mEq./L.)	Interstitial (mEq./L.)	Intracellular (mEq./L.)	
Sodium (Na+)	142	145	15	200
Potassium (K+)	5	4	157	90
Calcium (Ca++)	5	3	5	90
Magnesium (Mg++)	3	2	27	20
Chloride (Cl-)	104	116	4	200
Bicarbonate (HCO3-)	27	27	10	17
Protein (Prot-)	16	1	72	0
Phosphate (HPO4=)	2	3	100	26
Sulfate (SO4=)	1	2	18	22
Organic acids	5	5	0	50

*Adapted from Fluid and electrolytes, North Chicago, Ill., 1957, Abbott Laboratories.

Note that the electrolyte level of the intravascular and of the interstitial fluids is approximately the same and that sodium and chloride contents are markedly higher in these fluids, whereas potassium, phosphate, and protein contents are markedly higher in intracellular fluid. Normally most loss of electrolytes occurs through the kidneys, but with high fever or excessive perspiration 25 to 50 additional mEq./L. of both sodium and chloride may be lost through the skin and lungs.

excretion of potassium. Because of their rapid loss of water through the skin, infants normally lose more sodium than adults. They also tend to lose more potassium because more is freed by their rapid metabolism for growth, and its loss through the kidneys appears to be less finely controlled by hormonal action.[13]

The acidity or alkalinity of body fluids depends upon the concentration of the hydrogen ions (H^+) in relation to the concentration of the hydroxyl ions (OH^-) and is expressed as pH. A pH of 7 is a neutral solution. The normal body fluid is slightly alkaline (pH 7.35 to pH 7.45) and is maintained in a relatively stable condition by the "buffer systems" in the body. A buffer is a substance that can act as a chemical sponge, either soaking up or releasing hydrogen ions so that the normal ratio of acids to bases is maintained. There are several "buffer systems" in the body, but the carbonic acid–bicarbonate system is one of the most im-

portant clinically. Two types of carbonate are present in body fluids—carbonic acid (H_2CO_3) and bicarbonate (HCO_3^-). The ability of the body to keep the pH of body fluids within normal limits relies essentially upon maintenance of the normal ratio of one part of carbonic acid to 20 parts of bicarbonate. Since carbonic acid ionizes into a hydrogen ion (H^+) and a bicarbonate ion (HCO_3^-), and since bicarbonate ions plus water yield carbonic acid (H_2CO_3) and the hydroxyl ion (OH^-), the normal balance is maintained by removing from the body whichever ion, (H^+) or (OH^-), is in excess. The carbonic acid concentration is controlled by the lungs. The amount of carbon dioxide expelled is varied by the depth and rate of respiration. The bicarbonate concentration is controlled by the kidneys, which selectively retain or excrete bicarbonate depending upon body needs.

Replacement. A healthy person eating a well-balanced diet will easily ingest all the substances needed to maintain electrolyte balance. Any excess of electrolytes ingested will be excreted by the kidneys.

Fluid and electrolyte imbalance

Almost all medical and surgical conditions threaten the fluid and electrolyte balance. Excessive amounts of body fluid and the electrolytes contained therein may be lost through the skin due to profuse perspiration or to oozing from severe wounds or burns. They are lost from the gastrointestinal tract when profuse salivation, vomiting, or diarrhea occur and when the gastrointestinal tract is drained by intubation or purged with cathartics or enemas. In hemorrhage, body fluids and electrolytes are always lost. Fluids with their electrolyte constituents may be trapped in the body by conditions such as wound swelling, edema, ascites, and intestinal obstruction and therefore may not be available for normal processes. Any person under stress (emotional or physical) loses additional amounts of potassium through the kidneys because production of adrenocortical hormones increases. Potassium depletion is, therefore, common in all disease, injury, and surgery. When the respiratory system does not provide an adequate exchange of oxygen and carbon dioxide, serious electrolyte imbalance may ensue.

For clarity of discussion, imbalance of each ion and of body fluid will be considered separately. Actually, several imbalances occur simultaneously because of the interrelationship of body fluids and their electrolytes.

Excessive fluid loss. When too much fluid is lost from the body, *dehydration* occurs. As the blood loses its fluid, the plasma proteins remaining in it are concentrated, giving the blood a greater protein osmotic or *oncotic* (pull) pressure than the fluid in the interstitial spaces and in the cells. As a result, the interstitial fluid diffuses into the bloodstream. This process is a protective mechanism to prevent the blood volume from becoming depleted.

The symptoms of dehydration are flushed, dry skin with poor turgor; dry lips; a dry, coated tongue, abnormal thirst; sunken, soft eyeballs; and atonic muscles. If the cause of dehydration continues unchecked and

treatment is not given, anorexia, dyspepsia, and constipation develop as a result of inadequate fluids for gastrointestinal functioning. Normally about 8 liters of fluid are used daily for gastrointestinal fluids (Table 3), most of which is reabsorbed. As both intracellular and interstitial fluids decrease, cell function is impaired because food, oxygen, and waste products are diffused inadequately. The cells then release potassium, upsetting not only the potassium levels but the sodium levels of the body fluids and causing electrolyte imbalance, with all its symptoms.

If the blood volume cannot be replaced by mobilizing the reserve of extravascular fluids or if the loss of blood volume continues unchecked so that the volume cannot be maintained despite mobilization of extracellular reserves, the blood pressure falls. Renal function and vaporization then decrease, causing body wastes to be retained in the bloodstream, which disturbs the potassium-sodium and acid-base balances still further. The heat-regulating mechanism also is upset. Unless fluid and electrolyte treatment is begun at once, the patient may die. Because of his smaller water reserve, the baby quickly goes into shock from loss of blood volume.

In treating dehydrated patients, glucose and water often are given first to replace the water losses and to increase urinary flow. The urinary output must be normal for those electrolytes in excess of body needs to be excreted. Therefore, solutions containing electrolytes needed by the body are not given until the urinary output is adequate to regulate the amount to be retained. When renal function is adequate, isotonic sodium chloride usually is given. Additional electrolytes, such as potassium chloride and sodium bicarbonate, may be added to replace shortages of potassium and bicarbonate ions. If the patient can retain fluid given by mouth, fluids high in potassium content, such as fruit juices, and salty fluids may be ordered.

If plasma proteins are lost from the body, as occurs in hemorrhage, or if they are shifted from the blood to the interstitial fluid, the blood volume drops rapidly because fluid from interstitial spaces cannot be mobilized to maintain it; shock follows.

Table 3

Fluid composition of digestive juices*

	Approximate ml. of fluid (daily)
Saliva	1,500
Gastric juice	2,500
Intestinal juice	3,000
Pancreatic juice	700
Bile	500

*Adapted from Gamble, J. L.: Extracellular fluids, Cambridge, Mass., 1954, Harvard University Press. Note that approximately 8 liters of fluid are used daily for digestive purposes. Normally most of this fluid is reabsorbed. Some of each of the ions found in blood plasma is present in each of the fluids listed, but the individual concentration varies with each fluid.

Whole blood, plasma, or plasma expanders usually must be given to these patients to replace the protein loss before extensive fluid therapy is effective.

Fluid retention. Retention of abnormal amounts of fluid in the body usually is due to the retention of too much sodium chloride in extravascular fluid compartments. The salt holds water, causing tissue edema. Venous stasis causes fluid retention in tissues, especially in dependent parts such as the feet and legs. The hydrostatic (push) pressure in the engorged vessels is increased, pushing fluid with its sodium chloride from the bloodstream into the surrounding tissues and thus reducing the total blood volume. The kidneys then retain fluid and salt to bring the blood volume back to normal.

Adrenocortical hormones tend to favor sodium reabsorption, and, therefore, tissue edema can be expected in diseases in which abnormally large amounts of these hormones are secreted. Edema in patients being treated with ACTH and cortisone is caused by this action.

Fluid retention in body tissues also may be caused by overloading the vascular system with fluid, resulting in an increase in the hydrostatic pressure of blood. This increase may lead to general tissue edema. More important, if the increase in hydrostatic pressure is great enough to push large amounts of fluid from the bloodstream into the lungs, it rapidly leads to death from drowning in one's own fluids (pulmonary edema). The hydrostatic pressure in the pulmonary vessels normally is much lower than that in the general circulation, and therefore any increase in it is reflected rapidly in the lungs.

Overloading of the vascular system may be caused by giving too much fluid within a short period of time to a person who, due to circulatory or renal disease, cannot dispose of the surplus. Infants and young children also easily can be overloaded because they normally have little extravascular fluid reserve. Elderly people tolerate increases in blood volume very poorly since with inelastic vessels only relatively small increases in volume are needed to markedly increase the hydrostatic pressure.

Overloading of the vascular system also may be caused by increasing the oncotic (pull) pressure of the intravascular fluid by giving proteins so rapidly that the body cannot dispose of those that are in excess of its need. This overloading causes fluids to be pulled into the bloodstream from other body fluid compartments. The blood volume increases rapidly, neutralizing the oncotic pressure but increasing the hydrostatic pressure of the vascular system and the oncotic pressure of the interstitial fluid compartment. Fluid is then pushed into the tissues. Overloading the vascular system is a danger in giving fluids such as plasma, plasma expanders, albumin, and blood to any patient regardless of age or state of health.

Edema often is treated with diuretics, the action of which seems to be on the kidneys. Some, like the mercurial diuretics, block sodium reabsorption and, consequently, water reabsorption by the renal tubules. Some diuretic agents are partially or completely unabsorbable by the renal tubules and tend to carry sodium and water with them into the urine. When diuretics are given, large amounts of fluid are lost from the vascular system, increasing its oncotic pressure and causing it to pull fluid back into the bloodstream from the tissues. Potassium also is usually lost along with the sodium and the water.

Reducing the salt intake also may reduce edema, because the remaining supply of sodium seems to be needed to maintain the isotonicity of the blood and therefore is not available for holding water. If the edema is caused by venous stasis, elevating dependent body parts and applying supportive stockings promote venous return. These measures not only help to prevent the discomfort of venous disease but they also help to prevent fluid and electrolyte imbalance.

Overloading of the circulation is most often treated by phlebotomy (withdrawal of blood), and rotating tourniquets may be applied. If severe pulmonary symptoms are present, the administration of oxygen under positive pressure is started at once. (See the treatment of acute pulmonary edema, p. 328.)

Blood volume determination. Since maintenance of normal blood volume is essential to electrolyte balance and the prevention of shock, a blood volume determination may be made. This procedure often is done preoperatively so that normal blood volume can be restored if necessary. It also may be done to check on the effectiveness of fluid or blood therapy. A hematocrit reading usually is taken too, because it gives an index of the ratio of plasma to cells and thus indicates need for whole blood or for plasma or other fluid replacement only.

In making blood volume determinations, one of several substances, such as a harmless blue dye (Evans blue), albumin tagged with radioactive iodine (RISA), or red blood cells tagged with a radioactive substance such as radioactive phosphorus, may be used. A known quantity of one of these substances is injected intravenously, and blood samples are taken from the opposite arm at a specified time and are examined to determine how much the injected substances have been diluted. Evans blue or RISA is used to determine the plasma volume. Tagged red cells are used to determine the red cell mass. Using appropriate formulas, the entire fluid content of the intravascular compartment (red cells mass plus plasma) can be calculated from either the red cell mass determination or the plasma volume determination.

If blue dye is used, the patient should know that his skin may have a slight blue tinge for several days before the dye is completely excreted. It is excreted in the urine, which will have a bluish green color. Only tracer doses of radioactivity are given, and no special precautions are needed when these substances are used.

Electrolyte imbalances. No single electrolyte can be out of balance without causing some others to be out of balance also. This fact should be kept in mind while reading this section.

Imbalance of cations. Sodium, potassium, and calcium are all essential for the passage of nerve impulses. Whenever the concentrations of any of these cations are increased or decreased in body fluids, the increase or decrease is reflected in the stimulation of muscles by nerves. The muscles may become weak and atonic because of inadequate stimulation, or they may become somewhat spastic because of too much stimulation. A decrease in calcium concentrations in body fluids may cause the stimulus to be irregular, and muscles spasms may result. Gastrointestinal and cardiac symptoms so often produced by electrolyte imbalances result in part from changes in neural stimulation of the muscles of these systems.

With cation imbalances the distribution of body fluids frequently is upset. Abnormal collections of fluid probably cause some of the gastrointestinal symptoms such as nausea, vomiting, and diarrhea. Decreased amounts may cause anorexia, dyspepsia, and constipation. It is thought that edema of cerebral tissues may be responsible for headache, convulsions, and coma.

Sodium deficit. Whenever sodium is lost from the body fluids, they become hypotonic. Sodium loss from the intravascular compartment, therefore, causes fluid from the blood to diffuse into the interstitial spaces. As a result, the sodium in the interstitial fluid is diluted. In response to this reduction of the sodium concentration in the extracellular fluid, potassium moves out of the intracellular fluid. Therefore, the patient with sodium imbalance also is likely to have potassium imbalance.

Sodium depletion results most often from loss of lower intestinal fluids, as in severe diarrhea. Diarrhea in infants is extremely dangerous. They normally have large sodium losses through the skin, and therefore, when large amounts of sodium are lost through the bowel as well, their sodium supply quickly becomes depleted. Symptoms of sodium depletion also appear rapidly in patients with profuse ileostomy drainage. Losing large amounts of bile also depletes sodium stores.

Anyone who is perspiring profusely because of climate, exercise, or fever is losing large amounts of both sodium and water, and if he drinks too much water, he will develop a sodium deficit. Drinking an excessive amount of water at any time, even when no salt or water has been lost, will also produce a sodium deficit. Because of the inability of the kidneys to excrete the excess fluid as fast as it is being introduced, the blood volume increases, the isotonicity of the blood decreases, and fluid diffuses into the interstitial spaces in response to both the hypotonicity of the blood and its increased hydrostatic pressure. This diffusion in turn upsets the isotonicity of the interstitial fluid and pulls potassium from the cells. This type of sodium depletion (by dilution) is known as *water intoxication.*

The patient with a sodium deficit *(hyponatremia)* may have headache, muscle weakness, nausea, vomiting, abdominal cramps, and diarrhea. If salt is not replaced, convulsions may occur, reflexes disappear, and the patient may go into shock and die.

Sodium excess. If fluids are markedly limited or if extra salt is retained due to poor renal function or hormonal influences,

sodium may be concentrated in the body fluids *(hypernatremia).* Excess intravascular sodium causes fluid to be withdrawn from the tissues, resulting in dehydration. If fluids are not given to dilute the sodium and if excretion of sodium is not increased, extensive fluid and electrolyte imbalances will occur, causing manic excitement, tachycardia, and eventual death.

Potassium depletion. When cell metabolism is upset or when cells are damaged, potassium tends to move from the intracellular fluid to the intravascular fluid. Intracellular potassium also moves into the blood whenever the sodium level of the blood is reduced below normal levels. If the kidneys are functioning normally, potassium in excess of normal levels in the blood is excreted. This type of potassium shift rapidly depletes the body's potassium.

The patient who has a balanced diet withheld for several days, who is dehydrated, or who is given large amounts of parenteral fluids with no replacement of potassium develops potassium depletion. The parenteral administration of 5% glucose in water without the addition of potassium tends to dilute the potassium in the extracellular tissues. This dilution, in addition to the lack of a balanced diet and to potassium loss due to catabolism of body proteins, accounts for many problems of electrolyte imbalance in the postoperative patient. Patients who must eat a nutritionally inadequate diet or take no food for an extended period of time, or who are losing large amounts of fluid from the gastrointestinal tract, usually are given intravenous fluids containing proteins and electrolytes as well as glucose. Extra potassium in tablet form often is given to patients receiving ACTH and cortisone, because the adrenocortical hormones favor potassium excretion.

The practice of giving multiple enemas is becoming less common because it is now known that some of the enema fluid is absorbed and dilutes the potassium in the interstitial compartment, upsetting the balance between compartments. Solutions for hypertonic enemas may damage cells in the bowel mucosa, causing potassium loss.

The patient with potassium deficit *(hypokalemia)* has a reduction in nerve impulses to muscles. He often complains of generalized weakness. Paralytic ileus (p. 207) may develop, and the heart muscles may become weak, causing the circulation to slow down. The patient becomes apprehensive, and, without treatment, shock and death will ensue.

Potassium excess. As already stated, whenever there is severe tissue damage, potassium is released from the cells into the extracellular fluids. Since shock usually accompanies this damage, renal function is reduced and a high blood potassium level results *(hyperkalemia)*. There is great danger in giving extra potassium to any patient with poor renal function. If the patient is dehydrated or has lost vascular fluid, glucose and water or plasma expanders usually are given until renal function returns. Untreated adrenal insufficiency also is a contraindication for giving potassium. If the patient who has potassium intoxication needs a blood transfusion, fresh blood must be used. Cells in blood that has been kept for several days tend to release potassium during storage. If it is given, it may increase the patient's blood potassium level still further.

The patient with potassium intoxication develops spasticity of muscles due to overstimulation of them by nerve impulses. He complains of nausea, colic, diarrhea, and skeletal muscle spasms. The muscles later become weak because overstimulation produces accumulations of lactic acid in them and because potassium is lost from the muscle cells. If the condition is not controlled, overstimulation of the cardiac muscle will cause the heartbeat to become irregular and eventually stop. (See p. 99 for a discussion of the treatment of potassium intoxication.)

Calcium deficit. Patients with pancreatic disease or disease of the small intestine may fail to absorb calcium from the gastrointestinal tract normally, and they may excrete abnormally large amounts of calcium in the feces, thus reducing the blood level of calcium. Patients who have draining intestinal fistulas also lose calcium. In renal failure and when the parathyroid glands are removed, the level of calcium in the blood is reduced.

The patient who has calcium deficiency usually first complains of numbness and tingling of the nose, ears, fingertips, or toes. If he is not given calcium at this time, *tetany,* or painful muscular spasms, especially of the

feet and hands (carpopedal spasm), muscle twitching, and convulsions may follow. There are two tests used to elicit signs of calcium deficiency. *Trousseau's sign* is elicited by grasping the patient's wrist so as to constrict the circulation for a few minutes. If his hand goes into a position of palmar flexion (carpopedal spasm), he probably has a serious calcium deficit. *Chvostek's sign* is elicited by tapping the patient's face lightly over the facial nerve (just below the temple). A calcium deficit probably is present if the facial muscles twitch.

The specific treatment for a low blood level of calcium is the administration of calcium gluconate or calcium chloride intravenously or by mouth. (See p. 741 for treatment of hypoparathyroidism and p. 433 for treatment of tetany in renal failure.)

Calcium excess. A marked increase in the calcium level of the blood *(hypercalcemia)* may be seen in diseases with extensive bone involvement, such as metastatic malignancy and hyperparathyroidism. It also occurs in any patient who is immobilized. The excess calcium tends to be removed by the kidneys, which may cause renal stones to form. If additional calcium is not given, pathogenic fractures of bones may occur because they give up calcium to maintain the blood level within normal limits. The patient commonly complains of severe thirst and has polyuria. Gastrointestinal symptoms, including anorexia, nausea, vomiting, and constipation may also develop. Without treatment, the patient may become lethargic and confused, and he may become comatose. The only definitive treatment is removal of the cause.

Acid-base imbalance. Whenever the end products of metabolism cannot be removed from the body, the ratio of acid to base in the blood is upset. Specific symptoms of this problem center around respirations, since it is by increasing or decreasing them that control of the carbon dioxide level of the blood is varied. Acid-base imbalance always produces an imbalance of the body's cations as well. Therefore, symptoms of cation imbalance are seen in addition to the respiratory ones. Only respiratory symptoms will be considered here.

Bicarbonate deficit. In some conditions, such as uncontrolled diabetes mellitus and starvation, glucose either cannot be utilized or is not available for oxidation. The body compensates for this by using body fat for energy, producing abnormal amounts of ketone bodies. In an effort to neutralize the ketones (fatty acids) and maintain the acid-base balance of the body, plasma bicarbonate is exhausted. The resultant acid-base imbalance is known as *metabolic acidosis* or *ketoacidosis*. This condition can develop whenever the person does not eat a nutritious diet and his body fat must be burned. It rapidly develops in infants because they have minimal glycogen reserves. It also can develop whenever excessive amounts of lactic acid are produced due to strenuous muscle exercise or when oxidation takes place in cells without adequate oxygen, such as occurs in shock.[25] The patient in acidosis becomes dyspneic and has deep, periodic breathing. The hyperventilation represents an attempt to blow off carbon dioxide, thus compensating for the acidosis. If the condition is untreated, disorientation, stupor, coma, and death will occur.

Metabolic acidosis is controlled by giving intravenous solutions of sodium bicarbonate or sodium lactate. Sodium bicarbonate sometimes is given by mouth if it can be retained. Treatment of the condition precipitating the acidosis is then instituted.

Bicarbonate excess. When abnormally large amounts of hydrochloric acid and sodium chloride are lost through vomiting or drainage of the stomach, or when fluids high in potassium chloride are lost abnormally through biliary drainage, intestinal fistulas, or diarrhea, the result is an electrolyte imbalance in which there is an excess of base elements. This type of acid-base imbalance, which is known as *metabolic alkalosis,* is also caused by rapid ingestion of large amounts of sodium bicarbonate or carbonated drinks or the ingestion of these substances when renal function is impaired, when gaseous exchange in the lungs is inadequate, or when large amounts of carbon dioxide already have been lost during strenuous exercise.

In metabolic alkalosis, breathing becomes depressed in an effort to conserve carbon dioxide for combination with hydrogen ions in the blood to raise the blood level of carbonic acid. The administration of sodium chloride or ammonium chloride intraven-ously or by mouth helps to relieve metabolic alkalosis. If the condition is associated with loss of sodium chloride, potassium must be restored because it is lost with the sodium.

Carbonic acid deficit. When for any reason there is inadequate oxygenation of the blood despite normal pulmonary function, the lungs eliminate large amounts of carbon dioxide and thus lower the blood carbonic acid level. The condition caused by this extra loss of carbon dioxide is known as *respiratory alkalosis.* Overbreathing for any reason may cause it. Breathing is deep and rapid and the patient usually feels dizzy. Because there are too many free cations in the blood, they may be excreted through the kidney, leaving a deficiency. Large amounts of calcium are usually excreted in this condition. As a result of the cation depletion, tetany and convulsions may develop.

The treatment for respiratory alkalosis is oxygen administration. However, if the oxygen deficiency is caused by anemia, whole blood or packed cells are given.

Carbonic acid excess. Primary carbonic acid excess may occur in any medical condition that interferes with gaseous exchange in the lungs. This excess is known as *respiratory acidosis* or *carbon dioxide narcosis.* The symptoms are the same as those of metabolic acidosis, but the treatment is to increase the excursion of the lungs and thus to improve gaseous exchange. This objective is accomplished by using an intermittent positive-pressure breathing apparatus or by placing the patient in a respirator. Oxygen in high concentrations is never given because respirations may be sustained only by the low oxygen tension of the blood. (See p. 561 for a more complete discussion of treatment.)

Nursing care of patients with fluid and electrolyte imbalances

Important nursing functions include assisting the doctor in evaluating patients' fluid and electrolyte status, helping with replacement therapy and relief of symptoms, recognition and reporting of early symptoms, of fluid and electrolyte imbalances, and prevention of imbalances.

Determination of fluid and electrolyte balance. The nurse should learn the symptoms of fluid and electrolyte imbalances and observe her patients carefully for them. In addition, every acutely ill medical patient and every patient undergoing major surgery should have a chart of fluid intake and output that is thoroughly understood by nurses and all others who may give care to the patient. Space should be provided on this chart for recording the amount and kind of fluid intake and for recording urine output and identifying fluid losses from the less common routes, such as wound drainage. This record should be accurately kept and critically studied to determine if there is the expected ratio of intake to output. Any marked change in ratio should be reported to the doctor.

A well-hydrated person who is not losing fluids abnormally will excrete amounts of urine approximately equal to his liquid intake. Postoperatively, however, a person tends to lose slightly larger amounts of fluid than normal as "insensible water loss," and although he may have a fluid intake of 2,000 to 3,000 ml., he may have a urinary output of only 1,000 to 1,500 ml. a day. Because a baby loses so much fluid through his skin, there normally may be some discrepancy be-

tween his liquid intake and his urine output. Patients who are dehydrated and those who are losing large amounts of body fluids through perspiration, wounds, or the gastrointestinal tract also can be expected to have less urine output in relation to intake than normal. Urinary output in the adult should not fall below 900 ml. a day, however, and the total fluid lost from all routes should equal the fluid intake.

The intake record. The intake record should show the type and amount of all fluids the patient has received and the route by which they were administered. Unless a record of electrolyte replacement is needed, only the quantity of fluid taken by mouth is usually recorded. If it is needed, the kind of fluids must be recorded. A record of the solid food intake is likely to be needed as well. The ambulatory patient may be instructed to help in maintaining an accurate record of his fluid intake (Fig. 26).

Daily weight. Often a daily weight record is requested since it is a good indication of the onset of dehydration or of the accumulation of fluid either as generalized edema or as "hidden" fluid in body cavities. If the record is to be useful, the patient must be weighed on the same scale and at the same hour each day, and he must be wearing the same amount of clothing. Circumstances that may affect the weight should be kept as nearly identical as possible from day to day. Usually weights are taken in the early morning before the patient has eaten or defecated, but after he has voided. When extremely accurate measurements are needed, all clothing and even wound dressings are removed from the patient before he is weighed.

Urinary output. Urinary output should be recorded as to time and amount of each voiding. This record helps to evaluate renal function more accurately. If renal function is a major concern, as for instance in a severely burned patient, an indwelling catheter is used so that the amount of urinary drainage can be recorded every hour and fluid intake regulated accordingly. It has been said that nothing is more difficult to obtain in a modern hospital than an accurate record of urine output, and unfortunately this statement is often true. Conspicuous signs posted on the patient's chart and in the utility room

Fig. 26

Often the patient needs to be taught to measure and record fluid intake accurately.

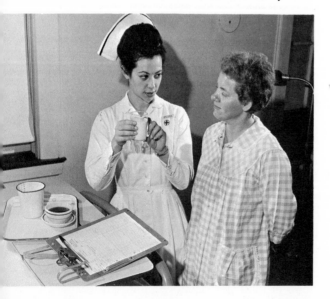

and bathrooms will help to prevent the discarding of urine before it is measured.

Wound drainage. If the patient has much drainage from a wound, the doctor may want the drainage measured. When the drainage is coming from a fistula in, for example, the biliary system or the pancreas, or is coming from an ileostomy, catheters or collection bags may be used so that accurate recording of the fluid loss is possible. At other times it may be necessary to weigh the dressings and any wet linen on a small gram scale prior to use, recording their weight as dry weight, and upon removal of dressings or linen, weighing them again. Fluid loss is the difference between the wet weight and the dry weight.

Other output. Electrolytes are lost in large amounts with vomiting, diarrhea, and gastric drainage. The amount and kind vary according to what type of gastrointestinal fluid is lost. For the doctor to determine the amount and type of fluid replacement needed, vomitus, gastrointestinal drainage, and liquid stools should be measured as accurately as possible and should be described as to color, contents, and odor. Gastric secretions are watery, a pale yellowish green, and usually have a sour odor. However, if the acid-base balance has been upset, gastric secretions may have a fruity odor because of the presence of acetone. Bile is somewhat thicker than gastric juice and may vary from bright yellow to dark green in color. It has a bitter taste and acrid odor. Intestinal contents vary from dark green to brown in color, are likely to be quite thick, and have a fecal odor. Any fluid used to irrigate nasogastric tubes should be subtracted from total drainage before it is recorded.

It is difficult to determine accurately the amount of water lost in the stools, but a description of their consistency and a record of the number of stools passed give the doctor an estimate. The color of stools should be recorded too. Because infants are likely to lose large amounts of water in their stools, daily records usually are kept for any baby who is ill.

Fluid aspirated from any body cavity such as the abdomen or pleural spaces must be measured. This fluid contains not only electrolytes and water but proteins also.

Blood loss from any part of the body should be measured carefully.

Diaphoresis is difficult to measure without special laboratory equipment. However, it may be important to estimate the loss of fluid by this route in some patients. Careful note of "heavy" perspiration and its duration should be made. If the clothing and linen become saturated, dry and wet weights may be taken as described in the discussion on wound drainage. Accurate recording of body temperature helps the doctor to determine how much fluid the patient needs, since fluid loss through the skin and lungs increases as the temperature rises.

Replacement therapy. The best way to restore water, electrolytes, and nutrients to the body is to give them by mouth (Fig. 27). When fluids can be tolerated by the

Fig. 27

The best way to replace fluids, electrolytes, and nutrients is to give them by mouth.

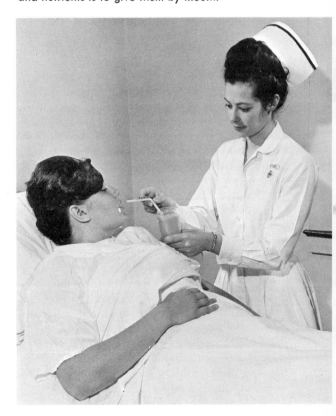

stomach but cannot be swallowed, a naso-gastric tube may be passed, and fluids containing all the essentials of a balanced diet may be given through it. Normal saline solution or plain water also may be given by slow drip through the tube to replace fluid loss.

If it is not possible for a patient to take food or fluid through the alimentary tract, the commonest method of replacement is by intravenous infusion *(venoclysis)*. A vein in the leg or arm usually is used for a venoclysis, but in babies a vein in the scalp or the femoral or the jugular vein may be used. Occasionally, an incision is made, and a polyethylene catheter is threaded into the vein, where it remains for several days. This incision is called a *cutdown*.

If for some reason fluid cannot be given by vein, such as because the patient is in shock and his veins are collapsed or because his circulatory system cannot withstand the direct introduction of additional fluid without becoming overloaded, physiologic solution of sodium chloride or solutions containing other electrolytes may be given into subcutaneous tissues *(hypodermoclysis)*. Infants and young children often are given fluids by this method. Elderly patients with severe cardiac disease may be given hypodermoclyses also, and they frequently are used for patients who are so restless that keeping a needle in the vein is difficult. In adults the fluid usually is injected beneath the skin of the thigh. In babies the thighs, scapular region, or abdomen frequently is used. Infants and young children also may be given fluid intraperitoneally. Normal saline solution or plain water sometimes is given by slow drip *(Murphy drip)* into the rectum, where it is absorbed quickly in most instances.

Fluids given by any route should be spaced throughout the twenty-four-hour period. Not only does this practice help to maintain normal body fluid levels, but it provides for better regulation of the electrolyte balance by the kidneys and prevents the end products of metabolism and toxic materials from being excreted in concentrated form. In this way the danger of renal damage, formation of calculi, and irritation of the lower urinary tract is reduced. In addition, fluid spacing prevents overloading of the circulation, which may result in dilu-

tion of body fluids, with resultant fluid and electrolyte shifts, the most serious of which causes pulmonary edema.

Concentrated solutions of sugar or protein should always be given in small amounts at a time and slowly, because they will pull fluids from the body to dilute themselves. Normal saline solution may cause fluid to diffuse from the tissues to equalize the concentrations of salt in the fluid compartments. Therefore, it, too, should be given slowly and in small amounts. If any of these concentrated solutions flow quickly into the vascular system, pulmonary edema can develop rapidly. Giving them rapidly and in large amounts into the alimentary tract causes the blood volume to drop, and if large amounts of fluid are needed to dilute the substance, irreversible shock can result. The "dumping syndrome," which sometimes occurs after a gastric resection (p. 657), is caused by this abnormal shift of fluid. Concentrated solutions sometimes are given intentionally to reduce cerebral edema (p. 888).

Giving large amounts of fluid either by mouth or parenterally is potentially dangerous even in a healthy person, and therefore, fluids of any kind should never be replaced faster than they are lost. Nurses should question the advisability of the rather common practice of speeding up the rate of flow of solutions given intravenously primarily to complete the treatment at a specified time. Every nurse should recognize the initial signs of pulmonary edema (bounding pulse, engorged peripheral veins, hoarseness, dyspnea, cough or pulmonary rales) and should observe closely for them in patients who are receiving concentrated solutions, those who must be given any intravenous solution rapidly, and those whose age or physical condition makes them special risks. At the first signs of increased blood volume, the rate of flow of the infusion should be greatly reduced and the doctor notified. Special care needs to be taken in giving fluids to infants, elderly patients with circulatory impairment, patients whose hearts are decompensated, those with renal impairment, and those who have had plasma shifts, such as burned patients and those with extensive tissue trauma from other causes. Patients whose plasma has

Table 4

Approximate division of total body fluid into compartments

Body fluid compartments	Liters of fluid	
	Lean adult weighing 100 pounds	Lean adult weighing 150 pounds
Intravascular (plasma)	2.8	4.2
Interstitial	8.4	12.5
Intracellular	22.3	33.3
Total	33.5	50.0

Note that the smaller the individual, the less fluid he has in each compartment and that plasma is reduced most markedly with decrease in size. The normal size and body type of the individual are considered when fluid replacement is ordered.

shifted need to be watched especially carefully after a few days because the plasma tends to shift back suddenly from the interstitial tissue to the bloodstream, producing an increase in blood volume, with resulting pulmonary edema (p. 328).

The size of the patient should be considered in giving fluids. The small person normally has less fluid in each body compartment, especially in the intravascular system (Table 4). He therefore becomes seriously dehydrated more quickly than a larger person and needs his fluid losses replaced more promptly. This prompt replacement is even more important in babies and young children. Because so much of their body fluid normally is extracellular, they have proportionately less reserve fluid in the cells from which to pull than a small adult has. In hemorrhage, for example, an adult who normally has only 3 liters of blood plasma and has bled extensively needs replacement of blood sooner than one who normally has 5 liters and has lost the same amount. A baby or child who has lost a proportionate amount needs even greater priority. The age of the adult must be considered, too. The inelastic vessels of an older person may prevent the best use of the remaining blood in supplying vital areas, and therefore, older people often tolerate blood loss poorly.

People with small or inelastic vascular systems also become overhydrated more easily. It is important to remember that a person who has had a large portion of his body, such as a limb, surgically or traumatically removed does not have the same-sized vascular system as previously.

Parenteral fluids. The nurse needs to know the common solutions used parenterally. Glucose, 5%, in distilled water is often used to maintain fluid intake or to reestablish blood volume. Ascorbic acid and vitamin B (Solu-B) are frequently added. Small quantities (1,000 ml. or less a day) of 5% glucose in saline may be used to maintain the sodium chloride level in the body, and potassium chloride may be added to maintain normal intake needs of potassium and to replace losses. A physiologic solution of sodium chloride usually is given only when sodium chloride has been lost in large amounts or when trying to reestablish the blood volume. One-sixth molar lactate solution may be ordered when sodium but not chloride needs replacement, and ammonium chloride solution may be used to replace chlorides without adding sodium. Balanced solutions containing several electrolytes may be used. Ringer's solution, Hartmann's solution (lactated Ringer's solution), Darrow's solution, and Tyrode's solution are examples.

Body needs for carbohydrates may be partially met by giving fructose or 10 or 20% glucose in distilled water. Since these

105

solutions are slightly hypertonic, there is some danger of their causing blood cell destruction.

There is no really satisfactory substitute for protein taken by mouth, but amino acid preparations (Aminosol) are being used rather widely. They have to be given slowly to prevent nausea, and in many patients they cause unpleasant side effects such as peculiar sensations of taste and smell. Whole blood, plasma, or plasma volume expanders can be given to substitute for blood protein loss and are used to reestablish normal blood volume and prevent shock (p. 90). Dextran is the most generally accepted plasma volume expander and has been stockpiled for emergency use in the event of major disaster, such as an atomic attack.

There is no satisfactory way to supply fat when it cannot be taken by mouth. Some intravenous fat substances such as Lipomul have been tried but the side effects have been so severe that their use has been largely discontinued. If such an infusion is given, it should be started very slowly (ten drops a minute) and gradually increased over a period of an hour to the rate prescribed by the doctor. The patient should be observed closely, and if any untoward symptoms develop, the infusion should be stopped and the doctor notified. The symptoms vary greatly, so that any complaint deserves attention.

Intravenous fluids containing electrolytes should be run slowly to allow the body to regulate their use. The patient should be watched carefully for signs of intoxication (excess of fluids or electrolytes). When solutions containing electrolytes are given, the nurse should observe the urinary output carefully and report any decrease in the amount of it to the doctor. Since the kidneys select the ions needed and excrete surplus ones, a normal output is significant. If she is planning the sequence of intravenous fluids, she should be careful to give hydrating fluids, such as physiologic solution of sodium chloride and glucose solution, first. Renal failure and untreated adrenal insufficiency are contraindications for the use of potassium. If these conditions are known or suspected to exist, the nurse should verify orders for its administration. Many doctors do not start in-travenous therapy for the day until chemical analyses of the blood have been reported.

The rate of administration of fluids usually is ordered by the doctor and will depend upon the patient's illness, the kind of fluid given, and the patient's age. An infusion is rarely run at a rate faster than 4 ml. a minute. If it is given continuously, or if it is given when there is impaired renal function or impaired cardiac function, it is rarely run faster than 2 ml. a minute. The usual rate for replacement of fluid loss is 3 ml. a minute.[14] This rate allows time for the fluid to diffuse into the extracellular fluid compartments and avoids overloading the circulation or raising the blood volume high enough to produce a diuretic effect. (For precautions as to the rate for concentrated solutions, blood, and blood products, see p. 104.) The nurse should realize that the various equipment for fluid administration may have varying numbers of milliliters per drop. This number must always be checked, since it is not the drops per minute but the milliliters per minute that are important.

It is imperative that the nurse check fluid bottles carefully for correctness of content and that she record accurately the fluids given. Too much fluid or too much of any of the electrolyte substances can be disastrous for the patient. The greatest care also should be taken to see that any needle that enters a vein has been sterilized by autoclaving to avoid its being contaminated by organisms (p. 708). (For details of equipment and nursing techniques needed in parenteral fluid administration, see a textbook on fundamentals of nursing.)

Patients who are receiving fluids intravenously should be observed frequently to check the rate of flow so that symptoms indicating the need to slow down, speed up, or stop the infusion may be noted. Signs of developing pulmonary edema should be watched for especially. The tissue at the site of the inserted needle should be checked at intervals for signs of infiltration. If infiltration occurs, the infusion should be stopped at once and plans made to restart it. Some solutions, such as those containing potassium, are very irritating and may actually cause tissue necrosis. When checking to see why an infusion is not running properly, the nurse should be extremely careful not to accidentally introduce air into the tubing. The air may act as an embolus when it reaches the bloodstream and cause death.

Food by mouth. The nurse needs to know which foods contain large and small amounts of various essential nutrients, minerals, and vitamins. When losses must be restored, the patient needs more than is required in the usual adequate diet. It is especially important to know which foods and fluids are high or low in potassium and sodium and which foods are complete proteins. Bananas, other fruits, all fruit juices, many fresh vegetables, coffee, and tea are relatively high in potassium and low in sodium content. Salty broths and tomato juice provide extra sodium but have a high potassium content. Meat, milk, and eggs all are complete protein foods and contain relatively large quantities of both sodium and potassium.[30] *Bridge's Food and Beverage Analysis*[18] and *Applied Nutrition*[30] are useful references, and the dietitian should be consulted as necessary.

The nurse frequently has an order to "force fluids." Since the amount required depends upon the size of the patient, the amount of fluid loss, and the circulatory and renal function, no standard amount can be given. Therefore, the nurse must make a judgment as to the desirable amount and inform members of the nursing team or family members who may be caring for the patient. If there is any question, the physician should be consulted. Adults who have no circulatory or renal malfunction usually are given between 2,500 and 3,000 ml. a day. Suggested amounts for babies and children are given on p. 82. Precautions should be taken so that the overzealous patient does not drink too much fluid in a day or that he does not take too much (three to four glasses) at one time. Excessive fluid intake may cause water intoxication (sodium depletion).

When many persons are ill, they find it difficult to eat or drink even though they are allowed to do so. There are many ways that the nurse can help the patient take adequate food and fluids by mouth and thus avoid the need for parenteral fluids. Fruit ades, tea, coffee, ginger ale or other soft drinks may be substituted for part of the water. Soup, bouillon, milk, eggnog, and cocoa provide both fluid and nutrients. Juicy fruits and other semisolid foods with a high fluid and nutrient content, such as custard, ice cream, or gelatin, may be more palatable than regular meals and plain water. Care must be taken, of course, that any substitutions are acceptable on the diet prescribed for the patient. If a fluid record is needed, the amount of fluid given in semisolid form should be estimated and recorded. A juicy orange, for example, contains about 50 ml. of fluid.

The techniques used in presenting food and fluids to patients may influence their consumption of them. Often a small amount of either food or fluid offered at frequent intervals is more acceptable than is a large amount presented less often. Giving some thought to serving foods that the patient likes may improve his appetite. For example, carbonated beverages may be better tolerated by patients who are nauseated, and consideration should always be given to the cultural and aesthetic aspects of eating (p. 116).

Gavage (feeding by tube). Water, a physiologic solution of sodium chloride, high-protein liquid foods such as Lonalac, or a regular diet that has been passed through a blender and diluted is often given by gavage to older children and adults. These fluids may be given as a slow, continuous drip, or 250 to 500 ml. may be given at spaced intervals. Infants and small children usually are given a prescribed formula equivalent in amount to their usual formula. The tube is left in place in older children and adults, but for babies and small children it usually is removed and passed for each feeding. (See p. 637 for the technique of passing the tube.)

Some special precautions need to be taken when food is given by gavage (Fig. 28). The nurse should be alert for aspiration of the feeding into the lungs. Coughing, choking, and cyanosis indicate aspiration, and if these symptoms occur, the procedure should be discontinued immediately. A small amount of water should always be given before the liquid food, because if the tube is displaced, aspirated water is less likely to cause serious trouble than the liquid food. Following the feeding, a small amount of water should be given to flush out the tube. Special care must be taken that high protein liquid foods are not given in too large quantities at once.

107

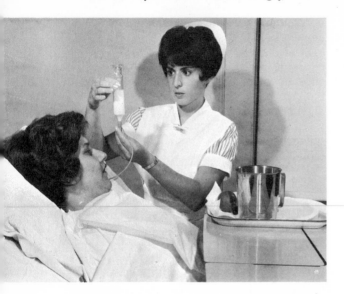

Fig. 28

Feeding a patient by gavage is a procedure requiring careful nursing attention.

Limiting protein intake prevents the pulling of excessive quantities of fluids from the bloodstream and thereby lowering the volume of circulating blood.

Relief of symptoms. Patients with fluid and electrolyte imbalances often have extreme thirst, nausea, and vomiting. These symptoms are distressing, and the nurse should know measures that can be used to give the patient relief.

Thirst. Thirst, the first and most insistent sign of dehydration, sometimes causes the patient more misery than an operation or the symptoms of a disease. It may develop even when fluids have been withheld only for a number of hours. If fluid is being withheld intentionally, thirst often is made more bearable by explaining to the patient why fluid is withheld and when he can expect to receive some.

Thirst usually is relieved rather readily by taking fluids. If fluids cannot be taken by mouth, the administration of fluids parenterally usually gives relief. It is often helpful to explain to the patient who is receiving an infusion that the procedure will soon give him some relief from his thirst.

Mouth care will allay some of the discomfort from thirst. This care should include cleansing the tongue and the use of cold mouthwashes. It may be necessary to repeat these procedures every hour. If the patient can be trusted not to swallow, he may be given water or ice chips to be held in the mouth and then expelled. Hard lemon candies (sour balls) often give relief even though they must be expelled. The chewing of gum helps some patients.

When fluids are not permitted, the temptation of a water pitcher at the bedside should be removed, and if the patient cannot be relied upon not to get up and drink at a water tap, special provisions, such as constant attendance or insistence on bed rest, may be necessary. Thirst sometimes compels the patient to obtain water if he can possibly do so.

Pronounced and continued thirst, despite the administration of fluids, is not normal and should be reported to the doctor. In the patient recently returned from surgery, this kind of thirst should make the nurse suspect internal hemorrhage, elevation of temperature, or some other untoward development. In the chronically ill patient it may indicate the onset of disease, such as diabetes mellitus, in which extra water is used by the kidneys to eliminate glucose in the urine. It also is a symptom of hypercalcemia.

Nausea and vomiting. Nausea and vomiting often are part of the body's response to insults to its integrity. They usually occur together, but occasionally, if the mechanism for vomiting is touched off by local pressure in the medulla, vomiting may be sudden and not preceded by nausea or any other warning sensation.

It is now known that there are two centers in the medulla involved with vomiting—the chemoreceptor emetic trigger zone and the vomiting center.[9] The vomiting center may be stimulated directly through the vagal or sympathetic nerves. Gastrointestinal irritants, distention or injury of any of the viscera, pain, and psychic trauma cause nausea and vomiting in this manner. Increased intracranial pressure may stimulate vomiting by direct local pressure. The vomiting center also may be stimulated indirectly through the chemoreceptor emetic trigger zone. Emetic agents such as morphine sulfate, meperidine hydrochloride (Demerol), ergot derivatives, digitalis preparations and metabolic emetic substances resulting from uremia, infection, and radiation produce this type of stimulation. Labyrinthine stimulation, the primary factor in the nausea and vomiting of motion sickness, which can occur in well people under unusual circumstances involving motion (as in seasickness, for example), is believed to pass through the trigger center too. It still is not clear by what route irritating gases, such as those used in anesthesia, affect the vomiting center nor what specifically causes vomiting during the first trimester of pregnancy. Toxic substances with an emetic effect probably account for vomiting later in pregnancy.

Nausea and vomiting always are distressing symptoms for the patient, but vomiting also can be a serious symptom. Prolonged and severe vomiting may interfere with nutrition, and it not only is a rather common symptom of electrolyte imbalance, but it may cause fluid and electrolyte imbalances. The act of vomiting produces a strain on the abdominal muscles, and in the postoperative patient it may cause wound separation, wound dehiscence, or bleeding. Vomiting is especially dangerous for anesthetized patients, persons in coma, and babies because they are likely to aspirate the vomitus into the lungs. This aspiration may cause asphyxia, atelectasis, or pneumonitis. It happens easily, too, in the elderly patient whose nasopharyngeal reflexes are less acute than those of a younger person.

Treatment of nausea and vomiting depends upon their cause. Drugs or toxic substances known to cause the trouble are usually stopped or eliminated, and fluid and electrolyte imbalances are treated. Most patients will have less vomiting if the emotional components of its cause are removed. Therefore, the nurse should try to relieve the patient's anxieties. Sedation may help to quiet the patient, and soluble phenobarbital often is ordered. Nausea and gagging sometimes are relieved by taking deep breaths through the mouth, and relief from these sensations may prevent vomiting. If the vomiting is due to irritants, such as anesthetic gases, letting the patient take water and then vomit may wash out the stomach and help prevent continued vomiting. Ginger ale and other effervescent drinks seem to have a remarkable effect in controlling postoperative vomiting and often can be taken and retained long before other fluids are tolerated. Effervescent fluids also may be effective in controlling vomiting from other causes, such as seasickness.

Antihistaminic drugs such as dimenhydrinate (Dramamine), meclizine hydrochloride (Bonine), and trimethobenzamide hydrochloride (Tigan) are used widely in control of motion sickness such as is encountered in air and sea travel. These drugs are effective prophylactically when taken about thirty minutes before the initial motion and then continued at regular intervals. They also are ordered with varying success in the nausea and vomiting associated with illness. Tigan in large doses has been quite effective in controlling nausea and vomiting postoperatively. All these drugs are available as rectal suppositories as well as for oral administration. Any of the antihistaminic drugs may cause drowsiness and dizziness, and the possibility of these reactions should be pointed out to persons who are taking them when traveling. They are especially dangerous to use when driving. When antihistaminic drugs are being used in the hospital, the patient must be watched carefully to prevent accidents such as falling out of bed.

The phenothiazine drugs given in relatively small doses are specific antiemetics, blocking the action of emetic agents at the trigger zone and thus preventing activation of the vomiting center.[9] They now are used frequently for postoperative patients and others with prolonged and severe vomiting not of vestibular origin. Many drugs in this category are on the market, and many of them are available for intramuscular injection. Some common ones used are prochlorperazine (Compazine), promethazine hydrochloride (Phenergan), and perphenazine (Trilafon). All these drugs have side effects of oversedation and hypotension, and therefore the hospitalized patient should be protected from accidents, and persons who are taking them at home should be warned about the danger. They should be given cautiously to patients whose blood pressure is already low.

Nausea and vomiting are profoundly affected by sights, sounds, and smells, and the nurse should try to protect the patient from such stimuli whenever possible. Some equipment used in caring for the sick, such as emesis basins, may be psychologically disturbing to patients. Even empty emesis basins are suggestive of vomiting and should be kept out of a patient's sight unless he actually is vomiting, and then it may be a comfort to have one conveniently placed. Emesis basins should be removed and emptied immediately after use. Relatives learning to care for a patient at home often need help in improvising equipment that will be psychologically acceptable. For example, they may be using a baby's potty as an emesis basin when an empty coffee can lined with paper might be less offensive. Some patients may become nauseated from seeing their dressings changed. If so, the nurse should try to distract their attention while this procedure is done. The sound of retching frequently makes even well people nauseated. Therefore, whenever possible, patients should be protected from others who are vomiting. Food odors, drug odors, and other odors that are part of a hospital setting also may contribute to nausea in the person who is ill. Even perfumes and strongly scented soaps may cause nausea. Rooms should be ventilated carefully during both the day and the night.

Prevention of fluid and electrolyte imbalance

There are many ways by which the nurse can help to prevent fluid and electrolyte imbalance in both the well and the ill. Teaching patients the principles of good nutrition and encouraging them to eat nutritionally adequate diets are very important ways.

Unless preventive measures are employed, many medical and surgical conditions and the techniques used to treat them may lead to fluid and electrolyte imbalances. There are some rather frequently encountered situations in which the nurse's attention to preventive aspects may lessen the possibility of the development of serious imbalances.

The patient with fluid loss from the gastrointestinal tract. Vomiting and diarrhea are common symptoms of many illnesses, and most people suffer from them from time to time. Sodium and some potassium are always lost, and chloride is lost in vomitus. As soon as fluids are tolerated, therefore, the patient who has had vomiting or diarrhea should be served salty broths and tea or another fluid high in potassium in order to replace the losses. This measure often keeps the patient from feeling so weak and exhausted. Dry soda crackers often are tolerated when fluids are not and can be used to replace sodium. Prompt replacement of both water and electrolytes is essential in babies since they have limited reserves. If vomiting or diarrhea persist for even a few hours and oral foods are not tolerated, they should have medical attention, since they may need intravenous replacement of losses.

A patient with a draining fistula from any portion of the gastrointestinal tract loses sodium, calcium, and some potassium. It is important, therefore, that his diet be supplemented. Extra milk will replace all the losses, and patients should be instructed to increase their milk intake somewhat above normal levels. For the body to use the calcium, of course, vitamin D also must be available, but most milk is now fortified with vitamin D. People with a permanent fistulous opening, such as an ileostomy, need to be especially careful to supplement sodium and potassium when vomiting, diarrhea, or fever adds to their already unusually large loss of electrolytes.

Many patients in the course of treatment have a nasogastric tube inserted and attached to suction drainage. Routine intravenous replacement usually is adequate to compensate for losses through this drainage, unless the patient has been allowed to take fluids by mouth or has had the tube irrigated frequently with water. Both of these practices, although they seem to be harmless because the fluid is removed immediately through the aspiration apparatus, stimulate the secretion of gastric juices. These juices, in addition to normal secretions with the stomach at rest, are aspirated and lead to electrolyte and sometimes even fluid imbalances. If irrigation of the tube is necessary, physiologic solution of sodium chloride should be used. Thirst is a problem for these patients, and measures must be taken to relieve it, but special precautions should be taken to be certain that the patient does not consume the fluid from ice chips or mouth rinses.

If there is an order for enemas until the returns are clear, the nurse should not give more than three enemas to the patient without consulting the doctor, since this treatment may result in electrolyte imbalance (p. 98). The practice of some people, especially those who are older, of taking daily enemas, especially if hypertonic solutions (detergents, for example) are used, should be discouraged. If an elderly person living at home complains of pronounced weakness without apparent cause, the nurse should ask whether he has been taking cathartics or enemas. If so, stopping this procedure, eating foods with high sodium and potassium content, and increasing the fluid intake may relieve the symptoms. Methods to combat constipation without purging should be taught (p. 120).

The patient with abnormal fluid loss through the skin, lungs, and kidneys. Any person who is perspiring profusely is losing sodium, and anyone who is hyperventilating because of fever, strenuous exercise, exposure to excessive heat, or other causes, such as acidosis, difficulty with oxygenation, or stress, is losing abnormally large amounts of carbon dioxide. In all the above situations, more fluid than usual is lost.

Even the well person who is perspiring profusely needs extra salt in his diet and should drink extra fluids, and some salty fluids should be given to any patient with a fever. Patients on salt-restricted diets and those with draining gastrointestinal fistulas are especially likely to suffer from sodium depletion. They should always be taught to increase their salt intake slightly whenever they perspire profusely. Patients who have hot packs applied to large areas of the body also lose sodium and water, although the loss may not be readily noticeable as perspiration. If they are able to take fluids by mouth, salty broths should be served to them several times a day. Attention to ingesting more salt and water than usual whenever a person is in situations of excessive heat, climatic or otherwise, may prevent heat exhaustion.

Patients who are hyperventilating for long periods of time, regardless of the reason, should have their fluid intake increased somewhat, because they are losing more fluid than usual through the lungs. Although this may not actually upset the fluid balance of the body in people with adequate renal function, it does cause the urine to become concentrated, which may allow waste products of metabolism, toxins, and minerals to pass through the kidneys without sufficient dilution. If this process continues for long, renal damage may occur. Babies and patients whose kidneys cannot conserve water because of disease will become dehydrated rapidly whenever more fluid than usual is lost by other routes.

Diuretics are administered to encourage excretion of sodium and water that are in excess of body needs. However, potassium, which may not be in excess, is lost also. Therefore, the nurse should encourage the patient who is receiving diuretics to eat foods that are high in potassium but low in sodium. Tea, coffee, and fruit juices are good sources of potassium, but the patient usually must limit fluids. Therefore, he should be advised to select most of his fluids from liquids containing potassium. Bananas and other fresh fruits also provide good sources of potassium without increasing the sodium or fluid intake. Diuretics eventually may cause sodium depletion, and therefore, the patient who is receiving extensive diuretic treatment should be observed for symptoms indicating it (p. 99). Since many patients receiving diuretics are at home, they should be taught to report symptoms of sodium depletion to the doctor.

Changes in the urinary output may forewarn of fluid and electrolyte imbalances. Therefore, persons with a urine output that greatly exceeds fluid intake and persons with oliguria should see a physician.

The patient with renal or circulatory impairment. Any patient with renal or circulatory impairment, such as may occur in shock, cardiac decompensation, or the constriction of blood vessels because of disease, may develop electrolyte imbalances. Sodium and water may be held in the tissues, the potassium level of the blood may rise, acidosis may develop from inadequate tissue oxygenation, and alkalosis may develop if the kidneys are unable to excrete waste products properly. The nurse should instruct patients with cardiac and renal impairment to avoid taking too much food containing sodium, potassium, or bicarbonate. They

111

should not drink carbonated beverages. Since many people take bicarbonate of soda or similar proprietary products, they should be told about the undesirability of this practice also.

Patients with renal or circulatory impairment can easily be overhydrated. The nurse should be especially aware of overhydration whenever intravenous fluids are being given, and she should consider it in planning "forced fluid" regimens for these patients.

The patient with respiratory impairment. Any change from the normal pattern of gaseous exchange or any impairment of cell oxygenation can cause acid-base imbalances. Overbreathing is a common cause of carbonic acid deficit in the blood. Because anyone tends toward alkalosis following strenuous exercise, carbonated drinks, which also contribute to alkalosis, should be omitted until the body has had time to regulate its acidity. Special attention should be paid to patients in respirators and to those who are receiving intermittent positive-pressure breathing to avoid respiratory alkalosis. If a patient complains of dizziness or shows any signs of muscle irritability, it is likely that the depth of respiration is too great, and the mechanical breathing apparatus should be adjusted. Nursing measures to reduce high body temperatures and anxiety help to prevent overbreathing in any patient.

Patients with diseases, such as emphysema, that limit lung excursion and therefore limit gaseous exchange should not take carbonated beverages or bicarbonate of soda. These substances tend to make the blood more alkaline than normal, and respirations are depressed in an effort to correct this imbalance. Depression of respirations is highly undesirable for these patients.

Any patient with symptoms of inadequate oxygenation or carbon dioxide retention requires medical treatment. Early recognition and treatment of the primary condition often prevents its becoming complicated by acid-base imbalance. Therefore, any person with symptoms suggestive of anemia, cardiac insufficiency, emphysema, asthma, or other obstructive diseases of the bronchioles should receive medical attention. Patients with symptoms of shock need care promptly.

The patient with hypercalcemia. One of the most serious consequences of hypercalcemia is the formation of renal stones. Therefore, any patients with this condition, regardless of its cause, should always be given generous amounts of fluid. Immobilization is a common cause of hypercalcemia, and the condition is seen frequently in patients with fractures and skeletal muscle paralysis. It can be prevented by helping the patient to exercise muscles in uninvolved parts of the body. This condition is an important reason for encouraging patients who are immobilized in a back-lying position to use a trapeze bar. It is also one reason for encouraging all patients who are able, to move about as much as possible and, with the use of side rails and other means, to engage in activities that require muscle action.

Because patients with marked hypercalcemia often are losing calcium from their bones, special care should be taken to prevent accidents that could result in fractures. Even the pressure used in giving a back rub must sometimes be avoided.

The patient with hypocalcemia. If the patient has a disease in which calcium is not absorbed from the gastrointestinal tract, he may have to be given calcium by parenteral routes. The patient with hypocalcemia should be observed carefully for signs of tetany (p. 100), and if they occur, replacement of calcium should be instituted. Any patient who is not absorbing calcium from the gastrointestinal tract will become constipated unless he pays special attention to increasing the fluid and the roughage content of his diet. The commonly used drugs Amphojel and Gelusil tend to block calcium reabsorption, and patients receiving them should be observed carefully for signs of hypocalcemia.

The effect of stress. Any stressful situation (physical or emotional) may precipitate a condition that leads to electrolyte and acid-base imbalances. Therefore, alleviation of anxiety, building up the patient's nutritional status preoperatively to increase his glycogen stores, and helping to restore nutrients to patients who are ill or who have had surgery are important aspects of nursing care and may be vital in preventing serious complications from fluid and electrolyte imbalances.

Maintaining body temperature

Life processes cannot continue at temperatures more than a few degrees higher or lower than the normal body temperature. Yet the body constantly generates heat by metabolism. The body must protect itself from this heat as well as against heat in the external environment. The body uses the same mechanisms to protect itself from both types of heat (p. 84).

Whenever the metabolism of the body is speeded up for any reason, provision must be made to dissipate the heat. If the heat is not dissipated, fever results. Babies and children, who normally produce a great deal of heat because of their very active metabolism, develop fevers rapidly when disease or stress demand additional energy expenditure, with the resultant release of heat. Because babies and young children still have immature heat regulatory mechanisms, measures to reduce fever need to be instituted more promptly than in adults.

References and selected readings*

1 Abbott, W. E.: Nutrition, body fluids, shock and burns, Surg. Gynec. & Obst. 116:141-146, Feb. 1963.

2 Anthony, Catherine P.: Fluid imbalances, formidable foes to survival, Am. J. Nursing 63:75-77, Dec. 1963.

3 Beeson, Paul B., and McDermott, Walsh, editors: Cecil-Loeb textbook of medicine, ed. 11, Philadelphia, 1963, W. B. Saunders Co.

4 *Bordicks, Katherine J.: Patterns of shock: implications for nursing care, New York, 1965, The Macmillan Co.

5 *Burgess, Richard E.: Fluids and electrolytes, Am. J. Nursing 65:90-95, Oct. 1965.

6 *Cohn, Howard D.: Hemostasis and blood coagulation, Am. J. Nursing 65:116-119, Feb. 1965.

7 Davenport, Rachel R.: Tube feeding for long-term patients, Am. J. Nursing 64:121-123, Jan. 1964.

8 Davis, Loyal, editor: Christopher's textbook of surgery, ed. 8, Philadelphia, 1964, W. B. Saunders Co.

9 *Downs, Howard S.: The control of vomiting, Am. J. Nursing 66:76-82, Jan. 1966.

10 Dunning, Marcelle F., and Plum, Fred: Potassium depletion by enemas, Am. J. Med. 20:789-792, May 1956.

11 Farr, Hollon W.: Fluid and electrolyte balance—with special reference to the gastrointestinal tract, Am. J. Nursing 54:826-831, July 1954.

12 Fenn, Wallace O.: The mechanism of breathing, Scientific American 202:138-148, Jan. 1960.

13 Fluid and electrolytes, North Chicago, Ill., 1957, Abbott Laboratories.

14 Gamble, J. L.: Extracellular fluids, Cambridge, Mass., 1954, Harvard University Press.

15 Harmer, Bertha, and Henderson, Virginia: Textbook of the principles and practice of nursing, ed. 5, New York, 1955, The Macmillan Co.

16 Jorgensen, H. E., and Schlegel, J. U.: Studies in metabolism of trauma—postoperative sodium retention, Surg. Gynec. & Obst. 108:339-342, March 1959.

17 *Levenson, Stanley M.: Current status of some aspects of parenteral nutrition, Am. J. Surg. 103:330-341. March 1962.

18 Mattice, Marjorie R.: Bridge's food and beverage analysis, ed. 3, Philadelphia, 1950, Lea & Febiger.

19 Moore, Francis D.: Regulation of the serum sodium concentration, Am. J. Surg. 103:302-308, March 1962.

20 Nelson, Waldo E.: Textbook of pediatrics, ed. 2, Philadelphia, 1964, W. B. Saunders Co.

21 Parenteral administration, North Chicago, Ill., 1959, Abbott Laboratories.

22 Parenteral nutrition, North Chicago, Ill., 1960, Abbott Laboratories.

23 Preston, F. W., and Henegar, G. C.: Use of intravenous fat emulsions in surgical patients, S. Clin. North America 39:145-159, Feb. 1959.

24 Seal, Anna L., and others: Symposium on injection therapy, Nurs. Clin. North America 1:257-307, June 1966.

25 *Simeone, F. A.: Shock: its nature and treatment, Am. J. Nursing 66:1286-1294, June 1966.

26 Snively, William D.: Sea within, Philadelphia, 1960, J. B. Lippincott Co.

27 Statland, Harry: Fluid and electrolytes in practice, ed. 3, Philadelphia, 1963, J. B. Lippincott Co.

28 Taylor, W. H.: Fluid therapy and disorders of electrolyte balance, Philadelphia, 1965, F. A. Davis Co.

29 U. S. Department of Agriculture: Composition of foods, agricultural handbook, no. 8, Washington, D. C., 1963.

30 Wayler, Thelma J., and Klein, Rose S.: Applied nutrition, New York, 1965, The Macmillan Co.

31 Weisberg, H. F.: Water, electrolyte and acid-base balance, ed. 2, Baltimore, 1962, Williams & Wilkins Co.

32 Williams, John A., and Frank, Howard A.: Transfusion therapy guided by blood volume determinations, Am. J. Surg. 103:325-329, March 1962.

33 *Wolf, Edith S.: The nurse and fluid therapy, Am. J. Nursing 54:831-833, July 1954.

*References preceded by an asterisk are particularly well suited for student reading.

5

Nutrition—a factor in nursing care

1 What nutrients, vitamins, and minerals are provided by each of the basic food groups?
2 Plan a well-balanced diet for a day for some cultural group living in your community.
3 If you were caring for a patient who was allergic to milk, how could you provide a well-balanced menu for him?
4 Talk to two or three patients about their food likes and dislikes. Try to find out if other members of their family have similar ones. Try to pinpoint the origin of these food likes and dislikes.
5 Check food prices in a local store and then plan a low-cost menu for a day. Indicate the cost. Plan a menu with the same amounts and including the same basic food groups without regard to cost. How much extra did you spend?
6 Keep a food diary for a day on a patient who is not acutely ill. What deficiencies in nutrition does he have?
7 Check the food intake for one day of two patients who have recently recovered from an acute illness or surgery but who are now on general diets. What foods did they eat? What deficiencies did they seem to have, considering that their protein and caloric intake should be greater than normal? Plan ways to help them improve their eating.
8 Keep a diary of your food intake for a day. How many calories did you consume? Compare this amount with the amount suggested for your age group.

Health is dependent upon good nutrition, and proper attention to nutrition not only helps prevent illness but also helps alter the course of the illness when it does occur.[16] Since nutritional needs can be met completely only by receiving an adequate intake of food, every nurse needs to know what foods should be eaten daily, and she needs to understand variations in caloric needs. Teaching the principles of good nutrition is an essential part of nursing.

Basic food needs

Good nutrition exists when calories, water, and the nutrients (proteins, carbohydrates, fats, minerals, and vitamins) are supplied in optimum amounts and are appropriately utilized by the body to meet its changing needs. For these nutrients to be made available to the body, the daily intake of food should include servings from the following four food groups*:

1. Dairy foods
   3 to 4 glasses of milk—children
   Smaller glasses for some children under 9

---

*Foods for fitness, a daily food guide, Washington, D. C., 1958, Institute of Home Economics, Agricultural Research Service, U. S. Department of Agriculture.

4 or more glasses—teen-agers
2 or more glasses—adults
Cheese, ice cream, and other foods made from
    milk can supply part of the milk
2. Meat group
    2 or more servings—meat, fish, poultry, eggs,
    or cheese—with dry beans, peas, nuts as
    alternates
3. Vegetables and fruits
    4 or more servings—include dark green or
    yellow vegetables; citrus fruit or tomatoes
4. Breads and cereals
    4 or more servings—enriched or whole-grain

The protein, mineral, and vitamin requirements are substantially met by the intake of these foods, and the caloric levels are approximately sufficient for an adult's normal basal metabolism. To meet energy and growth needs fully, additional foods may be selected from fats or sweets or from one or more of the four groups.[16]

The variance in caloric requirements depends on the body's metabolic rate. Anything that speeds up metabolism increases the calories needed. Age is an important factor in determining caloric needs because metabolism is much more rapid during periods of growth and during strenuous physical activity. Climate also affects the number of calories a person needs. The colder the climate, the more fuel must be burned to maintain the body's normal temperature. Sex, height, and body build all influence the use of calories. The person with a big frame and the muscular person require more calories. After puberty, men need more calories per unit of body weight than women. The caloric needs of both men and women, however, gradually decrease after the age of 25 and become sharply reduced after 45. While mental activity increases the metabolic rate very little, an intense emotional reaction causes a pronounced increase. Fever and infection always increase the metabolic rate, as do some other debilitating diseases. The most striking increase in metabolism produced by disease accompanies hyperthyroidism (p. 731). Table 5 outlines the caloric needs of the typically active person in the United States at various ages.

The essential nutrients are needed both in health and in illness. The majority of patients require no modification of the normal diet, other than perhaps an increase in calories, protein, vitamins, and minerals.

Table 5

Variations in the caloric needs of a typically active person of normal size in the United States*

Age (yr.)	Number of calories a day	
	Male	Female
0-1	Kg. X 115 ± 15	
1-3	1,300	
3-6	1,600	
6-9	2,100	
9-12	2,400	2,200
12-15	3,000	2,500
15-18	3,400	2,300
18-35	2,900	2,100
35-55	2,600	1,900
55-75	2,200	1,600

*Data from Food and Nutrition Board, National Academy of Sciences—National Research Council.
Note that after the initial growth period the caloric needs of men exceed those of women. However, 200 calories should be added during the second and third trimesters of pregnancy, and 1,000, if lactating.

Therapeutic diets are adaptations of the normal diet and are planned so that they maintain or restore good nutrition.

Effects of poor nutrition

Infections, injuries, and metabolic disturbances may lead to nutritional deficiencies even in the person whose nutrition is good if he is unable to eat sufficient food or if the disease increases the demand for most, if not all, the nutrients. As soon as stress, injury, or disease occurs, catabolism increases, causing loss of body protein (p. 82). In addition, if there are exudates or discharges, such as occur in ascites and draining wounds, as much as 50 grams of protein may be lost in a day,[10] and protein always is lost in hemorrhage. Depletion of body proteins can cause edema, and it inhibits wound healing, lowers the efficiency of the vital organs, prevents resumption of normal gastrointestinal activity, and delays the return of muscular strength. It is believed that renal and cardiac complications arising from infections and surgery also may be related to impaired nutrition. The effects of illness, injury, or surgery on people who are poorly nourished prior to its onset may be profound. Poor nutrition makes the person more susceptible to infectious disease, and it causes certain deficiency diseases, such as anemia, rickets, and pellagra.

Patients whose diets have been inadequate have poor wound healing, develop wound complications, and convalesce slowly. Lack of ascorbic acid has been proved to delay or prevent wound healing, and a deficiency of vitamin A is thought to interfere with normal epithelization. Vitamin B complex is an essential component for many vital physiologic processes, especially those related to utilization of foodstuffs. Therefore, if there is a deficiency of it, healing and return of vital functions are slow. Consequently, every effort is made to improve the nutritional state of patients before surgery. Whenever possible, improvement should be accomplished through diet, but if an adequate diet is not possible, or if the operation cannot be delayed, whole blood and infusions containing glucose, amino acids, vitamins, and minerals may be given before and during surgery. Efforts should be made to maintain the nutritional state of any postoperative patient or of any patient with tissue injury as well as possible and to restore it to an optimum state as soon as possible.

The emotional and social implications of food

The nurse should appreciate the universal emotional implications of food and how they may affect the patient who is denied food. Hunger is perhaps the most fundamental of all human drives and is the basic response to the instinct for personal survival. Food also represents association with other gratifying sensations. It is closely related to comfort and to companionship and belonging. In no primitive or civilized society is a gathering of human beings held for pleasant or convivial purposes without the serving of food. The infant learns to associate warmth, cuddling, safety, and belonging with food and thus with life. Withholding food, therefore, has meaning for the patient far beyond the actual denial of calories. It is probable that the denial of food, no matter how fully its purpose is explained to the patient and no matter how temporary he may know it to be, affects him much more profoundly than has been recognized. Deep-seated uneasiness may not be quickly put to rest by merely telling the patient that soon he may be able to have food.

Different foods have different meanings for different people. Cultural groups have developed feelings about and values for particular foods. A good example is the Thanksgiving turkey in our modern American culture. Some foods come to be associated with status, with whether or not an individual is a normal and accepted member of his cultural group. Some foods have negative cultural values for various groups. In one society of the past, green vegetables were considered "vulgar" and suitable for the common people but not for the nobility. Because of the importance of food in all societies, the list of foods that have significance in cultural groups is endless, and the resultant eating patterns may affect the nutritional state of people.

The nurse who is working with various cultural groups should learn their eating patterns and plan dietary intake around foods that are acceptable, as well as available, to the groups. Some common cultural eating patterns found in the United States are discussed in *Applied Nutrition*,[20] and suggestions for planning nutritious diets, normal as well as therapeutic, for these groups are given. The patient who is denied certain foods that have social, cultural, and emotional significance for him may suffer keenly, and if he is at home, he may fail to follow diet instructions.

In our American culture, complaining about food, especially food prepared in public eating places, is acceptable behavior. Patients often use complaints about food as an emotional outlet. It is important, therefore, for the nurse to try to decide whether a patient's complaints are legitimate or are being used as a means to obtain needed attention or to express dissatisfaction or frustration with other aspects of his progress, his treatment, or his nursing care. If the latter is true, additional attention should be given to the patient, or other changes should be made, if possible. In this way, neither his emotional state nor his nutritional state will suffer.

Specific nursing responsibilities for nutrition

The nurse should have the maintenance of good nutrition as one of her objectives in nursing care. This objective includes teaching the general public the principles of good nutrition and encouraging people to practice good eating habits, as well as seeing that patients receive and eat their prescribed diets. The nurse's interest in people, whether sick or well, and in their response to food, as well as her whole attitude toward nutrition, may greatly affect their acceptance or rejection of food.

Every nurse should be able to help people plan nutritionally adequate meals that will be acceptable economically and culturally, and she should know how to help patients plan for and prepare therapeutic diets, allowing for food likes and dislikes and cultural eating patterns. Exchange lists are available for many kinds of therapeutic diets and can be found in *Applied Nutrition*.[20] Although in most large public health agencies and hospitals a dietitian is available to as-

sist the nurse in this aspect of care, there are many situations in which there is no dietitian. The nurse, therefore, should know good references to use as guides.

Nutrition for the well

Malnutrition is erroneously considered by many to be a problem arising only in overpopulated and underdeveloped countries. Although it is true that the problem exists in these places, it also is very real in highly civilized countries where there is adequate food. Many people in the United States suffer from malnutrition despite the fact that this nation has the potential for the best nutrition in the world. Ignorance about basic nutritional needs and food sources that can provide essential nutrients is considered to be the primary reason for the unwise eating habits of people throughout the world.[5,1]

It is a commentary on the eating practices of the people of the United States that the best-fed group, with the exception of the armed forces, is in our federal prisons.[2] It is true that more leafy vegetables and more fruits are consumed than forty years ago. Yet wide consumption of food highly advertised but lacking in basic food value has proved that natural selection cannot be relied upon to ensure that each person will meet his nutritional needs in the best fashion. One study of adolescents and adults in the United States has shown that two out of three cannot select a well-balanced diet in a cafeteria, even when cost is no consideration. Misconceptions as to the nutritional value of foods seemed to play a part in the poor selection.[1]

Since the problem of poor nutrition is so widespread, and since good nutrition is basic to the maintenance of health, it becomes obvious that the nurse should take every opportunity to teach nutrition. She also should set an example of good nutrition for her own family and friends and for patients.

Eating patterns rarely affect only one person. More often, a family unit has similar patterns. Therefore, teaching aimed at the person who purchases and prepares the food may influence the dietary habits of the entire family. Young children are often good targets for instruction. Since their food patterns are not yet set, they usually are receptive to learning, and they often can have quite a persuasive effect on their elders. Beginning with the first contact with children, nurses in schools should stress good nutrition. Many nursery schools even have sessions on food. Students from grade school through high school who eat in the cafeteria or carry lunches should be helped with the proper selection of foods. The nurse who is teaching preparation for parenthood to high school students and the one working with new parents can teach them how to plan nutritious meals for a family. At this time she also has an excellent opportunity to stress the need for parents to set a good example of nutrition for their children. Their example is important because most food habits are learned in the family.

Eating habits are exceedingly difficult to change. The influence of habit and custom and of likes and dislikes has not been given enough consideration in the past. Particularly is this true of older people and foreign-born persons, whose cultural eating patterns have not been carefully considered. Many people, however, will and do make an earnest attempt to change food patterns, provided that they learn what changes to make and that these changes are not greatly out of keeping with their economic circumstances and their cultural and social values. Young mothers are often quite receptive to guidance on how to feed their families properly.

To teach nutrition, the nurse must know the basic essentials of proper eating that were described earlier. She also should know how caloric and nutritional intake should be varied with age and activity and be able to explain this variation to people. Nutrients needed vary somewhat with age as well as with circumstances. The need for dairy foods (calcium) decreases progressively after growth is attained. Additional calcium, however, is needed during pregnancy and when fractured bones are knitting. Iron in the diet becomes important for all persons after the first few months of life, but especially during adolescence and pregnancy. Vitamin D is essential throughout the growth period and at any time that bone must be replaced. Protein needs increase during growth, during strenuous physical activity, and during stress from any cause; at all ages they are proportionately greater for the male than for the female.[14]

Before she starts a teaching plan, the nurse should try to learn the eating practices of the person or persons she is to teach. They can be learned by asking about the kinds of food served in the home. A wife may be encouraged to talk about how she shops for food and how she prepares it. The husband and children may be asked about the type of food they usually have for meals. People also should be asked to list the food they eat for several days. The list should include not only the kind but the amount of each food eaten and the time it was eaten. By comparing the information concerning actual food intake with the nutritional needs of the person, based on his age, sex, body build, and occupation, the nurse should be able to determine in what way eating habits need to be changed. However, she is not ready to proceed until she learns about the amount of money allotted for food and the facilities for obtaining and preparing food. She also should try to find out any erroneous information the person may have about food, as well as any culturally determined practices in regard to food.

In teaching nutrition, as in any other teaching, the person must first be helped to want to learn. By using the diet history and comparing it to actual needs, the nurse may be able to help him recognize and identify the dietary problem. She then should begin to work with the problem as he sees it and hope gradually to help him see other, perhaps more important, implications.

Posters and pamphlets help a great deal in teaching people about nutrition, and excellent ones are available. Miniature copies of the poster *Basic Four Food Groups** and a pictorial guide such as *Guide to Good Eating*† or *Essentials of an Adequate Diet*‡ can be given to people. A young mother may be encouraged to hang the guide in the kitchen until she knows the groups well enough to

---

*Issued by the Bureau of Human Nutrition and Home Economics, Washington, D. C., 1957, U. S. Department of Agriculture.
†Prepared by the National Dairy Council, Chicago, 1964. (Also available in Spanish.)
‡Leaflet 425, Agricultural Research Service, Washington, D. C., 1958, U. S. Department of Agriculture.

plan her meals without using it. The leaflet *Foods for Fitness, Daily Food Guide** is helpful in determining caloric needs. Local health departments and voluntary community agencies are good sources of posters, pamphlets, and other visual aids in this field. Despite the use of visual aids, the nurse needs knowledge and imagination to help a person fit basic requirements into the foods he likes. She may suggest ways by which essential foods may be incorporated into mixed dishes if they are not otherwise acceptable. Above all, she must make her teaching practical. It is useless to recommend certain foods to people when it is obvious that the necessary money is not available. It also is fruitless to suggest special methods of preparation when the person lives in a boardinghouse and cannot prepare his own meals or when he has a job that requires travel so that he must eat in restaurants. The nurse should make some effort to know prices of foods in her own locality, and she should give people practical suggestions, such as buying foods in season, buying canned goods at special sales, buying suitable amounts of perishable foods, and taking advantage of special sales of surplus foods.

Nutrition for the ill

In caring for a patient, the nurse frequently acts as a liaison between him and the physician or the dietitian in matters relating to food (Fig. 29). She may observe and discuss with the patient his food likes and dislikes and relay the information to the dietitian. She often must interpret the reason for a prescribed diet to the patient, and she should assist all patients who are allowed to select their own diets, whether normal or therapeutic. Her assistance not only assures that nutritional needs are being met, but it provides an excellent opportunity to teach the patient good basic nutrition as well as the specifics of a therapeutic diet.

The nurse should note the daily intake of food of all patients under her care carefully enough to detect consistent deficiencies, and she should try to correct them either by substituting foods or encouraging the patient

*Issued by Home Economics Research, Agricultural Research Service, Washington, D. C., 1957, U. S. Department of Agriculture.

to eat those offered. Occasionally, a therapeutic diet is nutritionally deficient. If so, the doctor should be consulted because he may be unaware of the deficiency and may want to change the diet or to provide dietary supplements such as vitamins or minerals. A diet may be nutritionally adequate but cause complications because of its consistency. For example, a person who is on a bland diet for a long period of time may complain of distention and flatulence, since the emollient effect of this diet tends to decrease gastric secretion, slowing digestion, and its low roughage content tends to decrease peristalsis.

Some patients, because of their physical condition, should be cautious about certain foods or should include certain foods in their menus. For example, a person who has had his gallbladder removed need not necessarily be on a low-fat diet; however, a high-fat meal may cause him to be uncomfortable since there is no reserve bile to be poured out to assist in digestion of extra fat. A person who is on a constipating medication such as Amphojel needs to include more fluid, fruit, and roughage in his diet.

Fig. 29

The nurse helps the patient to understand and to accept her prescribed diet.

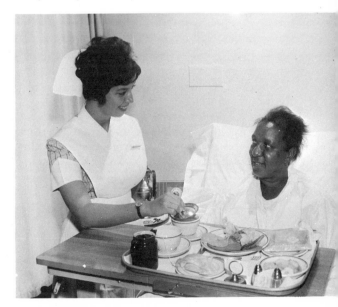

The daily elimination patterns of any patient may be altered by the sudden change from an active life to the inactive one of a patient. This problem may be overcome by increasing the intake of foods that provide bulk and that stimulate the intestinal mucosa, such as whole-grain cereals, raw fruits and vegetables, stewed fruits, and fruit juices, and by taking more fluids. Stewed prunes and prune juice are helpful to many patients. The nurse should learn the daily routine for each patient and should try to help him to be able to conform as nearly as possible to what is normal for him. If the patient has been accustomed at home to having the juice of a lemon in water before breakfast to stimulate a bowel movement, the nurse should try to see that he has it in the hospital. If, on the other hand, he drinks a cup of black coffee or some hot water, it should be provided.

If therapeutic diets are ordered for her patients, the nurse should know the purpose of the diets and the major adjustments in eating they represent for individual patients. Dietary prescriptions during illness may require changes from normal eating practices. It may be that the patient is served a well-balanced diet when he does not have a normal appetite and when he has not been accustomed to such a diet. The ingestion of new and unfamiliar foods and food mixtures in varying amounts may be necessary. Elimination from the diet of certain foods and food seasonings may be quite disturbing to some patients.

It is important to remind the patient who returns to work on a special diet that he may need to have it revised to provide more calories. If he feels weak, is losing weight, or has any other symptoms, he should consult his doctor at once. Persons with diabetes, for example, often find that although their diabetes was under control previously, they have difficulty upon returning to work.

Often the dietitian or the physican teaches the patient about his therapeutic diet. This teaching, however, does not relieve the nurse from responsibility. She must check to see that the patient and, if necessary, a family member are referred for instruction as early as possible and that they really understand the diet, will be able to obtain it, and are motivated to follow it. If not, further instruc-

tion and assistance may be needed in the hospital or the home or both. Sometimes, if money to buy food is a problem, or if the patient needs someone to prepare the food, the assistance of the social worker may be needed. Patients on therapeutic diets often need to have a nurse visit in the home to help them. If a patient is on home care, the nurse usually has the total responsibility for teaching the patient about his diet.

Appetite affects the inclination of anyone to eat, and it is affected by the environment in which food is served. Therefore, participation in making food attractive and in creating a suitable environment for eating is an important nursing function. No articles such as emesis basins should be about when food is served. Odors should be eliminated by thorough ventilation of rooms before meals, and no disturbing or painful dressings should be changed and no other treatments should be done either immediately before or after meals. A mouthwash shortly before meals makes food more palatable for some patients, and offering water so that patients confined to bed may wash their hands before eating is a desirable practice. Treatments and other activities should be planned so that food can be eaten as soon as it is served to prevent chilling of hot foods. Patients who are nauseated by the sight of large servings eat much more food if it is served in dainty portions. Supplemental food may then be needed. Children who are fussy eaters also are more likely to eat when given small servings. If the patient can be up, his appetite may improve if his meals are served away from bed and in an area such as the sun porch, where he may have the company of other patients. Group dining may be especially important in encouraging children to eat. Depending upon the patient's reaction, visitors should be encouraged or restricted during meal hours.

Irritability and apparent lack of cooperation are natural responses to food deprivations and should be understood and accepted by the nurse. She should relay facts learned about the patient's eating habits to the dietitian and the doctor. Adjustments can perhaps be made in the diet so that the patient will be happier. Members of the family can often prepare acceptable substitutes for desired foods or even prepare therapeutic diets in the home and bring them to the patient. This practice may be permitted by the physician if it is desired by the patient and his family, provided that therapeutic diet orders are followed. Diets should be planned to comply with cultural food patterns whenever possible. Seasoning is often prohibited in therapeutic diets and this prohibition sometimes is more disturbing than any other aspect. The nurse should be able to suggest alternates in seasoning.

Health problems directly related to diet

Diseases related to malnutrition

Malnutrition, or the deficiency of essential foods in the diet, causes serious health problems that are found throughout the world. All are preventable by attention to a well-balanced diet. Therefore, it is deplorable that because of ignorance these problems still exist, even in countries with enough food for adequate nutrition.

One of the most serious nutrient deficiency disorders is *acute protein malnutrition* (kwashiorkor). This disorder often develops in babies just after they are weaned. The children grow poorly, have poor muscle development and distended abdomens (ascites), and are weak and lethargic. They are very susceptible to infectious diseases and, consequently, often die at an early age. The disorder is caused by an inadequate intake of complete protein foods and can be cured by supplementing the dietary intake of complete protein.

Nutritional anemia is a rather common deficiency disease caused by failure to eat enough foods containing iron. It often is a problem of babies who are fed only milk. The problem does not arise until after the infant is 3 or 4 months of age, because he usually has adequate iron stores, obtained from his mother in utero, to last until then. However, if foods high in iron content, such as egg yolks and strained fruits, vegetables, and meats, are not added to the diet by the third or fourth month, anemia will develop. Nutritional anemia is fairly common in the elderly, many of whom do not eat enough protein. They tend to eat food high in carbohydrates, which may be less expensive, easy to prepare, and easy to eat (p. 406).

Failure to provide an adequate amount of either calcium or vitamin D or both in the diet of children may cause them to develop *rickets,* a disorder in which the bones fail to calcify normally. This disorder often causes the bones to become deformed (bow) and it may make weight bearing impossible. (See pediatric and orthopedic textbooks for a more complete discussion.) *Tetany* (p. 100) may develop at any age if not enough calcium is supplied in the diet.

Scurvy and *pellagra* are both vitamin deficiency diseases characterized by lesions of the skin and the mucous membranes. A deficiency of vitamin C causes scurvy; a deficiency of vitamin B causes pellagra. A deficiency of either vitamin A or vitamin B in the diet may cause *eye disorders* (p. 841). A deficiency of vitamin B also is a common cause of *peripheral neuritis* similar to that seen in pernicious anemia (p. 406). All these disorders are treated by providing foods high in the essentials found to be inadequate.

Obesity

Obesity is a major health problem in the United States. The emotional suffering caused by this condition is very great. In addition, statistics compiled by the Metropolitan Life Insurance Company show that excessive weight after the age of 45 years runs parallel with shortening of the life-span. They also show that our life expectancy after 45 years of age is not as good as that in some other countries. Our higher death rate is due to the degenerative diseases, and there is evidence that, with our high standard of living, many of us are literally eating ourselves to death. Cardiac disease is known to occur one and one-half times as often in those who are overweight. The overweight person is a greater surgical risk than the lean one, and often weight reduction is necessary before needed surgery can be done.

On the basis of life insurance statistics, the most nearly ideal weight to maintain throughout life is that which is proper at the age of 25 for one's height and body weight. The term *overweight* is applied to individuals who are 10 to 20% above desirable weight. This group is estimated to be approximately one-fifth of the population over 30 in the United States. The term *obesity* is applied to persons 20% or more overweight.[16] It is estimated that some 15 million people in the United States are obese.[17]

In most instances obesity is the result of the ingestion of more calories than are necessary to meet daily energy requirements. Although there are slight variations in the body's ability to extract maximum benefit from food consumed, it can be assumed that when people are overweight they are eating too much. The short, stocky person has a proportionately longer intestinal tract and may absorb food more efficiently than the tall, thin one, but if so, he probably needs less food. There are rare instances in which hormone balance interferes with normal metabolism and contributes to weight gain. Obesity resulting from disturbances of the thyroid or parathyroid gland accounts for less than 5% of the total incidence of obesity.[16] The nurse can safely emphasize to everyone that obesity is almost always due to the consumption of too many calories. If a person thinks that he is one of the rare exceptions, he should consult a specialist in medical illness and nutrition for a complete appraisal.

Many people gain weight during middle age simply because their energy output is lessened while their habits of eating are continued without modification as they go from young, active years to a more sedentary middle age. Women face the same problem as men. As their children grow up, they too often spend more time in sedentary activities and eating between meals.

This age group may not have given serious thought to the situation, or else these persons are not sufficiently motivated or well enough informed to make the small modifications that would keep them from gaining weight. For example, they may not realize that they can easily consume a full day's caloric needs in one meal. They may believe that if they eat practically no breakfast or lunch, they can eat as they please at dinner. The widespread practice of having a cocktail before dinner also adds substantially to the calories. Yet alcohol yields no essential nutrients.

A very large number of obese persons have serious psychologic problems. They may insist that they do not eat much, and they really believe that this is so. However,

in reality, they often eat large servings of the most fattening foods, and many of them snack almost constantly. Through food they seek to satisfy some very strong, compelling emotional needs that are not otherwise fulfilled. It is useless to advise such persons repeatedly about their eating habits and the consequences of these habits. Sometimes intense psychotherapy is beneficial if it is accepted by the obese person, but the results of even this treatment may be disappointing.

The public should be cautioned against wasting money on the many diet fad books that come on the market each year. People should be repeatedly reminded that there is no easy way to lose weight. It can be lost only by eating less, and once it is lost, the desirable weight can be maintained only by a continued practice of eating only as much food as the body can use. People also should be cautioned against rapid weight loss, since usually it is regained easily and quickly. There are indications that repeated weight gains and losses may cause greater stress to the body than constant obesity.[12] Before any stringent dieting is done, the person should be urged to seek medical advice, since severe caloric restriction and the consequent burning of body fat can be dangerous (p. 82).

Many studies are now being conducted on the effects of various types of diets, but usually a weight loss of not more than two pounds a week (achieved by a diet that has roughly 1,000 calories a day below what the person has been eating) is recommended. This diet allows for three good meals a day and can be used as a basis for dietary instruction. Sometimes, in addition to diet restrictions, the doctor will prescribe a medication such as amphetamine to increase metabolism and reduce appetite. If so, the patient should be watched carefully to avoid a drastic weight loss and inadequate nutrition. Personality changes or hypertension also may result; at the first signs of either the drug should be stopped. Occasionally, if obesity is an imminent threat to life, the patient may be hospitalized and given no food for one or two weeks (starvation diet). Water and some minerals and vitamin supplements are given. Patients having this treatment must be observed closely for signs of acidosis and other electrolytic shifts and for personality changes. If any of these complications arise, the regimen may have to be discontinued.

Clubs such as TOPS (Take Off Pounds Sensibly) have been organized throughout the country to help obese persons help each other with weight reduction. Summer camps for overweight teen-agers also have been instituted with some success.[15] Some Golden Age Clubs have organized weight-losing groups too.[12] Diet instruction is one of the aims of these groups. They also try to provide and encourage physical activity, and they serve as a social outlet.

The nurse should remember that obese persons often are malnourished. Many do not eat enough of the essential foodstuffs. Therefore, they usually are in need of instruction concerning good basic eating habits. The obese person also is often an inactive person. Physical activity programs, therefore, usually are indicated. Exercise should be started slowly and increased gradually but taken regularly.

Constipation

A frequent problem related to dietary intake is constipation. It is most often caused by inadequate fluid and roughage in the diet. It is a rather common problem among the older age group. The dietary intake appropriate to prevent constipation was discussed earlier in this chapter.

References and selected readings*

1 American public flunks on food fallacies, from Summaries of selected papers of 91st annual meeting, APHA, Nov. 11-15, 1963, Kansas City, Mo., Pub. Health Rep. **79**:242, March 1964.

*References preceded by an asterisk are particularly well suited for student reading.

2 Bortz, Edward L.: Nutritional deficiencies and premature aging, Second International Gerontological Congress, St. Louis, Sept. 11, 1951.

3 Burton, Benjamin T.: The Heinz handbook of nutrition, ed. 2, New York, 1965, Blakiston Division, McGraw-Hill Book Co.

4 Cooper, Lenna F., and others: Nutrition in health and disease, ed. 14, Philadelphia, 1963, J. B. Lippincott Co.

5 Fighting disease—the work of WHO, Dobbs Ferry, N. Y., 1962, Oceana Publications, Inc.

6 Fleck, Henrietta, and Munves, Elizabeth D.: Everybody's book of modern diet and nutrition, New York, 1959, Dell Publishing Co.

7 *Gerard, Ralph W.: Food for life, Chicago, 1952, The University of Chicago Press (Phoenix Books).

8 Gray, Florence I., and Little, Dolores E.: It's not just a matter of will power, Am. J. Nursing **61**:101-103, Nov. 1961.

9 *Kelly, Cordelia W.: Nurses, nutrition, and the general public, Am. J. Nursing **58**:217-218, Feb. 1958.

10 Krause, Marie V.: Food nutrition and diet therapy, ed. 4, Philadelphia, 1966, W. B. Saunders Co.

11 *Manning, Mary Louise: The psychodynamics of dietetics, Nursing Outlook **13**:57-59, April 1965.

12 *Mayer, Jean: Obesity control, Am. J. Nursing **65**:112-113, June 1965.

13 *Morris, Ena: How does a nurse teach nutrition to patients? Am. J. Nursing **60**:67-70, Jan. 1960.

14 *National Research Council: Recommended dietary allowances, National Research Council publication 589, Washington, D. C., 1958, revised 1963.

15 Peckos, Penelope S., and Spargo, John A.: For overweight teen-age girls, Am. J. Nursing **64**:85-87, May 1964.

16 Proudfit, Fairfax T., and Robinson, Corrine H.: Normal and therapeutic nutrition, ed. 12, New York, 1961, The Macmillan Co.

17 Shipman, William G., and Plesset, Marvin R.: Predicting the outcome of obese dieters, J. Am. Diet. A. **42**:383-386, May 1963.

18 *Spindler, Evelyn B.: Better diets for teenagers, Nursing Outlook **12**:32-35, Feb. 1964.

19 *Stare, Frederick J.: Good nutrition from food, not pills, Am. J. Nursing **65**:86-89, Feb. 1965.

20 Wayler, Thelma J., and Klein, Rose S.: Applied nutrition, New York, 1965, The Macmillan Co.

6

The patient with
disorders
of personality

**Study
questions**

1 Study the behavior of several selected patients on your ward. What impression do you receive of their mental health from observing their posture and facial appearance, their grooming, their bedside unit, and their relationships with other patients?

2 What provisions does your ward have for the safety of a patient who develops symptoms of mental illness? What is the policy of your hospital regarding care of such patients?

Personality means more than that one has a "pleasing personality" or a "difficult personality." It means all that a person is, feels, and does, either consciously or unconsciously, as manifested in interaction with his environment.[18] Man is a social being, and one of his basic needs is to feel secure and accepted by others in his social group. His entire life from birth to death, therefore, consists of a continuous series of adjustments so that his biologic and emotional needs can be met in socially acceptable ways. The person with a well-integrated personality has learned to make adjustments so as to live in relative harmony with his environment. The person with a personality disorder has failed in his adjustment to life in society, and therefore he has serious problems in interpersonal relationships. If his maladjustment is severe, he may attempt to seek security by retreating into a dreamworld where the realities of living need not be faced, or he may try to protect himself from others by aggressive or combative behavior. There are all degrees of maladjustment. Many people, although never learning to make adjustments readily, have achieved relative security within their particular environments. Additional stresses, such as those accompanying illness, however, may cause enough threat to their security to disrupt their personalities. Organic changes may cause disruption of even a basically well-integrated personality. Any person with personality disintegration has serious emotional problems and is classified as mentally ill.

Patients with personality disorders are often encountered in the medical and surgical units of general hospitals, and many general hospitals have set aside a few rooms with special safety provisions to meet the particular needs of emotionally disturbed patients. Anxiety, fear, and depression are normal reactions to illness. In persons whose personality is not basically well integrated, however, these symptoms may become severe and even progress to extreme behavioral symptoms such as panic or withdrawal. These symptoms are indications of attempts to escape from a situation that is untenable to them. Some patients who are physically ill suffer from psychoneuroses. They escape from the demands of society and gain needed attention through illness. Others become alcoholics or drug addicts in an attempt to relieve the anxieties produced by the problems of living. These people frequently develop physical ailments that necessitate medical or surgical treatment. Patients may develop acute organic or toxic psychoses as a result of medical or surgical illness.

When the mental illness is believed to be of short duration or does not require the facilities of a special hospital, the trend is toward housing the patient in the general hospital. Sometimes patients who are hospitalized for mental illness develop medical or surgical conditions that require temporary care in a general hospital. For example, a mentally ill patient being cared for at home who fractures a bone may need care on the surgical or orthopedic service of a hospital.

Basic courses in personality development help the nurse to understand the normal behavior of all her patients, but she needs specialized help in caring for persons with mental illness. If the hospital has a psychiatric division, it may be possible for the psychiatric nurses to consult with the medical and surgical nurses regarding the care of patients who are mentally ill. Since many hospitals do not have such experts available, however, nurses must depend largely upon their own knowledge and resources. When the nurse is assigned to care for patients with acute psychoses, she should refer to the many good textbooks and other references on psychiatric nursing. The following pages contain only a brief discussion of a few important principles or guides to follow in caring for patients with mental illness.

The patient's behavior

Behavior is an expression of personality. Actually, the behavior of the maladjusted person does not differ in kind from that of a so-called normal person. It differs only in degree.[18] Many patients with mental illness appear quite normal on casual observation and conversation, and it is only on more prolonged contact that abnormalities of personality may be evident. Consequently, the nurse needs to take time to know the patient for whom she is caring. On the other hand, the patient's interactions with others and his self-control may have deteriorated to a point where he is conspicuous. This type of behavior is most often manifested during an acute psychotic episode. It is seen fairly frequently on medical and surgical units because toxicity may precipitate delirium.

The nurse who for the first time encounters a patient in an acute psychotic episode may be truly unprepared for the behavior demonstrated. She has been accustomed, in her daily living and in her dealings with patients, to meeting persons who are able to face challenges to their security with a normal amount of assurance, thus keeping themselves in harmonious association with others. In the hospital the patient is expected to repress his fears, irritations, and aggressive impulses to a socially acceptable degree and to be a "good patient." Because the "normal" patient has a reasonably well-integrated personality, and because he anticipates a short stay in the hospital, he usually is able to live up to these expectations. The patient who has a severe emotional disturbance may be unable to control his emotional responses and may react freely and impulsively. He may be out of contact with reality at times, expressing bizarre ideas (*delusions*), and he may have false sensory perceptions (*hallucinations*). Hallucinations are usually auditory or visual, but they may be tactile, olfactory, or gustatory. The patient may also feel pain for no apparent reason. Regardless

125

of the unreality of these sensations, they are real to the patient. Hearing voices is very common, and patients often answer the voices or respond to the directions given by them. Tactile sensations usually are of crawling objects, and patients may try to flick them away or to run from them.

It is quite common for an emotionally disturbed person to be *severely depressed*. This depression is much deeper than that experienced in varying degree by normal people. It is described as a feeling of utter hopelessness or as a living death. The patient feels exhausted and is dejected in his posture, his facial expression, his gait, and his verbal reactions. He loses interest in his physical surroundings and his personal appearance. His appetite is poor, and constipation may develop. Although he may be quiet and lie for hours with eyes closed, the severely depressed patient seldom sleeps well. At times a depressed patient may become quite tense and restless, showing signs of agitation, such as pacing the floor and wringing his hands. He may be tearful and express feelings of inadequacy, unworthiness, and guilt. A depressed patient may mention and often contemplate suicide. Any severely depressed person who suddenly seems much better should be watched carefully, since this improvement often means only that he has decided on a means of escape that may be suicide. Studies have shown that the person contemplating suicide almost always shows warning symptoms in a desperate plea for help. He may talk about death or dying; get his affairs in order; ask to see business associates, family members, or friends; and if hospitalized, often make a point of saying good-bye to the nurse before she goes off duty or as she prepares him for sleep. Suicide claimed 10.8 lives per 100,000 population in the United States in 1964 (20,730 lives), and for every suicide committed it is estimated that six attempts are made.[33] In 1964 suicide was the fourth cause of death among people 25 to 44 years of age.[1]

The emotionally disturbed patient may be *hyperactive* (manic) or aggressive in his behavior. He may flit from one activity or one subject of conversation to another, and it may be impossible to hold his attention for more than an instant. Profanity and vulgarity are common, and the patient may be critical of the hospital and the personnel, as well as sarcastic and domineering. He has the exaggerated behavior of the noisy, demanding patient and may become irritated easily and express his irritation in assaultive behavior. Hyperactivity may become so pronounced as to cause exhaustion.

Suspicion (paranoid reactions) may be exhibited by some maladjusted patients. They may appear suspicious, critical, and watchful of every move others make, and they may question activities and refuse medications, treatment, and even food. At the same time they may feel persecuted and neglected if left out of any activity.

Some people with mental illness show *obsessive compulsive behavior*. They are compelled to follow certain rituals or behavior patterns that are far beyond the normal but that in some way serve to relieve inner tensions. For example, it is normal for many persons to count fence posts as they walk down the road. However, a compulsion neurosis is evident when a person cannot ever walk down a road without counting and touching each post. Ritualistic compulsions in such matters as bathing, washing hands, and dressing in certain sequence are common and, even when carried to great extremes, may sometimes be successfully concealed from the outside world.

The maladjusted person may become overconcerned and preoccupied with body function. This type of behavior is known as *hypochondriasis*.

Hysteria is an abnormal behavior pattern that has been recognized for centuries. Despite the lack of physical cause, the person may not be able to do such things as void or move a particular limb. He may have areas of numbness, lack of any of the special senses, or a variety of other physical complaints. He may have apparent convulsive seizures, although unlike the patient with a true convulsive disorder, he is not likely to injure himself during an attack.

Anxiety states are common among emotionally disturbed patients. The patient may have an abnormal fear of impending disaster, and this fear may be expressed in bodily signs such as flushing, tachycardia, and excessive perspiration. Although there may be no rational basis for his fear, it is very real to the patient and it cannot be dissipated by rational explanation. A word or two picked out of a statement made by his physician may serve as a basis for worries and fears. If anxiety becomes too great, *panic*—complete disorganization of behavior in the fact of overwhelming terror—may result. The patient then loses complete control of himself and is unable to perceive, communicate, or control motor actions. The environment is often misinterpreted, and the patient may try to escape from what he imagines is acute danger around him. This behavior may lead to physical injury such as may be sustained from falling out of bed, removing drainage tubes, or falling from an open window. The patient may not be intent upon suicide but may destroy himself as he attempts to flee from imagined danger unless special precautions for his safety are taken. The patient in a panic may attack hospital personnel in the belief that they are endangering his life. He acts quickly and impulsively and therefore should be watched most carefully.

General principles of nursing care

Basically the care needed by the mentally ill patient on a medical or surgical unit is no different from that needed by any other patient. He needs acceptance as a person, provision for physical needs, and provision for his safety. The nurse must accept the patient's exaggerated behavior, no matter how bizarre or preposterous it may seem to her, as being meaningful to him. She must realize that the patient is not being mean or uncooperative and must try to understand why it is necessary for him to behave as he does. Otherwise she may regard the patient as a problem, and her attitude cannot fail to be communicated either verbally or nonverbally to him. The patient is already insecure and probably is lonely and afraid. If the censure of the nurse is now added to that of society, his self-esteem is threatened even further.

Management of the patient's behavior

It is impossible to tell anyone exactly how to respond to a mentally ill patient. Indeed, no written words could ever transmit this skill which can be mastered only through practice. Certainly calmness and matter-of-factness combined with a genuine interest

in the patient and in trying to help him are positive qualities for the nurse to develop.

At all times, the nurse must avoid the temptation to develop a personal relationship with the patient. Her position is that of a nurse, or of a friend in the professional sense—of one who is interested and willing to listen and to help. She cannot take the place of the patient's family, and she should realize this fact. The patient may hope that the nurse can replace his emotional attachments to his family as he gropes for relationships that are satisfying and yet not too demanding. The inexperienced nurse may encounter serious difficulties and do real harm to the patient if she does not seek help from persons with more experience when patients become too dependent upon her.

The patient with mental illness benefits from calmness, consistency, and uniformity in his environment. Procedures should be explained to him calmly, and sometimes repeatedly, even though he may not appear attentive or concerned. Even the smallest details of necessary medical or surgical treatment should be explained before they are undertaken. The equipment used for procedures should be reduced to a minimum, but basic principles, such as aseptic technique used in changing dressings, should not differ from those used in good nursing anywhere. The patient must also be prepared for routine nursing measures; for example, when lights are to be turned out, a meal is to be presented, or a visit to the bathroom is to be made, the patient should be told what is going to occur.

Anything that increases the patient's anxiety may be harmful to him. The use of technical language and discussion of disease and technical procedures should be avoided. Subjects that appear to increase the patient's anxiety should be noted carefully, and mention of them should be made in the nurse's notes. Religion is commonly associated with anxiety or feeling of guilt. Sexual maladjustment is common in persons who are mentally ill. Mention of close members of the family may produce anxiety. Often the final failure in interpersonal relationships occurs in the family setting, among those whose acceptance was most valued by the patient. It is safest to let the patient volunteer the information he wishes. If he divulges personal

127

information, the nurse must let him know that his confidences will be kept and that his disclosures, regardless of their nature, do not lessen her opinion of him.

The nurse should be alert for changes in behavior indicating that anxiety is increasing and panic may develop. These may include failure to hear people speaking, muscular tension, perspiring for no observable reason, failure to make connections between details in conversation or conduct, headache, nausea, trembling, and weakness.[22] At this time action should be taken to help the patient release tension. Someone should stay with him, and if possible he should be removed from the situation that induces the increased anxiety. Activities such as walking, talking, counting, describing something, or playing a simple game reduce anxiety. It also helps to increase the patient's awareness of his surroundings.[22] If panic does occur, the patient can often be handled best by two people calmly approaching him, firmly but slowing addressing him, and leading him away from the situation. A number of people should not suddenly approach a greatly disturbed or active patient unless emergency measures are needed to protect him or others. The patient then should be placed in an environment as free from stimuli as possible, and someone should remain quietly with him until he becomes calmer. When he is left alone again, he should be assured of immediate response if he should need help.

It is useless to argue with the mentally ill person or to attempt to talk him out of his delusions by reasoning with him. He has lost the ability to understand the psychotic nature of his ideas or to see the fallacies in them. No attempt should be made to explain the patient's behavior to him. This belongs in the realm of psychotherapy. Very often the patient's behavior reflects his reactions to a life situation that has become unbearable, and by drawing his attention to his behavior the nurse may lose her effectiveness in helping to bring about his improvement.

A patient may ask the nurse to explain to him his false beliefs (delusions) and/or his false sensory perceptions (hallucinations). She should avoid doing so because she will only reinforce them in the mind of the patient. She may inform the patient that it would be more helpful for him to describe an experience to her again or more fully. She must be careful not to act as though it is unbelievable, but at the same time she should confirm for him only those parts that are realistic. She must never let the patient know that she knows anything about any past mental illness or his present problems. If she does let him know, the usefulness of her relationship with the patient will be destroyed.

Reassurance, in the general sense, should be avoided. Simply telling the patient that he is not going to die or that he is worthy of his family may do more harm than good, since it may destroy a picture of himself that it is necessary for him to have at the moment. However, reassurance in the sense of producing a calm, quiet, accepting environment is always of value. The patient should feel that he will not be censured or rejected because of his behavior. He should be given security by assurance of consistency of routine, of the conduct of others toward him, and of the limitations that are placed upon him. He may gain reassurance from consistency in the way in which he is encouraged to express negative feelings. He may show such feelings by disliking the nurse, for example. He may dislike the nurse without the fear of retaliation that would be present if he disliked his wife or any other close member of the family. Thus, hostility toward personnel may be a healthy sign and should be accepted as such by the nurse. Effort should be made to have the patient feel that his behavior is understood even though it may not be approved. The right of the patient to want to behave as he does is acknowledged. For example, the patient may have the right to want to hurl his water pitcher, but he should know that the staff will continue to prevent him from harming himself or others.

Restraints should be avoided, if possible, since anxiety is almost always increased by any kind of physical restraint, and real panic may be caused by their use. For this reason, psychiatrists usually try to control agitated patients by such means as warm baths, isolation in a quiet room, and drugs, and resort to physical restraints only if the patient's life or the lives of those around him are in danger. If restraints have been ordered and are to be used, it is imperative that enough help be available to carry the procedure through quickly once it has been started. In the general hospital an effective restraint can be made quickly by two persons holding a drawsheet at opposite corners and twirling it to form a soft rope. The sheet should never be prepared in the presence of the patient.

Physical care

When a patient in a general hospital becomes mentally ill, there is a tendency to become overconcerned with his behavior and to neglect his physical needs. It must be remembered that the patient needs good general nursing care, including mouth care, attention to cleanliness, and good grooming. Even if he is physically able to carry out these tasks for himself, he is likely to need help since he may be too preoccupied with his thoughts or with other activities to care for himself completely or safely. Patients with personality disorders have been known to lean against a hot radiator and sustain a severe burn or to step into a tubful of very hot water without flinching. Dressings must be changed and medications given. Often patients will not even ask for a bedpan or urinal or for medication for pain, and the nurse must be responsible for providing for these needs.

For some time before hospitalization the depressed patient may have eaten too little or improperly. He may refuse to eat, or he may hide his food to give the impression that he has eaten. The hyperactive patient may be too busy, frightened, or preoccupied to eat, yet he may require more than the usual amount of food. A careful record of *food* and *fluid intake* should be kept on all patients with mental illness. A record of *urinary* and *bowel elimination* is also necessary. The patient who is depressed often suffers from constipation, and the hyperactive patient may delay going to the bathroom because of his many preoccupations.

Medications are often refused by the mentally ill patient, who may be exceedingly clever at concealing the drugs not swallowed. Pills should be crushed and dissolved unless their bitter taste precludes this measure, because otherwise they can easily be held in the back of the mouth for some time and then expelled. A patient finds it much more difficult to retain fluids in his mouth, especially if the nurse remains to see that he takes several swallows of water after the medication. Serious problems in giving medications by mouth must be reported to the physician so that he may order another method of administration.

Sleep is necessary for the mentally ill patient but is sometimes hard to achieve. Plenty of sleep and good general physical health make it easier for him to face his problems and attempt to solve them. Patients with acute mental illness may require large doses of sedatives or tranquilizers, and even these drugs do not always succeed in producing sleep. Exercise outdoors, a quiet environment, a back rub or warm bath, and warm drinks are often surprisingly helpful.

Special needs of the depressed patient

The deeply depressed patient may require almost complete physical care to sustain him, and he may be almost totally unresponsive to any attempts to communicate with him. Nevertheless, the patient needs human contact both physically and interpersonally, even though he may seem oblivious to it. The observant nurse usually will be able to determine to some extent what type of activity or conversation seems to help a particular patient, and she must try to provide it. Overcheerfulness, overt solicitation, abruptness, or a dictatorial manner on the part of personnel usually is upsetting to depressed patients. A deeply depressed patient may be depressing to the nurse or other personnel caring for him. If so, personnel should plan their contacts with the patient so that they can provide continuity of care, prevent evident avoidance of the patient, and still retain reasonable emotional comfort themselves.

If there is just one person who consistently shows he or she cares for the patient, this fact may be enough to prevent him from coming to the point where he considers *suicide* the only means of escape from his untenable situation. Even though he is unable to ask for help openly, the depressed patient wants someone to be concerned about his welfare. He wishes to be protected from himself and his possible impulsive behavior. In contemplating suicide, he does not necessarily really want to die but to express the urgency of escape from an unbearable situation.

It is not true that persons who talk about suicide rarely attempt it. At least a third of those committing suicide talk about it or give some indirect indication of their intent. Mention of suicide intent by the patient should be taken calmly by the nurse but should be reported to the physician at once and recorded in the nurse's notes. The patient should immediately be given increased attention, with sympathetic and serious concern. By showing more concern for the patient, she indicates to him that he really matters. It is exceedingly important that the nurse not answer the patient in a way that appears to dare him to carry out his threat. Such a comment as "I know you don't mean that" leaves the patient with little choice but to carry out his threat to prove the seriousness of his statement.

Prevention of suicide or other injury requires alert attention on the part of the nurse. Pocketknives, objects such as nail files, razor blades, belts, drugs, and any pieces of equipment that might be used either impulsively or with premeditation must be removed. If the patient is known to be suffering from mental illness, such belongings should be removed on admission, as is done in mental hosiptals. Otherwise, they must be removed as inconspicuously as possible. If windows can be raised enough so that the patient could crawl through them, they must be equipped with "stop" devices to prevent complete opening, and occasionally protection over the glass is necessary. Doors must be fitted with locks that cannot be turned from the inside. Electrical fixtures must be out of reach of the patient who might attempt to electrocute himself by tampering with the socket or who might injure himself with glass from bulbs.

The physician is responsible for ordering constant observation if it is necessary because of the danger of suicide or of injury to others. The order, if issued, must be carried out to the letter. The newspapers bear testimony to many instances of patients leaping from windows or otherwise destroying themselves in the few brief moments when the nurse's back was turned. A decrease in the patient's tension should not cause a relaxation of vigilance, since decision on a plan of action may be its cause.

The nurse must find a way to observe the suicidal patient carefully and sympathetically without making him feel that she is hovering over him and that he is guarded or under constant scrutiny. The patient may resent constant observation, believing that he is being spied upon or that he is in danger from the observer. The least conspicuous way to observe a patient is by observing him in a group, but such an arrangement may not be feasible on the medical and surgical unit because of the patient's other illness. The nurse may appear to busy herself with a patient in an adjoining room while watching the mentally ill patient. Sometimes locating the observer outside the patient's room may cause the least annoyance. Efforts should be made to convey to the patient that he is being given special attention because the nurse cares about him and feels he needs her. When nurses consistently make a genuine and serious effort to find the best way to help a patient, their interest and concern may be crucial in keeping him alive.

Persons who have made unsuccessful suicide attempts are often admitted to general hospitals for emergency care. The immediate care depends upon the attempt made. Patients are frequently treated for barbiturate and other poisoning, severed arteries, and gunshot wounds. They must now face not only the original problem that precipitated the suicide attempt but the consequences of their act. Special care needs to be taken to avoid a repeated attempt, and psychotherapy usually is instituted. Family members, too, often need help in understanding and accepting the patient's problem. Sometimes they need the help of the doctor, a mental hygiene consultant, social worker, or member of the clergy in planning for the role they will take in the future in helping the patient.

Special needs of the patient with aggressive behavior

A patient with aggressive behavior is often overactive, and he fares best in a nonchallenging and nonstimulating environment. Noise should be kept at a minimum, and distraction and irritations of all kinds should be avoided.

The aggressive patient needs to be allowed to express his feelings in a calm, accepting atmosphere. Although he may be most annoying, he must not be allowed to feel that he is a nuisance or is unliked. He should not be prevented from verbalizing his annoyances, and no attempt should be made to talk him out of his attack or to defend the person or situation being verbally attacked. The patient should never be compared to other patients or to himself on previous occasions, as the comparison may make him feel rejected. Answers to questions should be simple and direct. The nurse should avoid encouraging stimulating conversation while still conferring a feeling of warmth and interest.

The aggressive patient may not respond favorably to direct requests. He usually is happier associating with quiet patients since his aggressiveness often calls forth aggression in others. Attempts should be made to channel the aggressive patient's energy into constructive activity, but he must be observed carefully to detect signs of approaching exhaustion and to prevent upsetting situations from arising because of the possibility of injury to the patient or others. A warm bath in a darkened, quiet room is sometimes helpful for the overactive, aggressive patient, and sedation may also be given.

Special needs of the psychoneurotic patient

The patient with a psychoneurosis requires infinite patience and understanding. He also needs careful, firm, and studied management. Usually he has told his physical symptoms endless times to numerous people and has worn out his welcome with all. The nurse should listen attentively for a reasonable time and should then try to direct the patient's conversation away from discussion of himself. She should not be trapped into implying that she thinks there is nothing wrong with the patient, and it is well to avoid discussion of any medical subject. Occupational therapy that can be undertaken at the bedside often helps divert conversation away from the patient and also may result in creative activity that earns recognition for him.

The nurse should watch for any attempts the patient may make to aggravate his physical ailment or to produce symptoms. So great may be his need to maintain an acceptable outlet for his problems through illness that he may go to surprising length to delay a cure. Patients have been known to drink hot water before an oral temperature is taken, tamper with their wounds in order to produce infection, deliberately take toxic drugs, and even subject themselves to needless operations. The nurse, however, should never under any circumstances assume that the patient is attempting to prolong illness. Such an assumption will be harmful to the patient. If suspicions that the patient is making deliberate attempts to delay his recovery are confirmed, it is important that the patient not be told directly of the nurse's knowledge of his attempts. To tell him would only embarrass him, increase his insecurity, perhaps cause him to find a new and less satisfactory outlet for his tensions, and delay any progress he may have made toward overcoming his psychoneurosis. Help of a psychiatrist is advisable.

Observations and recording

The nurse's notes are very important in the care of the mentally ill patient. She is around the patient longer than any other professional person, and she may be the only one who observes him during evening and night hours. Her recorded observations can be of great help to the psychiatrist in his management of the patient. These notes should be remarkable for their quality rather than their length, but it is best to err on the side of length rather than of brevity. They should contain actual expressions of the patient, using quotation marks and taking care that the words recorded are exactly those of the patient. Notes should be recorded immediately after significant conversation or behavior has been noted, so that details will be fresh in mind. Although the specialty of psychiatry has a complete vocabulary of its own, rather than to place labels such as delusions or hallucinations on the symptoms of the patient, it is better to write factual statements, such as "States over and over, 'I see men at the window, they are wearing red, they have come to kill me.'" The nurse's notes should also contain detailed accounts of what the patient does, such as "Sat at the window grimacing and

131

smiling for two and one-half hours this P.M.; keeps saying as he smiles, 'I'll be dead tomorrow.'"

Disorders not related to maladjusted personality

Organic and toxic psychoses

Organic psychoses are due to disease processes which have produced physical changes. Among the common causes of organic psychoses are neurologic syphilis, arteriosclerosis, and epilepsy with deterioration. Brain tumors, brain trauma, Huntington's chorea, and encephalitis are other examples of organic origins of mental illness.

Toxic reactions or *toxic delirium* may occur when high temperature is present or when toxins have accumulated in the body from disease (for example, nephritis). When such factors are the cause, the toxic reaction is *endogenous*. When psychosis results from a reaction to drugs such as bromides, anesthetics, and alcohol, the reaction is *exogenous*.

Toxic reactions are the most common of the psychoses seen in general hospitals. They usually come on suddenly and may disappear as quickly, particularly if the cause can be found and eliminated. Patients with toxic reactions almost always suffer from confusion, hallucinations, and delusions that usually cause fear and sometimes panic.

Specific disorders related to maladjusted personality

Functional psychoses

Functional psychoses have no demonstrable organic cause, though it is suspected that eventually one may be found. The emotional disorders that are commonly classified as functional psychoses include involutional psychotic reaction (involutional melancholia), manic-depressive reaction, schizophrenia (dementia praecox), and paranoia. Functional psychoses are rarely classified as distinct entities, since most patients have a mixture of reactions. Both schizophrenia and paranoia are very serious mental illnesses for which the patient usually needs long-term care in a special psychiatric facility. Patients with involutional melancholia and manic-depressive reactions have a fairly good prognosis for recovery from an at-

tack, but attacks tend to recur. If the nurse knows a patient has suffered from a functional psychosis, she should be alert for early signs of recurring emotional illness since mental health is taxed by physical illness.

Psychoneuroses

Patients with psychoneuroses are seen most often in general hospitals. This is because their behavior, although exasperating to the physician and to all who must help them solve their health problems, is seldom such that care in a mental hospital is necessary. The patient suffering from a psychoneurosis conforms to social standards and is able to appreciate the rights of others in a general sense. He is oriented as to time and place. However, in compromising his desires with social demands he has failed to make a satisfactory emotional adjustment and has escaped from the untenable demands of living by developing psychoneurotic behavior. This behavior may take the form of hypochondriasis, anxiety states, hysteria, or obsessive compulsive behavior. Although the patient may have a physical disease that may or may not be related to his basic emotional disturbance, the emotional problem is predominant and is the one that is really important to the patient. He is less upset by his symptoms than would be expected, and even when extensive diagnostic procedures and surgery are performed, he usually is surprisingly philosophic about the whole experience.

The nurse or anyone else caring for psychoneurotic patients should not assume that these patients are willfully sick. Unfortunately they are too often considered problems by members of the staff who lack the insight to recognize their need to be ill. The patient does feel real pain and discomfort even though no physical cause may be found. Psychoneurotic patients are large consumers of medical care and all related services. It is probable that the economic cost to society of this group of patients is greater than the cost for all the psychoses combined.

Alcoholism

Alcoholism is a disease that causes not only serious physical and emotional symptoms in the patient but disruption of families

132

as well. It is a public health problem of primary importance in the United States and in many other parts of the world. It is estimated that 70 million people in this country drink alcoholic beverages, and of these at least 5 million are alcoholics. An alcoholic as defined by the World Health Organization is a person who cannot control his drinking and whose drinking gets him into problem situations. Alcoholism is most common among men between 35 and 55 years of age, and the ratio of men to women alcoholics is 5.8:1. Although there is an increase yearly in the number of alcoholics, this increase probably reflects an increased size of the population and not an increased incidence of alcoholism.

The alcoholic as a hospital patient. The nurse in a general hospital is likely to be assigned the care of the alcoholic patient following a drinking bout during which he has sustained an injury or at a time when his physical ailments caused by alcoholism become so severe that treatment is necessary. Alcoholism is so common, however, that the patient may be admitted for a medical or surgical illness completely unrelated to his alcoholism, which may be unknown even to his physician. Or he may be admitted in coma and near death from acute alcohol poisoning. This discussion will consider only a few aspects of care related to general care and information about referring for treatment of alcoholism the patient whom the nurse may encounter either in the general hospital or outside the hospital.

Any patient in the hospital who is not known to be an alcoholic but who does not respond normally to preoperative medication, to anesthetics, or to sedatives should be observed carefully for signs of alcoholism. The alcoholic patient usually requires large doses of sedatives and anesthesia for effect, and he is likely to be overly excited and active as he reacts from anesthesia. The most apparent signs of chronic alcoholism that may be noted by the nurse are a tremor that is worse in the morning, and morning nausea. The patient feels "jittery," and were alcohol available, he would probably have a drink or two to "steady his nerves" before eating.

Alcohol may be prescribed for alcoholic patients during their hospitalization, particularly during an acute illness when reac-

tion to deprivation is severe. However, close observation is necessary because even the patient receiving alcohol as prescribed may be extremely resourceful in obtaining an additional supply. If a patient appears to be obtaining unauthorized alcohol, the physician should be notified. Any alcoholic patient admitted to the general hospital for an acute medical or surgical condition should be observed closely for signs of impending delirium tremens. Early treatment may prevent the development of an acute psychosis.

Regardless of the circumstances surrounding his hospitalization, the alcoholic patient often feels hopeless, guilty, and apprehensive. If his physical ailment is related directly to alcoholism, he is usually quite ill before he consents to be hospitalized. Often he wishes to talk to someone, but the person must be someone who seems to accept him as he is and to understand his probelm. The nurse caring for him needs to be patient and willing to listen. She should not appear critical of the patient or offer him specific advice but must try to make him feel that he is ill and that help is available. The patient is more likely to be able to accept help if he feels that he still has his self-respect.

Cause of alcoholism. There is no one cause of alcoholism, but alcoholics have been classified empirically into three groups: those whose alcoholism is a symptom of mental disease, those for whom alcohol is a physiologic poison, and those who develop from social drinkers. Persons in the latter group may appear well adjusted until some trouble arises to cause excessive drinking, or they may drift slowly and unknowingly into alcoholism. The alcoholic is likely to be basically insecure and to face realities with difficulty. Alcohol may become a means of escaping the demands of life. The person who is becoming an alcoholic tends to be untruthful about his drinking and to defend himself by rationalizations and pretenses. Alcoholism, like mental illness, is in no way related to social or economic class. It is equally common among the rich and the poor, the intelligent and the mentally limited, the successful and the unsuccessful. Usually alcoholism develops slowly, over a period of ten to fifteen years, until the person reaches a point where he "drinks to live and lives to drink." At this point he tends

133

to be irritable and unreasonable. He may lack judgment and develop physical as well as mental ailments.

Effects of alcohol. Alcohol contains calories but no vitamins, proteins, or minerals. It is absorbed rapidly from the stomach wall into the bloodstream. However, there is a limited rate at which body cells can use alcohol as food. Any taken in excess of the limit remains in the bloodstream, where it acts as a depressant and an anesthetic, which in turn slows down cellular metabolism. The anesthetic action of alcohol can have serious consequences. The margin of safety for the person anesthetized by alcohol is very small.[15] Unless stimulants are given, alcohol is removed from the stomach, and attention is paid to respiratory function, death may occur. Suctioning, oxygen, and constant nursing attention and observation may be needed.

The true alcoholic is more interested in alcohol than he is in food. The person who drinks a great deal may get as much as a third of his daily intake of calories from alcohol, and the alcoholic may get more calories from alcohol than from any other source. When he obtains the alcohol he wishes, he may become too intoxicated to eat or he may have no appetite for normal food. Alcohol is also the most common cause of acute gastritis that results in severe vomiting, which contributes to poor nutrition. Malnutrition may, therefore, contribute greatly to the alcoholic's physical and mental decline. The alcoholic may be in a general state of poor health with vitamin deficiency, anemia, liver changes, and debility. His resistance to infectious disease is low, and contact with infection is likely during severe bouts of drinking. Consequently he is often admitted to the hospital with infectious disease such as pneumonia or tuberculosis. Many alcoholics have neurologic symptoms (polyneuropathy) that may include severe pain in the legs and arms and burning of the soles of the feet. Foot drop and wrist drop may develop, and walking and use of the hands may be seriously limited or made impossible. Many alcoholics develop pellagra with its characteristic skin changes of redness, dryness, scaling, and edema. Both pellagra and polyneuropathy are due to vitamin deficiency and are treated

with massive doses of vitamin B complex. Weakening of the heart muscle and resultant heart enlargement ("beer heart") is believed to be caused largely by vitamin deficiency. Symptoms of acute heart failure may bring the patient to the hospital. Cirrhosis of the liver occurs often in persons who are alcoholic, and it is believed that the cause is primarily malnutrition—a lack of protein and perhaps other food constituents that are not contained in alcohol.

Chronic alcoholics often have personality changes and general deterioration of thinking processes. They may be emotionally unstable, suspicious, quick to take offense, and unpredictable in social and related situations. Serious impairment of memory may occur. Severe tremor, visual hallucinations, and marked loss of memory may develop even if nutrition has been adequate.[15]

Delirium tremens, an acute alcoholic psychosis, can occur when the confirmed alcoholic is denied a regular supply of alcohol, or it may develop when the patient is taking alcohol regularly. It may follow injury, infectious disease, anesthesia, or surgery and may develop in the patient who has not revealed his alcoholic status to his doctor. Delirium tremens is a serious mental illness and may cause the death of the patient. Signs of acute alcoholic psychosis include severe uncontrollable shaking and hallucinations. The patient often says that he sees insects on the wall and that rats or mice are on his bed and sometimes that they are biting him. He becomes extremely restless and apprehensive and perspires freely; sometimes true panic occurs. The treatment consists of tranquilizing drugs such as chlorpromazine (Thorazine), sedatives such as paraldehyde given rectally, intramuscularly, or by mouth, and a high-caloric and high-vitamin diet that may sometimes have to be given by nasogastric tube. The patient must be protected from physical injury, and signs of cardiac failure must be watched for carefully. ACTH and cortisone may be given. Recovery usually takes from one to two weeks.

Treatment. It is only when the patient truly desires and seeks helps with his alcohol problem that treatment is useful. The nurse frequently is the person present at the time the patient is most ready for help—when he has "reached the bottom" and is suffering from the embarrassment and discomfort of a physical misfortune brought on by his drinking. It may be at this time that he is a little more ready to face reality than he has been for some time in his recent past. The nurse's attitude toward the patient and her knowledge of facilities for treatment of alcoholism may be crucial in the life of the patient and for his family.

The objective of all treatment is to induce the patient to stop drinking alcohol. When the alcoholic does stop drinking, he can *never take one single drink* on any occasion without serious danger of relapsing. He is never considered cured, and abstinence is his only course. Sedatives and tranquilizers may be administered until he recovers from the nervous agitation and insomnia caused by the withdrawal of alcohol. Vitamins and a diet high in calories, proteins, and carbohydrates may be prescribed to improve nutrition and to help overcome weakness and fatigue. Psychotherapy may be helpful to the patient in overcoming the desire to drink.

The nurse should find out what facilities for the treatment of alcoholism are available in her community and how to refer a patient to these facilities. Most of the facilities do not require a physician's referral, and the patient simply presents himself. If the nurse encounters an alcoholic person in her community who is seeking help, she herself directs him to sources of help. If the patient is hospitalized, she would, of course, work through the physician in charge and often through the social worker with the physician's knowledge and approval. Alcoholics Anonymous (AA) is a group of self-acknowledged alcoholics whose only aim is to stay sober and to help other alcoholics gain sobriety. There are AA groups in most communities, and usually regular meetings are held. These groups are open to anyone who feels he has a problem with alcohol, and there are no charges involved. A complete listing of the available groups throughout the country, as well as literature describing the program, may be obtained from P.O. Box 459, Grand Central Station, New York, New York 10017. Local groups are listed in the telephone directory for each community. A phone call at any hour of the day or night will bring an AA member to see any alcoholic desiring help. In some communities there as subgroups of AA that also hold regular meetings. They include Al-Anon for the families of alcoholics, and Alteen for teenage children of alcoholics. Many communities have alcoholic clinics where medical and psychiatric help is available, and many industries now have medical and rehabilitation programs for alcoholics.

Drug addiction

While there is no general agreement on a definition for drug addiction, the World Health Organization has suggested the following: "Drug addiction is a state of periodic or chronic intoxication produced by the repeated consumption of a drug (natural or synthetic). Its characteristics include an overpowering desire or need (compulsion) to continue taking the drug or to obtain it by any means; a tendency to increase the dose; a psychological and gradually a physical dependence on the effects of the drug; detrimental effect on the individual and on society."* The drugs to which a person may become addicted are opium and its products such as morphine; synthetic substitutes for morphine such as meperidine (Demerol); barbiturates such as phenobarbital; other sedative drugs such as bromide, chloral hydrate, and paraldehyde; marihuana (Indian hemp), known colloquially as reefers; stimulant drugs such as cocaine; and the amphetamine type of drugs such as benzedrine.

Heroin, an opium derivative that quickly produces addiction, is the drug used most often by American addicts today. The user pays an average of five dollars for a dose that usually has been altered by dope peddlers so that it contains only about 2% pure heroin. Narcotic addiction is not considered to be as large a problem in the United States as alcoholism and schizophrenia. However, there is uncertainty as to the extent of the narcotic problem because many narcotic users are not known. The Federal Bureau of Narcotics reported 47,489 known users in 1962, with an increase of 6,840 new users each year between 1958 and 1962.[34] Approximately half of all addicts are young, male

---

*Expert Committee on Addiction-Producing Drugs: Seventh report (technical report series no. 116), Geneva, 1957, World Health Organization, pp. 9-10.

adults between the ages of 20 and 30 who began to use opiates in their middle or late teens. The typical addict lives in a large city, is a member of a minority group, has no vocation, and comes from the lower socioeconomic levels. He usually lives in the poorest area of the city and often has no close family ties.

Drug addiction is the expression of an emotional disturbance. The drugs usually are taken to compensate for some serious psychiatric or socioeconomic deficiency and are used to alleviate anxiety, depression, tension, insecurity, inadequacy, or helplessness. Most persons who become addicts are believed to have serious personality disorders, and the incidence is quite high among persons whose pattern of life does not conform in all ways to acceptable social standards. The incidence is high, also, among doctors and nurses, probably because the drugs are more available to them than to other groups of people. Occasionally a patient who must be given narcotics to control pain over a long period of time becomes an addict. It is rare, however, that addiction develops in those given narcotics for real pain, and the nurse should not let fear of the development of addiction keep her from administering prescribed narcotics to patients hospitalized and in severe pain.

Contrary to popular belief, the addict who is getting his drug regularly shows no signs of his addiction and may appear as a perfectly normal person to those around him. If he does not get the drug regularly, the addict usually will show signs of withdrawal. In narcotic addiction, they generally occur within six to twenty-four hours after the last dose of the drug was taken, and the first signs may be restlessness, irritability, and preoccupation. Other withdrawal symptoms may include diaphoresis, chills, nausea, diarrhea, marked tremor, coryza, and dilation of the pupils. Severe withdrawal symptoms may include tachycardia, elevation of temperature, increase in blood pressure, severe insomnia, and rapid respirations. Treatment consists of gradually withdrawing the drug while substituting other medications, as well as giving general symptomatic treatment.

In the United States, the addiction to narcotics has been considered a crime ever since the passage of the Harrison Narcotic Act in 1914. The treatment of narcotic addicts is under the jurisdiction of the courts and state and federal corrective agencies. The general feeling of the Council on Mental Health of the American Medical Association is that narcotic addiction should be considered and treated as an illness. The present methods of treating narcotic addicts are not satisfactory, and the incidence of relapse is high. The patient usually undergoes treatment at an authorized hospital. The narcotic drug to which he is addicted is stopped, and methadone, which is considered to be less addictive, is given. The amount of methadone is decreased gradually. The last dose usually is administered six to twelve days after admission to the hospital, depending upon the level of addiction. Then tranquilizers are given until they are no longer needed. The physical withdrawing from the drug usually can be tolerated fairly well when the patient is treated in this manner. However, the emotional dependence on the addicting drug remains, and the patient requires psychotherapy and rehabilitation.

Although patients receiving treatment for drug addiction usually are housed in special units of psychiatric facilities, the nurse on a medical or surgical unit may have patients who are drug addicts. The drug addict may develop any of the medical and surgical ailments that any other person may have. In addition, the drug addict, in an attempt to get drugs, may seek admission to a general hospital. He may complain of severe pain, such as that from renal colic or back strain, since these are disorders for which narcotics usually are given even before a specific diagnosis is made.

References and selected readings*

1 Accident Facts, 1964, Chicago, 1965, National Safety Council.

2 Anonymous: End of the line and the nurse and the alcoholic patient, Am. J. Nursing 62:72-75, Dec. 1962.

3 *Ayd, Frank J., Jr.: The chemical assault on mental illness, the major tranquilizers, Am. J. Nursing 65:70-78, April 1965; the minor tranquilizers, Am. J. Nursing 65:89-96, May 1965; the antidepressants, Am. J. Nursing 65:78-88, June 1965.

4 *Burd, Shirley F., and Marshall, Margaret A.: Some clinical approaches to psychiatric nursing, New York, 1963, The Macmillan Co.

*References preceded by an asterisk are particularly well suited for student reading.

5 *Cohen, Sidney, and Klein, Hazel K.: The delirious patient, Am. J. Nursing 58:685-687, May 1958.

6 Committee on Alcoholism and Addiction and Council on Mental Health, American Medical Association: Dependence on barbiturates and other sedative drugs, J.A.M.A. 193:673-677, Aug. 23, 1965.

7 Council on Mental Health, American Medical Association: Narcotics and medical practice, J.A.M.A. 185:976-982, Sept. 21, 1963.

8 *Davis, Anne J.: The skills of communication, Am. J. Nursing 63:66-70, Jan. 1963.

9 *Eiseman, B., Lam, R. C., and Rush, Benjamin: Surgery on the narcotic addict, Ann. Surg. 159:749-757, May 1964.

10 *Farberow, Norman, and Shneidman, Edwin S.: The cry for help, New York, 1961, McGraw-Hill Book Co.

11 *Fernandez, Theresa M.: How to deal with overt aggression, Am. J. Nursing 59:658-660, May 1959.

12 *Field, William E., Jr.: When a patient hallucinates, Am. J. Nursing 63:80-82, Feb. 1963.

13 *Gelber, Ida, and others: Drug addiction—A series of articles, Am. J. Nursing 63:53-71, July 1963.

14 Gregory, Ian: Psychiatry, biological and social, Philadelphia, 1961, W. B. Saunders Co.

15 Harrison, T. R., and others, editors: Principles of internal medicine, ed. 5, New York, 1966, McGraw-Hill Book Co.

16 Ludwig, Arnold M., and Levine, Jerome: Patterns of hallucinogenic drug abuse, J.A.M.A. 191:92-96, Jan. 11, 1965.

17 Mann, Marty: New primer on alcoholism, New York, 1958, National Council on Alcoholism, Inc.

18 *Matheney, Ruth V., and Topalis, Mary: Psychiatric nursing, ed. 4, St. Louis, 1965, The C. V. Mosby Co.

19 *McCarthy, Raymond G.: Alcoholism, Am. J. Nursing 59:203-205, Feb. 1959.

20 *McCown, Pauline P., and Wurm, Elizabeth: Orienting the disoriented, Am. J. Nursing 65:118-119, April 1965.

21 Mereness, Dorothy, and Karnosh, Louis J.: Essentials of psychiatric nursing, ed. 6, St. Louis, 1962, The C. V. Mosby Co.

22 *Newson, Betty, and Oden, Gloria: Nursing intervention in panic, emergency intervention by the nurse, no. 1, New York, 1962, American Nurses' Association.

23 *Neylan, Margaret Prowse: Anxiety, Am. J. Nursing 62:110-111, May 1962.

24 *Neylan, Margaret Prowse: The depressed patient, Am. J. Nursing 61:77-78, July 1961.

25 Noyes, Arthur P., and Kolb, Lawrence C.: Modern clinical psychiatry, Philadelphia, 1963, W. B. Saunders Co.

26 Parley, Kay: Supporting the patient on LSD day, Am. J. Nursing 64:80-82, Feb. 1964.

27 *Parry, Allen A., McNatt, Juanita, and Sahler, Sandra: Alcoholism and caring for the alcoholic, Am. J. Nursing 65:111-116, March 1965.

28 Roche Laboratories: Aspects of alcoholism, Philadelphia, 1963, J. B. Lippincott Co.

29 Scarpitti, Frank R., and others: Public health nurses in a community care program for the mentally ill, Am. J. Nursing 65:89-95, June 1965.

30 Shneidman, Edwin S.: Preventing suicide, Am. J. Nursing 65:111-116, May 1965.

31 Tallent, Norman, Kennedy, George F., Jr., and Hurley, William T.: A program for suicidal patients, Am. J. Nursing 66:2014-2016, Sept. 1966.

32 *Thomas, Betty J.: Clues to patients' behavior, Am. J. Nursing 63:100-102, July 1963.

33 U. S. Department of Health, Education, and Welfare: Monthly Vital Statistics Report: Highlights from the National Center for Health Statistics, March 23, 1966, Washington, D. C.

34 *Wilner, Daniel M., and Kassebaum, Gene G., editors: Narcotics, New York, 1965, McGraw-Hill Book Co.

7

The patient
who has
pain

Study questions

1 Review your notes on the nervous system. How are impulses carried to and from the brain? What are the anatomical terms used to describe nerve pathways?

2 Consult your notes on fundamentals of nursing and review the descriptive terms commonly used to describe various kinds of pain.

3 Review the analgesic drugs. What are the main classifications? Review the therapeutic benefit and potential hazard of each.

4 Study a patient in pain on your ward. Describe his physical and emotional reaction to pain. What are the physical causes of the patient's pain? Do any other factors seem to be involved?

Pain, although it warns us to move away from heat, cold, and sharp objects before injury occurs, and makes us aware of the presence of disease and tissue damage, is a two-edged sword. It usually influences us to seek medical attention, but fear of it may cause us to delay medical treatment. If the cause of pain cannot be located and relieved, its presence serves no useful purpose and it becomes harmful. Continuous, severe pain eventually causes physical and mental exhaustion and prevents the individual from functioning productively. Pain accompanies almost all illnesses, and perhaps no sensation is more dreaded by patients undergoing medical treatment or surgery.

Pain has never been satisfactorily defined or understood. It is an unpleasant feeling, entirely subjective, which only the person experiencing it can describe. It can be evoked by a multiplicity of stimuli (chemical, thermal, electrical, mechanical) but the reaction to it cannot be measured objectively. Pain is a learned experience that is influenced by the entire life situation of each person. What is perceived as pain and the reaction to that pain differ among people and sometimes differ in the same person from one time to another.

Care of patients suffering pain demands skill in both the science and the art of nursing. The nurse's responsibility is to make the patient as comfortable as possible physically and emotionally and to observe and report her findings so that they may help the doctor to make a correct diagnosis and to prescribe appropriate treatment.

Physiologic response to pain

There are two types of pain fibers: large myelinated fibers, which carry "fast pain" described as sharp or pricking, and much smaller nonmyelinated fibers, which carry "slow pain" described as lingering or burning pain. This difference in pain fibers accounts for the fact that sudden sharp or localized pain is experienced at once when one hits his thumb with a hammer and that a constant throbbing pain is experienced later in the entire extremity.

When pain fibers are stimulated, impulses travel along the sensory pathways of nerves and nerve plexuses to eventually enter the spinal cord through the dorsal root ganglia. Here some impulses may pass at once to motor neurons (a reflex response). Others pass through the lateral spinothalamic tracts to the thalamus, which in turn conducts them to the cerebral cortex, where the perception of pain takes place. (See Fig. 30.)

The simplest response to painful stimuli is the *withdrawal reflex,* in which impulses are conducted over the shortest nerve pathways from the place of injury to the spinal cord, where they synapse and travel back to local muscles as motor impulses. This reflex occurs when one accidentally touches a finger to a hot object and immediately withdraws the hand. *Visceral responses,* involving the vital organs and the glands of internal secretion, prepare one for "fight or flight." These responses account for the increased pulse and respiratory rates, dilated pupils, and muscle tension that often occur in sudden severe pain. The body is prepared for the possible need to flee from the cause of pain. Because blood supply is suddenly withdrawn from the viscera, nausea may also occur.

The sensation of pain

Cutaneous or surface injuries usually are more painful than injuries of deeper tissues, since the skin is richly supplied with sen-

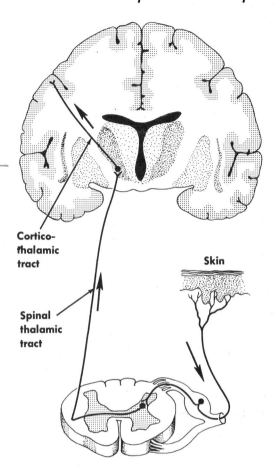

Fig. 30

Pathways of pain when the skin is the site of painful stimuli.

sory nerve endings. In surface injuries the intensity of the pain is usually proportional to the extent of injured tissue, but this is not always so, as is exemplified by the severe pain caused by herpes zoster (shingles).

The visceral organs have no sensory nerve endings, and therefore pain does not exist in normal viscera. It is believed that in diseased visceral organs, pain results from traction, pressure, and tension on parietal peritoneum or on mesenteric attachments.

The pain caused by a tension or pressure on the viscera may be described as aching, dragging, or boring. Muscle contractions may cause sensations described as cramping or spasm. Muscles that have peristaltic action frequently cause the pain to be stabbing. A sudden sharp, popping sensation is characteristic of rupture of a visceral organ.

Extensive tissue damage may occur before pain is felt from visceral disease. The viscera do not have pain fibers connecting with the spinal cord. Visceral pain is referred to surface areas that have pain fibers or to the spinal nerves supplying whole areas. Pain thus transmitted usually is not well localized because sensations originate from a wide area. In diseases affecting the viscera, other symptoms often precede pain, and the appearance of pain may indicate far-advanced disease.

Deep pain does not produce a body defense reaction (visceral response) similar to that which occurs when surface pain is experienced. Severe visceral pain, therefore, can cause shock. The patient becomes weak and prostrate. Blood pressure may drop, the skin may become cold and clammy, and nausea and vomiting may occur. Cardiac and kidney damage can follow, and, if the vital organs are already impaired by disease, even death may result.

Perception of pain

The perception of pain or the actual feeling of pain takes place in the cerebral cortex. It is known that a functioning frontal lobe of the brain is required to experience the full suffering and worry that result from pain. The reaction to the same stimuli differs widely among people and in the same person from one time to another because the final perception of pain depends more upon the interpretation in the cerebral cortex than upon the characteristics of the original stimuli. What the cerebral cortex interprets as pain will depend upon childhood training, previous experience, cultural values, religious beliefs, physical and mental health, knowledge and understanding, attention and distraction, fatigue, anxiety, tension, fear, state of consciousness, and the frequency and the intensity of pain impulses.

Newborn infants do not perceive pain because they do not have the experience to interpret this sensation. When the infant is about 6 weeks old, a condition such as colic causes him to scream with pain. The child seems, from that age on, to suffer pain as much as the adult and will respond by crying and withdrawing from the painful stimuli. Relating certain stimuli to the painful sensation is a learned experience, however, and the child will repeat certain activities that cause him pain until he perceives and interprets them as causing pain.

Atrophy of nerve endings, degenerative changes in the pain-bearing pathways, and decreased alertness may reduce the perception of pain in the elderly, and more stimulation may be required to evoke a response. Elderly persons, therefore, may fail to perceive tissue damage that normally would cause pain and thus alert a younger person.

The perception of a pain stimulus may be altered at many points by both normal and abnormal conditions. A pleasant environment, an enjoyable book, stimulating conversation, or other distracting activity of a pleasing nature may serve to lessen the sensation of pain. Tissue damage or inflammatory conditions at the site where the stimuli originate may increase or decrease the impulse. For example, slapping a person who has a sunburn may set off a far greater impulse than if the person were not sunburned. On the other hand, if the local nerve endings have been damaged by a severe burn, the patient may not respond at all to what would ordinarily be painful stimuli. Abnormal conditions within the spinal cord, such as inflammatory diseases, tumors, or injuries, may prevent transmission of nerve impulses. This may occur at either the spinal or the thalamic relay stations. The impulse may also be altered at either of these two relay stations by other activity going on simultaneously within the spinal cord. This probably accounts for the fact that sometimes bruises and cuts sustained during absorbing activities go unnoticed until the activity is over. Perception in the cortex may be influenced by abnormal conditions, such as inflammatory processes, degenerative changes, and depression of brain function, which may alter the original signal pattern. Anesthesia and analgesia also cause depression of sensory perceptions.

Pain threshold. The point at which a person first feels pain is called the pain threshold. It varies from person to person and may not be constant in the same individual from one time to the next because experience and physical and mental health also enter into its determination. Some authorities believe that the pain threshold and the threshold for tissue damage are the same. The sensation of pain often appears only a short time before actual damage to the tissue occurs.

The pain threshold or tolerance for pain may be raised by alcohol, drugs, hypnosis, warmth, rubbing, or distracting activities. Strong beliefs and faith seem to increase tolerance for pain, and it is sometimes difficult to judge how much pain a patient with deep faith is actually experiencing. Fatigue, anger, boredom, and apprehension may decrease one's ability to tolerate pain. The pain threshold also is lowered by persistent pain such as that which is sometimes experienced by patients with far-advanced carcinoma. A weak, debilitated patient usually tolerates pain less well than a stronger one, although increasing debility will eventually cause mental dulling, with a resultant decrease in pain perception.

Reaction to pain

Perception of pain is accompanied by reaction to pain. Reaction to pain is influenced also by such factors as past experience, conditioning, cultural values, and physical and mental health. Consequently, people will respond differently to the same stimuli. Some may accept the pain and be patient and resigned; others may become depressed and withdrawn. Some may be fearful, apprehensive and anxious, while others are tolerant and optimistic. Some weep, moan, scream, beg for relief or help, threaten to destroy themselves, thrash about in bed, or move about aimlessly when they are in severe pain. Others lie quietly in bed, and may only close their eyes, grit their teeth, bite their lips, clench their hand, or perspire profusely when experiencing pain.

Some people, by training and example, are taught to endure severe pain without reacting outwardly. American Indian men have rites in which they show their strength by the amount of pain they can endure. Such individuals probably would tolerate pain from disease or injury better than those from a culture in which free expression of feelings is encouraged. Persons from cultures in which health teaching and disease prevention are emphasized tend to accept pain

as a warning to seek help and expect the cause of pain will be found and cured.

Parents' attitudes toward pain may determine their children's lifelong reaction to pain. In the American culture, parents usually begin to teach their children what is expected of them in regard to courage and self-control about the age of 2 or 3 years. They try not to appear too concerned about minor injuries and usually encourage their children not to cry when they are hurt. Children try very hard to be brave, especially in the presence of other children. Boys particularly are expected not to cry when hurt, and girls who cry too easily are ridiculed.

The setting in which injury occurs may influence the external response to pain. Boys may feel, for example, that pain suffered from injury during a football game should be borne quietly, whereas pain resulting from an automobile accident may be expressed freely.

Fear influences pain. Morbid fear of a disease may intensify pain caused by it, or it may lead the individual to deny pain in his eagerness to believe that nothing is wrong. Anticipation of pain based on past experience often intensifies pain. For example, the child who enters the hospital for the last of several operations may react more vigorously to postoperative pain than he did on his first encounter with the sensation.

The personality makeup of a person also influences reaction to pain. A person who reacts hysterically to trying situations may find even a small amount of pain intolerable. People may sometimes use moderate pain as an escape from unacceptable life situations, or they may try to use it to control situations around them. This latter reaction is often demonstrated both in the hospital and in the home.

There is more reaction to pain in the night and early morning hours when the person's physiologic processes are at low ebb and there is little distracting activity. The patient's thoughts may easily turn to concern for himself and his loved ones, and his worrying may increase his reaction to pain.

Age affects the reaction to pain. The young fear it because it may represent an unfamiliar experience and frequently respond to it by crying. The older person may know what to expect and accept it, or he may be withdrawn and quiet while experiencing it because of emotional exhaustion.

Nursing care of the patient in pain

Observation

Patience, tolerance, gentleness, technical skill, and keen powers of observation are needed in giving care to the patient in pain. The nurse and the doctor are the two professional team members to whom the patient turns when pain is one of his major problems. Every report of pain should be responded to, and the patient should be observed carefully. Making judgments about the real cause of pain or ignoring the patient's and family's observations about the pain can result in emergency situations. In observing a patient in pain the nurse should evaluate the pain and the patient suffering from pain carefully. It is important that the nurse listen to the patient's interpretation of the pain he has. It is he alone who is experiencing the pain, and only he knows where it is located and how intense it is. His statements should be considered carefully and should not be minimized. The nurse should determine the exact location of the pain, its type, when it began, how long it has lasted, whether this is its first occurrence, and what circumstances immediately preceded it. She should determine whether it is constant or intermittent and whether it is relieved or made worse by medication, food, or rest. She should know whether it is affected by change of position or any other activity known to the patient.

Close observation of the patient often gives clues to the intensity of his pain. Pinched facies, drawn and wrinkled brows, clenched teeth, and tightened fists may indicate severe pain. Profuse diaphoresis and a rapid pulse also are valuable clues. The patient who is curled up in bed or who tosses about frequently is often in pain or at least is uncomfortable.

Observing the behavior of the young child who cannot yet talk is the only way to determine whether he has pain and where it is located. The child who tugs at his ear, doubles his body over and clasps his abdomen, or refuses to move a certain area of his body or permit it to be touched may be having pain in the area. Irritability and continuous crying that is unrelieved by the usual comfort measures should be reported to the physician. Parents may be asked about activities they have observed that appear to cause discomfort. When signs of pain are apparent, a close examination of the child's body should be made to rule out an injury or other obvious causes of his distress.

As the nurse gathers clues as to the presence of pain, she should observe the patient's emotional response to pain, but she should be careful not to let her own values and expectations affect her evaluation and interpretation of the patient's reaction. She should not minimize the pain of persons who report it with much vehemence and even noise, or the pain of those who do not reveal it readily. Either reaction may be acceptable in the patient's social and cultural setting. How the patient perceives and reacts to pain has been influenced by his whole life, and he cannot voluntarily modify this response very much. Regardless of the cause of pain or his behavior, his immediate need is for relief from pain. Knowing how the patient feels about pain helps the nurse initiate measures to make him more comfortable.

Relief of pain

After the nurse has made her observations and has interpreted the patient's reactions, she should decide on a course of action. If the pain is not a new or different one for this particular patient, she should try to relieve it with appropriate nursing care and/or the prescribed medication or treatment. If it is a new or different pain or if it does not respond to nursing care, she should report her observations and her action to the physician.

If after making objective observations of the patient's physical and mental reactions the nurse can determine no physical cause for the pain, she should not decide that the pain is not real. It is important for the nurse to remember that the patient *feels* the pain regardless of its cause. Recognition of this fact should guide her in care of the patient and prevent her from labeling patients and their families as complainers. There may even be situations in which the patient whose pain is largely based on emotional reactions is more in need of the nurse's interest and support than the one whose pain is largely caused by a physical ailment. At no time can the nurse let any patient in pain feel that she is lacking in sympathy and understanding of his problem, or that the time and effort spent in attempting to alleviate his pain are not worthwhile.

Every member of the nursing team who gives any kind of care to the patient in severe pain should have access to specific guides to his care. She should know why the patient is in pain, if the cause is known, what aggravates it, how he responds to it, and the special nursing techniques and nursing measures that have been found effective in helping him. The written nursing care plans should contain this information and should be kept up-to-date and available. Such individual and extremely important matters as how the patient responds to certain visitors, to his spiritual adviser, to food, to other patients, and to ways of moving him should be recorded.

Nursing measures

Raising the pain threshold. Anything that helps the patient relax raises his pain threshold. Reducing physical tension, unpleasant environmental stimuli, and emotional demands helps people relax. Activities that are pleasantly diversional to them also are relaxing.

Alleviating the family's concern. It is understandable that the family will be disturbed when the patient is in pain. Not only may he appear uncomfortable, but he may not respond in his usual manner to those about him nor relate appropriately emotionally and socially with people because his psychic energy is absorbed by the pain. Prompt attention to the patient's needs helps reduce the family's concern, and the patient's behavior should be interpreted as necessary to his family and friends with simple, clear explanations. Regardless of explanations, persons who are close emotionally to the patient may need extra time to accept the behavior, and they may need repeated explanations. However, reassurance of the family members is an essential part of the patient's care because they cannot help communicate their concern to him. This tends to make the patient increasingly tense, which in turn lowers his pain threshold. Helping the family understand the patient's behavior

often reduces the demands on the patient to try to relate as usual to them and may make him feel less guilty when he cannot respond acceptably.

Alleviating apprehension. The patient in pain is often afraid. Fear may be allayed in part by the nurse's calm, quiet manner and particularly by her demonstration of competence. Confidence in the persons who care for him is a tremendous help to the patient. It is a great comfort to the patient to know, for example, that the nurse will not be careless in her technique while giving nursing care and increase his pain or be so hurried that she forgets his medication as prescribed.

Sometimes preparation for pain helps to increase acceptance of it and in turn produces relaxation, which will decrease pain. An example is the benefit derived from special preparation for childbirth. Fear and irritability can sometimes be allayed by explaining to the patient why he has pain. This knowledge may let him relax somewhat and thereby lessen his discomfort. If he can be honestly told that the pain is probably of short duration, this should be done. Since pain usually is aggravated by activity, the nurse should explain to the patient why certain activities, such as moving postoperatively to prevent complications, are necessary. The nurse may be able to comfort the child who is frightened by his pain by holding him, rocking him, or talking to him. Older patients also may be comforted by having someone sit quietly with them, and some patients like the personal contact of holding another's hand.

Reducing emotional demands. Overtalkativeness and overoptimism are often annoying to the patient who has pain. This is particularly true when the patient knows or suspects that his prognosis is poor. Florence Nightingale gave the following advice on this subject:

But the long chronic case, who knows too well himself, and who has been told by his physician that he will never enter active life again, who feels that every month he has to give up something he could do the month before—oh! spare such sufferers your chattering hopes. You do not know how you worry and weary them. Such real sufferers cannot bear to talk of themselves, still less to hope for what they cannot at all expect.

143

Every effort should be made to place the patient with pain in a quiet location and reduce activity about him to a minimum. Plans should be made for a minimum number of persons to enter the room of the patient in severe pain. The patient cannot possibly learn to know and trust all the individuals who pop in and out of the average hospital room in the average hospital day. Unless some effort is made to control traffic in and out of his room, the patient may be afraid to relax and rest. The same principle applies to care of the patient in his own home, where the problem of neighbors is frequently a real one. The nurse, of all members of the health team, is in the best position to give attention to this real need of the patient. Some patients in pain welcome interruptions and distractions, whereas others prefer privacy and seclusion. The nurse should see that the patient's wishes are respected.

Reducing noise. Noise is troublesome to the patient in pain. Even the usual sounds accompanying normal living activities may become almost unbearable to the patient, and sudden unexpected sounds may be quite upsetting. The patient who, after continued effort, has been able to fall asleep often is very irritated when awakened by noise. The irritation and the fact that he has not slept long enough to relax often make it difficult for him to fall asleep again.

Providing spiritual strength. If no estimate can be made as to the duration of pain, the patient should be given encouragement that the problem will not become too great for him to accept with the assistance that is available. Many patients who have prolonged pain with no hope of relief can and do derive benefit from religious faith. This may help them to consider pain in a more positive way and thus make it more endurable for them. The nurse should help to make the appropriate religious adviser's service available to the patient.

Reducing painful stimuli. Care and treatment should be planned so that the patient in pain is moved about as little as possible and that rest periods between necessary activity are not interrupted. With careful planning it is usually possible to give an analgesic medication and allow time for it to take effect before procedures are performed and

to have sufficient help available so that such procedures as the removal of wound packing, an enema, a bed bath, and a change of bed linen can be done in definite sequence. It is distressing to the patient in pain to be moved, bathed, and have his bed linen changed only to find that an enema must be given or that he must be moved for a roentgenogram to be taken. The nurse cannot control all activity around her patient, but she can help a great deal by thoughtful planning for him.

With skill and adequate help, the nurse usually can move the patient without causing too much pain. Technique of handling the patient with generalized pain or a painful limb or part of the body is important. Support to painful parts of the body is essential. Supporting the trunk and limbs in good body alignment will prevent increasing the pain by unnatural pulling on muscles, joints and ligaments. A "turning sheet" is often useful in preventing uneven lifting or pull on patients with severe neck, back, or general trunk pain. Painful joints may be moved with less discomfort if they are placed on a pillow or otherwise supported rather than being lifted directly (Fig. 226). If there is tenderness or pain in the shaft of the bone, in muscles, or in large skin areas, the limb should be supported at the joints when the patient moves to prevent additional pain.

Binders, surgical belts, and girdles give support to the abdomen. Body casts, corsets, and braces are used to immobilize the vertebral column and thus decrease pain. A firm bed gives support and thereby lessens pain both when the patient is at rest and when he is moving. Traction, splints, casts, and braces are used to immobilize a painful part of the body such as an ankle. Special beds, such as the Stryker frame, the Foster bed, the CircOlectric bed, and the Bradford frame, allow movement with minimal handling of the body and thereby help lessen pain. If the nurse in caring for a patient in pain feels that any of these mechanical devices would benefit him, she should discuss the problem with the doctor.

Medication for pain. The nurse needs to know the precise effect on the body of drugs used in the treatment of pain. She must be aware of the time curve of their beginning effect, the height of their effectiveness, and their declining effect. She must also be aware of the possibility that the effects of the drug may vary according to the time of day they are administered and the physiologic status of the individual.

Narcotics. The opiates are drugs most widely recognized and used for the control of pain. Morphine and codeine are usually ordered. Synthetic narcotic drugs such as meperidine hydrochloride (Demerol) and methadone hydrochloride are also widely used. When given in therapeutic doses, narcotics act by depressing brain cells involved in pain perception without seriously impairing other sensory perceptions. They also affect to some extent the patient's feeling about pain and thus affect both physical pain and the reaction to it. In addition, the synthetic narcotic drugs have some antispasmodic action and thereby encourage relaxation.

The effects of narcotics vary with the physiologic state of the patient. The very young and the very old are quite sensitive to the effects of narcotics and require smaller doses to obtain relief from pain. The person of any age may be more depressed physically and emotionally by narcotics during the early morning hours (1 A.M. to 6 A.M.) than at any other time of the day and therefore should be watched carefully for untoward effects.

Narcotics cause lowering of the blood pressure and general depression of vital functions. This reaction can be an advantage in treating a condition such as hemorrhage, in which some lowering of blood pressure may be desirable. It may be a disadvantage in treating the debilitated patient, who may go into shock from an excessive dosage of a drug. The narcotic drugs are less likely to cause shock if the patient is up and moving about and taking food and fluids since these activities tend to maintain the blood pressure at a safe level.

Ataractic drugs. Ataractic drugs, or so-called tranquilizers, which affect the mood of the patient have been found helpful in the treatment of pain, particularly when given in combination with narcotics. This combination of drugs tends to separate the perception of pain from the reaction to pain. The sensation of pain appears less acute and therefore the reaction to it becomes less severe. When fear and apprehension appear to be the most striking features of the patient's reaction, the tranquilizers alone may be sufficient to help him relax. Prochlorperazine (Compazine) and chlordiazepoxide hydrochloride (Librium) are examples of commonly used tranquilizers. If these drugs cause lethargy and failure of normal response, this reaction should be reported to the doctor at once. The physiologic state of the person may cause a variance in response to these drugs similar to that seen with narcotics.

Analgesic drugs. One of the most useful of all analgesic drugs is acetylsalicylic acid (aspirin). This is the safest of the coal-tar products, and its continuous use over long periods of time has not been found injurious in any way unless excessive doses are taken. The specific action of acetylsalicylic acid on pain is not known. It does not cause clouding of the sensorium. Aspirin is often surprisingly effective when given with codeine, the combined effect being much superior to the use of either drug alone. Other coal-tar analgesics such as phenacetin and acetanilid may produce toxic effects after prolonged use. They should be used only under the direction of a physician despite the fact that they can be purchased without medical prescription.

Sedatives. Sometimes the patient needs a sedative drug instead of additional analgesics. This type of drug may permit him to become drowsy and relaxed enough for the analgesic to be effective. Phenobarbital, for example, often enables the patient to be comfortable with less narcotic drug than might otherwise be necessary. The patient with a severe emotional reaction to his illness will often get relief when analgesic drugs are interspersed with sedative drugs. This arrangement has been found useful when the narcotic or other analgesic drug does not seem to quite "hold" the patient for the desired interval. Small doses of phenobarbital appear to relieve most of the discomfort experienced by infants and small children when they have pain. The effect of sedative drugs, similar to narcotics, may be increased by the slowing down of physiologic response. In the presence of fever, they sometimes produce excitement rather than relaxation. This effect may occur in older patients as well. Because barbiturates may make the patient less aware of his surroundings, side rails and constant nursing supervision may be necessary to protect him from injuries such as falls.

Specifics for pain. Pain may be treated by drugs that help to relieve the cause of pain. For example, the belladonna group of drugs (atropine) or synthetic substitutes such as propantheline (Pro-Banthine), which cause relaxation of smooth muscle, may diminish the pain caused by spasm of the smooth muscles. If pain is due to impairment of circulation, drugs that dilate the blood vessels, such as papaverine, nitroglycerin, and tolazoline (Priscoline), may do more good than analgesic drugs.

Local application of drugs. Ointments, emollients, and liniments such as ethyl aminobenzoate and methyl salicylate (oil of wintergreen) may be applied locally to alleviate pain. Oil of clove, used for toothaches, is another example.

Placebos. Placebos are sometimes given to patients who appear to use pain as an attention-getting devise and to those who are being weaned from narcotics. They should never be used without a physician's order. The patient should be observed carefully to determine the placebo's effectiveness in controlling pain. The nurse's observations will help the doctor determine the best treatment for the patient. The patient should not know if a placebo has been found effective. Favorable response to a placebo should not lead the nurse to ignore complaints of pain, because the patient who responds to placebos is in great need of her interest and attention. The patient may also have a genuine new physical pain that needs attention.

Treatment for pain

Local applications of heat and cold often bring relief of pain. Hot sitz baths or a heating pad applied to the abdomen may relieve pain such as that caused by menstrual cramps. Hot gargles may relieve the pain of a sore throat, and an ice cap may be more effective than medication in relief of a headache. If pain in the abdomen is due to gaseous distention, removal of flatus by means of gastric and intestinal drainage, carminative enemas, or a rectal tube often gives more relief than the administration of analgesic drugs. Pain caused by an overdis-

tended bladder is relieved by catheterization.

Constant, relentless pain that cannot be controlled by analgesics (*intractable pain*) may be reduced or abolished by surgery. Interrupting sensory routes just before they enter the spinal canal (rhizotomy) relieves severe pain in the upper trunk. Severing the sensory nerve pathways within the spinal canal (spinothalamic chordotomy) relieves constant pain in the lower trunk. These procedures may be performed on certain selected patients (p. 916). For intractable pain in the lower leg caused by vascular occlusion or vasospasm, severing of the peripheral nerves may be necessary (p. 915).

Nursing application of medical treatment for pain

Nursing measures to lessen pain or to remove its cause should be considered before medications and treatments for pain are given. Medical treatment, however, should not be withheld when nursing measures alone are ineffectual. A doctor's order must be written for medications and other specific treatment.

Before giving medication for pain, the nurse should find out whether the patient is really in pain and in need of medication or whether his real need is for company, information, counsel, or acceptance. He also may need a treatment such as hot applications, gastric intubation, or catheterization more than medication. Knowing the patient as an individual, as well as understanding what disease condition he has and what treatment he has received, will help the nurse to give the appropriate medications or to seek new orders if she feels that they are needed.

So much emphasis has been placed upon the danger of drug addiction (and to be sure, the danger is very real) that nurses sometimes withhold narcotic drugs and allow patients to suffer more than is advisable. The patient in severe pain will not become addicted to narcotic drugs if they are given at frequent intervals for several days. Provided there are no physical contraindications, narcotics, when prescribed by the doctor, should be given to the patient with intractable pain as often as every three or four hours regardless of the possibility of addiction. However, before giving any patient an analgesic drug, the nurse should always determine whether the patient's pain is the same as that for which the drug was ordered. If it should be a "new" pain, analgesics may mask symptoms of disease that is undiagnosed.

Providing for independence, physical needs, and decision making

Decision making. Sometimes if the patient helps to make decisions regarding his care, he tolerates pain better. The nurse needs good judgment, however, in deciding when she should encourage the patient to make decisions. The patient may feel less helpless by making some decisions, or he may be too uncomfortable to want to be bothered. Pain may alter rational judgment so that the patient may not be able to make sensible decisions. If the nurse knows the patient's usual needs and anticipates necessary action, she can proceed without burdening the patient with decisons. However, if he desires, such matters as whether the bed should be changed before or after the nap or whether friends should be encouraged to visit can be decided by the patient. The patient may try to delay necessary moving and treatments. The nurse should know just how long moving should be delayed in the interest of comfort, rest, and benefit to the patient and how much damage will be done to the skin, the circulation, and other vital functions by not moving the patient or by not having him move enough.

Nutrition. Appetite is affected by pain. When one is in continuous pain, nothing, including meals, seems quite right. Care should be taken that foods the patient likes are prepared in a way that he likes. His appetite may be improved by small, attractive servings and by a sincere interest in his response to food. Foods that the patient does not like or that he believes disagree with him should not be offered to him. Very gratifying improvement in appetite has followed the control of intractable pain by surgical procedures that interrupt sensory pathways that transmit the painful sensation.

Mental outlook. When caring for the patient who is experiencing severe, continuous,

or intractable pain, the nurse must keep in mind the possibility of suicide. Pain is wearing and demoralizing, especially when it is difficult to control with drugs and when the patient knows or suspects that no permanent relief will be forthcoming. The patient may dread the danger of a growing dependence upon drugs, he may fear that drugs will no longer help, and he may be depressed by thoughts of being a burden and an expense to his family. He may appear to tolerate pain quite well but at the same time may be planning his own destruction. Plans for protection should be individually made for each patient and will depend on such factors as whether or not he is confined to bed. (For further discussion on patients who may contemplate suicide, see p. 129.)

References and selected readings*

1 Bergersen, Betty S., and Krug, Elsie E.: Pharmacology in nursing: ed. 10, St. Louis, 1966, The C. V. Mosby Co.
2 Best, Charles Herbert, and Taylor, Norman Burke: The physiological basis of medical practice, ed. 8, Baltimore, 1966, The Williams & Wilkins Co.
3 Breckenridge, Marian E., and Vincent, E. Lee: Child development, Philadelphia, 1965, W. B. Saunders Co.
4 Carlson, Anton J., Johnson, Victor, and Cavert, H. Mead: The machinery of the body, ed. 5, Chicago, 1961, University of Chicago Press.
5 Davis, Loyal, editor: Christopher's textbook of surgery, ed. 8, Philadelphia, 1964, W. B. Saunders Co.
6 *Hunter, John: The mark of pain, Am. J. Nursing 61:96-99, Oct. 1961.
7 *Kaufman, Margaret A., and Brown, Dorothy E.: Pain wears many faces, Am. J. Nursing 61:48-51, Jan. 1961.
8 Koch, Dorothy M.: A personal experience with pain, Am. J. Nursing 59:1434-1435, Oct. 1959.
9 Lewis, C. S.: The problem of pain, New York, 1962, The Macmillan Co.
10 *MacBryde, Cyril Mitchell, editor: Signs and symptoms ed. 4, Philadelphia, 1964, J. B. Lippincott Co.
11 *Mullan, John F., and Van Schoick, Mildred R.: Intractable pain, Am. J. Nursing 58:228-230, Feb. 1958.
12 *Nightingale, Florence: Notes on nursing: what it is, and what it is not, London, 1859, Harrison; reprinted by J. B. Lippincott Co., Philadelphia.
13 Sherman, E. David, and Robillard, Eugène: Sensitivity to pain in relationship to age, J. Am. Geriatrics Soc. 12:1037-1044, Nov. 1964.
14 Wang, Richard I. H.: Control of pain, Am. J. M. Sc. 112:590-607, Nov. 1963.

*References preceded by an asterisk are particularly well suited for student reading.

8

The patient
who is
incontinent

Study questions

1 Review the anatomy of the bladder, urethra, and lower bowel.
2 What products are formed when urine undergoes decomposition? How does this decomposition affect the skin? List some chemical substances that inhibit or prevent this action.
3 What is constipation? How may it be prevented and/or treated by diet? Review the mild cathartics and laxatives. Study the indications and contraindications for each. What is the therapeutic effect of glycerin suppositories? How should they be stored? How are they administered?
4 What is a fecal impaction? How may it be prevented and treated?
5 What foods are omitted or specially prepared in a low-residue diet?
6 What are the common drugs ordered for diarrhea? What is the therapeutic action of each?
7 How can decubiti be prevented? If they occur, what are accepted methods of treating them?

Incontinence, or involuntary expulsion of feces or urine, is probably one of the most distressing experiences patients can have. Many patients will find incontinence of any amount or frequency intolerable. The associations of thought and past experiences with excreta are very likely to be that excretory products are dirty and that incontinence is childlike and its occurrence is disgraceful. Recollection of childhood mishaps in learning control of elimination may be distressing and may cause an exaggerated reaction in adulthood. Acceptance of loss of control of excretory function will also depend a good deal upon the patient's regular habits of personal hygiene. If he is a very fastidious person, his distress usually will be greater. Most people demonstrate uneasiness both physically and emotionally when bladder and/or bowel control is lost even when they are very ill, and even if loss of control happens only once or very occasionally.

Urinary and fecal incontinence accompany many kinds of illness, and patients with this condition may be found at home and in every kind of health care facility. Some persons who have a long-standing problem of incontinence but are otherwise in relatively good health manage well and can continue working and carrying on a normal life. Unless meticulous care is received, however, skin irritations and even decubitus ulcers become additional problems to anyone who is incontinent.

Urinary continence

A person must have bladder sphincter control in order to have urinary continence. Such control requires normal voluntary and involuntary muscle action coordinated by a normal urethrobladder reflex. Understanding this coordinated sequence of nerve stimuli and muscle action will help the nurse to understand how continence is maintained. During the interval between voidings, the bladder outlet is elevated by the contraction of the levator ani muscle in the perineum, and the muscular walls of the bladder are relaxed. As the bladder fills with urine, involuntary nerve endings at the trigone are stimulated by the weight of the urine and the increased muscle tone of the bladder (Fig. 31). This stimulation causes the internal sphincter to relax, releasing urine into the posterior urethra. Stimulated by this action, the bladder muscles then contract preparatory to emptying the bladder. As these involuntary stimuli occur, some of the charges overflow to the pudendal nerve, which is a voluntary nerve from the sacral portion of the spinal cord. The stimulation of this nerve allows the central nervous system to send appropriate stimuli to the levator ani muscle, causing this muscle either to quickly and forcefully pull the outlet higher to prevent voiding or to lower the outlet to permit voiding. If any part of this complex function is upset, the patient is likely to be incontinent of urine.

Causes of incontinence

Patients with incontinence present baffling problems, and to solve them the nurse needs to know the physiologic causes of incontinence. This knowledge will help her determine whether functional rehabilitation of the bladder and bowel is possible, or if she should try to make the patient as comfortable and safe as possible, calling upon ingenuity in improvising equipment and in using the commercial appliances at her disposal. If the problem is a long-standing one, the patient or his family may have worked out a satisfactory solution. The nurse should find out if this is the situation. She may then continue the plan, with modifications if necessary. This approach will make transition from home to hospital or vice versa easier for the patient, his family, and the nurses who care for him.

Incontinence, which may be urinary, fecal, or both, has many causes. It may result from surgery performed to drain the urine or feces temporarily or permanently through an opening that cannot always be controlled. Examples of such surgical procedures are nephrostomy, ureterostomy, ileal conduit, cystostomy, ileostomy, cecostomy, and colostomy. Each of these procedures will be discussed in the chapter dealing with the diseases for which it is performed. Ureterostomy is not performed as frequently as it once was, but the nurse may still encounter patients who have had the procedure. Other causes of incontinence may be (1) disorders involving the central nerve pathways, resulting in loss of conscious control of the bladder and bowel functions, (2) spinal cord damage, resulting in loss of bladder and bowel reflex mechanisms, and (3) actual tissue damage of the bowel or bladder sphincters or of surrounding supportive tissue.

Causes of urinary incontinence

The five main causes of urinary incontinence are cerebral clouding, infections in the urinary tract, disturbance of central nervous system pathways caused by a lesion along their course, and local anatomic and physiologic changes due to age, disease, or trauma.

Cerebral clouding. Cerebral clouding is most common in the aged. In many instances the very elderly patient is incontinent of both urine and feces because of a lack of awareness of the need to empty the bladder or bowel. This type of incontinence is often not associated with any definite pathology, such as a cerebrovascular lesion, and patients often respond remarkably well to such simple measures as being helped out of bed and into a sitting position several times each day, which improves general circulation and increases awareness. Occasionally, ephedrine is given in doses of 25 to 50 mg. (⅜ to ¾ grain) three times a day to improve tonus and to increase alertness.

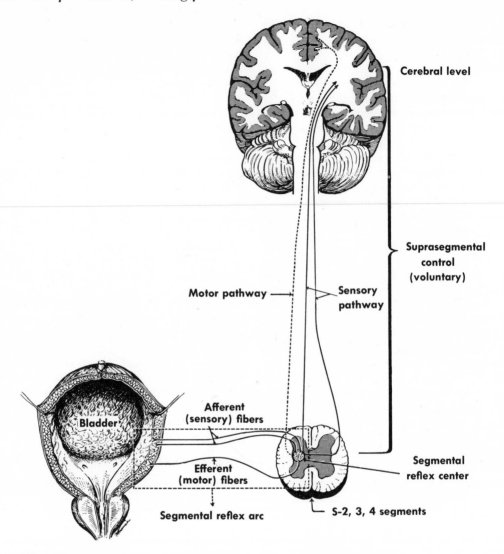

Cerebral level

Suprasegmental
control
(voluntary)

Motor pathway

Sensory
pathway

Afferent
(sensory) fibers

Bladder

Efferent
(motor) fibers

Segmental
reflex center

Segmental reflex arc

S-2, 3, 4 segments

Fig. 31

Normal nerve pathways involved in bladder function. (From Cordonnier, Justin J.:
Clinical urology for general practice, St. Louis, 1956, The C. V. Mosby Co.)

Cerebral clouding also occurs in the acutely ill patient, who may be so ill and so toxic that cerebration is dulled. He may not be able to think, or he may not have the energy to exercise voluntary control. This condition usually disappears at once with general improvement in the patient's condition.

A patient who is comatose is incontinent because he has lost the ability to control voluntarily the opening of the external sphincter. As soon as urine is released into the posterior urethra, the bladder contracts and empties. For this reason, patients sometimes void under anesthesia.

Infection. Infection anywhere in the urinary tract may lead to incontinence since bacteria in the urine cause irritation of the mucosa of the bladder and stimulate the urethrobladder reflex abnormally. This condition is quite common in elderly women who have relaxed perineal structures and subsequently poor emptying of the bladder.

The physician who is treating urinary incontinence determines whether or not there is infection of the urinary system before seeking other causes. Infection may be treated systemically with antibiotics and locally by instilling medication such as silver nitrate solution into the bladder at intervals. Specific causes of infection such as obstruction must be found and corrected (p. 453). Many elderly patients who are incontinent respond well to mobilization. Getting them out of bed and having them move about in an upright position, sit in a chair, and use a commode result in better emptying of the bladder and reduction of the infection. Urinary incontinence due to infection can sometimes be prevented in elderly patients by helping them out of bed regularly. This measure is primarily a nursing responsibility.

Disturbance of the central nervous system pathways. Incontinence due to loss of voluntary control may be managed in several ways. An *indwelling urethral catheter* may be inserted into the bladder. However, there are many disadvantages to the use of a urethral catheter, especially if it remains for a long time. As a foreign body, it causes irritation of the urethral and bladder mucosa, which in turn predisposes to urethritis and cystitis. Indwelling catheters not attached to a closed drainage system have proved to be a source of staphylococcal infection in the urinary tract.[2] When a urethral catheter is used, men may develop epididymitis because the ejaculatory ducts open into the prostatic urethra, and organisms easily enter at this point and proceed along the vas deferens to the epididymis. Since epididymitis is a painful and serious infection and frequently is complicated by vasoepididymal strictures, causing sterility, it is always best, if possible, to find means other than a urethral catheter to drain the bladder of a male patient. If a catheter must be used for several weeks, a cystostomy is frequently done. A cystostomy is a small suprapubic incision into the bladder through which a catheter is inserted. Because the peritoneum is not entered, the operation is a relatively simple one. Indwelling urethral

catheters are somewhat less dangerous for women because, having a shorter and straighter urethra, they are less susceptible to infection originating from traumatic catheterization. Prolonged use of a catheter in either sex may lead to the formation of bladder stones because the urine, instead of maintaining its usual acidity, becomes alkaline as a result of urinary tract infection. This alkalinity encourages inorganic materials found in the urine, especially calcium and urate crystals, to settle out and eventually form stones. A bladder that is drained continuously will eventually lose its muscle tone and its normal capacity. For this reason, when a urethral catheter or cystostomy tube is being used for a period of weeks to control incontinence in a patient who is expected to regain normal bladder function, it often is clamped and opened for drainage at regular intervals. Two to four hours is the usual interval. Sometimes a *tidal drainage apparatus* such as the McKenna irrigator is used to provide automatic filling and emptying. A disadvantage of this type of apparatus is that the patient must remain in bed.

If an indwelling catheter is being used, 3,000 ml. of fluid should be taken daily. This amount provides for internal bladder irrigation and assures that waste products are well diluted for excretion, thus lessening the chance of stone formation. A retention catheter should be changed about every ten days, since mineral deposits collect both within its lumen and at the point where it comes in contact with the bladder and urethra.

In catheterizing a patient, some organisms from the urethra are always introduced into the bladder, where the mucosa, if it is already irritated, is a fertile field for bacterial growth. Therefore, prophylactic doses of sulfisoxazole (Gantrisin) are usually ordered for most patients who have indwelling catheters. It is important that the catheter not be permitted to slip out accidentally. The more often a person must have a catheter inserted, the more likely he is to develop a urinary tract infection. To prevent a catheter from becoming displaced, the nurse should anchor it securely and attach the drainage tubing to the bed in such a way that the excess tubing is coiled on the mattress and

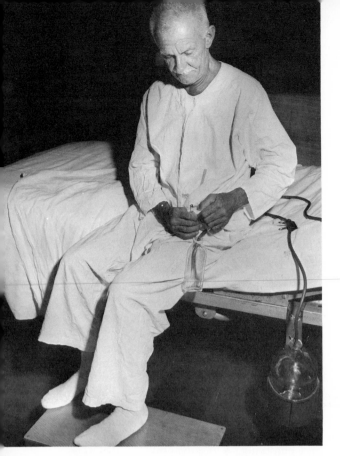

Fig. 32

The patient can be taught to detach the catheter from the large drainage bottle and attach it to an "up bottle." He is thus able to be more independent.

does not pull on the catheter. If the patient is up and about, the use of an "up bottle" prevents undue traction on the catheter (Fig. 32). If the patient is disoriented, he should be closely observed since he may seriously injure the bladder sphincters and the urethra by pulling on the catheter. It may be necessary to obtain an order for the use of mittens that make it difficult for the patient to grasp the catheter firmly.

Care must be taken that drainage is not inadvertently interrupted. Whenever a straight drainage system is being used, one should remember that it functions on the principle of gravity, so that the drainage collection receptacle must be placed at a level lower than the cavity being drained. Tubing should run straight from the mattress to the drainage bottle, and there should be no loops in the tubing. Leg urinals and "up bottles"

do not provide adequate drainage for a patient who is in a reclining position, but neither does the long drainage tubing used in bed provide adequate drainage for the patient who is up in a chair or walking about. The inappropriate use of either arrangement causes the tube to act as a cork, with resultant retention of urine and infection. Urine also may leak around the tube or other apparatus.

Because of the contraindications to the use of indwelling catheters, the resourceful nurse will usually try to control incontinence due to lack of voluntary control by other means.

In *toilet training* children, one takes them to the toilet at regular intervals to void. This same plan can be employed with an incontinent adult. People ordinarily void upon awakening, before retiring, and before or after meals. If a diuretic such as coffee has been taken, it is usually necessary to void about half an hour later. Using this knowledge, the nurse can begin to set up a schedule for placing the patient on a bedpan or taking him to the toilet. Then, if a record is kept for a few days of the times that the patient voids involuntarily, it is usually possible to determine the individual's normal voiding pattern. If the nurse carefully follows this schedule, the problem of incontinence should become minimal. It is important to know the amount the patient voids and to see that the bladder is not distended after voiding. Voiding in frequent small amounts may indicate that the bladder is overflowing as it becomes overdistended. The muscles are not contracting strongly enough to empty it completely. Gentle manual pressure applied downward and backward above the bladder will sometimes give the added impetus needed to stimulate the involuntary nerve pathways. Frequent voiding in small amounts is sometimes due to the pressure of a bowel distended with flatus or feces and can be relieved by the insertion of a rectal tube to release the flatus or by enemas.

Sometimes it is impossible to keep the patient on a voiding schedule. If so, a form of *external drainage* can also be used for a male patient because a watertight apparatus can easily be applied. A satisfactory method is as follows: Tie the closed end of a thin

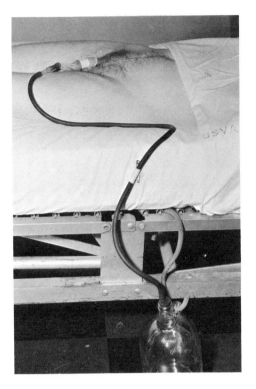

A

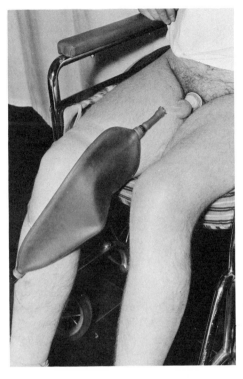

B

Fig. 33

Urinary incontinence in a man can be controlled by the use of an external drainage apparatus. **A**, The apparatus is arranged for the bed patient. **B**, The use of external drainage for the ambulatory patient. (Courtesy Medical Illustration Service, Veterans Administration Hospital, Hines, Ill.)

plastic or rubber penile sheath securely over one end of a large glass connecting tube; make a hole in the sheath so that the urine can drain into the connecting tube; carefully cleanse, shave, and dry the penis; pull the foreskin over the glans; invert the sheath and roll it onto the penis, leaving only about one-half inch between the meatus and the connecting tube. Secure the top of the sheath to the shaft of the penis with adhesive tape after tincture of benzoin has been applied to the skin. The adhesive should serve as a seal, yet not be tight enough to cause constriction in case of penile erection. The penis should be checked frequently for signs of skin irritation. The sheath should be changed and the skin thoroughly cleansed once every twenty-four hours.[3] (See Fig. 33.) External drainage apparatus, similar to that described, is now available commercially. Plastic incontinence urinals are available, but in using these there is great danger of skin irritation. Unless they are kept meticulously clean and aired daily, there is the additional problem of odor. External drainage may be used with an "up bottle" or leg urinal when the patient is ambulatory. Since it may be embarrassing and upsetting to a man to have a young nurse apply this type of drainage apparatus, someone else may need to do this procedure. If there is no male member of the nursing team, an older, more mature nurse may be called upon, or the patient's wife, brother, or son may be taught to care for this personal need. At other times the doctor may be willing to do this, or the patient may be able to do it himself.

Diseases such as cerebral embolus, cerebral hemorrhage, brain tumor, meningitis, or traumatic injury of the brain may permanently damage the original pathways that enable the patient to control voiding consciously. New pathways can usually be established if a persistent *retraining program* is carried out. As with the acutely ill or comatose patient, a voiding schedule is set up and strictly adhered to until gradually the patient again learns to recognize and react appropriately to the feeling of having to void. A successful program of this type, leading to complete rehabilitation, requires a mentally competent patient. Otherwise someone else must always remind the patient to follow the schedule.

Disturbance of the urethrobladder reflex. Any obstruction to the spinal nerve tracts above the sacral level of the spinal cord where the pudendal nerves synapse will cause incontinence. The obstruction prevents the transmission of the impulse to void to the central nervous system, and thus no conscious control is exercised. This form of incontinence may be seen in patients with cord injuries, cord tumors, tabes dorsalis, and compression of the cord from fractures of the vertebras, herniated disc, metastatic tumor in a vertebra, or postoperative edema of the spinal cord. This type of difficulty can result in two types of responses known as "neurogenic bladder." The bladder may be spastic, causing inability to retain any urine, or flaccid, causing the bladder to overflow periodically. Patients with neurogenic bladders have no way of knowing when they are going to void and are frequently embarrassed by this problem.

Incontinence due to neurogenic bladder can best be controlled by developing an *automatic bladder*—one that is trained to empty at regular intervals. A regular schedule of both intake and output is worked out with the patient by trial and error. Fluids are spaced in such a way that the bladder is filled and ready to empty at designated times. The schedule can be planned for the convenience of the patient and adapted to his living pattern. For instance, if he wishes to go out, the patient will limit fluids for several hours. Most patients limit fluids in the evening so that the bladder will be less likely to empty during the night. They should plan to force fluids to 3,000 ml.

within the twenty-four-hour period, however. This measure is necessary because neurogenic bladders seldom empty completely and infection and stone formation may occur. Since alcohol, the caffeine in tea and coffee, and the theobromine in tea and cocoa tend to stimulate the kidneys and upset the voiding pattern, it is wise to avoid them.

Patients may learn to recognize a full bladder by such systemic reactions as restlessness, sweaty or chilly sensations, or great abdominal discomfort. (Restlessness may also serve as a guide to the nurse in knowing when an unconscious patient should be placed on the bedpan.) If the patient has trouble starting to void, brushing motions over trigger areas such as the inner aspects of the thighs or over the bladder may stimulate micturition. Sometimes special positions such as one in which the patient leans forward will help, or it may be necessary to use the *Credé* method, which consists of exerting manual pressure over the bladder. This method may also be used to ensure more nearly complete emptying of the bladder.

It is important for both the patient and the nurse to know that this type of rehabilitation may take weeks and even months to accomplish. The patient often becomes discouraged by recurring accidental voiding and needs a great deal of encouragement. It is helpful if the patient is taught the physiology of voiding so that he can better understand and help in his rehabilitation. The rehabilitation of the patient with a neurogenic bladder is a complex undertaking. For a fuller discussion of this subject see specialized textbooks.[16]

Usually the patient will feel more secure if he wears some type of drainage apparatus in case of accidental dribbling. Men may wear an *incontinence urinal* (Fig. 34) or a *penile clamp* (Fig. 35), which mechanically compresses the urethral wall. Penile clamps usually are uncomfortable and must be released and repositioned every two hours to prevent circulatory obstruction. This procedure needs to be especially stressed to the paraplegic patient since he does not have sensation in the penis. Most patients who use clamps alternate them with an incontinence urinal and use the clamp primarily when they are going out.

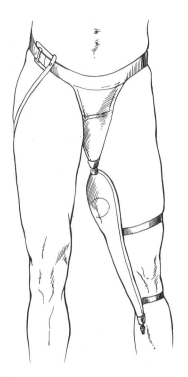

Fig. 34

An incontinence urinal. Note that it is supported by a strap about the waist and under the buttock and is connected to a drainage bag strapped to the leg. The stopper at the end of the drainage bag can be removed for emptying.

To improvise protection for the incontinent male patient, a shower cap can be used. Cut a hole near the elasticized edge big enough to fit around the penis. Bind the opening with adhesive tape to prevent tearing of the cap and skin irritation. Fill the inside of the cap with absorbent material placed in doughnut fashion. Then, slipping the penis inside, pin the edges of the cap together. If more support is needed, the cap may be pinned to a belt. This improvization may be used if skin irritation has resulted from the use of other external devices to collect urine. It may also be used following a perineal prostatectomy when every effort is being made to have the patient void normally. Methods that give more protection may decrease his efforts to achieve continence.

Protection for women with incontinence

presents an extremely difficult problem. At present the most satisfactory method is the use of perineal pads and plastic-lined pants (Fig. 36).

Tissue damage. Damage to the sphincters of the bladder from instrumentation, surgery, or accidents, scarring following urethral infections, lesions involving the sphincters, or relaxation of the perineal structures may cause urinary incontinence. The latter cause of incontinence is seen occasionally following childbirth. The problem is local in nature and does not involve the nervous system.

It is practically impossible to repair a sphincter that has been cut. If only the external sphincter has been damaged, the patient will be incontinent on urgency. A voiding schedule can be set up so that he will always void before the bladder is full enough to exert sufficient pressure to open the internal sphincter involuntarily. If only the internal sphincter is damaged, the patient may have no acute feeling of the need to void. Here, the problem is not one of in-

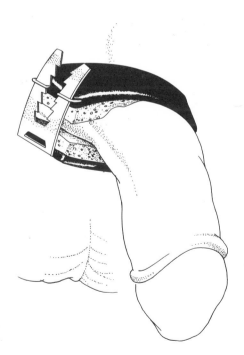

Fig. 35

Penile incontinence clamp. It should be applied at the base of the penis.

continence but of retention. To assure the regular emptying of the bladder, he, too, should use a voiding schedule. If both sphincters are damaged, the patient will be totally incontinent and will require permanent catheter drainage or the use of external protection.

Some conditions respond to treatment. For example, a levator ani muscle that is shortened by scar tissue, thus holding the bladder outlet at a downward angle and allowing a continuous dribbling or causing frequency of urination, may be treated surgically. Sometimes lesions may be surgically removed or improvements effected by plastic procedures.

Incontinence due to relaxation of the sphincters and the perineum presents serious problems. In men this condition may follow prostatic surgery or prolonged use of an indwelling catheter. In women it may follow childbirth, although some women who have had no children have relaxation of the perineum. Among adult women, 5.5% are reported to have poor control of the bladder outlet.[8] In both sexes old age may cause relaxation of the muscles and consequent incontinence. The patient with this type of problem is taught *perineal exercises*, which consist of contracting the abdominal, gluteal, and perineal muscles while breathing normally. These exercises can be explained by asking the patient to hold himself as he would if he needed to void very badly and there were no available facilities. Sometimes gluteal muscle tone can be increased by having the patient hold a pencil in the fold between the buttock and the thigh. Stopping and starting the urinary stream during voiding will give additional exercise. The patient should strive eventually to maintain a constant muscle tone. Although operations designed to tighten the muscles are sometimes attempted, the results are not always predictable. Much of the problem of incontinence due to a relaxed perineum in women can be prevented if perineal exercises are taught before and following childbirth. These exercises also may be included as part of the health teaching of any woman.

Another serious problem of incontinence occurs in women who have vesicovaginal fistulas. They may result from childbirth injuries or surgical injuries of the vagina or uterus. They also may occur after x-ray therapy for carcinoma of the cervix (p. 512).

Care of the skin of incontinent patients

Care of the skin is very important in incontinent patients. The perineal and genital areas should be thoroughly washed several times a day. Tub baths are preferable to showers. Washing the skin with soap and water will help prevent irritation and odor. Exposure to the air is beneficial. Since the acid or alkali in the urine will penetrate any ointment, ointments are useless in protecting the skin. If the skin becomes irritated, a heat lamp should be used for fifteen minutes after each bath. A zinc oxide powder, such as one used for babies, can be applied and may be helpful in reducing irritation. Cornstarch powder is often helpful in preventing itching.

Incontinence in children

If incontinence presents baffling problems in the care of adult patients, enuresis, or failure of children to gain and maintain urinary control, can sometimes be even more complex for parents to understand and manage. Overcoming this problem may be delayed until the child is in school, and then parents become anxious because teachers and others constantly bring it to their attention. Nurses can be particularly helpful to parents by understanding their emotional distress and by helping them to examine the circumstances in which the problem seems to have developed.

The infant is born with an automatic bladder that empties reflexly when filled to a certain point. When the nervous system is developed more fully, the child begins to learn voluntary control. Children between the ages of 1 and 2 years usually recognize imminence of micturition and can prevent voiding for a period of time. Day control is usually achieved more readily than night control. Children vary in the rate at which they develop voluntary urinary control just as they vary in other development, but by 4½ years of age, approximately 87.8% of all children have complete control.[11] At about 5 years of age most children have the ability to start the urinary stream at will and to stop midstream.[11]

It often is difficult to determine whether

the child with enuresis has a psychologic or a purely physical problem. The nurse who is helping the parents can often establish a description of the circumstances for a pediatrician's evaluation. Review of the development of normal bladder control for infants and children may help parents to remember details of events as they occurred for their child. The nurse also should learn about the child's total growth and developmental pattern from birth, including details of bowel control. If the problem developed after urinary control had been established, she should try to elicit the events in the child's family life and relationships preceding the onset of the problem. Questions regarding other children in the family and their development also may give clues.

If the problem seems to be a behavioral one, the parents can be helped to understand the problem and to work through a solution with the child. Bed-wetting may have been a problem for one or both parents, and their acceptance of this or their reaction to it may be quite different from the reaction of those persons who have not experienced it. In some instances the problem may be very complex, and the pediatrician may recommend psychiatric help for the family.

The child's problem, however, may be one of physiologic underdevelopment or actual pathology. Small bladder capacity is one of the most common causes of enuresis. The child may learn to compensate by drinking small amounts of fluid and emptying his bladder voluntarily at short intervals both in the daytime and during the night, but a training program with the objective of increasing the bladder capacity usually is more successful. A record of intake and output is kept for a few days to establish the usual pattern. The child then is encouraged to drink an increased amount of fluid during the day and to postpone voiding for as long as possible. If the child is old enough, it may be helpful to have him help keep the measurements since this participation may encourage him to try for larger capacities. The program should continue until the child has a bladder capacity of at least 250 ml., but preferably 400 ml., and this may take three to six months.

Bladder neck contracture, urinary tract infection, or other pathologic conditions may cause enuresis. The pediatrician will determine if a urologic examination is necessary.

Fecal incontinence

In fecal incontinence the anal sphincter may be relaxed, the voluntary control of defecation may be interrupted in the central nervous system, or messages may not be transmitted to the brain because of a lesion within the cord or external pressure on the cord above the sacral segments. The disorders causing breakdown of conscious control are identical with those affecting the bladder. Perineal relaxation and actual damage of the anal sphincter are often caused by injury during childbirth or during perineal operations. Relaxation usually increases with the general loss of muscle tone in aging. Perineal exercises similar to those used in urinary incontinence may help some patients.

If fecal incontinence is to be prevented, bowel training or a regular routine of stimulation of peristalsis and of going to the toilet should be carried out. Ordinarily the bowel is trained to empty at regular intervals. Once a day or every other day after breakfast is common. Food and fluids increase peristalsis, which many stimulate defecation. The taking of certain food or fluids may be associated with the accustomed time for defecation. For example, coffee or orange juice may provide the stimulus for some people. Most patients will be more relaxed and thus more likely to have a bowel movement if placed in as near the normal position as possible and if they have privacy. Glycerin suppositories (usually two are needed) help stimulate evacuation of the bowel; they should be inserted about two hours before the usual time of defecation. They should be lubricated with petrolatum and pushed well into the rectum with a gloved finger. If the patient is unconscious or has disease of the spinal cord, it may be necessary to use an enema or the laxative suppository, bisacodyl (Dulcolax). Usually about one quart of enema fluid is needed at one time to stimulate reflex peristalsis. Fluid is more easily retained if the patient is on his side. It may be necessary to pinch the buttocks together securely around the rectal tube to retain the fluid in the bowel, or to use a Foley catheter, inflating the balloon to help retain the fluid in the bowel. If a Foley catheter is used, insert it four inches into the rectum and then inflate the balloon with 30 or 40 ml. of fluid. After giving the enema, wait five minutes and then, with the patient on the bedpan or toilet, deflate the balloon. Patients may not get full results for one to two hours or longer following enemas, so they should be provided with protective padding.

Results from bisacodyl usually occur within a half hour. Care must be taken not to insert the suppository into a bolus of stool since it is then ineffective.

Sometimes it is possible for patients with cord lesions to develop *automatic* defecation. They may need to use a cathartic nightly, such as milk of magnesia, and to dilate the anal sphincter digitally, using a gloved finger. Manual pressure on the abdomen, rubbing toward the sigmoid and rectal areas, stimulates peristalsis. A diet that will form a soft stool should be given. The general welfare of the patient is benefited so much by automatic defecation that the time and energy expended to accomplish it are well spent.

Incontinent patients may have *diarrhea,* which may be a symptom of *fecal impaction.* The doctor usually makes a rectal examination, breaking up the impaction if necessary, and then an oil enema followed by a cleansing enema is given. Impaction is frequently a problem of the elderly, and the public health nurse often receives orders to loosen or break up the impaction. She should use lubricating jelly or cream on a gloved finger and gently remove feces from the lower rectum only. If the leakage continues despite enemas, and it is liquid in consistency, a rectal tube (28 or 30 Fr.) may be inserted into the rectum and anchored in the fold under the buttock with adhesive tape and attached to straight drainage. (See p. 444 for method of anchoring tubes.) If the diarrhea is not due to an impaction, one should look for other causes. A patient may find that certain foods cause him to have diarrhea. The nurse can help him analyze his diet and avoid foods that cause trouble. Emotional stress may also cause diarrhea, so it is important that it be reduced in any way possible. Diarrhea is a rather common reaction to medications, especially the antibi-

otics. Camphorated tincture of opium, bismuth subcarbonate, or kaolin may be given in an attempt to control the diarrhea. The camphorated tincture of opium slows down peristalsis, and the other two drugs have a soothing effect in the intestinal mucosa because of their coating property. These drugs are usually given after meals and after each loose bowel movement.

Uncontrolled urinary and fecal incontinence

Some patients will have urinary and fecal incontinence despite all efforts. The nurse must see that they are kept clean, odorless, and free from decubiti. Linen must be changed as soon as it is soiled. Newspaper pads covered with a piece of cloth can be used to protect bedding and furniture. Oilcloth and the newer plastic materials also can be used. Many commercial products of soft, absorbent cellucotton backed with light plastic are available. They come in a variety of sizes to be placed just under the buttock area or to cover approximately a square yard. Large rolls of absorbent cellucotton of several thicknesses can be purchased and then cut to the size desired.

Linen may be protected from soiling and the patient made more comfortable if pants made of some absorbent material backed with plastic are used (Fig. 36). A resourceful person may be able to improvise equipment that will be more comfortable and less costly than commercially manufactured pants. Zippers, snap-tape and ties, elastic, and a variety of fabrics and waterproof materials may be used. Cellucotton for padding is less expensive if purchased in large rather than small rolls. The commercial diaper service for adult patients is now becoming more available. It ensures a steady supply of dry, soft materials and spares the family from constantly searching for and making up improvised supplies.

Any padding used must be changed often, and the skin must be thoroughly washed and dried at each changing. If possible, the patient should be bathed in a tub of warm water at least once a day. Commercial preparations, such as methylbenzethonium chloride (Diaparene), that control odor of urine and to some extent lessen its irritating prop-

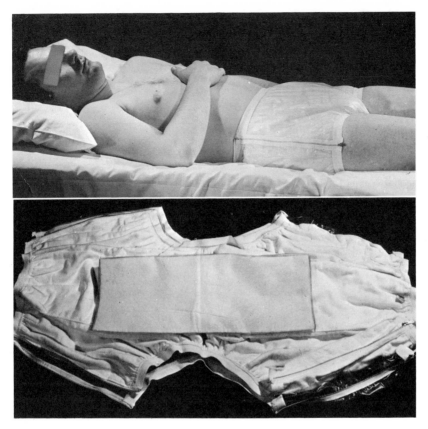

Fig. 36

Protective pants for the incontinent patient. The protective pads may be
disposable or washable. A cotton jersey liner must be worn under the plastic
pants to prevent excoriation of the skin, which must have special care.
(Courtesy Ferguson Manufacturing Co., Grand Rapids, Mich.)

erties are available. Zinc oxide powders also are beneficial to these patients. Deodorant sprays for use on dressings and linen are available, as are deodorants for deodorizing room air.

Elderly incontinent patients, particularly, may be helped to establish a definite time for defecation by using bisacodyl (Dulcolax) suppositories. By following such a regime, the patient can be saved the emotional stress of unpredictable movements and can have beter opportunities for socialization. In addition, the family members are saved time and linen usage is reduced.

Special bed arrangements are helpful for patients who are confined to bed for long periods of time. A *Bradford frame* with an opening under which a pan or urinal can be placed is helpful for a patient who is incontinent. A similar arrangement can be improvised by building the bed up with padding so that there is a depressed area in which a receptacle for drainage can be placed. This arrangement should be made so that the receptacle does not come in contact with the patient's skin. Sometimes, if the problem is expected to go on for years, a circular hole can be cut in the patient's mattress, the edges padded, and a funnel and collection bottle placed beneath the opening. A *Stryker frame, Foster bed,* or *CircOlectric bed* also can be modified to accommodate the incontinent patient.

If the patient can be up, his favorite chair

can be equipped with a commode seat. Special commode wheelchairs are also available, making it possible for the patient to be more comfortable and enabling him to mingle socially with others. Thus, he will probably be a happier individual and one with whom it is more pleasant to live.

References and selected readings*

1 Aaronson, Herbert G., and Boger, William P.: Incontinence in the elderly: an attempt at control, J. Am. Geriatrics Soc. 10:626-632, July 1962.

2 Adams, Ralph: Prevention of infections in hospitals, Am. J. Nursing 58:344-348, March 1958.

3 Barber, Knowlton E., Adams, John F., and Sosinski, Leonard D.: Control of incontinent urine by using external drainage, Am. J. Nursing 49:526-527, Aug. 1949.

4 *Buchwald, Edith, McCormack, Margaret, and Raby, Emilie: A bladder and bowel training program for patients with spinal cord disease, Rehabilitation Monograph III, New York, 1952, The Institute for Physical Medicine and Rehabilitation, New York University, Bellevue Medical Center.

5 Eckstrom, Sten: Urinary incontinence in old persons, Geriatrics 10:83-85, Feb. 1955.

6 Hirschberg, Gerald G., and others: Rehabilitation, a manual for the care of the disabled and elderly, Philadelphia, 1964, J. B. Lippincott Co.

7 Hurwitz, Sidney P., Jacobson, Edward B., and Kolman, Isadore I.: Preparation of an incontinence bag, J. Urol. 73:1103-1104, June 1955.

8 Kegel, A.: Physiologic therapy for urinary stress incontinence, J.A.M.A. 146:915-917, July 7, 1955.

9 Lapides, Jack: Stress incontinence, J. Urol. 85:291-294, March 1961.

10 *Morrissey, Alice B.: The procedures of urinary and bowel rehabilitation, Am. J. Nursing 51:194-197, March 1951.

11 Muellner, S. Richard: Development of urinary control in children, J.A.M.A. 172:1256-1261, March 19, 1960.

12 Muellner, S. Richard: Special problems of urinary control in patients with multiple sclerosis, J. Urol. 73:254-260, Feb. 1955.

13 *Robertson, Carolyn A.: Manual expression of urine, Am. J. Nursing 59:840-841, June 1959.

14 Rose, D. K.: Analysis of bladder and related renal symptoms in urinary obstruction and incontinence, West. J. Surg. 63:196-200, April 1955.

15 Rusk, Howard A.: Rehabilitation medicine, a textbook on physical medicine and rehabilitation, ed. 2, St. Louis, 1964, The C. V. Mosby Co.

16 Sawyer, Janet R.: Nursing care of patients with urologic diseases, St. Louis, 1963, The C. V. Mosby Co.

17 Saxon, Jean: Techniques for bowel and bladder training, Am. J. Nursing 62:69-71, Sept. 1962.

18 *Sister Regina Elizabeth: Sensory stimulation techniques, Am. J. Nursing 66:281-286, Feb. 1966.

19 Stafford, Nova Harris: Bowel hygiene of aged patients, Am. J. Nursing 63:102-103, Sept. 1963.

*References preceded by an asterisk are particularly well suited for student reading.

9

The patient
who is
unconscious

Study questions

1 As a result of your experience on the wards, list the equipment that you would need in preparing a room for the admittance of an unconscious patient.
2 Review your basic physical needs in a twenty-four-hour period. Do they differ from the needs of one who is unconscious? If so, how?
3 Review the following basic nursing procedures: mouth care, gavage, throat suction, enemas, and skin care.

Unconsciousness is an abnormal state resulting from disturbance of sensory perception to the extent that the patient is not aware of what is happening around him. Periods of unconsciousness may be momentary (the common faint or syncope) or may last for months (for example, following a serious motor vehicle accident in which extensive brain damage has been sustained).

The term unconsciousness is relative since there are many degrees or levels of unconsciousness: excitatory, somnolent, stuporous, and comatose. In *excitatory unconsciousness* the patient does not respond coherently but is easily disturbed by sensory stimuli such as bright lights, noise, or sudden movement. He may become excited and agitated at the slightest disturbance. This stage of unconsciousness is commonly seen in patients who are going under anesthesia or who are partially reacted from anesthesia. In caring for such a patient the room should be kept dimly lighted, the environment should be quiet, talking should be avoided, and any necessary moving of the patient or activity about him should be slow and gentle.

The *somnolent* patient is extremely drowsy and will respond only if spoken to directly and perhaps touched. This response is rarely more than a mumble or a jerky body movement in response to a stimulus.

The *stuporous* patient responds only to painful stimuli such as pricking or pinching of the skin. In deep stupor he may respond only to supraorbital or substernal pressure. This response may be a reflex withdrawal from the painful stimulus.

The patient in *deep coma* does not respond to any type of stimulus, and his reflexes are gone. He has no gag or corneal reflexes, and he may have an irregular pupillary reaction to light or complete loss of pupillary reflexes. The thermal, respiratory, or other vital regulatory mechanisms in the brain may be disturbed. In the presence of such a disturbance, the prognosis is poor.

Unconsciousness may be caused by systemic disease or toxemia affecting the brain. In vascular diseases such as cerebral hemorrhage or cerebral emboli there may be enough damage to brain tissue from anoxia to cause unconsciousness. The pressure of expanding lesions such as subdural hematomas and intracranial tumors also may cause unconsciousness. Other causes are head injuries with primary damage to the brain or pressure on the brain from swelling, drugs such as the barbiturates, alcohol, and anesthetizing agents. Unconsciousness is also seen in some functional diseases of the nervous system and in diseases such as epilepsy, in which there is a disturbance of brain physiology.

Nursing care of the unconscious patient

Although special care for the unconscious patient is directly related to the cause of the condition, general care does not vary with the cause. In this chapter, only the general nursing care will be discussed. Nursing problems related to unconsciousness in specific diseases are discussed in the appropriate chapters.

In caring for the unconscious patient, the nurse must make provision for meeting his physical and spiritual needs and his family's emotional and spiritual needs. The objectives of patient care are to maintain normal body function and to prevent complications that will hamper the patient when consciousness is restored. The nurse must remember that the patient cannot do anything for himself or even ask for help. He cannot, for example, change his position if he is uncomfortable, strained, or cramped. Nurses caring for unconscious patients should keep in mind the bodily needs they meet for themselves each day and should also recall the requests that conscious patients make for little extra comforts.

The patient who is unconscious because of anesthesia usually receives care in the recovery room. The critically ill, unconscious patient usually is cared for in the intensive care unit. When his condition stabilizes, he returns to the general pavilion.

The environment and the family

The appearance of the unconscious patient and of his surroundings is very important to the members of his family. Not being able to communicate with a loved one is very difficult for them. Seeing the patient looking comfortable in a room that is neat and pleasant helps members of the family to remain relatively composed. The room should be well ventilated, and the temperature should be kept at about 21° C. (70° F.). The very young and the very old patient may be more comfortable in a warmer temperature, 26° C. (80° F.). Since patients with depressed states of consciousness are often more disturbed in darkness, it is best to keep rooms well lighted at all times.[3] If a member of the family is remaining with the patient, a comfortable chair should be provided. He should be told where the rest room is, where he may eat, and where the public telephone is located. If the patient remains unconscious for a long time, other family members should be urged to share the time spent with him. Sometimes they can be encouraged to come only for short periods of time each day. They should be assured that they will be notified at once if there is any change in the patient's condition. The nurse should help them conserve their physical resources, for the patient who recovers after a period of unconsciousness needs much care and attention during convalescence.

Members of the patient's family frequently have many questions. If the nurse cannot answer them, she should refer the family to others who can. Explanations of treatments, such as would be given to the patient if he were conscious, should be given to members of the family. Explaining helps to allay some of their fears and helps them to understand and to feel they have a part in the patient's care. If the family wishes, the spiritual adviser should be called. He may help the patient and give the family comfort and emotional help. If religious medals are significant to the patient and his family, they may be attached to the head of the bed or secured in such a way that they are not lost. Often the patient wears a medal on a chain around his neck, and many hospitals do not require that it be removed unless necessary for a treatment or an examination such as a roentgenogram.

Hearing is probably the last of the critical faculties to be lost in unconsciousness. Upon regaining consciousness, many patients have reported conversations that were held near their beds, and many vividly recall conversations they heard when other faculties were obliterated by anesthesia. Conversation of persons close to the patient should be no different than if the patient were conscious. Members of the family and other visitors may need to be reminded of this fact. Because the patient may be able to hear, the nurse should tell him what she is going to do; for example, she should tell him if he is going to be moved onto his other side or given mouth care.

Physical care of the patient

Maintenance of an adequate airway. It is unsafe to leave an unconscious patient unattended if he is lying on his back because the tongue may fall back and occlude the air passages. When the patient is placed on his side or abdomen, a small, firm pillow rather than a soft one should be used under the head so that there is no danger of his becoming accidentally smothered as a result of his face being buried in the pillow. Since the patient is unable to blow or otherwise clear his nose, the nasal passages may become occluded with mucus. Cleansing or suctioning of the nasal passages of patients who have had brain surgery or who have suffered a head injury should not be done without a doctor's specific order, but in other instances the nose should be swabbed gently first with a moistened applicator and then with one lightly lubricated with mineral oil. If the mucous membranes of the nose and mouth

become unusually dry, a steam vaporizer is useful.

Excess mucus may need to be suctioned from the mouth or the nasopharynx. A No. 18 or No. 20 Fr. whistle-tip catheter may be used for this procedure. The mouth should be held open with a gag, and the suction should be shut off by pinching the tube or by leaving the Y valve open, if it is being used, until the tube is inserted. (See Fig. 42.) If the tube is to be inserted through the nose, it should be moistened with water. The mucus is aspirated by releasing the pinched catheter or covering the Y valve with the fingertip, rotating the catheter, and withdrawing it gently. A tracheotomy may have to be done to provide an adequate airway. (See p. 598 for care of patient having a tracheotomy.)

Maintenance of circulation. Circulation of blood is enhanced by muscle movement. The patient must not be left in a position that hampers circulation to any part of the body; for example, lying for any length of time with an acute angle bend at the knee joint will produce enough pressure on the popliteal artery and accompanying veins to hamper circulation to the lower leg. Reddened areas should be gently massaged, and they should be noted in the nursing care plan and in the nursing notes of the patient's chart so that they will receive special care. A definite routine for turning and for exercise not only improves the circulation and helps to maintain muscle tone but also helps to prevent hypostatic pneumonia or atelectasis. In addition, it maintains a normal range of joint motion and helps to prevent formation of vascular thrombi. Scheduled turning of the unconscious patient at specific intervals by an assigned team of nurse and/or auxiliary personnel assures maintenance of these physiologic functions. A checklist with the patient's name and the position changes needed at specific intervals is also useful. An alternating air-pressure mattress is helpful in preventing the development of decubiti.

Moving and position. A "turning sheet" should be used in moving an unconscious patient. It not only helps to maintain the patient's body alignment, by allowing the entire trunk to be moved at the same time, but also lessens the strain on the nurse's or attendant's back. A turning sheet is a large sheet folded lengthwise and then in half. It should be placed under the patient so that it reaches from above the shoulders to below the buttocks. The technique for placing a turning sheet under the patient is the same as for placing a drawsheet there. In preparing to turn the patient, remove the top bedclothes so that they will not be in the way and so that the alignment of the patient's body can be easily seen. Two nurses are needed to execute the turn—one on each side of the bed. Roll the sheet edges up close to the patient's body and grasp them firmly. (See Fig. 223.) Gently roll the patient onto his back, and then lift or pull him on the sheet toward the side of the bed opposite that to which he is to be turned. Bend the

Fig. 37

The nurse is preparing to give mouth care to an unconscious patient. Note that she has a padded gag to hold the mouth open. Note also that the patient is supported by pillows at her side and that her hand is curled about a hand roll with the thumb held in pronation.

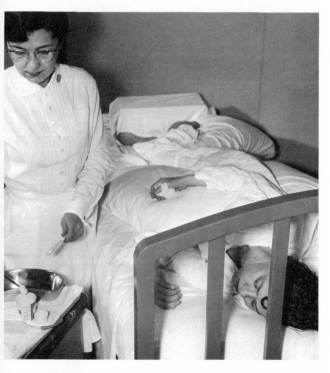

knee that will be uppermost after the patient is turned. The nurse who will be facing the patient after he is turned should then grasp the far side of the turning sheet and roll the patient toward her onto his side, pulling the hip and shoulder well under him. Check to see that the spine is straight, the neck is not bent, and the lower leg is straight. Place firm, plastic-covered pillows under the uppermost arm and leg. They should support the entire extremity and be of such a height as to prevent abduction or adduction of the arm or leg. The uppermost leg should be flexed with the knee at right angles to the hip. To prevent foot drop, the foot of the straightened leg should be firmly dorsiflexed against a foot block at scheduled intervals. The lowermost arm should be flexed at the elbow and placed palm up flat on the bed. The fingers of the hand that rests on the pillows should be allowed to curve gently over the edge of the pillow. The wrist, however, must be supported on the pillow to prevent wrist drop. The fingers should never be continuously hyperextended or tightly clenched, and sometimes it is advisable to maintain the hand in its position of function by placing a roll of 3-inch bandage in the palm and curling the fingers around it. If the thumb tends to fall forward, it may be supported in a position of common use by attaching a tab of cloth to the hand roll and using it as a supportive bandage (Fig. 37). If the unconscious patient is placed correctly in a side-lying position, a pillow to support his back is unnecessary.

If the patient does not move, all the extremities should be put through the complete range of joint motion at least twice each day. When he is turned each hour, the extremities on one side may be passively exercised. Such a routine assures passive exercise to all extremities. In turning the patient, extreme care should be taken to prevent strain on joints.

The patient may be turned directly onto his abdomen for short periods. When he is in this position, his feet should extend over the edge of the mattress to prevent pressure on the toes, and his head should be turned well to the side. Usually no pillow is necessary under the head, but a small one may be slipped under the abdomen to prevent excessive pressure on the chest. This is sometimes needed to relieve pressure on the breasts of women. Turning the unconscious patient is facilitated by the use of the Stryker frame or the CircOlectric bed.

Skin care. The unconscious patient should be thoroughly bathed with warm water each day. The skin should be briskly washed and dried to stimulate circulation. In some hospitals, patients who have been unconscious for some time are lifted into a bathtub several times a week since this measure seems to control the development of decubiti remarkably well. Three people trained in doing a three-man lift are needed for the procedure. Care must be taken not to injure the patient in moving him to the tub or to place undue strain upon the nurses. Shallow tubs at bed height with access on three sides are preferable but not essential.

If the skin is dry, it should be lubricated daily with lanolin or cold cream. Superfatted soaps may be used, or detergents may replace soaps. The feet should be lubricated each day since poor circulation from lack of activity causes the skin to become dry and the nails to harden and become horny. Alcohol is drying to the skin and should not be used. The fingernails and toenails should be short and clean. As the depth of unconsciousness becomes more shallow, many patients scratch themselves.

The hair should be neatly combed. If a woman's hair is long, it is usually more manageable and attractive in braids. If unconsciousness persists, the doctor may permit a shampoo, provided that the movement involved is not harmful to the patient. Shampoos should be given at least every two weeks to patients who are unconscious for long periods of time.

Mouth care. Since the unconscious patient tends to be a "mouth breather," the mouth often becomes dry. Therefore, mouth care should be given every two to four hours. Dentures should be removed and safely stored until the patient is fully conscious. The patient's own teeth should be brushed at least twice a day. A child's toothbrush is more easily used than an adult's. The inside of the mouth, the gum line, and the tongue should be inspected daily, using a flashlight and a tongue depressor, and the mouth should be cleaned thoroughly every two to four hours with glycerin and lemon juice or an aromatic alkaline mouthwash solution. (See Fig. 37.) The mouth will have to be held open with a gag, and it may be cleansed with a piece of gauze wrapped around a toothbrush or a tongue depressor. The nurse should never put her fingers in a patient's mouth because the gag or hold on the jaw may loosen and allow the jaws to close down on her fingers. A human bite may cause severe infection. The lips should be coated with a lubricant such as cold cream to prevent cracking.

Eye care. The patient's eyes should be carefully inspected several times a day. If they appear irritated, if the corneal reflex is absent, or if the lids are incompletely closed, they should be covered with an eye shield. If an eye shield is not available, a circle of transparent x-ray film, 9 cm. in diameter, may be used by slitting it to the middle and overlapping the edges of the slit to make a cone-shaped shield. All the edges of the x-ray film shield should be bound with cellophane tape to prevent irritation of the skin, and the shields may be held in place with cellophane tape. "Butterfly" adhesive strips may be used to close the eye. The doctor may order an eye irrigation. Physiologic solution of sodium chloride is often used. The eye should always be irrigated away from the inner canthus so that the return flow is away from the other eye. If the patient tends to open his eyes at intervals, there also may be an order for instillation of a drop or two of mineral oil or methyl cellulose, 0.5 to 1% solution, in each eye daily to protect the cornea from lint and dirt and to provide moisture and lubrication. Neglect of eye care may lead to drying of the cornea and eventual blindness.

Food and fluids. The comatose patient cannot be given fluids or food by mouth since he does not swallow normally and would surely aspirate fluid into the lungs. He may be fed by intravenous infusion or hypodermoclysis. Whereas protein and carbohydrates can be administered parenterally, fats are not yet being routinely administered intravenously, and it is therefore difficult to meet all his nutritional needs in this way. In most instances it is preferable to use a nasogastric tube and to give small amounts of liquid containing all essential foods. (See

p. 648 for preparation of these feedings.) Only about 100 to 200 ml. should be given, and this amount should be given every two to three hours. If the stomach is overfilled, the patient may vomit and aspirate with serious consequences. All feedings should be followed with about 50 ml. of water to clear the tube. The tube should be removed at least every five days and inspected. The distal end of rubber and plastic tubes becomes rigid and may traumatize the stomach mucosa.[6] Usually the doctor inserts the tube. If he does not, the nurse must be certain that she can perform the procedure without damage to the patient. After the tube is inserted, it is customary to test its placement in the following ways: by placing it under water and checking for the presence of air bubbles, which would indicate that it is in the lungs instead of in the stomach; by aspirating a little fluid to prove that it is in the stomach; by having a second nurse check to see if the tube is in the stomach before feedings are given; by inserting a small amount of clear water first, since it would cause the least harm if an error had occurred. For details of care of the equipment and of technique of this procedure, see textbooks on fundamentals of nursing. The patient who has a nasogastric tube inserted needs special care of the nose to prevent crusting and ulceration. (See discussion on common diagnostic tests and procedures, p. 647.) For patients requiring a slow, constant rate of delivery of food through the nasogastric tube, a mechanical pump is available. The pump may be adjusted so that it delivers from 40 to 200 ml. per hour of food into the stomach.

If the patient responds to verbal stimuli and has a gag reflex, fluids may be put into the back of the mouth through an Asepto syringe to which is attached about two inches of rubber tubing to obviate the danger of the patient's biting down on the glass tip of the syringe. He may have to be reminded to swallow each mouthful. Suction should be readily available in case he shows signs of choking. If signs of choking do occur, the nurse may have to apply pressure on the jaws to insert the suction tube.

Hyperthermia. When the heat-regulatory center in the hypothalamus is disturbed, the patient's temperature will rise suddenly. This is known as *hyperthermia*. It may occur after trauma to vital centers, and it often occurs in the last stages of chronic medical illness (such as uremia) when the body relinquishes vital controls prior to death. The temperature of any unconscious patient should be taken rectally every four hours, and, if it is elevated, it should be taken at least every two hours. Elevation of temperature may also be a sign of complications such as pneumonia, wound infection, dehydration, or urinary tract infection. The nurse should carefully observe the patient for any signs that might indicate the onset of complications.

When elevation of temperature is caused by the improper functioning of the heat-regulatory center, the nurse can help compensate for the loss of this natural control. If the temperature is over 38.4° C. (101° F.), some bedclothes should be removed, and sometimes the patient should be covered only by a sheet. Occasionally the patient's gown and sheet are removed and only a loincloth and breast covering are used. Aspirin may be dissolved and inserted through a nasogastric tube, or it may be introduced into the rectum as a suppository or dissolved in a small amount of water as a retention enema. The dosage for drugs given by rectum is usually double that given orally. Fluids may not be forced if the doctor feels that increasing fluid intake may increase intracranial pressure. If the temperature continues to rise despite conservative treatment, ice caps may be applied to the groins and axillas. Alcohol sponge baths often are ordered, and fans placed slightly to the side of the patient may be used to increase evaporation. If the fever still persists following this treatment, ice-water enemas may be given, and the patient may be packed in ice or placed in a tub of cool or cold water or on an ice mattress. (See discussion on hypothermia, p. 188.) In very hot weather he may be placed in an oxygen tent for its air-conditioned effect. The room should be kept cool so that body heat will be lost from the skin surfaces. If the patient's temperature goes over 40° C. (104° F.), it should be taken every hour until it returns to and remains at a lower level. Sometimes, if the elevation is due to increased intracranial pressure, a lumbar

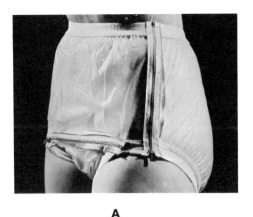
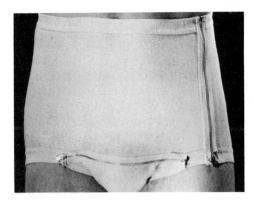

A   **B**

Fig. 38

A, Outside plastic pants for a woman. **B,** Cotton jersey liner for a man. Note that both the liner and the plastic outer pants open at the crotch so that the protective pads can be easily changed. (Courtesy Ferguson Manufacturing Co., Grand Rapids, Mich.)

puncture is done. Unabated high temperature eventually will cause death.

The family often becomes concerned lest the patient treated for hyperthermia develop "pneumonia." It must be explained that the fever is associated with the unconsciousness and is not related to infection, that the treatment the patient is receiving is the usual one for this complication, that there is little danger of pneumonia from chilling because the high temperature is keeping the patient warm, and that excessive bed covering will increase the temperature of even the normal person.

Hypothermia. The unconscious patient may have a temperature that is too low. This condition may occur when vital centers are depressed but control has not yet been lost. The unconscious patient who does not move produces less normal body heat and is likely to have a low temperature and to need extra covering. The nurse should feel the patient's feet to determine circulation in the extremities and to judge whether or not adequate external warmth is being supplied.

Problems of elimination. The unconscious patient often has both urinary and fecal incontinence. A Foley type of catheter or external drainage apparatus may be used to control urinary incontinence. If the use of

these devices is contraindicated, the nurse should try to determine the patient's normal voiding schedule and place him on a bedpan or put a urinal in place according to this schedule. The skin should be kept dry and clean to prevent decubiti and add to comfort (Figs. 36 and 38). The urinary output should be measured. If measurement is impossible because of incontinence, output should be estimated by recording each time the patient is incontinent and whether or not a large amount of urine was voided (p. 152).

The unconscious patient usually is given an enema every two or three days to help prevent fecal incontinence and formation of impactions. The patient who is fed through a nasogastric tube may be given juices that have a laxative effect, such as prune juice. Sometimes a mild cathartic, such as milk of magnesia, citrate of magnesia, psyllium hydrophilic mucilloid (Metamucil), a concentrate of senna (Senokot), or dioctyl sodium sulfosuccinate (Colace), is ordered and can be given through the nasogastric tube. In giving the enema, the nurse may need to hold the patient's buttocks together to prevent premature expulsion of the fluid, or she may insert an indwelling catheter and inflate the balloon to help retain the fluid in the bowel. When it is desirable for the enema to be expelled, the patient should be turned onto a bedpan, with special care taken to support the back and to prevent pressure damage to the skin from weight against the pan. A firm pillow protected with water-resistant material is best for this purpose. The lower abdomen should then be massaged gently from right to left. Sometimes it is necessary to siphon fluid from the lower bowel, in which case the enema may have to be repeated. The doctor may order bisacodyl suppositories (Dulcolax). A bowel movement usually occurs within half an hour after their insertion. Soap suppositories also may be used.

If the patient has a vaginal discharge, it should be reported to the doctor. Sometimes cleansing douches are ordered. The patient who is menstruating will need perineal care every few hours.

Prevention of accidents. Precautions should be taken to prevent accidents to unconscious patients. No external heat such as hot-water bottles or heating pads should be used. Padded side rails should be kept on the bed, since the patient might have a convulsion or suddenly move when not expected to do so. If a convulsion is anticipated, a mouth gag should be kept at the bedside. If a convulsion occurs, the gag should be inserted at the side of the mouth between the molar teeth, since the front teeth are easily loosened or broken. Manual pressure at the angle of the jaw sometimes makes it easier to open the mouth. The unconscious patient should be observed at least every half hour. If his condition is critical, he may need to be observed every fifteen minutes or to be attended constantly. Paraldehyde, 5 ml., or sodium phenobarbital, 30 to 60 mg. (½ to 1 grain), may be ordered for overactivity, excitability, or when seizures occur. Any patient who is unconscious and who receives sedation must be observed closely for signs of depression of vital functions. A certain amount of restlessness is desirable, as it encourages deeper respirations and the patient is more likely to move about in bed.[10]

If the patient is semiconscious, he may be placed in a chair twice a day. This improves circulation and prevents pulmonary and circulatory complications. To prevent him from falling, the nurse should apply a chest harness type of Posey belt or tie a twisted drawsheet about his waist and to the back of the chair. She must make certain that he is placed in as near a proper sitting position as possible. The spine should be straight, he should be sitting on his buttocks, and his feet should be flat on the floor. The head and arms will need to be supported. The reason for getting the patient out of bed should be carefully explained to the family members since they may feel that he is being treated poorly.

Observations

The nurse should make and record detailed observations of an unconscious patient. The diagnosis may be obscure, and the nurse who notes such things as stiffness of the neck and flaccid limbs or who carefully reports the course of a convulsion may provide the doctor with essential information. Observations over and above those made while giving patient care may be ordered. The doctor may wish the vital signs, the pupillary response, and the level of consciousness determined at periodic intervals. A rising blood pressure correlated with a slowing of the pulse rate is indicative of increasing intracranial pressure and should be reported at once. Any marked change in the character of the pulse or respirations or any decrease or increase in the level of consciousness should be reported.

The pupillary response is checked by opening the upper eyelid and flashing a light into the eye from the outer aspect inward toward the nose. Each eye should be tested separately. Irregular reaction of either eye or "fixed" pupils should be reported, since these responses suggest intracranial hemorrhage.

The corneal response is tested by the doctor. He will need a wisp of sterile absorbent cotton for this procedure. The patient who has lost the corneal reflex will not blink when the cornea is touched.

Convalescence

A patient may recover completely after being unconscious for several weeks. He will gradually return through the stages of unconsciousness, and he often first responds verbally to a familiar face or voice. Efforts should not be made to arouse him until the level of unconsciousness has lightened. He may be unable to speak, may be partially paralyzed, or may have other losses, and the rehabilitation program will be planned accordingly. If he has been well cared for while he was unconscious, so that decubiti, contractures, or blindness were prevented from developing, he should not have an extensive hospitalization period.

During convalescence, definite rest periods should be planned each day. If the patient becomes overtired, he will tend to regress. He will need the encouragement and security of knowing that family and friends are concerned and interested in his recovery. He also will need to be reoriented since his memory will be blank for the time immediately before and during unconsciousness.

Death of the patient

Many patients die without regaining consciousness. When death occurs, members of the family often need emotional support, since they are not only upset emotionally but also may be worn out physically. If the patient has been unconscious for some time, the sudden release of the tension of "not knowing" may cause some people to respond inappropriately. If this happens, they should be assured privacy and be protected from the embarrassment of having others aware of this reaction.

References and selected readings*

1 *Bardsley, Christine, and others: Pressure sores, a regime for preventing and treating them, Am. J. Nursing 64:82-84, May 1964.

2 Barron, James, Prendergast, John J., and Jocz, Martin W.: Food pump—new approach to tube feeding, J.A.M.A. 161:621-622, June 16, 1956.

3 Beeson, Paul B., and McDermott, Walsh, editors: Cecil-Loeb textbook of medicine, ed. 11, Philadelphia, 1963, W. B. Saunders Co.

4 Best, Charles H., and Taylor, Norman B.: The physiological basis of medical practice, ed. 8, Baltimore, 1966, Williams & Wilkins Co.

5 Brooks, Helen Louise: The golden rule for the unconscious patient, Nursing Forum 4:12-18, 1965, No. 3.

6 *Davenport, Rachael R.: Tube feeding for long-term patients, Am. J. Nursing 64:121-123, Jan. 1964.

7 deGutíerrez-Mahoney, C. G., and Carini, Esta: Neurological and neurosurgical nursing, ed. 4, St. Louis, 1965, The C. V. Mosby Co.

8 Eckenhoff, James E.: The care of the unconscious patient, J.A.M.A. 186:541-543, Nov. 9, 1963.

9 *Fuerst, Elinor V., and Wolff, LuVerne: Fundamentals of nursing, ed. 3, Philadelphia, 1964, J. B. Lippincott Co.

10 Luessenhop, Alfred: Care of the unconscious patient, Nursing Forum 4:6-11, 1965, No. 3.

11 MacBryde, Cyril Mitchell: Signs and symptoms, ed. 4, Philadelphia, 1964, J. B. Lippincott Co.

12 Meyers, Emma Mary: Nursing the comatose patient, Am. J. Nursing 54:716-718, June 1954.

13 Taylor, John C.: Decubitus ulcers, Nursing Science 2:293-310, Aug. 1964.

14 *Trowbridge, Lois K., and Trowbridge, William V.: Measures used in controlling central hyperthermia, Am. J. Nursing 53:1092, Sept. 1953.

15 Vanden Bergh, Richard L., and Davidson, Ramona Powell: Let's talk about death, Am. J. Nursing 66:71-75, Jan. 1966.

*References preceded by an asterisk are particularly well suited for student reading.

10

The patient
who has
surgical treatment

Study questions

1 What general reactions do you believe you would have if told that you must have an immediate operation? To whom would you wish to talk? Have you observed these reactions in any close member of your family? If so, describe them.
2 What general physical deficiencies can you identify that might necessitate delay of an operation?
3 What are safe and effective ways to cleanse the skin? Can the skin be made sterile?
4 Review the charts of several patients on your clinical unit who have received anesthetics. What kinds of anesthetics were used? How were they administered?
5 Talk to two patients on your clinical unit who have recently received anesthetics. Did they express fear? What vivid recollections do they have?
6 What is the significance to the circulatory system of a sudden drop in blood pressure?
7 Review the circulation of the blood and the physiology of respiration.
8 Consult your notes on fundamentals of nursing and review the dangers of prolonged bed rest. What techniques have you learned for helping patients to get into and out of bed? What safety measures should be taken in helping patients to get into and out of bed?
9 What disturbances of physiology can occur when the patient cannot take solids or liquids by mouth?
10 List the nursing measures you have learned that may assist a patient to void.

An operation with all its related experiences represents an upsetting ordeal for the patient and for his family—regardless of the circumstances under which surgery is performed. The impact of stress is severe when sudden illness or an accident force an ambulance ride to the hospital and immediate surgery. In a completely different way, it may be equally severe for the patient who must endure a period of observation and undergo numerous tests before surgery is done. The patient who must have repeated surgery also faces frustrations and fears that intensify his reactions.

No operation is minor as far as the patient and his family are concerned. An operation is always a major experience in the life of the patient and his family. Usually it is performed in a hospital, and although the patient knows that many wonderful things are done in hospitals, a hospital is still a place where one goes to have serious operations, and where one loses freedom of action and identity. In our society, also, many people die in the hospital. An operation is associated in the patient's mind with pain, and often with an anesthetic and its unpleasant side effects. It involves a physical encounter for the patient in which he is at a distinct disadvantage in that he cannot strike back or avoid the encounter in the usual fashion. An operation implies maiming or often loss of a part of the body, which is damaging to self-esteem and to the concept of self. In addition, surgery often raises fears of what will be found at operation and how it may change life for the patient and for his family.

The nurse is an essential member of the health team, which tries to make an operation a safer and more tolerable experience for the patient. She contributes by helping the doctor to know more about the patient and about his family. Sometimes the surgeon knows the patient and his family well. Many times he does not, and the public health nurse who visits the patient in the community, the nurse in the hospital clinic, the nurse on the scene at the time of an emergency, and the nurse caring for the patient in the hospital can help him by their keen observations of the patient and by their careful recording and reporting. The nurse can be helpful in developing educational materials that may make the entire experience of admission to a hospital and of the operation a smoother and easier one for the patient and for his family. The nurse contributes also in her technical skill, in giving physical care to the patient during the operative experience and in her sensitivity, alertness, and understanding of his entire situation. Some of the skills and abilities essential to her effective contribution are discussed in this chapter.

The purpose of care during the preoperative period is to prepare the patient, both physically and psychologically, to withstand the effects of anesthesia and surgery. The time allowed for this preparation depends upon the condition of the patient and the type of operation to be performed. It may be very short, or it may extend into weeks. The physician is primarily responsible for this preparation, but he relies upon the nurse for much assistance and delegates certain responsibilities to her. She can contribute substantially to the patient's physical and emotional welfare and can influence his preoperative progress. She should study the doctor's orders for preparation for surgery and carry out these orders in such a way as to provide the greatest possible comfort and safety for the patient.

She needs to draw upon her basic knowledge of the behavior of people and of normal physiology and the development of disease. In this way she can try to help the patient to accept the surgery anticipated, and she can make significant observations and refer them to the physician and to other appropriate persons.

Sociopsychologic preparation for surgery

Preparation for hospital admission

Preparation for surgery should begin as soon as the doctor makes a diagnosis and decides that an operation is necessary. From that moment on the patient and his family are faced with the decision of having this treatment and its many consequences. The doctor tells the patient and his family that the operation is necessary, explains why it must be performed, what will be done, and what the probable outcome will be. He discusses duration of hospitalization, cost, length of absence from work, and disabilities or residual effects that may be expected. An appointment for admission to the hospital is then made. The date for admission is influenced by the acuteness of the patient's illness, the hospital treatment needed preoperatively, and the amount of time the patient requires to make necessary arrangements regarding his family, financial matters, and work.

The patient needs to know when to arrive at the hospital, where to go, and what information to give. The admitting clerk will ask about his employment, insurance, and hospital plans. He should know that the business office can help him make arrangements for paying his bill and that he can consult a social case worker about family, financial, and convalescent problems. He should be told what toilet articles and clothing to bring with him. He will be interested in knowing the visiting hours and how his family may contact him. He should be encouraged to think through any problems that may arise and to plan for them. It is modern practice to permit a parent to accompany a child to his hospital bed, to remain with him during his first day and evening in the hospital, and on the morning of the operative day to be with him until he goes to the operating room.

Fear of surgery

Although patients may or may not express it, almost all of them have some fear of surgery. It can be a fear of the unknown, or it can be a fear based on something they have heard friends or relatives say about their operative experiences. They may have had personal contact with someone who died as a result of an operation. They may be afraid of the diagnosis. They may have fears about anesthesia, pain, disfigurement, disability, or death. The older patient often worries about becoming a burden to his family.

The nurse may be able to help the patient talk about his fears. She should be with him as much as possible and give him every opportunity to ask questions. If feasible, the same nurse or member of the nursing team should be assigned to care for the patient each day preoperatively so that he is really known by at least one person on the nursing staff.

The nurse can keep the patient and his family well informed and explain each procedure and examination (Fig. 39). She can inspire confidence in the nursing staff by a competent and unhurried manner. If it is

desirable, she can make arrangements for the patient to talk with other patients who have successfully recovered from similar operations. She can explain to the family the need for them to visit the patient frequently to show him that he is wanted and loved. Very often the patient has great confidence in his spiritual adviser and gains much comfort from speaking with him. If the patient wishes, the nurse can make arrangements for a visit from the hospital chaplain. If the patient shows signs of apprehension or depression by crying, withdrawing from others, refusing to eat, or not sleeping, the nurse should first attempt to obtain clues from the patient as to what meaning this behavior has for him and then consult with the physician.

The child should be told in simple language appropriate to his age and his developmental level what to expect before and after the operation and what the operative procedure will be (Fig. 40). The child, like the adult, should have individualized instruction. Sometimes the preparation should be gradual, and storybooks about hospitalization and anesthesia are available and are useful for parents to use. Unless the child is old enough to have developed a perspective

Fig. 39

The nurse supplements the doctor's explanation of the operation and postoperative care.

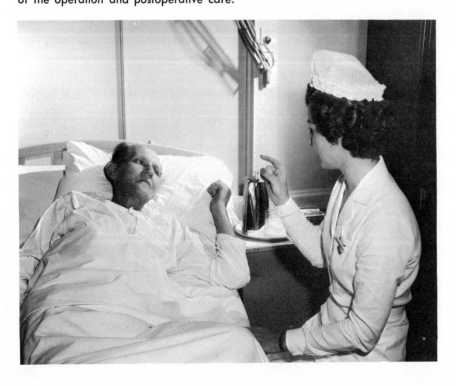

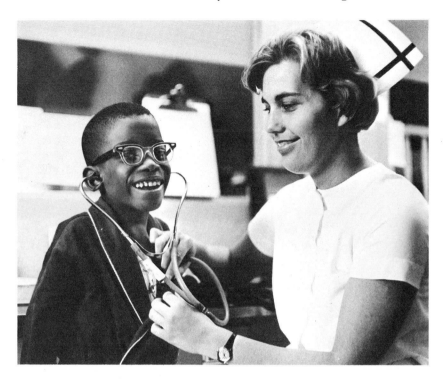

Fig. 40

Depending upon the child's age and development, he may be shown what it is hoped will be accomplished at operation. (Courtesy Muhlenberg Hospital, Plainfield, N. J.; photo by Warren R. Vroom.)

as to time, a small amount of factual information given shortly before the operation is best. Knowing too far ahead may only confuse the child, since his concept of time is immediate and he does not grasp the significance of a waiting period. Unnecessary and unpleasant details should always be avoided, but the child should never be told untruths. He should know that the experience will probably not be entirely pleasant, but the interesting and reassuring aspects of the situation should be stressed. The surgeon, for example, may tell the small boy that an operation on his foot "is going to help you run as fast as the other boys," or that an operation simply "is going to make you better." Placing a child in a room with other children usually helps him adjust to hospitalization more easily, and telling him (if it is true) that his mother will be at his bedside when he awakens helps a great deal to allay fear.

Preoperative information

The nurse should know what information has been given to the patient so that she can answer his questions intelligently. Many patients hesitate to ask the physician to repeat information and are often too upset to understand all they have been told or to ask questions. Thus they frequently turn to the nurse for clarification and reinforcement of such information. The nurse may also be questioned about the surgeon's competence, the number of people she has seen recover from a similar operation, and about the hospital. She should answer these questions factually and in such a way that the patient acquires confidence in the surgeon, the nursing staff, the hospital, and the outcome of the operation.

Some patients and their families are more frightened by what they do not know or by the unexpected than by what is explained to them and planned with them. Others function better not knowing and will say so if they are given the opportunity. Almost all persons, however, are apprehensive about the preparation for an operation and benefit from some explanation. The responsibility for giving preoperative instructions to the patient belongs primarily to the nurse who cares for him in the hospital. However, the nurses in the outpatient department, doctor's office, and public health agency also share this responsibility and should tell the patient as much as they can about the preoperative period. The patient and his family should be told how extensive the preoperative preparation will be and approximately how long it will take. The purpose of the physical examination, roentgenography, and other tests should be explained to them. The patient should be told about preoperative treatments such as shaving and preparation of the operative area, medications, the enema (if one is ordered), and why fluids and food will be withheld. He should know if he will awaken in a recovery room, if an oxygen tent, suction machine, or other equipment may be used, and if intravenous fluids will probably be given. He should be instructed in any special exercises that he must do postoperatively, such as coughing, contracting and relaxing the leg muscles, breathing deeply, and turning. He and his family should be told that frequent blood pressure recordings and other special observations and treatments are the rule, lest they be considered a sign of poor progress. He should be told that the doctor may think it best for him to be out of bed soon after surgery but that assistance in moving and walking will be given.

Sometimes when the patient is scheduled to remain in the hospital for only a few hours postoperatively, he and his family should be given instructions for postoperative care preoperatively in the home, clinic, or doctor's office. At this time the patient has not received medication to lessen his alertness, and a family member usually is present. These instructions should be reviewed with the patient and his family postoperatively.

The operative permit

The patient will be asked to sign an operative permit before undergoing surgery.

"The main purpose of this permit is to protect the physician and the hospital against claims of unauthorized operations and to guard the patient against unsanctioned surgery."* The patient should be made fully aware of the type of surgery to be performed. Usually the surgeon explains the operation at this time, and he may draw a diagram for the patient, explaining what will probably be necessary and any change in body function that it may entail. Sometimes the patient wishes to talk to a close family member before signing an operative permit. If so, the nurse should assist him in contacting the relative. If serious, extensive or disfiguring surgery must be anticipated, the patient may wish to leave the hospital for a short time to confer with relatives or attend to business affairs before he signs the permit. The nurse should realize that signing the operative permit is a very serious step for the patient that is taken much more easily when the nurse, by her interest in him and her manner, conveys warmth, friendliness, and sympathy for him at this time of decision.

Permission should be obtained for each operation and for every procedure that involves entering a body cavity, such as a thoracentesis or a cystoscopy. Written permission is safest and should be witnessed by the nurse, physician, or other authorized personnel. In an emergency, the surgeon may operate without written permission of the patient or his family, although every effort is made to contact some family member. Consent in the form of a telegram or letter or by telephone is permissible. If the patient is a minor, permission must be obtained from either parent or from his legal guardian. The signature of the husband or wife of a married minor is acceptable. An emancipated minor, that is, one who is married and/or earning his own living, can sign his own operative permit.

The nurse is usually responsible for seeing that the operative permit is signed and attached to the patient's chart when he goes to the operating room. The signature

---

*From Hayt, Emanuel, Hayt, Lillian R., Groeschel, August H., and McMullan, Dorothy: Law of hospital, physician, and patient, New York, 1958, Hospital Textbook Co.

should be obtained without pressure and before the patient receives sedation. The patient may refuse to undergo an operation, and it is his privilege to do so.

The nurse should note whether or not a permit has been signed at least a day before an elective operation is scheduled. If it has not been signed or if the patient is reluctant to sign it, she should notify the surgeon at once. The ultimate responsibility for obtaining the necessary permission for an operation rests with the surgeon.

Physical examination and preparation for surgery

Both surgery and anesthetics produce changes in the body, and the patient must be in the best possible physical condition to withstand these changes. The heart and the circulatory, respiratory, and urinary systems are depressed by anesthetics and therefore are carefully evaluated before surgery is attempted. A history of the patient's past and present illnesses is obtained, and a complete physical examination, including laboratory tests, is made to ascertain the patient's physical status and to discover coexisting diseases. Routine roentgenograms of the chest are taken to be sure that the patient does not have any lung disease that would complicate the operative course or be aggravated by anesthesia. Difficulties associated with inadequate oxygen supply through the lungs and of cardiac function are the ones most often encountered during anesthesia. If the patient is elderly, a measure of his vital capacity may be taken. This precaution is taken because it is sometimes difficult for the elderly patient to obtain enough oxygen, his rib cage having become firmer and alterations having occurred in all the tissues of the respiratory tract, particularly of the lung parenchyma (alveoli). Signs of any upper respiratory infection must be noted by the nurse and reported. Usually the surgeon prefers not to operate upon any patient of any age within one week of his having had symptoms of a cold or other upper respiratory infection.

The patient's urine is always examined preoperatively to detect the presence of urinary tract infection or of any other disease condition that may become a serious problem during and after the operation. For example, the presence of sugar may indicate diabetes mellitus; albumin or a low specific gravity may indicate chronic nephritis; and acetone, particularly in a small child, may indicate starvation and dehydration. Any of these conditions will alter greatly the treatment that is needed before, during and after surgery. Blood tests, such as a complete blood count, hemoglobin determination, and bleeding and clotting time determinations, will help ascertain whether or not the patient has a chronic infection or has signs of anemia or another blood dyscrasia. Any one of these conditions may produce difficulties during the operation or interfere with wound healing and thus prolong convalescence. If major surgery is anticipated, blood-typing and crossmatching, including determination of the Rh factor, is always done so that a transfusion of blood may be given at once if needed. If the patient is beyond middle age, a blood sugar test may be done to rule out the presence of mild or incipient diabetes, which, if present and untreated, may lead to such postoperative complications as delayed wound healing and infections. Determinations of blood volume are often made preoperatively so that blood and other fluids lost during the operation may be replaced more exactly and the dangers of shock and other complications minimized. Electrocardiograms are usually ordered for any patients who are likely to have cardiac disease and may be ordered routinely for all older patients.

When the preliminary examinations establish that there is a coexisting disease, a more intensive study is done. Although it is not always possible to cure existing diseases before surgery, knowledge of their presence will influence the care given to the patient in the preoperative period, during the operation, and postoperatively. For instance, efforts are made to bring cardiac diseases and diabetes mellitus under control prior to surgery or general anesthesia. Patients with bronchiectasis or emphysema are frequently treated with aerosol inhalations and postural drainage of the lungs for several days preoperatively. The nurse must see that all treatments are carried out and that the patient is prepared for all tests. She should assist with the tests when necessary and see that they are completed and that the results are reported before the operation is scheduled.

During the time that tests are being done and the patient is being prepared as fully as possible for the anticipated surgery, the nurse should observe him closely, get to know him, and report any significant findings to the doctor. An experience with sensitivity to a drug may not be reported by the patient when he talks to the doctor, yet may be mentioned to the nurse. The patient may have been taking tranquilizers without the doctor's knowledge. Because tranquilizers have been found to cause serious hypotension in some elderly patients both during and after anesthesia, many surgeons believe it is unwise to operate upon elderly patients who have been taking tranquilizers until at least two weeks have elapsed. Unless emergency surgery is necessary, most surgeons adhere to this rule.

Nutrition

The patient should be in the best possible nutritional state before undergoing surgery. Dehydration and poor nutrition at the time of operation have been found to influence adversely the operative prognosis particularly in infants and in elderly persons. When there is protein deficiency, wounds heal slowly and there is decreased resistance to infection. A lack of vitamin C retards wound healing. Excessive vomiting or diarrhea preoperatively will dehydrate the patient and cause electrolyte imbalance. Chronic illness and a poor appetite make a patient a poor candidate for any surgery. When emergency surgery must be done on patients whose nutritional status is poor, an intravenous infusion of fluid containing glucose is started before the patient receives an anesthetic.

Every effort is made to correct nutritional deficiency before surgery. A well-balanced diet will be ordered for the patient, and he may receive supplementary protein and vitamins. The nurse should always know how well the patient is eating and should consult with the physician about any problems that may arise. She should explain the importance of restoring and maintaining good nutrition and should encourage the patient to eat the proper foods. When he expresses

likes and dislikes or does not eat well, the nurse can ask the dietitian to talk to him so that satisfactory adjustments in his diet can be made. The patient's family may sometimes be permitted to bring him special foods that he particularly enjoys. When the patient cannot tolerate food by mouth, he is given fluids containing glucose, vitamins, and electrolytes parenterally. If marked protein deficiency exists, he may be given transfusions of whole blood or of blood plasma, and occasionally protein hydrolysates are given intravenously.

Care of the patient the day before operation

Preoperative orders

When the patient is ready for surgery, the physician writes orders for the immediate preoperative preparation. In many hospitals these orders cancel all previous ones. The nurse should consult with the physician at this time to see that the orders meet all the patient's needs. Care must be taken that orders for important treatments such as postural drainage, or for medications such as digitalis preparations and insulin or other hormones, are not inadvertently canceled. After the physician tells the patient and his family that the operation is scheduled, the nurse may begin preparing the patient. She explains the procedures and treatments that will be done and supplements the information given to the patient by the doctor.

Diet

Unless the patient is on a special diet, he may have a regular meal the evening before the operation. If the operation is scheduled late the next day or is going to be done under local or spinal anesthesia, the doctor usually permits a light breakfast and fluids up to six hours before the operation. If the operation is to be under general anesthesia on the following morning, fluids usually are permitted only until midnight, and the adult patient is told that he must not take anything by mouth after this time since there is danger that he may vomit while under anesthesia. If he vomits, he may aspirate stomach contents into his lungs. If the patient's mouth becomes very dry while waiting for surgery, a mouthwash may be used. If the nurse discovers that the patient has taken food or fluids immediately before the operation, she should inform the surgeon. He will either pass a nasogastric tube to empty the stomach or will delay the operation.

The child up to 7 or 8 years of age usually is given water and clear, sweet fluids such as fruit juice up to two to four hours before the operation, and sometimes hard candy is given a few hours before surgery. Differences in the physiology of the infant and the child from that of the adult make this measure necessary. A child's glycogen reserve in the liver is proportionately less than that of an adult, so that starvation is tolerated less well and signs of acidosis, such as acetone in the urine, occur frequently if special precautions are not taken. In the child a smaller proportion of the body fluid is in the intravascular compartment, so that changes in body fluids are less well tolerated. In addition, the nervous system of the infant is less well developed, so that alterations of body systems to meet sudden changes are less effective. More fluid is lost, too, through skin evaporation in the infant and child than the adult. This greater fluid loss results from the fact that although the infant's body weight is only approximately 5% of an adult's weight, his skin surface, from which evaporation is occurring constantly, is 15% of an adult's skin surface. Before major surgery is started on an infant, a phlebotomy or cutdown and insertion of a fine polyethylene tube usually is done on a vein so that fluids containing glucose and electrolytes can be given during and following the operation without interruption.

Because the body systems of the elderly patient are functioning at maximum capacity or with a very small margin of safety, the elderly patient also may require fluids containing glucose and electrolytes. This measure assures that vital organs such as the heart and the kidneys will not suffer for even a brief period without a constant supply of food.

Preparation of the skin

Thorough cleansing of the skin surrounding the operative area helps to reduce the incidence of wound infection. Although the skin can never be made completely free of bacteria, it can be cleansed so that when the incision is made, there are few bacteria present. The skin is usually scrubbed with soap and water and then shaved. The cleansing agent most commonly used is green soap, but a detergent agent, hexachlorophene, has been found to be very effective and is thought to be superior to green soap. It has antibacterial properties that have a cumulative effect. pHisoHex, which is a mixture of hexachlorophene in a synthetic detergent, is often used. Neither rinsing with water nor drying will remove hexachlorophene from the skin. Alcohol or ether (organic solvents) will remove it, however, and should not be used as a rinse.

Shaving the skin also lessens the likelihood of wound infections because it removes the hair to which bacteria may cling. Extreme care must be taken that the skin is not cut during shaving, because cuts are open wounds that can become infected. An autoclaved razor and a new blade should be used on each patient since it is believed that viral hepatitis may be transmitted through the use of inadequately sterilized razors in the preparation of the skin before surgery. The skin should be lubricated with soap, and the hair should be shaved in the direction in which it grows. The nurse should teach all personnel who shave patients the correct technique and the importance of not cutting the skin. Occasionally doctors permit patients to shave themselves. The nurse should check to see that the preparation is adequate. Many surgeons prefer to have the skin preparation done in the operating room immediately after the patient has been anesthetized. The patient is thus spared this sometimes embarrassing procedure, and there is less risk of infection.

Usually the surgeon leaves instructions as to how large a skin area he wishes to have prepared. In other instances, the nurse prepares an area specified by hospital procedure for a particular operation. The area to be prepared will be more extensive than actually required for the incision. Shaving of the skin usually is omitted in the infant and young child. When orders for preparation of the skin are written, the following areas are usually prepared for surgery.

Abdominal operations. If the patient is a woman, the skin from below the breasts to and including the pubic area is shaved. If the patient is a man, the skin from the nipple line to and including the pubic area is shaved. The umbilicus is cleansed with soap and water and any material collected there is removed.

Chest operations. The skin on the affected side from the spine to beyond the midline of the anterior chest and from the clavicle to the umbilicus is shaved.

Radical mastectomy. The skin from the spine on the affected side to beyond the midline anteriorly and from the clavicle to the umbilicus is shaved. The axilla and the arm on the affected side down to the elbow should also be shaved.

Rectal operations. The skin within a 6- to 8-inch radius around the rectum is shaved.

Gynecologic operations. The skin from the umbilicus to and including the pubic area and the perineum is shaved.

Kidney operations. The skin on the affected side from the spine to beyond the midline anteriorly and from the nipple line to the pubic area is shaved.

Neck operations. The skin from the chin to the nipple line and to the hairline of the face on both sides is shaved.

Head operations. The head usually is shaved in the operating room by the surgeon. Long hair should be saved and given to the patient or his family.

Other operations. Areas to be prepared for other operations will be specifically ordered by the surgeon. Operations for amputations and spinal surgery require preparation dependent upon the extent of the patient's disease and the preference of the surgeon.

Preparation of the bowel

Whether or not an enema is given preoperatively depends upon the circumstances as well as upon the personal preferences of the surgeon. If the patient has had a normal bowel movement the day before the operative day, and if the anticipated surgery does not involve the gastrointestinal tract and early mobilization is expected, it is now common practice to omit an enema preoperatively. Enemas are seldom ordered for children preoperatively. They are ordered to be given if the surgery to be done involves the gastrointestinal system or the pelvic, peri-

neal, or perianal areas. Any enema given should be effectual. If it is not, the doctor must be so informed. If the enema is to be given until the returns are clear, the nurse should ask the doctor how many enemas he wishes the patient to have. Too many enemas tire the patient, upset electrolyte balance, and irritate the rectal and bowel mucosa. Rest periods between enemas are beneficial to the patient, and enemas given slowly may produce better results and thus reduce the number necessary.

Sedation

It is important that the patient rest the night before the operation. Barbiturates such as Seconal, Nembutal, Amytal, and phenobarbital are ordered for this purpose and are usually effective. Small doses of sodium phenobarbital may be ordered for children. Barbiturates are given after all preoperative treatments have been completed. They sometimes cause the patient to become confused, and it is advisable to put side rails on the bed, especially if the patient is elderly. Chloral hydrate is sometimes given to older patients to avoid the confusion caused by barbiturates. The nurse should instruct the patient to call her during the night instead of getting out of bed if he wishes something. She should observe the patient frequently during the night, and if he cannot sleep, she should try to make him comfortable and spend as much time with him as possible. If a second barbiturate or any medication for pain is needed, it must be given at least four hours before the preoperative medication is due. This precaution will minimize any respiratory depression caused by the cumulative effect of these drugs. If it is too late to give the patient medication safely and if he is apprehensive or has pain, the doctor should be consulted.

Care of the patient on the day of the operation

On the day of the operation the nurse is chiefly concerned with observing the emotional state of the patient, checking his physical condition, safeguarding his belongings, and physically preparing him to receive anesthetics. She should visit him early unless he is sleeping. Fear may be allayed by explaining all procedures to the patient, and if the operation is to be delayed even for as short a time as one-half hour, the patient and his family should be so informed. The members of the family should be permitted to see the patient before the operation and to stay with him if they wish. A parent usually is encouraged to remain with the child. The patient may desire a visit from a chaplain on the morning of surgery. If the patient is very concerned about the operation and expresses fear about its outcome, the nurse should notify the surgeon or anesthesiologist. Patients who are extremely apprehensive tolerate surgery poorly, and the operation may have to be delayed or canceled.

Care on the morning of operation depends upon when the operation is to be done and the practices of each institution. Most surgeons, however, prefer that the patient not be disturbed in the morning until shortly before he is scheduled to go to the operating room. Usually a bath or shower is taken the evening before, and the patient can sleep through the early morning.

When the patient awakens or is awakened, his temperature is taken and any elevation is reported to the surgeon. The nurse observes the patient's respirations and his color and questions him about how he feels. Signs and symptoms of upper respiratory infections and expressions of new or different pain should be referred to the physician. Anesthetics and surgery aggravate such conditions and cause postoperative complications.

The patient should be given sufficient time to bathe, brush his teeth, and change to a hospital gown before he is called to the operating room. The woman patient is advised to braid her hair if it is long, and it can be secured with a bandana or towel to protect it from the anesthetic agents and from vomitus. Hairpins are removed because they may become dislodged and injure the patient's scalp and because they may cause sparks during administration of anesthetics. Since the nail beds are very sensitive to a lack of oxygen and some anesthetists check them for the presence of anoxia, the patient may be asked to remove nail polish. Religious medals or rosary beads taken to the operating room should be taped to the patient's wrist or secured to the bedpost. All jewelery and money should be taken

from the bedside and locked up. The patient is permitted to wear a wedding ring, but it should be taped or tied securely to the hand.

Most anesthetists prefer that dentures and removable bridges be removed before the patient goes to the operating room, since, as the muscles relax under anesthesia, these prostheses may fall away from the gums and drop back into the pharynx, causing respiratory obstruction. The removal of dentures also prevents their being broken accidentally. Dentures taken from the patient should immediately be put into a container in a safe place. Other prostheses, such as false limbs or eyes, should also be removed and placed in safekeeping.

The patient should void shortly before going to the operating room to prevent urinary incontinence due to muscle relaxation during the operation. An empty bladder permits the surgeon a better view of the abdominal cavity and decreases the chances of inadvertent injury to the bladder. Since restriction of fluids causes dehydration, the patient may not need to void immediately before surgery. Voiding during the preoperative night is sometimes recorded, for this may help determine whether or not catheterization is necessary. If the bladder must be kept in a collapsed state throughout the operation, an indwelling catheter is inserted and attached by tubing to a drainage system.

If the patient has pronounced varicosities, is elderly, and is to have an operation that may be time-consuming or that involves removal of any of the pelvic organs, elastic bandages (Ace bandages) may be applied to both legs and thighs before he goes to the operating room. This measure is believed to help prevent accumulation of blood in the veins of the lower extremities and to lessen the chances of the development of thrombophlebitis. It may also help to prevent shock by keeping blood that might otherwise collect in the veins in the circulating blood system.

Preoperative medication

A preoperative medication is given to the patient to reduce reflex irritability caused by pain, fear, and increased metabolic rate. This reflex irritability makes the induction of general anesthesia more difficult and decreases the effectiveness of the anesthetic agent. The preoperative medication also lessens the undesirable systemic action of the local anesthetic drugs. Examples of the medications given for these purposes are morphine sulfate, meperidine hydrochloride (Demerol), codeine sulfate, and the barbiturates such as soluble phenobarbital and amobarbital sodium (Amytal sodium). Sodium phenobarbital and very small doses of morphine or meperidine hydrochloride are most often ordered for children over 5 years of age. No narcotic is given to the younger child.

Atropine sulfate and scopolamine are given preoperatively to decrease the formation of mucous secretions in the mouth and respiratory passages and to prevent laryngospasm. While atropine and scopolamine have many similar effects in the body, scopolamine depresses the central nervous system when given parenterally and usually produces drowsiness, euphoria, relief of fear, relaxation, and amnesia. Scopolamine alone is the drug most often ordered for the infant and the child up to 5 years of age.[32]

In addition to sedative and analgesic drugs, antihistaminic drugs may be ordered for children to lessen postoperative vomiting. Occasionally antibiotics are given for prophylactic effect during the operation. They must be given exactly at the time specified so that their peak effectiveness will be during the height of the operation.

The nurse should give the preoperative medications at the scheduled time, since the full effect of these respiratory depressant drugs must be obtained before anesthetics may be given safely. The opiates have their maximum effect one hour to one and one-half hours after administration. In the event that the nurse cannot or does not give the medication when ordered, she should notify the surgeon and/or the anesthetist. They may decide to omit the medication or to give it intravenously. The maximum effects of the drug given by this route are reached in three to five minutes. After the medication is given, the patient should be carefully observed for signs of respiratory or circulatory depression caused by a sensitivity to the drug or by an overdosage. Because opiates make the patient feel drowsy, lightheaded, and unsteady on his feet, he should stay in bed after they are administered. If atropine

is given, the patient should be told to expect that his mouth will feel dry. The nurse should have completed all preoperative procedures before the medication is given. Rush, noise, and confusion should be avoided, and the patient's environment should be kept quiet until he is taken to the operating room.

Charting

The preoperative charting should be accurate and complete. It should contain information on the nurse's notes and the nursing care plan to provide a base line for observations and nursing care postoperatively. For example, if the patient has any irregular coloring of the nail beds or a slight cyanosis, the condition should be recorded because it would be significant postoperatively. If the patient is exceedingly restless and active preoperatively, his behavior should be recorded so that after surgery it may be understood better. The chart must also contain all the information that the surgeon and the anesthetist need at the time of operation. It is essential that the nurse chart the time the medication was given, the patient's temperature, pulse, and respiratory rate, the time he last voided, whether dentures were removed, and any treatments that were done. The operative permit should be attached to the patient's chart. All laboratory tests should be reported, and roentgenograms and charts of previous admissions should be available.

Transportation to the operating room

The patient is transported to the operating room in his bed or on a stretcher. He should be made comfortable and be protected from drafts. Cotton blankets should be used. Woolen blankets must be removed because they are a source of static electricity. Either before he leaves his room or in the operating room, the infant patient may be wrapped in cotton sheet wadding to conserve his body heat. Often the air-conditioning equipment in the operating room must be modified for the tiny patient.

The bed or stretcher should be inspected ahead of time to see that it is freely movable. The stretcher must have straps to protect the patient from falling. If the bed is used, a name tag must be used so that the patient will be returned to his own bed postoperatively.

The patient should be accompanied to the operating room by a nurse with whom he is familiar. There should be a minimum of delay, noise, and physical disturbance. The nurse should remain with the patient until she is relieved by a member of the operating room staff (usually the anesthesiologist), since the patient should not be left alone in this strange and sometimes frightening environment.

The patient's family

On the day of the operation the nurse should make time available when the closest relative can be alone with the patient for a short time. When the patient leaves to go to the operating room, the family's apprehension may increase. During this special time, members of the family will appreciate any comfort the nurse can give. If they so desire, they may wait in the hospital for the patient's return from the operating room. If there is a waiting room, they should be told its location. If they must leave immediately for work or home, they should be asked to leave their telephone number, given the telephone number and extension in the hospital, and told approximately when they should call to learn of the patient's progress. They should know whether or not the patient is likely to go to a recovery room and whether or not he may be visited there. Most hospitals do not permit relatives to visit the patient while he is in the recovery room, but they do allow a close relative to visit a patient when he is transferred to an intensive care unit or to the clinical unit. It is always advisable to urge that only one close family member visit the patient on the operative day. The family member should be told approximately when he may be able to visit and he should be prepared for the fact that the patient may be somewhat sleepy or unresponsive and that special equipment, such as suction or oxygen equipment, may be in use.

Use of anesthetics

Although the nurse should not administer an anesthetic, she should be able to answer a patient's questions about the anesthetic he is to receive, she should understand the preparation of the patient for anesthesia during the preoperative period, and she should know the effects of anesthetics so that she can help the patient recover from them quickly, safely, and without complications. She must also be able to assist the physician intelligently when he is administering regional anesthetics.

An anesthetic produces a loss of sensation in part or all of the body. If it also produces unconsciousness, it is called a *general anesthetic*. If it produces a loss of sensation in only a part of the body while the patient remains conscious, it is called a *regional anesthetic*.

General anesthesia is produced by inhalation of gases or vapors of highly volatile liquids or by injection into the bloodstream or introduction into the rectum of anesthetic drugs in solution. Certain drugs that produce general anesthesia, such as thiopental sodium (Pentothal sodium), do not always produce the complete muscle relaxation that is necessary for surgery. Other general anesthetics, such as ether, do produce surgical anesthesia but are very irritating to mucous membranes of the respiratory tract. Such irritation prolongs the introductory stages of anesthesia. Therefore, the patient may receive two general anesthetic agents during the course of the operation: one that quickly produces anesthesia, such as Pentothal sodium, and one that produces surgical anesthesia, such as halothane. Frequently a combination of inhalation anesthetics such as nitrous oxide and oxygen and cyclopropane may be used, depending upon the anesthesiologist's judgment of what is best for each particular patient.

General anesthesia affects all the physiologic systems of the body to some degree. However, it affects chiefly the central nervous, respiratory, and circulatory systems. The anesthetist judges the depth of anesthesia by the changes produced in these systems. These changes are used in describing the *stages of anesthesia*. Stage I extends from the beginning of the administration of an anesthetic to the beginning of the loss of consciousness. Stage II, often called the stage of excitement or delirium, extends from the loss of consciousness to the loss of eyelid reflexes. If the patient is very apprehensive or was not given premedication correctly or on time, this stage, usually of short duration, may last longer. The patient may become

181

markedly excited and struggle, shout, talk, laugh, or cry. Stage III, the stage of surgical anesthesia, extends from the loss of the lid reflex to cessation of respiratory effort. The patient is unconscious, his muscles are relaxed, and most of his reflexes have been abolished. Stage IV is the stage of overdosage or the stage of danger. It is complicated by respiratory and circulatory failure. Death will follow unless the anesthetic is immediately discontinued and artificial respiration given. The nurse may find that some patients recovering from the effects of general inhalation anesthesia pass through Stage II before becoming fully conscious and are very noisy and restless.

Regional anesthesia is produced by the injection or application of a drug such as procaine hydrochloride along the course of a nerve, thus abolishing the conduction of all impulses to and from the area supplied by that nerve. The patient experiences no pain in the operative area and remains awake during the entire procedure because the anesthetic affects a particular region only; it does not affect essential sensory function.

Choice of anesthetic

The choice of anesthetic is based upon many factors: the physical condition and age of the patient; the presence of coexisting diseases; the type, site, and duration of the operation; the personal preference of the surgeon, the anesthetist, or the patient; the skill of the anesthetist; and the effects of various agents and methods upon the patient. The anesthetist evaluates each patient carefully and chooses the anesthetic that is best for him. For example, ether is not given to a patient who has had a recent lung infection because the drug is irritating to the respiratory passages.

An apprehensive patient may not respond well to a regional anesthetic, and it can seldom be used for infants or young children. Infants and small children tolerate intravenous anesthesia less well than adults. They respond in some instances with depression of respirations. Because the blood pressure control of infants and small children is more labile than that of an adult, they are seldom given spinal anesthesia, which may lower the blood pressure. Spinal anesthesia, like regional anesthesia is also not practical for

children for psychologic reasons. Because cyclopropane affects cardiac conduction mechanisms it is used with the greatest caution and often only in combination with other anesthetics if the patient has cardiac disease.

Anesthesia and the patient

Patients have many anxieties and fears about anesthesia. They may be afraid of going to sleep and not waking up. They fear the unknown. They frequently express a dislike of ether because of previous experience with it, and they remember its pungent odor. They may worry that the anesthetic will not be effective and that they will feel pain during the operation. Many patients are concerned about the nausea and vomiting that may occur postoperatively as a result of the anesthetic. Some fear that they may talk while under the effects of an anesthetic and reveal facts that they do not want known. Others are frightened by the anticipation of having a mask placed over their face. Many do not want a spinal anesthetic because they do not wish to be awake during the operation.

Many fears can be dispelled if the patient and his family are given information about the anesthetic he is to receive. If the patient expresses concern about the anesthetic, he should be told that the anesthetist carefully studies each patient's physical condition and administers the anesthetic that is best for him. The patient does not always see the anesthetist, who may determine which agent is best by talking to the patient's surgeon and studying the patient's medical record. In most instances, however, the anesthetist visits the patient in the evening before or on the morning of the operation.

The nurse can assure the patient and his family that accidents resulting from the administration of anesthetics are exceedingly rare and that his chances of recovering from its effects are excellent. The patient and his family should be told that he will be watched carefully while he is under anesthesia and that he will not be left alone until he is fully recovered from its effects. The nurse can further explain that most anesthetizing agents are now administered in such a way that little vomiting occurs postoperatively. Very few patients talk while under anesthesia, and what is said is usually unintelligible, so that talking need not be of great concern to any patient. The nurse should relay any persistent anxiety of the patient concerning anesthesia to the physician or to the anesthetist.

Prevention of fire and explosion

Certain anesthetizing agents such as ether, ethylene, and cyclopropane are inflammable and explosive. Therefore, extreme precautions must be taken at all times so that electric charges are not produced to ignite or explode these agents. When the nurse enters the operating room for any reason, she should be aware of these dangers. She should dress according to operating room regulations, wearing conductor bands on her shoes to ground possible electric charges and using any other protection that is required. She should never approach the anesthetist or the head of the table, and she should never touch any of the anesthetist's equipment unless specifically instructed to do so.

General anesthesia

Inhalation anesthesia

Inhalation anesthesia is produced by having the patient inhale the vapors of certain liquids or gases. Oxygen is usually given with these anesthetics. The gas mixture may be administered by mask or be delivered into the lungs by a catheter or a tube that is inserted into the trachea or into the bronchi. The use of the catheter or tube is called *intubation* or intratracheal intubation. Intubation assures an airway that can be easily suctioned and that can be used to aerate the lungs when the chest wall is opened. Also, the tube fills the tracheal space so that aspiration of gastric contents cannot occur. Regardless of the skill of the anesthesiologist, a tracheal tube cannot help causing some irritation to the trachea. Because the child's trachea is smaller, edema may more easily obstruct the lumen. Therefore, signs of sudden respiratory difficulty are more likely to occur postoperatively in the child than in the adult. The child's respiratory pattern must be observed most carefully when a tracheal tube has been used,

and increased mucus or other signs of respiratory embarrassment such as cyanosis or difficulty in breathing must be reported to the doctor at once.

Ether. Ether is a volatile, inflammable liquid. It has a very pungent odor that is disagreeable to many patients. It is irritating to the mucous membranes of the pulmonary tract. This irritating quality prolongs the first and second stages of anesthesia. For this reason, a rapid-acting, nonirritating drug such as thiopental sodium (Pentothal sodium) often is used to produce sleep before ether is administered. Ether is a relatively inexpensive drug. It is used for many operations because it provides excellent muscle relaxation and has a greater margin of safety than some of the other anesthetic agents. Ether is generally not used for patients who have acute or chronic disease of the respiratory system, the liver, or the kidneys. Ether is considered to be the safest and best general anesthetic for infants and small children, although in some areas it is being replaced to some extent by halothane and methoxyflurane (Penthrane).

Recovery from anesthesia with ether may be prolonged, especially if a large amount of the drug was used. The patient will require constant supervision until completely awake. Because of ether's irritating qualities, large amounts of mucus may be present, in which case the patient must be suctioned frequently. Since vomiting often occurs after the administration of ether, the patient should be placed on his side to prevent aspiration of any vomitus. If the foot of the bed is elevated, gravity will aid the flow of mucus and vomitus from the throat and mouth. Before anesthesia is begun, mineral oil or a similar lubricant is dropped into the patient's eyes to prevent possible irritation of the eyes by ether. If an irritation does occur, a lubricant may be used postoperatively. Redness or blistering of the skin, which sometimes occurs around the site of the mask, is caused by the combination of ether, moisture, and pressure. This condition can be unsightly and uncomfortable for the patient. Petroleum jelly or other ointments may be applied as ordered to relieve discomfort. When the patient has recovered from anesthesia, he should be encouraged to breathe deeply and to cough productively to clear secretions from the bronchi. Since the odor of ether may be disturbing to others, patients recovering from anesthesia should not be close to other patients.

Nitrous oxide. Nitrous oxide is a nonirritating, sweet-smelling, nonflammable gas. It is used for operations that do not require deep anesthesia. Nitrous oxide is always given with proportionate amounts of oxygen. The patient becomes anesthetized quickly and recovers rapidly. This gas is used largely for dental surgery and as a preliminary anesthetic when ether is to be administered. It is relatively inexpensive. Patients who have hypertension and associated cardiovascular diseases or those with diseases of the respiratory tract tolerate nitrous oxide poorly. If an excessive amount of this gas is given, there is always the possibility of anoxia, and patients with cardiovascular and respiratory diseases tolerate a reduction in oxygen poorly.

Ethylene. Ethylene is a nonirritating, inflammable gas used for procedures not requiring deep anesthesia. Its odor is rather similar to that of ether, and may disturb some patients. Ethylene produces unconsciousness quickly, and recovery takes only two or three minutes. It is often used to produce sleep before ether is administered. Since ethylene must be given in high concentrations, oxygen must be concurrently given to prevent anoxia. Patients who have mild anoxia from pulmonary diseases or who have liver and renal diseases do not tolerate this anesthetic. Vomiting may occur after the administration of this drug, but little mucus is produced.

Cyclopropane. Cyclopropane is a highly inflammable and pleasant-smelling gas that quickly produces unconsciousness. The patient recovers rapidly from its effects because most of the gas is eliminated from the body about ten minutes after the anesthetic is stopped. It is not so potent as ether but does produce adequate relaxation for most abdominal surgery. Since it increases cardiac irritability and causes arrhythmias, it is contraindicated in all patients with cardiac diseases. The nurse should frequently check the pulse rate and rhythm for any irregularities that might occur as a result of the patient's having received this gas. Vomiting may occur postoperatively. Cyclopropane is highly inflammable and explosive. When it

is being administered, great care must be taken to prevent the production of any electric charge that might ignite it.

Vinyl ether. Vinyl ether is a highly volatile, inflammable liquid. Its vapor quickly produces unconsciousness, and recovery is rapid. It is usually used to produce sleep before ether is administered. It may also be used for minor surgical procedures in which deep anesthesia is not required—for example, in dental extraction or incision and drainage. This drug is expensive to use. It is irritating to the respiratory mucosa and causes a large amount of mucus to form, thus making frequent suctioning necessary. Its use is contraindicated in patients who have pulmonary diseases.

Halothane (Fluothane). Halothane is a highly potent, nonflammable drug. Its odor is not unpleasant, it is easily inhaled, and it is usually administered through special vaporizers with nitrous oxide and oxygen. Halothane is nonirritating and does not cause laryngospasm or irritate the pulmonary tract. Induction into and recovery from anesthesia is generally fairly rapid. Halothane can depress the circulation when high concentrations are given. Gastrointestinal discomfort in the postanesthesia period is minimal.

Methoxyflurane (Penthrane). Penthrane is a clear, colorless liquid with a characteristic odor. It is nonexplosive and nonflammable under normal conditions. Induction in Penthrane anesthesia is prolonged, and usually one of the quick-acting drugs such as thiopental sodium is given intravenously before its administration. Penthrane seldom causes nausea and is believed to be extremely low in toxicity. Because of its long-lasting effect, its use delays the patient's need postoperatively for an analgesic drug that may depress respirations.

Chloroform. Chloroform is rarely used because of its toxicity and narrow margin of safety. A very small amount can cause death. It may cause liver function derangement, cardiac depression, and serious biochemical disturbances. It produces anesthesia quickly and does offer excellent muscle relaxation, but it must be administered with great caution and skill.

Intravenous anesthesia

Thiopental sodium (Pentothal sodium) is the drug used most frequently for intravenous anesthesia. It produces unconsciousness quickly, and recovery is rapid. Pentothal sodium is used for brief, minor procedures such as dilation and curettage of the uterus and to produce sleep before an inhalation anesthetic is administered. If a patient is very apprehensive about the operation, Pentothal sodium is sometimes given in his room before he goes to the operating room. It may also be given to relieve severe, prolonged convulsive states. Because of its depressing effect upon the respiratory system of children, its use in pediatric surgery is limited.

Patients who have received this drug should be watched carefully for laryngospasm. Signs of laryngospasm are restlessness, apprehension, stridor, retraction of the soft tissue about the neck, and cyanosis. The nurse should notify the physician when these signs begin to develop, for the patient may require an emergency tracheostomy. If large amounts of Pentothal sodium have been used, the patient may sleep for a long time and should be observed for signs of respiratory depression, such as shallow, slow respirations. The blood pressure should be checked frequently because it may fall suddenly. Patients who receive this drug often have generalized muscle twitching. The cause of this condition is not known, but if it continues for any length of time, it should be reported. Pentothal sodium is detoxified in the liver and excreted by the kidneys. Therefore, patients with diseases of the liver or kidneys may not tolerate this drug.

Rectal anesthesia

Some drugs can be given rectally to produce anesthesia, analgesia, or amnesia. Occasionally thiopental sodium is used. *Tribromoethanol* (Avertin) is a drug also given for these purposes. This clear, colorless, non-irritating liquid is instilled into the rectum, where it is absorbed. Since dosage is based on body weight, the nurse must weigh the patient carefully and record his weight accurately. Tribromoethanol induces sleep but, if major surgery is planned, must be followed by a drug that produces a deep anesthesia.

The patient who has received Avertin may remain unconscious for some time after its administration, since the rate of its elimination from the body varies with each patient. Depression of respirations is common, and the patient should be placed in a position that enables him to breathe freely. When the patient does awaken, he is very drowsy and should be protected from injury by the use of side rails on the bed. Since hypotension may also occur, the blood pressure should be taken frequently. Avertin is detoxified by the liver and eliminated by the kidneys and, therefore, is contraindicated in patients with liver or kidney disease. It is not given to patients who have pulmonary tract infections or diseases of the heart and other circulatory disturbances. Elderly and cachectic patients tolerate Avertin poorly.

Regional anesthesia

Regional anesthesia is used for treatments, diagnostic measures, examinations, and surgery. The nurse usually assembles the equipment necessary for the administration of the drugs used to produce regional anesthesia. She assists the physician during the procedure and observes the patient for reactions to the anesthetic or to the procedure.

The drugs used to produce regional anesthesia are usually called *local anesthetics.* Examples are procaine, cocaine, tetracaine (Pontocaine), dibucaine (Nupercaine), butacaine sulfate (Butyn sulfate), and piperocaine (Metycaine). When these drugs are absorbed into the bloodstream, they cause stimulation of the central nervous system and depression of the heart. Care, therefore, is taken that they are given in a localized area and in the smallest dose necessary to produce anesthesia. A barbiturate is usually given before the drugs are administered to reduce their action on the central nervous system. Epinephrine may be added to the solution of local anesthetic drugs to produce vasoconstriction in the area of the injection. Vasoconstriction tends to reduce the rate of absorption, to extend the length of anesthesia, and to reduce hemorrhage.

The nurse must observe the patient carefully for signs of excitability, twitching, pulse or blood pressure changes, pallor of the skin, and respiratory difficulties. At the first signs of these toxic reactions, an intravenous injection of a short-acting barbiturate such as Pentothal sodium should be ready for the physician to administer. Oxygen may also be necessary, and it is important that an airway be maintained. If the reaction is due to an idiosyncrasy to the drug, circulatory failure may occur, and emergency measures such as artificial respiration must be started. Patients should be questioned regarding any previous sensitivity to these drugs, and skin tests are usually advocated before their administration.

Recently regional anesthesia of the limbs has been achieved by injecting an anesthetizing agent such as chloroprocaine into a vein in the limb to be anesthetized. A tourniquet is applied to the limb to prevent the distribution of the anesthetizing agent throughout the body.[16,24]

Topical anesthesia

Topical anesthesia is accomplished by applying or spraying a local anesthetic drug such as cocaine directly on the part to be anesthetized. It is used for diagnostic procedures or treatments of the nose and throat, and it may be used for minor skin operations.

Infiltration anesthesia

Infiltration anesthesia is accomplished by the injection of the anesthetic drug directly into the area to be incised or manipulated. This method is used for minor procedures (incision and drainage, thoracentesis). Another method of infiltration anesthesia is the *nerve block,* in which the drug is injected into the nerve a short distance from the site of the operation. This method may be employed in tonsillectomies or plastic or dental surgery.

In a *saddle block,* the drug is injected into the dural sac at the third and fourth lumbar interspace and affects the perineal area, a band around the body from the pubis to the umbilicus, and the legs, partially or completely. When a *caudal block* is done, the drug is injected into the caudal canal lying below the cord and affects the nerve trunks that supply the body from the umbilicus to the toes.

Spinal anesthesia

Spinal anesthesia is accomplished by the injection of a local anesthetic drug in solution into the subarachnoid space, where it acts upon the nerves as they emerge from the spinal cord. Depending upon the type of anesthesia desired, the injection is made through the second, third, or fourth interspace of the lumbar vertebras. Anesthesia is quickly produced and provides good relaxation of muscles.

Spinal anesthesia is used for surgery of the lower limbs, lower trunk, and lower abdomen and sometimes for surgery in the upper abdomen such as removal of the gallbladder. It is not used for operations on the upper part of the body because it can cause paralysis of the diaphragm and other muscles of respiration. With spinal anesthesia the patient may be conscious of pulling sensations throughout the operation but he experiences no pain. Occasionally a feeling of faintness and nausea occur; these symptoms may be of psychic origin. One of the limitations of spinal anesthesia is that the patient is awake during the operation, although the preoperative medication may make him quite unaware of his surroundings. A screen restricts his vision in the operating room, and a towel may be placed over his eyes. The conversation and activities of the members of the operating room staff should be carried on with his consciousness in mind. It is a nursing responsibility to remind other members of the team that the patient is awake if topics that might disturb the patient are discussed. Another limitation of this type of anesthesia is that it may cause hypotension during the operation. Drugs such as ephedrine hydrochloride may be given if a drop in blood pressure occurs.

Following spinal anesthesia, the patient should be kept flat in bed with a pillow under his head. Since sensation may not return to the anesthetized area for an hour or two, the nurse must see that the patient sustains no injuries such as burns from hot-water bottles during this time. He will need to be turned, and he should not be placed in a strained or unnatural position that might cause him later discomfort. The nurse must always be alert for signs of respiratory or circulatory depression. Although the patient is conscious, his blood pressure, pulse, and respirations should be checked frequently. Although hypotension may occur as a result of relaxation of the vascular bed, the patient should not be placed in the position for shock until a physician gives the order. There is a danger that the anesthetic may travel up the spinal canal and affect the diaphragm.

Although some physicians permit the patient complete freedom of movement immediately after the operation, other physicians request that the patient remain flat in bed for six to twelve hours following spinal anesthesia to reduce the possibility of a "spinal" headache. This headache is thought to be due to leakage of spinal fluid from the puncture in the dura or to sterile chemical meningitis. It usually occurs twenty-four hours after the puncture and is more common in women than in men. It may last several days, and occasionally it persists for weeks or months. The nurse should not suggest the possibility of this complication to the patient. If it does occur the patient complains of a throbbing, pulsating headache that is aggravated by a change in position. He should remain flat in bed and move about as little as possible. An ice bag may bring relief. To lessen discomfort, analgesics and sedatives should be given as ordered.

When the effects of the anesthetic wear off, the patient occasionally complains of a backache. His pain may be the result of the position in which he was placed on the operating table or of the insertion of the needle at the time of the puncture. The complaint is treated symptomatically, and heat applied locally often brings relief.

Muscle relaxants

Certain drugs such as *d*-tubocurarine chloride (curare) and succinylcholine chloride (Anectine) relax skeletal muscles. They are adjuncts in anesthesia and are given when anesthetics that are to be used do not provide sufficient relaxation of the abdominal muscles. These drugs cause respiratory depression or paralysis, and the patients must be watched very carefully for signs of respiratory difficulty during and after their administration.

Hypothermia

Refrigeration anesthesia—local hypothermia

Refrigeration anesthesia refers to the lowering of the temperature of only a part of the body, such as a limb. It is used largely to produce surgical anesthesia prior to amputation of a limb affected by arteriosclerotic gangrene. Elderly, debilitated patients and patients who have diabetes are most likely to be treated with this anesthesia. Advantages of this method are that physical shock to the patient is minimal, no inhalation anesthesia is required, and the lowered temperature reduces cell metabolism.

Fluid and food are permitted up to the time of surgery. Because the patient is usually experiencing pain and the weight of the ice makes him more uncomfortable, a barbiturate or narcotic is usually administered before the procedure is initiated.

If crushed ice is to be used to anesthetize the limb, extra plastic sheets are placed under the patient to protect the bed. Approximately one-half hour before the ice is applied, ice bags are placed around the limb at the sites where the tourniquets will be applied to reduce local sensitivity to them. The tourniquets are used to prevent chilling of the rest of the body by curtailing blood flow out of the affected extremity. After the tourniquets are applied by the doctor and secured with clamps to prevent their slipping, the limb is covered with crushed ice. A metal trough or plastic sheet can be used to contain the ice, support the limb, and protect the bed. Provision should be made for drainage of melted ice by elevating the head of the bed on blocks so that water may drain down into a receptacle. Anesthesia is obtained in about one and one-half hours if only the lower leg is involved and three hours if the entire limb is to be anesthetized. The refrigeration equipment is removed in the operating room. Duration of anesthesia by this method is approximately sixty minutes.

Another method for producing anesthesia in an extremity is the use of a special electric refrigeration unit consisting of coiled tubes that are wrapped around the extremity. This unit is thermostatically controlled and is set at 4.5° C. (40° F.) during induction and surgery. This method is more convenient than the cracked-ice method.

The nurse should supplement the doctor's and/or the anesthetist's explanation of the procedure to the patient and to his family.

She should move the affected limb as carefully and gently as possible, work quickly, and arrange for someone to stay with the patient until he goes to the operating room. Emotional reaction to the need for an amputation may be further aggravated by general illness and pain, which increase the patient's uneasiness if he is left alone.

General hypothermia

Hypothermia refers to the reduction of body temperature below normal with resulting reduced oxygen and metabolic needs. It is possible by this means to reduce metabolic needs 50 to 70%.[29] This reduction has enabled surgeons to perform heart surgery, vascular surgery, and neurosurgery that formerly were not possible because of hemorrhage and threat to metabolic needs of vital structures such as the brain, the heart, and the kidneys. The temperature range usually used is between 32° C. (89.6° F.) and 26° C. (78.8° F.). Depending upon the amount of cooling, hypothermia is referred to as mild, moderate, or deep. Hypothermia is now being used widely for a variety of illnesses when extremely high temperature occurs. For example, patients with neurologic disease causing a high temperature may be kept in a state of relatively mild hypothermia (30.6° to 35° C. or 87° to 95° F.) for as long as five days.

If hypothermia is to be used as an adjunct to anesthesia during surgery, the patient usually is given meperidine hydrochloride (Demerol) and atropine sulfate forty-five minutes to one hour before the procedure is to start. After the patient has been anesthetized, an intratracheal catheter is inserted. It is used to inflate or deflate the lungs if the chest wall is opened or to administer oxygen if respirations are depressed by hypothermia. Provision is made for monitoring temperature readings from different parts of the body, preferably the esophagus and the rectum, by placing electric thermometers in those areas. In addition, the heart is monitored with an electrocardiograph to detect cardiac arrhythmias produced by lowered temperatures, and the brain is monitored with an electroencephalograph to detect cerebral anoxia. The temperature is then lowered by one of the following methods. The care of the patient at this time is under the supervision of the operating room team.

Ways of achieving general hypothermia. *External hypothermia* may be produced by applying crushed ice around the patient, by totally immersing the patient in ice water, or by exposing him to the cooling effects of special blankets. When the cold bath is used, a tub is partially filled with water and crushed ice at a temperature of approximately 10° C. (50° F.). After being anesthetized, the patient is placed in a tub until the desired hypothermia is reached. He is then lifted up to the operating table. When the cooling blankets are used, the patient is placed on and covered by body-sized vinyl pads that contain many coils. The pads are connected to a reservoir filled with alcohol and water, a pump that fills the coils and circulates the solution, and a unit that will heat or cool the solution to a preset temperature. (See Fig. 41.)

Extracorporeal cooling, a method of bloodstream cooling, consists of removing the blood from a major vessel, circulating it through coils immersed in a refrigerant, and returning it to the body through another vessel. Bloodstream cooling is the fastest method for producing hypothermia and is used primarily for patients who are undergoing surgery. The patient is given heparin to prevent the blood from clotting during the procedure.

Internal hypothermia is another method of achieving a lowering of the temperature. Drugs such as chlorpromazine hydrochloride (Thorazine) and promethazine hydrochloride (Phenergan) or meperidine hydrochloride (Demerol) are given intravenously or intramuscularly. This combination of drugs is referred to as the *lytic cocktail.* The chlorpromazine hydrochloride affects the thermal regulating mechanism and the Phenergan and Demerol are sedatives. All tend to reduce shivering. A reduction in temperature of only about 4° usually is achieved, but this amount may be crucial in determining the outcome for the patient undergoing surgery or suffering from a dangerous degree of hyperpyrexia.[29]

Rewarming the patient. Rewarming of the patient at the conclusion of the operation or the end of the treatment is accomplished by partially immersing him in tepid or warm

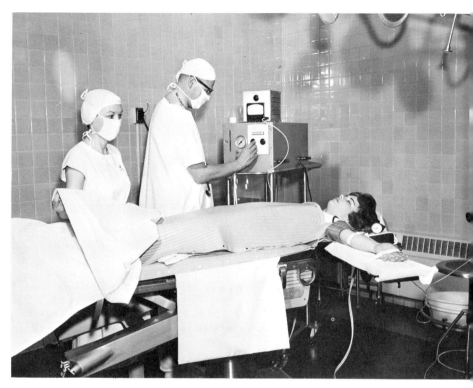

Fig. 41

Hypothermia can be produced by means of a cooling blanket. Cold alcohol and water are circulated through the coils by a pressure pump. (Courtesy Gorman-Rupp Industries, Inc., Bellville, Ohio.)

water, by heating the solution in the circulating blanket, or by diathermy. If the temperature has been lowered only a few degrees, he may be permitted to return slowly to his normal temperature without assistance. Usually rewarming procedures are stopped when the temperature is within one or two degrees of the normal. Care is taken to prevent burning the patient during the warming until his temperature reaches 32° C. (89° F.), at which time consciousness usually returns. The patient's temperature, pulse, and blood pressure are checked frequently, and any changes should be reported at once to the physician.

There may be some so-called temperature drift upward as rewarming occurs. The temperature control mechanism is more labile than normal after hypothermia, and a sharp rise in temperature may occur.

Nursing care of patients having prolonged hypothermia. If he is conscious, the patient who is to have hypothermia for an elevation of temperature needs reassurance that the procedure will not be too uncomfortable. Because the treatment is relatively new and

is often erroneously conceived by the laity, the patient may have fears and apprehension that should be reported to the doctor so that he can answer specific questions that may be causing worry. When hypothermia is to be continued for several days, any of the external methods for producing hypothermia may be used. Before the procedure is started, the patient is given a complete bath, and a thin coating of oil or cream may be applied to the skin. A cleansing enema may be ordered. While the temperature is being lowered to the desired level and for as long as the procedure is continued, the patient is observed constantly. Any irregularities of pulse, temperature or blood pressure must be reported at once. It is expected that all of these vital signs will lower gradually. If they rise, drop too suddenly, or fluctuate, the doctor should be notified. The temperature is monitored by a rectal thermometer to determine whether or not a desired temperature (usually between 30° and 32° C. or 86° and 89.6° F.) is maintained throughout the treatment.

Shivering is a complication of hypothermia that should be avoided because peripheral vasoconstriction is accompanied by an increase in body temperature, circulation rate, and oxygen consumption. Usually shivering occurs when the temperature is lowered to 30° C. (86° F.). To prevent shivering, chlorpromazine hydrochloride (Thorazine) usually is given before the treatment is started and is repeated as often as every two hours if shivering continues. Since urinary output is decreased when the body temperature is reduced to 32° C. (89° F.), a retention catheter (Foley type of catheter) is inserted before hypothermia is started so that output can be measured accurately. Intake must also be measured carefully and recorded. Because the gag and other reflexes may be depressed, food and fluids are not given by mouth. Fluids containing glucose and electrolytes are given intravenously and usually through a polyethylene catheter that has been sutured into a vein. Depending upon the method being used to produce hypothermia, the patient may be fed by means of a nasogastric tube. The patient's skin must be observed for signs of pressure, edema, and discoloration. He should be turned at least every two hours, and footboards and pillows should be used to prevent strain on joints and to maintain proper body alignment. Often the patient is placed on a CircOlectric bed to make possible a complete change in position. Good oral hygiene is necessary, and dried secretions should be removed from the nares. If corneal reflexes are diminished and eye secretions reduced, the eyes may need to be cleansed and covered to protect them as described on p. 165.

The cooling agent is removed at the termination of hypothermia, and regular blankets are applied. The patient is usually allowed to warm at his own rate. The temperature must be observed carefully as it approaches normal, and blankets must then be removed. The thermometer is removed when the temperature becomes stable.

Immediate postoperative nursing care

The immediate postoperative period is a critical one for the patient. He must be watched carefully until the effects of the anesthetic have worn off, his reflexes have returned, and his vital signs are stable. The nurse is largely responsible for the care of the patient at this time, and she must be prepared to meet his specific needs as they arise. Her first responsibilities are to make certain that the patient has a clear airway until his pharyngeal reflexes have returned, to prevent and to be alert for any circulatory depression, to remain with the patient until he is rational and oriented, and to protect him from any physical injury.

It is the practice in most hospitals to have all patients taken to a recovery room where they can be given undivided attention as soon as surgery is completed. All the equipment that may be necessary is available in a recovery room: oxygen, suction machines, sphygmomanometers, infusion fluids, shock blocks, airways, emergency medications, respirators, side rails, and provision for cardiac massage. Ideally, recovery rooms are located on the same floor as the operating room or in its immediate vicinity. If there is no recovery room, the nurse prepares the patient's unit with as much equipment as may be needed. In either instance, the bed is made according to hospital routine. Details may vary, but it is usually prepared so that the patient can be easily returned to it and so that it is protected from any drainage or emesis that may occur. The patient is placed directly into his bed from the operating table or is transferred very gently onto a stretcher. The move should be done with a lift sheet or by the three-man lift so that all parts of the patient's body are supported. The patient should be accompanied to the recovery room or to his room by the anesthetist and another member of the operating room professional staff because of the danger of respiratory embarrassment or the aspiration of vomitus en route.

The nurse in the postoperative unit assumes the responsibility for the care of the patient after she receives a report on the patient's condition from members of the operating room staff. The nurse in the operating room can contribute to better care for the patient both in the recovery room and on the clinical unit. She does so by sharing pertinent information about the operative course so that the nursing staff are able to observe the patient more intelligently and make sounder judgments about the nursing care he needs.

Maintenance of aeration

The most desirable position to ensure *maintenance of an airway* depends upon the size and condition of the patient, the anesthesia used, the operation performed, and the amount of experienced nursing care that is available. Ideally, the patient should be in a position so that he can breathe normally with full use of all portions of his lungs and so that vomitus, blood, and mucus can drain and will not be aspirated. The back-lying position with head hyperextended permits the fullest expansion of the lungs and is the least likely to dislodge an airway. It is a dangerous position, however, from the standpoint of danger of aspiration of vomitus or mucus. It is never used if the patient is partially awake and an airway has been removed. If vomiting occurs, the patient is likely to aspirate unless the *whole body* is turned. Turning the patient's head when his chest and shoulders remain in the back-lying position is useless. If there is the *slightest* evidence of nausea, if the patient is a large adult who cannot be turned quickly by the staff available, or if the staff available is not adept at detecting the earliest signs of awakening or nausea, the patient should be placed on his side. The side-lying position usually is used after an airway has been removed and if there are any signs of gagging or vomiting. It somewhat diminishes the chest expansion, but this disadvantage can be minimized by turning the patient frequently and by raising the flexed upper arm and placing it on a pillow. The prone or face-lying, position or the semiprone position provides excellent drainage from the throat, and it is believed that because the tongue falls forward, there is less irritation of the pharynx and less tendency to vomit.[42] This position is used routinely for children following a tonsillectomy. Chest expansion in this position is maintained by placing a pillow under the abdomen. Limitations of this position are that it is difficult to take the patient's blood pressure

and observe for vital signs such as pupillary reaction. It also is difficult to turn an adult quickly into a satisfactory position for immediate suctioning if it becomes necessary.

A metal, rubber, or plastic airway is often left in place following the administration of an anesthetic to keep the passage open and to keep the tongue forward until the pharyngeal reflexes have returned. This tube should be removed as soon as the patient begins to awaken since its presence is irritating and leads to vomiting.

When the tongue is relaxed from anesthesia, it may fall back and prevent free passage of air. This condition can be prevented by holding the patient's jaw up and forward or by placing him on his side. If it should occur, however, the nurse should turn the patient over onto his side or onto his abdomen with his head hanging down over the side of the bed. This position will bring the tongue forward. If it is not possible to turn the patient, the nurse can open his mouth by pushing at the angle of the jaw with her thumbs and have someone insert a padded tongue depressor between the back teeth. The tongue can then be brought forward by grasping it with a piece of gauze or with a clamp.

Excessive secretions in the nasopharynx, trachea, and bronchial tree also may obstruct the airway and interfere with respirations. These secretions are usually caused by the anesthetic, by other drugs that have given, or by irritation to the mucosa of the throat and trachea from intubation or suctioning. They are removed from the posterior pharynx with a catheter (Fig. 42). If a Y connecting tube is used, the suction machine is turned on and the catheter inserted to the lowest point to be aspirated. The open end of the Y tube is then closed with a fingertip to create suction, and the catheter is rotated slowly and withdrawn gradually. This method prevents trauma to the posterior pharynx and/or trachea and prevents buildup of pressure within the catheter. If the secretions are in the tracheobronchial area and cannot be reached by the catheter, intratracheal suctioning must be done, and sometimes a tracheostomy is necessary.

Air inhaled normally is at approximately 32° C. (80° F.) with 35% humidity. Upon exhalation it is 38.4° C. (98° F.) with almost

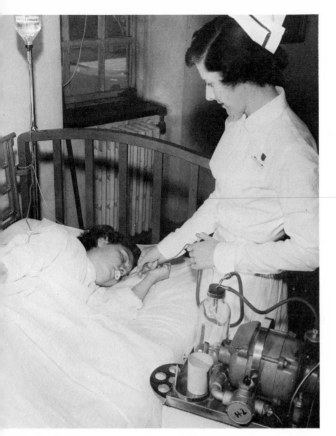

A

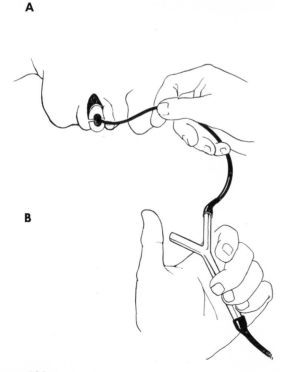

B

Fig. 42

A, Suctioning the unconscious patient. **B,** The Y tube valve, which is left open until the catheter is inserted and in place. The Y opening is then occluded with the fingertip and the secretions are aspirated.

100% humidity.[39] This normal physiologic process by which heat and moisture are lost is well tolerated by most people in good health but causes complications in persons who may be dehydrated, who may have irritation of the respiratory passages from drugs and trauma, or who may not have been breathing normally during surgery. Humidity of the air breathed should be increased postoperatively to keep secretions soft, facilitating their removal, and to prevent dry air from further irritating the already irritated respiratory passages.

Because, after general inhalation anesthesia, almost all patients have decreased pulmonary expansion and areas of atelectasis, both of which result in retained secretions and poor aeration of the alveoli, humidity and oxygen usually are given postoperatively. Commercial machines that give a fine mist of moisture in the oxygen (e.g., Hydrojets and DeVilbiss ultrasonic humidifiers) are available. Moisture can be directed close to the patient by means of a hood, or it can be spread about the entire room. Mucolytic agents and detergent or "wetting" agents such as tyloxapol (Alevaire), sodium ethasulfate (Tergemist), which contains iodine, and Suprenone may be given with the oxygen. However, there is not a unanimity of opinion as to their value. If signs of bronchospasm occur, bronchodilators, such as epinephrine hydrochloride (Vaponefrin) and epinephrine (Adrenalin), and hydrocortisone or prednisolone may be used. Occasionally it is necessary to use a portable respirator such as the Bird respirator to maintain adequate ventilation of the lungs postoperatively. There are attachments on portable respirators so that they can be used with tracheostomy and intratracheal tubes.

Maintenance of circulation and prevention of shock

As soon as the nurse is certain that the patient's airway is clear, she should check his blood pressure and pulse. Moving the patient from the operating room table to his bed, reaction to drugs and anesthesia, loss of blood during the operation, and postoperative bleeding all will cause circulatory changes that may result in lowering of the blood volume. Shock resulting from lowered blood volume must be prevented because the liver, kidneys, brain, heart, and other vital organs do not tolerate long periods of anoxia. The blood pressure should be taken frequently until it reaches a satisfactory level and remains there. The pulse is also checked for rate, volume, and rhythm. When the blood pressure drops, the pulse rate usually increases, pulse volume becomes thin and thready, and the skin becomes cold, moist, and pale. The physician should be notified at once if there is a change in blood pressure or if any arrhythmias develop. Blood, plasma, or other intravenous fluids usually are ordered to increase the blood volume. Oxygen may be given to increase its concentration in the available circulating blood. The position for shock, unless contraindicated, may be used to help increase the blood flow to vital organs.

Protection from injury

Following anesthesia, side rails are usually placed on the bed and are left until the patient is fully awake. Although the patient is constantly watched, it is possible for him suddenly to turn and throw himself from the bed. Hot-water bottles, heating pads, or heat lamps must be used with care while the patient is unconscious, so that burns do not occur. If infusions are being given, the patient's arm should be secured so that the needle does not become dislodged and cause injury. Physical restraints are seldom used if the patient is restless. Instead, the nurse should remain with the patient and guide his movements so that he does not hurt himself. The patient should be turned frequently and be placed in good body alignment to prevent nerve damage from pressure, and muscle and joint strain due to lying in one position for a long period of time. The patient under anesthesia has complete muscle relaxation with loss of sensation and is unable to indicate discomfort. The nurse must be constantly aware of this when moving or turning him.

Additional considerations during reaction from anesthesia

The nurse must check the patient's dressing for any drainage or bleeding. She should also look for tubes of any kind and connect them to the drainage system ordered. Infusions should be checked and added to as ordered. The doctor's order sheet must be checked for other instructions, treatments, and medications.

There should be complete and accurate charting about the postoperative course so that the nurse who continues care has a complete picture to which to refer as necessary. All medications, fluids, and treatments that the patient receives during this time must be recorded so that there will be no duplication that might prove harmful to the patient.

The nurse can ascertain the return of reflexes and the consciousness of the patient by asking him his name and other questions that would indicate he is oriented to time and place. The patient may be returned to his room as soon as his blood pressure is stable, if he is breathing freely, is not vomiting, and is fully awake.

General postoperative care

The patient and his family

The nurse in the clinical unit should show the greatest consideration of the patient's family during the time that he is in the operating room and the recovery room. If the operation has been completed, if the surgeon was delayed in starting the operation so that the patient's return to the unit will be delayed, or if the patient is expected to return to the unit in a short time, the family should be so informed. Information that can be shared with the patient's family helps to lessen their anxiety.

The nurse should know what operation was performed and what pathology was present so that she can plan the nursing care accordingly. She needs to know what information was given to the patient and to his family so that she will be able to answer their questions intelligently. The patient and his family frequently are too upset to hear or to understand all that the surgeon tells them, and they often ask the nurse for repeated explanations. Most surgeons discuss the results of the operation with the family immediately after surgery and also visit the patient, telling him briefly what was found and reassuring him about his condition. The surgeon often tells the family when a malignancy is found at operation, but he usually does not tell the patient at once. He may tell the patient that a tumor or growth was found and removed.

Immediate postoperative needs

When the patient returns to the unit postoperatively, the nurse should immediately check his blood pressure, pulse, respirations, dressings, drainage tube, and state of orientation. If the vital signs are relatively stable and there are no indications of hemorrhage or abnormal drainage, she should wash his face and hands, give him mouth care, rub his back, change his gown and bed linen as needed, and change his position, providing support for all dependent parts. A pillow usually is placed under his head, and if general chest or abdominal surgery has been performed, the head of the bed may be raised to a low Fowler's position. If necessary, medication for pain should be given. Since the patient may still be affected by sedation and anesthesia, side rails should be placed on the bed. They provide a firm support to which the patient may hold in order to turn or move himself more easily. After being made comfortable, the patient usually wishes to see a member of his family for a few minutes. This visit not only comforts the patient but reassures the family.

Most surgeons and most pediatricians believe that sedative and analgesic drugs in small, carefully measured doses should be given to children postoperatively to prevent pronounced pain and restlessness. Despite this measure, some children tamper with the wound. Usually a clean wound can be covered with enough adhesive to ensure protection, but children are sometimes remarkably ingenious at removing drains and tubes. Therefore, arm restraints must be used occasionally, and jacket or tie restraints are used by some hospitals. If a parent who is care-

fully instructed and who is equipped emotionally to help the child remains with him postoperatively, the need for restraints is often obviated. In many hospitals a parent may remain with the child in the pediatric units, and this practice is becoming more common when children must be placed in adult units postoperatively.

Since some types of restraints have caused strangling and death of the child, they must be used with the greatest caution. The nurse must apply the restraint correctly and must use it only when absolutely necessary and when it has been approved by the medical and administrative staffs of the hospital. The need for restraints and the panic that causes children to struggle when they are used can be reduced by careful explanation to the child both preoperatively and postoperatively and by understanding nursing attention postoperatively.

A small child can be prevented from tampering with a wound in the lower abdomen by fastening the hospital gown securely at the back, placing a cradle over the child's upper body, and then bringing the lower part of his gown up over the cradle and fastening it with safety pins. The small child cannot then reach around the cradle, and yet he is spared the aggravation of having his hands restrained. The cradle can be made secure by tying it at intervals to the rails or sides of the crib or small bed.

Sometimes keeping a child flat in bed is difficult, and special jacket restraints must be used. If drainage tubes are necessary and must be attached to bottles, the child may be cared for more easily on a frame, such as a Bradford frame.

Complications and their prevention

Much of the nursing care postoperatively is concentrated upon the prevention of complications, and this care should be started as soon as the patient returns from the operating room. The nurse should know what complications can develop, how she can help prevent them, and their early signs and symptoms.

Respiratory complications

The most common respiratory complications are bronchitis, atelectasis, and pneumonia. *Bronchitis* is an inflammation of the bronchi. *Atelectasis* is the blockage of air to a portion of the lung, causing this portion to fail to expand. *Pneumonia,* a bacterial infection, often follows atelectasis. Signs and symptoms of these complications usually develop within twenty-four to forty-eight hours after surgery. There is usually a rise in the patient's temperature and in his pulse and respiratory rates. He may or may not complain of chest pain, cough, or difficulty in breathing. Cyanosis may occur, and the patient may be restless and apprehensive. These complaints should be brought to the doctor's attention immediately.

Although most patients experience some respiratory irritation following intubation and inhalation anesthesia, respiratory complications most frequently occur in patients who smoke heavily, who suffer from chronic respiratory diseases such as bronchitis or bronchiectasis, or who are very young, elderly, debilitated, or obese. They are most likely to occur after high abdominal operations when prolonged inhalation anesthesia has been necessary and vomiting has occurred during the operation or while the patient is recovering from anesthesia. Gastric contents are known to be extremely irritating to the lungs, and most patients who aspirate vomitus postoperatively develop respiratory complications.

If postoperative patients are kept on their sides or in a semiprone position until they are fully awake, have the respiratory passages suctioned when necessary, are turned frequently, and are encouraged to breathe deeply and to cough productively, respiratory complications often can be prevented. Even after awakening from anesthesia, the back-lying position is not advisable for the elderly patient sleeping soundly under sedation or for any patient with a history of sinusitis or chronic postnasal drip, since there is danger of aspiration of infected material from the nasopharynx.

Following inhalation anesthesia, bronchial secretions usually are increased. Unless the mucus is removed, the bronchioles will become obstructed and atelectasis will occur. The lungs may be inadequately aerated because of incomplete excursion of the chest. Preoperative and postoperative medications, anesthesia, and shock tend to depress respira-

tions. Tight abdominal dressings or binders tend to inhibit normal action of the abdominal muscles and the diaphragm, causing the lung bases to remain uninflated. In the elderly patient, firming of the rib cage and loss of elasticity of chest structures increase this problem. Surgical trauma, especially after high abdominal operations, may lead to injury of fibers of the phrenic nerve, causing the diaphragm to become flaccid and relaxed. Pain in the incision or fear of pain may prevent the patient from fully expanding his chest cavity on inspiration. The patient then tends to have shallow respirations and to compensate for the restricted intake of air by breathing rapidly. Any factors that limit the full expansion of the lungs encourage the development of atelectasis because the ability to expel bronchial exudates is decreased. As the air is absorbed behind the occluded bronchioles, further exudates and consolidation of this portion of the lung usually occurs. This condition is known as pneumonitis, or inflammation of the lung.

Turning. If the patient lies in one position with continuous pressure from his weight against the chest wall, proper ventilation and drainage of secretions on that side of the chest are not possible, and atelectasis can develop. Atelectasis can be prevented by changing the patient's position frequently while he is on bed rest. Turning and changing of position provide for better ventilation of the lungs by encouraging deep respiration and drainage of secretions. The patient should be turned at least every two or three hours. His position may usually be rotated in the following manner: side, back, side, abdomen. When turning is restricted by the nature of the operation, he should be moved within the specified limitations. Although turning may increase pain in the incision, the nurse can use techniques that will cause as little discomfort as possible, such as turning the patient in one smooth movement. This procedure can be accomplished by three nurses working in unison or by one nurse using a lifting sheet. When the patient is able to cooperate in turning, the nurse can help him to first move his head and trunk to the side of the bed and then move his buttocks and lower extremities. The patient then is in a good position to roll onto his side or abdomen. Good body mechanics should be used to protect both the patient and the nurse from injury, and the nurse should not attempt to move a helpless or very heavy patient without assistance. When the desired position is attained, the patient should be placed in good body alignment with all dependent parts supported to prevent pull on the incision and unnatural strain on muscles and joints. Pillows placed against the back and abdomen and between the legs may make the patient more comfortable in a side-lying position. Unless contraindicated by the type of anesthetic used or surgery performed, the head of the bed should be elevated slightly. The schedule for turning the patient should be interrupted only when he is out of bed for several hours at a time and should be discontinued only when medical examination indicates that his lungs are clear and expanding fully. Roentgenograms may be taken to verify the return of the lungs to normal function.

Deep breathing and coughing. When the patient coughs productively, he expels any mucous secretions blocking the bronchi. Deep breathing often causes the patient to cough, and it assures complete ventilation of the lungs. All postoperative patients therefore, are asked to breathe deeply and to cough at least every two hours. During the first few hours postoperatively the doctor may wish the patient to breathe deeply and cough every fifteen minutes. Unless specifically contraindicated, deep breathing and coughing should be done routinely by all patients who have had a general anesthetic. Coughing may be contraindicated in a few situations, such as following brain, spinal, or eye surgery, but deep-breathing exercises should be done.

The patient can be taught abdominal breathing, in which he relaxes his abdominal muscles as he breathes in and thus causes his diaphragm to go down, and contracts his abdominal muscles as he breathes out and thus draws the diaphragm up. The nurse can determine whether or not he is breathing correctly by placing her hand lightly on his abdomen as he breathes. This type of breathing permits the diaphragm to descend fully and the entire lung to expand. If there are secretions in the bronchi, deep breathing will stimulate coughing and expectoration of the mucus. The patient should

be asked to do the breathing exercises at frequent intervals himself.

Since most patients find coughing painful after surgery, they need encouragement and assistance. Some surgeons advocate the administration of narcotics before coughing is begun. Narcotics decrease the cough reflex, however, and heavily sedated patients should be encouraged to cough more frequently. The nurse can best assist the patient to cough by placing her hands firmly on either side of the incision and exerting pressure. She can also splint the operative area with a drawsheet or towel. (See Fig. 133.) Such splinting prevents excessive muscular strain around the incision. If the patient must remain flat in bed while he coughs, restraining bedclothes and pillows should be removed from around the chest. If he is permitted to sit up in bed, a pull rope attached to the foot of the bed will help him assume and maintain a sitting position while coughing. The patient should be encouraged to cough deeply and productively. If the first attempt is not successful, he should rest and then try again. If he is unable to cough productively and if his attempts only lead to fatigue, the physician may use intratracheal suction to stimulate the cough reflex, or a bronchoscope may have to be passed to remove pulmonary secretions. A Bird respirator or one of several postoperative ventilating machines may be used to assist the patient who cannot cough effectively. Humidity as already described is also used to help liquefy tenacious secretions and facilitate their expectoration.

It is often exceedingly difficult to induce children to breathe deeply and to cough. A variety of games, such as blowing ballons, soap bubbles, feathers across a table, or colored water from one bottle to another (Fig. 43), may be used to encourage children to breathe deeply and to cough.

Coughing at regular intervals should be continued until the lungs are clear of all secretions. The doctor determines the condition of the lungs by auscultation, percussion, and roentgenographic examination.

Circulatory complications

The formation of clots in the veins of the pelvis and the lower extremities is a fairly common and a potentially serious postopera-

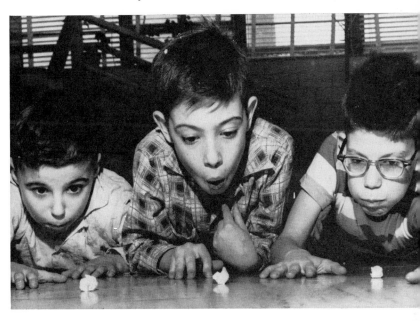

Fig. 43

A variety of games, such as blowing wads of paper across the room, may be used to get children to breathe deeply and to cough. (Courtesy Today's Health, American Medical Association, Chicago, Ill.; UPI Photo.)

tive complication. It is thought to be due to impairment of the venous flow of blood and to trauma or irritation of walls of the veins. Additional factors related to anesthesia and surgery may play a part in the development of this complication following an operation. Although this has not been proved, most surgeons feel that early ambulation helps to prevent the development of venous complications. This conviction, along with the knowledge that moving freely and getting out of bed soon after an operation is beneficial to all body systems, accounts for the emphasis on early ambulation for almost all operative patients. Venous stasis occurs in the lower trunk and extremities as a result of muscular inactivity, of postoperative respiratory and circulatory depression, and of increased pressure on blood vessels from tight dressings, intestinal distention, and prolonged maintenance of a sitting position. Other contributing factors are obesity, cardiovascular diseases, debility, malnutrition, foci of infection, and old age. Vascular complications occur much more frequently in adults than in children, although they can and do occur in adolescents. Varicose veins predispose to the development of vascular complications. In an effort to prevent this development, it is now routine practice in many hospitals to have all elderly patients and those with evidence of varicosities wear elastic bandages (Ace bandages) when in bed and when walking for the first time. They should be applied smoothly either from the foot to the groin or from the foot to the knee, and are removed and reapplied daily.

Phlebothrombosis and *thrombophlebitis* are the most common circulatory complications. The two terms are sometimes used interchangeably and may be difficult to distinguish since inflammation almost always follows the formation of a thrombus as well as the obstruction of a blood vessel. The term phlebothrombosis usually designates a clot formed in one of the larger veins without inflammation of the vein and sometimes giving no symptoms. Postoperatively it often forms in a vein of the foot or the calf, where it may cause pain upon dorsiflexion of the foot (Homan's sign). However, pain does not always occur. The thrombus is soft,

197

is loosely attached distally, and it's free end floats in the blood. As it enlarges, it, or a portion of it, may break loose from its attachment and may be carried by the bloodstream to the lungs, heart, or brain and cause a sudden fatal embolism. A common site for an embolism to lodge is the lungs (pulmonary embolism), where it causes sudden sharp, upper abdominal or thoracic pain, dyspnea, shock, and frequently death (p. 573). Because of the danger of dislodging a clot, even if the patient has no symptoms, the nurse should never massage the muscle portion of a postoperative patient's limbs without a doctor's order. If she notes a patient massaging his leg, she should question him about his discomfort and report it to the doctor. If the patient complains of pain in the foot, the calf of the leg, or the thigh upon walking, he should be put to bed at once and advised to keep the limb quiet, and the doctor should be notified.

In thrombophlebitis the clot develops and becomes firmly attached to a vein wall and increases until it occludes the lumen of the vein. It is believed to occur most often in vessels irritated or inflamed by pressure or other factors. It occurs in either deep or superficial veins, where it is accompanied by pain and local tenderness. If a superficial vein is involved, thrombophlebitis can be noted as a reddened line along the vessel route and feels firm on gentle palpation. If it forms in the femoral or iliac veins, the entire limb becomes swollen, pale, and cold. There is usually exquisite tenderness along the course of the vein. The swelling and coldness are caused by lymphatic obstruction and arterial spasm. The patient's temperature often rises. If the thromboplebitis is confined to the saphenous vein, the accompanying edema is not so marked, but pain and tenderness are just as severe, and heat and redness can be noted along the inflamed vein. The development of the thrombi prolongs the patient's convalescence. He is confined to bed, and intensive treatment is begun (p. 384).

Postoperative exercises and early ambulation. Nursing measures to attempt to prevent thrombus formation should be initiated at once after the operation. Bed exercises and early ambulation are known to minimize the effects of venous stasis caused by bed rest, and they usually are contraindicated only in the presence of thromboembolic diseases or after vascular surgery such as anastomosis of a blood vessel. Specific exercises for the upper extremities are not usually necessary since the patient uses his arms in eating, bathing, combing his hair, and reaching for articles on his bedside stand or overbed table. (For specific exercises when needed, see p. 809.)

Exercises of the lower extremities are particularly important in the prevention of venous stasis and should be performed until the patient is up and walking about several hours a day (Fig. 44). He should be taught to bend his knees, to lower them, and to push the backs of the knees hard against the bed. The nurse can slip her hand under the popliteal area and have the patient push hard against it. The same thing can be accomplished by having the patient alternately contract and relax his calf and thigh muscles. This should be done at least ten times, and a brief period of rest should follow each contraction and relaxation. The cycle is contract, relax, rest. Leg exercises should also include flexion, extension, adduction, and abduction of the leg, and extension, flexion, and rotation of the foot. A footboard placed at the bottom of the bed, against which the foot can rest in the normal walking position and against which the patient can push firmly, will help prevent foot drop and provide additional exercise. Whenever possible, the patient should lie on his abdomen for one-half hour two or three times a day to prevent blood from pooling in the pelvic cavity. This position also prevents contracture at the hip joint. Until he is permitted out of bed, he should have supervised exercise at least every four hours, but he should be encouraged to do the exercises more frequently than scheduled and to move his legs about in bed as much as possible. The bed should be made so that the bed linen does not restrict the patient's movements. If the patient is unable to do these exercises actively, they should be done passively by the nurse.

If the patient has responded well to surgery and does not show excessive fatigue, ambulation usually is started within twenty-four hours after surgery. At first he should walk only a short distance, and he should

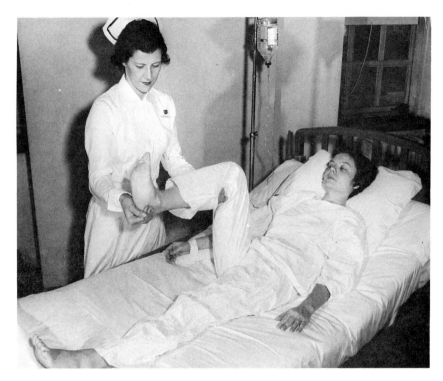

Fig. 44

not be pushed beyond his physical ability. The distance walked should be increased each time, and usually the patient is encouraged to walk two or three times a day. When the patient becomes tired he should return to bed.

The nurse should assist and supervise the patient in getting out of bed and walking until he is able to do this without difficulty or danger of injury to himself. Early ambulation should not consist of sitting in a chair at the bedside, since this posture may cause increased stasis of blood in the lower extremities. If the patient is permitted to sit in a chair, he should be advised to stand up frequently and walk about. When he is sitting, he should elevate his legs on another chair to prevent pooling of venous blood in the lower extremities. The legs should be supported from the knees to the ankles, but there should be no pressure against the popliteal area.

Most patients are more confident if there are two people to help when they get up for the first time. However, by using good body mechanics, one nurse can help most postoperative patients out of bed for the first

Supervising the postoperative patient in bed exercises. Here the nurse assists the patient as she bends the knee and dorsiflexes the foot.

time without injury to herself or to the patient. The nurse should walk close beside the patient and link her arm with his so that his palm is up and her palm is down. If the patient becomes weak, the nurse can then slide her arm up into the patient's axilla and, by moving her outer leg to the side, provide herself with a wide enough base of support to balance the patient against her hip until help arrives.

When the nurse helps the patient up for the first time, she should appraise his condition carefully to see what problems are involved. The aged patient usually has difficulty getting up because of stiff joints and muscle weakness. Patients who have arthritis or arteriosclerosis or who have been on prolonged bed rest may need time to become ambulatory. They should sit on the edge of the bed and dangle their feet for short periods before walking is attempted.

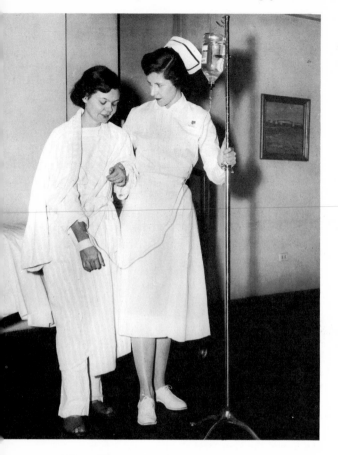

Fig. 45

The patient who is receiving an infusion can be assisted to be ambulatory.

Their progress may be slow, and they should be observed with special care for signs of fatigue. They may need assistance longer than most patients. The fact that any patient is to be out of bed at intervals should never be taken by the nurse as a sign that he is able to care for himself.

Young children usually recover quickly from the effects of surgery and often sit up and walk around in their cribs without urging. Older children occasionally are fearful of injuring the operative site and must be encouraged to leave bed and to move about freely.

Treatments need not interfere with helping the patient out of bed. If the patient is receiving an infusion, his arm can be secured

to an arm board, and the bottle of infusion fluid can be hung on a movable pole that can be pushed along by the nurse as the patient walks (Fig. 45). Permission is usually given by the physician to clamp off nasogastric tubes for a short period of time. Urethral catheters and other tubing can be attached to small, portable drainage bottles.

Pain in the incision is a common postoperative complaint. The patient often becomes aware of this pain as soon as he awakens from anesthesia. It usually lasts twenty-four to forty-eight hours after surgery, but it may continue longer, depending upon the surgery performed, the pain threshold of the patient, and his particular personality. Most of this pain arises from trauma to the somatic nerve fibers in the skin. It is sharp and localized. Muscles and fascia are also supplied with somatic nerve fibers, and extensive dissection or prolonged retraction of these tissues will produce deep, long-lasting pain. Pain in the operative area may be aggravated by skin sutures, tight dressings, swelling of the incision during healing, and the presence of infection or hematomas in the wound. Continuous and severe pain can produce anxiety, restlessness, sleeplessness, anorexia, and irritability. Its presence can also prolong convalescence since it may interfere with return to activity.

It is not always possible to prevent the occurrence of pain, but it can be alleviated so that the patient is relatively comfortable. Patients who have had adequate preoperative instructions and who have confidence in the surgeon, in the nurses, and in the outcome of the surgery usually have less postoperative pain than the apprehensive patient because they have less tension. Infants and young children usually recover from symptoms of pain more quickly than older people. Pain can be relieved by nursing measures and/or by the administration of narcotics. The patient's position often aggravates wound pain by causing pressure or pull on the incision. A change of position, elevation of the head of the bed, loosening of restraining sheets, and support of dependent parts of the body may give relief. Dressings that are binding or casts that are too tight should be reported to the doctor so that they can be loosened or removed.

In addition to making the patient as comfortable as possible, it may be necessary to give a narcotic. If the patient has real pain, most surgeons feel that narcotics should not be too strictly withheld during the immediate postoperative period. Before a narcotic is given, however, the nurse should decide whether the patient's pain is a reasonable result of the operation or whether it is a new development. The latter must be reported to the physician. The nurse should also check the patient's vital signs. Since most narcotics depress the respiratory center, the patient's respirations should be above fourteen per minute before these drugs are administered. Narcotics, especially meperidine hydrochloride (Demerol), cause the blood pressure to drop. Therefore, if the blood pressure is low or unstable, they should not be given without consulting the doctor. A very drowsy patient should not receive a narcotic because it will further depress his respirations and activity. Since young children and aged patients usually do not tolerate narcotics well and have a high pain threshold, these drugs should be given to them in small doses and as infrequently as possible.

When the nurse decides that the need for a narcotic is justified, she should give the medication as ordered to keep the patient comfortable. Narcotics can be given every four hours during the first twelve to thirty-six hours postoperatively without danger of addiction. Narcotics, however, besides causing respiratory and circulatory depression, may cause urticaria, restlessness, nausea, and vomiting. Therefore, the patient should be observed for any untoward reaction. A patient who has received a narcotic shortly before getting out of bed to walk should be supervised closely since the action of the drug may cause him to become dizzy or faint. The need for narcotics should decrease after forty-eight hours, and continuous, severe pain after this time should be reported to the physician.

Care of the wound

Most surgical wounds are clean, closed wounds that heal rapidly with a minimum of scarring. After the incision has been sutured, the incised skin surfaces are quickly glued together by strands of fibrin and a thin layer of clotted blood. Plasma seeps onto the surface, forming a dry protective crust. There should be a very small amount of serous drainage from such a wound, and after a few hours all seepage onto the dressing should cease.

Occasionally surgeons leave an operative wound uncovered, believing that healing progresses best when the wound is exposed to air. Usually, however, for psychologic reasons and to prevent trauma, the wound is covered in the operating room with a dry sterile dressing. Medicated sprays such as Rezifilm form a protective, transparent film on the skin and are being used as dressings over clean incisions. The film lasts three to four days, may be removed with acetone, or will form flakes and peel off eventually. This type of dressing is particularly useful in covering wounds in children.

Drains may be inserted at the time of surgery to allow fluids such as bile, pus, and serum to drain from the operative site and prevent the development of deep wound infections. They may exit directly from the incision or through a separate small incision known as a stab wound. The nurse should check with the doctor or look on the operative sheet to determine the exact location of drains so that she will know the type and amount of drainage to expect. Drainage from stab wounds may be profuse, and a catheter that can be attached to low suction may be used as the drain.

If there is no drainage, the dressing does not need to be changed until the sutures are removed. The wound is weakest during the third to sixth day after surgery. After this time there is union of deep tissues as a result of fibroplasia and collagen deposition. Increase in wound strength progresses rapidly from the sixth to the fourteenth day and then continues slowly for some months. Although wound union is only relatively firm until after the sixth postoperative day, the sutures permit the patient to cough, turn, and get out of bed without danger of wound separation. It is important for the patient to know this fact. Otherwise he may be reluctant to participate in such activities for fear of harming the incision. Skin sutures (black silk thread, fine wire, or metal skin clips) are removed from abdominal wounds on about the seventh postoperative day, from neck and face wounds on about the third to the fifth postoperative day, and from wounds of the extremities on the eighth to tenth postoperative day. Retention sutures made of heavy wire and placed deep into muscle tissue usually are not removed until the fourteenth to the twenty-first postoperative day. Most patients become apprehensive when they know the sutures are to be removed. They may be told that they will have little, if any, pain during the procedure. Unless there is some seepage of fluid after the sutures are removed, a dressing is not necessary, and the area may be washed.

The most exact attention to good aseptic technique is essential in caring for all wounds since organisms can be introduced from the environment into wounds, including those already infected. (For the correct technique in changing dressings, see texts on fundamentals of nursing.) Care must be taken that a drain is not inadvertently removed when the dressings are changed. Neither must the drain be permitted to slip into a deep wound, where probing, with possible trauma to the wound, might be needed to remove it. Thin drains, such as Penrose drains, are usually anchored with a large safety pin that cannot enter the wound opening. A piece of gauze dressing is placed under the pin to keep it from direct contact with the skin about the wound. Using Montgomery straps simplifies changing the dressings and eliminates the repeated removal of adhesive tape from the skin. If the drainage is irritating to the skin, the skin should be washed frequently with soap and water and a protective ointment such as zinc oxide or a protective spray such as Rezifilm applied. The character and amount of drainage should be recorded, and any change in the amount, color, or consistency should be reported to the surgeon. The patient should be told the reason for the drainage so that he does not become alarmed when he sees it on the dressing or on his gown. Drains are shortened gradually and are removed when the drainage has diminished sufficiently. The opening caused by the drain heals in a few days.

Hemorrhage from the wound

Although hemorrhage from the wound is most likely to occur within the first forty-eight hours postoperatively, it may occur as late as the sixth or seventh postoperative day in apparently normal wounds, and after a much longer time if the wound is infected. Hemorrhage occurring soon after operation may be due to the slipping of a ligature or the mechanical dislodging of a clot, caused, for example, by vomiting after a tonsillectomy. Hemorrhage may also be caused by the reestablished blood flow through vessels that, if the patient's blood pressure was low or if a tourniquet was used during the operation, were not noticed and properly obliterated. Hemorrhage after a few days may be due to sloughing of a clot or of tissue, to infection, or to erosion of a blood vessel by a drainage tube.

The nurse should inspect every postoperative dressing frequently. If bright red blood is present, she should outline the area with a pencil so that the rate of increase can easily be determined, and she should report it to the doctor. The dressings then should be checked at fifteen-minute intervals or oftener to determine the rapidity of bleeding, and the patient should be observed for other signs of hemorrhage, such as fall in blood pressure, rise in pulse and respiratory rates, restlessness, pallor, weakness, and cold, moist skin. If the bleeding is profuse, the nurse should apply a pressure dressing until the doctor arrives and remain with the patient. Her actions should be efficient, and she should remain calm so that the patient is not unduly alarmed. She should take the patient's blood pressure in order to help the doctor to determine the extent of the hemorrhage. The nursing staff should gather equipment that the doctor may need, such as infusion fluid, material for drawing blood for typing and crossmatching, shock blocks, and dressing equipment. The doctor usually treats a wound hemorrhage by applying pressure on the wound to occlude the bleeding vessels and, if necessary, administering a blood transfusion to replace blood loss. A hemostatic gelatin sponge, such as Gelfoam, soaked in saline solution is sometimes used to control wound bleeding. The sponge is applied to the bleeding site, and pressure is exerted for two to four minutes. It is left in place and, over a period of several weeks, is absorbed. As absorption occurs, drainage from the wound may appear dark, and pieces of black material may be on the dressing occasionally.

When severe wound hemorrhage occurs, the patient is taken immediately to the operating room, where the wound is opened and the bleeding vessel ligated. If a preoperative medication is ordered, the nurse should check to see when the last narcotic was given. Under pressure of the emergency, there is danger that the patient may receive an overdose of narcotic, thus causing respiratory and circulatory depression and prohibiting the administration of an anesthetic. Since the patient often becomes frightened by the hemorrhage and the subsequent emergency procedures, the nurse should make every effort to reassure him and to keep noise, confusion, and technical discussions at the bedside to a minimum.

Infection

Wound infections are fairly common postoperative complications. The causative organisms often are staphylococci and streptococci and are usually introduced into the wound. Wound infections are more prevalent in debilitated and obese patients possibly because the blood supply to the site of operation may be impaired. From three to six days after surgery the patient begins to have a low-grade fever, and the wound becomes painful and swollen. The nurse should be alert for purulent drainage on the dressing. She should report complaints of persistent pain in the incision to the physician, who may change the dressing to inspect the wound. If spontaneous drainage of the wound does not occur, and if there is definite evidence of infection, the surgeon may choose to open a portion of the healed incision to facilitate drainage. Wound discomfort usually disappears when this procedure is done. The nurse usually is asked to change the dressings as necessary.

A culture may be made of the fluid obtained from an infected wound, and the administration of appropriate antibiotics is started either before or when the report of culture growth is obtained. For superficial wound infections, sterile, hot, wet dressings may be ordered. (See fundamentals of nursing texts for the procedure.) Sometimes infected wounds have to be irrigated or have

packing that must be changed at intervals (p. 70).

Dehiscence and evisceration

Wound disruption *(dehiscence)* is a partial to complete separation of the wound edges. Wound evisceration is protrusion of abdominal viscera through the incision and onto the abdomal wall. These complications often are brought to the nurse's attention by the patient's complaint of a "giving" sensation in the incision or of a sudden, profuse leakage of fluid from the incision. Upon inspection, the dressing will be found to be saturated with clear, pink drainage. The wound edges may be partially or entirely separated, and loops of intestine may be lying on the abdominal wall. (See Fig. 46.) These complications may occur at any time through the fourteenth postoperative day, but they usually occur between the sixth and the eighth day. They are thought to be due to cachexia, anemia, advanced age, hypoproteinemia, dehydration, infection, or excessive vomiting, retching, and coughing.

If the nurse discovers either of these complications, she should put the patient to bed in a low Fowler's position and caution to him not to cough. She should try not to alarm him, but he should be told to remain quiet

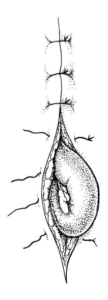

Fig. 46

Wound evisceration.

and not to eat or drink anything until the doctor has seen him. While awaiting the doctor's arrival, the nurse may apply warm, sterile dressings over the protruding viscera to keep the serous membrane from becoming dry if this is the policy of the hospital. Otherwise, she should apply a sterile towel or sterile dressings and secure them loosely with a scultetus binder or adhesive tape. She should then assemble the equipment that the doctor will need, such as dressing equipment and infusion fluid. The patient's blood pressure, pulse, and respirations should be taken to determine if he is in shock.

The treatment for wound dehiscence and wound evisceration is immediate closure of the wound under local or intravenous anesthesia. Since the patient is likely to be in shock, he is taken to the operating room in his bed, and preoperative medication usually is not given. These serious complications are potential threats to the patient's life, involve a second operation, and prolong convalescence, although usually the wound heals surprisingly well following the secondary closure.

Return of urinary function

If the patient is well hydrated, urinary function usually returns within six to eight hours after surgery. Although 2,000 ml. of intravenous solution usually is given on the operative day, the first voiding may not be more than 200 ml., and the total urinary output for the operative day may be less than 1,500 ml. The small amount of urinary output, in relation to fluid intake, is due to the loss of body fluid during surgery and to perspiration, hyperventilation, and vomiting. As body functions stabilize and fluid and electrolyte balance returns to normal, however, the ratio of intake to output should also return to normal. This process may take about forty-eight hours, and during this time a record is kept of the intake and the time and amount of each voiding. If the urinary output is less than 500 ml. in twenty-four hours, this fact must be reported to the doctor, since the decreased urinary output may be due to renal failure caused by shock or a reaction to the anesthetic or other drugs.

Occasionally, after extensive surgery in elderly patients or other patients who have shown signs of shock immediately following surgery, a retention catheter (Foley type of catheter) is inserted before the patient awakens from anesthesia. Urine is then recorded in a calibrated bottle, and the surgeon may wish to be notified if the output is less than 30 ml. per hour. This decrease in output may indicate impending renal failure, which should be prevented by immediate measures to raise the patient's blood pressure. Measures might include giving whole blood, blood volume expanders, and other fluids and drugs such as levarterenol (Levophed).

Some patients are unable to void after surgery and may thus experience severe discomfort. The difficulty may be due to the recumbent position, nervous tension, the remaining effects of anesthetics such as tribromoethanol (Avertin) or of spinal anesthetics that interfere with bladder sensation and the ability to void, the use of narcotics that reduce the sensation of bladder distention, the pain caused by movement onto the bedpan, or pain at the site of operation if it is near the bladder or urethra. Inability to void is a common occurrence following operations on the rectum or colon and following gynecologic procedures, since the innervation of the bladder musculature may be temporarily disturbed, and local edema may increase the difficulty. Voiding may be facilitated by nursing measures such as forcing fluids, placing the patient on the bedpan at regular intervals, running the water in the sink while the patient is on the bedpan, pouring warm water over the pelvic area, and assuring the patient of privacy. Male patients need the same consideration as to privacy when they are attempting to void following an operation. Most patients are able to void if they are helped out of bed and can use a commode. If these measures are not effective, the doctor may order catheterization. Because of the emotional trauma to the young child, the possibility of reproductive tract infections in men, and the danger of urinary infection to all patients, the doctor may delay catheterization longer than the usual eight hours postoperatively in the hope that the patient will void normally. If the bladder is palpable over the pubic bone and suprapubic pressure causes discomfort, however, he usually orders catheterization to prevent stretching of the vesical wall. Marked and prolonged distention of the bladder may cause infection of the urinary system and atony of the bladder muscles, resulting in inability to void later. If the patient must be catheterized repeatedly after an operation, a Foley catheter usually is inserted into the bladder, the patient is given sulfisoxazole (Gantrisin), and fluids are forced.

Occasionally a patient voids frequently but in small amounts. This condition is known as "retention with overflow." The overdistended bladder expels just enough urine to relieve the pressure within it temporarily. The condition should be reported to the physician, who will probably order the patient catheterized for residual urine. Since a large volume of residual urine is a good medium for bacterial growth, a Foley catheter may be left in place for several days. Otherwise, catheterization usually is done every six to eight hours until the residual urine left in the bladder after voiding is less than 50 ml.

Postoperative urinary tract infection can usually be avoided by emptying the bladder completely at each voiding, preventing bladder distention, and using sterile, nontraumatic technique when catheterizations are necessary. Staphylococcal infection of the urinary tract, a common complication of catheterization, is thought to be most often caused by poor technique in doing the procedure. Patients who must be on prolonged bed rest, who have had urinary tract infections in the past, who are elderly, or who have had operations on the pelvic organs are especially prone to bladder and kidney infections. Special attention should be given to the amount and quality of their urinary output, and they should drink at least 3,000 ml. of fluid a day unless this measure is contraindicated by age or by cardiac or renal dysfunction (p. 431). Symptoms such as a burning sensation in the bladder and urethra during or after urination, frequency, chills, fever, malaise, and anorexia may be indicative of urinary tract infection and should be reported to the doctor.

Return of gastrointestinal function

Following surgery, gastrointestinal functions returns to normal more quickly if the patient's usual diet can be resumed at once. Fluids (not chilled) and food are often given as tolerated after the patient has reacted fully from the anesthesia and all sensations of nausea and vomiting have passed. There is some evidence that iced fluids tend to cause gaseous distention and distress. Most children can take clear fluids the evening of the operative day and a soft diet the day after surgery. With careful attention to giving suitable fluids and foods by mouth in frequent small amounts, the need for parenteral fluids may be obviated. There is general agreement that the best way to supply essential foods to all patients is by mouth, and some surgeons believe that the patient should eat solid food because mastication promotes flow of saliva, which aids digestion and stimulates the stomach to empty. This process, in turn, stimulates peristalsis in the lower tract. Discomfort from accumulation of flatus and the need for enemas and other treatment for distention and constipation can probably be reduced further by the patient's moving about freely in bed and by early ambulation. Ingestion of solid food also helps to prevent the occurrence of nonepidemic parotitis, a painful inflammation of the salivary glands that occurs occasionally in debilitated patients who have poor mouth hygiene and who also may be dehydrated. If the patient has had operative treatment of a fracture of a bone, surgery of the chest, or a simple herniorraphy, for example, food usually is given as tolerated. No patient, however, should be urged to eat solid food for a day or two following anesthesia and surgery. Urging solid food when the patient has no appetite may cause vomiting, which will give pain and distress and may lessen the desire to eat.

Since a quick return to good nutritional status speeds wound healing, the patient should be encouraged to eat a well-balanced diet as soon as he can tolerate one. It is estimated that a caloric intake of 50% more than the basic caloric requirement for the individual is needed to provide for energy expended in early ambulation and for reparative processes.[25] An attractive, well-balanced general diet should be served, and the patient should be allowed to select what appeals to him. After even a few days of enforced starvation, the patient may be somewhat indifferent to food. It may take two or three days on a well-balanced general diet to overcome this condition, brought on, in part at least, by lack of food. Special surgical diets usually are ordered only after gastric or bowel surgery. Special diets for medical conditions, such as diabetes mellitus or cardiac insufficiency, should be resumed as soon as possible after surgery.

When surgery has been performed on the gastrointestinal tract or on the closely related organs within the abdomen, fluids and foods are not given until peristalsis returns. Usually a nasogastric tube is inserted and left in place for approximately twenty-four hours if surgery has been done on the gallbladder, and for approximately two to four days if an operation has been performed on the stomach. A nasogastric or a Miller-Abbott tube may be inserted and left in place approximately two to five days if surgery has been done on the small or the large bowel. These decompression tubes, attached to suction, remove flatus that may cause tension on the operative site or fluids and secretions that may accumulate. Because these tubes remove secretions containing electrolytes and because they cause general discomfort, they are removed as soon as possible. While they are in use the patient is given nothing by mouth, and he is given fluids intravenously that contain foods and electrolytes to meet, as nearly as possible, his daily needs and to restore losses caused by use of the decompression tube. However, it is impossible to meet metabolic needs fully by giving fluids parenterally. By using modified gastric tubes (Abbott-Rawson or Olander-Puestow) it is possible to decompress the stomach as necessary following gastric surgery and yet supply liquid feedings into the jejunum.[13] The use of these tubes thus provides better nutrition. The greatest care should be taken that tubes used for decompression do not cause further nausea, since it increases the danger of serious postoperative respiratory complications. (For care of the patient having gastric or intestinal decompression, see p. 639.)

The patient who is taking no fluids or foods by mouth should have frequent mouth care. If he is receiving sufficient fluids intravenously, thirst should not be a problem. Chewing gum or sucking on small pieces of hard candy or ice often helps to allay thirst and makes the patient's mouth feel better.

The return of normal peristalsis is verified when the doctor hears bowel sounds upon auscultation. The passage of flatus by rectum or a spontaneous bowel movement also indicates the return of peristalsis and should be reported to the doctor. When peristalsis returns, the patient usually is given clear fluids first. If he tolerates them well, he can usually progress rapidly to other foods.

Vomiting

Postoperative vomiting is one of the most distressing problems that the patient encounters. In addition to the discomfort it causes, severe vomiting or retching can be harmful to the operative wound. Usually it is due to the effects of anesthetics such as ether, to an accumulation of fluid in the stomach, or to eating food or drinking water before peristalsis returns. Psychologic factors also contribute to vomiting postoperatively. It is not unusual for the patient who expects to vomit postoperatively to do so.

To prevent danger of aspiration, the patient who is vomiting should lie on his side. He should be advised not to take food or fluid for several hours and to lie quietly in bed. The emesis basin and soiled bed linen should be removed, and mouth care should be given. When vomiting has subsided, sucking on chips of ice, taking sips of ginger ale or hot tea, or eating small amounts of dry, solid food may relieve nausea. Sometimes, trimethobenzamide hydrochloride (Tigan), an antiemetic, may be administered.

Persistent postoperative vomiting is usually a symptom of pyloric obstruction, intestinal obstruction, or peritonitis. This type of vomiting tires the patient, puts a strain on the incision, and causes excessive loss of fluids and electrolytes. Projectile vomiting of gastric contents occurs in the presence of pyloric obstruction. In intestinal obstruction, the vomitus is fecal in nature, and it usually flows continuously and effortlessly from the patient's mouth. If persistent vomiting occurs, a nasogastric tube is passed, and the stomach is lavaged. The tube may be left in place and attached to a suction apparatus to keep the stomach empty. The patient is not given anything by mouth, and intravenous fluids containing electrolytes are administered to replace the fluid and electrolyte loss.

Hiccoughs

Hiccoughs interfere with eating and sleeping and are among the most exhausting postoperative complications. The exact cause of postoperative hiccoughs is not known, but it is known that dilation of the stomach, irritation of the diaphragm, peritonitis, and uremia each causes either reflex or central nervous system stimulation of the phrenic nerve. Fortunately, hiccoughs are not a common postoperative complaint. They usually disappear within a few hours. The doctor may order such a simple measure as having the patient breathe his own carbon dioxide at five-minute intervals by inhaling and exhaling into a paper bag held tightly over his nose and mouth. Carbon dioxide inhalations, using 5% carbon dioxide and 95% oxygen, may also be given for five minutes every hour. If dizziness occurs, they should be discontinued, since an overdose of carbon dioxide may cause convulsions and coma. Aspiration of the stomach will stop hiccoughs caused by gastric dilation. Chlorpromazine hydrochloride (Thorazine) is used to treat mild cases of hiccoughs. If the hiccoughs are persistent and do not respond to these treatments, local infiltration of the phrenic nerve with 1% procaine may be necessary, or in extreme cases surgical crushing of the phrenic nerve may be done.

Abdominal distention

Postoperative distention is a result of an accumulation of nonabsorbable gas in the intestines caused by handling of the bowel during surgery, by swallowing of air during recovery from anesthesia and as the patient attempts to overcome nausea, and by passing of gases from the bloodstream to the atonic portion of the bowel. Distention will persist until the tone of the bowel returns to normal and peristalsis resumes. It is experienced to some degree by most patients after abdominal and renal surgery.

"Gas pains" are caused by contractions of the unaffected portions of the bowel in an attempt to move the accumulated gas through the intestinal tract. The patient complains of discomfort, and if the distention is high in the abdomen, he may have

difficulty in breathing. High distention may be due to stomach dilation and can be relieved by aspiration of fluid and gas from the stomach with a nasogastric tube. Ambulation often stimulates the return of peristalsis and the expulsion of flatus. Gas in the lower bowel may be removed by a lubricated rectal tube inserted into the rectum. This tube should be inserted just past the rectal sphincter and should be removed when ordered. If necessary, it may be used every four hours. Heat applied to the abdomen in the form of a hot-water bottle, heating pad, or flaxseed poultice may be ordered in conjunction with the use of a rectal tube. Small carminative enemas of milk and molasses or of glycerin, magnesium sulfate, and water sometimes are ordered to stimulate the expulsion of flatus. If the distention progresses and the flatus is not expelled after forty-eight hours, a *paralytic ileus* is suspected. This condition is the complete absence of bowel tone and is caused by the anesthetic, by a generalized infection such as peritonitis, or by other causes. The patient is given nothing by mouth, and nasogastric suctioning is started and continued until peristalsis returns.

Defecation

A careful record should be made of when the patient passes flatus after an abdominal operation and when a bowel movement occurs. The first spontaneous bowel movement usually occurs four to five days after surgery and indicates that normal gastrointestinal function has returned. Unless there are symptoms of fecal impaction or intestinal distention, no attempt is made to hasten bowel evacuation. The patient who is eating normally, drinking adequate fluid, walking about, and going to the bathroom routinely will usually have a bowel movement without an enema. When an enema seems necessary, a small soapsuds enema usually will stimulate defecation. If the patient is constipated, an oil retention enema followed by a soapsuds enema may be necessary.

While caring for the postoperative patient, the nurse should question him about the expulsion of flatus or the occurrence of a bowel movement, since a delay in bowel evacuation beyond four or five days postoperatively may be a symptom of paralytic ileus or intestinal obstruction.

Postoperative diarrhea may occur. Since it may be caused by a fecal impaction, it should be reported to the physician. If the patient has severe burns of the buttocks or has undergone extensive rectal or pelvic surgery, bowel movements may be intentionally delayed for several days by the administration of lead and opium pills, paregoric, or bismuth subcarbonate by mouth.

Preparation for discharge from the hospital

Preparation of the patient for discharge from the hospital is an important part of his nursing care postoperatively. Plans for discharge may have been discussed and begun preoperatively, but most of the teaching, arrangements, and preparations are done after surgery. The patient, his family, and the members of the health team responsible for the care of the patient during his hospitalization should participate in the long-range planning.

As a result of the early resumption of ambulation and a nutritious diet, most patients regain their strength rapidly, and the average hospital stay following surgery is less than two weeks. During this time the patient and his family should be prepared for any care that must be given at home, and any necessary arrangements for convalescent care should be completed several days prior to discharge. The patient should be helped to become as self-sufficient as possible before being discharged so that he does not have to depend any more than necessary upon the assistance of relatives and friends.

Soon after surgery the nurse should consult with the doctor regarding the anticipated discharge plans for the patient. She should know his ability to participate in the care to be given at home, the interest and the desire of the family to help, and the home situation and its facilities. Whenever possible, both the patient and a member of his family should be taught all treatments and exercises that must be done at home. Sometimes arrangements should be made for a member of the family to come to

the hospital to observe and perhaps practice procedures, to talk to the dietitian, to consult with the doctor, to discuss problems with the social case worker, and to plan with the nurse about home care. The patient and his family should have ample opportunity to ask questions.

The nurse should try to anticipate any problems that might arise and help the patient and his family plan for them. For example, if a colostomy irrigation must be given and there are no bathroom facilities, extra equipment will be necessary so that it can be done in the room available. If the patient is reluctant or unable to give himself an injection, some member of the family must be taught how to give injections, or arrangements must be made for a public health nurse to give them. If the patient does not understand English, an interpreter may be needed to explain diets, medications, or treatments. If dressings are needed, the patient should be given a forty-eight-hour supply to take home if a family member has not been to the hospital and obtained what is needed. The patient and his family should know where in the community they may obtain dressings and other materials they may need. If treatment of almost any kind is to be done at home, it is advisable for the nurse to discuss with the doctor and with the patient the advisability of having a public health nurse visit the patient in his home soon after he leaves the hospital. A written referral should be made, and the report returned by the public health nurse helps the nurse in the hospital to learn how effective her teaching of the patient has been.

If the patient lives alone, has no relatives, or is unable to be cared for by his family, he may have to go to a nursing home. Arrangements for admittance to another hospital or to a nursing home for further treatment or for terminal care often take time. Since there is usually a long waiting list, the arrangements should be begun as soon as the decision is reached by the doctor, the patient, and the family.

On discharge the patient is given an appointment for a follow-up examination in the doctor's office or in the outpatient department of the hospital. This appointment is usually for one or two weeks after discharge. The nurse should make sure that the patient understands the importance of returning for the medical examination and that he can make arrangements to come in at this time.

With modern surgical techniques the wound is well healed by the time of discharge from the hospital. Therefore, the convalescent period usually is relatively short, and most patients may return to their usual activity and occupation within two to four weeks postoperatively. During this time the patient should rest when he becomes tired and should increase his activity gradually. Usually the patient returns to the doctor for a follow-up examination about two weeks after he leaves the hospital. At this time the doctor checks the healing of the wound and the patient's general physical condition. Depending upon the outcome of this examination and the type of work the patient does, the doctor will decide when it will be desirable for him to resume his usual activities.

References and selected readings*

1 *Adams, Ralph: Prevention of infections in hospitals, Am. J. Nursing 58:344-348, March 1958.

2 *Adriani, John: Anesthesia for infants and children, Am. J. Nursing 64:107-110, Aug. 1964.

3 Adriani, John: Some new anesthetic agents, Am. J. Nursing 61:60-62, May 1961.

4 Alexander, Edythe Louise, and others: Care of the patient in surgery, ed. 4, 1967, The C. V. Mosby Co. (In press.)

5 Artusio, Joseph F., and Mazzia, Valentino D. B.: Practical anesthesiology, St. Louis, 1962, The C. V. Mosby Co.

6 Beal, John M., editor: Manual of the recovery room, ed. 2, New York, 1962, The Macmillan Co.

7 Benson, Clifford D., and others, editors: Pediatric surgery, vol. I, Chicago, 1962, Year Book Medical Publishers, Inc.

8 *Bird, Brian: Psychological aspects of preoperative and postoperative care, Am. J. Nursing 55:685-687, June 1955.

9 *Breckenridge, Flora J., and Bruno, Pauline: Nursing care of the anesthetized patient, Am. J. Nursing 62:74-78, July 1962.

10 Calvert, D. G.: Inadvertent hypothermia in pediatric surgery and a method for its prevention, Anesthesia 17:29-45, Jan. 1962.

11 *Cantor, Alfred J., and Foxe, Arthur N.: Psychosomatic aspects of surgery, New York, 1956, Grune & Stratton, Inc.

12 *Case, Thomas C., and Giery, R. A.: Surgery in patients between 80 and 100 years of age, J. Am. Geriatrics Soc. 12:345-349, April 1964.

13 Cole, Warren, and Mason, James H.: Surgical aspects. In Cowdry, E. V., editor: The care of the geriatric patient, ed. 2, St. Louis, 1963, The C. V. Mosby Co.

14 Cullen, Stuart C.: Anesthesia: a manual for students and physicians, ed. 6, Chicago, 1961, Year Book Medical Publishers, Inc.

15 Davis, Loyal, editor: Christopher's textbook of surgery, ed. 8, Philadelphia, 1964, W. B. Saunders Co.

16 Dickler, Donald J., Friedman, Paul L., and Susman, Irvin C.: Intravenous regional anesthesia with chloroprocaine, Anesthesiology 26:244-245, March-April 1965.

17 Egbert, L. D., Laver, M. B., and Bendixen, H. H.: The effect of site of operation and type of anesthesia upon the ability to cough in the postoperative period, Surg. Gynec. & Obst. 115:295-298, Sept. 1962.

18 Fisher, B., Fedor, E. J., and Smith, J. W.: Temperature gradients associated with extracorporeal perfusion and profound hypothermia, Surgery 50:758-764, Nov. 1961.

19 Fuerst, Elinor, and Wolff, LuVerne: Fundamentals of nursing, ed. 3, Phliadelphia, 1964, J. B. Lippincott Co.

20 *Glenn, Frank: Surgical care of the aged, J. Am. Geriatrics Soc. 10:927-931, Nov. 1962.

21 *Goulding, Erna I., and Koop, C. Everett: The newborn, his response to surgery, Am. J. Nursing 65:84-87, Oct. 1965.

22 Gross, Robert E.: The surgery of infancy and childhood, Philadelphia, 1953, W. B. Saunders Co.

23 Hale, Donald F., editor: Anesthesiology, Philadelphia, 1963, F. A. Davis Co.

24 *Harris, William Hamilton, Slater, Eliot M., and Bell, H. Michael: Regional anesthesia by the intravenous route, J.A.M.A. 194:1273-1276, Dec. 20, 1965.

25 Hayes, Mark A.: Postoperative diet therapy, J. Am. Dietet. A. 35:17-18, Jan. 1959.

26 Hayt, Emanuel, and others: Law of hospital, physician, and patient, New York, 1958, Hospital Textbook Co.

27 *Hershey, Nathan: The patient's consent, Am. J. Nursing 62:99-101, Sept. 1962.

28 Hershey, Nathan: Whose consent is necessary? Am. J. Nursing 62:94-95, Oct. 1962.

29 Hickey, Mary Catherine: Nursing care for patients in hypothermia. In Technical innovations in health care: nursing implications, no. 3, New York, 1962, American Nurses' Association.

30 *Hickey, Mary Catherine: Hypothermia, Am. J. Nursing 65:116-122, Jan. 1965.

31 Kay, Brian: Recent advances in pediatric anesthesia, S. Clin. North America 44:1595-1609, Dec. 1964.

32 Leigh, M. Digby, and Belton, M. Kathleen: Pediatric anesthesiology, ed. 2, New York, 1960, The Macmillan Co.

33 Leithauser, D. J., Gregory, Louis, and Miller, Stella M.: Immediate ambulation after extensive surgery, Am. J. Nursing 66:2207-2208, Oct. 1966.

34 Linton, Robert R.: Venous thrombosis, pulmonary embolism, and varicose veins, J.A.M.A. 183:198-201, Jan. 19, 1963.

---

*References preceded by an asterisk are particularly well suited for student reading.

35 Modell, Walter, editor: Drugs in current use, 1966, New York, Springer Publishing Co., Inc.

36 *Newton, Kathleen, and Anderson, Helen C.: Geriatric nursing, ed. 4, St. Louis, 1966, The C. V. Mosby Co.

37 *Nugent, G. Robert, and Graves, Nancy: Prolonged hypothermia and nursing during prolonged hypothermia, Am. J. Nursing 60:967-970, July 1960.

38 Redo, S. Frank: Surgery of the ambulatory child, New York, 1961, Appleton-Century-Crofts.

39 Sandove, Max S., and Cross, James H.: The recovery room—immediate postoperative management, Philadelphia, 1956, W. B. Saunders Co.

40 Sawyer, Janet R.: Nursing care of patients with urologic diseases, St. Louis, 1963, The C. V. Mosby Co.

41 Scully, Harold F., and Martin, Stevens J.: Anesthetic management for geriatric patients, Am. J. Nursing 65:110-112, Feb. 1965.

42 Shaw, Wallace M.: Positional control of immediate postanesthetic vomiting, Anesthesiology 26:359, May-June 1965.

43 Simeone, F. A.: Shock, Am. J. Nursing 66:1286-1293, June 1966.

44 *Stahl, William M.: Major abdominal surgery in the aged patient, J. Am. Geriatrics Soc. 11:770-780, Aug. 1963.

45 *Wang, Kwo Chen, and Howland, William S.: Cardiac and pulmonary evaluations in elderly patients before elective surgery, J.A.M.A. 166:993-997, March 1, 1959.

46 Warren, Richard: Surgery, Philadelphia, 1963, W. B. Saunders Co.

47 *Webb, Watts R.: Management of pulmonary complications, Hosp. Med. 1:16-22, Oct. 1965.

48 Wright, Irving S.: The treatment of thrombophlebitis, J.A.M.A. 183:194-198, Jan. 19, 1963.

11

The patient
needing
plastic surgery

Study questions

1 What reaction does the average person have when he encounters someone with a facial abnormality? What types of work would probably not be available to the person with such a deformity? List as many recreational activities as you can that would be difficult or impossible for a person who has a marked deformity of the right hand.

2 Review the anatomy of the skin. How does skin differ from granulation tissue? Describe how new skin forms at the edges of a wound. On what does the elastic quality of skin depend?

3 What is meant by an autoimmune reaction?

4 Review the procedure for using sterile, moist compresses.

Plastic and reconstructive surgery has been attempted for centuries. Surgery of this kind was done before the era of the Roman Empire. Hindu records describe some very good results from efforts to alter deformities caused by disease or other misfortune. In the sixteenth century, Italian surgeons did remarkable work in plastic surgery, and there was interest in the emotional aspects of facial deformities. The discovery of anesthetics and of the cause of infection enabled surgeons to make strides in this field. Disfigurements resulting from World Wars I and II challenged the imagination of surgeons so that new techniques were developed.

There is every reason to believe that plastic and reconstructive surgery will become a more important part of medical care as time goes on. The main purposes of such surgery are to restore function, prevent further loss of function, and cosmetically improve the defects caused by deformities present at birth, disease, or trauma. Plastic surgery such as skin grafting may be done as an emergency measure in severe burns. Occasionally, plastic surgery may be done purely for cosmetic improvement.

Although medical science has made progress in learning the causes of some developmental anomalies—for example, it has been learned that German measles contracted during the first trimester of pregnancy may cause anomalies in the infant—it is not possible at the present time to prevent the occurrence of many defects at birth. Many birth defects, such as cleft lip and cleft palate, require plastic and reconstructive surgery. The cause of cancer is still unknown, and extensive surgery will continue to be used until a better method of treatment is discovered. Following surgical treatment for this disease, plastic and reconstructive surgery often is necessary. Trauma such as that sustained in automobile accidents often necessitates plastic and reconstructive surgery, and it seems likely that the number of people requiring such treatment will increase. Plastic and reconstructive surgery is often needed following loss of skin and scarring from burns. *Keloid tissue,* the thick, weltlike masses of overgrowth of scar tissue that occur particularly in Negroes, often requires plastic surgery. Posttraumatic scars in which subcutaneous tissues are separated from or are adherent to underlying structures such as bone may be corrected by plastic surgery.

Many of the procedures in reconstructive surgery overlap with plastic surgery, and surgical treatment of the patient often is assumed by several medical specialists. The dental surgeon, the ear, nose, and throat specialist, and the plastic surgeon may all work together, for example, in treatment of the child who has a cleft lip and a cleft palate.

In doing reconstructive surgery, the doctor may use, in addition to the patient's own tissues, inert materials and tissues from other human beings. Inert substances must meet several criteria. They must not be irritating or contribute to the development of cancer, they should be an appropriate consistency for their intended use, and they should not deteriorate or change their shape and form with time. A very large variety of substances have been used in the past, including wax, metal, ivory, and bone that has been rendered inert by boiling. In recent years plastic materials such as Teflon and silicone have been used extensively, since they appear to be nonirritating and they retain their form indefinitely. Best results seem to be achieved

when the plastic material forms a framework around which the body develops its own cells. Teflon, a plastic tetrafluoroethylene homopolymer can be used as a woven material, as thread, or as felt. As a tightly knitted tube, it is now widely used as a substitute for a portion of a defective artery that has been resected.

For many years reconstructive procedures have been attempted in which the tissues of other human beings are used. To be successful, these operations require adequate surgical treatment. Furthermore, the grafted tissue must grow and carry on normal function. In recent years great strides have been made in the technical aspects of transplanting tissues, and it is well within the realm of possibility that any organ of the body, including perhaps even the brain, may be transplanted in the future. Less success has been achieved in inducing the body to "accept" and make a part of itself the tissue it receives. Long ago it was observed that skin grafts taken from another human being appeared to do well for a short time. Eventually, however, and usually within four to fifteen days, they underwent changes and died. It is believed that the graft from another person (homograft) acts as an antigen, causing the host to produce antibodies and to develop a sensitivity to it. When a second homograft is used, it is rejected more quickly than the first, thus substantiating the belief that a sensitivity is produced. Many questions regarding the autoimmune reaction are not yet answered, and results of studies on experimental animals have not always been entirely consistent. Until medical science solves the riddle of the autoimmune reaction and learns how to deal with it, the transplantation of body organs and any tissue from one person to another will be fraught with hazards. The least difficulty is encountered with tissues, such as the cornea of the eye, that have a very limited blood supply. Attempts are made to combat the body's sensitivity by giving so-called immunosuppressive drugs. With the use of these drugs, grafted tissues have survived for years in some instances. Azathioprine (Imuran) and 6-mercaptopurine are given at the time of operation, and if rejection threatens, actinomycin C and prednisone are given in large doses.

General nursing care

The nurse has two important functions relating to patients needing plastic and reconstructive surgery. She should direct persons who may benefit from plastic procedures to appropriate medical care, and she is an important member of the team that cares for the patient undergoing plastic and reconstructive procedures.

Helping the patient to receive appropriate care

Many people do not know that it is possible to correct a congenital defect. Some parents may delay seeking medical care for a child with a defect due to a congenital anomaly because of their own guilt feelings. They may hope that somehow, miraculously, the child will "outgrow" the condition. Often they do not realize that the normal development of the child depends upon early treatment of some conditions. A defect may interfere with the use of a part of the body, so that normal growth does not take place. This result follows the principle that form follows function; for instance, a child's deformed and therefore unused hand does not grow at the same rate as the hand that is used normally. Contractures of joints and atrophy of muscles occur with disuse, thus increasing the defect and handicap; for example, facial asymmetry can result from contractures in the neck that prevent uniform action of the muscles of both sides of the face even though the muscles themselves are not affected.

Parents need to know that healthy emotional development in the child is dependent upon normal physical appearance. When a defect is allowed to persist, there may be emotional maladjustment that will affect the child's whole life. For example, conspicuous patches of brightly discolored skin present at birth and known as birthmarks or portwine stains are quite common. These stains, particularly if they are on the face or neck, cause the child great emotional distress and sometimes lead to serious personality maladjustment. Yet many people do not know that they may sometimes be effectively treated by tattooing.

A patient's emotional reaction to a deformity or defect must not be underestimated. One's pride in himself, his ability to think well of himself, and to regard himself favorably in comparison with others are essential to the development and maintenance of a well-integrated personality. Every person who has a defect or a handicap, particularly if it is conspicuous to others, suffers from some threat to his emotional security. The extent of the emotional reaction and the amount of maladjustment that follows depend upon the individual's makeup and upon his ability to ward off emotional insults. Disfigurements almost invariably lead to disturbing experiences. The child who has webbed fingers may be ridiculed at school; the adolescent girl who has acne scars may be a wallflower at school parties; and the young man with a posttraumatic scar on his face may be refused a salesman's job. Under any of these circumstances it is not unusual for the individual to withdraw from a society that is unkind. The defect may be used to justify failure to assume responsibility or to justify striking out against an unkind society by such reactions as becoming a "problem child" or, in some extreme cases, a criminal.

Plastic and reconstructive operations may require repeated and long hospitalizations that may place serious financial strain upon the patient and his family if they must assume responsibility for the major part of the expense. Clinic nurses, public health nurses in the community, social workers, and welfare agency personnel can help in preparing the patient for this problem and in helping him to meet it. If the patient is an adult, leaves from employment, financial support while undergoing treatment, and plans for convalescent care and rehabilitation are examples of problems that must be faced in many instances. The patient should be encouraged to discuss his problems freely, since their solution does affect his medical treatment.

Many parents do not know that financial resources are available to cover costs of plastic and reconstructive surgery for children. Every state in the country has a plan for medical care of crippled children. This program is partially supported by matching funds from the federal government, administered by the Children's Bureau of the Department of Health, Education, and Welfare, which was created soon after the first White House Conference on Child Care, held in Washington, D. C., in 1912. Children and adolescents up to 21 years of age with defects requiring plastic and reconstructive surgery are eligible for care under this plan. If the nurse encounters a child who might benefit from medical treatment, she should first ask members of the family if they have a family doctor with whom she can discuss the matter. If the family has no personal physician, the local hospital may conduct a clinic or may recommend a physician designated to care for eligible children in the area or the state. Small community hospitals may not have clinics of their own but may refer patients to larger hospitals or special clinics in nearby cities. In larger communities, the school nurse is usually well informed about available resources.

Preparation for surgery

It is believed that any plastic and reconstructive surgery for an obvious defect is justified if it helps the patient to feel he has a better chance for recognition among his fellowmen. The plastic surgeon may reshape a nose or repair a deformed hand so that an emotionally stable person will have more assurance among others. However, it is foolish to assume that reconstructive surgery alone will correct a basic personality problem. It has been learned that some people blame an apparently trivial physical defect for a long series of failures in their lives when the major defect lies within their personalities. Because of this possibility, the patient is usually carefully studied before surgery is planned. It is necessary to know what the patient expects the operation to accomplish before the doctor can decide whether or not such expectations are realistic and whether or not surgery should be done.

It is necessary to learn about the social standards and cultural mores of the community in which the patient lives and his adjustment to them. His economic contribution as a citizen and as a member of a family, his characteristic pattern in interpersonal relationships, and whether or not he has previously sought medical treatment for the particular problem should be known. The

social worker is often called upon to assist the surgeon in his efforts to learn as much as possible about the patient. By observing and reporting the patient's behavior at home, in school, in the clinic, upon arrival in the hospital, and during preparation for the operation, the nurse can help the surgeon in his study of the patient. Sometimes the help of specialists in psychology and psychiatry is sought. Before surgery, the doctor will tell the patient what probably can be done and what changes are possible. It is important that the nurse know what the patient has been told so that she can increase the patient's confidence in his surgical treatment and can avoid contributing to misunderstandings and misinterpretations.

The patient who is admitted to the hospital for plastic and reconstructive surgery may have extensive scarring and deformity and may be exceedingly sensitive to scrutiny by the people he encounters. On the other hand, the patient may have little apparent deformity, and it may be difficult to understand what brought the seemingly well person to the hospital for surgery. The nurse cannot possibly know what the disfigurement means to the individual patient and should avoid judging whether or not surgery is necessary. The nurse may be inclined to concentrate her efforts on the more physically ill patients. Yet it is important for her to learn about each patient who is to have plastic surgery and to assure him of her interest.

The patient should be in the best possible physical condition before plastic and reconstructive surgery is begun. When the plans are made for elective surgery, the patient may be advised to eat a diet high in protein and vitamins for a short time prior to coming to the hospital because good nutrition is thought to help in the "take" or healing of the graft. Hemoglobin and clotting times are usually determined, and many surgeons request that the blood protein level be assayed, because a normal blood protein level has been found necessary for satisfactory growth of grafted tissue.

The wound that is to receive the graft must be free from infections that would delay healing, lead to more scar tissue formation, or cause death of the graft. Infection is treated by the administration of antibiotics and by the use of warm soaks and compresses. A sterile physiologic solution of sodium chloride is the solution most often used. Before skin grafting is attempted, any dead tissue that is adherent to the wound is removed by debridement; otherwise this tissue will interfere with the graft's healing.

The *donor site* (the area from which skin is to be taken) is shaved and scrubbed with soap and water or with a detergent solution the evening before surgery, and this cleansing may be repeated the morning of operation. Strong antiseptics are avoided because they may irritate the skin. If the *recipient site* (the area that is to receive the graft) is not an open wound, it is cleansed in the same way.

It is important to explain to the patient the measures used to prepare him for surgery, and he should be prepared for the postoperative experience. It must be repeatedly explained to him that the immediate results may not meet his expectations. Postoperative tissue reaction may distort normal contours, suture lines may be reddened, and the color of the newly transplanted skin may differ somewhat from that of surrounding skin. The patient may become alarmed and discouraged if he has not been prepared for the normal appearance of skin grafts and reconstructed tissue immediately after surgery. Preferably he should not see the operative site until it is well healed. If it is not possible to remove all mirrors to prevent the patient from inspecting the results of facial surgery, dressings may be left on longer than necessary to cover wounds. Members of the patient's family should also know what to expect so that they will not be unduly worried and so that they can give support to the patient if apprehension occurs.

Special procedures for contractures

Plastic surgeons make excellent use of the natural elastic quality of the normal skin. Operations known as a Z-*plasty* and a Y-*plasty* are often done. Scar tissue can often be removed, and the Z-shaped or Y-shaped incision enables the surgeon to undermine adjacent skin, draw the edges together, and cover the defect without using skin from another part of the body (Fig. 47). These procedures are naturally limited by the size of the scar and its location, since elasticity of skin varies in different parts of the body. Z-plasty and Y-plasty procedures are suitable for such locations as the axilla, the inner aspects of the elbow, and the neck and throat. They are not so useful in treating defects on the back or on the palmar surfaces of the hand because the skin in these areas cannot be undermined and stretched.

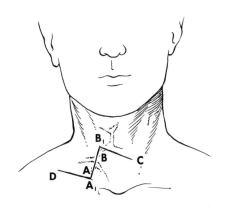 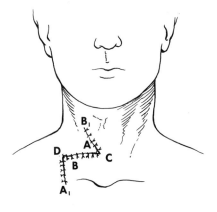

Fig. 47

By means of Z-plasty operations, scar tissue can be removed and defects can be covered without the need to transplant skin.

Types of grafts
and related nursing care

Nearly all plastic and reconstructive surgery requires moving tissue from one part of the body to another. The moved tissue, or graft, is known as an *autograft,* and skin, bone, cartilage, fat, fascia, muscle, or nerves may be taken. Tissue transplanted from another person is called a *homograft (allograft).* It can be obtained from living persons, or it can be taken from persons shortly before death. Tissue taken under the latter circumstances can be used only if cancer or an infectious disease was not present. The use of homografts may be necessary when the patient's condition is poor and autografting is impossible. For example, the patient may be in shock but require the covering of large burned areas by grafted skin. Homografts survive only about one to three months and will then die and slough or be absorbed and replaced by the host's own developing tissues. They are used only as temporary grafts. Heterografts (xenografts) consist of tissue from another species. They are rejected by the recipient and are rarely used. The transplant acts as an antigen, and the body forms antibodies against it that prevent growth and function of the graft. When bone, cartilage, or blood vessels are obtained from sources other than the patient, it has been noted that they do not become part of the patient's body but act as a framework around which the body usually lays down cells of its own. The homograft is then gradually absorbed over a period of time.

Plastic surgery may be done by means of free grafting—cutting tissue from one part of the body and moving it directly to another part. It may also be done by leaving one end of the graft attached to the body to provide a blood supply for the graft until blood vessels form at the new place of attachment. The surgeon selects skin for grafting that is similar in texture and thickness to that which has been lost. He studies the normal lines of the skin and its elasticity to avoid noticeable scars. Scar tissue contracts with time, and in normal circumstances this process is good because it produces a complete closure of the line of injury. However, in some cases scar tissue may contract in such a way that surrounding tissues are pulled out of normal contour, and distortion may result. The plastic surgeon is an artist as well as a surgeon, and he studies cosmetic and many other aspects of the patient's problem before he decides upon the type of graft or plastic procedure that will be most effective.

Free grafts

Free grafts are those that are lifted completely from one part of the body to another. There are several kinds of free grafts, and each has its advantages and its limitations. *Reverdin grafts,* or *pinch grafts,* grow easily and can sometimes be used to cover wounds that have been recently infected, such as those that result from varicose ulcers. In such a graft, the skin at the donor site is picked up with a needle, and tiny pieces, about 0.5 cm. in diameter, are removed by means of a razor or sharp knife and placed on the recipient site about 1.5 cm. apart. Because the full thickness of skin is taken, the grafts regenerate epithelium around their edges until finally they coalesce on the recipient surface. The donor site, on the other hand, regenerates new skin around the edges of the small wounds left when the grafts were taken. Pinch grafts are easy to obtain, and if a few of them die and slough, no serious damage has been done. The disadvantages are that the resultant skin has a bumpy, unattractive appearance, and there are permanent small scars at the donor site. This graft is now seldom used.

Ollier-Thiersch grafts, or *razor grafts,* are thin layers of the outer skin that are removed from the donor site (usually the front of the thigh) by a long, razorlike knife or by a dermatome. The use of these grafts is limited because they contract easily, often become shiny and discolored, and have poor wearing qualities. Their advantages are that they will often live on bony and tendinous areas where blood supply is poor, they can be taken in large pieces to cover large defects, and new skin regenerates quickly and without scarring at the donor site. Razor grafts are often used to replace mucous membrane in reconstructive surgery of the mouth and vagina. These grafts may be taken from another person (homografts) to cover large burned areas and reduce the loss of body fluids. Within a few weeks they die, and can then be removed and replaced by a split-thickness graft from the patient.

The *split-thickness graft* is very widely used. This graft consists of the outer layer and part of the middle layer of skin. It does not wrinkle, contract, and become discolored as easily as the razor graft, yet the donor site is able to regenerate completely because the deeper layers of skin are not removed. Split-thickness grafts can be used to cover almost any part of the body. They can be cut in large pieces with a dermatome that is set to ensure a uniform thickness of the graft, and these large pieces can then be cut into small pieces (Fig. 182).

Wolfe's grafts, or *full-thickness grafts,* include all three skin layers and are used mainly to cover small areas where matching skin color and texture are important, as on the face. One disadvantage of the Wolfe graft is that only a moderate-sized piece of full-thickness skin can survive as a free graft under the best of circumstances because blood supply cannot become established quickly enough to provide essential nutrition. For nourishment these grafts depend entirely upon existing lymph until their own blood supply can be established. It takes at least two weeks for blood supply to become established, although it is usually possible to tell within a week whether the graft is going to survive. If the graft dies, the skin is irretrievably lost to the body, since regeneration of skin at the donor site is not possible. Surrounding skin at the donor site is usually undermined so that the skin edges can be brought together, and grafting of the donor site is not necessary. This means that full advantage may have been taken of the elastic quality of the skin, and another graft probably cannot be taken from the same place for some time at least.

Skin flaps and sliding grafts

When a large and deep defect is to be covered, a skin flap may be used. *Sliding, rotating,* and *pedicle* are terms used to identify various types of grafts that are never removed from a source of blood supply. Flap grafts may include skin, subcutaneous tissue, and sometimes fat and cartilage or bone. If the location of sites on the body permits, as, for example, the hand against the abdomen, the graft may be released from the donor site on three sides

that are then sutured into the recipient site. This graft is known as a *primary* graft.

When the edges of the graft are sutured together to form a tube, the graft is known as a pedicle, or *suitcase-handle* graft. This modification is often made when the skin is to travel a considerable distance, because the danger of infection is much less than if it were open. Tissues such as fat and cartilage can also be easily transferred within the tube. This type of graft might be used to cover a defect on the back of the neck with skin from the abdomen. For example, the piece of skin taken from the abdomen may be grafted to the wrist. Then, when circulation is safely established there, the attachment on the abdomen may be released and attached to its final location on the neck. The attachment on the wrist is maintained until circulation is established in the neck, at which time the graft is freed from the wrist and the tube opened and sutured into place to cover the defect. Circulation from the new attachment is often tested by putting a rubber-covered clamp or tourniquet about the pedicle close to its oldest attachment and noting the color and warmth of the pedicle at intervals of from ten to fifteen minutes. Usually it takes from three to six weeks for new blood vessels to become established. These grafts are less likely to die than are free grafts, but strangulation can occur from pressure, and tissue can be lost from infection. Pedicle grafts are often taken from the abdomen, where fat and subcutaneous tissue are available, to support skin areas of the body that are subject to pressure, such as the heel, the sole of the foot, and the palm of the hand. The piece of skin taken is fairly narrow, and adjacent skin is undermined so that edges can be sutured together. When this wound has healed, a small gauze dressing is usually placed between the pedicle and the suture line to keep the area dry and free from the accumulation of dead skin.

Postoperative medical and nursing care

The life of the patient is not usually at stake in plastic surgery, but time, discomfort, and economic and emotional factors are involved. Sometimes a procedure that is not successful cannot be repeated because neces-

217

sary skin is lost and too much scar tissue may have formed. Moreover, the patient undergoing extensive reconstructive surgery has usually suffered a great deal both physically and emotionally. His ability to cope with the disappointment of unsatisfactory results may be limited.

In addition to general supportive nursing care and care of any patient who has had an operation, the nurse has special responsibilities for the success of the procedure in care of the patient following plastic surgery. Maintaining pressure dressings as requested, preventing infection of grafted areas, and applying compresses to stimulate circulation to the graft all require meticulous nursing attention.

Care of the operative areas

A graft must be in constant contact with the underlying tissue in order to attach itself and to grow. Anything that comes between the undersurface of the graft and the recipient area, such as a discharge caused by infection, excess serous fluid, or blood, will float the graft away from close contact and may cause it to die. To prevent floating, some surgeons insert tiny drains at strategic spots along the edges of the graft, or a small catheter is inserted on the edge of the graft under the recipient skin and attached to suction to remove the fluid.

If the recipient site is a clean wound with no infection, the graft usually is sutured with many fine sutures to hold it in place and in contact with the normal skin adjacent to it. If the recipient site is known to be infected, only a few scattered sutures or no sutures at all may be used.

A wide variety of materials are used as dressings. The choice depends upon the kind of graft and the surgeon's preference. Gauze impregnated with petroleum jelly or bismuth tribromophenate (Xeroform) are most often selected. Silver foil may also be used. Often the graft is covered with a piece of coarse-mesh gauze that is anchored to the adjacent skin edges with an elastic bandage (Elastoplast) to give firm, gentle pressure and to immobilize the area. The first dressing may be covered with a compress of sterile normal saline solution and then protected with Pliofilm or another waterproof material. A continuous pressure is necessary to keep the graft adherent to the recipient bed, but pressure should not be so firm as to cause death of the graft. Marine sponges, rubber sponges, cotton pads, and mechanic's waste may be applied as outer dressings by the doctor to provide the amount of pressure he wishes. Occasionally the sutures anchoring the graft at the skin edges are left uncut and brought over a pressure dressing to hold it firmly against the graft. The nurse should be certain that dressings do not become loosened so that pressure is reduced and that the patient does not lie on these dressings or in any other way increase the pressure on them. When flap grafts are used, slings and casts may assure immobilization and help to keep parts of the body in the correct relationship for healing (Fig. 48).

Some surgeons believe that grafts are stimulated in their effort to establish blood supply by the use of warm, moist compresses, and sterile normal saline solution is usually ordered for this purpose. The greatest care must be taken that infection is not introduced when compresses are being changed and moistened. The nurse must remember to wash her hands before handling dressings or changing compresses and must follow the most meticulous technique so that infection does not occur. She must be careful, too, not to traumatize the newly grafted skin. The temperature of the compress solution should not be over 40.5° C. (105° F.), and compresses should be applied with sterile forceps. Compresses may sometimes be covered with a sterile petroleum jelly dressing and moistened by gently directing fluid from a sterile Asepto syringe under the edge of the dressings. Sterile tubes with tiny openings (Dakin's tubes) may also be placed through the outer compresses to provide a means of moistening the inner dressings without disturbing them and without introducing infection.

The patient may be placed on an oscillating bed in order to improve circulation to the graft as well as to help prevent circulatory complications such as thrombophlebitis. Some physicians prescribe vasodilating drugs such as tolazoline hydrochloride (Priscoline), nicotinic acid, papaverine hydrochloride, and alcohol in a further attempt to produce vasodilation at the recipient site.

When split-thickness grafts have been

used, the donor site (often the anterior surface of the thigh) may be a greater source of discomfort to the patient than the recipient site. This area is covered with impregnated gauze (usually Xeroform), and a firm outer dressing is applied and anchored with Elastoplast bandage that does not encircle the thigh lest it hamper circulation. This dressing usually is not changed for two weeks. A more recent method of treatment is to cover the area with one firm layer of gauze anchored firmly at the edges and leave it exposed to the air. It is believed by some surgeons that healing occurs faster with this method and that there is less danger of death of the deeper skin layer, which must develop the new outer skin layer.[13] Analgesic drugs such as dextropropoxyphene hydrochloride (Darvon), acetylsalicylic acid (aspirin), and meperidine hydrochloride (Demerol) may be needed for pain and should not be withheld during the first few days postoperatively.

The nurse should observe the dressings at both the recipient and the donor sites for drainage and bleeding. She should make sure that they are secure and that they have not become too tight because of local edema, thus interfering with circulation. Inner dressings on the recipient site are changed by the surgeon from one to twelve days after the operation, and it is usually possible to know then whether or not the result of the operation is satisfactory. Sutures may be removed at this time.

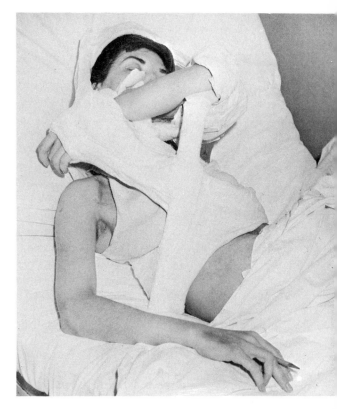

Fig. 48

Plastic operations sometimes require the patient to be in extremely awkward positions. Eating, mouth hygiene, and communicating with others are problems in caring for this patient. Note the pencil used for communicating.

Care of the patient requiring a cast

The patient who must be in a cast for one or more stages of plastic and reconstructive surgery requires special care. Sometimes it is helpful preoperatively for the patient to assume the position that will be necessary for the next stage of the procedure so that he may become accustomed to a posture that may cause tedious strain on joints and muscles. Immediately after application and frequently thereafter, the cast must be examined for cracks or breaks that will interfere with support for the graft, and it must be carefully checked to make certain that no excessive pressure is being exerted. Pillows can be used to give support and to lessen strain on body parts. Sometimes overbed bars and side rails help

the patient to shift his position if he has one free arm and is otherwise able to do so. The patient who is in an extensive cast for several weeks must be reminded to do muscle-setting exercises for limbs in the cast and to exercise actively the limbs that are not confined.

Arrangements should be made for the patient to see what goes on around him. Sometimes this is made possible by changing his position in bed or the position of the bed in the room. In some instances putting the patient "head to foot" in the bed is helpful. A mirror may be attached to the bed and arranged at such an angle that the patient can see at least a part of the room if his head, neck, and shoulder movements are restricted by a cast.

General care of the patient requiring lengthy hospitalization

Occupations must be planned to keep the patient busy and to keep his mind off his discomfort. If he cannot engage in handwork, then passive activities such as listening to the radio, reading, and watching television should be arranged. Even the patient who appears to be in a very complicated cast and in an awkward position can be placed on a stretcher or wheeled in his bed to a solarium or to other locations where he may have a change of scene and engage in some activity with others. Members of the patient's family should be encouraged to visit him as much as possible and to try in every way to help him maintain his community relationships that have been temporarily interrupted by his hospitalization.

The nurse may also help the patient to think along constructive lines in regard to what he will do when surgery is completed. Since a long period of rehabilitation is sometimes necessary, it is important to keep the patient in the best possible physical condition so that he will be ready to undertake specific rehabilitation activities and not require corrective therapy for disabilities acquired during hospitalization. For example, the patient who is having extensive skin grafting for a large traumatic wound on one leg should not be found to have foot drop on the unaffected limb when reconstructive procedures are completed.

The patient may tire of the hospital menu and may need to be encouraged to eat a well-balanced diet to promote healing of the graft, to reduce the chance of infection, and to maintain muscle strength during hospitalization. If he is on bed rest for a long time, it is important that bulk food be eaten in sufficient quantities to help elimination and that plenty of fluids be taken so that complications of the renal system do not develop.

Tattooing

Tattooing has been found useful in plastic surgery for changing the color of grafted skin so that it more closely resembles the surrounding skin. This treatment is usually given on an ambulatory basis. Pigment is carefully selected and blended with the normal skin coloring by a skilled technician who then impregnates the grafted skin, using a tattooing needle. The procedure is painful, since no anesthetic is used. Sometimes the patient is given a sedative such as phenobarbital or is instructed to take such medication approximately one hour before coming to the clinic or the doctor's office. Prior to the tattooing, the skin is cleansed with a gauze sponge moistened with alcohol or normal saline solution. There may be a slight serous oozing from the skin, and it should be left to dry and crust. Sometimes a piece of sterile gauze can be placed over the tattooed area, and an ice bag may be applied if severe discomfort follows the treatment.

Tattooing is usually done in several stages. The amount done at one time depends upon individual circumstances, such as the location of the part treated and the emotional reactions of the patient. For example, treatment of the skin close to the eye is often quite painful and is extremely trying for the patient. Therefore, usually only a small amount of tattooing is done at one time. Children may be given a general anesthetic for treatment around the eyes. Grafted skin may change in color with time, so tattooing done for the purpose of changing the color of grafted skin may have to be repeated.

Port-wine stains that are too large to treat by excision and grafting have also responded to this method of treatment with excellent results. The whole area may be treated at one time and the treatments repeated so that the color changes slowly. This is a tedious procedure if the stain is large and dark but, finally, in some cases the stain is barely apparent to the casual observer.

Dermal abrasion

Pockmarks, scars from acne, and certain other disfiguring marks may be removed from the skin by abrasive action. The variable results depend upon the type and extent of the condition, but there is usually noticeable improvement in the patient's appearance. Preoperatively the patient is prepared by the doctor for the degree of improvement to be expected so that his expectations are realistic. He is also informed about the face bandage he may wear, postoperative swelling, discomfort, crusting, and the erythema which may persist for several weeks. The procedure is done under local or general anesthesia, depending on the size of the area to be treated, the individual patient, and the preference of the doctor. It may be done in the clinic, the doctor's office, or the hospital, again depending on the extent of the procedure and the preference of the physician. Hospitalization is necessary if a general anesthetic is used.

The skin is first cleansed with soap and water or a detergent and then with alcohol or an antiseptic such as benzalkonium chloride. Ethyl chloride or other, less flammable, spray anesthetics, such as Frigiderm, are used most often for local anesthesia. After the skin preparation has been completed, the skin is stretched and its superficial layers are removed either by sandpapering or by using an abrasive machine (Dermabrader). If the procedure has not been extensive and oozing is slight, the area may be left uncovered. Usually it is covered either with an ointment or by moist compresses moistened with an antiseptic solution such as benzalkonium chloride and then by a pressure dressing that covers the entire face except for the eyes, nose, and mouth. Prepared dressings that adhere less readily to the skin surface, such as Telfa dressings, are also used.

If the patient has had a general anesthetic, he must be turned to his side to prevent the dressing from becoming wet or contaminated in the event of vomiting or excessive salivation. The dressing should be checked for signs of bleeding, and the patient must be observed for signs of respiratory embarrassment, which may be caused by pressure from the dressing. A pressure dressing usually is removed after forty-eight hours, and the patient is discharged to return to the doctor's office or the clinic. Washing the face and shaving are seldom permitted until all the crusts have fallen away, but some physicians permit the patient to wash his face gently with a mild soap as soon as the dressing has been removed. If the patient's face feels dry after healing has occurred, gentle lubri-

cation with substances such as cold cream usually is advised. Dermal abrasion may be done in stages. At least two weeks and often longer may intervene between treatments.

Maxillofacial surgery

Maxillofacial surgery is a specialty requiring a surgeon with unusual preparation and nurses with special knowledge and experience. Maxillofacial surgery received impetus as a result of the injuries sustained in World War II and the increase in radical surgery now being done for malignancies of the face. The surgeon works closely with the dental surgeon and with the specialist in problems of the nose and throat. Preventing infection, ensuring an airway, and providing nourishment for the patient are some of the greatest nursing problems. (For details of nursing care, see p. 603.)

The emotional reactions of patients who undergo extensive maxillofacial surgery are severe, and one of the biggest nursing problems is attempting to keep up the patient's morale. The patient may be helped by seeing someone else who has undergone a similar operation with a good result and who has made good adjustment. When damage has been so great that reconstruction with living tissue is impossible, it is sometimes possible to construct prosthetic parts of the face that are so true to natural color and contour that they are not easily detectable. For example, a side of the nose may be replaced by a prosthetic part that is colored to match the patient's skin and disguised with marking to resemble skin.

Birth defects

Birth defects can occur in any part of the body. Providing they are treated at the proper time in the child's life, most of them can be improved a great deal by reconstructive procedures and some can be corrected entirely. The most important nursing responsibilities lie in helping to place children with birth defects under specialized medical care. These responsibilities are discussed in the first part of this chapter. Anomalies of the urogenital system are fairly common and are discussed in Chapter 19 and more fully in

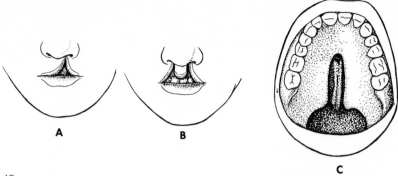

Fig. 49

Cleft lip and palate. **A,** Single cleft of lip. **B,** Double cleft of lip. **C,** Cleft of posterior palate.

pediatric nursing texts and specialized medical texts on these subjects. Musculoskeletal anomalies and deformities are among the more common anomalies and are discussed fully in specialized nursing texts on orthopedic nursing.

Cleft lip and *cleft palate* are among the most common birth defects (Fig. 49). Cleft lip usually is repaired surgically as soon as possible and sometimes when the infant is only a few days old. A second operation often is necessary but does not imply that the first one was not successful. A cleft palate is a much more difficult defect to treat than a cleft lip. It is repaired as early as possible, depending upon the extent of the defect and the condition of the child. Most specialists believe that it should always be repaired by the time speech is attempted. The many nursing problems that are encountered in teaching mothers to feed and care for an infant with this defect and that the nurse needs to know to care for a child who has had a cleft lip or cleft palate repaired are included in pediatric nursing texts and current periodicals and will not be included here.

Cosmetic surgery

The most common operation for purely cosmetic effect is removal of some of the cartilage from the ears in order to flatten them against the head. This procedure is relatively simple for the plastic surgeon and requires only a short hospitalization.

Rhinoplasty, or reconstructive surgery of the nose, is another common cosmetic operation. Bone and cartilage may be removed from the nose if it is irregular, or they may be inserted if defects such as saddle nose are being corrected. A local anesthetic is often used for these procedures unless it will interfere with a study of contours during the operation. In this case, an intravenous or a rectal anesthetic may be used. The incision is usually made at the end of the nose inside the nostril so that it is not conspicuous. A nasal splint made of plaster, tongue blades, or crinoline may be used for protection. Immediately after the operation there will be ecchymosis and swelling around the eyes and nose. Ice compresses and an ice bag may be used to help prevent these reactions. The patient must anticipate waiting several weeks before evaluating the final result of the operation.

Meloplasty is commonly called "facelifting." An incision is made at the hairline, and excess skin is separated from its underlying tissue and removed. The remaining skin is pulled up and sutured at the hairline, thus removing wrinkles and giving firmness and smoothness to the face. A gentle pressure dressing is then applied and left in place for approximately a week. This procedure is sometimes repeated at intervals of five years or more.

Attempts may be made occasionally by plastic surgeons to partially remove wrinkles by injecting chemical substances under the skin.[8]

Mammoplasty can be done to improve the appearance of a woman's breasts. Some women develop conspicuously large and pendulous breasts that they wish to have reduced in size. Large breasts are embarrassing to some women and make it difficult for them to participate in sports, maintain good posture, and buy clothes that fit. Such women often respond to reconstructive surgery remarkably well. Cosmetic surgery of the breast may also be done to make unusually small breasts larger. A variety of plastic materials may be used for this procedure.[1]

Reconstructive surgery of the breast is usually major surgery and requires the use of general anesthetics and a hospital stay of about two weeks. Pressure dressings are kept in place for about a week postoperatively. The patient is advised to wear a firm, supporting brassiere both night and day for several months after surgery. It is important that the fit be such that firm, constant support is provided when the patient is in the prone position. If the patient cannot make necessary adjustment in brassieres she already owns or cannot buy satisfactory ready-made brassieres, she may need to have some especially made. Large department stores usually provide this service.

References and selected readings*

1 Baker, Thomas J.: Cosmetic surgery for small breasts, Am. J. Nursing 61:77-78, June 1961.

2 Converse, John Marquis, and others: Symposium on reconstructive plastic surgery, S. Clin. North America 39:259-530, April 1959.

3 Conway, Herbert: Skin grafts—the techniques, Am. J. Nursing 64:94-97, Nov. 1964.

4 Davis, Loyal, editor: Christopher's textbook of surgery, ed. 8, Philadelphia, 1964, W. B. Saunders Co.

5 Edwards, Benjamin F.: Endoprostheses in plastic surgery, Am. J. Nursing 64:123-125, May 1964.

6 Iverson, Preston C., and Staneruck, Isabella D.: Dermal abrasion and nursing care after dermal abrasion, Am. J. Nursing 57:860-864, July 1957.

7 *Kallaus, Jane: The child with cleft lip and palate: the mother in the maternity unit, Am. J. Nursing 65:120-123, April 1965.

8 Litton, Clyde: Chemical face lifting, Plast. & Reconstruct. Surg. 29:371-380, April 1962.

9 Longmire, William P.: A current survey of clinical experience in tissue and organ transplantation, S. Clin. North America 45:407-421, April 1965.

10 *Macgregor, Frances Cooke: Some psychological hazards of plastic surgery of the face, Plast. & Reconstruct. Surg. 12:123-130, Aug. 1953.

11 Macgregor, Frances Cooke, and others: Facial deformities and plastic surgery, Springfield, Ill., 1953, Charles C Thomas, Publisher.

12 McDermott, Margaret M.: The child with cleft lip and palate: on the pediatric ward, Am. J. Nursing 65:122-125, April 1965.

13 Moyer, Carl A., and others: Surgery—principles and practice, ed. 3, Philadelphia, 1965, J. B. Lippincott Co.

14 *Nayer, Dorothy D.: Skin grafts—the patient, Am. J. Nursing 64:98-101, Nov. 1964.

15 *Newton, William T.: The biologic basis of tissue transplantation, S. Clin. North America 45:393-406, April 1965.

16 Richardson, S. A.: Some social psychological consequences of handicapping, Pediatrics 32:291-297, Aug. 1963.

17 Ripley, Ione L.: The child with cleft lip and palate: through his years of growth, Am. J. Nursing 65:124-127, April 1965.

18 Stark, Richard B.: Plastic surgery, New York, 1962, Harper & Row, Publishers.

*References preceded by an asterisk are particularly well suited for student reading.

12

The patient
needing special
continuing care

Study questions

Study questions

1 Review the case histories of patients on a medical or surgical ward in your hospital. What proportion has a chronic illness as either primary or secondary diagnosis? What proportion has more than one chronic condition? What age group is affected most by multiple diseases?

2 Consult your notes on social and community health aspects of nursing, and review what you learned about the facilities for care of the chronically ill patient in your immediate community. What is the total patient capacity of these facilities, and what percentage of the total population of the city or town could hope to receive care from them if necessary? How are these facilities supported financially?

3 What kinds of patients do you think are most in need of rehabilitation? Select a patient from one of the hospital wards to illustrate rehabilitation needs.

4 From what you have learned of anatomy, outline in detail the physical movements necessary in order to rise from a sitting position in a chair to a standing position. Describe how you would assist a patient to a standing position while allowing him opportunity to help himself.

Prevention and control of chronic diseases is one of the major health problems in the United States today. The incidence of chronic diseases and mortality from chronic diseases have increased since the beginning of the nineteenth century, with the most rapid increase occurring in recent years. This increase has been brought about by a number of developments, one of the first of which was general improvement in sanitation, which led to reduction of many infections that, prior to this time, had cut short the lives of many persons at a relatively early age. A pronounced reduction in the deaths that were caused by the acute communicable diseases and by infections came about as organisms became better known, immunizations against many of them were developed, and drugs to combat many organisms were found. In 1900 the leading causes of death were pneumonia and influenza, tuberculosis, and those diseases classified as gastritis. Today the leading causes of death are diseases of the heart, malignant neoplasms, and vascular lesions of the central nervous system.

There has been a tendency among health workers to equate chronic disease with old age. While it is true that most elderly people have one or more chronic diseases, chronic disease is common in the younger age group, which is increasing proportionately more rapidly than the older age group. The life-span at all age levels has increased, and the number of people in each age group has increased as the population as a whole has grown. Predictions of the number of persons who may be afflicted with chronic illness in the future must be based upon predictions of population growth based on fertility rates. Fertility rates, however, have been found to be quite unpredictable and do not change as might be expected. For this reason the Bureau of the Census makes two sets of predictions based on fertility rates—one that supposes a high level of fertility, and the other a lower level. On either basis the predictions are that by 1980 the largest proportion of the population will consist of persons 5 to 19 years of age.[21] Based on these predictions and present figures, it is estimated that by 1980 there will be 39.5 million more people than at present who will have one or more chronic conditions, and that 24.4 million of these will be under 35 years of age.[21]

Extent and effect of chronic illness

According to the National Health Survey, 73.8 million have one or more chronic conditions. The National Health Survey list of chronic diseases included asthma, allergy, tuberculosis, severe bronchitis, sinusitis, rheumatic fever, arteriosclerosis, hypertension, heart disease, cerebral vascular accident and other vascular conditions, hemorrhoids, gallbladder or liver disease, gastric ulcers, kidney stones, arthritis, prostate disease, diabetes mellitus, thyroid disease, epilepsy or convulsions, spinal disease, cancer, chronic dermatosis, and hernia.

About 17 million people, or 10% of the total population in the United States, are limited in normal activities by a chronic condition. In this group 5 million persons are under the age of 45 years, 6 million are 45 to 65 years of age, and 6 million are 65 years and older.[39] Heart conditions, arthritis, rheumatism, and visual impairment were reported to be among the chief causes of limitation of activity. Of the total number limited in activity, 3.9 million are unable to carry on their major activity (to work, keep house, or go to school); 10.2 million have limitations of some kind but could still carry out major activity; and 5 million have limitations but not in their major activity. The remaining 54.5 million have no limitations.[57]

Many of the chronically ill were found to be limited as to mobility. About 900,000 of the 73.8 million were confined to their homes; 1 million could not get around at all without the help of another person, and 2.8 million had difficulty getting about without help. The remaining 69 million had no limitation in mobility.[57]

The inability to work or to move about influences greatly the kind of medical treatment and health supervision needed by persons who have chronic illness. Some need only periodic medical examination and perhaps continuing treatment with drugs. Others may require complete physical care. Some have a disease that progresses very slowly without remissions, while others may have episodes of acute illness and then seem comparatively well for a time. Each person requires thorough consideration to determine the stage of his illness and the course his disease is likely to take. To help the patient appropriately, the nurse should be able to distinguish between these phases of illness.

Differences between acute illness and chronic illness

An acute illness is one caused by a disease that produces symptoms and signs soon after exposure to the cause, that runs a short course, and from which there is usually a full recovery or an abrupt termination in death. Acute illnesses may become chronic. For example, a common cold may develop into chronic sinusitis. A chronic illness is one caused by disease that produces symptoms and signs within a variable period of time, that runs a long course, and from which there is only partial recovery. The symptoms and general reactions caused by chronic disease may subside with proper treatment and care. This period during which the disease is controlled and symptoms are not obvious is known as a *remission*. However, at a future time the disease becomes more active again with recurrence of pronounced symptoms. This is known as an *exacerbation* of the disease. A chronic disease is characterized by remissions and exacerbations and slowly progressive physical changes. Many emotional, social, and economic implications of chronic illness will be mentioned later in this chapter.

Acute exacerbations of chronic disease often cause the patient to seek medical attention and may lead to hospitalization. Distinction must be made between acute illness and an acute phase of a chronic illness. The needs of a patient who has an acute illness may be very different from those of the patient with an acute exacerbation of a chronic disease. For example, a young person may enter the hospital with complaints of fever, chest pain, shortness of breath, fatigue, and a productive cough. If the diagnosis is pneumonia, the patient usually can be assured of recovery after a period of rest and a course of antibiotic treatment. However, if the diagnosis is rheumatic heart disease, and if the patient is being admitted to the hospital for the third, fourth, or fifth time, the reassurance needed will not be so definite, clear-cut, or easy to give. In this instance it will be necessary for the nurse to begin planning care that will extend beyond the period of hospitalization, taking into consideration many aspects of the patient's total life situation. The concerns of the patient who has had repeated attacks of illness will be very different from the concerns of the one who has a short-term illness.

The nurse needs to be aware of patients who are admitted to the hospital with an acute illness but who also have an underlying chronic condition. For example, the elderly patient who enters the general hospital with pneumonia may receive treatment for the pneumonia and recover from his illness. However, he may still be hampered by the arteriosclerotic heart disease and arthritis that he has had for years. These two chronic conditions may have been aggravated by the acute infection, or the patient's return to his former activity may be hindered by joint stiffness resulting from enforced bed rest and inactivity. The nurse who considers the patient's several diagnoses can help in preventing new problems associated with his chronic illness.

Early detection of chronic illness

Relatively little is known about how to prevent chronic illness. Predisposing characteristics or habits that help to identify the person likely to develop a particular chronic disease have been studied extensively. By altering habits of eating, rest, activity, or smoking, the course of certain chronic diseases, such as emphysema or cardiac disease, may be changed. Unfortunately, many chronic conditions begin without the individual's awareness of significant physiologic changes. An important step in prevention is early detection of these changes.

Screening programs and periodic health examinations are two methods that have helped to identify persons who are "high risks" and considered more likely to develop certain chronic diseases. Simple tests are offered to all citizens of the community or to selected groups, such as workers in industry, children at school, women, or men. Some of the more familiar screening tests are chest x-ray examinations to detect heart disease, cancer, or tuberculosis; urine or blood sugar tests to detect possible early signs of diabetes; and blood pressure determinations to detect hypertension.

Screening tests may be offered to apparently well persons who have no particular symptoms. Often in the course of interviews with persons coming to these screening programs, signs and symptoms of chronic illness are obvious to the interviewer although the person has either attached no meaning to them, ignored them, or attributed them to some other cause. Careful questioning about daily activities frequently uncovers discomforts such as joint pains, backaches, swelling of the ankles, shortness of breath, and other signs that may indicate early and chronic disease.

The interview accompanying a screening test can be as important in detection as the test itself. If the nurse is responsible for planning screening programs, she should try to ensure the inclusion of an interview as part of the program. Ideally, the nurse as well as the physician should participate in the interviews. Conferences scheduled with parents in order to discuss their children offer ideal circumstances and opportunity for the nurse in the hospital clinic or community agency to offer counseling, health guidance, health appraisal, and appropriate referral for diagnosis.

Screening tests differ from diagnostic tests in that the latter are used either to establish the presence of disease or to rule it out. The nurse should know the diagnostic facilities available in her community and should encourage the public to use them. Earlier medical treatment is now sought by families who carry medical, hospitalization, or group health insurance, but most persons need help in understanding the importance of early detection.

Nursing care of the chronically ill

The care of the chronically ill today is focused on prevention and reduction of disability, and on enabling the person to remain a socially functioning individual in every respect. Some of the disability seen among the chronically ill might have been prevented if prompt, aggressive, suitable medical and nursing care had been available at the onset of illness. Many of the difficulties that limit the chronically ill may not have been caused by the disease but may have developed because the patient was immobilized at the onset of disease.

Keeping the patient's body in good alignment, maintaining muscle tone, and preventing contractures are physical measures that every nurse must bear in mind constantly as she works with a patient. A careful plan of rest and activity helps to preserve physical resources and to make the day purposeful. If assistance is needed, the nurse or a trained aide can help the patient with the activity.

Much was said in Chapter 1 about the nurse's knowing and understanding herself as a person as well as understanding her patient. This concept is particularly important in caring for the chronically ill patient. Before a nurse can help a patient to help himself, she needs to distinguish between her values, standards, and goals, and those of the patient. In day-to-day contact with a patient who is making little or no progress, the nurse may be tempted to make plans for his future because of a sincere interest in helping him. This is particularly true when the patient is about the same age as the nurse. She may feel that something must be done to speed progress. Helping the patient to help himself—for example, in getting out of bed independently—is progress (Fig. 50). She may become frustrated by the feeling of wanting to do something or wanting to see some marked change. However, she needs to recognize that care of the chronically ill patient requires a slow-

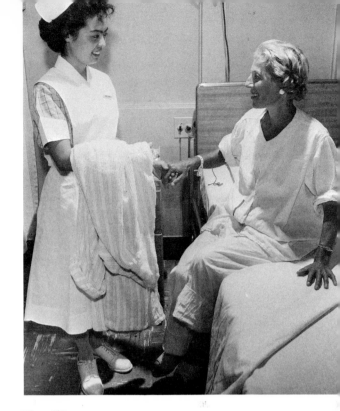

Fig. 50

The use of the Hi-Lo bed permits the patient to get out of bed with minimal assistance.

moving, persistent pace with possibly little or no change for a long time. The patient's physical and mental condition must be maintained at its present level or improved, and effort must be made to further his progress and to encourage his and his family's acceptance of his condition. His eagerness and readiness to progress will be determining factors of his future. The "doing" in the care of the chronically ill patient is not always an active, physical "doing" with the hands. Many times the maintenance of a positive approach and attitude and a demonstration of real interest are the greatest help to the patient.

Nursing care of chronically ill patients requires alertness of feeling, seeing, and hearing. Continued warmth and interest are necessary to the well-being of a chronically ill person. Very often it is the nurse who helps the patient change and become highly motivated. It may be taxing to listen to the same person and to say the same things day after day, but the nature of chronic illness may require this attention,

227

and the way in which the nurse responds will convey warmth and interest. The world of a chronically ill person, whether he is in the hospital or elsewhere, becomes narrowed and circumscribed. He treasures and is interested in those things and those people who are close about him. His conversations may be largely about himself, his immediate environment, a few close objects, and the persons who are close to him. Although he is confined to bed and to his room, others can keep him up-to-date on outside news. Many patients welcome hearing about outside events, but others may not be able to think beyond themselves. Newspapers, magazines, radio, and television help patients to keep up their interest in others and in outside world events. Creating something with their own hands also helps some patients (Fig. 51).

Public libraries in many communities provide facilities for disabled persons. Ceiling projectors for books, books of current interest printed in large type, and recordings of books and music are often available on loan. Volunteer workers may act as readers both in hospitals and in homes (Fig. 52). Many libraries have elevators and ramps that make library facilities available to the person who is unable to climb stairs, and may make taking a person to the library in a wheelchair possible. The publication *Books for Tired Eyes** should be of interest to nurses.

Some communities have organized "friendly visiting programs" in which volunteer workers go to the hospital or the home to provide companionship and to do errands for patients. The nurse should evaluate the advisability of such a plan, and sometimes the physician should be consulted. "Visitors" are not advisable for all patients and should be selected carefully. Often the nurse can help the visitor to give appropriate help to the patient.

Since medical diagnoses do not accurately reflect the physical capacity of the chronically ill person, the use of a *physical profile system* may be instituted as a guide for those working with the patient.[30] The patient is graded considering six categories: (1) physical condition, such as cardiovascular, pulmonary, gastrointestinal, genitourinary, endocrine, or cerebrovascular disorders; (2) upper extremities, including shoulder girdle, and cervical and upper dorsal spine; (3) lower extremities, including pelvis, and lower dorsal and lumbar sacral spine; (4) sensory components relating to speech, vision, and hearing; (5) excretory function, including bowels and bladder; and (6) mental and emotional status. The grades for each of these categories range from 1 to 4. Grade 1 indicates no unexpected difficulty. Grade 2 indicates a minor difficulty that does not preclude normal life activity but that may require occasional medical supervision. Grade 3 indicates a difficulty that requires medical and/or nursing supervision but that does not prevent limited activity. Grade 4 indicates severe impairment requiring constant and complete care.

The nurse should assist in making the evaluation of each patient and in interpreting it to others who may care for him or who may be making plans with him. The Patient Information Guide for the Nurse, included in Chapter 1, can be useful to the

Fig. 51

Occupational therapy provides the patient with purposeful activity. Interest shown by the nurse encourages the patient to complete the project.

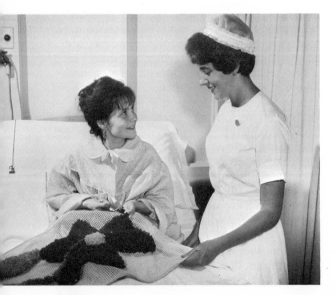

---

*Published by the American Public Library Association.

nurse in carrying out this responsibility. The nurse can use the guide in planning for nursing care, both immediate and long term, and will find it useful in assisting the family to make realistic plans for the patient's care. Since a chronic condition is not static, reassessment should be made at regular intervals to indicate improvement or regression.

Recognizing what is meaningful to the patient is one of the first steps toward helping him to help himself. Personal needs become of paramount importance to the chronically ill patient. Meeting these physical needs provides a way for the nurse to convey to the patient her interest in his progress and welfare. By helping the patient to take his own bath, to attend to toilet needs, and to groom himself, the nurse can give him some sense of accomplishment and help him to maintain his self-esteem. Helping him to be dressed appropriately is important. Patients who are in their homes or in substitute homes should be encouraged to dress in regular, comfortable street clothing rather than in pajamas or gowns. Visitors coming into the home and members of the family who constantly see them dressed for bed think of them as sick and are reminded of the illness. Seeing them dressed as they ordinarily would be helps to maintain normal attitudes, relationships, and expectations. An appropriately dressed housewife seated in a wheelchair and paring vegetables is much more conducive to ordinary, cheerful conversation with neighbors than one who is dressed in a gown, robe, and slippers and sitting with her hands idle.

Activity with a purpose, no matter how small the activity may be, is desirable for the chronically ill person. One may hear the patient say to friends that he does not have time to visit because he has to take care of the plants, do personal laundry, or perform some other task that may seem unimportant to the casual observer. Actually, to the patient these jobs may appear to be the most important in the world.

The chronically ill patient and his family

Most patients with a chronic or long-term illness can be cared for at home and ac-

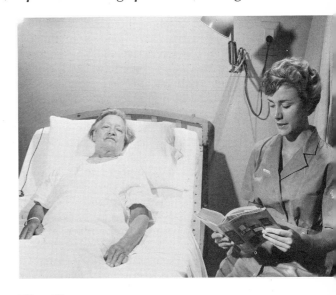

Fig. 52

Volunteers can often be recruited to read to disabled patients.

tually prefer to be at home, where family and friends are close by and where they can still contribute something to family life. They all require medical supervision. The arrangements that can be made vary greatly, and depend upon the patient's needs and the facilities available. Many patients are ambulatory and during remissions are able to visit their local clinic. Others manage with visits from their personal physicians and with a periodic diagnostic work-up done in the office or with the assistance of a technician who goes into the home. Public health nurses from voluntary and official agencies help the chronically ill in their homes. Many chronically ill persons with disabilities also visit special rehabilitation units of hospitals or outpatient centers for daily or periodic instruction and practice in physical skills and job training.

The nurse who visits the home to assist the patient and/or family member to accomplish daily care will need to give special attention to helping the family understand the patient. The chronically ill patient is very often misjudged by even the closest members of his family because of lack of understanding. The nurse needs to help the patient's family to understand his limitations and his necessary restrictions. Both the patient and his family may benefit from association with others who have had similar experiences. Patients and their families often meet together in organized groups to share experiences. For example, there are organizations for patients who have an ileostomy and for patients who have multiple sclerosis. There has been a recent growth of such groups because of the increase in chronic illness and because people are reluctant to accept the isolation that chronic illness may impose.

Marked changes often take place in family living as a result of chronic illness. Families often find themselves drawn closer together, and new relationships develop. For example, when it is suddenly learned that the mother has a heart condition, the husband and teen-age children may rally to assist in household chores. All seem to work together with a special purpose in mind. On the other hand, families may drift apart and be incapable of helping one another. Chronic illness may threaten an individual's basic emotional stability, and the whole situation may be unbearable to others. Sometimes the patient's emotional needs may not have been apparent to the family early in the illness, but when such needs develop and grow obvious, relatives feel inadequate in the situation. The length of the illness, periodic hospitalization, increased financial burdens, and emotional and social burdens are sometimes more than families can withstand. Public assistance is accepted by many families, whereas others find it degrading. Many persons struggle on their own to assume the full financial burden and consequently expose other members of the family to lower standards of nutrition, housing, and care. Many times relatives move in with one another, arguments develop, and family ties are strained or broken. Some accept public and other assistance without reservation and make little attempt to help themselves.

The effects upon patient and family are numerous and varied. Usually the patient and the family as a whole will respond in a manner similar to that in which they have reacted to problems in the past. However, the first impact of the disability may nearly immobilize both the patient and his family. For example, a person who is almost totally helpless as a result of an accidental spinal cord injury may seem to have no interest in learning ways to help himself. His family may react in the same way and be of little help to him. At this time both the patient and his family need interest and support from professional persons. With this reassurance the patient may learn that he can do some activities, such as bathing part of his body and combing his hair. This small success may be stimulating enough to strengthen his motivation so that he and his family may make amazing strides in thinking through and working out future problems themselves.

The nurse should think of each chronically ill person as someone who must live his life although his problems may seem insurmountable to her. She should recognize that many times life has meaning for the patient even though it may not be apparent to her. Nurses with this understanding can help make the patient's life more satisfying and can influence positively the attitudes of the family, her co-workers, and the public.

The cost of disability

Every effort should be made to prevent disability in any person who has a chronic illness. Disability can be devastating to the individual, his family, and the community, and it takes its toll in the nation's productivity. Most individuals who are unable to work must be supported by others, either from private or from public funds.

There are 2 million adults between the ages 18 and 64 years who are unable to work because of chronic disabilities.[21] There are an additional 3.5 million who are partially limited in ability to work. About 800,-000 of the totally disabled persons are now receiving benefits under the Social Security Administration's Old-Age, Survivors, and Disability Insurance Program. An additional 400,000 disabled persons receive public assistance from the Aid to the Permanently and Totally Disabled Program.

The death rate of the disabled population is high. For persons under 50 years of age, the death rate is ten times that of the total population between the ages of 25 and 49 years. The death rate for disabled persons between the ages of 50 and 54 years is higher than that for all persons in the general population who are 75 to 84 years of age. Two-thirds of the disabled persons are men.

The ability of the individual family to pay its own way is determined in part by which member of the family becomes disabled. Studies show that if the wife is disabled, the family suffers less economic deprivation. Economy is only one consideration; each disabled person and his family are subjected to great personal and emotional losses.

Rehabilitation

Rehabilitation has been defined by many persons, and each definition seems to express the particular viewpoint of the person or organization offering it. "Rehabilitation is an adjustment to living"[32] is one simple definition. An expanded definition is as follows: "Rehabilitation is the process of assisting the individual with a handicap to realize his particular goals, physically, mentally, socially, and economically."[32] The purpose or extent of rehabilitation ranges from employment or reemployment for the handicapped person to the more limited achievement of developing the ability to give his own daily care. This latter accomplishment can be just as important to the individual as earning money and may represent his greatest life achievement. This might be true, for example, for a person who was born with a severe physical handicap such as cerebral palsy.

Success in learning to adjust to living with a disability will depend on motivation, intelligence, heredity, and environment of both the patient and the persons who are trying to help him. The rehabilitative process, as any form of education, is involved as deeply in the motives and purposes of the teacher as in those of the learner.[52]

The person with a disability, whether it is obvious to others or unrecognizable to them, should not be viewed from the standpoint of his disability alone. Usually his greatest need is for comprehensive health services and continuing care. *Comprehensive care* has been defined as "care that is provided to the patient according to his needs in an appro-priate, continuous, and dynamic pattern."[41] Accommodating the plan of care to the patient is the essence of comprehensive care.

The nurse in rehabilitation

The concepts of comprehensive nursing care and of rehabilitation can be considered synonymous. Helping the patient and his family to help themselves is an integral part of nursing care. The nurse who is working with patients who have disabilities has a responsibility to see that disability from disease is limited as much as possible and that a rehabilitation program is planned and implemented. She should be alert to the prevention of complications, to the early recognition of symptoms of exacerbations or complications, and to the prevention of deformity. The nurse should teach the patient and his family, and if necessary his employer, about his limitations and the rehabilitative expectations.

Much of what the nurse does in the rehabilitation process is no different from the nursing care she gives all patients. The assistance that she will be able to give the patient and his family will depend also upon her ability to understand her own feelings and behavior and those of the patient, his family, and other professional team members. Chapter 1 includes a discussion of these basic understandings. The patient must often learn and practice special physical techniques to strengthen muscles and to improve mobility. Such measures as physical exercise to improve walking, activities to improve self-care abilities, and the use of protheses often require the physical and occupational therapists to have special knowledge and technical skills. The nurse plans and works cooperatively with the therapist so that she can help the patient to use these physical techniques in activities of daily living.

One of the most important aspects of giving continuing care to a patient with a disability is the nurse's own attitude, perseverance, and expectations. Improvement may be slow and the patient may reach a "plateau" in his progress. Such a time can be critical for the patient because he may become discouraged and not wish to continue with his program of care. The nurse's encouragement can often sustain the patient so that he will not regress in any respect until some improvement is noted.

Teamwork in rehabilitation

The number of professional people required to assist the patient and his family with rehabilitation will vary. Most often the patient, his family, the doctor, and the nurse can work out a practical plan. If a patient's problems are complex, a social worker and perhaps a psychiatrist may be necessary. Specific physical limitations of the patient may require the services of a psychiatrist, physical therapist, occupational therapist, or speech therapist. If learning a new type of job is a part of the patient's adjustment, a vocational counselor may be needed. Teamwork requires that each member of the group be able to use his special knowledge and skill and understand the value of his contribution to the patient's care. In addition, each team member needs some understanding of each of the other professional persons' functions and contributions.

One of the cooperative efforts of the team is to thoroughly evaluate the patient and the abilities he has to use. Based upon this assessment, the patient and the team devise a plan to help him readjust, compensate, and learn new ways of managing self-care and living. In Fig. 53 a rehabilitation team consisting of a psychiatrist, an occupational therapist, and a student physician, as well as a doctor, a nurse, and a social worker, review a patient's problem.

Patient motivation

The most important contributions to his rehabilitation are made by the patient himself. The patient, the doctor, the nurse, the social worker, and sometimes others planning together can arrive at the best goal for his future, but the patient's attitudes, acceptance, and direction of motivation are the most important considerations. If he cannot accept his disability, whatever it may be and however extensive it may be, attempts at rehabilitation usually are hindered. The patient is the person who really makes the

Fig. 53

The team approach to rehabilitation is essential. Here the patient, the doctor, the nurse, the social worker, the occupational therapist, the psychiatrist, and a student physician review a particular problem.

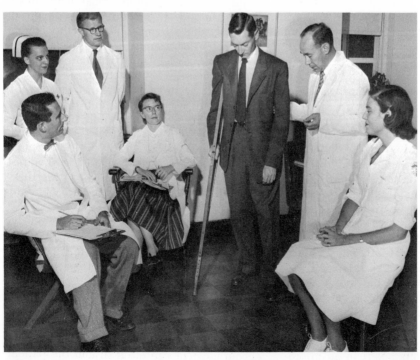

decisions, and he changes within himself at his own pace. If he is agreeable to suggestions but makes little or no effort to try them, one should question if he really has accepted the suggestions.

The patient's behavior from day to day in small ways can be the first indication of the direction of motivation. For example, if he makes every effort to resume normal daily activities such as feeding himself, bathing, and dressing, one can be quite certain that he is a person with a sincere desire to be independent. As he becomes ready for more advanced activities, such as ambulation and work in the occupational therapy shop, he needs continuing genuine interest and support from the nurse and others. As obstacles present themselves, he may be able to accept them and eventually overcome them. However, there are some patients who, when faced with an added burden, cannot accept it and give up trying. Those who are truly motivated toward helping themselves seem never to give up and find ways of accomplishing activities that professional personnel might believe impossible.

Special services for rehabilitation

Patients with very complex problems of rehabilitation may need to receive care at specialized centers for rehabilitation, or care at home may be combined with visits to a day rehabilitation center. Rehabilitation centers and services have developed quite rapidly since World War II. There are various types of centers: teaching and research centers (centers located in and operated by hospitals and medical schools), community centers with facilities for inpatients, community outpatient centers, insurance centers, and vocational rehabilitation centers. In addition to centers that provide multiple services for the physically disabled, there are specialized centers for rehabilitation of the blind, deaf, mentally ill, and mentally retarded. Most centers offer a wide range of services that usually fall into three areas:

MEDICAL AREA
Physical and medical evaluation
Physical therapy
Occupational therapy
Speech therapy
Medical supervision of appropriate activities

PSYCHOSOCIAL AREA
Evaluation
Personal counseling
Social service
Psychometrics
Psychiatric service

VOCATIONAL AREA
Work evaluation
Vocational counseling
Prevocational experience
Industrial fitness of programs
Trial employment in sheltered workshops
Vocational training
Terminal employment in sheltered workshops
Placement

Advantages of organized programs. Patients participating in organized programs of therapy have an opportunity to see and be with others who have similar or more extensive disabilities. Often they progress more rapidly when they realize that others have similar difficulties and are overcoming them. Group therapy often arouses a competitive spirit, and a formerly reluctant person may become willing and diligent. On the other hand, the nurse, doctor, and therapist need to be alert to those patients who have the opposite reaction. A patient who sees others advance in activity while he either does not improve or progresses very slowly may become so discouraged that he gives up trying.

Activities are scaled so that the individual can see his own progress in comparison with his beginning abilities. Patients may take an active interest in keeping their own scores. After a program of therapy has been planned and is scheduled as to time of day, the patient can help to keep himself on the schedule by having a copy of it at the bedside. The nurse can help him gradually to assume more and more responsibility for getting himself ready for scheduled activities.

A master plan of activities for all patients on the unit can be a useful device for nurses, doctors, and therapists. The plan can be kept in a central place on the unit and should list name, activity, and time of activity for each patient. This type of plan is helpful, too, when a patient's progress is to be reevaluated.

A public program for vocational rehabilitation has been serving the nation since 1920 in a partnership between the states and the federal government. Services for disabled persons are provided by state divisions of vocational rehabilitation. The federal government, through the Vocational Rehabilitation Administration (VRA), administers grants-in-aid and provides technical assistance and national leadership for the program. Opportunities and services are available in each of the fifty states, the District of Columbia, and Puerto Rico. All persons of working age with a substantial job handicap resulting from either physical or mental impairment are eligible for help or assistance. The purpose of this service is to preserve, develop, or restore the ability of disabled persons to earn their own living. The individual services offered are medical care, counseling and guidance, training, and job finding. Thirty-six states have separate rehabilitation programs for the blind. Application for such services can be made to the Vocational Rehabilitation Administration or to the agency in the state for serving the blind.

Patterns and facilities for continuing patient care

It is impossible to include here all of the many facilities that provide continuing patient care. Only those programs that have been developed or emphasized recently will be considered.

Outpatient care. The term ambulatory care is used interchangeably with the term outpatient care. Patients who are able to come to a patient care facility outside their own homes very often attend outpatient clinics. The number of patients receiving care solely in the outpatient service has increased tremendously and is still growing. A good outpatient service constitutes one of the most important elements of the hospital's contribution to community health. Many patients receive all their medical care under these auspices, whereas others come only for diagnosis or follow-up care. Increased use of outpatient emergency services is one of the most rapidly developing practices at the present time.

Home care. Until fairly recently, the home was the place where medical treatment was given. Well-to-do patients rarely thought of going into a hospital, and they received the services of a private physician in their own home. The family was responsible for the day-to-day care. Poor families were among the first persons to use hospitals. The philosophy of home care can be traced as far back as 1796, when the Boston Dispensary provided medical care to the sick poor. One of the first institutions to study and demonstrate the advantages of continuous medical care for patients at home was the University Hospital in Syracuse, New York, in 1940. The Montefiore Hospital Home-Care Program in New York City is a more recent example of provision of adequate health services in the home. Their services started in 1947, and within a year the New York City Department of Hospitals initiated similar programs in five city hospitals. By 1950 eleven additional New York City hospitals offered this service. In 1960 some thirty cities had forty-five coordinated home care programs, caring for approximately 5,000 patients.[22] By 1965 there were some sixty coordinated home care programs in the United States.

One of the most obvious reasons for the development of home care programs was to provide care to patients with long-term illnesses who did not need the around-the-clock services of an institution and yet might be too ill to go to an outpatient service. Caring for patients at home is what the patient and his family often want, and it also releases hospital beds for use by acutely ill patients.

The coordinated home care program provides comprehensive patient care for persons who otherwise might not receive it. The specification that the program is coordinated means that it is centrally administered and, through coordinated planning, evaluation, and follow-up procedures, provides physician-directed medical, nursing, social and related services to selected patients at home. This program can be offered either by a hospital or by a community center (e.g., a local health department).

Most patients have been in the hospital before referral to home care and often have had short hospital stays for acute exacerbations or complicated treatments interspersed with periods at home. This service provides care that could not be equaled easily in institutional care. Not only does the patient have the security of knowing that he is counted as a part of the hospital census and will receive continuing care, but he also has the satisfaction of being cared for in his own environment by a group of professional people who know him, his family, and his total situation.

Home care is not the solution for all patients. The present trend is toward smaller dwellings, and adequate space for the patient and other members of the family may be at a premium. The choice of home care or institutional care will depend largely on the desires of the patient and his family. Despite many inconveniences, some families wish to have the patient with them. The family's understanding of the patient and his situation and their ability to assist one another will make a great difference. Not only may space be inadequate, but many times it is impossible to have a member of the family in attendance with the patient during the day. Members of the family who work cannot afford to sacrifice jobs to stay with the patient. However, many families find it easier financially to have the patient at home and are able to make satisfactory arrangements even though the facilities are limited.

Some communities now provide portable meals (meals on wheels) for homebound chronically ill patients. Most programs provide one hot meal daily and unheated food for at least one other meal. The cost differs widely (from a few cents to $2 per day) and depends on the services offered, such as special diets, and on the sponsorship of the plan. Volunteer groups frequently act as delivery messengers. The local public health nursing service usually participates actively in the plan by selecting suitable patients and by being a resource for the workers who encounter health problems on their "rounds." This service alone often makes it possible for a chronically ill person to remain at home.

Homemaker services. Homemaker services have developed with the increased use of home care plans. These services are increasingly in demand in many communities, and may be sponsored by a public or voluntary health or welfare agency that employs personnel to furnish "homemaker" service to families with children and to the person who is convalescing, aged, or acutely or chronically ill. Women are trained to assist in homes in which the mother or other responsible family manager is temporarily unable to carry her usual responsibilities because of illness or absence.

Institutional resources. Many patients and families have to resort to institutional care for the patient because their own facilities are not suitable, no member of the family can be in attendance during the day, or the kind of care needed by the patient requires close professional supervision. A vast or a limited selection of outside facilities may be available, depending on the community. The types of homes include chronic disease hospitals, convalescent homes, rest homes, homes for the aged, and nursing homes.

Foster homes. Care in foster homes is a relatively new service that is now being widely used in many communities. Carefully selected families volunteer to take chronically ill persons into their own homes and provide the nonprofessional care that is needed. The family is paid either by the patient or his family, from public funds, or by some social agency. The plan is primarily for those patients who have no family and who cannot live alone, but who neither desire nor need institutional care.

References and selected readings*

1 Allan, Scott W.: Rehabilitation—a community challenge, New York, 1958, John Wiley & Sons, Inc.

2 Allgire, Mildred J., and Denney, Ruth R.: Nurses can give and teach rehabilitation, New York, 1960, Springer Publishing Co., Inc.

3 Areawide planning of facilities for rehabilitation services, Report of the Joint Committee of the Public Health Service, publication no. 930-B-2, Washington, D. C., 1963, U. S. Department of Health, Education, and Welfare.

4 *Brackett, Mary E.: The community: nursing in tomorrow's health services, Nursing Outlook 11:650-653, Sept. 1963.

5 *Brown, Frances Gold: Who said care of long-term patients is routine? Am. J. Nursing 62:58-61, May 1962.

6 Bryant, Zella: Report on nursing care of the sick at home, Public Health Service publication no. 901, Washington, D. C., 1962, U. S. Department of Health, Education, and Welfare.

7 Chapman, A. L.: Considering the aged, Pub. Health Rep. 74:333-337, April 1959.

8 Clague, Ewan: Employment outlook for the handicapped, Pub. Health Rep. 76:923-924, Oct. 1961.

*References preceded by an asterisk are particularly well suited for student reading.

9 Cockerill, Eleanor, and Margolis, H. M.: The concept of disability, J. Chron. Dis. 3:167-169, Feb. 1956.

10 Commission on Chronic Illness: Chronic illness in the United States—care of the long-term patient, Cambridge, Mass., 1956, Commonwealth Fund by Harvard University Press.

11 Council on Medical Service, Committee on Aging: Report on conferences on aging and long-term care, Chicago, 1965, American Medical Association.

12 *Dahlin, Bernice: Rehabilitation: fact or figure of speech? Nursing Outlook 12:34-37, Nov. 1964.

13 Do it yourself again—self-help devices for the stroke patient, New York, 1965, American Heart Association.

14 Gordon, Gerald, editor: Proceedings: Conference on Medical Sociology and Disease Control, New York, 1966, National Tuberculosis Association.

15 Guidelines for the practice of nursing on the rehabilitation team, New York, 1965, American Nurses' Association.

16 *Hanna, Patricia: Rehabilitation of patients in nursing homes, Nursing Outlook 12:56-59, Nov. 1964.

17 *Hurd, Georgina Greene: Teaching the hemiplegic self-care, Am. J. Nursing 62:64-68, Sept. 1962.

18 *Kottke, Frederic J., and Anderson, Eleanor M.: Deterioration of the bedfast patient, causes and effects and nursing care, Pub. Health Rep. 80:437-451, May 1965.

19 *Kurtagh, Cathryn H.: Which bed to buy, Am. J. Nursing 58:208-210, 1958.

20 Larson, Carroll B., and Gould, Marjorie: Calderwood's orthopedic nursing, ed. 6, St. Louis, 1965, The C. V. Mosby Co.

21 Lilienfield, Abraham M., and Gifford, Alice J., editors: Chronic diseases and public health, Baltimore, 1966, The Johns Hopkins Press.

22 Littauer, David, Flance, I. Jerome, and Wessen, Albert F.: Home care, hospital monograph series no. 9, Chicago, 1961, American Hospital Association.

23 *Madden, Barbara Williams, and Affeldt, John E.: To prevent helplessness and deformities, Am. J. Nursing 62:59-61, Dec. 1962.

24 Mead, Sedgwick: Rehabilitation. In Cowdry, E. V., editor: The care of the geriatric patient, ed. 2, St. Louis, 1963, The C. V. Mosby Co.

25 Mercita, Sister Mary, and others: Rehabilitation, a series of articles, Nursing Outlook 10:580-603, Sept. 1962.

26 *Morris, Ena M.: Choosing a nursing home, Am. J. Nursing 61:58-61, Jan. 1961.

27 Morrisey, Alice B.: Rehabilitation nursing, New York, 1951, G. P. Putnam's Sons.

28 *Morrisey, Alice B., and Zimmerman, Muriel E.: Helps for the handicapped, Am. J. Nursing 53:316-318, March 1953; 53:454-456, April 1953.

29 *Morrisey, Alice B., and others: Rehabilitation, a series of articles, Am. J. Nursing 62:58-71, Sept. 1962.

30 *Moskowitz, Eugene, and McCann, Cairbre B.: Classification of disability in the chronically ill and aging, J. Chron. Dis. 5:342-346, March 1957.

31 Myers, Julian S.: An orientation to chronic disease and disability, New York, 1965, The Macmillan Co.

32 National Health Forum: Changing factors in staffing America's health services, New York, 1954, National Health Council.

33 Naylor, Martha Ball: Nursing care of the chronically ill, Hospital Topics 39:27-30, Oct. 1961.

34 Needs of the long-term patient, Chicago, 1964, American Medical Association.

35 *Newton, Kathleen, and Anderson, Helen C.: Geriatric nursing, ed. 4, St. Louis, 1966, The C. V. Mosby Co.

36 Nursing homes increasing but still in short supply, Am. J. Nursing 63:79, July 1963.

37 Park, Wilford E., and Moe, Mildred I.: Rehabilitation care in nursing homes, Pub. Health Rep. 75:605-613, July 1960.

38 Phillips, Elisabeth Cogswell: Meals a la car, Nursing Outlook 8:76-78, Feb. 1960.

39 Program guide nursing service; nursing care of the long-term patient, Department of Medicine and Surgery, G-8, M-2, part V, Washington, D. C., 1963, Veterans Administration.

40 Questions and answers on health insurance for the aged, medical and related aspects of the new program and how it will operate, Social Security Administration, Washington, D. C., 1965, U. S. Department of Health, Education, and Welfare.

41 Ryder, Claire F.: The chronic disease era, J. Mississippi Med. Ass. 4:96-101, March 1963.

42 Saunders, Ethel, and Swinyard, Chester A.: The public health nurse's role in rehabilitation, Nursing Outlook 9:426-427, July 1961.

43 Schreiber, Frederick C.: Dental care for the long-term patients, Am. J. Nursing 64:84-86, Feb. 1964.

44 Sheps, Cecil G., and Bachar, Miriam E.: Emerging patterns of practice, Am. J. Nursing 64:107-109, Sept. 1964.

45 *Sister M. Willa: Nursing in rehabilitation, J. Nurs. Educ. 4:15-23, April 1965.

46 Sister Regina Elizabeth: Sensory stimulation techniques, Am. J. Nursing 66:281-286, Feb. 1966.

47 *Skinner, Geraldine: The nurse—key figure in preventive and restorative care, Hospitals 35:52-56, Jan. 1961.

48 *Smith, Louise C.: Factors influencing continuity of nursing service, New York, 1962, National League for Nursing.

49 Speir, Hugh B.: Characteristics of nursing homes and related facilities, Public Health Service publication no. 930-F-S, Washington, D. C., 1963, U. S. Department of Health, Education, and Welfare.

50 *Stoeckle, John D., and others: Medical nursing clinic for the chronically ill, Am. J. Nursing 63:87-89, July 1963.

51 Survey of coordinated home care programs, Public Health Service publication no. 1062, Washington, D. C., 1963, U. S. Department of Health, Education, and Welfare.

52 Talbot, Herbert S.: A concept of rehabilitation, Rehabilitation Literature 22:358-359, Dec. 1961.

53 Terry, Florence J., and others (Deborah MacLurg Jensen, editor): Principles and technics of rehabilitation nursing, ed. 2, St. Louis, 1961, The C. V. Mosby Co.

54 Terry, Luther L.: Health needs of the nation, Pub. Health Rep. 76:845-851, Oct. 1961.

55 The expanding role of ambulatory services in hospitals and health departments, Bull. New York Acad. Med. 41:1-158, Jan. 1965.

56 U. S. Department of Health, Education, and Welfare, Office of Vocational Rehabilitation: New hope for the disabled, Washington, D. C., 1956.

57 U. S. Department of Health, Education, and Welfare, Public Health Service: Health statistics—chronic conditions causing limitations of activity, National Health Survey, 1959 to 1961, series B, no. 36, Washington, D. C., Oct. 1962.

58 Weeks, Lewis E., and Griffith, John R., editors: Progressive patient care, an anthology, Ann Arbor, Mich., 1964, University of Michigan.

13

Nursing in accidents, emergencies, and disaster

Accidents

Study questions

1 Based on reports in the daily papers, list what you believe to be the most common causes of accidents.
2 What provisions are there in your hospital for the reporting of accidents within the hospital? What action is taken when an accident occurs? By whom is the action taken?
3 What are some precautions taken in your unit to prevent accidents to patients?
4 List potential accident hazards that are found in the average home.
5 What is the civil defense program in your hospital, in your community, and in your state?
6 What are the common causes of accidents to older patients?

The accident death rate in the United States has risen from 95,300 in 1957 to 101,000 in 1963. The cost to the nation of these accidents, in which 10,100,000 persons suffered disabling injuries, including wage loss, medical care, claims, and property damage, is estimated to be at least 16 billion dollars.[1] This figure does not record in any way the tremendous suffering and loss in social contribution of the injured, many of whom spend months and years seeking total or partial rehabilitation.

Accidents are the leading cause of death for persons 1 to 24 years of age and the second cause for those 25 to 44 years of age. From the ages of 45 to 64, accidents rank in fourth place. After the age of 65 accidents rank sixth as a cause of death, being exceeded by heart disease, vascular lesions of the central nervous system, cancer, arteriosclerosis, and pneumonia.[1] These figures are shocking since accidents are, for the most part, preventable and require only public education and individual caution for their control. This is in sharp contrast to cancer, which is among the three top causes of death in all age groups from 5 years of age on, but which is, to a much greater extent, beyond our control.

Prevention of accidents

Prevention is the keynote to success in dealing with the problem of accidents. Accident control has been acknowledged as a major public health goal, and the American Public Health Association has an active subcommittee on accident prevention. In 1955 this subcommittee made a survey and prepared a report entitled "Suggested Home Accident Prevention Activities for Health Departments." Some communities have local citizens committees that have been helpful in conducting surveys of accident hazards in homes.

Teaching accident prevention and participating in programs for accident prevention are responsibilities of all members of the health team, including doctors, nurses, health educators, and others. The nurse is an essential member of this team. Her influence can be felt in many areas, since she is represented in schools, in industry, in the home, in the hospital, and elsewhere in the community. Space does not permit a detailed description of the many ways in which a nurse can contribute in this important health field, but a few examples will be given for some areas. Many references are available. The nurse can turn to the National Safety Council, which has a monthly publication, *Home Safety Review,* and a yearly bulletin, *Accident Facts.* An excellent way for the nurse to keep informed in this field is to read regularly the *Statistical Bulletin* of the Metropolitan Life Insurance Company. She can contact her local health department for health education materials and for information on other sources, such as the many excellent publications on accident prevention prepared by life insurance companies and industrial organizations. Engineers are often invaluable resource people for consultation on structural hazards at home and in the community. The safety committee in the nurse's own hospital or public health agency may be of help. Finally, she must use her own resourcefulness and imagination in preventing accidents.

Home and community

The nurse can help in accident prevention whether she is actively practicing nursing in a hospital or in a community nursing agency or whether she is a full-time mother and homemaker. Lay individuals and lay groups often turn to her for assistance and guidance in learning of community needs and of how they may best contribute in accident prevention. She should be able to point out good sources of general information on the national level, such as the reports of the National Safety Council. The local or county health department, the local police department, the visiting nurse association, the welfare and health council, or similar agencies are all good sources of help. The nurse should assure the layman that his voice will be heard provided it is directed to the right authorities, and she may point out that groups have a stronger voice than individuals. Parent-teacher associations, various religious and social organizations, and many other groups are interested in the problem of accident control. Efforts should be made to use existing agencies and groups and to work with them in order that the sincere efforts of small groups of enthusiastic citizens will not be dissipated. Phases of accident prevention that should be of community interest include the following: how accident prevention can be taught in the public school, how better control and inspection of homes for the aged may be fostered by law, how rigid enforcement of driving regulations can be enforced, how better street lighting and wider use of light signals at busy intersections can be brought about, how regular checking and inspection of all cars can be done, and what laws pertaining to fireproof features in buildings are needed.

Accidents in and about the home cause almost one-third of all accidental deaths each year. Falls account for about half the number, and fires, burns, and poisonings account for most of the remainder. Many aged persons who fall do so when walking from room to room. Some fall because of slippery floors, loose rugs, poor lighting, scattered toys, and other conditions that could have been corrected. A fair number of fatal home accidents occur as a result of the recently intensified "do it yourself" movement. People are falling from roofs, windows, high ladders, and steps, and are being fatally burned or otherwise injured while using solvents and cleansing agents without proper knowledge of their hazards. The number of electrical appliances used in the home has increased the danger of electric shock and of fire from overloaded circuits. Each year the consumption of cigarettes increases, and many persons die in fires caused by burning cigarette ashes left on furniture or rugs and by cigarettes that are dropped as the smoker falls asleep. More rigid control measures are needed to prevent death in the home from escaping gas. More caution should be taught to persons living in rural areas who use gas to heat their homes and who are not prepared to care for equipment that is not functioning properly.

The public health nurse may be called upon to evaluate the patient's home for accident hazards prior to his leaving the hospital. Very often such patients are those with physical disabilities. This kind of request provides the nurse with an ideal opportunity to teach not only the patient but also members of his family about general accident prevention as well as specific measures for the safety of the patient.

Hospital

In the hospital the nurse should take an active part in accident prevention. The doctor looks to her to help devise means to protect each individual patient from accidents. The hospital administrator depends upon her for suggestions on how the hospital can be made a safer place for patients. Every nurse should be on the alert for accident hazards and should use her initiative in suggesting ways to prevent them. She should submit her suggestions verbally or in writing to her nursing supervisor so that they may go through appropriate channels to persons who can put them into general use.

The danger of accidents to hospital patients has increased in recent years. The turnover of patients is much more rapid, and the patient has less time to adjust to his new environment. Early ambulation of patients has added to accident hazards. Most important is the great increase in the proportion of elderly patients. Many are in their eighties and even their nineties. An infinite number of improvements could be made in general hospitals that might reduce accidents, and they vary with each situation. For example, handrails should be installed in the corridors of medical and surgical units, where patients now walk about each day. Stools should be placed in showers, beside tubs, and in washrooms. Chairs with arms should replace the straight, armless ones sometimes used.

Careful study of nursing practice and of the quality of nursing care may reveal good suggestions for accident prevention. For instance, one large hospital* analyzed a group of accidents in which patients fell out of bed. The two main causes of the falls were attempts to climb over the side rails and attempts to reach for a bedpan or other piece of equipment on the bedside table when the table or the bed had free-rolling casters. Obvious solutions seemed to be the use of Hi-Lo beds and the removal of casters on beds and bedside tables. The change to Hi-Lo beds must be made gradually, since few hospitals can afford to replace all beds at once.

Study of the patients who attempted to climb over side rails showed that most of them were aged and that many had received barbiturate sedation. Again, measures for prevention of accidents seemed obvious. Aged patients should be placed in Hi-Lo beds and in a location where they will have frequent observation. After having slept for sixty years in a low bed, they cannot remember that they are in a high hospital bed; like Rip Van Winkle, they awake to find many changes. Fewer sedatives should be given to elderly patients than to younger ones. It is better to rely upon nursing measures such as a warm drink, a back-rub, a cheerful word, attention to ventilation, and control of noise to ensure a good night of sleep.

The danger of accidental injury or death from fire must be constantly borne in mind by all hospital personnel. If smoking is permitted in patient units, the nurse should caution patients who smoke to be careful and should be on the alert for signs of lack of caution. Many hospitals no longer permit smoking except in a sitting room, porch, or solarium. If the patient has physical and/or emotional limitations that make his conduct unpredictable, and if the doctor

---

*Unpublished study, The New York Hospital–Cornell Medical Center.

240

feels that he should be permitted to smoke, the nurse or an auxiliary nursing staff member should remain with him while he smokes. Conscientious participation by all nurses in regular fire drills is necessary in case a fire should occur.

Emergency care

Every nurse should be conversant with the general principles of first aid and, if a physician is not present, should be prepared to assume leadership when accidents occur. First aid is defined as immediate and temporary care given the victim of an accident. Some general principles have application to most accident situations. The nurse can teach these principles to patients and to their relatives. Booklets such as *When the Unexpected Happens** should be useful in helping the public learn the practical steps in first aid.

In the following discussion a distinction will be made between the first aid given by the nurse at the scene of an accident and the nursing care she may give or help to give in the hospital. Usually, standing orders guide her actions in schools, industries, and public health agencies. Emergency treatment of medical emergencies, including postoperative shock, pulmonary embolism and edema, heart attack, convulsions, cerebrovascular accident, and severe burns, will be considered in chapters relating to the body systems involved.

Emergency management in general

The first thing to do when an accident occurs is to stop for a moment and remember to keep calm and to think before acting. The nurse may then step forward and identify herself as a nurse to the patient and onlookers and take the patient's pulse. This act will establish the nurse as a person of experience, *reassure* the patient, and lessen his shock if he is conscious. Untrained yet overzealous individuals can be helpful when

*Prepared by the John Hancock Mutual Life Insurance Co.

diplomatically asked to report the location and nature of the accident by telephone to the local police department and doctor, and to stop traffic or direct people away from where the patient lies. Usually it is best for the police to call the ambulance.

If the patient is conscious, talk to him, minimizing his injuries and assuring him that help is on the way. Make a careful but rapid examination to determine the nature of the injuries. Indications of breathing difficulties are checked first, then bleeding, fractures, and other injuries in that order. If artificial respiration is indicated, start it without delay. Because physical shock accompanies all traumatic injuries, keep the patient lying down and warm if circumstances permit (a blanket under the patient preserves body heat and sometimes may be pushed under the patient with a long, flat stick), and continue to reassure him. Moving the patient should not be attempted until the nurse has a clear idea of the extent of the injuries. If the patient may be moved, clear and firm directions should be given to persons willing to help.

Breathing

The best way to tell whether or not the patient is breathing is to watch the movement of the chest and the nostrils and to feel for flow of air from the mouth or nose. Any obstruction to breathing must be removed at once, and if the patient vomits, his head must be turned to one side. His head should be tilted backward to attempt to enlarge the airway to the trachea, but the tongue must be kept forward to prevent its obstructing the air passage. If the patient is not breathing, artificial respiration should be started at once.

The accepted method of artificial respiration at the present time is mouth-to-mouth or mouth-to-nose breathing.[4] First, any foreign matter in the victim's nose and mouth must be removed with a finger or a finger covered with cotton material. The procedure is then as follows:

1. Tilt the victim's head back and pull or push the jaw into a jutting-out position.

2. If the victim is a small child, place your mouth over his mouth and nose and blow gently. If the victim is an adult, open your mouth wide and place it over the vic-

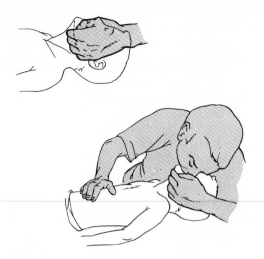

Fig. 54

The correct method of mouth-to-mouth breathing. Note that the victim's chin is held forward.

tim's mouth while pinching his nostrils, or close his mouth and place your mouth over the victim's nose; blow vigorously.

3. Remove your mouth, turn your head to the side and listen for return rush of air.

4. If there is no air return, check position, turn the victim quickly on his side, and slap him between the shoulder blades to loosen foreign matter. Return him to the back-lying position and remove any material from his mouth or nose. (See Fig. 54.)

For a child the rate of blowing should be approximately twenty times per minute, blowing shallowly. For an adult it should be twelve times per minute, blowing vigorously. A piece of gauze or other material such as a handkerchief can be placed between your mouth and the victim's. With vigorous blowing, this does not diminish the air blown into the victim's lungs much.

Artificial respiration should be continued until the patient has started to breathe or has been pronounced dead. It may be continued for four or more hours. Although a few gasping breaths on the part of the patient are most heartening to the person giving artificial respiration, they should not be taken as an indication that artificial res-

piration can be stopped. Patients may take one or two breaths and then stop breathing again. The patient must be watched carefully for at least an hour, and assistance must be given as needed. A cyanotic and then deep red flush will suffuse the entire face when breathing is resumed.

External cardiac massage is now considered an emergency procedure and has been found to be more satisfactory than internal massage in restoring heart action in some patients. Nurses and others who have had special preparation in this procedure may save lives by taking immediate action in the interval before a doctor arrives. Very often nurses working in special cardiac units, in intensive care units, or in industry become very skilled in the procedure and are expected to use their own judgment in beginning cardiac massage. At this writing, however, there is still much controversy about persons other than physicians doing external cardiac massage. Nursing practice acts approved by the state or by individual hospital policy may prohibit nurses or others from doing the procedure under any circumstances. Obviously, no nurse should ever attempt the procedure unless she has had special training in the techniques employed.

The usual steps in cardiopulmonary resuscitation are usually carried out as follows and require the presence of two persons (Figs. 55 and 56). First, place the victim face up on a hard surface. Check the carotid artery for pulse, the pupils for dilation, and the breathing for signs of respiration; then check the sternum to locate the xiphoid process. Next, tilt the head back to ensure an open airway and give five to six deep breaths either mouth-to-mouth or mouth-to-nose; then recheck the pulse. If there is no pulse, start cardiac massage by placing the heel of one hand just above the xiphoid process, with fingers spread and raised, and the other hand upon the first one; press down firmly, depressing 1½ to 2 inches. Repeat this procedure five times, once per second, maintaining the ratio of one mouth-to-mouth respiratory excursion to five depressions. Check the pupils for dilation frequently. If no pupillary contraction occurs after five minutes, it is usually considered useless to continue cardiopulmonary resuscitation.

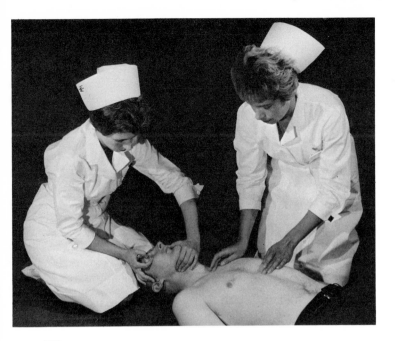

Fig. 55

Cardiopulmonary resuscitation. One nurse is
checking for carotid pulse and dilation of the
pupils while the other nurse locates
the xiphoid process.

Fig. 56

Cardiopulmonary resuscitation. As one nurse
does mouth-to-mouth breathing, the other applies
external rhythmic pressure to the sternum.
Note the first nurse's hand under the patient's
neck to maintain hyperextension.

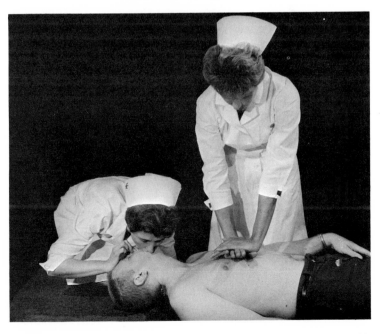

Hemorrhage

Bleeding may be external or internal. Severe external bleeding must be treated at once. Quickly run your hands over the entire body surface. Any pronounced bleeding will have saturated the clothing and can be noted in this way. Cut or tear away the clothing and expose the wound. Cover the wound with several layers of sterile dressing or the cleanest material available. Apply pressure over the dressing with the extended hand. Elevate an extremity that is bleeding. Most bleeding can be controlled in this way, but bleeding from a cut artery may require the use of pressure on a major blood vessel over a bony prominence (Fig. 57). Digital pressure is most effective when three fingers are used rather than the thumb or only one finger.

A tourniquet may be used in the case of multiple injuries or if bleeding will not stop by using the other methods. The tourniquet should be at least 1 inch wide, and it should never be made of a material that might cut the flesh (such as a rope or a wire). Tighten the tourniquet just above the wound, tight enough to stop the bleeding but no tighter. Once the tourniquet is applied it should be released by a physician, no matter how long it has been in place. A notation should be made and attached to the patient, giving the location of the tourniquet and time of application. A large T on the forehead, made with a lipstick, identifies the patient as having a tourniquet on.

Internal bleeding may be identified by a weak, rapid pulse, thirst, and sighing respirations. If internal bleeding is suspected, keep the patient flat and quiet and apply ice packs if materials are available.

Fracture

It is best not to move the patient or the part when a fracture is suspected. Nerves, blood vessels, and other tissues may be damaged, and pain and shock will increase. Fractures of the skull usually are accompanied by loss of consciousness, unequal pupil dilation, heightening color of the face, and, in the case of a fracture at the base of the skull, by bleeding or draining serous fluid from the nose and/or the ears. Only loose, fluffy dressings may be used on bleeding head wounds, as pressure on the damaged area may increase pressure on the damaged brain.

Fractures of the extremities very often will be pinpointed by the conscious patient. Fractures should be suspected if the limb is out of alignment, edematous, or very painful. A compound fracture should be covered loosely with a sterile dressing and a tourniquet placed, but not tightened, above the wound.

Moving the patient. If it is necessary to move the patient before medical help arrives, the fracture's extremity must be immobilized, if possible, in the position of injury before the patient is moved. Immobilization may be accomplished by the use of splints. Splints may be improvised from a variety of materials, such as pillows, pieces of board, and rolled-up newspapers. Even rifle barrels, golf clubs, and tennis rackets have been used by resourceful persons. A heavy magazine

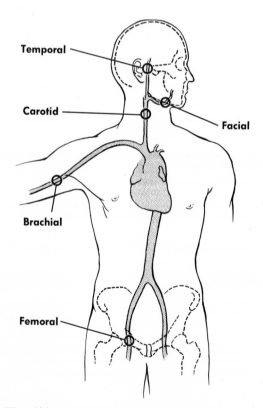

Fig. 57

The pressure points—locations at which large blood vessels may be compressed against bones to help control hemorrhage.

Temporal

Carotid

Facial

Brachial

Femoral

makes an excellent splint for the wrist. Lacking even this, many pages of the daily newspaper serve almost as well.

Before the patient is moved, the splints should be prepared and all persons who are to help must know what to do and how to work together. If the fracture is within a joint, the entire limb may be very carefully supported, placed upon a splint such as a pillow, and bandaged securely. If the fracture is in the shaft of the bone, traction and countertraction will usually be needed. One person may support the part above the fracture and one may exert a steady, firm pull until the splint has been applied and secured with improvised bandages above and below the site of fracture. Enough bandages should be used to secure the splint and immobilize the whole limb. In some instances (for example, when strong muscle pull is involved, as in fracture of the femur), a steady pull away from the body must be maintained.

No matter how expertly the emergency care has been given, improper handling and careless transportation often add to the severity of the original injuries, increase shock, and, frequently, endanger life. Various carriers can be used in emergencies, but the stretcher is the preferred device. Stretchers may be improvised from blankets, coats, poles and cloth, or rigid sheets of wood. At least three but preferably four people should work together as gently and steadily as possible to lift an injured person onto a stretcher. The fourth person works opposite the other three and places his hands under the thighs and shoulder of the injured person and assists in raising him. While the patient rests on the knees of the three members of the team, the fourth person places the stretcher under the patient.

Fracture of the spine. All questionable injuries to the back, even in the absence of signs of paralysis, should be treated as for fracture of the spine. Paralysis in the unconscious person may be determined by pinching or pricking the toes or fingers with a pin or other sharp object. The patient with injury to the spine requires the most exact care in handling if he must be moved. Forward or backward bending of the spine must not be allowed to occur, since it may cause pressure on the spinal cord and

immediate death. A door makes the best temporary splint. It takes at least six persons working in perfect harmony to move the patient safely. The patient with a fracture of the neck or of the lower spine should not be rolled if he is lying on his back. He should be slid carefully sideways onto the board or splint. One person kneels at the patient's head and, holding the head securely with his hands under the jaws, exerts a firm, steady pull. A second person supports the patient's feet, again exerting a firm, steady pull. The other members of the team draw the patients body onto the stretcher or splint. At no time must his head be allowed to bend forward, backward, or to the side. His head and body must move as one piece, and there must be very firm support under his shoulders so that sagging, which will cause forward-bending of the neck, cannot occur. If the patient is found lying on his face, he is usually rolled very carefully onto his back and onto the splint. Again, traction is applied to his head so that his spine is kept straight, and forward or backward bending is avoided. A folded blanket is laid on the splint at the level of the thoracic spine before the patient is placed on it so that the normal position of the spine is maintained when the patient is in a back-lying position. (For hospital care of patients with fractures, see p. 831.)

Other injuries

Puncture wounds of the chest must be covered immediately, and manual pressure must be applied to seal off the opening. Penetrating objects must be left in place, supported and padded until medical attention can be obtained.

The patient found unconscious

If a person is found unconscious either in his home or on the street, he should be examined for signs of having bitten his tongue, as so often happens in convulsions, and for a fruity odor to the breath, which may indicate diabetic acidosis. Patients subject to convulsions and those with diabetes mellitus are usually advised to carry identifying information on their persons. The odor of poisons such as phenol and iodine and of alcohol can be detected on the breath. When

245

an odor of alcohol is detected, it should not be assumed that the cause of unconsciousness has been determined. The environment should be carefully inspected for evidence of the cause of the patient's condition, and the patient should be examined for signs of injury, particularly of the head. No attempt should be made to give anything by mouth to an unconscious person. A doctor should be called and immediate arrangements should be made to get the patient to a hospital. Unconsciousness with marked decrease in respirations is common in patients with morphine and barbiturate poisoning and in carbon monoxide poisoning. Artificial respiration may be given while awaiting arrival of an ambulance.

Bites

Animal bites

The most common animal bites are those of dogs and cats. Dog bites are particularly dangerous, since dogs are the most common carriers of the deadly disease hydrophobia, or rabies. Cat bites are likely to cause infection because the cat's mouth contains many pathogenic bacteria and because the long, sharp teeth make a deep wound that may become sealed off. Human bites easily become infected because of the very high bacterial count in the human mouth.

The first-aid treatment for all animal bites is extremely thorough washing with soap and hot water for five to ten minutes. Running water should be used. Tetanus toxoid and/or antitoxin may be given. If the bite is deep and if the animal is suspected of having rabies, the wound must be made to bleed and may even be probed, depending upon circumstances and how soon medical aid will be available. Strong caustic medications should not be applied. Detergent solutions, however, have been found to be very effective in cleaning wounds from animal bites. The wound should be covered with a piece of sterile or clean gauze, and the advice of a doctor sought at once. He will decide whether or not treatment for rabies is necessary. The offending animal should always be kept alive until the advice of a doctor has been obtained. If it is a household pet and the circumstances indicates that the bite was

accidental, the animal will usually be confined and observed for a week to ten days. If the animal must be killed immediately for the protection of others, the brain should not be damaged and must be sent to a laboratory for examination. If an animal suspected of having rabies is at large, the police department and the health department must be notified at once.

Rabies. Rabies is a fatal acute infectious disease caused by a filtrable virus that travels along nerve pathways to the brain. The disease has been known for centuries. In the twentieth century B.C. the Eshnunna code of ancient Mesopotamia set forth strict regulations about the obligations of dog owners who let mad dogs bite persons, thereby causing death.[17] Rabies is most commonly acquired from dogs, but it can be carried by any animal that nurses its young. In the United States it is fairly common in dogs, cats, rats, cows, skunks, foxes, and even bats. The economic loss from rabies among cows is significant, even though the cow is not a common source of the disease in man.

Infection always occurs through an open break in the skin caused by the bite of an infected animal. Clothing gives some protection, since the animal's teeth are wiped by the garments. Because the saliva is infectious for several days before the onset of symptoms in the affected animal, it is exceedingly important that all suspected animals be caught and kept under inspection for ten days. If the animal shows symptoms that are strongly suggestive of rabies and is destroyed or dies, its brain is sent to a laboratory for examination. The presence of Negri bodies in the brain of an animal is conclusive evidence of rabies.

Acute rabies can be prevented in man by the *Pasteur treatment.* Some persons who are exposed will not contract the disease. However, since the disease is always fatal if it develops, the treatment is always given if the offending animal is known or suspected to have rabies. If bites have been sustained about the head, the injections will very likely be started at once, since the incubation period seems to be shorter than when the bite is on other parts of the body. Antirabies treatment is usually given if the animal has escaped and is suspected of having rabies.

The Pasteur treatment, which is painful

and expensive, consists of an injection of antirabies vaccine daily for fourteen to twenty-one days. These injections may cause severe local reaction and sometimes evoke serious and even fatal complications. Death occurs often enough to make rigid control of wandering animals imperative. Furthermore, since a series of injections of antirabies vaccine gives protection for a maximum of only six months, a child might have to have more than one series in a year. It is recommended that two additional injections be given if a questionable bite is received later than three months after a series of injections has been given. If six months have elapsed since the Pasteur treatment was given, the complete series must be repeated.[43] Passive immunization is now attempted by giving hyperimmune antiserum. To be effective, it must be given within seventy-two hours of exposure to the disease and is usually given in combination with the vaccine.

The control of rabies is a public health responsibility. The police and health departments must be notified at once if a rabid animal is thought to be at large. In England and the Scandinavian countries the disease has been almost entirely eliminated by rigid enforcement of laws that prohibit allowing dogs to run about unleashed. Rabies could be controlled by compulsory vaccination of all dogs and cats kept as household pets, capture and confinement of stray animals, and destruction of wild animal reservoirs of infection under the supervision of wildlife experts. Annual vaccination of all dogs is required in some states and counties. Recent improvements in the vaccine have resulted in the decision in one state (New York) to permit dogs to run loose twenty-one days after inoculation, whereas formerly, a period of thirty days was required. How long the immunity lasts following vaccination is not known for certain. Immunization in man is thought to last about a year and in animals up to thirty-nine months.

The public should know that not all rabies-infected animals are "mad." There are two types of rabies. In one type the animal may be restless, barking, and biting. In the other, so-called "dumb" rabies, the animal may be quiet and stay close to its master. In the latter type, paralysis, which begins in the throat and lower jaw, may lead the animal's owner to suspect that something harmful has been swallowed. If he tries to investigate the trouble, some of the highly infectious saliva may enter an abrasion on his hand.

Another name for rabies is *hydrophobia*. The incubation period of the disease in man is from ten days to more than a year.[6] The involvement, as in animals, is in the central nervous system. The disease is ushered in with a few days of melancholia, depression, pain at the site of the animal bite, and a feeling of impending danger. Acute symptoms (difficulty in swallowing, excessive salivation, muscle spasm, often maniacal fear, difficulty in breathing, and convulsions) then appear. A terrific, painful spasm of the muscle of deglutition, occurs when there is an attempt to swallow water—hence the name hydrophobia. Even the mention of water is often enough to bring on an attack. Aerophobia is also present, and convulsions can be produced by a draft of air on the skin.

The nursing care of the patient with acute rabies is difficult but of short duration. Most patients die from heart failure or respiratory difficulty within three or four days of the acute onset of symptoms. The patient is restless, irritable, and fearful, with episodes of uncontrolled fear and mania alternating with periods of calm. Every effort is made to keep the patient quiet. The room is darkened, and noises in the halls outside the room should be eliminated. Side rails are placed on the bed and are sometimes padded to help prevent injury during episodes of uncontrolled thrashing about. Sedatives, including chloral hydrate, morphine, and the barbiturates, are given. Anesthetics may be given intravenously. Fluids may be given intravenously, and it is important to bandage the arm securely on a board to prevent injury in the event of a convulsion or an attack of mania while a needle is in the vein. The head of the bed is sometimes lowered in an attempt to facilitate drainage of saliva, and often suctioning must be used. The nurse should wear gloves when giving immediate care, and some authorities believe that doctors and nurses caring for a patient with rabies should receive antirabies serum. Relatives of the patient must be prepared for the fact that the patient cannot talk. Sometimes the visits of relatives bring on severe painful muscle spasm in the throat of the patient, who is usually conscious up to the time of death, even though he is unable to speak.

Insect bites

Insect bites are more serious in children than in adults. Multiple bites have caused serious systemic reaction and even death of children. If the reaction is severe or prolonged, medical aid should be sought at once. The bites of wasps and bees are among the most common of insect bites and occasionally cause serious and even fatal reactions. A poultice of sodium bicarbonate and water often gives relief, since formic acid is present in the material injected by these insects. A weak solution of household ammonia also decreases pain and is safe to use.

A tick is best removed by holding a lighted match to it, thereby causing it to withdraw its mouthpiece. Sudden removal of a tick will result in its mouthpiece being left in the skin. A drop of turpentine placed on the insect is also effective and without fire hazard. Ticks are the vectors of Rocky Mountain spotted fever and Colorado tick fever. If the person bitten lives in an area where these diseases are endemic, the advice of a doctor should be sought.

Mosquito bites are important because one species of mosquito (*Anopheles*) is active in the transmission of malaria and encephalitis and because the bites of mosquitoes and similar insects sometimes cause troublesome infections. The greatest danger of infection is in elderly persons with poor circulation in whom bites on the legs may lead to infected ulcers that heal with extreme difficulty. The best treatment for the nuisance and discomfort of mosquito bites is prevention, largely by avoiding highly infested areas and wearing protective clothing when one must be exposed. A mosquito net worn over a broad-brimmed hat when outdoors and the use of a large net canopy when sleeping provide good protection. Draining of swamps where mosquito larvae live helps in some areas. Oil of citronella and many trade preparations are useful as repellents, but none are completely effective. Lotions containing calamine and phenol

help to allay the itching and discomfort accompanying the bites.

The bites of poisonous spiders and other poisonous insects such as scorpions are treated in a manner similar to treatment of snakebite.

Snake bites

There are four kinds of poisonous snakes in the United States. Three of them, the copperhead, the cottonmouth moccasion, and the rattlesnake, belong to the group known as pit vipers and are distinguished by a pit resembling a second nostril between the eyes and the nostril and by a broad, flat, triangular head. Everyone should know the kinds of poisonous snakes found in the part of the country in which he lives and how to recognize them. The copperhead is named for its color, is about 3 feet long, and is found in the eastern and southern states. The cottonmouth moccasion is grayish in color and blends with its surroundings. It is found in marshy country in the southeastern states. Rattlesnakes are probably to be found in every state in the United States and are responsible for the largest number of bites and the largest number of deaths. One antivenin is effective for all pit vipers. The fourth poisonous snake, the coral snake, is small and brilliantly colored. It is found in North Carolina and other southern states, particularly around the Gulf of Mexico. The snake is shy and seldom bites, but its venom is deadly and affects the nervous system. No specific antivenin is prepared for the bite of the coral snake, but the cobra antivenin kept in most zoos is effective.

Poisonous snakes in North America will almost always move away when disturbed and will not bite unless suddenly molested without warning. Snakebites can often be prevented by wearing high leather boots and thick trousers when walking through snake-infested areas. Heavy gloves should be worn and the greatest care taken when climbing, because hands may be placed on ledges that cannot be seen, and reptiles, often sun themselves on rocky ledges.

The bite of a poisonous snake is distinguished by two fang marks above the horseshoe-shaped array of tooth marks. Immediate severe pain and swelling distinguish the bite of a poisonous snake from that of a nonpoisonous one, even when swelling and discoloration are so sudden as to make the fang marks impossible to see. The wider the space between the fang marks, the larger the snake (sometimes unseen) and the more intensive the treatment should be.

The first-aid treatment for snakebite is the immediate application of a tourniquet just above the bite. This tourniquet should not be tight enough to prevent venous return in deep vessels but should be tight enough to prevent superficial circulation of blood and lymph, thus stopping absorption of the poison. In severe cases, if swelling appears above the tourniquet, the tourniquet is reapplied above the level of edema, or a second tourniquet may be used. Incision into the bite must be made immediately, and the cut should be made in the direction of nerves and blood vessels to prevent injury to them. A pocketknife or any sharp instrument, sterilized if possible by flaming with a match, can be used. If emergency snakebite equipment* is not available, suction must be applied by mouth. This procedure is safe since the venom is not poisonous if swallowed. Suction should be continued constantly for at least thirty minutes and then for fifteen minutes out of each hour until medical aid is found. The patient should lie quietly to lessen circulatory flow and absorption of the poison. Since shock may develop from the poison, he should be kept warm. Medical aid should be sought at once. About 15% of the persons bitten by poisonous snakes die without treatment.[4] If a snakebite kit is available, antivenin should be given at once. If a physician is not available or is delayed, whoever is at the scene should inject at least half of the ampule into the tissue around and above the bite and the rest intramuscularly in any part of the body. Warm fluids can be given. Alcohol is contraindicated since it may speed up the absorption of venum. Signs of poisoning are palpitation, weakness, shortness of breath, nausea and vomiting, and dimness of vision. Occasionally the venom from the

snake is injected directly into a blood vessel and fatal reaction may occur within fifteen minutes.

When the patient who has been bitten by a snake arrives at the hospital, the nurse should anticipate that stimulants such as strychnine and caffeine may be ordered. Intravenous infusions of glucose and physiologic solution of sodium chloride may be ordered for those patients who are dehydrated, who have low blood pressure, and in whom liver damage is suspected. Tetanus toxoid is usually administered, and antibiotics are given to combat infection. Since there is horse serum in antivenin, a reaction may be anticipated in some patients who have been treated at the scene of the accident. Usually skin testing for sensitivity to horse serum is done before additional antivenin is used in the hospital. Occasionally, massive sloughing of tissue occurs following snakebite. This type of wound heals very slowly and in severe cases may necessitate amputation.

Poisoning by drugs and chemicals

More than four-fifths of all fatal accidents from poisoning occur in the home. Poisoning is the third-ranking cause of home accidents among people of all ages.[1] In small children, poisoning usually results from accidental ingestion of poisonous substances. In adults it commonly occurs from not checking medications and from suicide attempts. Most large cities now have poison centers in the emergency departments of hospitals where emergency information and supplies are kept. This program is sponsored by health departments and is under the supervision of specialized pediatricians. These centers act as resources for physicians and provide immediate telephone directions to citizens.

Barbiturates are most often recorded as the cause of accidental death by poisoning. Their consumption has increased so tremendously in the last three decades that serious thought is now being given to much stricter supervision of these products. Many states now have laws prohibiting the dispensing of barbiturates without medical prescription. The nurse should discourage the public from injudicious use of barbi-

---

*Snakebite kits contain a suction cup, tourniquet, razor blade, iodine, ampule of antivenin powder, vial-syringe of sterile distilled water, and instructions.

turates and should urge safekeeping of these drugs where they will not be accessible to children. Acetylsalicylic acid (aspirin) and petroleum products also are sources of poisoning for many children.

Drug cabinets, kitchen cupboards, and laundry closets are the places from which poisons most often are taken. Strychnine poisoning from eating rodent poisons or laxatives containing strychnine occur quite often. Disinfectants such as phenol, iodine, bichloride of mercury, and cresol are easily taken by children if these substances are not locked away. Bromides and sleeping and tranquilizer tablets left on bedside tables and in handbags are a potential source of trouble. The "do it yourself" movement has brought more paints, solvents, dyes, stains, turpentine, bleaches, and paint removers into the home, and suburban living has increased the danger of poisoning from insecticides. The public constantly needs to be reminded to keep poisons of all kinds conspicuously labeled, stored in cupboards, separate from foods, and placed out of the reach of children. Most manufacturers list the constituents of their products on the outside of the container. Some do not. People should be encouraged to buy only those products whose contents are noted on the container, since medical treatment in the event of accidental poisoning may be delayed while the doctor attempts to learn what poison must be dealt with.

First-aid treatment in poisoning consists of trying to find out what poison was taken, diluting the poison, removing it from the stomach if possible, and getting in touch with a doctor. Lives have been saved by quick commonsense treatment while awaiting the doctor. For example, if bichloride of mercury, a deadly poison, can be removed from the stomach within fifteen minutes, the patient will usually live. On the other hand, when a strong acid such as phenol or a strong alkali such as lye has been taken, further damage and even rupture of the esophagus may be caused by vomiting. If strychnine has been taken, convulsions may be brought on by vomiting. If in doubt, give something bland by mouth and seek a doctor.

When poisoning is suspected, first examine the mouth of the patient for signs

of burns and for any poison that can be removed and saved for study. Note the breath for an odor such as that of kerosene or phenol. The poison can be diluted by giving large amounts of fluid by mouth, provided the patient is conscious and able to swallow. Do not try to remember the specific antidote for each poison, but if the container is nearby, naturally one would read the label for the antidote recommended. Give milk, egg, soap and water, plain water, soda and water, mustard and water, or other fluid that is on hand. The important thing to do is to give plenty—usually six or seven glasses—and then produce vomiting by tickling the back of the throat. After a few minutes, repeat the process. If it is known that an alkaline substance has been taken, give an acid such as vinegar or lemon juice. If an acid has been taken, give an alkaline substance such as baking soda or starch and water. After the stomach has been washed out thoroughly, give a bland liquid such as milk. Then get in touch with the doctor, who will give directions as to what to do next and may suggest that a saline laxative be given.

In the hospital the nurse need not know the specific antidote for each poison. The emergency wards of most general hospitals have a list and keep the common antidotes, as well as equipment for washing out the stomach, on hand. A few of the more common poisons and their antidotes are given in Table 6.

Good nursing care of the acutely poisoned patient may make the difference between a favorable and a fatal outcome. The patient should be kept warm and watched extremely carefully for changes in physical signs such as rapid, thready pulse, respiratory changes, cyanosis, diaphoresis and other signs of collapse, shock, or impending death. Changes must be reported to the physician at once. Pulse rate, respirations, and blood pressure reading should be recorded every fifteen minutes for several hours. Nausea, vomiting, and abdominal pain should be noted, and all vomitus should be observed for signs of blood and should be saved for study. Stools and urine must be checked for abnormal constituents such as blood. Intravenous infusions that

Table 6

Common poisons and their antidotes*

Poison	Antidote
Mercury and heavy metals	Milk and egg albumin
Barbiturates	Amphetamine sulfate and caffeine
	Picrotoxin
Arsenic	BAL (2,3-dimercaptopropanol)
Lead	Calcium in large doses
	Milk
Alkaloids (strychnine, quinine, nicotine)	Potassium permanganate 1:10,000 by mouth
Cyanide	Sodium nitrite and sodium thiosulfate intravenously

*From Gold, Harry, and others: Cornell conferences on therapy, vol. 4, New York, 1951, The Macmillian Co.

have been ordered must be administered at the prescribed rate.

When poisoning has resulted from an overdose of opiates, barbiturates, bromides, or other sedatives, efforts must be made to keep the patient awake. A cup of strong coffee may be given every hour if it can be swallowed and retained. Strong coffee may also be ordered to be given as a retention enema. It is not good treatment to walk the patient about, since this simply tires him and may cause complete exhaustion. The artificial kidney may be used in an effort to speed up excretion of the drug (p. 434).

If the patient has marked depression of respiration, oxygen may be given, and sometimes a respirator is used. A suction machine should be on hand at all times, for sometimes deep suctioning of the bronchial tree is necessary in an effort to prevent pneumonia. If the patient is unconscious, his position must be changed every hour, and he should be turned completely on alternative sides to provide drainage from each bronchus. Occasionally, the head of the bed is lowered to encourage drainage of bronchial secretions. Death from barbiturate poisoning is likely to be delayed. Many patients live two or three days before death occurs. Death from poisoning by gas, however, is much more sudden. The patient who is in the hospital recovering from carbon monoxide poisoning must be observed very carefully for the first twenty-four hours. Some patients who appear to have responded favorably to artificial respiration and oxygen die of heart failure several hours after some level of consciousness has been restored.

The person who has been known to take poison in a suicide attempt presents additional nursing problems. Such a patient must not be left alone under any circumstances. He should be in a room whose windows are equipped with bars or stops if one is available. Upon awakening, the patient has not only his original problem to face but also the discomfort and the emotional impact of learning that he has failed in his suicide attempt. Patients in these circumstances have been known to jump out of a window when it was not thought possible that they had the strength to get out of bed. Others have attempted to electrocute themselves or to carry out their original aim of self-destruction by other means. The routine precautions used for mentally ill patients should be observed (p. 129).

Food poisoning

Acute food poisoning. Each year a large number of people, many of whom eat away from home, suffer acute gastrointestinal upsets due to food poisoning. Acute food poisoning, until recently termed cholera morbus and ptomaine poisoning, is usually caused by a toxin produced by certain strains of staphylococci. This toxin causes immediate irritation to the gastrointestinal tract, hence the name enterotoxin. Illness is not caused by eating foods that are simply "old" and that have been subject to bacterial action. In many parts of the world (for example, in England, where "seasoned" game is popular), "spoiled" foods are ingested without harm. Pathogenic organisms must be present and active to produce disease. Cooking will destroy the organisms and stop the production of enterotoxin but will not destroy the poison that has already been formed.

Acute food poisoning can be prevented by rigorous enforcement of sanitary practices in eating establishments and by teaching the public to take sensible precautions, particularly when eating in restaurants and attending picnics during hot weather. Staphylococci are carried on the hands of workers and inadvertently deposited on food. Food handlers should not be allowed to work if they have even minor infections on their hands or if they do not meet requirements for washing the hands. Foods that are handled and allowed to remain without refrigeration before being cooked or eaten are the most dangerous. For example, chicken that has been removed from the bone and left for some time before creamed chicken is prepared, potatoes that have been peeled and left standing before potato salad is prepared, and seafood that has been removed from the shell by hand some time before being eaten all provide excellent opportunities for the pathogenic organisms to produce enterotoxin.

Signs of acute food poisoning include salivation, cramping, nausea, vomiting, and diarrhea. Signs and symptoms usually appear from one to six hours after eating the offending food, the length of time depending upon the amount of food eaten and the amount of enterotoxin present. In severe cases there may be lassitude, headache, dehydration, rapid pulse, and prostration. Treatment may be the same as for drug poisoning, although a laxative is seldom given since the contents of the gastrointestinal tract are largely evacuated. Usually

fluids such as tea, boiled milk, and broth are tolerated within a short time. If diarrhea is severe, drugs such as bismuth and camphorated tincture of opium are ordered, and fluids may be given intravenously.

Mushroom poisoning. Poisonous mushrooms are the most common cause of death from poisoning by food. It is best to teach the public that there is no sure way to tell whether or not a wild mushroom is safe to eat. All mushrooms found in the free state should be looked upon with suspicion, and only those grown under cultivation should be eaten. Deaths occur each year from the consumption of mushrooms by persons who either thought they were experts in determining a safe variety or else listened to other so-called experts.

Signs and symptoms of mushroom poisoning are severe abdominal pain, nausea, vomiting, diarrhea, and prostration occurring usually within one-half hour to twenty-four hours after eating the mushroom. The first-aid treatment should be the same as for drug poisoning: give fluids and induce vomiting, keep the patient warm, and notify a doctor at once. One ounce of magnesium sulfate may be given in water by mouth, and enemas can also be given to speed any poison still in the intestinal tract out of the body.

In the hospital, the care is symptomatic. Fluids are given intravenously. The position for shock and suctioning may be ordered, and side rails are used if convulsions occur. Moist compresses may be ordered if lacrimation is excessive. The patient should be attended constantly, since he is fearful of death.

Botulism. Botulism is a very serious form of food poisoning caused by a neurotoxin produced by an anerobic, spore-forming organism, the *Clostridium botulinum.* Improper home canning is often the cause of the poisoning, since the spores can resist several hours of ordinary cooking. Even intermittent cooking is not considered safe. People should not can any foods at home unless pressure-cooking methods are used. Agricultural colleges in most states distribute booklets on home canning, and the nurse should encourage their use. The neurotoxin, unlike the enterotoxin produced by a strain of staphylococcus, is destroyed by cooking.

It is not destroyed by mere heating. Foods should be cooked for ten to fifteen minutes, depending upon the density of the solid food, before they are safe to eat.

There is no emergency first-aid treatment suitable for botulism poisoning except to notify the doctor at once and to make preparations to move the patient to a hospital. If the symptoms are severe, the patient may not tolerate being moved. All persons who are suspected of having eaten the contaminated food should be reached, for it is in early treatment of persons least affected that the best results are obtained. Symptoms usually appear within twelve to thirty-six hours after ingestion of the food, and their severity depends upon the amount of infected food eaten. There may be constipation, lassitude, headache, and double vision. Nausea and vomiting are often absent. As further damage to the nervous system occurs, there are difficulty in swallowing, lowered voice, and finally inability to talk or to swallow and muscular incoordination. Treatment consists of supportive care and the administration of large doses of antitoxin. Antitoxin cannot undo damage that has been done, but it helps to prevent further damage. The mortality rate from botulism in the United States is approximately 65%, with patients usually dying within three to sixteen days of the onset of symptoms. Fortunately, this poisoning is now quite rare.

Nursing the victim of botulism poisoning includes keeping the patient quiet, usually in a darkened room. Other aspects of nursing care are similar to those described for patients with mushroom poisoning.

Reactions to the sun's heat

Sunburn. Sunburn can occur even when the sun cannot be seen, since rays are able to filter through clouds. Reflection of rays from water increases the danger of burning. The best prevention for sunburn is careful, gradual exposure to the sun's rays and avoiding the midday hours, when the rays are hottest. Some trade preparations, such as those containing para-aminobenzoic acid, are helpful in keeping out harmful rays, and olive oil, cocoa butter, and many creams and ointments are useful. Compresses of magnesium sulfate or sodium bicarbonate may be used to ease discomfort from sunburn. If chills, fever, edema, or blistering occur, the advice of a doctor should be sought.

Heat cramps. Heat cramps are sudden muscle pains caused by excessive loss of sodium chloride in perspiration during strenuous exercise in hot weather. The best treatment is prevention by taking extra salt when severe exertion is anticipated. The immediate treatment consists of salty fluids and foods by mouth, extra water, and rest for a few hours.

Heat exhaustion. Heat exhaustion is vasomotor collapse due to inability of the body to adequately supply the peripheral vessels with sufficient fluids to produce the perspiration needed for cooling and yet meet vital tissue requirements. The condition usually follows an extended period of vigorous exercise in hot weather, particularly when the person concerned has not had a period of acclimatization. The symptoms are faintness, weakness, headache, and sometimes nausea and vomiting. The skin is pale and moist. Heat exhaustion can often be prevented by taking extra salt and extra fluid during hot weather and by tempering physical activity during very hot weather. Emergency treatment consists of lowering the patient's head, preferably by placing him with the head lower than the body. He should be in the coolest spot available. Fluids should be given, and preferably they should contain salt. If the attack has been severe, the patient should rest for several hours before resuming activity.

Heatstroke (sunstroke). Heatstroke is a serious condition requiring immediate emergency treatment. It is due to a failure of the regulating mechanism of the body that controls perspiration. The person undergoing vigorous exercise in intense heat may perspire profusely for some time and then become dehydrated and fail to produce sufficient perspiration to maintain normal body temperature. The skin is dry, hot, and flushed in contrast to the pale, moist skin of the person suffering from heat exhaustion. The patient becomes confused, dizzy, and faint, and may quickly lose consciousness.

There is probably no greater medical emergency than heatstroke. Without treatment almost 100% of heatstroke victims will die, but with prompt and vigorous treatment almost as many will recover. The patient must be moved to the shade, preferably to a cool room, and a doctor must be notified at once. The patient's temperature should be taken as soon as possible. Treatment to reduce the temperature must be started immediately. The best method of doing this is to place the patient in a tub of cold water and to massage the skin vigorously to bring more blood to the surface for cooling. Spraying the body with cold water from a garden hose is often effective. Ice should be placed on the head and cold drinks given by mouth if the patient is conscious and can swallow. Pouring cold water on the patient and fanning him helps in the absence of tubs and sprays. If the elevated temperature is allowed to persist, serious permanent damage is done to the brain and the entire nervous system. A temperature of 40.5° C. (105° F.) or more means that treatment is essential. Treatment should be continued until the temperature has been lowered to 39.9° C. (102° F.), and it must then be checked carefully for several hours for sudden rise. The patient should respond when the temperature lowers. Failure to do so may indicate that brain damage has occurred. Patients do not recover from heatstroke as quickly as from heat exhaustion. Often there is faulty heat regulation for days and a lowered tolerance to heat for years and sometimes for the rest of the patient's life. The person who has had heatstroke should be advised to plan his living so that repeated long exposures to heat are avoided.

Frostbite

Frostbite occurs most often on the nose, cheeks, ears, toes, and fingers. Sometimes the patient will not know that he has been frostbitten since he cannot see the part, although it will feel numb and will appear white upon inspection. The frozen parts should not be rubbed with snow or cold water as was formerly thought desirable, because if this is done, the frozen crystals of body fluid will traumatize cell walls and may cause serious damage to them. Good first-aid treatment consists of taking the

patient to a warm room, keeping him warm, and giving him warm drinks. Alcohol is sometimes recommended. The frozen part should be thawed as quickly as possible by immersing it gently in warm, but not hot, water or by wrapping it in warm blankets. Massage must be avoided because it damages tissues. The use of direct heat in any form, such as placing the part near a warm stove, is harmful because it increases metabolism, thereby taxing blood supply demands that are already seriously reduced. When the part thaws, the patient should be advised to exercise it gently. Blisters that form should not be disturbed. As thawing occurs, pain may be severe. Aspirin may be given for the pain. The patient should be taken to a doctor or a hospital as soon as possible. The care for frostbite is then similar to that needed in vascular disease of the extremities. Efforts are made to decrease the oxygen needs of the tissues while healing takes place, to improve blood supply by the use of drugs, and to prevent infection if there are open lesions. Some tissues may eventually die and have to be debrided as healing occurs.

Frostbite can usually be prevented by better attention to the clothing worn out-of-doors in intemperate weather. It is more likely to occur in the aged and debilitated person or the one with poor circulation. In the colder states of the United States it also occurs fairly often among teen-agers who conform to local styles in regard to clothing, such as no hats or covering for the ears.

Asphyxiation

The common causes of asphyxiation are inhalation of carbon monoxide gas, inhalation of fumes from burning buildings, drowning, and electric shock. If carbon monoxide or toxic fumes are encountered, it is useless to hold a cloth over the nose, as is so often done by persons who enter burning buildings. While this procedure may screen out some smoke and smoke particles, it does not screen out carbon monoxide or other toxic fumes. The victim of carbon monoxide or other toxic gas poisoning should be moved at once into fresh air, and artificial respiration should be started. Emergency aid, including a pulmotor, should be sent for.

The victim of drowning should be placed on his back with his chin forward. It is not necessary to elevate his feet in an attempt to drain water out of the respiratory passages. The important thing to do is to begin artificial breathing while other aid is being sought. Nothing takes the place of artificial respiration.

Electric shock accidents become more numerous as man puts up more electric wires to operate equipment in his home and at work. Immediate first aid consists of removing the person from contact with the live wire, with the rescuer being careful to avoid contact with the electric charge. The rescuer must never have direct contact with the body of the victim because the charge may be transmitted. He should use a long, dry stick and stand on a dry board. Also, asbestos or some other material or heavy, dry gloves should be used when moving the victim away from the wire. Artificial respiration should be started at once and a doctor summoned. Artificial respiration should be continued even when there is no evidence of response. Some patients have responded after as long as several hours.

Foreign bodies in the eye

The eye should not be rubbed when a foreign body has entered it. Hands should be thoroughly washed before attempting first-aid measures. The inner surface of the lower lid should be examined first. If the foreign object is not there, then gently bring the upper lid down over the lower lid (many foreign bodies lodge on the undersurface of the upper lid). If this is not effective, lavage the eye, using an eyecup, a medicine dropper, or a drinking glass. This measure often suffices to wash away the offending material. The patient can usually feel and tell approximately where the irritation is. If it appears to be under the upper lid, the lid should then be inverted. The procedure is as follows. Prepare an applicator by anchoring a shred of clean cotton on a toothpick and moistening it with tap water. Then, preferably standing behind the patient, grasp the upper lashes

firmly and invert the lid over a match, pencil, or other convenient object. Standing behind the patient is favored by some nurses because it allows for better control if he should jerk and permits one to use a sidewise approach to the lid with the applicator, again avoiding danger if the patient should move quickly. The exact method used depends upon individual manual dexterity and right- or left-handedness.

If the foreign body is on the cornea and is not removed by irrigation, or if marked irritation remains but no foreign object is seen and removed, it is best to close the eye, cover it with a piece of cotton, and anchor the cotton with tape such as cellophane tape. The patient should then seek a doctor at once. Foreign bodies embedded in the cornea can lead to serious consequences because of the danger of infection and ulceration. They should never be removed by the uninitiated. Metallic objects are of particular danger because rusting, which is extremely irritating to the eye tissues, may occur.

Chemicals accidentally introduced into the eyes should be washed away with copious amounts of plain water. Many persons whose vision could have been saved by this simple remedy are now blind. Use a cup or glass and pour the water from the inner to the outer part of the eye. The eye must be held open since the patient will not be able to do this himself. Sometimes it is best to put the victim's head under a faucet if one is available and to use large amounts of running water. A drinking fountain is ideal for this purpose. An eyecup does not ensure diluting the chemical sufficiently and should not be used. Lavage should be continued for several minutes, and after fifteen minutes the procedure should be repeated. The patient should then be taken at once to a doctor.

Foreign bodies in the ear

When a foreign object has entered the ear canal, the first thing to do is to attempt to identify it. In this connection the outer ear is held up and back in an adult and down and out in a child. This straightens the ear canal and makes it possible, with good lighting, to see as far as the eardrum. The patient must be cautioned not to try to dislodge the object since such an attempt may push it farther into the ear. Children must be constantly observed and may need to be restrained. Occasionally, the foreign object (for example, a wad of material or cotton) may be removed with tweezers if it can be readily seen and has free ends. Some authorities believe that it is permissible in first-aid treatment to attempt to get behind the object with a bent hairpin, but this practice may be dangerous in the hands of the uninitiated. Irrigation of the ear is often a fruitless practice, since it seldom dislodges a foreign body that is firmly anchored. If the object turns out to be a bean, a pea, or any other substance that swells, irrigation may cause further damage. The best procedure is to take the patient to a doctor.

The best treatment for insects in the ear is to drop a little oil or strong alcohol into the ear canal. Water should not be used because it makes the insect more active, which will increase pain. Insects can sometimes be enticed out of the ear canal by a flashlight held to the ear. The light from matches should not be used because of the danger of burns.

Foreign bodies in the nose, throat, and esophagus

Foreign bodies in the nose are usually placed there by children during play. If they are visible, one may attempt to remove them with a fine forceps or a pair of tweezers. If a foreign body has passed into the posterior nose or pharynx, it is best to take the patient to a doctor.

Food and other material may become lodged in the throat and interfere with breathing, necessitating emergency treatment. The best procedure is to place the patient on his face, with the head lower than the feet, and to slap him briskly between the shoulders. Children may be treated by picking them up by their heels, which usually suffices to cause them to cough and dislodge the foreign object.

Surprisingly large objects can pass the larynx and go into the trachea and bronchi. Sometimes they cause immediate respiratory difficulties, whereas at other times the aspirated object (a peanut, for example) may remain in the lungs for some time and lead to a mistaken diagnosis of asthma or cause an abscess before it is discovered. The procedure for removal of these objects is discussed on p. 538.

Foreign objects that lodge in the esophagus are usually fish and chicken bones. The symptoms of choking and discomfort are very distressing. First aid consists of keeping the patient as quiet as possible and encouraging him not to swallow or struggle to dislodge the object. A doctor should be notified at once. Foreign objects in the esophagus are removed relatively easily by means of esophagoscopy. There is danger of fatal mediastinitis following perforation of the esophagus by a foreign object, and antibiotic drugs are given to prevent it.

Disaster nursing

Disaster nursing has become increasingly important because of the occurrence of a relatively greater number of natural disasters such as hurricanes and floods in recent years and because each year finds nations of the world with larger and more powerful means of mass destruction. The main differences between damage caused by atomic attack and that caused by other major disasters, such as severe explosions, are extent of damage and the spread of radioactive substances. In the following discussion, consideration will be given particularly to nursing preparation for, and conduct during, disaster resulting from atom bombing. Emphasis will be placed upon the principles of disaster nursing that remain relatively constant from year to year and that apply, in varying degrees, to all major disasters. It is a foregone conclusion that information confined within the covers of a book cannot possibly be completely up-to-date. However, pamphlets are released at frequent intervals by national, state, and local agencies responsible for keeping professional workers and the public informed about new dangers that may have to be faced, and they include changes in methods of treatment and management in the event of disaster.

The nurse cannot begin too early in her professional preparation to think seriously of her own particular responsibility in national disaster. In general this responsibility consists of knowing what overall plans are being made on national, state, and local levels and how she may best fit in with these plans. She should help the public to learn some simple facts that may save lives, and she should understand what will be encountered in the event of bombing and what services she may be required to give. The professional nurse will be looked to by others for leadership and guidance in time of disaster. She is a member of the largest single professional group in the health field and will, therefore, be in contact with many people. Her sphere of activity covers a wider range than that of members of most other professional groups who will be in positions of leadership. In time of disaster her duties will include direct care of the sick and injured, the teaching of lay persons to care for themselves and others, administrative duties, supervision of practical nurses, medical aides, and other workers, and assistance in the field of sanitation and disease prevention. Decentralization of cities and relocation of perhaps millions of people will present challenges to all health workers because there will be interruption of sanitary controls for milk and water and for the disposal of wastes.

Overall plans

Overall disaster planning for a country as large as the United States is a major undertaking and is dependent upon public and private organizations working in close cooperation with each other. The Division of Health Mobilization, under the United States Department of Health, Education, and Welfare, is the official national agency concerned with all aspects of national defense. Within this administration are several divisions, such as the Medical Care Division, which has a nursing branch. Some functions of the Division of Health Mobilization are to encourage states to establish civil defense commissions, to furnish part of the funds needed for supplies, and to arrange for civil defense forces from one state to aid those of another state in the event of bombing within its boundaries. This Division works closely with other groups, including other governmental departments such as the Department of Agriculture, the military services, other divisions of the United States Public Health Service, the American Medical Association, the American National Red Cross, the American Hospital Association, and the national nursing organizations. It serves regional, state, and local civil defense organizations in a guidance capacity. Specific activities include helping to prepare literature and helping to develop courses for professional groups such as doctors, dentists, and nurses. It also sponsors the assembling of improvised hospitals, each of which will be able to care for over two hundred patients. These hospitals will be located close to probable target areas. It is assigned the responsibility for assembling such essential equipment as transfusion sets, dressings, plasma and blood volume expanders, and drugs and equipment to determine radiation contamination (survey meters, dosimeters, and dosimeter readers). The state civil defense commissions carry out similar functions on a state level, providing supplies and developing plans for training professional workers as well as for educating the public. Responsibility for civil defense within states is usually delegated to the state health department. Local communities may have their own organization, the Emergency Medical Service.

Certain highly populated cities and industrial areas throughout the country have been designated as target areas because they are most likely to be attacked. Communities near these target areas have been designated as support areas, and in the event of an attack their medical forces will go immediately to the assistance of the attacked area without direction from the state. Additional help will be sent as needed by the state and is termed state-directed aid. If further help is needed, the Division of Health Mobilization will direct aid from other nearby states.

Every nurse should learn about the Emergency Medical Service in her community. This information can usually be obtained by enrolling in courses in medical and nursing aspects of medical defense offered by the local civil defense organization. Here, her knowledge can be tested to some extent in practical experience. Membership in local units of the National League for Nursing and the American Nurses' Association is important as a means of learning of new developments in disaster nursing. Local organizations of the two associations, sometimes assisted by the state, may sponsor and conduct institutes and refresher courses for their members. The professional nurse may contribute to lay education and refresh her own knowledge by teaching courses sponsored by the Division of Health Mobilization and the American National Red Cross (for example, home nursing and first-aid courses and courses for nurse's aides).

The nurse's attendance at local civil defense meetings is valuable for her and for others. She should not, however, offer her services as a plane spotter or a Geiger count checker, for instance. The reason is simply that her special training in care of the injured will be so badly needed if disaster occurs that she will not be available for duties that can be handled by nonnurses. She should know specifically where and how she reports in the event of disaster and should be prepared to go quickly. Most nurses who work in general hospitals should be quite well oriented by their institutions. The Joint Committee on Accreditation of Hospitals now requires that all hospitals wishing to qualify for accreditation have a written plan for their institutions in the event of disaster. It is probable that in the future there will be more detailed planning within general hospitals and better orientation of the professional members of the staff for their particular assignments.

Nurses who are not attached to a hospital or an emergency medical unit should listen for radio instructions and proceed immediately to the nearest assignment depot in the area in which they happen to be. Nurses who live a considerable distance from their place of regular work should know the location of the assignment depot and of secondary-aid stations in their living area. Married nurses should make some provision for care of their children so that they may make themselves available in the shortest possible time.

The nurse who reports in time of disaster and for emergency drills should not wear a uniform. It has been suggested that a canvas apron with six pockets in the front be worn over slacks and blouse or sweater.[32] The nurse should carry her personal identification as a nurse and wear a Civil Defense armband if she has one. In addition, it is advised that she have with her a flashlight with batteries, bandage scissors, a dozen safety pins, a hypodermic syringe and needle, indelible pencil, matches, a small package of tissues, a small notebook, and lipstick for skin marking.

Educating the public for protection

Everyone should know the basic rules for self-protection in the event of sudden enemy attack, how to prepare for disaster, and how to protect oneself immediately following a bombing. The nurse should include this information in teaching health education to all patients and in all her contacts with laymen.

The American public is strangely apathetic about learning to cope with the hazards that will be present in atomic disaster. Despite the thousands of booklets and pamphlets distributed on the subject and the pages in the daily papers devoted to a description of the proper courses of action, the average citizen does not know the most fundamental steps that may be necessary for his survival. Just as the patient often delays going to the doctor when he fears cancer lest his suspicions be confirmed, so he fails to heed the constant public reminders of what he should know to help assure his survival.

Many pamphlets give simple but complete explanations and rules to go by in preparation for disaster and during disaster. *Survival Under Atomic Attack*, a pamphlet released by the United States government, is excellent for the average layman.

Families living in or near target areas should set aside materials for an emergency. These materials should include two flashlights, a battery radio, a first-aid kit, canned food to last two weeks, bottled and canned fluids, a can opener, a bottle opener, spoons, newspapers, and paper dishes. A large bottle of drinking water should be stored (ideally several gallons) and changed weekly. In addition, a container of water should be available for washing in case anyone is exposed to radiation dust, since water may suddenly be cut off or contaminated. A garbage can with a tight cover and a pail for human wastes is necessary.

Every citizen should have a transistor (battery) radio that can be used in a national emergency. The radio should be turned on and instructions awaited if a bombing is threatened. Windows and doors should be closed and blinds drawn, all electric equipment except the radio should be turned off, and pets should be brought indoors. The family should then proceed to the basement. Many people fear that they may be trapped in the cellar, but it has been shown that this danger is much less than that which will be encountered by staying above ground in the event of an atomic bombing. When a bomb is known to have been exploded, the family should remain in the basement until advised by radio that it is safe to go outdoors.

It is important to know what to do when at work or out-of-doors at the time of a bombing. Despite the tremendous fear of radiation in this country, by far the greatest number of deaths and severe injuries in an atomic bombing will come from blast and heat. The following three rules, if followed, will save many lives:

1. Try to put a wall between yourself and the bomb, judging that the bomb will be dropped in the most industrialized area. Even a ditch or a gutter is better than no protection.

2. Fall flat on your face, bury your face in your arm, and if possible pull something over your head and hair.

3. Stay there until things are quiet. Do not rush out to look around. Explosive radiation lasts about a minute after a bomb has exploded and may easily affect persons within a mile of the center of the attack unless they have been quite well protected.

Lingering radiation is due to the presence of many fine particles of "ashes" or leftover fission products that may remain in the vicinity of the bombing for an indefinite time. These particles usually rise high in the air and spread over a wide area and may not be concentrated enough to do harm to persons a few miles from the site of the bombing. Lingering radiation dust is extremely difficult to remove from houses, and it is advised that windows broken by the blast be covered with a blanket or cardboard to prevent as much dust as possible from entering the house. If a large amount of radiation dust is present, some will undoubtedly filter into the house. If the explosion occurred underwater or if water reservoirs were exposed to large amounts of radiation dust, the water will be seriously contaminated. So far there is no known simple or effective method for decontaminating such water, and if a major bombing occurs, the water supply may present an extremely serious problem, although the use of shale, coagulant, and settling gives promise of effectiveness. Persons who are at home should draw water immediately and put it into covered, clean containers, because the water in the immediate mains will not be contaminated by radioactive substances and may suffice for emergency needs. Thereafter it is not advisable to use water from taps until advised by radio of its safety. Even if water is not contaminated by radioactive substances, it may be contaminated by bacteria following damage to sewer systems. Bacterial contamination can be overcome by boiling the water, but boiling will not remove radioactive contamination.

Although radiation is a real danger following a bombing, it should not prevent one from assisting others. Anyone who is out in the open shortly after a bombing should keep his head and other parts of the body covered. Upon coming into the house, he should shed his outer clothing, including his shoes, at the doorway and should scrub thoroughly with soap and water. If possible, he should then be checked for the amount of radioactive contamination still present, particularly on exposed parts of the body, and the scrubbing process should be repeated if necessary.

The public is urged not to telephone during a disaster. The radio will give instruction for the precautions and cleanup measures that are necessary for each vicinity. A safe rule to follow if in doubt, however, is to err on the side of caution. Food that has been uncovered during a bombing should be discarded. Food in wrappers is safe, though the outer wrappings should be carefully removed and discarded. The outsides of cans, as well as utensils, furniture, and any equipment that has not been in tightly closed cupboards or drawers, should be washed thoroughly.

The public should know that mass evacuation of cities may seriously affect water and other sanitary facilities. Foods and fluids of all kinds should be cooked if there is any doubt about contamination. Disaster conditions often threaten mass epidemics of diseases such as typhoid. It may be that persons living in target areas will soon be urged to receive immunization against typhoid and tetanus so that it will not be necessary in time of a national disaster. Personal identification, which includes blood type, may also be encouraged for persons who live in target areas.

Immediate services in event of bombing

Patients whom the nurse will encounter in disaster will not differ very much from those seen in her everyday practice. It will be the numbers of injured and the severity of the injuries that will be different, as well as the conditions under which she will work. It is estimated that one atomic bomb could kill 80,000 persons and wound 80,000 more. Of the injured it is estimated that approximately 12,000 will be in shock, 12,000 will suffer radiation illness, 27,000 will be severely burned, and 13,000 will have fractures, open wounds, and crushing injuries. It is almost impossible to think in these numbers and to plan how work can be carried out with the confusion and tensions that will be present. Major obstacles will be dislocation of transportation, communication, light, and water supply.

It must be understood by all nurses that tremendous adjustments in basic thinking will have to be made if an atomic bombing should occur. It will not be possible even to begin to do all that might be desirable for everyone. Whatever is best for the largest number must be done. The dying should be made as comfortable as possible, but the available facilities must be used for those whose possibility of survival is best. Some careful techniques will have to be discarded, and the nurse will have to rely

heavily upon her knowledge of basic principles rather than specific procedures. She will have to improvise and use whatever is available. For example, one syringe may have to be used for several patients, with only the needle being changed. She must remember that prompt action will save many lives. Those who are available to help will be less likely to suffer emotional reactions if they are kept busy with definite tasks. In the first few hours of disaster, treatment will have to be routine and simple. Much of it will have to be performed by unskilled workers, whereas nurses will have to do many things usually done by physicians. Perhaps the nurse's ability to keenly appraise the physical condition of people will be her greatest asset in time of disaster. She is the only person with this skill with the exception of the physician. For example, by observing a group of patients, she will be able to determine quickly which one is not responding to fluid therapy, which must be constantly attended lest he attempt to remove an artificial airway, and which is responding well and can tolerate being moved.

All nurses should serve willingly where most needed in time of disaster. There will not be time for consideration of choices and probably not even time to use all skills to the best advantage. It is hoped that physicians will be in charge of all aid stations. It is possible, however, that a nurse may have to take charge until a doctor arrives. Nurses will be assigned from their designated assignment depots to secondary-aid stations, permanent hospitals, improvised emergency hospitals, and holding stations. Secondary-aid stations are established at designated places outside target cities as part of preparation for disaster. First-aid stations will be determined by groups sent out from the secondary-aid station after the bombing. Permanent hospitals will be hospitals in the target city that are suitable for use. Improvised emergency hospitals will be temporary facilities set up in school buildings, garages, or any other place with suitable space at a considerable distance from the bombed area.

Stretcher teams will go from the first-aid station, give first aid, and bring the wounded to the secondary-aid station, where the important function of sorting and identifying casualties is done. This function is called *triage*. Classification for treatment has been listed in four priorities as follows:

Priority I—Persons requiring outpatient care only

Priority II—The moderately injured and ill, whose chances of recovery are good following immediate definitive treatment

Priority III—The injured and ill whose chances of recovery are not jeopardized by delayed definitive treatment

Priority IV—The critically injured or ill, who require extensive, complicated, time-consuming or material-consuming procedures, and the persons who are beyond help

The doctor should be responsible for triage and should decide which patients should receive immediate treatment, which should be sent to secondary-aid stations, and which should be sent to remote stations. He should also determine which should be transported by litter and which may be treated as "walking wounded." If no doctor is available, a nurse will have to substitute. She should follow the general rules taught in all first aid: treat suffocation, severe hemorrhage, shock, severe wounds, burns, fractures, and dislocations in that order. Judgment in estimating the severity of the injury must be used along with this rule. Treatment will not usually be given at the triage station, but each patient will be tagged and the injuries noted on the tag. Priorities in triage may change, depending upon the help and facilities available and upon individual patients' responses.

Injuries may be any of the following: injury caused by blast of the nuclear weapon, traumatic injuries resulting from flying parts of physical structures, burns from the initial bombing or from the heat from explosions, radiation injuries from explosive radiation, or poisoning from nerve gas or other poisons. Emotional reactions will also occur.

In first-aid stations and secondary-aid stations nurses may be called upon to do things usually done by physicians, such as prescribing medications, starting intravenous infusions, giving anesthetics (if she has had some preparation), suturing lacerations, debriding wounds, applying pressure dressings, dressing burns, applying and readjusting splints, and directing the disposition of patients. It is to be hoped that the nurse will not be so occupied with medical procedures that observing patients for changes in vital signs is neglected. She may also be needed to search for and help persons who are injured and in need of care yet who are too frightened to leave their homes or places of hiding.

Morphine has been stockpiled in disposable Syrettes, each containing 30 mg. (½ grain). Penicillin in oil has also been stockpiled, and chlortetracycline hydrochloride (Aureomycin), 250 mg., and oxytetracycline (Terramycin), 250 mg., are available. Dried plasma has been stocked in containers ready for the addition of sterile distilled water and normal saline solution. Sodium citrate has been stocked in powdered form, ready for use by addition of unsterile water. This solution is given by mouth to persons who can take fluids orally.

Shock. Shock will be a major problem, particularly in the first few hours following the explosion, and should sometimes have first priority in treatment, sometimes even taking precedence over hemorrhage. Shock will probably be due to trauma that may or may not have caused external laceration. Blood loss may be external or internal and may be due to crushing injury or fluid loss from burns. Shock may be partially prevented and controlled by stopping hemorrhage, giving medication for pain if the patient is not already in shock, splinting fractures before moving patients, covering burns, dressing open wounds, preventing loss of body heat, and giving fluids by veins, by hypodermoclysis, or by mouth. The lower limbs should be elevated above the level of the trunk.

Hemorrhage. The care of the patient with hemorrhage will not differ from that given in any emergency situation. Once applied, a tourniquet is not removed until a nurse or doctor checks the patient for cessation of bleeding. Removal of the tourniquet must be done where facilities are available to control the bleeding. Whenever a tourniquet is applied in the field or in a first-aid station, a large T is marked on the forehead of the patient with a skin pencil. He then will receive priority in transportation to a secondary-aid station.

Burns. Patients burned in disaster have been classified into three groups: the hopelessly burned, the severely burned, and the moderately burned. Attention in disaster will be given first to the severely burned, since the hopelessly burned will not be expected to survive. Treatment includes prevention of infection by giving antibiotics, alleviation of pain, and replacement of body fluids. A special burn dressing has been stockpiled in large quantities as part of civil defense emergency medical supplies. It consists of a cellulose pad covered with a layer of cotton and faced with extremely fine gauze. The gauze is placed next to the burn, and the dressing is then held in place with a tensile yarn roller bandage, included in the burn package. Burn dressings are provided in two sizes. When applying dressings, it is important to bandage the neck loosely, never to leave two skin surfaces in contact, to cover the burned area completely, and to avoid overlapping of the cellulose dressing, since an overlap may cause uneven pressure. The pressure of the outer yarn bandage should be firm, gentle, and even. (For further details in care of patients with severe burns, see p. 791.)

Wounds, lacerations, and fractures. Many patients will have open chest wounds, wounds of the face and neck, and penetrating abdominal wounds, as well as fractures of the skull and other bones of the body. Abdominal viscera must be kept moist. If sterile water or normal saline solution is not available, plasma or even unsterile water may be used to moisten dressings applied over the protruding viscera. No penetrating objects or debris should be removed, the patient should not be given fluids by mouth, and he should be sent at once to a secondary-aid station.

Open chest wounds can sometimes be closed by applying wide adhesive tape (three-inch) in a crisscross fashion. A small, dry dressing should be placed over the opening, and the adhesive tape should extend approximately four to six inches on each side of the wound so that good traction can be obtained and so that the wound can be kept airtight. If the patient is having

difficulty in breathing, he should be placed on his injured side, with the head and shoulders elevated. If he does not have difficulty in breathing or injury to contraindicate this, he should be placed in shock position, with the body flat and lower limbs elevated about 45 degrees.

Severe wounds of the mouth and jaw often cause obstruction of breathing after an hour or more when swelling occurs. Under no circumstances should tight bandages or slings be applied to severe wounds of the jaws, mouth, or throat, since they may cut off passage of air as edema occurs. Patients should be transported in a face-down position. In some instances it is safest to insert an airway before the patient is moved. Airways are stocked in the supplies for emergency medical units.

Blood clots and obstruction must be removed before an airway is used. The airway is inserted by directing it along the tongue, with the concave side down, and by moving it carefully back and slightly from side to side until the guard comes in contact with the teeth. It is then tied in place or anchored with adhesive to prevent its slipping out in transit.

Some debridement of large open wounds is necessary to prevent infection. Even with large doses of antibiotics, infection cannot be prevented if much dead tissue is left. The nurse who is not familiar with suturing or who does not have suture equipment may make excellent use of strips of adhesive tape to hold wound edges together. Pieces of adhesive tape are notched and folded over in the center portion and are applied so that the center part passes over the wound. This center portion is flamed before the adhesive tape is applied. Adhesive tape of any width can be used, depending upon the location and size of the wound. The skin must be dry, and usually several strips, or "butterflies," are used (Fig. 58). Wounds on the lips and other parts of the face are often very satisfactorily cared for in this way. Skin clips can be used easily by nurses who are not familiar with the technique of suturing.

The care of fractures is similar to that necessary in any accident situation, with the exception that many patients with fractures will also have severe burns and may

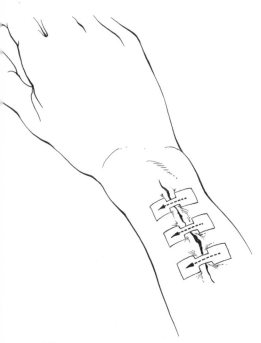

Fig. 58

The use of "butterfly" adhesive strips to approximate the skin edges in a laceration of the forearm. Note the irregular wound edges and the placement of the adhesive. Arrows indicate the direction of pull used to partially close the wound.

be suffering from radiation effects or other injuries. The enormous number of persons with fractures will make the need for improvised equipment very great. Pieces of wood from destroyed buildings, doors, canes, umbrellas, ironing boards, and magazines are a few of the materials that may be used.

Obstetric emergencies. A bombing disaster will cause many women to abort and many to deliver their babies prematurely. They will be sent to the secondary-aid stations to be delivered, and the nurse may be the only professional person available. No materials have been stockpiled for this situation, and the nurse or person in attendance will have to improvise to the best of her ability. A shoelace, a piece of string, or a piece of bandage may have to be used to tie the cord. A lay person may be called

upon to check the fundus for an hour or more, and the patient may then be treated as a "walking wounded" and returned to her home or sent to a permanent hospital. It is very important that the mother and baby be identified. Identification bands for both mother and baby can be made of cloth, and information on each should include the name of the father, the address, the sex of the baby, and the time and place of birth. If at all possible, the baby should be kept with the mother. If the delivery has been such that there is danger of infection, an antibiotic may be given.

Radiation. Radiation injury may come from gamma rays and neutrons released as the explosion occurs (*initial* radiation). This type of injury is most likely to affect persons who had insufficient protection between themselves and the blast and who have suffered severe burns and flash injuries. It can come also from irradiated strontium, which is part of the mushroomlike cloud that rises and is dispersed widely (*fallout*). Strontium (strontium-90) will be acquired by inhalation, by ingesting foods with external contamination or containing the radioactive substance, or by drinking water that has been contaminated.

Radiation illness probably will not become apparent until several hours or even days after exposure. Persons affected may have nausea, vomiting, and malaise within a few hours of exposure. Since it may be difficult to distinguish the person with early and severe radiation illness from the one with severe emotional reaction, all persons suspected should have immediate bed rest and should be sent as quickly as possible to a hospital where treatment can be given as necessary. More detailed descriptions are available in recent specialized publications.[25,30]

If the exposure has been lethal, severe vomiting and diarrhea will occur within a few hours. Since the entire body may be exposed in an atomic bombing, the reactions that occur first probably will be systemic and may cause death while no skin reaction or other external reaction is evident. Other symptoms of severe radiation illness are severe inflammation and sometimes sloughing and hemorrhage of the mucous membrane of the mouth and throat, hemorrhage spots under the skin, and loss of hair. A severe leukopenia quickly follows exposure to large amounts of radiation.

There is no specific treatment for radiation illness. The patient needs the same care as the one who receives radiation treatment for a specific illness (p. 283). This care may include rest, antibiotics, protection from superimposed infection, blood transfusions, fluids and electrolytes, and a bland diet that is high in calories.

Nerve gas damage. Nerve gases are the substances that are most likely to be used in chemical warfare. They are colorless to light brown, and can be released in either liquid or vapor form. They have a slightly fruity odor or else are odorless. If inhaled in large amounts, they may cause death within a few minutes by producing overstimulation of the centers of respiration and circulation. Symptoms include excessive salivation, constriction of the pupils, dimness of vision, pain in the eyeballs, coryza, cyanosis, coughing, circulatory disturbances, and convulsions. Atropine sulfate should be given at once in large doses (1/30 grain or 2 mg.). It has been stockpiled in tablets of this strength. Clothing should be removed and the skin washed with sodium bicarbonate in water. If sodium bicarbonate is not available, plain water should be used. Since clothing is highly contaminated by liquid gas, care should be taken to avoid contamination of others with such clothing. The victim of nerve gas poisoning should be hospitalized as soon as possible.

Emotional reactions. The stresses and strains placed upon all who survive a major disaster are almost beyond our imagination, so that it is almost impossible to think through the problems and to plan for care. The emotional reactions will affect the doctor, the nurse, and all others giving aid, as well as all other survivors. Members of the medical and related staffs will be less likely to show signs of emotional effects than others because they will have more knowledge of what is happening and will be busy. The American Psychiatric Association has outlined the major types of reactions that are likely to occur and has suggested methods of management.

1. Normal reaction. There may be a nor-mal reaction of tremor, profuse diaphoresis, pallor, and nausea that soon disappears.

2. Acute panic. This reaction is one of the most serious of the reactions and must be dealt with immediately, since in time of crisis it is acutely "contagious." It has been demonstrated repeatedly that in times of disaster one person in panic can set off a chain reaction and cause untold damage. The person in panic is devoid of judgment and is inordinately but not purposefully active. He cannot be reasoned with and makes wild attempts to flee. Horses in panic have been known to rush back into a burning barn and be killed, and such behavior is not too different from that of human beings in panic. Panic must not be confused with rapid exit from a point of danger. This is sensible, provided it is orderly and purposeful. The person in true panic must be restrained, usually by force, and should be firmly held by medical aides until he can be removed to a place where his influence upon others will not be dangerous. Persons who have experienced disaster should be segregated from those who have not, since they may easily become panicky at threat of further disaster.

3. Depressed reactions. Persons who have depressed reactions will be slowed down or numbed. They will sit and stare into space and will be completely oblivious to what is going on around them. These patients must be protected, since they will not move to help themselves.

4. Overly active response. The persons will be very active, possibly joking inappropriately or laughing hysterically, be unable to concentrate on one job, and be a disturbing influence upon the person in command of the location.

5. Severe bodily reactions. The person may not be able to use a limb and may have nausea and vomiting as a result of fear of radiation exposure.

In management of patients and others who are suffering from emotional effects, the nurse should apply the basic principles of psychiatric nursing. She must remember that there will be serious limits to what she can do. She should observe each patient and decide what can be done in the particular situation and what is best for the patient and the group. It is useless to argue with the patient, to expect him to stand up better under strain than he has done, or to imply that any of his beliefs or physical limitations are not real. Kindness and gentleness are important. Most patients with emotional reactions are afraid, and they respond to a genuine kindly interest in them and an honest attempt to understand how they feel. Patients should be kept busy if at all possible. The patients in panic must be restrained, the dazed ones given routine things to do in as quiet an environment as possible, and the overly active ones assigned to tasks that require moving about. Patients with an imagined major physical defect can often help with a task with which their imagined problem does not interfere, such as writing identification tags if they believe that their lower limbs are affected.

Chlorpromazine has been stockpiled for use by medical workers primarily and may be used to treat those who have severe or prolonged emotional reactions. This drug relieves nausea and vomiting, releases tension, and lessens anxiety.

The most important point in nursing management and in prevention of emotional reactions is the poise and conduct of the nurse herself. Just as one person in panic can upset a crowd, so one calm, collected person can quiet a group.

References and selected readings*

1 *Accident Facts, Chicago, 1965, National Safety Council.

2 American Medical Association: Summary report on national emergency medical care, Chicago, 1959, American Medical Association.

3 *American Nurses' Association: Nursing in disasters, Am. J. Nursing 60:1130-1133, Aug. 1960.

4 *American Red Cross: First aid textbook, ed. 5, Washington, 1962, American National Red Cross.

5 Anderson, Gaylord W., Arnstein, Margaret G., and Lester, Mary R.: Communicable disease control, ed. 4, New York, 1962, The Macmillan Co.

6 Beeson, Paul B., and McDermott, Walsh, editors: Cecil-Loeb textbook of medicine, ed. 11, Philadelphia, 1963, W. B. Saunders Co.

7 Costa, P. James, and Dews, Mary Jane: Mushroom poisoning and nursing care, Am. J. Nursing 56:998-1000, Aug. 1956.

8 Crawford, Ora E.: Eye injuries in a chemical plant, Nursing Outlook 3:447-449, Aug. 1955.

9 *Creighton Helen, and Armington, Sister Catherine:

The bite of a stray dog, Am. J. Nursing 64:121-123, July 1964.

10 Denton, Frances H.: Police and firemen help prepare students for disaster nursing, Nursing Outlook 9:28-29, Jan. 1961.

11 Division of Health Mobilization, Public Health Service: The role of the nurse in national disaster, publication no. 1071-1-5, Washington, D. C., 1965, U. S. Department of Health, Education, and Welfare.

12 *Dolman, C. E.: Botulism, Am. J. Nursing 64:119-124, Sept. 1964.

13 Gold, Harry, and others: Cornell conference on therapy, vol. 4, New York, 1951, The Macmillan Co.

14 *Goldstein, Joseph D., and Werley, Harriet H.: Care of casualties caused by nuclear weapons, Am. J. Nursing 56:1576-1582, Dec. 1956.

15 Gordon, John E., editor: Control of communicable disease in man, ed. 10, New York, 1965, The American Public Health Association.

16 *Green, Josephine M.: Emergency care of the obstetric patient, Nursing Outlook 6:694-696, Dec. 1958.

17 Harrison, T. R., and others, editors: Principles of internal medicine, ed. 5, New York, 1966, McGraw-Hill Book Co.

18 Hollister, William Gray: Some mental health aspects of civil defense for public health workers, Am. J. Pub. Health 46:1275-1282, Oct. 1956.

19 Holthaus, Louise Sharko: Cooperation to prevent home accidents, Am. J. Nursing 56:1160-1162, Sept. 1956.

20 *Kummer, Sylvia B., and Kummer, Jerome M.: Pointers to preventing accidents, Am. J. Nursing 63:118-119, Feb. 1963.

21 *Lindsey, Douglas: The case of the much-maligned tourniquet, Am. J. Nursing 57:444-445, April 1957.

22 *Lindsey, Douglas: Effective emergency splinting, Am. J. Nursing 56:1120-1124, Sept. 1956.

23 *Lueth, Harold G.: Meeting disaster, Am. J. Nursing 56:1135-1138, Sept. 1956.

24 *Magnussen, Ann: Who does what—in defense, In natural disaster, Am. J. Nursing 65:118-121, March 1965.

25 *Mahoney, Robert F.: Emergency and disaster nursing, New York, 1965, The Macmillan Co.

26 *Manheimer, Dean I., and others: Fifty thousand child-years of accidental injuries, Pub. Health Rep. 81:519-533, June 1966.

27 *Mendelson, Janice A.: Sprains and strains, Am. J. Nursing 61:45-50, June 1961.

28 Miller, Russell R., and Johnson, S. Roger: Poison control now and in the future, Am. J. Nursing 66:1984-1987, Sept. 1966.

29 *Mushlin, Harry R.: Drugs and food for the disaster shelter, Am. J. Nursing 64:116-119, Oct. 1964.

30 Nabbe, Frances Crouch: Disaster nursing, Paterson, N. J., 1961, Littlefield, Adams & Co.

31 Neal, Mary V.: Disaster and mass casualty nursing, Nursing Outlook 8:225-226, April 1960.

32 New York State Department of Health: Supplement to the guide for nurses, emergency treatment and techniques in aid stations, Feb. 1956, V-C-1.

*References preceded by an asterisk are particularly well suited for student reading.

33 *Parrish, Henry M.: Incidence of treated snakebites in the United States, Pub. Health Rep. **81**:269-276, March 1966.

34 *Pearce, Marion G.: Emergency service for the poisoned, Am. J. Nursing **63**:116-117, March 1963.

35 *Peszczynski, Mieczyslaw: Why old people fall, Am. J. Nursing **65**:86-88, May 1965.

36 *Phillips, Elisabeth Cogswell: A nurse with many jobs, Nursing Outlook **6**:580-583, Oct. 1958.

37 *Ridgway, James M.: The nurse in disaster medical and health programs, Nursing Outlook **5**:41-42, Jan. 1957.

38 Sandick, Herbert: Emergency care of the injured, Am. J. Nursing **62**:93-96, Dec. 1962.

39 *Scheffler, Gustave L.: The nurse's role in hospital safety, Nursing Outlook **10**:680-682, Oct. 1962.

40 Schrogie, John J.: Training in cardiopulmonary resuscitation, Pub. Health Rep. **80**:68-74, Jan. 1965.

41 *Skellenger, William S.: Treatment of poisoning in children, Am. J. Nursing **65**:108-112, Nov. 1965.

42 *Steele, James H., and Carroll, L. Dorothy: Animal diseases transmissible to man, Nursing Outlook **4**:156-161, March 1956.

43 *Steele, James H., and Lester, Mary R.: Rabies and rabies control, Am. J. Nursing **58**:531-536, April 1958.

44 *Stewart, Richard D.: Poisoning from chlorinated hydrocarbon solvents, Am. J. Nursing **67**:85-87, Jan. 1967.

45 *Sullivan, Catherine M., and Eicherly, Elizabeth E.: Civil defense in a nuclear age, Am. J. Nursing **65**:121-125, Nov. 1965.

46 *Sullivan, Catherine M., Elliman, Virginia B., and National League for Nursing: What price survival, the bridge between, disaster and mass casualty nursing, Nursing Outlook **8**:128-135, March 1960.

47 U. S. Department of Health, Education, and Welfare: Education for survival, Washington, D. C., 1957, U. S. Government Printing Office.

48 When the unexpected happens, Boston, 1956, Health Education Service of the John Hancock Mutual Life Insurance Co.

49 Whitney, John M.: National medical civil defense planning and requirements, J.A.M.A. **160**:1195-1201, April 7, 1956.

50 Wilson, William J.: Heat injury, Am. J. Nursing **60**:1124-1125, Aug. 1960.

51 Wright, William H.: How one poison control center works, Am. J. Nursing **66**:1988, Sept. 1966.

14

Nursing in neoplastic disease

Study questions

1 Review the differences between benign and malignant tumors. What are the important characteristics of malignant growths? How are tumors classified, and how are they usually named? What features of a growth help to determine the degree of malignancy? What is meant by metastasis, and how does it occur?
2 Review the principles and techniques used in medical aseptic technique (isolation).
3 What facilities, such as home care programs and hospitals for chronically ill patients, are available in your community for care of the patient with cancer in the terminal stages?
4 What is the physical law of inverse-square?
5 Review the gonadal and pituitary hormones. What preparations of male and female hormones are often given? How are they administered?

The professional nurse can take a very active part in the prevention and control of cancer, as well as in the care of patients who have the disease. She may contribute to the prevention of cancer as she works in industry. She may do case findings in the community and educate the public to report early suspicious signs to competent physicians. She may give care to patients hospitalized for treatment of cancer. She may be a team member in a research center. She may assist the patient's family in giving him terminal care at home or help persons who give such care in nursing homes.

Cancer is a disease that is much publicized and greatly feared in our society. However, the nature of many nursing functions foster a close feeling on the part of the patient toward the nurse, and as a result she often is the recipient of confidences when fear or other emotions keep patients from seeking help from other persons. The nurse should examine and perhaps alter her own feelings about cancer if she is to be alert to signs of the disease and be effective in helping the patient to secure medical attention.

Fear of cancer must be faced squarely and can be dealt with intelligently only by using current knowledge of prevention, control,

Table 7
Cancer status chart: leading sites*

Site	Estimated new cases 1965	Estimated deaths 1965	Danger signal (when lasting longer than two weeks see your doctor)	Safeguards	Comment
Breast	63,000	27,000	Lump or thickening in breast	Annual checkup; monthly breast self-examination	Leading cause of cancer death in women
Colon and rectum	73,000	43,000	Change in bowel habits; bleeding	Annual checkup, including proctoscopy	Considered a highly curable disease when digital and proctoscopic examinations are included in routine checkups
Kidney and bladder	30,000	14,000	Urinary difficulty; bleeding, in which case consult your doctor at once	Annual checkup with urinalysis	Protective measures for workers in high-risk industries are helping to eliminate one of important causes of these cancers
Lung	55,000	50,000	Persistent cough, or lingering respiratory ailment	Prevention: Heed facts about smoking; annual checkup; chest x-ray	Leading cause of cancer death among men, this form of cancer is largely preventable
Mouth, larynx, and pharynx	21,000	10,000	Sore that does not heal; difficulty in swallowing; hoarseness	Annual checkup, including larynx	Many more lives should be saved because mouth is easily accessible to visual examination by physicians and dentists
Prostate	34,000	16,000	Urinary difficulty	Annual checkup, including palpation	Occurs mainly in men over 60; disease can be detected by palpation and urinalysis at annual checkup
Skin	85,000	5,000	Sore that does not heal, or change in wart or mole	Annual checkup; avoidance of overexposure to sun	Readily detected by observation and diagnosed by simple biopsy
Stomach	21,000	18,000	Indigestion	Annual checkup	A 40% decline in mortality in twenty years, for reasons yet unknown
Uterus	44,000	14,000	Unusual bleeding or discharge	Annual checkup, including pelvic examination and Papanicolaou smear	Uterine cancer mortality has declined 50% during last twenty-five years; with wider application of Papanicolaou smear, many thousand more lives can be saved

*From 1966 cancer facts and figures, New York, 1965, American Cancer Society, Inc.; reprinted by permission of the American Cancer Society, Inc.

Table 7

Cancer status chart: leading sites—cont'd

Site	Esti-mated new cases 1965	Esti-mated deaths 1965	Comment
Leukemia	18,000	14,000	Leukemia is a cancer of blood-forming tissues and is characterized by abnormal production of immature white blood cells. Acute leukemia strikes mainly children and is treated by drugs that have extended life from a few months to as much as three years. Chronic leukemia strikes usually after age 25 and progresses less rapidly.
			Cancer experts believe that if drugs or vaccines are found that can cure or prevent any cancers, they will be successful first for leukemia and the lymphomas.
Lymphomas	21,000	16,000	These diseases arise in lymph system and include Hodgkin's disease and lymphosarcoma. Some patients with lymphatic cancers can lead normal lives for many years.

and treatment. To be effective in helping patients and their families, the nurse needs mature attitudes and reactions. Optimism is essential; every experienced nurse can recall striking exceptions to the usual response to treatment. She also needs knowledge of the disease and of its treatment, and a knowledge of the community resources available to persons who have cancer.

Facts about cancer

About 550,000 persons in the United States are diagnosed as having cancer each year. Cancer ranks second only to heart disease as the cause of death in the United States. In 1964 there were an estimated 290,000 deaths from cancer.[36] The number of deaths per 100,000 population in the United States rose from 112 in 1930 to 151 in 1964.[3] The increase is undoubtedly due in part to the fact that more people live to an age when cancer is likely to develop. Since the death rate from infections has been lowered because of the use of antibiotic drugs, and since many deaths from communicable dis-

ease in childhood have been prevented by immunization, the life-span has been lengthened. Except for cancer of the lung, the death rate for cancer, when adjusted to the age distribution of the population, shows little change.[3]

The incidence of cancer is highest in the middle years of life. Although it is the leading cause of death among women 30 to 40 years of age, in 1964 more men than women died of cancer, the ratio being approximately 55 men to 45 women.[3] More than one-half of all cancer deaths occur among persons under 65 years of age. Cancer occurs relatively frequently in children and in young adults. It now follows accidents as the leading cause of death in the age group from 4 to 25 years. Since the leukemias and Hodgkin's disease have been statistically included with other forms of cancer, a more realistic picture of the incidence of malignant disease in children is possible.

Although, in general, cancer is no respecter of race or social status, there are some variations with regard to race and sex as well as age. Some of these variations cannot be explained, but others seem to have at least a partial cause. For example, there has been a marked decrease in the incidence of cancer of the stomach in the United States during the past twenty years, whereas cancer of the stomach has increased in the Soviet Union. The reason for this variation is unknown. The tremendous increase in the incidence of, and mortality from, cancer of the lung among men in the United States, particularly among those who smoke heavily, has been shown conclusively to be associated with the use of cigarettes.

Although the incidence of cure of cancer has not improved materially over recent years, there is reason to believe that the rate of cure could be improved substantially if there were earlier recognition and more complete reporting of early signs. Success in treatment of many cancerous lesions, such as those of the esophagus, stomach, and lung, awaits better and more sensitive diagnostic aids to detect the lesions in their early stages. In some parts of the body, such as the skin and the cervix, early recognition and prompt treatment of suspicious lesions are possible and often result in permanent cure of early cancerous lesions. The death rate from cancer involving the female genital tract has dropped substantially in the past twenty years, and there is ample evidence that the use of the Papanicolaou test to detect lesions of the cervix before symptoms develop has made early treatment of cancer of the cervix yield a high rate of cure.

Characteristics of tumors

Normal tissue contains large numbers of mature cells of uniform size and shape, each containing a nucleus of uniform size. Within each nucleus are the chromosomes, a specific number for the species, and within each chromosome is *deoxyribonucleic acid* (DNA). DNA is a giant molecule whose chemical composition controls the characteristics of *ribonucleic acid* (RNA), which is found both in the nucleoli of cells and in the cytoplasm of the cell itself, and which regulates cell growth and function. When ovum and sperm unite, the DNA and RNA within the chromosomes of each will govern the differ-

entiation and future course of the trillions of cells that finally develop to form the adult organism. In the development of various organs and parts of the body, cells undergo differentiation in size, appearance, and arrangement, so that the histologist or the pathologist can look at a piece of prepared tissue through a microscope and know the portion of the body from which it came.

A *malignant* cell is one in which the basic structure and activity have become deranged in a manner that is unknown and from a cause or causes that are still poorly understood. It is believed, however, that the basic process involves a disturbance in the regulatory functions of DNA. It is known that the DNA molecule is affected by radiation in certain instances, and it is speculated that it may be affected by other things also.

A characteristic of malignant cells that can be observed through a microscope is a loss of differentiation, or a *likeness* to the original cell (parent tissue) from which the tumor growth originated. This loss of differentiation is called *anaplasia*, and its extent is a determining factor in the degree of malignancy of the tumor. Other characteristics of malignant cells that can be seen through a microscope are the presence of nuclei of various sizes, many of which contain unusually large amounts of chromatin (hyperchromatic cells), and the presence of mitotic figures (cells in the process of division), which denotes rapid and disorderly division of cells. These are some of the criteria used to grade malignant tumors. A Grade I tumor is the *most* differentiated (most like the parent tissue) and therefore the *least* malignant, whereas Grade IV is the least differentiated (unlike parent tissues) and has a high degree of malignancy. These classifications are useful to the doctor in knowing whether or not the tumor may be expected to respond to radiation treatment as well as in planning all other aspects of the patient's treatment. Usually the tumor composed of less well-differentiated cells (highly malignant) responds best to radiation because the immature (malignant) cells are more sensitive to radiation than the normal body cell. For this reason, a tumor can be treated with radiation without destroying normal tissue around it.

Malignant tumors have no enclosing capsule, and thus they invade any adjacent or surrounding tissue, including lymph and blood vessels, through which they may spread to distant parts of the body to set up new tumors (*metastases*). Unless completely removed or destroyed, they tend to recur after treatment, and their continued presence causes death by replacing normal cells and by other means not fully understood.

There is a great deal of difference in the rate of growth of malignant tumors. Occasionally one grows so slowly that it can be removed completely after a long period of time. This characteristic accounts probably for the good results obtained in a few circumstances even when treatment has been delayed. No doctor, however, ever relies upon this possibility to justify delay in treatment. Occasionally a malignant tumor grows slowly for a long time and then undergoes change, and the rate of growth increases enormously.

Cancer was recognized in ancient times by skilled observers who gave it the name cancer (crab) because it stretched out in many directions as the legs of the crab. The term is somewhat general and is used interchangeably with malignant tumor or malignant neoplasm. It denotes a tumor caused by abnormal cell growth. Forms of cancer are found in plants and in other animals as well as in man.

Malignant tumors may arise from any or all of the three embryonal tissues from which all other tissues are formed. These embryonal tissues are as follows: (1) the *ectoderm*, from which arises the skin and the glands within it, and the entire nervous system including the eyes; (2) the *mesoderm*, from which develop the muscles, bones, fat, cartilage, and other connective tissue; and (3) the *entoderm*, from which develop the mucous membrane lining and the cellular elements of the respiratory tract, the gastrointestinal tract, and the genitourin-

Table 8

Types of tumors

Type of cell or tissue	Benign tumor	Malignant tumor
Epithelium		
Skin, outer layers	Papilloma	Squamous cell carcinoma
Skin, pigmented layer (melanoblasts)	Nevus	Malignant melanoma
Glandular epithelium	Adenoma	Adenocarcinoma
Muscle	Myoma	Myosarcoma
Connective tissue		
Fibroblast	Fibroma	Fibrosarcoma
Cartilage	Chondroma	Chondrosarcoma
Bone	Osteoma	Osteosarcoma
Fatty tissue	Lipoma	Liposarcoma
Endothelial tissue		
Blood vessels	Hemangioma	Hemangiosarcoma
Lymph vessels	Lymphangioma	Lymphangiosarcoma
Nerve tissue		
Neuroglia	Astrocytoma	Glioblastoma
Medullary epithelium		Medulloblastoma
Lymphoid and hematopoietic tissue		
Lymphocytes		Lymphosarcoma
		Lymphatic leukemia
Myelocytes		Multiple myeloma
		Myeloid leukemia

ary tract, as well as the cellular elements of other internal organs such as the liver and the spleen.

The term *carcinoma* denotes a malignant tumor of epithelial cells, and the term *sarcoma* denotes a malignant tumor of connective tissue cells. When a malignant tumor contains all three types of embryonal tissue, it is called a *teratoma*.

Benign or nonmalignant tumors are composed of adult or mature cells growing slowly and in an orderly manner within a capsule, not invading surrounding tissues, causing harm only by pressure, remaining localized and not entering the bloodstream. Benign tumors do not recur upon removal and cause death only by their pressure on vital structures within an enclosed cavity such as the cranium.

Tumors derive their names from the types of tissue involved (Table 8), but classification of malignant tumors is difficult since many contain several types of cells and may have benign tissue incorporated within them as well. They are named also for general characteristics of the tumor. The scirrhus carcinoma, for example, is a common malignant tumor developing in the breast and is so named because of the large amount of fibrous connective tissue surrounding the active cells, giving a firmness to the tumor that is detectable when it is palpated.

Research

Although a tremendous amount of money and research effort goes into attempts to learn the cause and true nature of cancer, as yet the cause of the disease is unknown. However, each year more is learned about cell behavior and cell growth, and it is expected that eventually the actual cause of abnormal cell growth probably will be found.

Cancer research workers are active in a variety of fields, and it finally may be shown that several factors act together in the development of abnormal cell growth. Many years ago it was observed that skin cancers developed in men who were employed to sweep the chimneys in English homes in which coal was burned in fireplaces. It was then learned that when the suspected substance (methylcholanthrene)

contained in the sweepings was repeatedly painted on the ears of experimental animals, cancer developed. Then it was noted that this carcinogen was somewhat similar in chemical structure to some of the hormones. This observation led physicians to experiment with removal of the ovaries in women who had cancer of the breast and later to give male hormones to men who had developed cancer of the prostate. Hormone treatment is used at the present time for many forms of cancer in both sexes, and although it does not cure the disease, it sometimes retards the activity of abnormal cell growth to a remarkable degree.

There appears to be a genetic factor involved in the predisposition to develop cancer and in the determination of the part of the body attacked. This factor has been conclusively demonstrated in experimental animals by repeated breeding of mice from cancerous and noncancerous strains. A strain of mice has been developed in which almost all the mice develop breast cancer, an indication that heredity may affect the tendency to develop cancer, although many other factors may be involved. Evidence obtained through animal experimentation does not necessarily prove that human beings react in the same way, but it raises the possibility that they may do so.

The possibility that viruses may contribute to the development of cancer has been raised repeatedly and is undergoing intensive study at the present time. In the animal laboratory it has been demonstrated that some substance in the milk of the mouse from a carcinogenic strain can be transmitted to the young who ingest this milk. In a high proportion of cases, baby mice from a noncarcinogenic strain, put to nurse immediately at the breast of a mouse from a carcinogenic strain, will later develop cancer.

It is believed that certain chemical compounds may have cytotoxic (toxic to cells) effects that contribute to the development of cancer. It is known that certain toxic damage to cells, such as is caused by repeated exposure to substances containing radium, can cause cancer. It is also known that cancer may follow chronic irritation to any part of the body. Examples are cancer of the lip in pipe smokers and cancer of the skin over the bridge of the nose or behind the ears in people who wear glasses.

Prevention and control

Prevention and control of cancer depend largely upon use of present knowledge to avoid those conditions that are known to predispose to the development of the disease, and to educate the public to have thorough periodic physical examinations and to seek attention promptly if any signs of cancer appear. The nurse is important in any program for prevention and control of cancer. Charles S. Cameron, the medical and scientific director of the American Society for the Prevention of Cancer, once said: "If cancer control is to make the progress so urgently called for, the nurse will have to assume more and more responsibility, as a community-minded citizen, for the development of broad cancer education programs among the general public. The success of control measures depends in large measure on developing a public with higher awareness, better understanding, and a more constructive attitude toward the disease."*

Prevention. Sources of chronic irritation that may lead to cancer should be avoided. Effort is being made in industry to protect workers from coal-tar products known to contain carcinogens. Masks and gloves are recommended in some instances, and workers are urged to wash their hands and arms thoroughly to remove all irritating substances at the end of the day's work. Industrial nurses participate in intensive educational programs to help the workers understand the need for carrying out company rules that may help to prevent cancer.

There are many ways to prevent irritation that may lead to cancer. It is possible that cleanliness of the skin is helpful, particularly for persons who live and work in highly industrial environments where the soot content in the air is high. Prolonged exposure to wind, dirt, and sunshine may lead to skin cancer. Skin cancer on the face and hands is particularly frequent among farmers and

cattle ranchers who have fair complexions and who do not protect themselves from exposure.

Any kind of chronic irritation to the skin should be avoided, and moles that are in locations where they may be irritated by clothing should be removed. Shoelaces, shoe tops, girdles, brassieres, and shirt collars are examples of clothing that may be a source of chronic irritation. Glasses, earrings, dental plates, and pipes that are in repeated contact with skin and mucous membrane may contribute to cancer. Chewing food thoroughly is recommended to lessen irritation in the throat and stomach. Cancer in the mouth is sometimes associated with rough jagged teeth and by the constant irritation of tobacco smoke. The habit of drinking scalding hot or freezing cold liquids is thought to be irritating to the mouth and to the esophagus. Indiscriminate use of laxatives is thought to have possible carcinogenic effects upon the large bowel.

Encouraging women to breast-feed their babies, if there are no contraindications, may contribute to the prevention of cancer of the breast. Cancer of the breast is reported to be unknown among Eskimo women and to be relatively rare among Japanese women. Both groups practice breast feeding, and it is believed that this factor may be responsible for the favorable record, although the relationship is still unproved.

There is now no question that excessive smoking is linked with the increased incidence of lung cancer. More and more reports are appearing that incriminate moderate and heavy cigarette smoking as a predisposing factor in the development of lung cancer, which now causes ten times as many deaths each year as it did thirty years ago. In the United States approximately one hundred deaths from cancer of the lung occur each week among men, and it is now believed that more than 75% of these deaths may be definitely attributed to excessive cigarette smoking.[3] An enormous amount of interest and effort is being made by both private and public agencies concerned with the health of the public to alert everyone to the dangers of cigarette smoking. As of January, 1966, federal law requires that all packages containing cigarettes carry a label warning of the danger in their excessive use. The re-

---

*From A cancer source book for nurses, New York, 1950, American Cancer Society, Inc.; reprinted by permission of the American Cancer Society, Inc.

cently organized National Interagency Council on Smoking has prepared educational materials for use by teachers and school administrators. These materials, and films such as *Point of View,* produced by the National Tuberculosis and Health Association, attempt to influence teen-agers not to begin smoking, and to urge teachers to set a good example to schoolchildren by not smoking. Nurses have a responsibility, both as citizens in their communities and in their professional capacity in a hospital or any other agency, to interpret to people of all ages the seriousness of the implications of smoking and should set an example of good health practice by not smoking.

Air pollution caused by smoke, industrial fumes, and exhaust from motor vehicles may also be a contributing factor in the rapidly increasing incidence of cancer of the lung. It is known that air pollution contributes to other respiratory illness (p. 558).

Control. More widespread knowledge of cancer and a more positive attitude toward the disease are essential for the control of the disease. Despite all the public announcements that have been made in the last few decades, there are still people who think of cancer as a disgraceful disease that must be hidden from others. Cancer is talked about in whispers by many people who look upon it as a punishment for past sins, a shameful disease, or a disgrace to the family. This attitude stems partly from the fact that cancer, in its terminal stages, often is a painful and demoralizing disease that is sometimes accompanied by body odor and other signs of physical decay that are deeply etched upon the consciousness of friends and relatives. Actually there is no characteristic odor of cancer, although diseased tissue that breaks down and becomes infected with odor-producing organisms will be as unpleasant as any other infected wound. The essential point—so often missed by the public—is that this tragic situation is by and large an unusual one.

Some people fear cancer and shun persons who have the disease because they believe it is contagious. Scientific speculation on the possibility that a virus may be the cause has added to this fear. At this time there is no conclusive evidence that a virus or any other communicable agent contrib-

utes in any way to the development of cancer.

The positive aspects of cancer should be emphasized. It is estimated that approximately one-third of the persons for whom a diagnosis is made are cured by medical treatment. Another third could perhaps be cured by medical treatment if diagnosed early enough. Only a third, therefore, have cancer occurring in locations in which the disease advances beyond permanent medical aid before sufficient signs appear to warn the patient of trouble. In spite of these facts, however, some patients think it is useless to report symptoms early, since they believe that if they do have cancer, they cannot be cured.

Early signs and symptoms. Everyone should know the seven danger signs of cancer and should report them immediately to his physician: (1) any sore or lesion in the mouth or anywhere else in the body that does not heal within two weeks, (2) a lump or mass in the breast or anywhere else in the body, (3) any unusual bleeding or discharge from any body orifice, (4) any change in size, color, or appearance of a wart or a mole, (5) persistent indigestion or difficulty in swallowing, (6) persistent hoarseness or cough that does not clear up within two weeks, (7) any change in normal bowel habits. It should be emphasized in all health teaching that any of these signs should be investigated medically but also that their occurrence does not necessarily mean that the patient has cancer.

A very common misconception that leads the patient to ignore symptoms is a belief that a disease as serious as cancer must be accompanied by weight loss. Weight loss is usually a late symptom of cancer, yet the patient often remarks, "I wasn't losing weight so I thought nothing serious could be wrong." Another reason for neglect of cancer is that it may not cause pain, and, again, the patient takes the absence of pain as a sign that his indisposition is minor. It must be repeatedly emphasized to the public that pain is not an early sign of cancer and that cancer may be far advanced before pain occurs.

All people should know the most common sites of cancer. In women they are the breast, the uterus (cervix), the skin, and the gastrointestinal tract. (See Table 7.) All women should be taught to examine their breasts each month immediately after the menstrual period. Women past the menopause should designate a day on their calendars regularly for this examination. Such self-examination (Fig. 185) is a much better method of detecting early cancer than is an annual physical examination. (See p. 804 for details of self-examination of the breast.)

Women of all ages should know the importance of reporting any abnormal vaginal bleeding or other discharge occurring between menstrual periods or after the menopause. (See p. 508 for details of early symptoms of cancer of the female reproductive system.)

All women over 35 years of age should have a pelvic examination annually, and a cervical smear should be taken for testing by the Papanicolaou method. The nurse should encourage all women to visit their doctor regularly for this test and to request that the test be done if it has inadvertently been overlooked by the physician. The Papanicolaou test represents an enormous step forward in the early diagnosis of cancer of the cervix. It is also useful in diagnosing cancer in other parts of the body, such as the lungs. The value of the test lies in the fact that abnormal malignant cells that are sloughed off in the early stages of a cancer of the endothelium may be identified from secretions about the lesion. The sloughing of these particular cells usually occurs before the lesion has invaded the deeper structures, and if the test is done early, the cancer may be diagnosed and removed before metastasis occurs.

The most common sites of cancer in men are the skin, lungs, gastrointestinal tract, and prostate gland. All men 40 years of age and over should have an annual physical examination that includes search for diseases in these locations. In many cancer-detection clinics, proctoscopic examinations are done on all men 35 years of age or over because of the high incidence of cancer of the lower bowel in men of this age group.

Facilities for education and care. The nurse needs to teach that there is no quick or certain cure for cancer. Despite all the public education and all efforts of the medical profession to control the extravagant claims of a few unethical practitioners, there are still some people who rely on quick "cure" remedies prescribed by quacks. The best hope for cure of cancer lies in immediate medical attention if danger signs appear. If a person who suspects he has cancer has no private doctor or feels that he cannot afford one, he should report to his local health department and seek referral to a suitable hospital or to a local cancer-detection clinic. The state or local branch of the American Cancer Society will have complete directives on facilities as to location, services available, and financial arrangements.

In dealing with a patient who has delayed seeking early medical treatment, the nurse must give hope and encouragement to him and his family. Sometimes guilt, a feeling of hopelessness, or a fatalistic attitude will cause further delay in pursuing a suggested course of medical diagnosis or treatment.

The nurse should know of sources of information and help for persons who have cancer. There is one large national voluntary organization, the American Cancer Society, Inc.,* which has branches in all states and in eleven major cities. It was organized in 1913 as the National Society for the control of Cancer with the major objective of combating the fear, shame, and ignorance that were outstanding obstacles in the early treatment of the disease. The huge organization, which receives large annual bequests and gifts, has expanded its functions and now has several objectives. It finances research to seek the cause of cancer and to develop better methods of treatment. It publishes booklets and pamphlets for the use of doctors and nurses, and it stimulates better preparation of professional people in the care of patients with cancer by sponsoring institutes and programs for special groups. Information about booklets and pamphlets may be obtained by writing directly to the main office of the Society or to the state or local offices.

In addition, the American Cancer Society has a division known as the Women's Field Army, which strives constantly to educate the public. It works intensively through magazines, women's clubs, insurance com-

---

*Headquarters: 521 W. 57th St., New York, N. Y.

panies, state departments of health, and medical and nursing organizations in an effort to reach all the population with the educational message of how cancer may be prevented and controlled. Through the Women's Field Army, a large amount of literature for the laity is prepared and distributed annually. Also, many excellent films for use in public education are made available.

The American Cancer Society also performs services for patients and their families. Branches in most communities provide assistance for cancer patients who cannot afford to pay for adequate care and for those who, although they can presently afford to pay, will eventually leave their families medically indigent. Depending on how much local support is given to the Society, the services may include dressings, transportation to and from clinics and doctors' offices, special drugs such as expensive hormones, blood, prostheses, and the loan of expensive equipment such as hospital beds. In some communities, homemaking, visiting nurse, and rehabilitation services are also provided. Of the money collected, 60% remains with the local chapter for the community's use. Patients and their families should know about these services before their own resources are depleted, and local citizens should be urged to support the Society generously. Many of these agencies do not use the term cancer in their title so that patients who do not know their diagnosis may be safely referred to them.

In addition to the American Cancer Society, some large cities have other voluntary organizations that serve only cancer patients; for example, Cancer Care, a large voluntary organization in New York City, confines its activities solely to the tremendous needs of patients with advanced cancer and to the needs of their families. The nurse who works in a small community or a rural area may learn of the resources available to cancer patients through her local or state health department.

Lists of available films for both professional and lay use can be obtained from the American Cancer Society and from state and local health departments. Some insurance companies, such as the Metropolitan Life Insurance Company and the John Hancock Insurance Company, prepare very useful pamphlets on control of cancer and the care of persons who have the disease. These pamphlets are useful to nurses in conducting health education programs and in teaching relatives of a patient with cancer how to care for him.

Federal recognition of the need to give intensive assistance to educational programs in cancer was evident in 1926, when Congress proclaimed April of each year as National Cancer Control Month. In 1937 the National Cancer Institute was created within the National Institutes of Health. This Institute, with generous support from the federal government, conducts an extensive program of research in the field of cancer.

General nursing care

A sound personal philosophy and an objective, positive attitude toward the disease based on real knowledge will help the nurse who is caring for the patient with cancer. She should be able to give encouragement, support, and hope to the patient and to his family. Although she should have compassion, she should avoid inspiring false hope. She must try to understand the fears experienced by the patient as he awaits diagnostic procedures or other treatment—fear of hospitals, fear of pain, fear of radical surgery with mutilation, fear of expense that cannot be met, and fear of death, with all that it means to him. In working with the patient, the young and inexperienced nurse should not hesitate to turn to her instructor, head nurse, or supervisor with problems that appear too great for her to handle alone.

A nurse's kindly interest in the patient as an individual often helps him. Many patients must undergo extensive diagnostic examination and surgery in large medical centers a long distance from their homes. Some patients have reported that, although they were confident that they were in "good medical hands," such confidence did not make up for the feeling that they were not always known as individuals. They needed desperately to feel that at least one person knew and understood them as individuals. Some patients experience near panic at the thought of their loved ones' coming to visit and being unable to locate them. The nurse who works with the patient in the community, in the small hospital, or in the doctor's office can help the patient by preparing him for what he may experience in the large center. In most instances it is best for the patient to be accompanied by a relative or a close friend. It should also be recognized that even a patient in familiar surroundings may feel very much alone when awaiting diagnostic tests or surgical treatment for known or suspected cancer.

The nurse should find out whether or not the patient has been told that he has cancer. She should know quite specifically what he knows so that he may not be upset by conflicting impressions. He may receive several different answers to the same questions from doctors, nurses, social workers, physical therapists, and others, or he may receive no answer to his questions. This is one of the most upsetting experiences for patients in today's busy hospitals. It is unfortunate in any situation, but it is doubly so when a threat of cancer hangs over the patient. Some hospitals have partially overcome this problem by having regular meetings of all the members of the professional staff at which the information given to each patient is reviewed by the professional team members. The nursing group taking care of patients with cancer should be careful in their communications with each other and should plan a consistent approach so that the patient's daily care will proceed as swiftly and with as little stress to him as possible.

The emotional climate produced during the period of diagnostic examination and initial treatment is very important in determining whether or not the patient will continue diagnostic examination, treatment, or repeated follow-up care after discharge. The care he receives in the hospital may shape his attitudes toward his disease and may determine whether or not he can return home and either care for himself or be cared for by his family. An important nursing function in care of the patient with cancer is building up his faith in the doctor and in the clinic or the medical center where he receives care. The patient needs to feel certain that everything possible is being done for him and that new measures will be tried if there is any promise of their being helpful.

Members of the medical profession differ in their opinions as to whether or not the patient with cancer should be told the diagnosis. Decision usually depends upon the patient, his family, and the physician. The present trend is toward telling the patient he has cancer, although studies show that fewer than 50% of physicians tell their patients.[28] Many spiritual advisers recommend telling the truth. However, some patients obviously do not want to know the diagnosis. They may ask and then answer their own question negatively. Some do not ask for the diagnosis because they do not wish to have confirmed what they already suspect. Some insist on knowing the diagnosis and are preoccupied with every detail of their progress and treatment in a detached but completely abnormal fashion. Finally, there are some who wish to know the facts and who can accept them in a realistic way. Some physicians prepare the patient over a period of time and tell him the complete truth when they feel it is best to do so. Psychologic reactions depend upon the emotional makeup of the individual and are as varied as man's ability to face stresses and threats throughout life. Since disclosure of the diagnosis lies entirely with the discretion of the doctor, the nurse cannot tell the patient or his family. She can, however, refer to the doctor any questions, misinformation, or apprehensions that the patient or his family have expressed to her. This will often help the doctor to decide what course of action seems best. Any sudden severe depression or expressed thoughts of suicide should be reported at once. Often a patient's fears are communicated to a nurse long before he summons the courage to question the doctor.

The patient needs something to keep him occupied while he is awaiting completion of diagnostic tests and treatment and between steps of treatment such as surgery or x-ray therapy. Usually he fares best in a room with other patients, where there is more going on and less time for introspective thought. Most patients are able to concentrate only on conversation, music, newspapers, and light games at this time. Some patients may like to do work with their hands, such as crocheting, or working with leather. If there is no occupational therapy department from which supplies may be obtained, the nurse may arrange for members of the patient's family to provide them.

The family also needs to keep busy while awaiting the results of diagnostic tests and the outcome of surgery or of other treatment. One woman, upon learning that her husband had far-advanced carcinoma, went home immediately and made his favorite cake, even though he was in the hospital and unable to enjoy it. Psychologic relief may sometimes come from keeping occupied with usual daily activities. Anxious relatives also receive satisfaction from doing things that the patient would do if he could, thus preserving parts of cherished routines. Taking the dog for his daily walk is an example. Members of the family often need direction in their activity when they have just learned that a loved one has cancer. They may need to talk over immediate and long-term plans with someone not close to the family situation. The nurse can sometimes be this listening person. At other times she should refer the family to a social caseworker, who will help them talk through and think through a course of action.

Surgical treatment

The best treatment for cancer at the present time is complete surgical removal of all malignant tissues before metastasis occurs. Surgery must often be extensive and may require adjustment for the patient beyond that needed in many other conditions. The patient with cancer does not have the privilege of electing surgery, as he may in some diseases. This fact alone makes him feel trapped and seriously threatened. He does not have time to accustom himself gradually to the idea of how the surgery may change him and how it may affect his way of life. The patient must often face the prospect of mutilating surgery with only the hope and not the certainty that it will cure the cancer and save his life. He may be more concerned about his family than he is about himself. Obviously he needs sympathy and understanding when he and his family are attempting to accept the news and the immediate surgical treatment that the surgeon recommends. The operative procedures and nursing care for cancer involving the par-

ticular systems are discussed in the appropriate chapters and will not be included here.

Radiation

Ionizing radiation consists of electromagnetic waves or material particles that have sufficient energy to ionize atoms or molecules (that is, remove electrons from them) and thereby alter their chemical behavior.[39] In large-enough amounts it destroys the cells. Radiation is used medically for diagnosis, treatment, and research.

General facts about radiation

Every living thing from the beginning of time has been exposed to small amounts of radiation from the sun and from certain natural elements in the earth, such as uranium, that emit gamma rays in the process of their decay. This is called *natural background radiation*.[39] No problem regarding radiation existed until after 1895, when the roentgen-ray (x-ray) machine was developed and became widely used in diagnosis of disease. The development of this machine was followed by the discovery of radium and the use of both radium and x-rays for treatment of diseases such as cancer. With developments in the field of nuclear energy, it has been possible to produce radioactive isotopes of a number of the elements, although only a few of them, such as gold, cobalt, and phosphorus, have medical application at the present time. The problem of over-exposure and possible harm to patients and to the personnel caring for them has increased greatly with the increased use of x-rays in diagnosis and treatment and the more recent wide use of radioisotopes in diagnosis and treatment. Also, radiation in the environment resulting from atomic testing has become a widely feared and much debated subject in the United States and in many other parts of the world.

No one really knows how much exposure to radiation is safe for persons working with patients and for patients having repeated x-ray films taken for various purposes. Relatively small amounts of exposure have produced serious damage in experimental animals, but man has not lived through enough generations of relatively high exposure for conclusive evidence of safe levels to be obtained. It is reasonable to assume that the less exposure one has the better. This does not mean that a patient receiving radiation treatment should not receive adequate nursing care. There are ways in which the nurse can protect herself from exposure, and most hospitals have procedures and guides for persons who care for patients receiving radioactive materials. The nurse should familiarize herself with the procedures used in the hospital in which she is located.

The ionizing effect of radiation upon the body cells remains, so that exposure is cumulative throughout life. Exposure of the entire body enormously increases the amount of radiation received. For this reason, all of the body except the part being treated is protected from exposure when relatively high doses are given for therapeutic purposes.

The National Committee on Radiation Protection has accepted 5 R (roentgens, or units of measurement) per year as the maximum of exposure considered safe for well people over 18 years of age.[24] The United States National Academy of Sciences and the United Nations have estimated that the average person receives a total of 3 to 5 R from background radiation between birth and 30 years of life. They also estimate that additional exposure for medical and dental work probably doubles this amount in the Western world. The amount of exposure the patient receives from a series of x-ray films taken for diagnostic purposes depends upon the machine used and the technical skill involved. Usually the fluoroscopic examination entails more exposure than the roentgenogram. To prevent excessive exposure with fluoroscopy, the doctor allows time for his own eyes to adapt to the darkened room so that he can then observe the patient with a lower intensity of the machine. The exposure of the average nurse working in a hospital and occasionally assisting a patient while a roentgenogram is taken is almost negligible.

Systemic reactions to excessive radiation exposure are leukopenia, leukemia, and sterility or damage to the reproductive cells. Leukemia is an occupational disease among radiologists, with one study showing that its incidence was nine times higher among radiologists than among other physicians.[24] Because of the increased risk, badges are worn by persons whose daily work exposes them to radiation. The badge, which contains photographic film capable of absorbing radiation, is developed each month. A darkening or blackening of the film indicates excessive exposure. Personnel who are becoming overexposed are removed, at least temporarily, from direct contact with radiation.

Because of the possible danger to the fetus, particularly between the second and sixth weeks of life, roentgenograms are seldom taken on pregnant women at this time. If they must be taken, the lower abdomen is protected carefully. Also, pregnant women usually are not employed in x-ray departments or in caring for patients receiving radioactive materials internally.

If the nurse works where she is exposed to x-rays repeatedly or cares for patients receiving radioactive substances, she must take some responsibility for learning how she may protect herself and others from too much exposure. She should read the patient's chart and should understand fully the kind of treatment he is receiving, and she should then learn, if she does not already know, the behavior of the particular kind of radiation with which she is working.

The radiation used medically consists of alpha, beta, and gamma rays. Alpha and beta rays cannot pass through the skin. Therefore, exposure to them must come from taking them into the body through the mouth by careless handling of drainage or body wastes and by not washing hands thoroughly after touching any materials that may be contaminated. Gamma rays, however, have been found to penetrate several inches of lead, although lead shielding offers a considerable degree of protection. X-rays, which are similar to gamma rays, require lead protection.

Radiation can be delivered to the patient by exposure to rays externally (*external radiation*), either from an x-ray machine or from cobalt-60, which has been made radioactive artificially, or by placing material from which radiation emanates, such as radium, radon seeds, radioactive cobalt (Co^{60}), or radioactive gold (Au[198]), within a body cavity or within the tissues (*sealed internal radiation*). Another way to give internal radiation is to administer radioactive materials intravenously or orally, so that they are distributed throughout the body (*unsealed internal radiation*).

Radiation delivered externally (including x-rays) can do harm to persons working with the patient *only during* the time that the patient is being treated. This is true also of the radiation from some radioactive substances used for other methods of treatment, as will be described later. Patients with internal radiation who emit gamma rays, however, may expose other persons to radiation for varying periods of time, and the time one can be exposed safely to the patient is important in planning care. The time interval required for the radioactive substance to be half dissipated is called its *half-life* (Table 9). This period varies extremely widely, but as the end of the half-life is reached, danger from exposure decreases.

There are three ways by which exposure to radiation can be controlled. These are *time, distance, and shielding*. All emanations are subject to the physical law of *inverse-square*. For example, if a person stands 2

Table 9

Characteristics and uses of some commonly used radioactive agents*

Radiation source	Half-life (where applicable)	Rays emitted	Appearance or form	Method of administration	Source of contamination or exposure (amount depends upon rays emitted, dosage and time, distance and shielding)
X-ray	—	Gamma	Invisible rays	X-ray machine	Rays
Radium	1,600 years	Alpha Beta	In needles, plaques, molds	Interstitial (needles)	Rays
		Gamma		Intracavitary (plaques, molds)	Rays
Radon	4 days	Beta Alpha Gamma (low intensity)	In seeds	Interstitial (seeds)	Rays
Cobalt (Co⁶⁰)	5 years	Gamma Beta	External (cobalt unit)	Machine (tele-therapy)	Rays
			Internal (needles, seeds, molds)	Interstitial (needles, seeds)	Rays
Iodine (I¹³¹)	8.08 days	Beta Gamma (low intensity)	Clear liquid	By mouth	Vomitus Urine Feces Rays (with large dosage)
Phosphorus (P³²)	14 days	Beta	Clear liquid	By mouth, intracavitary, intravenous	Vomitus Cavity drainage
Gold (Au¹⁹⁸)	2.7 days	Beta Gamma	Purple liquid	Intracavitary	Cavity drainage Rays
Iridium (Ir¹⁹²)	74 days	Gamma (low intensity)	In needles, wires, seeds	Interstitial	Rays
Yttrium (Y⁹⁰)	2.7 days	Beta	Encased rods	Interstitial	Rays

*For a more complete list, see National Bureau of Standards: A manual of radioactivity procedures, Washington, D. C., 1961, U. S. Department of Commerce.

feet away from the source of radiation, he receives only one-fourth as much exposure as when standing only 1 foot away. At 4 feet he receives only one-sixteenth of the exposure. Therefore, increasing the distance from the emanations decreases the exposure. When a patient such as an infant must be held for x-ray treatment, the nurse or person who holds him must be careful to keep at arm's length or as far away as possible and to avoid having any part of her body in the direct path of the rays. Lead-lined gloves and a lead apron, which act as a shield to reduce exposure, should be used by anyone who attends patients during x-ray treatment or during examination by fluoroscopy.

Time, distance, and shielding are the three ways by which exposure to radiation can be controlled. When the nurse knows the kind of substance used, the kind and amount of rays it emits, its half-life, and its exact location in the patient and considers these facts in relation to control of exposure, safe and adequate care for the patient can be planned.

Radiotherapy and cancer

Radiotherapy is the term used when forms of radiation are employed in the treatment of disease. Radiotherapy has been used in the treatment of cancer for a little over fifty years, whereas surgery has been used for hundreds of years. The principal radiation agents used are x-ray, which consists of electromagnetic radiation produced by waves of electrical energy traveling at a very high speed, radium, which is a radioactive isotope occurring freely in nature, and the artificially induced radioactive isotopes produced by bombarding the isotopes of elements with highly energized particles in a cyclotron. One of the most useful of these radiation agents is radioactive cobalt (cobalt-60, irradiated cobalt), which is now used in external radiation therapy. Because of its lower cost it is largely replacing radium for sealed internal use.

Radiotherapy is effective in curing cancer in some instances. In other instances it controls the cancer cells for a time. Because it may deter the growth of cancer cells, it may relieve pain even when extension of the disease is such that cure is impossible. Radiotherapy is based upon the known fact that malignant cells are more sensitive to radiation than normal cells. Therapeutic doses of radiotherapy are calculated to destroy or delay the growth of malignant cells without destroying normal tissue.

To many people, radiotherapy and cancer are synonymous. It is natural, then, that the patient may react with panic to news that this treatment is necessary. Sometimes the patient is told that the treatment is necessary "to cure a growth that may become cancerous if not so treated." Often he does not really believe this statement. The nurse should give the patient who is about to receive radiation therapy a chance to talk. She should find out how he feels about the treatment and, if necessary, she should ask the doctor to discuss it further.

Because radiation therapy often causes depression of the hematopoietic system and in turn a low white blood cell count, the patient should be protected from infection. If the patient is at home and receiving treatment on an ambulatory basis, he and his family should be cautioned to avoid persons with upper respiratory or other infections. In the hospital he should never be in the same room with patients who have these conditions. Antibiotic drugs may be ordered by the doctor and given prophylactically both during and following a course of treatment.

External radiotherapy. The patient who is to have x-ray or radioactive cobalt therapy needs explanation so that he will know what to expect before, during, and after the treatment. He may have heard that the treatment causes nausea or skin "burns or irritation." If he asks about these problems, the nurse should explain that with the carefully controlled dosages now given they seldom occur, or she should refer the question to the doctor. Usually patients are not told of these possible complications unless they occur. The nurse's course of action must depend upon her knowledge, her experience, and her judgment. The patient should know that he will be placed on a table in a room by himself and that the equipment, although somewhat similar to what he has probably seen during a routine x-ray examination, will be larger and more complicated. He should know that the radiologist or the radiotherapist will be stationed outside the room, will observe him throughout the treatment, and will communicate with him if he wishes. He must be told how he can assist by remaining in the exact position in which he is placed so that the rays will be correctly directed. He should be told that the treatment will not be painful.

In giving treatment, rays can be directed at the tumor from several different angles so that normal tissue has a minimum of exposure. The areas through which rays pass are known as *ports*. Different ports may be used on different days, or the position may be changed at intervals during a daily treatment so that only a certain amount is given through each of several ports. The patient may be placed on a rotating device such as a rotating chair so that, although the tumor mass receives the full dose of radiation, skin areas receive less exposure.

The patient may be curious as to how many treatments he will receive. It is best not to give a definite answer. Radiation dosages may be difficult to estimate accur-

ately if the growth is deep within the body. Sometimes treatment must be discontinued because of local skin reaction or other reasons. Thus the patient who has been told the number of treatments planned to assure successful recovery may become depressed when treatment is discontinued. The patient also becomes concerned if he learns he is to receive more treatments than were originally planned. If he shows apprehension, the doctor should be notified so that he may give needed reassurance.

Skin preparation for external radiation therapy includes removal of any ointment and dressing and thorough cleansing of the skin. This procedure usually is followed by an alcohol rub. After this preparation, nothing should be used on the skin. The area to be treated is usually outlined by the radiologist at the time of the first treatment. Occasionally a small tattoo mark is used instead of the conspicuous skin markings when treatment is given to exposed parts of the body. Marks must not be washed off until the treatment is completed because they are important guides to the radiologist (Fig. 59). If the patient is ambulatory, he is instructed not to wash the skin in the area being treated or remove the marks.

Fig. 59

When the bath is given, care must be taken not to remove skin markings used to guide the radiologist in giving x-ray treatment.

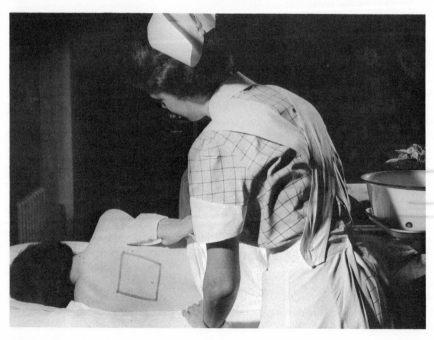

Sponge bathing of other parts of the body must replace showers and tub baths. A vegetable fat or oil may be ordered to protect the affected skin.

Medicated solutions or ointments and even powders that may contain heavy metals such as zinc are not permitted on the skin until the series of treatments is completed because they may increase the dosage. Starch may be used instead of powder.

When treatment is directed toward abdominal organs or any deep tissues, there is almost always some skin reaction. There may be itching, tingling, burning, oozing, or sloughing of the skin. The term "burn" should never be used in referring to this reaction since it implies incorrect dosage. Reddening may occur on or about the tenth day, and the skin may turn a dark plum color after about three weeks. The skin may also become dry and inelastic and may crack easily. Usually, the radiologist should be consulted about the appropriate care. The area may be cleansed gently with sterile mineral oil, but crusts should not be removed. Lanolin or petroleum jelly may be used to protect the area, and healing ointments containing vitamins A and D and healing oils such as codliver oil may be used if breakdown of superficial tissues occurs. Healing usually starts approximately in the fifth week of treatment and should be complete about a month later.

Ointments are best applied by spreading them on a piece of sterile gauze and fastening the gauze to the patient's clothing. If this procedure is not possible, dressings may be bandaged loosely or anchored to good, healthy skin outside and beyond the treatment ports. If tape must be used instead of bandage, cellophane tape should be used instead of adhesive tape because it is less irritating to skin. In removing dressings the greatest care must be taken to pull toward the middle of the area and thus avoid any pull on affected skin. Dressings should be loose to permit circulation of air and to avoid pressure on the skin.

Because the skin exposed to radiation treatment may become irritated and break down easily, it should be protected from constricting clothing or friction of any kind. For example, the patient receiving treatment to the trunk should not wear a girdle, a garter belt, or a constricting trouser or skirt belt during the period of treatment and for several weeks thereafter. During the period of treatment, the patient should avoid excesses of heat and cold to affected skin surfaces. Hot-water bottles and ice caps should not be used, and exposure to the sun should be avoided. Some doctors advise that no water be used on the skin for at least two weeks after the completion of treatment.

If the radiation dosage has been high and blanching or discoloration of the skin has resulted, the doctor may advise the patient to avoid exposure to temperature changes for several years. The patient may have to take much cooler baths or showers than formerly, and he may have to avoid sunbathing or any other extreme of temperature. If x-ray treatment has been given to a woman's face, she must be cautioned regarding the use of cosmetics to cover discolored skin. They may contain heavy, irritating oils and should not be used until the doctor believes they are safe.

When treatment must be given to any part of the head, women patients may ask about the danger of loss of scalp hair and men about loss of beard. Whether or not hair will return after falling out depends upon the amount of radiation received. Specific questions should be referred to the physician. Attractive scarves and wigs are useful for women patients who must receive large doses for palliative purposes, with permanent baldness resulting, or until such time as the normal hair returns.

Gastrointestinal reactions to radiation therapy are more common when treatment includes some part of the gastrointestinal tract or when the ports lie over this system. The patient may have nausea, vomiting, anorexia, malaise, and diarrhea. This difficulty is not discussed with the patient before treatment is started because it is thought that the power of suggestion may contribute to symptoms. However, almost all patients who receive moderate or large doses of radiation have these symptoms in varying degrees. Liver extract, vitamin B, and intravenous solutions of glucose in physiologic solution of sodium chloride are used for nausea, anorexia, and dehydration. Pyridoxine (vitamin B_6), dimenhydrinate

(Dramamine), chlorpromazine (Thorazine), and trimethobenzamide hydrochloride (Tigan) relieve symptoms in some patients. Camphorated tincture of opium (paregoric) may be used to control the diarrhea, but drugs such as bismuth subcarbonate are not given because they contain a heavy metal that will increase radiation dosage.

Many patients find that resting just before meals and lying down immediately after eating help to control nausea and vomiting. Frequent small meals instead of the usual three per day should also be tried. Some patients find that it helps to avoid food for two or three hours before and about two hours after each treatment. Sour beverages and effervescent liquids may also prevent nausea. Usually breakfast is the meal best tolerated. Therefore, it should be substantial, and the patient should be encouraged to eat as much as possible. Problems related to radiation therapy in specific locations are discussed in the appropriate sections of this book.

Internal radiotherapy. Whether or not the patient receiving internal radiation will be isolated and the nursing time with him restricted depends upon the amount of radioactive material used, its location, and the kinds of rays being emitted (Table 9). Special precautions may be taken if more than a tracer-diagnostic dose has been given. The patient may be placed in a single room, and a sign on the door designates him as one who is not permitted to receive visitors. The nurse and all who come in direct contact with the patient for any length of time may wear an isolation gown and rubber gloves and a film badge under the gown to determine the amount of exposure received. Occasionally, no direct contact with the patient is permitted. If so, the patient's room must be equipped with an intercommunication system and all supplies he may need during his isolation. The room should have a window through which the patient can be observed and through which he can see other people. It should have a telephone so that he can talk to family members if he is able and wishes to do so. Food and other items the patient desires or needs usually are passed into the room through a special porthole.

It is important to explain the routine to the patient and the reason for the precautions that are to be taken. He is being kept in his own room for the period of isolation so that danger of contamination to others is minimized and so that his reaction to the radioactive substance can be studied and controlled. He should know that isolation is temporary, and he should be told specifically when restrictions will be removed. The nurse explains to him that she will be available for anything he needs but that she will work quickly while in the room and will remain only long enough to carry out essential nursing activities. She should assist him in notifying relatives and close friends of the time when he cannot receive visitors.

The patient should know how the radioactive substance he takes is eliminated lest he fear that he will be dangerous to other people indefinitely and become panicky about social isolation or about the possibility of harming his loved ones when he returns home. He should have a radio or television in order to keep in contact with outside happenings, and a communication system between the patient's room and the nurses' station helps. The patient needs to see the nurse too, however, and if treatment permits, she should speak to him from the open doorway. If isolation is complete, she should come to the observation window frequently and speak to him via the intercommunication system.

There are many things the nurse can do to add to the patient's physical and emotional comfort during the period of restricted nursing contact. Before treatment is given she should survey the environment. Are the bed and bedside table in the most convenient location for self-help? Can any arrangement be made so that the patient may draw his own blinds or curtains? Are extra covers readily available? Does the patient have reading material and is the lighting adequate and conveniently located? Are plants and flowers receiving care, and is it possible to arrange their location so that the patient may care for them himself if he feels able?

Before treatment requiring a period of precaution or isolation is started, the patient should have a complete bath so that bathing may be omitted for a few days. The bed should be made with clean linen and all personal linen should be fresh. If the patient is very ill and requires help in turning and moving, a turning sheet may be placed under him so that nursing staff can turn him and raise him in bed in a shorter time and with less close contact. Sometimes a laxative or an enema is ordered to obviate the need for an enema or attention to bowel elimination for a few days. If treatment requires lying still in a specified position, measures for comfort should be anticipated. For example, if the patient is receiving treatment to the cervix and must lie on her back, a small pillow should be provided to use against the curve of the back *before* fatigue and discomfort become a major problem. This measure helps to lessen the nursing time needed to massage the patient's back and to assist her with any very slight change of position that may be permitted.

Trips made in haste into the patient's room are disturbing to him psychologically because they imply that he is not acceptable to others. The nurse should list in her mind the things she wishes to observe in the patient, such as toxic signs, fluid intake and output, appetite, and emotional reactions. The nurse who plans thoughtfully might deliver a letter, a telephone message, an ice cap, fresh water, and the newspaper and make her observations in much less time than the one who plans less well and must make several trips into the patient's room. Social isolation for the patient by too infrequent visits to him must be avoided when possible. Brief communication with him from an open doorway is permissable, often to assure him that he has not been forgotten.

Many patients anticipate cure from radioactive isotopes. The nurse can learn what the patient understands about the treatment as she gives care and should report any misunderstandings on his part to the physician.

Sealed internal radiotherapy. Radium, a naturally occurring radioactive isotope, and cobalt and iridium that have been made radioactive artificially, are used to deliver sealed internal radiotherapy to certain malignant lesions that can be expected to respond to this kind of treatment. These radioactive substances may be used in the form of molds, plaques, needles, wires, special applicators, or ribbons that are carefully placed and left

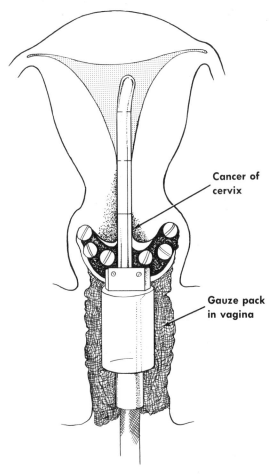

Cancer of cervix

Gauze pack in vagina

Fig. 60

Ernst applicator in place for treatment of cancer of the cervix. Note the gauze packing in the vagina to help maintain the applicator in position.

in position for a specified length of time (Fig. 60). Emanations from the radioactive substances may also be sealed in tiny gold tubes (seeds) and left indefinitely within the tissues into which they are inserted (Fig. 61). The half-life of the seeds is much less than that of the substances from which their emanations came (Table 9). Radium is extremely costly, and its use is being replaced with the use of radioactive cobalt and other radioactive materials.

A fairly common site for the implantation of seeds is the mouth. Plaques and molds

285

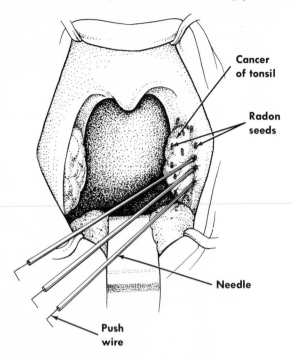

Cancer
of tonsil

Radon
seeds

Needle

Push
wire

Fig. 61

Radium emanations may be sealed in tiny gold
tubes (radon seeds) and left indefinitely within
the tissues into which they are inserted.
This schematic drawing shows insertion into
the tonsil.

also are used for lesions in the mouth. (For
the nursing care of patients having treatment in this location, see p. 627.) Sealed internal radiation also is used widely in
treatment of cancer of the cervix (p. 512).

Safe practice for the nurse caring for a
patient receiving sealed internal radiotherapy depends upon the principles of time,
distance, and shielding. Radioactive materials for sealed internal therapy usually are
kept in a lead-lined container in the radiology department and are inserted into the
patient in the operating room. They should
never be touched with bare hands. When the
nurse handles these products, she should
use a pair of forceps at least 14 inches long
and should hold the radioactive materials at
arm's length and above waist level. A pair of
forceps is usually placed in the patient's
room so that direct handling can be avoided

if the radioactive implant should become
dislodged.

Sealed radioactive material often is reused. Upon removal from a patient the radioactive material should be cleansed and returned to the radiology department in a
lead-lined container at once so that it may be
safe from accidental handling or loss. Even
if it is not to be reused, it is returned in a
lead-lined container. To prevent accidental
loss in cleansing, radioactive material is
cleansed in a basin of water instead of in
an open sink. If a brush must be used, it
must be grasped with forceps so that close
contact with the material is avoided.

Exposure is sometimes termed *external* in
that it can occur only by direct contact with
the encased radioactive substance. It cannot
result from contact with linen, vomitus, or
urine, or from touching the patient. Knowing
where the radioactive material is implanted
helps the nurse to plan activities of care. If,
for example, the substance is in the patient's
mouth, there is less exposure if one stands
toward the foot of the bed. If it is in the
uterus or bladder, standing at the head of
the bed is safer.

Sloughing of tissue and subsequent hemorrhages are complications that must be
considered when radiation is used in any
form. Hemorrhage is not mentioned to the
patient, but if he is ambulatory, he is told
that he should report to the doctor at once
should any sloughing of tissue occur.

Unsealed internal radiation. Unsealed internal radiation is delivered to the patient by
mouth as an "atomic cocktail" or as a liquid
instilled into a body cavity. Exposure for
persons caring for the patient can result
from direct contact with emanations from the
substance in the patient (*external exposure*)
or from contact with the patient's discharges
that contain the radioactive substances (*internal exposure*). It may be inhaled, ingested, or absorbed through the skin. The
exposure varies with each of the substances
used, and safety for the nurse and for other
persons caring for the patient depends upon
a thorough knowledge of the substance used
and its action within the body. Many times,
if only tracer doses (very small amounts) of
radioactive substances are used, as is often
done for diagnostic purposes, no precautions
are necessary.

286

The substance used most often at the present time are radioactive iodine (I^{131}), radioactive phosphorus (P^{32}), and radioactive gold (Au^{198}). None of them cures cancer, but they sometimes control the disease to some extent and lessen pain. They are used in selected cases of cancer along with other forms of treatment, such as surgery and x-ray therapy.

Radioactive iodine is a clear liquid with a half-life of 8.08 days. Originally it was hoped that it might destroy malignant cells in the thyroid gland, but results of its use have been disappointing because malignant thyroid cells do not concentrate iodine as well as normal thyroid cells. Therefore the treatment of the original tumor in the thyroid gland or its areas of metastasis with radioactive iodine is not effective. However, it is often used in conjunction with surgical removal of the thyroid gland. Radioactive iodine is also used extensively in the study and diagnosis of disease of the thyroid and to treat hyperthyroidism. Also, researchers are experimenting with it in other diagnostic tests. Radioactive iodine–tagged albumin has proved useful in locating tumors in the brain, and it is frequently used to determine blood volume.

In diagnostic procedures, a tracer dose of the radioactive iodine either is taken by mouth or is injected intravenously as radioactive iodine–tagged albumin. The scanner (Geiger-Müller counter), an instrument that is very sensitive to radioactivity, is then passed over the body to locate areas that have retained the radioactive substance. The tests may be dependent upon the percentage of the dose picked up (blood volume) or upon the rate of excretion (hyperthyroid studies).

When used for treatment, radioactive iodine is given in larger amounts. Most of the radioactive iodine is eliminated through the kidneys, but small amounts will be present in sputum, vomitus, perspiration, and feces. Special precautions are needed only for the urine, which usually is collected in a lead-lined container. It is transported daily on a special cart to the radioisotope laboratory, where it is stored until it can be disposed of safely. An indwelling catheter may be inserted before the radioactive iodine is given, and it may be released at intervals to drain directly into the container. If the insertion of a catheter is not considered advisable, patients may be instructed to empty their urinal or bedpan directly into the container. It is important that all urine be collected carefully, because it is the quantitative determination of the amount of radioactive substance excreted that determines when the patient may be removed from isolation. The nurse should find out the approved procedure in her hospital to safely care for any urine that may be spilled on the floor accidentally.

No linen or equipment should be removed from the room until it is monitored with a Geiger-Müller counter for contamination. If the isolation gown and linen show contamination, they are placed in a special container labeled "radioactive" and stored in lead containers in the isotope laboratory, or they are burned. Dishes are washed thoroughly and then monitored, or else paper dishes are used and then burned. In some institutions the dishes are sent to the kitchen if the monitor reading is less than 6 milliroentgens (mR) per hour. If the nurse's skin should become contaminated, she should wash it thoroughly with soap and water and monitor it. If contamination remains, washing should be continued until monitoring shows that additional cleansing is not necessary. Because washing is essential to prevent or to lessen contamination, the patient must be in a room that has running water.

When the patient is removed from isolation, all equipment is monitored and carefully scrubbed by attendants who have been instructed in safe methods by persons who are in charge of the administration of the radioactive substance. It is then remonitored. The room is aired until monitoring shows that radioactivity is negligible and that the room is safe for any other patient. Airing takes at least twenty-four hours.

Radioactive phosphorus (P^{32}) is a clear liquid with a half-life of fourteen days. It is used in the treatment of polycythemia vera and leukemia. It may be given intravenously, orally, or directly into a body cavity. Sources of contamination are vomitus and seepage from wounds. There is no danger from external exposure because the beta rays emitted by this substance are absorbed by the patient's body. Vomitus and dressings are placed in a lead-lined container and taken to the radioisotope laboratory for disposal. Care of contaminated equipment and the procedures used when staff members are exposed by contamination on the skin are similar to those described for radioactive iodine contamination.

Radioactive gold (Au[198]) is a purple liquid with a half-life of 2.7 days. It is used largely for treatment of cancer of the lung that has caused effusion into the pleural cavity and for peritoneal ascites due to generalized carcinoma. It is injected into the body cavity, and the patient is turned every fifteen minutes for two hours so that the radioactive gold will be spread evenly within the cavity. In addition to beta rays, the substance emits gamma rays, so that special isolation precautions may be necessary to prevent external exposure.

If a purple stain appears, it indicates that some of the radioactive gold is escaping from the wound or the site of injection. Wearing rubber gloves, the nurse should apply dressings over the site of injection or the seeping wound. Linen that has been in contact with the wound or the site of injection should be placed in a special container clearly marked for care in the isotope laboratory or other facilities provided by the hospital. Dressings and cleansing tissue should be burned immediately or sent for disposal in special containers to the isotope laboratory.

The patient who receives radioactive gold is usually terminally ill. If he dies soon after receiving Au[198], a notation that the patient was receiving radioactive gold immediately before death should be made on a tag, and the tag should be conspicuously placed on the body for the protection of the coroner and the mortician. If the nurse has any questions about precautions that should be taken, the doctor in charge of radioisotopes in the institution should be consulted.

Antineoplastic drugs

The research in drugs for cancer has been disappointing. Although there are several types of drugs used, they have severe limitations and are used largely as palliative measures when metastasis occurs and all other means of treatment have failed. Severe toxic reactions and profound changes in metabolism and in endocrine balance often accompany their use. Most of the drugs used are still experimental. Therefore, the nurse must not only give particular attention to the physical discomforts of the patient but must also be alert for signs of toxicity of the drug being given. If possible, she should find out something about the nature of experimental drugs being given, and she must report toxic signs accurately.

Hormones. It is believed that hormones may determine the time of development or "trigger" the growth of a malignant tumor providing other factors within the cell are present, and it is also believed that they may be necessary for the continued growth of certain tumors of the secondary sexual gland tissues. Attempts to alter the hormonal influences on the tumor consist of either removing the glands producing the hormones (the ovaries, testicles, and adrenal glands) or the endocrine gland controlling their secretion (the pituitary gland), or negating the action of these respective hormones by giving their antagonists. Thus, women who have carcinoma of the breast with metastasis may be given a male hormone such as testosterone, and men having carcinoma of the prostate may be given a female hormone such as stilbestrol. These persons may also be given large doses of hormones of their own sex to prevent stimulation of the pituitary gland and to prevent their own sex glands from producing the hormone.

The antimetabolites. These drugs presumably retard cancer cell growth by interfering with metabolism within the cell. They include the *folic acid antagonists* such as aminopterin and amethopterin (methotrexate), given by mouth for carcinoma of the uterine lining (choriocarcinoma) and the testicle, the *purine analogues* such as 6-mercaptopurine, given by mouth in acute leukemia in childhood, and the *fluorinated pyrimidines* such as 5-fluorouracil, given intravenously for carcinoma of the colon and the ovary. All these drugs are quite toxic and may cause anemia, bone marrow depression, leukopenia, and severe gastrointestinal symptoms.

Alkylating agents. This group of drugs

acts presumably by reacting with certain molecules within the malignant cell and inhibiting its activity and growth. Nitrogen mustard is the most widely used of these preparations, all of which are highly toxic to the gastrointestinal tract and to the hematopioetic system, thereby limiting their usefulness. Others frequently used are triethylenemelamine (TEM), chlorambucil, and dimethanesulfonoxybutane (Myleran). For details of these and newer or related drugs, the nurse should consult recent pharmacology textbooks.

Alkylating agents are given in infusions or perfusions. They all cause local skin reactions, and rubber gloves should be worn by persons preparing and administering them. Care needs to be taken to prevent any of the drugs from coming in contact with the patient's skin. If such an accident occurs, the area should be washed at once with copious amounts of water.

Since the alkylating agents usually cause nausea and vomiting a few hours after injection, mealtime should be planned so that it does not coincide with the height of the reaction. Care to prevent infection, similar to the care discussed under treatment of patients receiving radiation therapy, is often used.

Infusion. The alkylating agents and some of the antimetabolic drugs may be given as an intravenous infusion for their general suppressive effect upon an advanced malignancy. More recently they have been given in this way at the time of surgery for their suppressive effect on any malignant cells that might be released into the circulation or remain at that time. They may also be given by infusion along with radiation therapy in order to hasten or increase its effect.

Perfusion. By means of several variations of a fairly recent procedure known as perfusion, it is now possible to deliver a large dose of one of the alkylating agents directly to a tumor. *Arterial perfusion* differs from the usual intravenous method only in that the drug is introduced under pressure and inserted into an artery flowing directly into the area to be treated. Thus the full strength of the drug reaches the tumor before it enters the general circulation and is distributed throughout the body. Complications to be watched for are hemorrhage from the artery at the site of injection, either during or after the treatment, and renal failure. If a lesion in the head is being treated, temporary baldness may occur on the affected side several weeks after treatment and may be most distressing to the patient. Ulceration of the mouth also occurs and makes frequent mouth care necessary. It may become a real challenge to find enough suitable foods to maintain the patient's nutrition.

In the special technique known as *extracorporeal perfusion,* or *isolation perfusion,* a portion of the body to be treated may be isolated in its blood supply from the rest of the body during the time of treatment. This measure makes it possible to give much larger doses more directly to the tumor than would be tolerated if they were introduced into the general circulation. For example, a tumor of the lower limb can be treated by applying a tourniquet to the upper portion of the thigh. The drug is injected directly into an artery leading to the tumor, and venous blood is removed from the area being treated through a catheter circulated through an oxygenator to provide oxygen, and then returned under pressure to the artery. After the drug has been circulated for the prescribed length of time, the blood in which the drug was circulated may or may not be replaced by a fresh transfusion, depending upon the condition of the patient, the amount of drug used, and its toxicity.

If the tumor to be treated is in the abdomen or lower pelvis, an abdominal operation may be required, and the entire procedure becomes much more difficult. The blood supply to the cancerous area is isolated and blocked from systemic circulation by means of pneumatic tourniquets and clamps to prevent distribution of the drug throughout the body. Catheters are inserted into the artery and vein supplying the area to be treated, and the agent is introduced through the arterial catheter as near to the tumor as possible. The venous catheter is attached to a pump oxygenator that provides for oxygenation of the blood and pumps it back into the arterial system through the arterial catheter. This procedure is essential for tissue viability. (See Fig. 62.) When the treatment is complete and fresh blood has been supplied by transfusion if necessary, the vessels are unclamped,

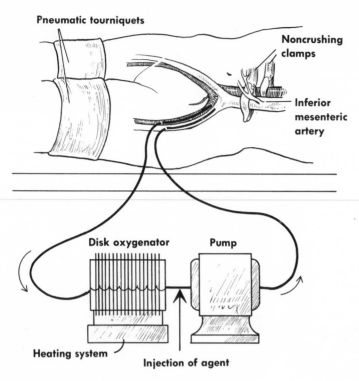

Fig. 62

Extracorporeal perfusion into a pelvic tumor.
(From Sawyer, Janet R.: Nursing care of patients
with urologic diseases, St. Louis, 1963,
The C. V. Mosby Co.)

catheters and tourniquets are removed, and
the surgical wound is closed.

Postoperative concerns are related to the
local tissue tolerance and the amount of
leakage of the agent used. Local tissues can
be permanently damaged, and thrombosis
and phlebitis may occur at or near the sites
of treatment. Reactions of significance appear
as tanning, erythema, or blistering of skin
over tissues that have been perfused. These
reactions resemble toxic reactions to radiation. The toxic effects of leakage may cause
bone marrow depression, and infection such
as septicemia can occur. The general signs of
circulatory disturbance that sometimes occur
after cardiac surgery should be watched for
and reported promptly if they occur (p.
355). Renal function must be checked carefully. Following extracorporeal perfusion of
an extremity, color and warmth of the ex-

tremity must be observed. Pain in the extremity is a danger sign and often indicates
that there has been severe tissue damage.

The patient who undergoes perfusion procedures needs thoughtful care and encouragement. Usually his disease is advanced
and the procedure is only palliative, although
it is done only when there is reasonable assurance that metastasis has not spread
throughout the body. Sometimes the patient
develops lesions elsewhere after the growth
seemed to be controlled satisfactorily by
perfusion.

Care of the patient
with uncontrollable cancer

When all possible surgery and maximum
radiation therapy have failed to control
cancer, the patient and his family have
many special problems. They need encouragement and help in living as normally as
possible, in planning for the late stages of
the patient's illness, and in adjusting to
death and its implications for the family.

Before the nurse can help the patient and
his family, she must have developed a ma-

290

ture philosophy that allows her to accept death as an eventual reality for everyone. This philosophy may not be acquired overnight. Study, reflection, contemplation, experience, and constant effort to enlarge one's perspective all help the nurse to work effectively with the patient and his family in facing the crisis of death. Textbooks in fundamentals of nursing,[15] the many excellent references in these texts, and readings at the end of this chapter may help the nurse develop her own working philosophy about death. Patients of all ages are often quite realistic and accept the probability and even the certainty of death with surprising equanimity. Family members may be less accepting. The nurse should be careful that she does not inject her own uncertainties and failure to accept death into the patient's and his family's thinking.

At the present time there is a great deal of discussion concerning whether or not the patient who has uncontrolled cancer should be told. The feeling is increasing among religious workers, students of social psychology, and psychiatrists that the patient should be told. The statement often made by physicians, "Can the patient stand to know?" may eventually be changed to, "Can the patient stand not to know?" There is evidence that to many persons the uncertainty of not knowing their situation is much more upsetting than knowing the truth. There appears to be no relationship between telling the patient and increase in suicide. In one study the reverse was true.[28]

Despite general feelings on the subject, the final decision to tell or not to tell the patient that he has uncontrollable cancer and is going to die rests with the physician. The majority of physicians still do not tell their patients. One detailed study[28] indicates that their reasons are related much more to their own attitudes and emotional reactions than to facts. The nurse may help by discussing with the doctor the reactions of the patient and the feelings he expresses, but she must acknowledge the physician's final responsibility. It is her responsibility and sometimes her real challenge to accept this situation and work effectively for the ultimate benefit of the patient, within the seeming limitations it may impose.

The patient who knows he has cancer with uncontrollable metastasis often asks about the length of time he may expect to live. Since life is precious to every normal person, it is safe to assume that this question is on every patient's mind even though he may not ask it directly. Although no absolute answer can be given, the doctor can give the best estimate of life expectancy, and such questions should be referred to him. The nurse must know what the doctor tells the patient since the patient may also ask her or mention what the doctor has said, and she should be prepared to clarify misunderstandings. Very occasionally there is a mistake in diagnosis, or the disease is in some way arrested for a long time. If the patient assumes that one of these occurrences may take place in his case, the nurse should not try to help him face probable reality. She must, however, avoid encouraging false hopes. Many patients accept their prognosis philosophically, with the hope that a cure for cancer will be found before their disease is far advanced. Some patients are better able to accept the situation if their religious faith can be strengthened. The nurse must encourage the patient and his family to live each day as fully as possible without looking too far ahead. Sometimes patients with cancer have few symptoms and are able to carry on quite well until shortly before death. It is useless for them to concern themselves with problems that may not arise.

Patients with uncontrollable cancer should resume their regular work if they can possibly do so, for work makes them feel as though they are still an active part of their group and worthy of the approval of others. It was said many centuries ago that employment is man's best physician, and this concept applies particularly to persons whose existence is seriously threatened by cancer. Social activities and all experiences associated with normal family life should be continued whenever possible. There is probably no better service the nurse can give to the patient with uncontrollable cancer than to help him to continue in any way she can. Family members often need guidance in seeing the patient's need to live as normally as possible. Sometimes the patient appears almost unduly concerned with the details of some aspect of his immediate treatment and almost oblivious to his entire problem. Such a patient senses that success with the immediate treatment is his only way to remain up and about or carrying on as well as he is at that time.

The patient with uncontrollable cancer often worries about whether or not he will have severe pain and whether or not such pain can be alleviated. He should know that medical science now has several ways of controlling pain. Hormones, radiation therapy, and a number of analgesic drugs are available and helpful in most instances. Synthetic substitutes for the opiate drugs make it possible to alternate drugs so that their benefit is not lessened by tolerance and so that toxic reactions can be avoided. Members of the patient's family are sometimes told of operations that can be performed if pain becomes too severe to control by other means (p. 915).

The patient may be haunted by fear of brain involvement, loss of mental faculties, and the possibility that he may become completely helpless and dependent upon others. By these fears he expresses one of man's basic wishes—the wish to leave the world with as much dignity as possible. The nurse should urge the patient and his family to discuss such fears with the doctor. The patient may feel that the doctor is too busy and that his questions are too trivial to justify the use of the doctor's time. Such questions, however, are not trivial at all, and a satisfactory answer to them adds tremendously to the patient's peace of mind. Metastasis to the brain in persons who have other metastases is somewhat rare, and some patients suffer more from fear of damage to the brain than is justified. The patient should know that good general hygiene, good nutrition, being up and about for part of each day, and doing deep-breathing exercises with attention to posture all help to prevent helplessness. A positive approach to all problems certainly shortens the time of helplessness and makes the patient more content.

At least half of all deaths from cancer occur in the patient's home. Planning for home care of the patient without completely disrupting the rest of the family takes the concerted efforts of many people. The patient must always be consulted, and his wishes should be respected in the early stages of the disease. In the final stages, he is too ill to be bothered or concerned with making decisions. In the hospital, the doctor, the social worker, and the nurse must work together with the local community nursing agencies, such as the American Cancer Society, to ensure continuity of care from the hospital to the home. The principles governing suitability for home care are similar to those for any patient receiving home care, although the patient with cancer may not live as long as many others with chronic long-term illnesses. The patient must be under medical supervision; it must be possible to give the care he needs in his home, he must want to be home, his family must want him home and be able to assist with care, and the home facilities must be suitable. (For further details on home care, see p. 235.)

References and selected readings*

1 Accident Facts, 1964, Chicago, 1965, National Safety Council.

2 *Alston, Frances, and others: Perfusion, Am. J. Nursing 60:1603-1607, Nov. 1960.

3 American Cancer Society, Inc.: 1966 cancer facts and figures, New York, 1965, American Cancer Society, Inc.

4 *American Cancer Society, Inc.: A cancer source book for nurses, 1963, American Cancer Society, Inc.

5 Barber, John C., King, Hartung, and Mason, Marie Jay: Cancer rates and risks, Washington, D. C., 1964, U. S. Department of Health, Education, and Welfare.

6 *Barckley, Virginia: What can I say to the cancer patient? Nursing Outlook 6:316-318, June 1958.

7 *Best, Nelliana: Radiotherapy and the nurse, Am. J. Nursing 50:140-143, March 1950.

8 *Boeker, Elizabeth H.: Radiation safety, Am. J. Nursing 65:111-116, April 1965.

9 Boyd, William: A textbook of pathology, ed. 7, Philadelphia, 1961, Lea & Febiger.

10 *Donaldson, Sarah H., Fletcher, William S., and Nowak, Patricia Ann: The treatment of cancer by isolation perfusion and nursing care in isolation perfusion, Am. J. Nursing 64:81-88, Aug. 1964.

11 *Downs, Howard S.: The control of vomiting, Am. J. Nursing 66:76-82, Jan. 1966.

12 Ellison, Rose Ruth: Treating cancer with antimetabolites, Am. J. Nursing 62:79-82, Nov. 1962.

13 Fitzpatrick, Genevieve Manfredonia, and Shotkin, Jane McDonald: Pelvic perfusion, Am. J. Nursing 61:79-81, June 1961.

*References preceded by an asterisk are particularly well suited for student reading.

14 *Fox, Jean E.: Reflections on cancer nursing, Am. J. Nursing **66**:1317-1319, June 1966.

15 Fuerst, Elinor, and Wolff, LuVerne: Fundamentals of nursing, ed. 4, Philadelphia, 1964, J. B. Lippincott Co.

16 *Geis, Dorothy P.: Mother's perceptions of care given their dying children, Am. J. Nursing **65**:105-107, Feb. 1965.

17 *Karnofsky, David A.: Cancer quackery: its causes, recognition and prevention, Am. J. Nursing **59**:496-500, April 1959.

18 *Kasley, Virginia: As life ebbs, Am. J. Nursing **48**:170-173, March 1948.

19 *Kautz, Harold D., Storey, Robert H., and Zimmerman, Albert J.: Radioactive drugs, Am. J. Nursing **64**:124-128, Jan. 1964.

20 *Kegeles, S. S., and others: Survey of beliefs about cancer detection and taking Papanicolaou tests, Pub. Health Rep. **80**:815-823, Sept. 1965.

21 *Kyle, Sister M. Willa: The nurse's approach to the patient attempting to adjust to inoperable cancer—effective therapeutic communication in nursing, Clinical Session 8, 1964, American Nurses' Association.

22 Lee, Marjorie Mackay: The nurse in cancer epidemiology, Nursing Outlook **6**:160-162, March 1958.

23 *Levine, Lawrence A.: Intra-arterial chemotherapy, Am. J. Nursing **64**:108-110, March 1964.

24 *Lieben, Jan: The effects of radiation, Nursing Outlook **10**:336-338, May 1962.

25 *Moore, Condict: Smoking and cancer of the mouth, pharynx and larynx, J.A.M.A. **191**:283-286, Jan. 25, 1965.

26 *Moore, George E.: Cancer: 100 different diseases, Am. J. Nursing **66**:749-756, April 1966.

27 Nealon, Thomas F., editor: Management of the patient with cancer, Philadelphia, 1966, W. B. Saunders Co.

28 *Oken, Donald: What to tell cancer patients: a study of medical attitudes, J.A.M.A. **175**:1120-1128, April 1, 1961.

29 Pearson, Olaf H., and Lubic, Ruth Watson: Adrenalectomy and hypophysectomy and nursing care after adrenalectomy and hypophysectomy, Am. J. Nursing **62**:80-86, April 1962.

30 *Regan, Peter F.: The dying patient and his family, J.A.M.A. **192**:82-83, May 24, 1965.

31 *Rhoads, Paul S.: Management of the patient with terminal illness, J.A.M.A. **192**:77-82, May 24, 1965.

32 Robbins, Stanley L.: Textbook of pathology with clinical application, ed. 2, Philadelphia, 1962, W. B. Saunders Co.

33 Sandberg, Avery A., and Yamada, K.: Chromosomes and cancer, CA **15**:58-74, March-April 1965.

34 Tansley, Doris A.: The young wife with choriocarcinoma, technical innovations in health care: Nursing implications, no. 4, New York, 1962, American Nurses' Association.

35 U. S. Department of Commerce, National Bureau of Standards: Safe handling of radioactive materials, handbook 92, Washington, D. C., March 9, 1964.

36 U. S. Department of Health, Education, and Welfare, Communicable Disease Center: Morbidity and mortality, advance report, Jan. 14, 1966.

37 Vanden Bergh, Richard L., and Davidson, Ramona Powell: Let's talk about death, Am. J. Nursing **66**:71-75, Jan. 1966.

38 Warren, Richard, editor: Surgery, Philadelphia, 1963, W. B. Saunders Co.

39 Warren, Shields: Ionizing radiation and medicine, Scient. Am. **201**:154-176, Sept. 1959. (Entire issue devoted to radiation, including articles on what it is, its circulation in the body, and how it affects the cell, evolution, and the whole animal.)

40 *Zaino, Constantino: Eliminating the hazards from radiation, Am. J. Nursing **62**:60-61, April 1962.

15

Nursing in communicable diseases

Study
questions
1 Plan a teaching program to encourage new parents to have their babies receive the recommended immunizations.
2 Plan a teaching program to encourage the public to participate in (a) typhoid immunization, (b) influenza immunization.
3 If you were working in an immunization clinic, what conditions that would contraindicate vaccination against smallpox should you bring to the attention of the doctor? What would contraindicate a person's receiving immunization for influenza? Poliomyelitis? Measles?
4 What is the danger of giving immunizing agents that are prepared from chicken or duck embryos? What question should the patient be asked in order to avoid the possibility of an untoward reaction?
5 What is the danger of giving antibodies in horse serum? What is the procedure that should be followed prior to injecting this type of solution?
6 Active immunization might be described as "giving one a small local infection." Review the signs and symptoms of local infection in various age groups (Chapter 3). Describe to the mother what type of reaction she can expect from a smallpox vaccination of her baby. What type of reaction would her little boy, who is 7 and being revaccinated, be likely to have? How would you explain to the mother why the two children have different reactions to the same inoculation?
7 What are the most common means by which diseases are transferred from one person to another? How are they transferred from animals to man?
8 What are some of the provisions of the sanitary code in your community and of the laws in your state that protect against communicable disease?
9 Look up the characteristics of the agent causing (a) scarlet fever, (b) mumps, (c) hepatitis, (d) malaria, (e) trichinosis, (f) Rocky Mountain spotted fever, (g) ringworm. On the basis of the information, plan the isolation measures, if any, needed to control spread of the disease. Where would you look for the source and how could it be controlled?
10 Assume that there has been an outbreak of food poisoning in a school. What is the most probable source? What measures would help to reduce the possibility of a recurrence?
11 If there was an outbreak of diarrhea in a nursery, what precautions would you take? Why?

A communicable disease is an illness that is caused by an infectious agent *(pathogen)* or its toxic products. The pathogen may be transmitted directly to a susceptible person *(the host)* by an infected person or animal, or it may be transmitted through an intermediate animal host (a vector) or something in the inanimate environment contaminated by it, such as the milk or water supply. The origin of the infectious agent is known as *the source.* In order for disease to occur, the pathogen must be present in the environment and it must be able to be transmitted to a person susceptible to it. It also must be virulent enough to overcome the body's defenses against it. The prevention and control of communicable disease either in an individual or in a community depend upon application of knowledge of the interdependence of the host, the infectious agent, and the environment. Alteration in any one of these factors may cause disease or allow it to occur.

Since the turn of the century, significant changes have occurred in the prevention and control of communicable diseases. Increased knowledge about causative organisms, development of immunizing agents, and more successful treatment with the introduction of antibotics have changed the nature and extent of the problem in many countries, including the United States. However, there are many countries throughout the world where communicable disease still constitutes a major health problem.

The Communicable Disease Center of the United States Public Health Service has classified communicable diseases in the United States into three categories. Category A includes diseases that requires only constant surveillance. Much of the natural history of these diseases is known, and if preventive measures are applied regularly, the diseases occur infrequently and when they do occur, there are control measures for immediate use. This group includes such diseases as cholera and malaria. Category B includes diseases occurring more frequently and requiring more intensive application of preventive measures. This group includes such diseases as brucellosis and tuberculosis. Category C is the largest and most important. In this group of diseases, effective preventive measures still need to be developed. Diseases such as infectious mononucleosis and salmonellosis are included. For the United States there are 50 communicable diseases occurring in these categories: 7 in category A, 11 in category B, and 32 in category C.[18]

Although regional variations in occurrence of communicable disease may be caused by differences in causative factors, perhaps the greatest variation is related to the application of measures for prevention and control. One of the primary objectives of the World Health Organization (WHO) is to improve and standardize measures of disease prevention and control throughout the world. Its Epidemiological Intelligence Service in Geneva, Switzerland, receives immediate notification of outbreaks of communicable disease throughout the world and, therefore, is able to warn countries of impending epidemics (massive outbreaks of disease). It also gives them advice as to control measures. *The Weekly Epidemiological Record* has been published by this group (originally part of the League of Nations) since 1925.

With the increase in speed and amount of travel to all parts of the world, the possibility of the spread of communicable diseases to new areas or to areas presumed safe has become great, and relaxation of surveillance or of application of controls can cause drastic changes in the occurrence of communicable diseases. Thus, the use of measures for the general promotion of health as well as specific methods of prevention and control needs continued emphasis.

Progress in prevention, control, and treatment of communicable diseases has produced changes in nursing responsibilities. Today education of the public about control of communicable disease is a primary responsibility. Not only must the nurse help to ensure that the gains of the past fifty years are maintained by teaching sanitary practices in the home, interpreting community efforts in sanitation, and encouraging immunization against diseases for which this protection is available, but she must interpret to the public new and needed controls and thereby gain support of programs for communicable disease control. This teaching may be done at the bedside of the hospitalized patient, in the clinic, in the school, in the patient's home, or in other community settings and is every nurse's responsibility. The nurse also may direct the investigation of persons suspected of having contracted communicable disease, and of their relatives, friends, or other contacts, and she may care for or teach others to care for persons who are ill with communicable disease.

Principles of communicable disease control

Agents that cause communicable diseases

The agents that cause communicable diseases in man depend, at least partially, on man for the proteins essential for their life cycle and, in the process of obtaining them, produce disease in him (p. 55). These disease-producing agents may be classified as helminths (worms), protozoa, fungi, bacteria, rickettsiae, and viruses. The following is a list (not complete) of diseases produced by specific organisms in each category.

Bacteria

Brucellosis
Chancroid
Cholera
Diarrhea of the newborn
Diphtheria
Gas gangrene
Gonorrhea
Meningococcal meningitis
Pertussis
Plague
Pneumococcal pneumonia
Staphylococcal infections
Streptococcal infections (scarlet fever)
Syphilis
Tetanus
Tuberculosis
Typhoid and paratyphoid fever
Yaws

Rickettsiae

Q fever
Rickettsial pox
Rocky Mountain spotted fever
Typhus

Protozoa

Amebic dysentery
Kala-azar
Malaria
Trichomonas vaginitis

Fungi

Blastomycosis
Candidiasis
Histoplasmosis
Monilial vaginitis
Ringworm
Thrush

Helminths

Filariasis
Hookworm
Pinworm
Schistosomiasis
Tapeworm
Trichinosis

Viruses

Chickenpox
Common cold
Diarrhea of the newborn
Encephalitis
German measles
Hepatitis (infectious and serum)
Herpes zoster
Influenza
Lymphogranuloma venereum
Measles
Mumps
Poliomyelitis
Psittacosis
Rabies
Smallpox
Trachoma
Yellow fever

The nurse should know the communicable diseases that are prevalent in the region in which she works and become thoroughly acquainted with the characteristics of the agents that cause them. This knowledge will guide her in helping with control measures.

Planning for control of the spread of communicable disease

The principles basic to invasion of human beings by pathogens are outlined on p. 55. They should be reviewed in conjunction with this section.

In planning control measures it is important to know about the *physical characteristics* of the agent—that is, whether it can live outside the human body, whether it can remain inactive for periods of time and still exist *(sporeformers)*, whether its activity is seasonal or climatic in nature, whether it requires passage through an intermediary host (*in* which it lives), such as a mosquito, in order to complete its life cycle, and whether it needs an intermediary agent (*on* which it lives), such as a tick, louse, or flea, in order to spread. This information gives clues that will aid in looking for the source of the infectious agent and in determining the appropriate control measures. For example, if the source is environmental, such as water or flies, controls need to be exerted over these factors. However, if the disease is spread by human beings via "droplets" of mucus or via hands, the infected persons must be isolated. Sometimes, in order to control the disease, the original environmental source may need to be eliminated and the infected persons isolated. For example, an outbreak of typhoid fever originating from the milk supply must be controlled in this way.

Knowledge of where the organism obtains its food and reproduces—*its biologic characteristcs*—provides a guide in determining who may be susceptible to attack. Viruses, for instance, feed on deoxyribonucleic acid (DNA), a giant molecule found in the nucleus of living cells, and consequently can live only on healthy cells. Viruses, therefore, rarely complicate diseases that cause tissue breakdown. On the other hand, bacteria can live on cells that are broken down, and bacterial diseases frequently attack tissue that has been damaged already by disease, infection, or trauma. Many infectious organisms can live only on specific tissues or produce disease only after reaching these tissues. Others require specific conditions, such as the absence of oxygen or the passage through an intermediary agent, for reproduction. Some organisms, although they reproduce in man, can be transferred to other people only by a vector. Medical treatment often is based on decreasing the organism's ability to use food. Antibiotic drugs, hyperbaric oxygen, and hypothermia all operate on this principle. If an intermediary host or a vector is essential, elimination of it will bring the disease under control.

If one knows the source of the pathogen and how it gets into the body (*portal of entry*), on what tissue it reproduces, and how it leaves the body (*portal of exit*), necessary isolation procedures or reverse precautions can be used. The purpose of isolation is to prevent the passage of the pathogen causing the communicable disease from infected persons to others. Because individuals can carry infectious organisms in and on their bodies without having disease themselves, it is essential that susceptible people be protected against passage of these organisms to them. This is the purpose of reverse isolation procedures, which are described in detail on p. 61, and it constitutes the basis for health teaching of such measures as handwashing and sanitary procedures related to food, water, sewage, vermin, and insects, such as flies and mosquitoes. Sanitary codes have been established by law to control potential environmental sources of infection, such as food, water, and sewage. The pasteurization of milk and the determination of the bacterial count of public water supplies and swimming facilities are examples of measures required by the codes.

Prevention of the spread of highly virulent organisms is exceedingly important. Knowledge of the *chemical characteristics* of the pathogen gives clues as to its virulence. Organisms that produce toxins usually cause serious disease that is difficult to control because the toxin is spread throughout the body by the bloodstream. Methods of artificial immunization against these organisms are being sought constantly, and as they become available, the public should be urged to use them. Chemical characteristics also influence the viability of the pathogen (its resistance to destruction). Knowledge of this viability is essential for determining adequate decontamination processes.

It would be impractical in a book of this type to try to discuss each communicable disease in relation to its control. The American Public Health Association publishes a manual* containing the facts about the common communicable diseases occurring in the world. It is a valuable addition to every nurse's bookshelf. Because of the rapid reproduction of pathogens, genetic mutations that change the characteristics of the organisms appear rather frequently, and therefore it is important to use current information in the control of communicable disease. Information on any communicable disease found in the world can be obtained from the Epidemiological and Vital Statistics Reports of the World Health Organization.

Whether or not the infectious agent gets

---

*Control of communicable diseases in man, American Public Health Association, 1790 Broadway, New York, N. Y.

a foothold in a new host depends upon the host's response. The organism may not be allowed entrance to the body, or if it enters, it may be overcome by the body's defenses. (See p. 55.) If the majority of the population is unfamiliar with the control of an infectious organism, it may spread from person to person and cause an epidemic.

Immunization

It is sometimes possible and desirable to enhance the body's defenses against disease-producing organisms artificially. This is known as *immunization,* and immunization programs have played and continue to play a primary role in the control of infectious disease throughout the world. The body can be stimulated to produce antibodies against some specific diseases without actually having the disease *(active artificial immunity).* Temporary protection sometimes can be provided by injecting antibodies produced by other persons or other animals into the bloodstream of a human being *(passive artificial immunity).*

Active immunity. Active immunity can be acquired by artificially injecting small numbers of weakened or dead organisms of specific types or modified toxins from the organisms into the body. This procedure is known as *inoculation.* A long-term antigen-antibody response similar to that described on p. 57 is produced without the person's having the infectious disease. This method is highly effective and desirable in preventing infectious disease. If 90% of the population is protected against organisms that require continued passage through human beings in order to reproduce and live, the disease caused by the organism can be virtually eliminated because there are too few susceptible hosts for the organism to thrive. Smallpox has been eliminated from the United States in this way. This type of protection of a group is called *herd immunity.* It is ineffectual, however, against organisms, such as tetanus bacilli, that can exist independently of man, and each person must be immunized to be protected. If the disease is one not prevalent in the environment, such as smallpox in the United States, or is not spread from person to person by direct contact, such as tetanus, the inoculation must be repeated at regular intervals to maintain

protection (p. 299). This inoculation is called a *booster dose,* and usually one-tenth of the original inoculating dose is sufficient.

An inoculation causes a histamine response. Local symptoms of inflammation (redness, tenderness, swelling, and sometimes ulcerations) appear at the site of the injection, and symptoms of widespread tissue involvement (slight febrile reactions, general malaise, and muscle aching) for a day or two are common. The initial inoculation produces delayed symptoms because tissues must become sensitized. There is an accelerated and less severe systemic reaction to subsequent inoculations because antibody production is stimulated at once. The local reaction also is less severe than that following the initial inoculation because the organisms have less opportunity to produce inflammation.

An inoculating substance containing a disease-producing organism is called a *vaccine.* It is produced in the laboratory by exposing the pathogens to heat, cold, chemicals, or repeated cycles of growth to decrease their ability to produce disease while still retaining their ability to stimulate antibody production. Organisms that are not killed but only made less virulent are called *attenuated organisms.* Vaccines for poliomyelitis (Sabin vaccine), rabies (Pasteur treatment), yellow fever, and the new measles vaccine are prepared from organisms that have been weakened by repeated cycles of growth in laboratory animals. The bacilli that cause typhoid, paratyphoid, cholera, plague, whooping cough, and influenza are injected after being killed by heat, as is the Salk vaccine for poliomyelitis. In some cases the body also will manufacture antibodies against a virulent pathogen if it is exposed to a less virulent pathogen with similar characteristics. For instance, an injection of cowpox virus will produce an active immunity against the smallpox virus. The vaccine for tuberculosis (BCG) is made from an attenuated bovine strain of the bacillus. The procedure of introducing vaccine into the body is called *vaccination.*

An inoculating substance containing a modified toxin of a specific pathogen is called a *toxoid.* It is produced in the laboratory by treating the toxin chemically so that its toxicity is decreased but its antibody-producing properties are maintained. Diphtheria toxoid and tetanus toxoid are widely used, and streptococcus and staphylococcus toxoids are available.

Immunization programs. Active artificial immunization now is available against many of the common and virulent bacilli and viruses. Every person should be encouraged to avail himself of the protection advised by health officials in his local area. He also should be advised to keep a permanent record of the date of each immunization.

In the United States, the Public Health Service recommends that all children be immunized against diphtheria, pertussis (whooping cough), tetanus, smallpox, poliomyelitis, and measles. The injections are started when the baby is 3 months old, and 0.5 ml. of DPT, a combination of diphtheria, pertussis, and tetanus vaccines, is given monthly for three months and followed by a reinforcing dose a year later. To be certain of immunity to tetanus, a booster dose of toxoid every three years throughout life is recommended. Then, if an injury is sustained, a booster injection of tetanus toxoid will protect against tetanus. If the injured person has not received a booster dose within five years, he may be given 1,500 to 5,000 units of tetanus antitoxin and 0.5 ml. of fluid tetanus toxoid. (See p. 77 for precautions in giving antitoxin.)

Vaccination against smallpox is done at 6 to 12 months of age. This vaccination should be repeated at least every five years, especially now that rapid travel to all parts of the world has increased the possibility of coming into contact with the smallpox virus.

Immunization against poliomyelitis may be started when the infant is 6 weeks of age or older. Salk vaccine is now rarely used, but the nurse should be familiar with the schedule by which it is given to help parents determine whether their children had a complete course. This is essential for protection. Two injections of Salk vaccine are given one month apart, a third injection seven months later, and a booster dose in a year. Immunization with oral Sabin vaccine is now recommended. To provide maximum protection it should be started two or three months before the "polio season." Trivalent oral vaccine (Orimune), which contains Sabin strains types I, II, and III, is usually given.

Two drops of the vaccine are taken orally either on a cube of sugar, in a small amount of distilled water, or with a spoonful of corn syrup. Two doses are given eight weeks apart, and a booster dose is recommended in two to four years or under threat of an epidemic. In infants the total vaccine series should be repeated at 10 to 12 months of age. Three oral doses of monovalent poliovaccine may be given to infants one to two months apart in the following order: type 1, type 3, and type 2. Approximately one year later a single booster dose of a trivalent preparation is administered.[1,2]

Measles vaccine is not given until the child is 9 months old because antibodies from the mother make it unnecessary. At present the number of injections and the time intervals vary according to the type of vaccine used. Both killed and attenuated forms are available. However, the Schwarz strain, a new one-injection vaccine, is most commonly used.

Immunization to protect against other disease is given on a selective basis; that is, groups with a high risk are immunized. It is highly recommended that because of the ever present dangers of natural or atomic disaster, with the possible contamination of water and food supplies, all people maintain immunity against typhoid and paratyphoid fever. This immunity is initiated by giving three injections of the vaccine at two-week intervals and can be sustained by a biennial booster dose. Because of the prevalence of influenza and its potential of producing death, especially among older persons, United States Public Health Service officials suggest immunization against influenza. Initial protection is obtained by giving two injections of the vaccine two months apart beginning in October or November. Infants and children up to 5 years of age are given three small doses, the first and second doses two weeks apart and a third dose two months later. Yearly booster doses are needed to maintain immunity.

In 1966 the United States Public Health Service announced that a new vaccine against German measles (rubella) had been developed. It is presently being tested for its safety and effectiveness.

Passive immunization. Antibodies produced by other persons or by other animals such as the horse, cow, and rabbit can be introduced into the bloodstream of a person to protect him against attack by a pathogen. This protection is *temporary,* usually lasting only a few weeks, and stimulates no production of antibodies by the recipient. It is called *artificial passive acquired immunity.* Artificial passive immunization is given to a person who has been exposed to a disease and has no natural or artificial active immunity. It usually is given before the disease develops, but it may be given to modify the symptoms of a disease. However, for effectiveness after the disease has developed, it must be administered early, before extensive damage to body tissues has occurred. Passive immunization usually is reserved for situations in which the disease would be detrimental to the person. For example it is rarely given to prevent a disease such as chickenpox or mumps in children because they are at an optimum age for the body to produce antibodies with minimal histamine response. On the other hand, an adult exposed to the same disease often would be given antibodies because adults may have a severe histamine response. Immunization is given to all age groups exposed to pathogens that cause serious diseases such as hepatitis, poliomyelitis, diphtheria, tetanus, or rabies. Antivenins, which are given to people bitten by poisonous snakes or black widow spiders, also are passive immunologic products.

Products used for passive immunization may be specific to the disease. Antitoxins and immune animal and human serums are examples. The whole blood of a patient who has recently recovered from a disease against which antibodies are produced also may be used. Antitoxins are available for diphtheria, tetanus, botulism, gas gangrene, and the venom of snakes. Immune animal serum is available against the *Haemophilus influenzae* virus and rabies; human immune serum is available for mumps, measles, pertussis, poliomyelitis, and tetanus.

Gamma globulin, or immune serum globulin (pooled serum), is widely used in an effort to produce temporary immunity in persons who have been exposed to communicable diseases for which no substance containing specific antibodies or antitoxin is available. The serum globulin from many donors is pooled to produce the gamma globulin used. The rationale is that someone among the donors will have had the diseases and will have developed antibodies against them. The globulin fraction of the plasma is believed to carry the antibodies, and because it is known not to transmit the virus of hepatitis, it is considered safe to use. Gamma globulin may be given to children who have been exposed to scarlet fever; however, it is usually given to children exposed to poliomyelitis or measles and not immunized against these diseases, since it tends to make the disease less severe. It also is given at the same time as one of the live virus vaccines for measles (the Edmonston strain) to lessen the severity of reaction to the vaccine. It may be given to people who have been exposed to infectious hepatitis, and it is given to men who have been exposed to mumps, in an effort to prevent the complication orchitis (inflammation of the testicle). It also should be given to women who have been exposed to German measles in the first trimester of pregnancy because this disease is known to cause congenital anomalies during the first three months of fetal development. However, a new specific active immunizing substance has recently become available, and it is hoped that the substance will be safe and effective in immunizing women of the childbearing age, as well as children, against German measles.

The nurse's responsibility in immunization. Probably the greatest responsibility of the nurse in immunization programs is to teach the public the advantages of immunization and encourage widespread participation in programs recommended by the local public health officer. A survey of the United States in September, 1963, revealed that 60% of children from 1 to 4 years of age had not completed diphtheria-pertussis-tetanus immunization; 40% had not been vaccinated against smallpox; and 32% had not received adequate immunization against poliomyelitis, although immunization almost always is available free of charge.[24] In teaching it is advisable to provide the public with the following information: against what disease protection is being given, why immunization is desirable, and when booster doses should be obtained. The relative safety of the immunization and the advantages of immunization early in life should be stressed.

The nurse is responsible for screening patients prior to immunization because there are some contraindications to receiving certain immunizing substances. Those that are prepared in chicken or duck embryos may cause an allergic reaction in persons who already are allergic to eggs. Many people are allergic to horse serum, and substances containing horse serum, such as tetanus antitoxin, should never be given unless a small amount of the substance has been injected intradermally (a sensitivity test) and after twenty minutes produces no "hive" reaction about the injection site (p. 77). It is inadvisable to give a smallpox vaccination to any child at the time he or any of his brothers or sisters have an open skin lesion because there is danger of accidental infection of the other lesions, causing vaccinia, the disease produced by cowpox virus. Active immunologic products should not be given while a person has a cold or other infection because the histaminic reaction from the immunization will be greater than usual. Children with histories of allergy often are not given routine immunization against diseases for which there is herd immunity, because the danger of severe allergic response to the immunization is greater than the danger of contracting the disease. These children should be immunized against diseases such as tetanus, however, and immunization is achieved by giving the vaccine or toxoid in tiny doses over a period of several weeks or months. The package inserts accompanying the immunologic product should always be read carefully to determine the indications, precautions, and side effects.

Before the person leaves the clinic, he or his family should be instructed as to the expected effects and told to contact his doctor or to report to a hospital emergency room if any other symptoms develop. He should be cautioned not to scratch any lesion produced by an inoculation. If a severe local reaction, with redness, swelling, and tenderness occurs, the doctor may order the application of hot, wet dressings. If the lesion is open, these dressings should be sterile.

When antitoxins, antiserums, or antivenins are given, the patient should be kept under observation for twenty to thirty minutes. Symptoms of severe allergic response (p. 77) usually will appear within that period of time.

Controlling contact with communicable disease

Communicable disease sometimes can be controlled by limiting the contacts of infected persons with others and by identifying potential susceptible hosts so that they can be protected prophylactically. The nurse often is called upon to help with this measure.

All patients with known infection should be isolated as necessary to decrease the possibility of their infecting others. When there is a known epidemic of airborne disease, such as influenza, scarlet fever, or poliomyelitis, health officials may close public meeting places such as schools and theaters in an attempt to minimize the spread of the disease by persons who are in the incubation stage. The nurse often must interpret this restriction to the public and try to gain their cooperation. Without it, groups may continue to gather, and spread of the disease will not be halted. During this period the public also should be urged to practice good general hygiene in relation to rest, food, exercise, and fresh air so that optimum resistance to infection is maintained. Keeping rooms well ventilated and with air moderately humid and avoiding chilling also may deter invasion by airborne pathogens.

Sometimes an infected person has a serious communicable disease such as tuberculosis or syphilis that he may have transmitted to persons with whom he has been in close contact. To ensure that these persons (the *contacts*) receive early and adequate treatment, and to prevent their infecting others, the nurse may be asked to help trace them and encourage them to seek medical attention. This procedure, requiring the utmost tact, is described on p. 528.

Mass screening often is done to identify groups that have a high risk of contracting diseases such as scarlet fever, diphtheria, and tuberculosis because they have no resistance to the disease-producing organism. The *Schick test* is done to detect susceptibility to diphtheria, and the *Dick test* is done to detect susceptibility to scarlet fever. A prescribed amount of toxoid is given intradermally on the forearm. A positive reaction (a red, indurated area at the site of injection appearing in twenty-four to forty-eight hours and lasting four or five days) to either of these tests indicates susceptibility to the disease. Artificial active immunization should be given to persons with a positive Schick test, and persons with a positive Dick test should try to avoid contact with people who have scarlet fever. If they become exposed, they should seek medical attention at once. Usually antibiotics are given. The *tuberculin test* can be done by various techniques. A positive reaction to this test indicates that the person at some time has had contact with the tubercle bacillus, but it does not indicate that he has had active tuberculosis. However, positive reactions in children under the age of 2 years usually indicate active disease. (See p. 549 for a complete discussion of this test, the prophylactic measures used for persons whose reaction is negative, and the further screening of those who have positive reactions.) The nurse working in the community often is asked to teach the public about the need for this type of screening, and the public health nurse frequently is responsible for scheduling screening clinics in her community at regular intervals. The nurse may read and record the test results, and she is responsible for directing persons who need further treatment or follow-up to the proper facilities and for explaining the need for this continued care to them.

Nursing the patient with a communicable disease

General care. In general the nursing care of a patient with a communicable disease is the same as that needed by anyone with a generalized infection (p. 65). Rashes and skin lesions frequently accompany such childhood diseases as measles, chickenpox, and scarlet fever. Care of wounds, which may be involved, is described on p. 67.

Isolation. The patient with a communicable disease may require medical aseptic techniques (*isolation*). In planning care, therefore, the nurse first needs to determine the characteristics of the pathogen with which she is dealing to determine whether or not the patient needs to be isolated and, if so,

what type of isolation is needed. The determining factor is the method by which the pathogen is spread from person to person. A patient with tetanus, for example, need not be isolated because the organism can be passed to others only by injection deep into a wound. On the other hand, aseptic precautions must be used with a patient who has gas gangrene as long as the wound is draining, because the pathogen is in the drainage and can be transferred by the hands, clothing, and bedding to other patients with wounds or to personnel who may have breaks on the skin of their hands or elsewhere.

Any patient who is isolated for a communicable disease should have his own thermometer. If the disease is one such as infectious hepatitis, in which safe terminal disinfection of the thermometer is not possible, it should be discarded when no longer needed for the patient. If the pathogen is spread by urine, feces, sputum, vomitus, or wound drainage, gown protection is needed by persons in close contact with the patient. Food trays and linen should be isolated. The hands should be protected with gloves if the organism is the type that enters the body through a break in the skin (for example, the bacteria that cause gas gangrene). If the organism is passed in the excreta, precautions may need to be taken in disposing of it. With most urban sewage disposal, no disinfection is needed. Occasionally, the excreta must be placed in containers containing chlorinated lime for twenty-four hours before disposal in common facilities. The local health officer can be consulted about the adequacy of sewage disposal. Contaminated dressings should be burned at once. Disposable containers should be used for sputum, and the container, all tissues, and solid food waste should be wrapped securely and burned. If the organism is passed through blood, all needles and syringes used for parenteral injections, such as hypodermics and venipunctures, and all razors should be autoclaved immediately after use. Preferably, disposable equipment should be used; and discarded in closed containers. All of the equipment in the room must be terminally disinfected and then cleaned before being used for others.

If the disease is caused by airborne pathogens, as in scarlet fever or measles, the door of the room must be kept closed and the room well ventilated. All persons entering for any reason should wear a cap to cover their hair, a dry, double-thickness, muslin face mask, and a protective gown. A mask made of six layers of 42 by 42 mesh or the new 3 M disposable mask, made of nonwoven fabric, and preshaped to fit well against the face but not touching the nose or mouth, may also be used.[20] All material that has been in the room is treated as isolated.

If the pathogen is spread by "droplets" or sputum, as in pneumonia, the patient sometimes is taught simply to turn his head and cover his nose and mouth when he coughs. Persons attending him do not wear masks, which allows the patient to see the face of persons in his room, perhaps making him feel less isolated. However, anyone in close contact with the patient, doing such tasks as bathing him or making his bed, should wear a protective gown (Fig. 63). The room should be kept well ventilated. A room that has an air conditioner with a filter is desirable.[20] All food trays and linen are isolated, and terminal disinfection of all equipment is necessary.

If the pathogen is found in excreta or drainage and can be passed to others by food or through open wounds, flies that might transmit the infection to others must be prevented from entering or leaving the patient's room. If the pathogen must pass through a vector in order to complete its life cycle and be transmitted to human beings, as, for example, the pathogen that causes malaria passing through the anopheles mosquito, then protecting the patient with mosquito netting is the only precaution needed—and this only if he is in an area where there are anopheles mosquitoes.

In caring for any patient with a communicable disease requiring isolation, careful and thorough hand washing after any contact with the patient or the equipment in his room is mandatory. (For special techniques of isolation procedure, see fundamentals of nursing texts.)

Prevention of complications. Many of the communicable diseases commonly prevalent today are caused by viruses. Special care should be taken to protect patients with

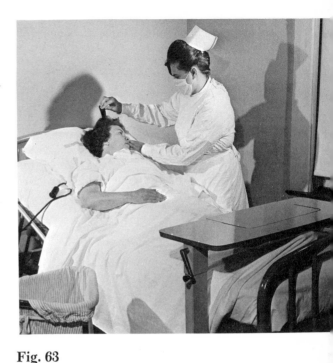

Fig. 63

When giving direct care to the patient who is on medical isolation, the nurse wears an isolation gown and often a mask.

viral diseases from exposure to bacteria, because cells damaged by viral infection invite bacterial invasion. Because bacterial complications frequently accompany viral diseases, and because bacteria are prevalent in hospitals, doctors may prefer to treat patients with viral diseases at home. Antibiotics may be given prophylactically in an attempt to prevent serious complications from occurring. Ear infections, meningitis, and encephalitis of bacterial origin are common complications of measles, and staphylococcal pneumonia is a common sequela of viral influenza.

Toxin-producing bacterial diseases, such as streptococcal sore throat, scarlet fever, rheumatic fever, and diphtheria, frequently cause serious secondary disease of the heart or kidneys. Patients with these diseases usually are given antibiotics and are kept relatively quiet until the blood sedimentation rate returns to normal.

Home care. Unless the pathogen is highly

contagious, patients with communicable diseases frequently are cared for at home. The public health nurse often is asked to teach the mother or some other family member how to care for the patient and how to protect herself and other family members; other nurses may be consulted by friends and neighbors about protection. The same principles apply in the home as in the hospital. A smock or coverall may be used to protect the clothes, and a mask can be improvised from any closely woven, absorbable white material, or disposable ones can be bought at a pharmacy. All liquid wastes can be flushed down the toilet. Garbage and other wastes from the room should be burned. Dishes should be boiled for ten minutes before washing. If the laundry must be isolated, it can be boiled for ten minutes and then washed. When the patient has recovered, the room should be thoroughly aired. Depending upon the type of illness, the walls, floor, and furniture may need to be washed well with a detergent or disinfectant and warm water. If materials that cannot be washed, such as books and toys, have been contaminated, leaving them in the sun and air for twenty-four to forty-eight hours usually provides sufficient protection.

References and selected readings*

1 *Ager, Ernest A.: Current concepts in immunization, Am. J. Nursing 66:2004-2011, Sept. 1966.

2 American Academy of Pediatrics: Report of the committee on the control of infectious diseases, ed. 14, Evanston, Ill., 1964, American Academy of Pediatrics, Inc.

3 Anderson, Gaylord W., Arnstein, Margaret G., and Lester, Mary R.: Communicable disease control, ed. 4, New York, 1962, The Macmillan Co.

4 *Benenson, Abram S.: Why does smallpox still exist? Am. J. Nursing 62:77-79, Sept. 1962.

5 Benson, Margaret E.: Handwashing—an important part of medical asepsis, Am. J. Nursing 57:1136-1139, Sept. 1957.

6 *Carroll, L. Dorothy: Problems in acute communicable disease control, Nursing Outlook 2:593-595, Nov. 1954.

7 Control of communicable disease in man, ed. 10, New York, 1965, The American Public Health Association.

8 Cramblett, Henry G., and Crews, Jeanette: The current status of influenza vaccine, Am. J. Nursing 63:78-80, Oct. 1963.

9 Douglas, Gordon W.: Rubella in pregnancy, Am. J. Nursing 66:2664-2666, Dec. 1966.

10 DuBois, Rene J.: Bacterial and mycotic infections of man, ed. 4, Philadelphia, 1965, J. B. Lippincott Co.

11 *Fighting disease—the work of WHO, Dobbs Ferry, N. Y., 1962, Oceana Publications, Inc.

12 Gell, P. G. H., and Combs, R. R. A., editors: Clinical aspects of immunology, Philadelphia, 1963, F. A. Davis Co.

13 *Getting, Vlado A., Food-borne diseases, Nursing Outlook 2:364-367, July 1954.

14 Horsfall, Frank L., and Tamm, Igor: Viral and rickettsial infections of man, ed. 4, Philadelphia, 1965, J. B. Lippincott Co.

15 *International quarantine, World Health, p. 24, Feb. 1964.

16 Kempe, C. Henry, and Benenson, Abram S.: Smallpox immunization in the United States, J.A.M.A. 194:161-166, Oct. 11, 1965.

17 *Krugman, Saul: Rubella: new light on an old disease, J. Pediat. 67:159-161, Aug. 1965.

18 Leavell, Hugh Rodman, and Clark, E. Gurney: Preventive medicine for the doctor in his community, ed. 3, New York, 1965, McGraw-Hill Book Co.

19 *Lefson, Eleanor, Lentz, Josephine, and Gilbertson, Evelyn: Contact interviews and the nurse interviewer, Nursing Outlook 10:728-730, Nov. 1962.

20 Ripley, Richard L., and O'Grady, Francis: Airborne infection, New York, 1961, The Macmillan Co.

21 *Rogers, Fred B., editor: Studies in epidemiology, New York, 1965, G. P. Putnam's Sons.

22 *Roueche, Berton: Eleven blue men, New York, 1953, Berkley Publishing Corp.

23 Scinchetti, Lea A.: Immunological agents, ed. 2, 1965, Skyline Publishers, Inc.

24 Statistical abstract of the United States, 86th annual edition, Washington, D. C., 1965, U. S. Government Printing Office.

25 *Steele, James H., and Carroll, L. Dorothy: Animal diseases transmissible to man, Nursing Outlook 4:156-161, March 1956.

26 *Steele, James H., and Lester, Mary R.: Rabies and rabies control, Am. J. Nursing 58:531-536, April 1958.

27 *Telfer, James: Communicable disease—challenge from abroad, Nursing Outlook 12:50-53, Sept. 1964.

28 Top, Franklin H.: Communicable and infectious diseases, ed. 5, St. Louis, 1964, The C. V. Mosby Co.

29 World almanac and book of facts for 1965, New York, 1965, New York World-Telegram & The Sun.

30 World Health Organization: International sanitary regulations, ed. 2, Geneva, Switzerland, 1961.

*References preceded by an asterisk are particularly well suited for student reading.

Nursing related to specific medical and surgical care

16

The patient
with
cardiac disease

Study questions 1 Diagram the main chambers of the heart and the adjacent blood vessels. Trace the flow of blood through these structures, and review the normal physiology of the cardiovascular system.
2 What drugs improve, regulate, or stimulate heart action? How are these administered?
3 What is the normal daily intake of sodium chloride. What common foods are high in salt content?
4 Review the nursing care needed by a patient receiving oxygen.

More people in the United States are affected, directly or indirectly, by cardiac disease than by any other illness. It is difficult to determine the exact prevalence of cardiac disease (and the associated vascular conditions such as cerebrovascular disease and peripheral vascular disease) in a community or in the entire country. Diagnostic techniques have not yet been developed that can be used in mass screening for all types of cardiovascular disease. Many persons do not know that they have heart disease until severe symptoms develop.

In 1964, out of a total 1,798,051 deaths in the United States, more than half of them, or 973,182, were caused by cardiovascular diseases and 699,861 by heart disease.[65] Cardiovascular diseases cause more deaths than all other causes combined. Thus, at the present time it can be safely predicted that unless some remarkable events occur to change the present trend, at least one out of every two persons alive in the country today will die of cardiovascular disease.

Deaths caused by cardiac disease vary with age. Congenital malformations of the heart and closely related vascular system are the cause of over 90% of the deaths from these causes in children under 5 years of age, and of more than one-third of persons 5 to 24 years of age. By far the most common

307

cause of death from heart disease after the age of 25 years is ischemic heart disease (coronary artery disease).

Despite some advances in prevention and treatment, the incidence of heart disease continues to be high. Approximately 10 million persons in the United States, including 500,000 children, have heart disease.[58] Most of the advances in treatment deal with amelioration of heart disease and not with removal of its causes.[63] Research efforts continue in attempts to find effective drugs, but results from use of the drugs now available have not always been beneficial over long periods of time. For example, widespread use of antibiotics has produced drug-resistant strains of bacteria and drug-resistant persons. Drugs used to lower the cholesterol levels in the blood, and perhaps reduce the incidence of coronary artery thrombosis thereby, are not wholly satisfactory, and some new drugs that produce vasodilation in animal studies have not proved helpful to man. Heart surgery is publicized widely and is valuable treatment at times, but at present it is practicable in less than 1% of all patients with heart disease.[58]

Prevention

Although at this time a "cure" is not usually possible for patients with heart disease, development of the disease can be prevented in many persons, and many of those who have heart disease can be helped to live happy, useful, and long lives. Immunization against acute infectious diseases such as diphtheria, scarlet fever, and measles and control of infections through selectively used antibiotics have contributed much to the decreased incidence of infectious complications such as pericarditis, endocarditis, and myocarditis. The incidence of syphilitic aortitis has decreased due to early case findings and prompt treatment. State health departments now provide physicians with gamma globulin for women in the first trimester of pregnancy who have been exposed to German measles in an effort to prevent congenital heart disease or other malformation of their babies. Immunization against German measles may soon be possible since a vaccine has been developed that appears to be effective.[20]

Since streptococcal infections are frequently complicated by rheumatic fever with heart involvement, educational programs stressing the importance of early and adequate treatment of these infections have been directed at the medical professions and the general public. The incidence of rheumatic heart disease is being decreased markedly by vigorous educational and prophylactic programs. Through the joint efforts of local heart associations and local health departments, penicillin for prophylactic use has been made available at a reasonable cost to families who have children with rheumatic heart disease. Since dental extractions and surgery may activate a bacterial infection in the heart, efforts have been made by dentists and surgeons to prevent bacterial endocarditis in persons with known diseases of the heart. Antibiotics are usually given prophylactically before and following surgery.

Unfortunately, at the present time there are no certain measures that can be taken to prevent ischemic heart disease (coronary artery disease), which is by far the most prevalent disease of the heart in the United States today. Some measures that may possibly prove to be preventive in the future are discussed later in this chapter.

Research in prevention

Although the causes of many types of heart disease are not yet known, extensive epidemiologic studies and research are being carried on currently in an attempt to determine preventive measures. Organizations such as the American Heart Association are financing research to uncover further information on the causes of heart disease and to develop new methods for its treatment. As part of the National Institutes of Health, supported by the federal government and under the United States Public Health Service, the National Heart Institute is conducting an intensive study on the cause, control, and treatment of heart disease. Vital statistics are being studied carefully in an attempt to discover whether such factors as sex, occupation, constitutional makeup, ethnologic background, or dietary patterns are associated with certain types of heart disease. Grants have been made to study the effects of new drugs on the heart, to perfect techniques that will make cardiac surgery possible for more patients, and to study the mechanisms by which heart diseases affect the tissues. Future studies of many people in their own home and community setting, to learn how diet, living practices, and many other aspects of living affect heart disease, will require the help of nurses who are particularly skilled in working with people.

The report of the President's Commission on Heart Disease, Cancer, and Stroke points out the need for research and education in these areas and the need for health services by patients with these conditions. It recommends the establishment of a national network of regional centers for research, teaching, and patient care. Certain phases of the program are now before Congress in the form of legislative proposals.[40]

The nurse in prevention. The informed nurse can play an important part in public education concerning heart disease, in the prevention of heart diseases, and in case finding. She is often in a position to observe symptoms that may be significant in the detection of heart disease, or she may pick up clues of significant symptoms from details of family history. Frequently, it is the alert nurse who can help persons with undiagnosed heart disease to obtain medical attention.

A fatalistic attitude about heart disease and a conviction that nothing can be done about heart attacks, which "just happen," prevent many persons from reporting early signs of heart disease to their physicians. Since early medical treatment could often prevent or delay progress of the condition, this is doubly unfortunate. Persons who are unfamiliar with the symptoms often ignore them or attribute them to some other cause. Nurses can help to prevent the development of serious heart disease by teaching the public the early signs of possible heart disease and by urging prompt referral to physicians when they occur. For example, attacks of shortness of breath or unexpected dyspnea on exertion, feeling of pressure in the chest, awakening in the night with consciousness of heart action or distress, and discomfort resembling indigestion that is relieved by sitting up are reasons to see a doctor even though the cause may be found to be trivial.

Most persons have read magazine articles about anginal attacks with pain. They should be taught that pain is *not* a common sign of coronary artery disease. Dyspnea and signs of cardiac decompensation are much more often found. Many elderly persons hesitate to report symptoms because they believe that nothing can be done for them because of their age. Again, this idea is very seldom accurate. A friendly interest on the part of the nurse and her assurance that medical care can be helpful will often lead them to seek medical treatment. By working closely with the parents of children with rheumatic disease, nurses can help them to care for the children and encourage them to cooperate with medical follow-up and with long-term programs for prevention of recurrences.

The nurse can also offer counsel that may prevent cardiac complications as a result of other illness or of a variety of other causes. For instance, she should impress upon parents the importance of seeking medical care for children with diseased tonsils and carious teeth. She can advise parents to have children immunized against infectious diseases. She can encourage people with infectious disease to stay in bed and to have medical care. She can encourage people to have an ECG as part of their physical examination, when the physician suggests one. She herself should set an example of good hygienic practices by avoiding undue mental strain, obesity, and lowered resistance due to poor dietary habits, lack of rest, and irregular patterns of living.

The nurse needs to understand the many fears to which patients and families might be subject, so that she is able to help them to a clearer understanding of the positive aspects of the situation. One of the biggest problems to be met in educating the public on heart disease is overcoming fear. Awareness of the fact that the heart is necessary to life makes most people view heart disease differently from diseases of such organs as the kidneys or the liver. Much of the publicizing of heart disease from magazine articles, television programs, and films depicts the fatality more than the control of the disease. Although public education measures are intended to motivate people to have physical examinations and to use discretion in eating, exercising, resting, and checking symptoms with their doctor, they create threats for some people. Some persons who are told that their symptoms are suggestive of heart disease, when diagnostic tests prove nothing, often continue to worry and cannot accept the fact that nothing is wrong. The person who has had one heart attack may live in fear of another and be prevented from resuming his place as a useful member of society. Others cannot find work because employers are afraid to hire them. Heart associations, health departments, and insurance companies spend large sums of money each year for educational publications on heart disease in an attempt to overcome these problems.

The nurse needs to face realistically any fear she may have about heart disease before she can give good care to patients and families. She needs to help others see the positive side of the picture, such as the fact that many who have heart attacks recover almost completely and are able to live relatively normal lives. She should try to gain their cooperation in following medical advice, helping them to see how they themselves can participate in keeping well. Much of this ability stems from the nurse's own confidence in, and her realistic approach toward, treatment of heart disease.

Some families in which a member has heart disease live in fear of a repeated heart attack, particularly because they realize that they do not know what to do in such an emergency. The nurse should know the signs and symptoms of heart diseases and also the kind of emergency care the patient's family can give. Family members usually can be taught to act wisely in an emergency if the doctor and the nurse are explicit and certain of what should be done. Some families find little consolation in being told to call an ambulance or to call the police, but if they also know the position in which to place the patient and perhaps how to administer medication, they will react better in an actual emergency. Although emergencies may be expected, the nurse should help the patient who has cardiac disease and his family to develop a wholesome attitude toward his condition so that they can lead relatively normal lives and not live in constant expectation of disaster.

Diagnostic procedures

Signs and symptoms

Heart diseases are diagnosed by the clinical signs and symptoms. Laboratory tests and an x-ray examination are helpful mainly in confirming the diagnosis, determining the course of the disease, indicating complications, showing residual effects, and predicting the results of treatment. The nurse can help in the diagnosis by carefully observing and recording signs and symptoms as she works with the patient. The character, as well as the rate, of the *pulse* is important. The pulse may be markedly irregular, or there may be a regular irregularity that recurs in the same pattern. The pulse may be abnormally rapid or unusually slow. The heartbeat and the radial pulse may not be the same, since sometimes the heart beats ineffectually, and little blood is pushed out into the arteries. The *respirations* may be labored, and this difficulty may be increased by certain positions or activities. The patient may have *pain* in his arms, chest, neck, upper back, shoulders, or epigastrium. It is important for the doctor to know the location and type of pain, as well as the activity that caused it. The patient's *color* and its relationship to activity, position, dyspnea, and pain should be observed. The presence of *edema* of the tissues and increase or decrease of edema related to activity, position, or fluid and salt intake should be recorded. Many of these signs and symptoms are subtle and will be missed if one is not especially looking for them.

The nurse may assist with some of the procedures. In addition, she helps to prepare the patient for special examinations and laboratory tests by explaining what will be done and why it must be done. Explanations should lessen the anxiety and fear that can impede the recovery of the patient with heart disease.

Blood analysis

Blood count. A complete blood count is made on all patients with heart disease. In bacterial endocarditis an anemia persists as long as inflammation is active. The blood count, therefore, guides the doctor in determining when the patient's physical activity can be increased. The red blood cell count and the hemoglobin level are observed carefully in patients with heart disease that involves intracardiac shunts, for such observations enable the doctor to determine how well the blood is being oxygenated. Adequate oxygenation of the blood is a major problem in cardiac disease. If there has been a myocardial infarction, which causes death of a portion of the heart muscle, the white blood cell count is usually elevated, because necrotic tissue anywhere in the body will cause leukocytosis.

Blood sedimentation rate. A determination of the blood sedimentation rate is ordered for many patients with heart disease. It is used to follow the course of acute rheumatic heart disease, infectious disease of the heart, and acute myocardial infarction.

Prothrombin time determination. A prothrombin time determination is a blood test that indicates the ability of the blood to form intravascular clots. This test may be done routinely on all patients with heart disease, especially if there is reason to believe that blood clots may form within the blood vessels or the chambers of the heart. Patients who are being given anticoagulant drugs, such as bishydroxycoumarin (Dicumarol), warfarin sodium (Coumadin sodium; Prothromadin), or a combination of heparin and one of these drugs which lower the prothrombin level, to prevent intravascular blood clotting must have daily prothrombin time determinations to determine how much of the drug should be given each day. It is the nurse's responsibility to see that the blood is drawn and sent to the laboratory. Patients who are on smaller, maintenance doses of anticoagulant drugs may have prothrombin time determinations made at longer intervals.

Blood urea nitrogen test. A blood urea nitrogen test (BUN), used to determine kidney function, is usually made to learn whether kidney function is disturbed as a result of impaired cardiac output or as a result of other causes.

Serum cholesterol. Serum cholesterol tests usually are made in order to determine the cholesterol level in the blood. People with a high cholesterol level are known to have a high incidence of coronary artery disease, although the relationship that may exist is not clearly understood. (See medical texts.) The normal levels are considered to be between 150 to 280 mg. per 100 ml. of blood.[2]

Urinalysis

A urinalysis is made to learn if there is albuminuria or some other abnormality. Albuminuria may occur in patients with heart failure and in those whose heart disease is complicated by kidney damage. It often is present in patients with hypertension and shows that stress is being placed upon the kidneys.

Enzyme tests

A transaminase (serum glutamic oxalocetic transaminase, or SGOT) test is helpful in diagnosing acute myocardial infarctions. The normal range for this test is 6 to 40 units per milliliter of serum. After an acute myocardial infarction, the level may rise to as high as 500 units and then usually returns to normal four to seven days after the infarction. Levels above 500 do not occur following an infarction but are indicative of hepatic disease. This test is also used in the diagnosis of skeletal muscle disease. Another test sometimes used to determine myocardial necrosis is the enzyme test known as the *lactic dehydrogenase* (LDH) test. LDH consists of five components or isoenzymes. Numbers used to designate them are 1, 2, 3, 4, and 5. Elevated levels are observed in almost all patients within a few hours of the occurrence of an infarction.

Electrocardiogram

An electrocardiogram (ECG or EKG) is a record of the electric activity of the heart muscle. On the electrocardiogram, certain drugs such as digitalis and quinidine produce changes similar to those seen in disease. Therefore, if the patient is receiving such a drug, the electrocardiologist should be so informed.

Three or more electrodes, or leads, are placed against the patient's skin on the extremities and the thorax and then connected by wires to a recording galvanometer. They are usually placed on both forearms, on one or both lower legs, and over the precordial area, but many variations may be ordered. A special electrode jelly is rubbed onto the portion of the skin on which the lead, a small strip of metal, is strapped. The patient lies down or sits while the electrocardiogram is made, and he should be relaxed. If it is his first ECG, an explanation of the procedure should be given. If the patient is hospitalized, a technician may come to the bedside to do this procedure. The recording machine may be brought to the bedside, but in some institutions the wires are plugged into special wall outlets that transmit recordings to a central location, or "heart station."

The nurse should understand the ECG in order to be able to explain the procedure to the patient and to understand the significance of the tracings (Fig. 64). The electrical currents spreading in a wavelike pattern over the heart proceed in an orderly cycle if the heart beat is normal. The cycle normally begins with impulses from the sinoatrial (SA) node. The SA node controls the heart rate and is the pacemaker. However, any part of the myocardial tissue has the ability to initiate impulses and may take over under abnormal circumstances.

The initial impulse spreads from the SA node through the muscles of the atria causing them to contract, and is directed obliquely to the atrioventricular (AV) node, then down the bundle of His, spreading along the left and right branches to reach the terminal fibers, the Purkinje system. The Purkinje fibers spread throughout the muscles of the ventricles, and the ventricles contract as the electrical impulse reaches this last point. There is then a period of muscular rest while the ventricles fill with blood, and then the cycle is repeated.

For purposes of recording and reporting, the five wave deflections described above

have been designated P, Q, R, S, and T in the electrocardiographic testing. They are recorded by using the electrodes (leads) placed on the surface of the body. These electrical forces of the heart are transmitted to the body surface, and the deflections can be recorded on the galvanometer. The flow of electrical forces spreads in several directions and must be recorded in different planes. The three major planes, or leads, are obtained by attaching the electrodes to the right arm, the left arm, and the left leg. If a cardiac monitor is being used, a single lead, equivalent to lead II, is used. The majority but not all arrhythmias can be detected by this lead.

The graph paper used for recording is divided into vertical lines, designating time, and horizontal lines, which measure voltage. Thus the P wave represents the electrical impulses from the SA node and the spread through the atria. If these waves are normal in size and shape (Fig. 64), one can assume that the impulse began at the SA node. If the waves are absent or unusual in shape, the impulse began outside the SA node.

The *P-R interval* is designated as the period between the start of the P wave and the beginning of the QRS complex. It indicates the time it takes for the original impulse to reach the ventricle and initiate contraction. The latter may be referred to as *depolarization*. During this time (usually not exceeding 0.2 second), the impulse has passed through the atria and the AV node. If the time exceeds 0.2 second, a conduction delay is considered to have occurred in the AV node. If the P-R interval is shorter (less than 0.1 second), then it may be that the current reached the ventricle through a

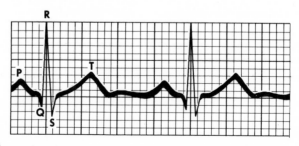

Fig. 64

A normal electrocardiogram.

shorter-than-normal path. (This is termed the Wolff-Parkinson-White syndrome.)

The *QRS complex* consists of 3 waves, an initial downward deflection (Q wave), a large upward deflection (R wave), and a second downward wave (S wave). These waves reflect the time necessary for the impulse to spread through the bundle of His and its branches. This impulse usually takes less than 0.12 second. An increased amount of time indicates that the ventricle has been stimulated in a delayed, abnormal manner, such as in a bundle-branch block.

The *S-T segment* is the time interval between completion of depolarization and repolarization (recovery) of the ventricular muscles. If there is injury to the muscle, as in myocardial infarction, the S-T segment may be elevated or depressed.

The *T wave* is the recovery phase after contraction (repolarization). If this is abnormal usually because of tissue injury or ischemia, the T wave may be inverted.

The ECG does not show the actual physical state of the heart or its function. If the electrical forces are disturbed by the pathologic process, then usually the ECG will be abnormal. Its most important diagnostic use is the identification of abnormal rhythms and coronary heart disease. Since the rhythm may be normal even in the presence of serious heart disease, a single electrocardiogram often is not significant, and repeated tracings may be necessary before evidence of disease can be detected. Electrocardiograms may also be done at intervals to follow the course of disease. These repeated examinations may be upsetting to the patient who does not understand why so many must be made.

Roentgenogram of the chest

A roentgenogram of the chest may be taken to determine the size and shape of the heart and the aorta. Calcifications in the pericardium, heart muscle, valves, or large blood vessels also can be visualized in such an x-ray film, which is sometimes called a *cardiovascular film*.

Special tests

Special procedures and tests may be ordered to gain additional information concerning certain heart diseases. If known infection is present or if the patient has a transient fever of unknown origin, a *blood culture* is usually made in an effort to learn the causative organism and the antibiotic that will be most effective in treating it. Multiple blood cultures are ordered for patients who have suspected endocarditis. The most scrupulous attention to aseptic technique must be observed in any procedure in which a blood vessel is entered. The nurse has a major responsibility because she prepares equipment and assists during the procedure. Some procedures may be done, for example, in the x-ray department, where the nurse and the doctor are the team members most aware of the aseptic precautions that are necessary.

Venous pressure. Venous pressure is the pressure exerted by the circulating blood against the venous walls. It is elevated in congestive heart failure, in acute or chronic constrictive pericarditis, and in venous obstruction caused by a clot in a vein or external pressure against a vein, as when the jugular vein is manually compressed. The measurement of venous pressure is particularly helpful after open heart surgery in detecting hypervolemia, hypovolemia, and cardiac tamponade.[15] The normal venous pressure ranges from 60 to 120 mm. of water. To test it, the following equipment is necessary: a 10 ml. syringe, a No. 19 needle, a manometer, a three-way stopcock, sterile normal saline solution, a tourniquet, a solution such as benzalkonium chloride, and sponges to cleanse the skin. The patient lies or sits so that his arm is supported at a level with his heart. He may be flat in bed with the arm outstretched on the bed, or if he must remain in a sitting position, the arm can be supported slightly below shoulder level with pillows. He should be comfortable and relaxed. A stopcock is attached to the hub of the syringe, and with the needle attached to one side of the stopcock, 5 ml. of sterile normal saline solution are drawn into the syringe. The doctor then does a venipuncture, drawing 2 or 3 ml. of blood into the syringe. The manometer is attached to the other side of the stopcock, the tourniquet is released, the blood and saline mixture is run into the manometer, and then the stopcock to the vein is opened (Fig. 65). The pressure is recorded when the level of the fluid stabilizes in the manometer. The nurse assists by encouraging the patient, placing and

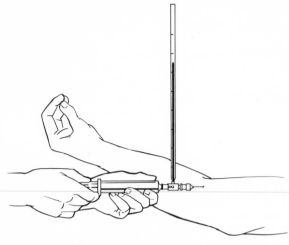

Fig. 65

Technique used to determine venous pressure.
Note the stopcock placed between the syringe
and the needle, and the saline-blood
mixture rising in the manometer.

holding the manometer, and recording the
readings.

Circulation time determination. Circulation time is tested in order to determine the
amount of time it takes a patient to taste
a substance, such as sodium dehydrocholate
(Decholin sodium), injected intravenously.
The normal arm-to-tongue time is fifteen
seconds or less. Circulation time is prolonged in congestive heart failure. To do
this test, the following equipment is necessary: a stop watch, a sterile 5 ml. syringe, a
No. 19 needle, a tourniquet, an ampule of
Decholin sodium, sucrose, or calcium chloride, a solution such as benzalkonium
chloride, and sponges to cleanse the skin.
The nurse should explain carefully to the
patient his part in this test, and she may
be asked to record the time interval between
the injection of the drug and the time that
the patient tastes it. Special variations on
this test may be used.

Angiocardiogram. An angiocardiogram is
a roentgenogram of the heart and its vessels made after the intravenous injection of
a radiopaque substance. It outlines the
chambers of the heart and the large blood
vessels and enables the doctor to see how
these chambers function. The meal preceding the x-ray procedure is omitted, and the
patient is given a sedative such as phenobarbital sodium about one-half hour before
going to the x-ray department. The sedative
helps to alleviate apprehension. After injecting a local anesthetic, the doctor makes a
skin incision over the antecubital vein and
then inserts a No. 19 needle, attached to a
syringe, into the vein. The dye is forced
rapidly into the vein, and a series of roentgenograms are taken as the solution flows
through the heart, pulmonary vessels, and
aorta (Fig. 66).

Some patients are sensitive to drugs containing iodine, such as sodium acetrizoate
(Urokon sodium) and iodopyracet (Dio-
drast), which may be used as the radiopaque substance. Nausea is a frequent untoward reaction, and urticaria, dyspnea, or
severe anaphylactic reaction may occur. If
the patient has a history of asthma or other
allergic reactions, this test is seldom done.
Any systemic reaction to the drug usually
occurs immediately, and an antihistaminic
drug, such as tripelennamine hydrochloride
(Pyribenzamine) or epinephrine (Adrenalin), and oxygen should be readily available.

Leakage of the dye outside the vein may
cause irritation and sloughing of tissue.
Thrombosis of the vein at the site of the
injection may occasionally occur. When the
patient returns from the x-ray department,
the incision should be checked for bleeding
and irritation. The vein will be tender, and
the patient may have difficulty bending his
arm. He should be reassured that this condition is temporary and will probably disappear within twenty-four hours. If irritation
or thrombosis of the vein occurs, warm
sterile compresses are usually ordered.

Selective arteriography. Selective visualization of the aorta and its major arterial
systems now enables the physician to study
a particular vessel closely. For example, in
a patient with renal hypertension, the renal
arteries can be studied down to the very
fine intrarenal branches. The physician can
study the pathologic anatomy of the coronary artery and its branches and by this
means may plan a course of treatment that
is best for the particular patient.

The patient is prepared with an explanation of the procedure by the doctor and re-

ceives nothing by mouth on the day the procedure is to be performed. An antibiotic drug is usually given as a prophylactic measure against infection during the treatment. Some form of barbiturate or a tranquilizing drug is given to help relieve anxiety. Local anesthesia only is used. The patient is placed on a special fluoroscopic table, and test roentgenograms are taken to make certain that the position is correct for best visualization of the vessels to be studied.

Usually the femoral artery or the brachial artery is used. The site of puncture is infiltrated with procaine hydrochloride, and the technique of entry to the artery is known as the *percutaneous catheter replacement technique.* A special needle is inserted, and a long, flexible spring guide is passed through the needle for about 15 cm. At this point the needle is removed, and an arterial catheter is threaded over the spring guide into the artery. The guide and the catheter are advanced until the desired position is reached, and then the guide is withdrawn. A few milliliters of a radiopaque substance are injected through the catheter so that the tip of the catheter can be seen under the fluoroscope, and at the same time the patient is observed for signs of sensitivity to the radiopaque substance, such as chills, tremor, or dyspnea. Since the radiopaque substance is eliminated very quickly by the kidneys, rapid films are taken by means of a special camera that makes it possible to take four to six pictures per second. This type of film is known as a *cinefluorogram.*

Upon completion of the examination by means of films, the catheter is withdrawn, and manual pressure is applied for about five minutes. A pressure bandage is applied, and the patient is returned to his room. Usually the pressure bandage is removed in approximately half an hour, and an Ace bandage is applied firmly. After forty-eight hours this bandage may be removed and a small strip of adhesive tape used.

Providing that the patient has no local or systemic reactions to the examination, he may be up and about within two hours of returning to his room. Blood pressure readings are taken every fifteen minutes for the first two hours, and the puncture site is checked for bleeding. Chance of hemorrhage from the puncture site is much greater than would be the case if a vein had been opened. If bleeding does occur, the nurse should apply pressure firmly with thumb or fingertips an inch above the site of bleeding, and the doctor must be notified at once.

Cardiac catheterization. Cardiac catheterization is the procedure of passing a catheter into the heart to better study heart function. Cardiac catheterization, once limited to study of the right side of the heart, has been improved and is now used to study the left side of the heart also. Right cardiac catheterization is done when congenital heart disease is suspected, but it may also be used to evaluate certain acquired heart conditions, such as mitral stenosis and valvular incompetence. Blood samples and blood pressure readings are taken, electrocardiographic studies are done, and roentgenograms of the right heart chambers and the pulmonary arterial circulation are made. The doctor who obtains the patient's written permission should explain the procedure to him. The nurse should reinforce this explanation as necessary, and she must know what the doctor tells the patent, since often the latter is not told exactly what will be done lest he become unduly anxious. Even with careful explanation most patients are apprehensive. The meal prior to the procedure is withheld. A sedative such as phenobarbital is given the evening before and the morning of the procedure, and an antibiotic drug such as penicillin may be given the day before, the day of, and the day following the procedure. Young children usually are given a general anesthetic. For adults a local anesthetic is injected over the vein to be used. A cutdown similar to that for an angiocardiogram is done, usually using the antecubital vein.

A sterile radiopaque catheter similar to a ureteral catheter, but 100 to 125 cm. in length, is passed into the incision in the vein and through the vein into the superior vena cava, through the right atrium and the right ventricle, and into the pulmonary artery. The course of the catheter is followed by fluoroscopy, and roentgenograms may be taken at any point. An electrocar-

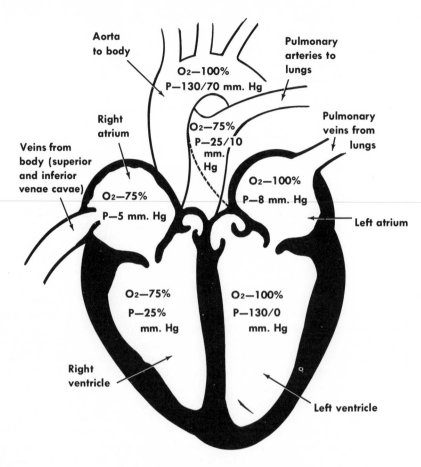

Fig. 66

The pressure readings and the concentration (percentage of saturation) of oxygen in the chambers of the heart and the major blood vessels entering and leaving the heart.

diogram is monitored on an oscillograph, and pressures can be checked regularly. As the catheter is passed through the various vessels and cardiac chambers, samples of blood are taken to study the oxygen content, and blood pressures are recorded (Fig. 66). When there is an interatrial septal defect, the oxygen content is higher in the blood of the right atrium than in the superior or inferior vena cava. In certain heart conditions, such as pulmonary or mitral stenosis, the pressure readings within the heart may be elevated three to four times above normal.

The patient has no pain during a right cardiac catheterization, but he usually is extremely alert and anxious. He may feel the passage of the catheter, and he may complain of a feeling of warmth and of a fluttering sensation around the heart. He also may have a tendency to cough as the catheter is passed up the pulmonary artery. When he returns from the special x-ray room, he is usually quite exhausted and needs rest since the procedure takes from one to three hours. He may resume his regular activity as soon as he desires, but his pulse is usually taken every fifteen minutes for one hour and then every half hour for three hours. Tachycardia or arrhythmia should be reported to the doctor. The temperature may be slightly elevated for four to six hours after the procedure, and the patient may complain of some discomfort at the site of the cutdown. It should be checked at hourly intervals for several hours to note any bleeding or inflammation. If a local thrombophlebitis occurs, it is treated with warm, moist compresses.

In studying the left side of the heart, there is a choice of method. By means of a special bronchoscope, a needle is passed through the wall of the left main bronchus directly into the left atrium, or the left ventricle may be entered directly through the chest wall by a needle puncture at the apex of the heart. If aortic stenosis is absent, the left ventricle can be catheterized in retrograde fashion through the aorta. The catheter is passed into the femoral artery, up the aorta, around the aortic arch, and down the ascending aorta to the aortic valve. The catheter is then guided into the left ventricle.

Risks during cardiac catheterization are slight, although complications can occur. Cardiac arrhythmias, thrombophlebitis, and local infection are the most common complications. Right cardiac catheterization may be done in the radiology department, but left cardiac catheterization usually is done in the operating room. Direct puncture of the heart may cause pneumothorax, severe arrhythmia, or hemopericardium.

Memory of the experience often is vivid, and the patient can describe in detail what was done. This ability to recall so vividly may be due to the amount and size of the equipment that is used, the number of personnel needed to do the procedure, fear of the catheter and its placement in the blood vessels and heart, the anticipation of something going wrong, and thoughtless discussion by persons performing the procedure. The time required for the catheterization may also have affected the patient. The patient's tension is increased by lying rather still for three hours or more while procedures are done, by instructions given back and forth among physicians and technicians, by changes in voice tones of personnel, and by equipment noises. If the patient is allowed to talk about his reactions, his preoccupation with them may be at least partially relieved.

Ballistocardiogram. When a ballistocardiogram is ordered, the patient is placed on a special table that is so delicately balanced that any vibration of the body, caused by the systolic ejection of blood from the heart into the aorta and pulmonary arteries, can be recorded by a machine attached to the table. There is no special preparation for this test. The patient simply lies quietly on the table. He may be aware of the vibrations and may be startled by them. The ballistocardiograph, a relatively new apparatus, is thought to be more sensitive in some instances than an electrocardiograph, but it gives a very different kind of information.

Graphic procedures. Many other tests have been and are being developd. Two of them are phonocardiography, which produces an electrical record of the heart sounds, and electrokymography, which produces a record of the border movements of the heart.

Classification of heart diseases

Heart diseases may be divided into two general groups: those that are acquired after birth and those that are congenital. Acquired disease may affect the heart either suddenly or gradually. There may be damage to the heart from bacteria, chemical agents, or diminished blood supply. For example, inflammation may cause scarring of heart valves, muscle, or outer coverings, all of which may impair the heart's function. Any changes in the coronary vessels supplying the heart muscle may decrease its efficiency. Congenital heart disease follows an abnormality of structure caused by error in fetal development.

Heart disease may also be classified according to a specific cause, such as rheumatic fever, bacterial endocarditis, or hypertension. It may be classified according to anatomic change, such as valvular scarring, or according to a physiologic abnormality, such as arrhythmia.

Since cardiac insufficiency (leading to congestive heart failure) and cardiac arrhythmias are the cause of many of the symptoms commonly associated with various cardiac diseases, these conditions will be discussed before the specific diseases.

Nursing related to specific medical and surgical care

Congestive heart failure

Physiology

The amount of blood the heart pumps to all parts of the body varies with body activities. Under normal conditions the heart and blood vessels adjust the flow of blood to body needs, and usually the heart is not worked to capacity. Moderate activity such as sitting, standing, or walking places only nominal demand on the heart. However, when the pumping action of the heart is decreased because of some impairment, the heart may have to work to capacity to meet even modest demands.

In congestive heart failure the heart is unable to receive its normal flow of blood from the venous system and to pump out the required amount through the arterial circulation. The left ventricle does not empty completely into the aorta, and the blood that would normally enter the right atrium from the superior and inferior venae cavae cannot do so. Pressure rises in the venous circulation, and the organs and tissues that are normally drained by the veins become congested with the blood that is flowing slowly against increased pressure. The left ventricle, meanwhile tries to do extra work to pump this blood, and it becomes enlarged. This process is usually a gradual one, occurring over a period of months or years. Congestive heart failure is also known as *cardiac decompensation, cardiac insufficiency, heart failure,* and *cardiac incompetence.*

Congestive heart failure is often classified as right-sided or left-sided, according to the side of the heart at fault. Most often it begins in the left ventricle and later becomes a combination of left-sided and right-sided failure. Heart failure may temporarily disappear as soon as the mechanisms causing it are rectified. It may be present for the rest of the patient's life and require continuous care and medication; or, despite treatment, it may quickly become worse and cause death.

Symptoms

The symptoms of heart failure are caused by the accumulation of fluid throughout the body and by an inadequate blood flow to body tissues. *Edema,* which is an excessive amount of fluid in the extracellular tissues and body cavities, is a common symptom of congestive failure. It may occur in the legs, the liver, the abdominal cavity, the lungs, the pleural spaces, or other parts of the body. When the heart becomes an inefficient pump, venous stasis occurs and venous pressure increases. Because of this, fluid remains in the venous system rather than circulating normally to the kidneys, where the excess sodium would be excreted. If the patient consumes more sodium in his diet than can be excreted, the excess is stored in the body. Sodium is a water-fixing ion; that is, it holds water to prevent body fluids from becoming too salty. Therefore, the more salt in the body, the more water will be retained. Some of this fluid passes into the interstitial spaces and causes generalized edema.

In *right-sided heart failure* the right ventricle cannot effectively propel into the lungs the blood returning to it from the inferior and superior venae cavae through the right atrium. This causes the blood to dam back into the veins of the systemic circulation and leads to edema in the lower extremities. This edema is of the pitting type (can be depressed by touching) and is nontender. It is known as dependent edema and almost always disappears at night, when the legs are not lower than the rest of the body. As the edema becomes more pronounced, it progresses up the legs into the thighs, scrotum, abdomen, and sacrum. If the tissues become too engorged, the skin may crack, and fluid may "weep" from the tissues. The liver may also become engorged with blood, causing it to enlarge and producing tenderness in the right upper quadrant of the abdomen. As the venous stasis increases, increased pressure within the portal system often forces fluid through the blood vessels into the abdominal cavity. This is known as *ascites.* As much as 8,000 or 10,000 ml. (8 to 10 quarts) or more of serous fluid may accumulate in the abdominal cavity, and, unless removed by a paracentesis, the accumulation may cause severe respiratory distress as a result of elevation of the diaphragm.

In *left-sided heart failure* the weakened left ventricle of the heart cannot effectively pump into the arterial circulation the oxy-

318

genated blood coming from the lungs through the pulmonary veins into the left atrium. This causes the blood to dam back into the pulmonary vessels so that serous fluid is pushed out into the pulmonary tissues, causing *pulmonary edema* and *pleural effusion.* The fluid may be present in the lower interstitial tissues of the lungs, in the alveoli of the lungs, in the bronchioles, or in the lower pleural cavity. *Dyspnea,* or shortness of breath, is an early symptom of left-sided congestive heart failure. It is caused by a decreased vital capacity because of the fluid level in the lungs. Dyspnea may occur or may become worse only on physical exertion, such as climbing stairs, walking up an incline, or walking against a wind, since these activities require increased amounts of oxygen. Sometimes dyspnea occurs upon lying down. This type is called *orthopnea.* When the patient is lying flat on his back, there is decreased vital capacity, and the blood volume to the pulmonary vessels is increased. Patients with orthopnea often must sleep propped upright in bed or in a chair. Although orthopnea may occur immediately after lying down, it often does not occur until several hours later, when it causes the patient to wake up with severe dyspnea and coughing. This condition is known as *paroxysmal nocturnal dyspnea* and is probably triggered by such things as a nightmare, a noise, or a full bladder, which causes the output of the right ventricle to be increased for a short time and increases the need for oxygen.[2]

In cardiac failure the patient may have periods of apnea and *hyperpnea* (Cheyne-Stokes respirations). Often an insufficient amount of oxygen is carried by the blood to the brain. Oxygen insufficiency makes the respiratory center in the brain insensitive to the normal amounts of carbon dioxide in the arterial blood, and respiration ceases until either the carbon dioxide content in the arterial blood increases enough to stimulate the respiratory center or until the oxygen level in the blood drops to a level that is low enough to stimulate the respiratory center. The carbon dioxide content of the arterial blood is also decreased by the periods of overbreathing. Periodic overbreathing often begins as the patient goes to sleep, and decreases as sleep deepens and

ventilation decreases.[2] Morphine sulfate may relieve Cheyne-Stokes respirations because it slows the respiratory rate. Usually the doctor does not prescribe high concentrations of oxygen for this condition because they would prevent the reflex stimulus caused by low oxygen content in the blood, which is actually what stimulates the patient to start to breathe again and to build up carbon dioxide.

Pulmonary edema caused by left-sided heart failure may be very severe, and moist rales (moist breath sounds) sometimes may be heard across the room. This condition is known as *acute pulmonary edema.* The patient is extremely dyspneic, is apprehensive and struggles for breath, has a persistent cough and may expectorate frothy or even blood-tinged sputum, is usually cyanotic, and his heart pounds rapidly. Acute pulmonary edema is a medical emergency, since, if it is not immediately treated, the patient may "drown" in his own secretions. Treatment will be discussed more fully later in this chapter.

A persistent hacking cough and expectoration of mucoid material are frequent symptoms of left-sided heart congestion. They are usually caused by the congestion of the lungs and bronchi. Cardiac pain is not common in congestive heart failure, although some patients develop discomfort in the chest upon lying down. This discomfort is often described as a "heavy feeling" or a "feeling of pressure" and arises in patients with a diseased heart that is sensitive to a deficiency in the oxygen content in the coronary circulation because the blood is less completely oxygenated when the patient is lying flat than when he is sitting, standing, or even walking.

Fatigue is a common sign of congestive failure and is one of the earliest signs to develop. The patient notices that he becomes tired following activities that ordinarily would not tire him. This fatigue results from the impaired circulation of blood to the tissues and from the consequent lack of sufficient oxygen and nutrients for the needs of the cells. In addition, the slow-moving blood does not carry off wastes with sufficient speed to permit the muscles to regain their power.

Because of the edema, weight loss may

not be noticed in patients with congestive heart failure. Often 5 to 10 kg. (6 to 22 pounds) of fluid may be retained. The patient, however, may have lost much muscle tissue because of inadequate nutrition. On reduction of the edema, he may appear as emaciated as a patient with an advanced malignancy.[2]

Medical treatment and nursing care

Medical authorities[2] state that the principles of treatment for congestive heart failure are to bring back into balance the demand for blood and the supply of blood and to remove and thereafter to prevent the accumulation of excess fluid and excess blood volume when the output of the heart cannot be made to meet normal requirements of the body. These objectives are accomplished by reducing the requirements of the body for oxygen, by increasing the cardiac output, and by eliminating the edema.

Rest. Physicians do not agree on the amount of rest the patient should have or the activity permitted. The nurse should be certain that she knows what each doctor wishes for his patient. (See later discussion concerning special rest provisions for the patient with a myocardial infarction.) The body's oxygen requirements can best be reduced by providing the patient with both physical and mental rest. The patient with congestive heart failure is usually kept in bed until he is free from the signs and symptoms of the disease; that is, until the heart rate has been slowed, venous engorgement has disappeared, dyspnea and orthopnea have lessened, pleural effusion, ascites, and generalized tissue edema have decreased, and the liver has become smaller and is no longer tender. The time required may be days, weeks, or months. If the attack is mild, with only edema of the legs or minimal signs of pulmonary edema, the patient may be treated on an ambulatory basis with only a regimen of less activity and more rest than usual. If the attack is severe, however, a program of strict bed rest may be maintained for some time.

Rest may be difficult to provide, and sometimes it takes the ingenuity of all persons concerned to obtain it for the patient. Providing rest is one of the major responsibilities of the nurse in caring for the patient who is acutely ill with congestive heart failure. A restless, anxious, disturbed patient cannot rest, and the nurse must employ measures that will help such a patient to relax.

The patient's environment is very important. In many hospitals, where intensive care units or coronary units are available, the patient who is seriously ill will be under the constant surveillance and attention of an especially skilled team of nurses and physicians. However, many institutions do not have special facilities, and the patient will receive care in the usual patient room accommodations. If possible, he should be in a room alone, where the atmosphere of quiet and relaxation can be maintained. Many patients relax better if a close family member stays with them.

Almost every patient in cardiac failure is extremely apprehensive and anxious, both about his own physical condition and about the welfare of his family. Many times the doctor feels that it is best to tell the patient what he wishes to know, because an explanation will often quiet him. Visitors should be prohibited with the exception of close family members. However, if their presence disturbs the patient, the doctor or nurse should explain the situation to the family and gain their cooperation. In any case the family should be kept well informed of the patient's condition. Members of the family should be encouraged not to worry him, but mention of daily problems should not be avoided since he may suspect that information is being withheld. No news often is worse than bad news, and the patient may imagine that conditions are much worse than they are.

The nurse should listen carefully to the patient to find out what concerns him and makes it difficult for him to rest. She should visit the acutely ill cardiac patient often in order to give him a chance to mention worries that are interfering with rest and sleep. Evening and night hours may be particularly stressful if the patient is worried. It may help if he can be in daily contact with a social worker to whom he can talk about his family, his job, and his plans for the future. Although the social worker will not make extensive plans with him at this time, she often can take care of immediate problems and thus help to relieve his mind.

Visits from a spiritual adviser may be quieting to some patients. Visits from other patients who are progressing satisfactorily from the same condition sometimes give reassurance. Reading, watching television, and listening to the radio for short periods of time may be relaxing for some patients. Others find these activities very distracting, so that provisions for patients should be made on an individual basis. Occupational therapy that does not require extensive arm movements and that is not so intricate as to tire the patient may be a valuable pastime as the patient improves.

Weighing the patient. Although careful records of intake and output are kept on most patients with cardiac failure, the doctor often relies more heavily upon the patient's changes in weight to estimate his progress and his response to prescribed diet, drugs, or other forms of treatment. The patient's weight should be carefully recorded upon admission, after which time the doctor orders how often he wishes the patient weighed and what procedure can be used. Some hospitals have large scales on which a stretcher can be placed; the patient may be moved to the stretcher by other persons, without exertion on his part. Other hospitals have portable scales that can be brought to the bedside easily.

Sedatives. The patient should have adequate sleep, and it is better for him to sleep at night and to be awake during the day. Cardiac patients are likely to be apprehensive during the night. Pentobarbital sodium, 0.1 Gm. (1½ grains), at bedtime and repeated if necessary, or phenobarbital, 30 to 60 mg. (½ to 1 grain), may be ordered by the doctor. Whiskey, 30 to 60 ml. (1 to 2 ounces), at bedtime may be ordered to increase the effectiveness of the barbiturates. For older patients and for patients with renal damage, paraldehyde by mouth, by rectum, or by intramuscular injection may be necessary. Chloral hydrate or sodium bromide may also be used. If the patient is unable to sleep, time should be taken to talk with him, and nursing measures such as rubbing his back and straightening the bedclothes may help him to relax. It is usually impossible to give warm milk because of fluid and salt restrictions, but if this measure seems desirable, it may be possible

to plan with the dietitian to include warm milk in the patient's diet. Sometimes other warm fluids may be given when milk is not permitted.

If dyspnea under sedation is marked, if the patient complains of pain, or if he is very restless and anxious, the doctor may order morphine sulfate, 10 mg. (⅙ grain). If necessary, the drug may be given as often as every four hours for two or three days. The nurse should give it before the patient becomes agitated, since worry and excitement normally cause constriction of the blood vessels, which increases the heart rate. Although a normal heart can accommodate to an increase in pressure and activity, the diseased heart may be overburdened by it. Some patients are allergic to morphine sulfate and develop nausea and vomiting. The doctor may then order meperidine hydrochloride (Demerol) or pantopium (Pantopon).

Position in bed. A comfortable position in bed can best be determined by the patient. Since no two patients are alike, the nurse must be guided by the patient's habit patterns and his symptoms in finding a position that is most conducive to rest. Most patients with congestive heart failure are more comfortable and can breathe more easily with the head of the bed elevated in a high Fowler's position. A pillow may be placed lengthwise behind the shoulders and back in such a manner that full expansion of the rib cage is possible. The patient who is in proper position for comfortable breathing will also be in correct body alignment. A foot block may help to prevent the patient from slipping toward the foot of the bed. Patients who must be in a high Fowler's position are usually more comfortable and have less pull on their shoulder muscles if pillows are used to support the lower arms. A small pillow slipped under the small of the back also may make the patient more comfortable. If the patient must remain upright all the time, his position may be changed occasionally by allowing him to rest his head and arms on pillows placed on an overbed table pulled up close to him (Fig. 67). Both the pillows and the table should be tied to prevent them from slipping. Side rails should be kept on the bed to give the patient something firm on

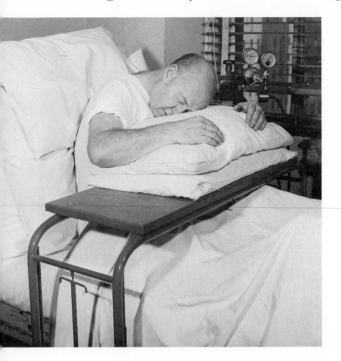

Fig. 67

Pillows placed on the overbed table provide a comfortable support for the patient who must sleep in a sitting position.

which to hold during changes of position and to prevent accidents.

Oxygen. The patient with congestive heart failure may be more comfortable and rest better in an oxygen tent, since oxygen helps to relieve the dyspnea and cyanosis by providing a higher concentration of oxygen in the bloodstream. In cardiac failure the oxygen content of the bloodstream may be markedly reduced because of the less effective oxygenation of the blood as it passes through the congested lungs. There is danger, however, in giving too much oxygen. The nurse must report to the doctor at once if Cheyne-Stokes respirations occur, because they may be due to too much oxygen in the blood.

If pulmonary edema is severe, a high concentration of oxygen under pressure may be given by means of a positive-pressure mask. This helps to prevent further transudation of serum from the pulmonary

capillaries by exerting pressure on the pulmonary epithelium during expiration. The doctor must determine the concentration of oxygen, the desired pressure, and the frequency of use. Fifty to 100% concentrations of oxygen are usually given at a pressure of 3 to 4 ml. of water, and later, although the oxygen is continued, the positive pressure may be used only every one to four hours for a short period of time. The patient receiving this treatment needs attention to the skin where pressure from the mask may cause irritation. The skin should be massaged, sponged, and powdered between treatments if they continue for some time. The nurse must protect the patient with pulmonary edema from *any* exertion since any activity increases the body's need for oxygen.

Activity. Restricted physical activity is necessary for the patient with congestive heart failure, and the nurse should find out from the doctor how much activity the patient may be allowed. Some patients are not even permitted to turn or to feed themselves. Because dependence on nursing personnel for even these simple tasks is disturbing to some patients, the tasks should be carried out without apparent rush, and the patient's needs should be anticipated so that he will not have to ask for help. If it is evident that the patient simply cannot accept complete dependence on the nursing staff, the doctor should be consulted. Occasionally it is better to let the patient do some things for himself.

Most patients with heart failure are not allowed to bathe themselves, and while they are acutely ill, they should not be disturbed more than is necessary for their safety and comfort. If special attention is given to the back and to bony prominences, a partial bath may suffice for several days. The patient's head often cannot be lowered to change bedclothes; thus, when the lower sheets need changing or tightening, he may need to be supported in an upright position while the head of the bed is lowered and made. The sheets are more easily changed from the top to the bottom than from side to side. If the patient is permitted to use a commode once a day, the bed can be changed at this time. Occasionally it seems best to have several people lift the patient to a stretcher and support him in a sitting position while the bed is completely changed.

If the patient must remain on complete bed rest, he should move his legs about occasionally and tighten and relax his leg muscles, to help prevent phlebitis and muscle wasting. While the patient is being bathed, the joints should be put through the complete range of motion (Figs. 2 to 4). When the patient is acutely ill, this procedure should be done by the nurse while the patient remains passive. Later, when he is convalescing, he is taught to do the procedure without help. The patient also may be encouraged to breathe deeply five to ten times every one or two hours to expand the lungs and help to prevent hypostatic pneumonia.

Skin care. Since there may be generalized edema, special skin care should be given to the patient. The patient may be thin, malnourished, or elderly. Bony prominences should be inspected carefully for any signs of irritation and should be massaged frequently. The elbows should be observed carefully, and a lubricant should be applied to the skin, since irritation often occurs, especially if the patient must be kept in high Fowler's position. Patients also easily develop decubiti in the sacral region because of continual pressure and the edema caused by the upright position. Only light, plastic, waterproof materials should be used for protecting the mattress. Soft tissue areas are not massaged without an order from the doctor. It is best to use an alternating air-pressure mattress or a sponge-rubber mattress, but if neither type is available, pieces of sponge rubber are very helpful when placed under areas receiving pressure.

Feeding the patient. The nurse should try to make mealtime as pleasant an occasion as possible. Few people like to be fed, and the appetite of a patient with heart failure may be poor. During the acute stage of congestive failure, the diet should be soft or liquid, and the foods served should be easily digested. The work of the heart is increased during digestion, since blood is needed by the digestive tract for its functions. Several small meals a day may be better tolerated than three large meals. When the patient is allowed to feed himself, his appetite may improve as his morale improves with the feeling that he is making progress toward recovery.

Defecation. It is advisable for the patient with cardiac disease to avoid straining at defecation since it places an extra burden upon the heart. The feces are kept soft by giving daily a mild cathartic such as milk of magnesia, a mild bulk cathartic such as psyllium (Metamucil), or a stool-softening agent such as dioctyl sodium sulfosuccinate (Colace). If an oil enema is necessary, it should be given with a small rectal tube inserted only three to four inches. Most patients dislike using the bedpan, and the effort required to get onto the pan and to maintain a satisfactory position on it often puts a real strain on the heart. Some doctors prefer that the patient slide off the bed onto the commode to have a bowel evacuation. The desirability of using a commode depends upon the size of the patient and his condition. Commodes raised to bed height, so that little moving is necessary to get the patient onto them, are now available. The patient with cardiac disease should not be left alone when on the commode or a bedpan, although the nurse or attendant may leave the room or step outside the curtain to give privacy. The patient should never be made to feel hurried.

Ambulation. Ambulation for the patient recovering from acute congestive heart failure is started slowly to avoid overburdening the heart and to determine how much activity the heart can tolerate without again showing signs of failure. The regimen varies according to each patient and according to the doctor's orders. Even older patients who are acutely ill may be put on a modified schedule of bed rest after only a few days to prevent the development of circulatory or other complications. The doctor may wish them to be out of bed in a chair for several hours a day.

The usual procedure for ambulation is to have the patient dangle his legs from the side of the bed for fifteen minutes twice a day. He then may progress to sitting in a chair at the side of the bed twice a day for gradually increasing periods of time. When dangling, the patient should have support at his back and a chair on which to place his feet if he so desires. If being up in a chair is tolerated well by the patient, walking is then permitted. It should also be increased very gradually and should be closely supervised. The patient may tolerate only a few steps around his room the first few times he walks. The activity permitted is increased slowly, and most patients are fairly self-sufficient before discharge from the hospital, usually having climbed stairs, taken a bath or shower, and performed all the activities of daily living.

The patient should be observed closely during his progress in ambulation. The nurse should be alert for signs of fatigue, increased pulse rate, and dyspnea. If at any point the patient shows that he cannot tolerate the activity, or if he shows signs of distress, he should return to bed. If he is at all dyspneic, the head of the bed should be elevated. The doctor should be consulted before further ambulation is attempted. The plan for ambulation should be explained to both the patient and his family. They should understand that if activity tires the patient excessively, it may be curtailed. Overactivity can produce physical and mental setbacks that delay ultimate recovery. In the early stages of ambulation it is important to begin stressing to the patient the importance of rate of activity, that is, the demand on the heart is decreased when a normal activity is performed more slowly than before.

Digitalization. When digitalis, one of its derivatives, or a drug with similar action on the heart muscles is given to a patient with heart failure, the cardiac rate decreases and the contraction of the heart muscles become stronger, increasing the cardiac output and thereby producing improvement of all symptoms of heart failure. Over a period of twenty-four to forty-eight hours, the doctor may order that the patient with congestive heart failure be given an amount of digitalis that will slow the ventricular rate to between 70 and 75 beats per minute. This amount of digitalis is called a *digitalizing dose*, or the *optimum therapeutic dose*. In some instances this amount of digitalis may approach the toxic level, and the nurse should watch the patient carefully for symptoms of toxicity. She should observe for slowing of the pulse, irregular rhythm, loss of appetite, nausea and vomiting, mental confusion, and yellow discoloration of the conjunctivas and the skin. She should be especially alert for these symptoms when the heart and circulation return to normal under treatment because the full effects of these drugs will then be realized. Since digitalis preparations have a cumulative effect and are slowly eliminated, early recognition of toxic symptoms and discontinuance of the drug will decrease their severity and duration.

After the optimum therapeutic dose has been determined, the patient is placed on a daily maintenance dose of digitalis. The selection of a particular preparation of this drug is determined by the rapidity of action desired, the route by which it is to be given, and the response of the patient.

Before a digitalis preparation is given, the pulse rate should be taken. If the radial rate is below 60, the apical rate should be taken. If this rate also is below 60, the drug should be withheld until the doctor has been consulted. The pulse rate of patients with cardiac disease should always be taken for a full minute since the pulse may be irregular. The patient who is being digitalized usually is placed on recorded fluid intake and output, and, if possible, he is weighed before treatment is started and daily thereafter. A record of daily weight is a helpful guide to the doctor in determining whether edema is being decreased. The weight should be taken at the same time each day, preferably early in the morning, since it is more accurate before the patient has eaten or has had a bowel movement. The patient's color, the amount of edema, and the amount of dyspnea should also be observed and recorded. When the color is otherwise normal, cyanosis may be noticeable in the nail beds, the earlobes, and the lips.

The nurse should be familiar with the usual dosage of the digitalis preparation being given. Since these preparations are very potent and thus are given in small units, an overdose is extremely serious. Many of the preparations have similar names, and some come in milligram doses whereas others come in gram doses. An error between 0.1 Gm. and 0.1 mg. might mean that the patient would be given 1,000 times the dose ordered.

Powdered digitalis, or the whole leaf digitalis, is a potent oral preparation to which many patients develop toxic reactions. Usually 1.5 Gm (22 grains) of the drug are given in divided doses over a period of twenty-four to forty-eight hours in order to achieve initial digitalization. The usual maintenance dose is 0.1 Gm. per day. If any toxic symptoms appear, such as loss of appetite, nausea and vomiting, a drop in the pulse rate below 60, development of an irregular rhythm, headache, malaise, drowsiness, blurred or colored vision, or hallucinations, the drug is stopped, and the patient is kept quiet with sedatives. Potassium chloride may be given intravenously if the patient has potassium deficiency. When the digitalis has been eliminated from the body, treatment may be resumed.

Several types of purified glycosides of digitalis have been developed for use when the patient cannot tolerate powdered digitalis. The effects are the same, but the speed of action and the rate of elimination are different. Although the toxic symptoms are the same, severe toxicity is less likely to occur.

Digitoxin is a glycoside of digitalis. It may be ordered under the following names: Purodigin, Digitaline nativelle, Crystodigin, and Unidigin. Digitoxin is excreted slowly. The usual digitalizing dose is 1.5 mg. (1/40 grain) given over a period of twenty-four to forty-eight hours. The maintenance dose is 0.1 or 0.2 mg. (1/600 to 1/300 grain) a day. This drug may be given either orally or intravenously.

Lanatoside C (Cedilanid) is also a purified glycoside of digitalis. It comes as an oral preparation only, and the usual maintenance dose is 0.5 mg. (1/120 grain) a day.

Deslanoside (desacetyl-lanatoside C; Cedilanid-D) is a glycoside of digitalis for intravenous use. An initial dose of 1.2 to 1.6 mg. (1/50 to 1/40 grain) is usually given, followed by a maintenance dose of 0.2 to 0.6 mg. (1/300 to 1/100 grain) each day.

Digoxin (Lanoxin) is a purified glycoside of digitalis that produces effects more rapidly than does digitoxin. It is also eliminated more rapidly. It may be given either orally or intravenously. The average digitalizing dose is 4 mg. (1/16 grain) orally or 0.5 to 1.5 mg. (1/120 to 1/40 grain) intravenously. The maintenance dose both orally and intravenously is 0.25 to 0.75 mg. (1/250 to 1/90 grain) daily. If any of the drug infiltrates into the tissues during intravenous injection, sloughing may occur since digoxin is a tissue irritant. Heat should be applied to the infiltrated area immediately to encourage absorption of the drug into the bloodstream.

Digalen is very similar to digitalis. It can be given both orally and intravenously. The usual maintenance dose is 0.5 to 1 U.S.P. unit three times a day.

Digilanid is a drug that has an action similar to that of digitalis. It can be given orally, rectally, intramuscularly, and intravenously. Two to four tablets (0.67 to 1.33 mg.) are given by mouth daily until the patient is fully digitalized, and then one or two tablets are given daily as a maintenance dose.

Digifolin is also a form of digitalis leaf. It can be given orally and intravenously. Until the desired effects are obtained, 0.8 U.S.P. unit is given daily.

Gitalin (amorphous) (Gitaligin) is excreted more slowly than digoxin but more rapidly than digitoxin. It is given by mouth, and two or three tablets are given daily for three or four days or until 4 to 6.5 mg. (1/15 to 1/10 grain) have been given. The daily maintenance dose is then usually 0.25 to 0.75 mg. (1/250 to 1/90 grain).

Ouabain (g-strophanthin) is the drug often used for emergency treatment of patients with congestive heart failure. It acts very rapidly when injected intravenously or intramuscularly, but it is quickly excreted. Therefore, it is not suitable for a maintenance drug and usually is used in conjunction with some other digitalis preparation. Usually no more than 0.5 mg. (1/120 grain) of this drug is given daily because of its potency.

Treatment with diet. Edema is most effectively controlled in patients with heart failure by restriction of sodium intake. The degree of restriction depends on the severity of the failure. In mild failure the doctor may order that sodium be restricted only to 1 to 2 grams per day.[31] The normal diet contains 3 to 6 grams of sodium per day. This diet is essentially normal except that no extra salt is added to prepared foods. If this measure does not control the edema, however, salt may be restricted to as little as 250 mg. of sodium chloride a day. Because it is difficult to maintain an adequate protein intake on a sodium-restricted diet, a very low-sodium milk, such as Lanalac, may need to be used to supplement the diet. Since the vitamin B intake may also be inadequate because of low protein in a sodium-restricted diet, vitamin supplements are usually ordered. A diet with a very low sodium content is unpalatable, and special efforts should be made to use other seasonings. If the patient does not have kidney involvement, the doctor may permit the use of salt substitutes such as potassium chloride. (See p. 359 for suggestions for making sodium-restricted diets more palatable.) If the patient is on diuretic drugs, sodium may not be limited below 3 to 5 grams because of the danger of sodium chloride depletion in the blood (p. 99).

Fluids are often limited to 1,800 ml. a day for patients with congestive heart failure. Such patients may have only about six glasses of fluid a day in addition to fluids contained in food. Soups are usually not served because they tend to make the patient thirsty. Watery foods also must be restricted because they may appreciably increase the fluid intake. If the patient finds this degree of fluid restriction intolerable, the nurse should be sure that foods that might make him more thirsty are not being served, that fluids are spaced throughout the day, and that he is given frequent mouth care, using an iced mouthwash.

Some physicians feel that fluids need not be limited as long as the patient is on a restricted-sodium diet and is receiving diuretics and digitalis. They feel that under these circumstances fluids actually act as a diuretic and are beneficial in helping to remove fluids from the tissues. The nursing care would then be adjusted to this theory, and fluids would be forced.

The reason for diet and fluid restrictions should be explained to both the patient and his family so that the patient does not become unduly upset and so that the family does not bring him food or fluids that are unacceptable. The patient often must continue the diet and fluid restrictions after discharge from the hospital. Therefore, when he feels better, mealtime may be used to teach him about the type of foods he may include in his diet at home. If he does not eat well, efforts should be made to find food preparations that he will eat in order to maintain normal nutrition.

Diuretic drugs. If restrictions of sodium and fluids and the administration of digitalis do not appreciably relieve the tissue edema and the pulmonary edema, the doctor may order diuretic drugs. A diuretic also may be used to give prompt relief to the patient who is in acute distress because of severe edema of the tissues. Any patient who is receiving a diuretic drug should be weighed daily. If the patient is at home, arrangements will need to be made to provide scales, and the patient or his family must be taught to record the weight daily. Usually the drug is prescribed to be given during the early hours of the day so that the height of the diuretic effect does not fall within normal sleeping hours and disturb sleep unduly.

The organic mercurial diuretics are considered probably the most effective and are widely used, although chlorothiazide (Diuril) and its derivatives are now being used more often. Mercurial drugs are available for use orally, intravenously, intramuscularly, and subcutaneously. The intramuscular route is usually preferred. Rare deaths due to ventricular fibrillation following intravenous injections of these drugs have been reported.[3] The mercurial drug may be given every second or third day or weekly, depending upon the individual patient. As much as 1 to 2 liters of fluid may be excreted during the day of the injection. The patient may complain of local discomfort at the site of the injection. Discomfort may be relieved by hot applications to the area, which hasten the absorption of the drug.

The patient who is receiving any mercurial diuretic over a long period should be watched for signs of toxic reactions to the mercury such as stomatitis, gingivitis, increased salivation, diarrhea, albuminuria, hematuria, and skin eruption. He may also complain of flushing and have febrile reactions to the drug. Toxic signs must be reported to the doctor at once.

Some patients receiving mercurial diuretics may have toxic signs caused by sodium, calcium, or potassium depletion, since sodium, calcium, or potassium may also be lost in large amounts through the kidney while its reabsorptive powers are depressed by the mercurial diuretics. Nausea, vomiting, fever, and cramps in the calves of the legs and in the stomach can be due to sodium depletion. Potassium depletion causes extreme weakness and symptoms of paralytic ileus. Calcium depletion may cause the patient to develop tetany, with muscle spasm. Skin rashes may also occur. The patient who is receiving both diuretic drugs and digitalis needs to be watched closely for toxic reactions to digitalis since toxicity occurs much sooner if the serum potassium is low. If a reaction to a mercurial preparation occurs, the doctor will institute measures to replace the depleted electrolytes. Reactions often can be prevented by giving the patient a little more salt in his food (if medically approved) and by encouraging him to take food and fluids high in potassium and calcium. Another form of the drug often can be substituted later without untoward reactions.

Mercurial diuretics may be given in combination with *ammonium chloride,* which is a diuretic now seldom used alone. It has an acidifying effect that enhances the potency of the mercurial drugs because, in an effort to prevent acidosis, the sodium from the tissues unites with the chloride to neutralize it, mobilizing both the salt and the water for excretion by the kidney.[2] Ammonium chloride in enteric-coated tablets may be given on the two or three days prior to, and on the day of, the administration of the mercurial preparation. For the best results it should then be omitted for a day or two. The usual dosage is 6 to 10 Gm. a day given in four doses.[2] Ammonium chloride should be taken after meals or with food since it may cause gastric irritation. Neither the mercurial drugs nor ammonium chloride are usually prescribed by the doctor if the patient has signs of kidney damage, since serious electrolyte imbalance may occur.

A widely used mercurial drug is *meralluride injection* (Mercuhydrin injection). It contains organically combined mercury and theophylline and is given intramuscularly or intravenously. The addition of theophylline increases the diuretic effect by improving absorption and also decreases irritation at the site of injection.[3] The dosage is usually 1 to 2 ml. *Mercaptomerin sodium* (Thiomerin sodium) is a mercurial preparation that can be given subcutaneously and has,

therefore, the advantage that patients or their family members can learn to give the drug. It causes little pain upon injection but may cause local reactions such as edema. The injection should be given quite deeply to avoid injection into subcutaneous fat. Since the drug deteriorates at room temperature, the patient receiving it at home must be cautioned to keep it in the refrigerator. Thiomerin is now available to be used in rectal suppository form.[3] *Chlormerodrin* (Neohydrin) is a form of mercurial drug that can be taken orally, although it is seldom prescribed if edema is severe. The average dose is 55 to 110 mg. (¾ to 1½ grains) daily. Many other mercurial preparations are now available.

Chlorothiazide (Diuril) is a relatively new and effective oral diuretic. It inhibits the reabsorption of sodium from the glomerular filtrate by the kidney tubules and thereby causes less reabsorption of water and other electrolytes. It is often given in two doses of 0.5 to 1 Gm. (7½ to 15 grains) daily, although only one daily dose may be given. The drug is effective for about twelve hours.

Many other drugs allied to chlorothiazide are now available and are described in pharmacology texts. Chlorothiazide and the related drugs cause loss of potassium, and for this reason the doctor may order that potassium be given parenterally or orally and that potassium in the diet be increased by having the patient take more high-potassium foods, such as fresh fruit and fruit juice, daily. Toxic signs are not common, but blurring of vision, dryness of the mouth, dizziness, muscle cramps, skin eruptions, and agranulocytosis have been reported. Large doses may lead to acidosis due to excretion of bicarbonate and may be contraindicated if the patient has renal disease.

Acetazolamide (Diamox) is a preparation that depresses the renal tubules, promoting excretion of the bicarbonate ion rather than the chloride ion. It is given orally once a day in doses of 250 to 500 mg. and remains active for six to eight hours. It often is given every other day, being alternated with a mercurial preparation. This drug may make the patient drowsy, and he may complain of numbness and tingling in the face and extremities.

Spironolactone (Aldactone) has a diuretic

effect by blocking the action of aldosterone, a hormone that acts by increasing the retention of sodium and the excretion of potassium. It has been given in combination with other diuretics to lessen the excretion of potassium. This drug is given orally in doses of 3 Gm. (45 grains) daily. It is slow in its action, and toxic signs have been reported, particularly in patients who have hepatic or renal damage.

Occasionally, xanthine derivatives are used as diuretics. They act by increasing the rate of sodium elimination from the kidneys. *Theobromine calcium salicylate* and *theophylline ethylenediamine* (aminophylline) are the drugs most often used. Theobromine usually is given in doses of 0.5 Gm. (7½ grains), and 0.25 Gm. (4 grains) of aminophylline may be given. Aminophylline may be given orally, rectally, or intravenously. Xanthine derivatives given orally cause gastric irritation and therefore should be given with food. These drugs may be used if smooth muscle relaxation is also desired; for example, they are often prescribed for patients who have angina pectoris to help relax the smooth muscles of the coronary vessels.

To relieve an abdominal ascites or a pleural effusion, sometimes it is necessary for the doctor to aspirate fluid. This is done through an abdominal paracentesis and a thoracentesis, respectively. (For the nursing care of patients undergoing these procedures, see texts on fundamentals of nursing and pp. 714 and 571.)

Acute pulmonary edema

Acute pulmonary edema is a medical emergency in patients with heart disease. It is caused by additional or prolonged strain on an already damaged heart, with resultant failure. Either physical or emotional exertion can precipitate pulmonary edema. Cardiac output is decreased and serous fluid under pressure is pushed back through the pulmonary capillaries into the alveoli. Fluid rapidly reaches the bronchioles and bronchi, and the patient begins to drown in his own secretions. Acute pulmonary edema also may follow such conditions as inhalation of irritating gases, cerebrovascular accident, fractures of the skull, too rapid

administration of plasma, serum albumin, whole blood, or other intravenous fluids, and barbiturate or opiate poisoning. Severe dyspnea, cyanosis, and restlessness are usual symptoms.

The patient with suspected acute pulmonary edema should be placed in bed in a high Fowler's position, and the doctor should be summoned immediately. He usually orders morphine sulfate, 15 mg. (¼ grain), to be given at once to quiet breathing and to allay apprehension. It may be given intravenously since circulatory collapse may hinder its absorption from the tissues. Aminophylline usually is given because it helps to increase the cardiac output and to lower the venous pressure by relaxing the smooth muscles of the blood vessels and because it relieves bronchial spasm. Digitalization usually is started immediately. Either ouabain or deslanoside is used because of the quick action of these drugs. Since it is dangerous to give either of these drugs if the patient is routinely taking digitalis, the nurse should try to ascertain from the patient or his family whether he takes any heart medicines, and she should inform the doctor of her findings. Oxygen under pressure is usually ordered to prevent further escape of fluid from the pulmonary capillaries into the lungs. A mercurial diuretic also may be given.

The doctor may order rotating tourniquets to relieve acute pulmonary edema. The tourniquets are placed on three of the extremities at a time, thus reducing the amount of blood that must be circulated by the overtaxed heart. (See Figs. 68 and 69.) Every fifteen minutes, in clockwise or counterclockwise order, one tourniquet is removed and placed on the extremity that has had no tourniquet on it. In this way the vessels of each extremity are occluded for forty-five minutes at a time, and then the tourniquet is released from the extremity for fifteen minutes. The fourth tourniquet should be applied before one is removed. Care must be taken that no tourniquet is left on longer than forty-five minutes lest the tissues be permanently damaged, and the tourniquet should not obliterate arterial pulses in the extremity. The use of a prepared diagram and time schedule kept at the patient's bedside helps ensure the proper changing of the tourniquets. This procedure may be done by either the doctor or the nurse, and it is continued until the acute pulmonary edema subsides. If the patient is alert, the procedure should be explained to him. He may need a narcotic to make him less conscious of the pressure of the tourniquets and of the uncomfortable sensation in the extremities caused by venous engorgement. If the procedure must be continued over a long period, the skin should be watched carefully for beginning signs of irritation from pressure. The tourniquet may be placed over the patient's gown or a towel to prevent damage to the skin. If the extremity does not readily return to normal color on release of the tourniquet, the doctor should be informed. When treatment is to be discontinued, one tourniquet is removed at a time, according to time intervals, until all tourniquets have been removed. Sometimes, if the patient is not in shock, the doctor will remove 500 to 800 ml. of blood by a *phlebotomy*. The decrease in the amount of circulating blood decreases pulmonary engorgement. This procedure is similar to that for taking blood from a blood donor.

Home care. If possible, patients with acute pulmonary edema are hospitalized. However, if it is impossible to move them from their homes, improvisations can be made to care for them adequately. Oxygen can be obtained from fire stations or ambulances for emergency use, and hospitals or medical supply houses will provide equipment for continued use. Other sickroom equipment usually can be borrowed from the local public health nursing agency. The local health department office often knows where equipment is available. The patient can be put in a high Fowler's position in the home by use of an inverted straight chair placed on the bed and padded with blankets and pillows. Six-inch blocks placed under the legs of the bed to raise the height make it easier to care for the patient, although side rails should then be used. The patient with acute pulmonary edema needs continuous nursing care. The nurse will need to assist the family in learning to provide parts of the patient's care, if possible, and she may help them to secure a nurse who will remain in the home during the critical period. As the patient improves, his care will be that of

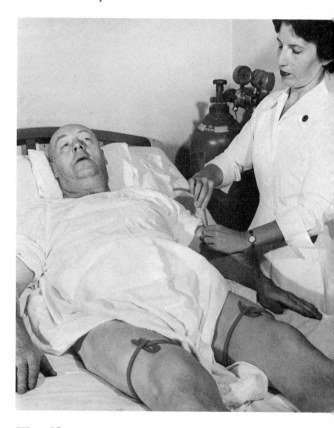

Fig. 68

Here the tourniquets are being applied in a clockwise order. The nurse has removed the tourniquet from the right arm and is applying it to the left arm.

any patient with heart failure. Continuing care can be planned by the patient's physician, the public health nurse, and the family.

Cardiac arrhythmias

Cardiac rhythm, the sequence of heart beats, is normally controlled by the sino-atrial node, sometimes called the "pacemaker." The stimulus initiating the beat arises in the sinus node located in the right atrium spreads over the atria, inducing their contraction, and then spreads over the atrioventricular bundle to stimulate simultaneous contraction of both ventricles.[2] Both the rate and the rhythm of the heartbeat are usually regular but may vary under cer-

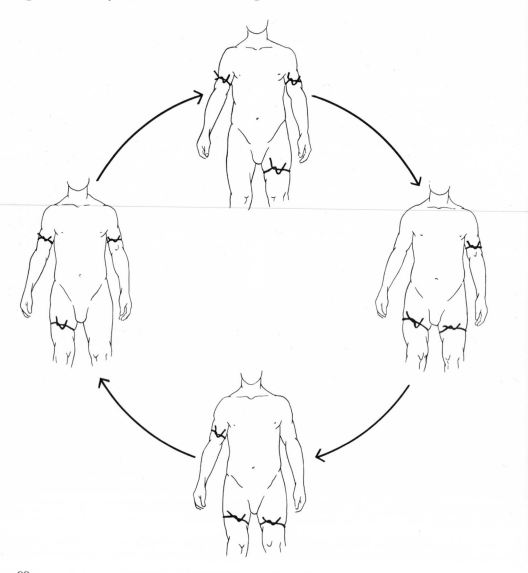

Fig. 69

Clockwise method of removing and applying rotating tourniquets.

tain circumstances. These variations may be a normal physiologic response, may have no clinical importance, or may be a symptom or a complication of organic heart disease. Although some arrhythmias do not cause any symptoms, they are noticeable to the patient and cause apprehension. He may describe the sensations as a "flutter," a "turning over" of the heart, "pounding" or "palpation" of the heart, or "skipping" of the heart. He often feels weak or faint. If he

feels his pulse, he may be aware that it is very rapid and irregular or perhaps very slow. Patients with extremely slow pulse rates, however, are less likely to have symptoms.

Patients with cardiac irregularities should be urged to seek medical attention. If, after a thorough examination, the doctor finds nothing organically wrong, the patient should be urged to live normally.

Cardiac irregularities in patients with organic heart disease should be reported to the doctor immediately, since they may become incompatible with life. The pulse rate of a patient with cardiac disease should be taken by a professional nurse for a full minute several times a day to note any marked increase or decrease in the rate, the presence of alternating strong and weak beats (pulsus alternans), coupling of beats (two together followed by a pause), or other irregularities in the rhythm. Abnormal rates and rhythm in a patient with heart disease often mean that the ventricle is not pumping adequate blood into the systemic circulation to take care of body needs. Congestive heart failure may then occur.

Sinus tachycardia

The most common rhythm disturbance of the heart is sinus tachycardia. It is characterized by a heartbeat of more than 100 contractions per minute, and is a normal physiologic reaction to exercise, fever, fear, and excitement, or any other condition in which the basal metabolism is increased, thus necessitating a greater supply of blood. For example, tachycardia is common in patients with fever, anemia, pulmonary tuberculosis, rheumatic fever, hyperthyroidism, myocardial infarctions, congestive heart failure, and hemorrhage. The patient may be unaware of the speeded-up heart rate, or he may complain of palpitations. The doctor may order sedatives to relieve annoying symptoms. When the underlying cause is corrected, the heart rate returns to normal.

Sinus bradycardia

In sinus bradycardia the heart rate falls to 60 beats per minute or slower. A heart rate as slow as this is common in young adult men and in athletes. Bradycardia also normally occurs during sleep. It may also occur in patients with brain lesions and in patients receiving digitalis because of the drug's action in slowing the heartbeat. On withdrawal of digitalis, the heart rate will return to normal. There is no treatment of bradycardia other than removal of the cause.

Heart block

In heart block, normal stimuli arise in the sinoatrial nodes, but they are blocked or delayed on their way down the atrioventric-

ular bundle. The passage of a stimulus from its point of initiation in the atrium to the ventricle normally takes less than 0.2 second.[2] If there is any interference in its passage, the ventricles do not contract as expected, and thus a heart block has occurred. It may be only partial or it may be complete. The patient with complete heart block may have no symptoms once the block is established because, although no impulses from the atria reach the ventricles, the ventricles have adjusted by setting up their own rate. This rate is usually very slow (30 to 40 beats per minute). During the period before complete block occurs, however, the patient may have symptoms known as the *Adams-Stokes syndrome*. He may faint and have convulsive seizures, and on exertion he may feel dizzy and weak. This syndrome may be treated by giving Adrenalin 1:1,000 (0.5 to 1 ml.) during acute seizures and then ephedrine sulfate, 20 to 30 mg. three times a day. A newer preparation frequently used is isoproterenol hydrochloride (Isuprel), 10 to 15 mg. (1/6 to 1/4 grain) tablets, administered sublingually. Isuprel has a stimulating effect on the heart, resulting in better conduction of electrical impulses, an increased ventricular rate, and improvement of blood circulation. When the block is due to an acute inflammatory disorder, as in acute rheumatic fever, steroids may be given. There is some evidence that steroids given intravenously may promote normal conduction in patients with acute myocardial infarction who develop heart block.[2] Doctors usually advise patients with heart block to avoid strenuous exercise but otherwise to lead normal lives. Heart block in a patient with arteriosclerosis or a myocardial infarction is indicative of progressive heart damage.[2]

Pacemaker. The electric pacemaker is an electrically operated mechanical device that stimulates ventricular heart action. It can be adjusted to stimulate the ventricular contractions either constantly and at a normal rate or else only when normal impulses are not forthcoming or fall below a rate set by the doctor. The machine can also be set solely to monitor the heartbeat. If the heart stops beating while it is being monitored, an alarm will sound and the pacemaker will send two charges of electricity through the heart at eight-second intervals. The medical

331

staff, responding to the alarm, will then decide whether further stimulation is necessary. The electric pacemaker may be used as an emergency measure in event of sudden heart block, as a safety measure following cardiac surgery, or in medical illness when it is suspected that heart block may occur.

A special paste is applied to the skin, and the electrodes from the machine are placed across the anterior chest and secured under a rubber strap fastened about the chest. The skin beneath the electrodes should be kept clean and dry, and the paste is renewed every two or three hours to prevent burning of the skin, since the paste dries in that time. The position of the electrodes is changed daily by the doctor. The greatest care must be taken in turning the patient lest the electrodes become loosened. The patient on whom this device is used usually is critically ill and needs constant nursing attention. He needs repeated reassurance when he becomes aware of his condition and of the significance of the machine.

Another method of regulating the heart rate externally is by stimulation of the right ventricular endocardial surface by means of a cardiac catheter placed into the jugular vein. A battery pacemaker is then worn about the neck. A cardiac catheter without lumen and an electrical wire with metal tip are passed into the jugular vein to the right ventricle. When satisfactorily placed, the catheter is sutured to the skin to prevent displacement. With the unit working satisfactorily, the patient may be discharged to his home and return every month or when necessary for battery check and/or change, fluoroscopy to determine the position of the catheter, and an electrocardiogram.

Another method of regulating the heart rate is the use of needles that may be inserted under the skin as electrodes or inserted into the heart through the chest wall and connected by wires to an external pacemaker. Needles also may be placed in the myocardium at the time of surgery and connected by wires brought out through the skin to the external pacemaker.

The maintenance and operation of the electric pacemaker is the responsibility of the physician, but the nurse must understand its use and be able to care for the patient when it is used. A continuous high-pitched beep is heard as the electrical activity of the heart is picked up and amplified. It serves to inform the persons in attendance that the equipment is working properly. In contrast, most alarms sound a steady, loud buzz if anything is wrong. Portable pacemakers are now available for use by patients who need this apparatus for long periods but who otherwise need not remain at bed rest in the hospital (Fig. 70).

The patient is usually quite apprehensive when being weaned from the machine and again needs almost constant nursing attention and repeated reassurance for a time.

External pacemakers are unsatisfactory for long-term use because infection will travel along the electrode wires. Several types of implantable (internal) pacemakers are available. One type uses mercury cells as its source of power and is estimated to last five years.[14] The unit, which is encased in Teflon, is implanted in the subcutaneous tissues of the chest or other adjacent areas of the body. Its electrode wires extend through the chest wall the electrodes are implanted in the myocardium, usually the left ventricular wall[32] (Fig. 71). Another type of implantable pacemaker is a tiny, self-contained, transistorized unit measuring 6 cm. in diameter and 1.5 cm. in thickness (Fig. 72). The internal pacemaker delivers from 8 to 15 volts to the heart muscle at regular intervals and may last for as long as five years. Batteries or cells in the set can be replaced without disturbing the electrodes by making a small surgical opening in the tissue directly over the pacemaker.

Any patient who uses an internal pacemaker should have careful medical and nursing supervision. If the patient returns home, a referral to the public health nursing agency in his community is often needed. Many patients do surprisingly well with this seemingly complicated form of treatment. Occasionally, however, any part of the equipment may act as a foreign body and cause local or systemic reaction. The patient who develops any pain or tenderness at the point of insertion or of attachment of any piece of the equipment, or who develops an elevation of temperature or any other general symptoms should be advised to contact his doctor at once.

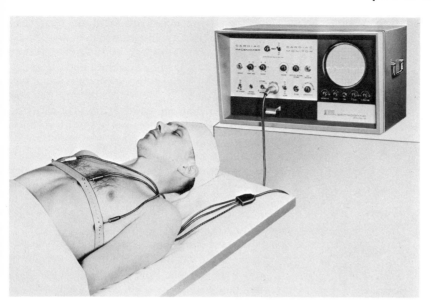

Fig. 70

The pacemaker is an electrically operated mechanical device that stimulates ventricular heart action. (Courtesy Electrodyne Co., Inc., Norwood, Mass.)

Sinus irregularity

In sinoatrial block, the sinus node pauses momentarily, causing an interruption in the discharge of impulses over the atria and into the ventricles. This interruption is caused by increased activity of the vagus nerve and may be precipitated by quinidine, potassium salts, or digitalis.[2] It may also follow stimulation of an oversensitive carotid sinus by sudden turning of the head, pressure of a tight collar, or bending forward. The heartbeat will be irregular, and if no stimuli are discharged for several seconds, the patient may faint. This condition may be treated with such drugs as atropine sulfate, tincture of belladonna, ephedrine, and phenobarbital. Sometimes the carotid sinus must be denervated to relieve the symptoms.

Ventricular and atrial premature contractions

The irregularity in rhythm of both the atria and the ventricles gives similar symptoms, but atrial arrhythmia occurs more

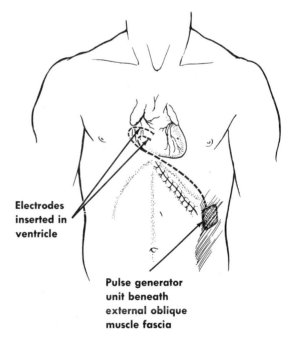

Electrodes inserted in ventricle

Pulse generator unit beneath external oblique muscle fascia

Fig. 71

The pacemaker may be implanted subcutaneously in the upper abdominal area and the electrodes directed through the diaphragm into the myocardium of the heart.

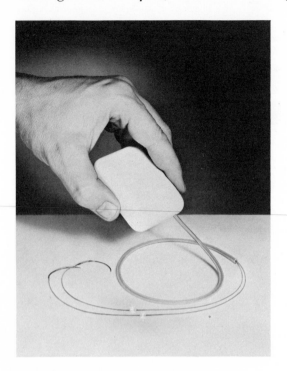

Fig. 72

Implantable pacemaker; the entire unit
is implanted within the body where electrodes
go to the heart muscle. Note the size
of the pacemaker. (Courtesy Electrodyne
Co., Inc., Norwood, Mass.)

often in young persons, whereas ventricular arrhythmia occurs more often in older persons. In both conditions there is a premature contraction of the chamber due to abnormal stimuli. The beat is coupled, and the patient is often aware of the irregularity, complaining of palpitation and "flutter." He may have a "catch" in his throat and a cough. This premature beat may occur only occasionally, it may occur in a regular pattern, or there may be several beats in sequence. Atrial and ventricular arrhythmias may be of no significance, or they may be associated with organic heart diseases such as mitral stenosis and coronary artery disease. Triple bromides, 1 Gm. (15 grains), or other sedatives may be given three times a day to relieve intolerable symptoms. The patient taking this drug should be warned that he will be drowsy and therefore should neither drive

on long trips nor work with or near machinery or in any situation where his safety depends upon alertness. A rash may occur, and the drug is then discontinued. If sedation fails to relieve the symptoms in a patient with atrial arrhythmia, digitalis may be given. The patient with ventricular arrhythmia, however, is often not digitalized since the irritability of the ventricle may be increased, thereby causing greater irregularity in the heartbeat. Quinidine sulfate is sometimes given to patients with this condition.

Paroxysmal tachycardia

Paroxysmal tachycardia may be either atrial or ventricular in origin. Atrial paroxysmal tachycardia is seen more frequently in young people, and ventricular paroxysmal tachycardia is seen more frequently in older patients. An attack is often precipitated by the consumption of large amounts of alcohol, by excessive smoking, by a gastrointestinal upset, or by an acute infection.[2] Both forms are characterized by a sudden onset of rapid, regular heartbeats. The rate frequently increases to over 150 beats a minute. The patient complains of palpitation and flutter of the heart, feels weak and faint, and is short of breath and apprehensive.

Patients often arrest attacks of atrial paroxysmal tachycardia by holding the breath, inducing vomiting, bending forward, or pressing on the carotid sinuses. The latter is dangerous and should be done only by a doctor. He may suggest that the patient try the other measures himself. If the attack persists over an extended period of time, the patient is put to bed, and the doctor may order digitalization and sedation. The treatment for ventricular paroxysmal tachycardia is bed rest and quinidine sulfate. This treatment terminates the fibrillation and restores normal rhythm. The doctor may also order *procainamide hydrochloride* (Pronestyl hydrochloride), which decreases the irritability of the ventricular muscle and, when given orally, acts in thirty to sixty minutes. If given intravenously, it must be given very slowly, and the blood pressure must be taken as it is administered. If hypotension occurs, the rate of administration must be slowed down. The usual oral dose is 1 Gm. (15 grains), followed by 0.5 Gm. (7½ grains) every four to six hours. If untreated, this condition can lead to ventricular fibrillation and death.

Fibrillation

Atrial fibrillation is a common irregularity of cardiac rhythm. It usually is associated with organic heart diseases such as rheumatic heart disease, mitral stenosis, and myocardial infarction, but it may follow the injudicious use of alcohol, excessive smoking, large meals, or anesthesia.[2]

The sinus node no longer controls the rhythm of the heart, the atria no longer contract in coordination, and there is a complete irregularity of the ventricular beats. The atria may receive as many as 400 to 600 stimuli a minute, but the ventricles rarely contract more than 130 to 150 times a minute, since not all the stimuli are carried over the atrioventricular bundle, and the ventricles do not respond to all the impulses that are sent through. When the ventricle contracts at a very rapid rate, there is little blood in the ventricle when systole occurs, and not enough blood is pumped into the aorta with each beat to produce radial pulsation. This accounts for the pulse deficit (the difference between the apical pulse and the radial pulse). The pulse deficit represents wasted cardiac energy.

The patient whose heart is fibrillating usually is put to bed and given either digitalis or quinidine sulfate. Digitalis acts by blocking the impulses that pass from the atria to the ventricles, increasing the interval between the heartbeats so that the ventricles will contain more blood before they contract. *Quinidine sulfate* restores the normal rhythm by increasing the rest period of the atrial muscles. The doctor may order the pulse rate to be taken before quinidine sulfate is given. If there has been a marked slowing of the rate, the drug should be withheld and the physician consulted. The usual dose of quinidine is 0.2 to 0.4 Gm. (3 to 6 grains) by mouth. It may be repeated every four hours for two to three days. When quinidine is first given, the patient should be watched carefully for toxic signs since many persons are allergic to it. If he becomes flushed, complains of ringing in the ears, or becomes nauseated or faint, or if the pulse rate increases, the drug should be withheld until the doctor is consulted.

In the patient with a diseased heart there is also the danger that the sudden return to a regular atrial heartbeat may cause emboli to break away from the atrial walls. Thrombi are likely to have formed there while the blood has been pumped inadequately.

The nurse often is asked to record the apical-radial pulse rate several times a day so that there will be an indication of how well the patient is responding to treatment. In taking an apical-radial pulse rate, one nurse counts the apical beat, using a stethoscope, while a second nurse simultaneously counts the radial rate. One must be responsible for indicating the beginning and ending count so that results will be accurate. As the patient improves, the apical beat should gradually decrease and strengthen until each beat is carried through to the radial artery and the two rates are the same.

In *ventricular fibrillation* the coordinated contraction of the ventricles is replaced by rapid, irregular twitching of the ventricular muscles.[2] Continued ventricular fibrillation is incompatible with life, since these twitchings do not force enough blood into the systemic circulation to meet body needs. Ventricular fibrillation is often the cause of sudden death in patients with coronary artery disease and during or after the administration of some anesthetic agents. This condition is known as *cardiac arrest* and requires immediate and drastic emergency measures. The doctor may give procainamide hydrochloride intravenously, or he may give it directly into the heart muscle to stop the fibrillation. Cardiac massage may be done.

Artificial respiration is used first since it may be sufficient to revive the patient. If the patient takes several deep breaths but a pulse cannot be detected in the major vessels, external cardiac massage usually is started by the doctor. If two persons are present, artificial respiration is given by one.

Cardiac massage

External cardiac massage. External cardiac massage is the rhythmic compression of the heart between the lower sternum and the thoracic vertebral column. As pressure is applied, blood is forced out into the systemic and pulmonary circulation. With re-

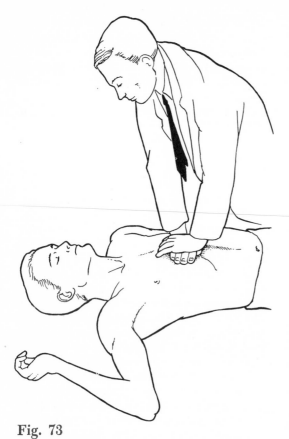

Fig. 73

Physician doing external cardiac massage.

laxation, the heart refills with venous blood. The doctor either kneels or stands to one side of the patient and applies pressure with the heel of his hand to avoid pressing on a large area of the chest wall and possibly damaging or breaking the ribs (Fig. 73). The rate of compression and relaxation is usually 60 to 80 beats per minute. The patient's body should be supported by a firm mattress or board (floor when necessary) to provide the proper resistance when pressure is being applied to the sternum. (See p. 242.)

The nurse should keep the patient area clear of persons not helping with treatment. Usually, two nurses working together can keep drugs ready and assist in the observation of blood pressure and femoral pulse as well as obtain any additional equipment required. One nurse should check carefully for signs of return of pulse in the carotid or

femoral arteries. Constriction of pupils, occasional respiration, movement of the body, and improved color are signs of general improvement.

The most common complications of external cardiac massage are fracture or cracking of the ribs. If medications are injected into the heart, signs of pneumothorax should be watched for carefully. They include chest pain and dyspnea. Other possible accidents are hepatic hematoma or rupture and fracture of the sternum.

Many hospitals have a prepared team of personnel, including doctors, nurses, anesthesiologists, and technicians, who can be called upon to give immediate and complete care when cardiac arrest occurs. Most hospital wards are equipped with a cardiac arrest tray or have access to a specially equipped cart on which all necessary items are available. Equipment needed includes an electrocardiograph, a defibrillator, a laryngoscope, a variety of endotracheal tubes, a venous cutdown set, fluids for intravenous use, a suction machine, oxygen, and a tracheotomy set. The drugs usually given are epinephrine 1:1,000 for direct intracardiac injection, sodium bicarbonate (44 mEq.) to combat acidosis, and calcium chloride, 10% solution, to improve myocardial tone.

External cardiac massage is now considered an emergency procedure. Formerly it was a medical procedure and could be performed by physicians only. Nurses and other persons who have received special preparation in this procedure may save a life by taking immediate action as well as summoning a doctor. If nothing is done for the patient until the doctor arrives, it may be too late to save the person's life, or extensive brain damage may have occurred. Very often, nurses working in special cardiac units or intensive care units become very skilled in this procedure and are expected to use their own judgment in beginning cardiac massage. Nursing practice acts approved by the state or by individual hospital policy may prohibit nurses or other persons from taking the initial steps for cardiac massage. At this writing there is still much controversy about persons other than the doctors doing cardiac massage.

Open cardiac massage. In this seldom used method of cardiac massage, the chest cavity is surgically incised directly over the heart, the ribs are spread apart, and the heart is massaged with the hands or stimulated with an electric current. A 100-volt alternating current with an amperage of 1.5 is used. An electrically operated defibrillator and pacemaker may be used; the defibrillator stops the irregular heartbeat, and the pacemaker then restarts heart action. A combination machine, which acts as a defibrillator as well as a pacemaker and monitor, may be used. Occasionally a patient is saved by the use of open cardiac massage, but it must be employed within three minutes after the cessation of cardiac function.[47]

Specific diseases of the heart

Hypertensive heart disease

An estimated 17 million adults in the United States were found to have definite hypertension and 10.5 million adults to have hypertensive heart disease during the recent Health Examination Survey.[34] Hypertension is one of the most common causes of heart diseases, and it affects all age groups. However, prevalence of both hypertension and hypertensive heart disease rises with age. The patient is said to have hypertension when the resting systolic blood pressure reading is consistently over 160 mm. Hg, the diastolic pressure is over 90 mm. Hg, and any of the symptoms of hypertensive disease are present.[2] The elevation of the diastolic pressure is of greater significance than that of the systolic pressure. The diastolic pressure more closely indicates the pressure exerted on the arterial walls by the circulating blood exclusive of the additional pressure caused by the contraction of the left ventricle, the pulse pressure. In hypertension there is increased peripheral arteriolar resistance. The constricted systemic arterioles offer greater resistance to the flow of blood from the arteries into the capillaries and veins. The arterial pressure rises to compensate for this increased resistance. The cardiac output remains normal in volume, but blood must be pumped by the heart at an increased pressure to counteract resistance and thus maintain flow. Two pathologic changes occur in time. The walls of the arterioles thicken, and the left ventricle, which has to work increasingly harder to

push against the resistance, becomes hypertrophied. Eventually, the left ventricle may no longer be able to pump the blood out of the heart adequately, and congestive heart failure develops. Inadequate blood supply through the coronary arteries may cause symptoms of angina pectoris, or acute myocardial infarction may occur.

Hypertension may be present for years before the patient has any symptoms. Since no prevention or specific treatment is known, doctors feel that it is best only to tell patients that they have a tendency toward high blood pressure and to reassure them that it may not cause any difficulties for many years. Until symptoms appear, follow-up examinations may be suggested for only every six months to a year. No restrictions are placed on activity, except that young people are encouraged to participate in individual sports instead of group sports lest they feel impelled to overexert themselves so as not to let down their teammates. Moderation in all activities should be the rule, as it should be for all people. Excess in food, alcohol, tobacco, tea, and coffee should be avoided, and adequate rest should be obtained. If the patient has a tendency to become overly tense, he should be encouraged to talk to someone who will listen to his problems—a medical doctor, a member of his family, a friend, a minister, a nurse, a social worker, or a psychiatrist. The doctor may discuss the problem with members of the family to obtain their cooperation in freeing the home environment of tension-creating situations, since emotional upsets increase the constriction of the already narrowed arterioles.

One of the first symptoms of hypertension may be headache. There may be fatigue, dyspnea upon exertion, failing vision, or symptoms of uremia. When tissues beyond the constricted arterioles receive too little blood, or when a constricted arteriolar wall ruptures, symptoms appear. The heart, the brain, the kidneys, and the eyes most often give rise to symptoms. The patient may have loss of vision, have a cerebral vascular accident or a peripheral arterial embolism, or develop kidney or heart failure.

A variety of laboratory tests may be made on patients with hypertension in an attempt to determine the cause. Complete kidney and endocrine studies often are done. If the cause cannot be found, the status of the heart, eyes, kidneys, and nervous system are determined and recorded on the patient's record as a guide in evaluating the course of the disease.

If the cause of the hypertension can be determined, and if it is amenable to treatment, curative treatment is started. The treatment of essential hypertension and of hypertension caused by irreversible changes is usually palliative, and it may be divided into medical therapy and surgical therapy. The purpose of both types of treatment is to decrease the blood pressure, thus delaying the onset of serious complications. Sometimes the patient may be hospitalized, but often he is treated on an ambulatory basis.

Medical treatment. Bed rest may lower the blood pressure slightly, and it is usually part of the initial treatment of a patient with severe symptoms of hypertension. Sedatives such as phenobarbital are often given to relieve tension and to foster rest. Some long-term sustaining measures for adequate rest and relaxation may be needed. Often patients with hypertensive disease are hard-working, driving, and ambitious in their everyday life. They constantly push themselves in activities. Modifications in their daily habits of work, exercise, and rest are advisable along with prescribed medications.

The doctor makes a very careful selection of drugs to treat hypertension. Caution is necessary not only because of the particular stage of the person's illness but also because of the possible side effects of some of the drugs. An ideal antihypertensive drug should decrease the resistance of the arterioles and lower the blood pressure. It should not decrease the output of the heart. However, no drug with these ideal effects is available.

Even with the mildest of drugs, side effects occur. The nurse should give patients the opportunity to discuss symptoms in general and should select those which may be due to the particular hypertensive drug the patient is taking. Often such symptoms occur, but the patient or members of his family attribute them to his general ill health, his age, or possibly his personality. One of the more serious side effects is mental depression. Other patients may become

increasingly tense. The significant symptoms to look for are described with the following specific drug treatments.

Rauwolfia serpentina (Raudixin) or partially purified fractions from it, such as alseroxylon, may be used in treating mild or moderate forms of hypertension. *Alseroxylon,* 4 mg. orally, is usually given at bedtime each day. It takes several weeks to obtain a maximum effect from this drug, and severe hypotension is not likely to occur. Both the systolic and the diastolic blood pressures are lowered. The drug is thought to act by depressing the hypothalamus and central sympathetic centers and by stimulating parts of the parasympathetic nervous system. Dizziness and headache are relieved, but the patient often complains of nasal congestion in the morning. This congestion is relieved by antihistaminic drugs. Since alseroxylon may make the patient drowsy, he should be cautious while driving or working around machinery. The appetite is stimulated, and the patient may gain weight. Since the stimulation of the parasympathetic nerves causes increased bowel motility, nausea, vomiting, and diarrhea may occur. The side effects of the drug subside readily on reduction of dosage or withdrawal, but the hypotensive action continues for several weeks. Marked mental depression may necessitate stopping the drug. *Reserpine* is a purified alkaloid of rauwolfia serpentina. Some of the trade names for this drug are Serpasil, Rau-Sed, and Reserpoid.

Hydralazine hydrochloride (Apresoline) is used for patients with moderate or early malignant hypertension. It is thought to reduce the blood pressure by acting on the midbrain and by inactivating some of the pressor substances found in the blood. It increases the blood flow through the kidney, but this action is often transient. The drug is given orally in gradually increasing doses. The patient is usually started on 40 to 50 mg. of the drug a day, given in divided doses. The dosage may be increased to as much as 800 mg. a day. While the patient is receiving this drug, his blood pressure should be checked frequently. Nausea, vomiting, headache, tachycardia, tingling of the extremities, malaise, nervous tension, depression, and hypotension on standing may be toxic reactions. Any of these symptoms should be reported to the doctor. Although the depression is often very distressing for the patient, the doctor may decide not to discontinue the drug, since with continued treatment the depression seems to decrease.

Pentolinium tartrate (Ansolysen), mecamylamine hydrochloride (Inversine), and chlorisondamine chloride (Ecolid chloride) are potent hypotensive drugs that produce ganglionic blockage. These drugs inhibit the transmission of nerve impulses through both the sympathetic and the parasympathetic ganglia, preventing vasocostriction and thereby causing an increase in blood flow and a drop in blood pressure. Pentolinium tartrate is given either intravenously or subcutaneously. The usual dosage is 0.5 to 10 mg. (1/120 to 1/6 grain) intravenously or 1 to 15 mg. (1/60 to 1/4 grain) by mouth every six hours. Toxic signs of this group of drugs for which the nurse should watch include signs of hypotension, blurring of vision, faintness and transient nausea, constipation, and retention of urine.

The chlorothiazide derivatives so widely used as diuretics have also proved effective in the treatment of hypertension. Usually the patient loses weight even though he may not have appeared to have edema. Although few toxic reactions have been reported, skin reactions, thrombocytopenia, and jaundice may occur. When the drug is stopped, there may be an abrupt rise in blood pressure. Thus, careful recording of blood pressure and observations for other signs of relapse should be made.

Alkavervir (Veriloid) is a potent antihypertensive agent that causes a dilation of the arterioles and constriction of the venous vascular beds. It causes a prompt lowering of the blood pressure, and it slows the heart. It should be given only under the direct supervision of a physician, since bradycardia, severe hypotension, respiratory depression, and collapse may result.[3] The blood pressure and pulse rate should be taken frequently. If the blood pressure falls too rapidly, if the pulse becomes irregular, or if vomiting occurs, the drug should be stopped. The patient may complain of epigastric burning and an increased flow of saliva. Usually 9 to 15 mg. (⅛ to ¼ grain) of alkavervir are given daily in divided doses.

Protoveratrine A and B (Veralba) is a drug used to lower the blood pressure of patients with tachycardia, renal failure, or convulsive episodes. The patient should be hospitalized during treatment with this drug. Usually 0.5 mg. ($\frac{1}{120}$ grain) is given by mouth after meals and at bedtime. The drug may also be given intravenously or intramuscularly. The patient may complain of flushing and excessive salivation, and he should be checked carefully for cardiac arrhythmia and hypotension. Complaints of substernal pain and chest tightness should be reported to the doctor, and the drug should be withheld until he has examined the patient.

Diet. Sodium-restricted diets are sometimes ordered for patients with hypertension. Patients with associated renal disease and heart failure are often placed on this regimen. Two types of diet are commonly used: The 2 or 3 gram sodium diet and the rice diet (Kempner diet). The rice diet contains less than 0.5 gram (7½ grains) of salt, only 20 grams of protein, and little fat. For six weeks the patient may have only rice, fruit, and sugar. Other foods are then gradually introduced. Unless this type of diet relieves their symptoms, few patients will maintain it. Since there is no evidence that this regimen slows down the progress of hypertension, doctors rarely order it until symptoms appear. In the summertime, patients on this diet may need to take extra salt to prevent sodium depletion. If they develop abdominal or leg cramps, weakness, nausea, or vomiting, one should suspect that more salt is needed for normal body processes. A low-caloric diet may be ordered for obese patients, and patients with symptoms of hypertension are usually advised to limit the use of alcohol, tobacco, tea, and coffee.

Surgical treatment. Bilateral resection of some of the sympathetic fibers (sympathectomy) may be done to block stimuli to the blood vessels they innervate. The vessels, in turn, dilate, increasing the flow of blood through the body and lowering the blood pressure. However, a sympathectomy does not always give the desired result in the patient with hypertension. Now that drugs to lower blood pressure are available, the operation is seldom done for hypertension.

If coarctation of the aorta is suspected as

the cause of hypertension, an aortogram may be made to determine the location and nature of the obstruction. This type of lesion can be corrected surgically, providing relief of hypertension in the upper part of the body. Another cause of hypertension amenable to correction by surgical treatment is an abnormality of the arterial circulation of one kidney. This vascular abnormality may be congenital or acquired. Renal arteriograms make definite diagnosis possible, and removal of the affected kidney or correction of the vascular abnormality may cure the hypertension. Endocrine neoplasms such as tumors of the adrenal gland produce large amounts of epinephrine or norepinephrine and may cause intermittent or constant arterial hypertension. Removal of the tumor may bring about a cure of the hypertension.

Ischemic heart disease
(coronary artery disease)

Ischemic heart disease is the number one health problem of our times. Of the 699,861 deaths from heart disease in 1964, 545,499 were due to ischemic heart disease.[65] In the same year, 198,202 persons died of cerebrovascular accidents, 15,923 of rheumatic heart disease, and 57,443 of heart disease due primarily to hypertension.[65]

There are indications that ischemic heart disease is increasing. The crude death rate from coronary disease in the United States rose from 7.9 per 100,000 population in 1930 to 290 per 100,000 population in 1963. It is believed that a substantial part of this increase is not due to changes in age distribution, better reporting, improved methods of diagnosis, or changes in terminology but represents a real increase in coronary artery disease.[26] Deaths from ischemic heart disease appear to be higher in the United States than in some other countries. It is also believed that lesions leading to ischemic heart disease are developing at an earlier age. For example, it was found that 77.3% of young men of the average age of 22 years who were killed in the Korean War had gross pathologic changes in the coronary arteries, and 10% had evidence of advanced disease.[26] Ninety percent of the persons who develop symptoms of ischemic heart disease are between the ages of 40 and 70 years.

The incidence is much higher in men than in women until the menopause is reached, and then women appear to quickly lose their poorly understood immunity.

Coronary artery disease is caused by a narrowing or obstruction of the coronary arteries, resulting in a reduction of blood supply to the myocardium. In most instances, atherosclerosis and general arteriosclerosis cause the narrowing and/or obstruction in the coronary arteries. As atherosclerosis develops, yellowish, fatty material composed largely of cholesterol is gradually deposited as plaques along the walls of the arteries, causing them to become fibrotic, thick, calcified, and narrowed in their lumen. This condition may cause a temporary anoxia of the myocardium, such as occurs in angina pectoris, or it may cause a complete obstruction of the blood supply to a portion of the myocardium, such as occurs in myocardial infarction. The resultant damage to the heart muscle may cause severe cardiac complications such as congestive heart failure and arrhythmias, or it may cause cardiac standstill and immediate death. If the obstruction is only slight, the blood supply may not be reduced significantly and the disease may by asymptomatic. Autopsies on patients who died from other causes frequently show a slight obstruction in their coronary arteries.

Symptoms of congestive heart failure may develop in persons who have had mild symptoms of ischemic heart disease or in those who have had an acute coronary attack with myocardial infarction if the heart muscle has been seriously damaged.

Although an enormous amount of research (both epidemiologic and in the laboratory) is being conducted in order to learn the cause of ischemic heart disease, at the present time the cause is unknown. Certain characteristics, however, have been singled out as being common in persons who have or who will develop coronary atherosclerosis. They include (1) family history of coronary artery disease, (2) hypertension, (3) a high level of blood serum cholesterol, (4) gout, (5) diabetes, (6) overnutrition, or obesity, (7) excessive smoking, (8) muscular build with heavy bones, and (9) sedentary existence.[45]

Individuals who have most of these conditions are considered to be "high risk" for coronary heart disease. These characteristics of the high-risk group have been studied intensively, and summaries of some investigations are included in current texts.[26] One of the most comprehensive studies conducted (in Framingham, Massachusetts, under the sponsorship of the National Heart Institute) attempted to outline the observations and determinations by which risk of heart attacks can be expected. These findings consider age, the level of serum cholesterol, blood pressure, ECG abnormalities, vital capacity, and cigarette smoking. The study showed the following: A man in his fifties has four times the risk of attack as a man in his thirties. A man with a serum cholesterol level above 240 mg. per ml. of blood has more than three times the risk of a man with a serum cholesterol level below 200 mg. An individual with systolic blood pressure greater than 160 has four times the risk of one with systolic pressure of less than 120. An individual with an abnormality of his ECG has two and one-half times the risk of one with a normal ECG. An individual with a low vital capacity has approximately twice the risk of one with a high vital capacity, and one who smokes has almost twice the risk of the nonsmoker.

Prevention of coronary artery disease.
The nurse has a very real responsibility to contribute to the prevention of coronary artery disease by general health education of people. It appears likely that good health practices established in childhood in regard to diet, exercise, and not smoking can contribute to better health in later years and perhaps to the prevention of coronary artery disease. Formation of habits or the established patterns of behavior in regard to food and exercise are developed in the younger years and can persist during a lifetime. Poor habits well established are difficult to change, and coronary artery disease may be advanced when adulthood is reached. If teen-agers and young adults can be convinced that they should stop smoking, their risk would be lessened, and they would help materially in setting a good example to younger children. There seems to be increasing evidence that exercise is important in the prevention of coronary artery disease, and there is general agreement that regular moderate exercise contributes to good general health and better functioning of many body systems. Yet many people in the United States do not exercise at all. Teen-agers should plan to obtain in young adulthood a somewhat modified form of the exercise they receive in the usual school activities. Our present way of life, in which we ride to work in automobiles, spend working hours sitting down, in many cases, and then spend evenings sitting in front of a television set, may need modification to allow for more exercise.

Persons who have had physical examinations and who may have some evidence of coronary artery disease can often benefit from changing health practices, and it is a nursing function to help them make changes. Even if damage already done cannot be reversed, further damage may be prevented or delayed.

Because there is much interest in the association of coronary artery disease to a high-fat diet, the nurse may be asked for information about this relationship by the general public and her patients. At the present time there is a great deal about this subject that is uncertain, controversial, or unknown. An enormous amount of research is presently under way. In addition to the laboratory work, studies are being made of the eating patterns of large units of the population, so that some definite evidence of the relationship of diet to coronary artery disease may be forthcoming in the near future. Until more facts are known, however, it is a nursing responsibility to counsel people to avoid dietary fads, because these fads are expensive and may result in dietary deficiencies.

To date it has not been definitely proved that *any* food has *any* effect upon the development of arteriosclerosis, atherosclerosis, and coronary artery disease. There are some facts or circumstances, however, that appear to indicate that there may be some relationship between diet and coronary artery disease: (1) The national dietary average for fat consumption is at an all-time high in the United States, with approximately 40% of our dietary calories being derived from fats, (2) studies show that populations that consume low-fat diets generally have been found to have lower blood serum cholesterol levels than those consuming high-fat diets, and there seems to be a strong correlation between high-fat consumption and the death rate from coronary heart disease, and (3) it is known that the atheromatous lesions of atherosclerosis contain free cholesterol, that certain dietary constituents have been found to increase the concentration of blood cholesterol, that blood cholesterol level is lowered when fats containing a high proportion of polyunsaturated fatty acids (especially linoleic acid) are substituted for the more saturated fats, and that a high-fat meal induces hypercoagulability of the blood for several hours.

Cholesterol in the body comes from two sources: it can be taken into the body directly as food (eggs and butter are high in cholesterol) or it can be manufactured by the liver. Approximately 0.8 gram of cholesterol is manufactured by the liver each day to be excreted with bile salts into the intestines to participate in the digestion and absorption of fats. The average amount ingested daily in a normal diet is 1 gram. The complex process by which cholesterol is manufactured, distributed, and eliminated is not very well understood, although it is widely believed that the inherited endocrine system plays a definite part because of its effect on the metabolic processes. Studies have shown that when a large amount of saturated fat is eaten, the cholesterol level in the blood tends to rise. It has also been found that the blood cholesterol level is lowered when saturated fats in the diet are replaced by unsaturated fats.

On the basis of these findings, many physicians believe it is advisable to reduce the total caloric intake, limit the amount of fat consumed, and substitute polyunsaturated fats for the more saturated fats in the diets of those individuals who have signs of coronary artery disease. Many believe that the amount of fat in the diet should provide approximately 25% of the total calories (in contrast to the present 40%) and that these calories should come largely from polyunsaturated fats. Examples of saturated fats are hydrogenated shortenings, butter, lard, and animal fats. Examples of unsaturated fats are corn oil, cottonseed oil, peanut oil, and certain fish oils. Foods that are low in cholesterol or contain no cholesterol are fruits, vegetables, cereals, bread, syrup, egg white, fish, very lean meats, soup stocks made without fat, and skimmed milk.

It should be emphasized that rigorous change in diet should be avoided in the light of the evidence now available. Some capable clinicians believe that evidence is still so conflicting that no dietary changes should be made at this time; others believe that changes should be made when cholesterol levels are high, evidence of coronary artery disease persists, or a myocardial infarction has occurred. Still others reason that if such measures are useful and possibly help to prevent further attacks in the case of persons already affected, they should be instituted as preventive measures long before any changes can be detected. The American Heart Association has endorsed a policy recommending some modification in diet to lower the consumption of saturated fats for everyone.

Recently, scientists have been studying with increasing interest the part that sugars may possibly play in the development of atherosclerosis. It has been noted that during the last seventy years there has been a marked decrease in the total carbohydrate intake of people in the United States but a dramatic increase in the use of refined sugar. This increase appears more pronounced than the increase in consumption of saturated fats.[26] At the present time this finding probably has no health education implications for nurses beyond the fact that the sugars consumed in large amounts as candy, ice cream, and sweet desserts contribute to dental decay and to obesity and should be avoided. Fresh fruit can be substituted in many instances.

Angina pectoris. Angina pectoris is a serious cardiac disorder. Although it is usually caused by atherosclerosis of the coronary vessels, the incidence of angina pectoris is high in patients with hypertension, diabetes mellitus, thromboangiitis obliterans, polycythemia vera, periarteritis nodosa, and aortic regurgitation due to syphilis or rheumatic heart disease. It is characterized by paroxysmal retrosternal or substernal pain, often radiating down the inner aspect of the left arm. The pain is often associated with exertion and is relieved through vasodilation of the coronary arteries by means of medication or by rest. It is believed to be caused by a temporary inadequacy of the blood supply in meeting the needs of the heart muscle. The location and severity of the pain vary greatly, but the same pattern recurs repeatedly in a given individual. The frequency and severity of the attacks usually increase over a period of years, and less and less exertion may cause pain. No matter how mild the attacks, they may be complicated at any time by acute myocardial infarction, cardiac standstill, or death. The diagnosis of angina pectoris may be confirmed by electrocardiograms taken at rest, after exercise, or preferably during an attack.

Treatment. Treatment of the patient with angina pectoris is based on the symptoms and is individualized for each patient. The success of the treatment in achieving a comfortable and worthwhile existence for the patient depends upon educating him to live within his limitations, being guided by the pain. The nurse, as well as the doctor, should participate in the teaching program. Since the patient often is not hospitalized, the nurse in the doctor's office or in the clinic carries the major nursing responsibility for helping the patient with angina pectoris. He is taught to cease effort immediately upon experiencing pain, and to rest for several minutes after the pain has subsided. *Nitroglycerin tablets* placed under the tongue and allowed to dissolve in the saliva before swallowing often relieve the pain by causing vasodilation of the coronary arteries. Usually tablets containing 0.4 mg. (1/150 grain) of the drug are prescribed. Effects should be noticed in two or three minutes, but if pain persists, the dose may be repeated two or three times at five-minute intervals. Other nitrate preparations are available, but most patients prefer nitroglycerin since it is less expensive and causes fewer side effects. Perles of *amyl nitrite* come in 3 ml. doses and are preferred by some patients because the action is immediate. The perle is crushed into a handkerchief, and it should be inhaled no more than three times. Nitrite preparations cause flushing of the skin because of capillary dilation. The pulse and respirations increase, and the blood pressure may fall slightly. Many patients develop severe headaches from the use of nitrites. This difficulty can usually be overcome by decreasing the dosage. Some patients use nitroglycerin prophylactically when they have no choice but to undertake some activity that usually causes pain. The action lasts for about one-half hour. The patient with angina pectoris should always carry a nitrite preparation with him. He may use it freely since the effects do not decrease with usage, and it is not habit-forming. Many patients are reluctant to use the medication for various reasons and must be encouraged to do so by careful discussion of their objections.

A xanthine preparation such as theophylline ethylenediamine (*aminophylline*) or theobromine may be given three or four times a day to produce a prolonged vasodilation. Since these preparations frequently cause nausea and vomiting, they should be given after meals or with food.

Diet. If the attacks of anginal pain are precipitated by eating, six small meals taken at evenly spaced intervals, rather than three average meals, may give relief. If the patient is overweight, a low-caloric diet may be prescribed. The doctor may suggest that the patient drink 15 to 30 ml. (½ to 1 ounce) of brandy or whiskey several times a day to dilate the blood vessels. Doctors usually advise the patient to smoke very little if at all.

Activity. Most patients with angina pectoris can tolerate mild exercise such as walking and playing golf, but exertion such as running, climbing hills or stairs rapidly, and lifting heavy objects causes pain. The pain is likely to be invoked more easily in cold weather since the vessels normally constrict to conserve body heat. When the patient with angina pectoris must be exposed to the cold, he should err on the side of being too warmly clad. It is unwise for him to sleep in a cold room, and walking against the wind and uphill should be avoided because these activities increase the work load of the heart and cause pain.

Since excessive emotional strain also causes vasoconstriction by releasing epinephrine into the circulation, emotional outbursts, worry, and tension should be avoided. The patient may need continuing help in accepting situations as he finds them. The family, the spiritual adviser, business associates, and friends can sometimes help. An optimistic outlook helps to relieve the work of the heart. Many patients who learn

343

to live within their limitations live out their expected life-span in spite of the disease. Helping a patient to adjust to living with this disease can be most rewarding for the family, the patient, the doctor, and the nurse. Fear of impending catastrophe is almost a characteristic of anginal pain, and many patients believe each episode of pain is a "heart attack." Therefore, reassurance and education are extremely important.

Acute myocardial infarction. Acute myocardial infarction is caused by sudden blockage of one of the branches of a coronary artery. It may be extensive enough to interfere with cardiac function and cause immediate death, or it may cause necrosis of a portion of the myocardium, with subsequent healing by scar formation or fibrosis. A *coronary thrombosis,* in which the blood supply is interrupted by the formation of a thrombus in the coronary artery, may occur. *Coronary occlusion* is a more general term because it includes other causes of blockage of a coronary artery. Blockage may be caused by sudden progression of atherosclerotic changes or by extended constriction of the arteries. Myocardial infarction usually follows an acute occlusion of a coronary artery.

Acute myocardial infarction is the most common cardiac emergency. The mortality rate for a first attack is about 20%.[12] The patient typically complains of a sudden, severe, crushing or viselike pain in the substernal region. This pain may radiate into the left, and sometimes the right, arm and up the sides of the neck. At other times it may simulate indigestion or a gallbladder attack, with abdominal pain. The patient often becomes restless, gets up and paces about the room, throws open the windows, or has a sudden urge to have a bowel movement. He often feels that he is dying, and his skin becomes ashen and clammy. He may become dyspneic and cyanotic and show signs of severe shock. The pulse is usually rapid, and it may be barely perceptible. The blood pressure usually falls, and the patient may collapse.

The major objective in caring for the patient who has had an acute myocardial infarction is to provide him with physical and mental rest. The damaged heart may be able to maintain basal activity, but additional strain may cause it to fail. The patient is usually kept in bed for three or four weeks, and then, if the sedimentation rate has returned to normal and if he has no complications, he may gradually return to normal activity. During this period a collateral circulation has had a chance to develop, and the necrotic tissue in the myocardium has healed, forming a fibrotic scar. The convalescent period for most patients following a coronary occlusion is two or three months.

The doctor usually orders morphine sulfate or meperidine hydrochloride (Demerol) to be given at frequent intervals until the pain is relieved. If the patient is at all dyspneic or cyanotic or has severe pain, oxygen usually is given. If pain continues, the doctor may order theophylline ethylenediamine (aminophylline) or papaverine hydrochloride. Since both of these drugs relax smooth muscle, they help to dilate the coronary vessels.

To decrease the possibility either of further extension of the thrombus or of embolic complications, the patient who has had a myocardial infarction is usually given an anticoagulant, such as bishydroxycoumarin (Dicumarol), for three or four weeks. While he is receiving this drug, the doctor will order a periodic prothrombin time determination. The dosage of the anticoagulant is based on this determination. The prothrombin time is maintained at approximately thirty seconds, or 10% of normal.[2] If the prothrombin time should drop below 10%, there is danger that the patient will bleed profusely from minor cuts such as shaving nicks or from gum injuries sustained while brushing his teeth. Hematuria may also occur. The nurse should be alert for any signs of excessive or unusual bleeding and report them to the doctor. If bleeding should occur, the patient may be given vitamin K or a small blood transfusion.

Within the first twenty-four hours the temperature may become slightly elevated, and leukocytosis occurs. It is unusual for the temperature to be over 38.5° C. (101° F.), and any further elevation should be reported to the doctor because it may be caused by a complication such as a pulmonary infarction. The fever and leukocytosis are normal reactions to tissue necrosis.

To confirm the diagnosis, the blood sedimentation rate and the transaminase level of the blood serum are determined, and an electrocardiogram is made. The electrocardiogram may show no changes for several days but then usually shows changes indicative of a myocardial infarction. The blood sedimentation rate and transaminase level are elevated, and the blood cholesterol level often is elevated. (See p. 311.)

The prognosis of a patient who has had an acute myocardial infarction is always guarded until about four weeks after the attack. There is danger of such complications as pulmonary or systemic embolism, cardiac rupture, cardiac standstill, ventricular fibrillation, irreversible shock, and acute pulmonary edema. The first two weeks are considered the most dangerous, and patients who survive the third week usually recover from the attack.[2] The degree of residual disability cannot be predicted, however, and some patients are permanently incapacitated with severe angina pectoris or congestive heart failure. Many patients may return to normal or near normal activity, and perhaps 60 to 80% of patients who have recovered can return to some employment.

"*Armchair care*" may be ordered for the patient who has had a myocardial infarction. The rationale behind this treatment is that the work load upon the heart is lessened by the person's being in an upright or semiupright position. It has been shown that a larger blood volume tends to "pool" in the pulmonary vessels when the patient is in a prone position, and it is believed that this condition may increase strain on the heart that may be relieved by permitting more blood to flow into the lower extremities, as when the patient sits up.

The provision of armchair care does not imply that rest for the patient is less important or that activity is permitted. The patient must be lifted very carefully into a comfortable armchair for the length of time designated by the doctor. Since getting out of bed has been found to be an activity that requires a large amount of energy under normal circumstances,[39] the nurse and the persons helping her must not allow the patient to do anything for himself. He must be cautioned repeatedly to relax and to let the nursing staff do the lifting and moving,

and he must be helped to relax by the calm and confident way in which they go about moving him. When in a chair, the patient must be protected from chilling, and he must be observed closely. Sometimes a low footstool is used to elevate the feet slightly, and some patients are more secure and comfortable with a light restraint, such as a loose drawsheet, across the front of the chair to give them security when they relax and sleep.

General nursing care. The patient who has had a coronary occlusion needs the best possible nursing care. The nurse must anticipate his needs so that he can rest. She must keep the environment conducive to rest and help the patient to obtain peace of mind. All the aspects of nursing care discussed under congestive heart failure and suggestions for the rehabilitation of cardiac patients in general and for the patient with angina pectoris in particular should be considered in caring for the patient who has had a myocardial infarction. The patient is likely to be quite apprehensive, perhaps for the rest of his life, and he may have many vague complaints. The nurse should listen carefully to his complaints. The symptoms may be caused by anxiety, or they may herald complications. Abrupt onset of severe apprehension, changes in the cardiac rate or rhythm, changes in blood pressure, and symptoms suggestive of congestive failure or embolic activity should be reported to the doctor at once.

Since the patient who has a myocardial infarction is quite likely to be in the prime of life and to have become ill suddenly, the nurse should anticipate that he may have many worries and concerns related to his business and to his family. It is often better for the patient if he is allowed to make some arrangements or at least told what arrangements are being made. The family, a business partner, or the social service worker may be able to give the help needed so that the patient can be more relaxed. The decision in this regard, however, is the doctor's. He often orders rather heavy sedation for the patient who seems exceedingly upset over business or personal matters.

The myocardial necrosis usually heals within six to eight weeks. Therefore, the patient should remain on limited activity for the duration of this period. Bed rest may not be necessary, but vigorous activity must be avoided. The program varies with each patient. Hill and stair climbing are usually some of the last activities in which the doctor permits the patient to engage, because they add to the work load of the heart substantially. Walking is considered a desirable exercise, and increased distances can be walked daily. This activity also helps to combat the weakness and fatigue that results from muscle disuse. Sometimes the patient is allowed to do too much for himself and to return to activity too quickly because unless he has complications, he may appear quite well. His appearance may also make it more difficult for the family to comprehend fully the seriousness of the situation and the very real possibility of repeated attacks or death for the patient who does not respect his condition and live in moderation both physically and emotionally. Sometimes, on the other hand, the patient is needlessly made an invalid for the rest of his life. Since there is evidence that exercise is beneficial in myocardial disease, return to work may be much better for the patient than a long period of enforced inactivity and leisure. It has been found that more myocardial infarctions occur during leisure hours than at work.[12]

Before the patient is discharged, he and his family should have been instructed concerning appropriate activities, how to follow a pattern of living in moderation, and how to recognize when activity or emotional strain is too great. The patient should know that if he should have any further symptoms, rest is of prime importance and that the doctor should be contacted at once. He should remain under close medical supervision, and he should follow the doctor's suggestions and instructions. More than half of the persons who have an acute attack of coronary artery disease can return to full employment and are better and happier in so doing. Recurrences, however, are frequent, and only approximately 50% live more than five years beyond the first attack.[2]

Subacute bacterial endocarditis

Subacute bacterial endocarditis is a serious complication of heart diseases. Organisms in the bloodstream invade the heart. The valves are most often involved, being covered with vegetations or products of bacterial degeneration. During healing after active infection, the cardiac valves may become scarred, resulting in functional difficulty and eventual heart failure, although the infection itself is cured. The most common organism affecting the heart is the streptococcus, and its invasion is usually preceded by rheumatic involvement of the cardiac valves or by a congenital heart anomaly. Diseased teeth and gums also seem to predispose to subacute bacterial endocarditis.

The patient usually has recurring bouts of fever and malaise, often dating from an attack of grippe. He may have petechiae (small capillary hemorrhages) in the conjunctiva, in the mouth, and on the legs, and his fingers are often clubbed if the infection occurs in the presence of congenital heart anomaly. If the disease is untreated, it progresses rapidly, and death may follow within one or two months of onset as a result of emboli to the lungs, kidneys, brain, or spleen or as a result of heart failure. Ninety percent of patients with subacute bacterial endocarditis can now be cured by the administration of massive doses of penicillin and/or other antibiotics. It is important to obtain the organism by blood culture prior to treatment in order to aid in selection of proper antibiotics. Treatment is usually continued for two to six weeks, and the patient is kept on bed rest during this time and for some time afterward. Prevention of bacterial endocarditis by early and adequate treatment of infections, especially streptococcal infections, and by the administration of prophylactic doses of antibiotics to patients with known heart disease before and after tooth extractions and operations is extremely important.

Cardiovascular syphilis

Cardiovascular syphilis usually occurs from fifteen to twenty years after the primary syphilitic infection. Since the highest incidence of primary syphilis is among persons in their early twenties, patients with symptoms of cardiovascular syphilis are usually over 35 years of age. If the primary infection is not treated, approximately 10% of persons affected will develop syphilitic aortitis or aneurysm.[2]

It is the aim of health organizations and

medical personnel to treat all persons with syphilis before they develop cardiovascular disease or any of the other complications of late syphilis. Primary syphilis can be arrested. However, once syphilis has affected the aorta and the valves of the heart, little can be done except to treat the patient symptomatically. The treatment of primary syphilis is discussed on p. 524.

In cardiovascular syphilis the spirochetes attack the aorta, the aortic valve, and the heart muscle. The portion of the aorta nearest the heart usually is affected, and the elastic wall of the aorta becomes weakened and bulges. This bulge is known as an aneurysm. As the aneurysm grows, it may press on neighboring structures, such as the intercostal nerves, and cause pain. Aneurysms may also be present without symptoms. Evidence may be discovered on x-ray examination. There is a possibility that the aneurysm may rupture as it increases in size, and the patient is encouraged to avoid excessive and strenuous activities that might cause a sudden increase in the pressure exerted against the bulging vessel. Surgical resection of the aneurysm can sometimes be done (p. 380).

Syphilis may also attack the aorta more diffusely, causing aortitis. The aorta becomes dilated, and small plaques containing calcium are laid down. Patients may complain of substernal pain associated with exertion due to constriction at the orifices of the coronary arteries. Thrombi may develop along the aorta, causing death. An embolus or myocardial infarction may develop.

The spirochete may also attack the aortic valve, causing it to become scarred. This causes aortic insufficiency, and the patient may have a bounding pulse and a high systolic blood pressure because of the extra effort demanded of the ventricles to pump blood into the systemic circulation. Heart failure eventually occurs.

The use of penicillin in the treatment of the patient with cardiovascular disease is thought possibly to prolong life, since penicillin destroys any active organisms and permits healing to occur. Treatment at this stage, however, will not restore damaged aortic tissue or damaged aortic valves, and extensive scarring may occur. The patient with cardiovascular syphilis should be given guidance in planning his activities of daily living and in selecting work that places the least possible burden on the damaged heart and aorta. In certain cases of aortic insufficiency, surgery is possible. A more complete discussion can be found in recent publications.

Rheumatic heart disease

Rheumatic heart disease is so closely related to rheumatic fever that some consideration of rheumatic fever will also be given here. For details of the development and the treatment and nursing care of rheumatic fever with joint involvement, see p. 921. Rheumatic heart disease may be acute, occurring during an acute attack of rheumatic fever, or it may be chronic and give symptoms many years after the acute infection. Probably somewhat less than 10% of patients with rheumatic fever develop rheumatic heart disease, and about one-half of those with rheumatic heart disease have mitral stenosis.[14] It is possible for rheumatic fever and rheumatic heart disease with mild symptoms to go undiagnosed, or the disease may be subclinical, with no noticeable symptoms occurring. Thus, years later the discovery of rheumatic heart disease is made. Careful recall of illness in childhood may include a recollection of "growing pains," confirming the likelihood that the patient had rheumatic fever with acute rheumatic heart disease during childhood.

About 20 to 40% of persons who have acute rheumatic heart disease are disabled or have life shortened from this cause. The nurse should understand rheumatic fever—its origin and its consequences—so that she can help either to prevent the rheumatic infection or to prevent the development of the complications of heart disease.

Acute rheumatic fever with clinical symptoms follows from 0.3 to 3% of hemolytic streptococcal infections.[56] The streptococcal infection that leads to rheumatic fever is usually caused by group A streptococci, and almost always it is the respiratory system that is first affected. The severity of the infection and complications are usually greater in persons who are undernourished and who live in crowded urban households. Approximately one-half of all streptococcal infections do not give rise to symptoms, and the only accurate way to detect presence of infection is to take a throat culture.

Rheumatic fever is still one of the most important infections of childhood. Although mortality and morbidity rates for the disease have decreased, it is difficult to estimate the true incidence. Not all states (39 in 1964) require reporting of rheumatic fever or of streptococcal infections. Available statistics show an increase in streptococcal infection and scarlet fever from 147,502 in 1955 to 402,334 in 1964.[66] Part of this increase, however, may be due to better procedures for reporting these infections. The rates for rheumatic fever are highest among persons who have recently moved from rural to urban living.[56] Susceptibility to rheumatic fever has a definite familial tendency, but patterns vary. It is probable that both environment and heredity contribute to susceptibility.

About 90% of first attacks of rheumatic fever occur among persons 5 to 15 years of age.[57] The age of greatest risk is 8 to 10 years. It is relatively rare for an attack of rheumatic fever to occur before the age of 2 years or after 25 years of age.[56] Since immunity is not developed by an attack of rheumatic fever, attacks of the disease can recur. Streptococcal infections precipitate recurrences in 25 to 50% of children with a past history of the disease. Approximately 20% of patients have a recurrence within the first five years after the initial attack, but the likelihood of recurrence decreases with age. Recurrence is relatively rare after 20 years of age.

Acute rheumatic heart disease is an acute inflammatory reaction. It may involve (1) the lining of the heart, or endocardium, including the valves, resulting in scarring, distortion, and stenosis of the valves, (2) the muscle of the heart, or myocardium, where small areas of necrosis develop and heal, leaving scars (Aschoff bodies), or (3) the outer covering of the heart, or pericardium, where it may cause adhesions to surrounding tissues. The development of symptoms of chronic rheumatic heart disease in later life depends upon the severity of the damage and other factors.

Prevention. Rheumatic heart disease cannot be prevented unless its precursor, rheumatic fever, and in turn its precursor, group A hemolytic streptococcal infection, are prevented. Learning that group A hemolytic streptococcal infections precede rheumatic fever has led to treatment that has greatly reduced the incidence of rheumatic fever, but *primary prevention*—the prevention of streptococcal infections—still needs particular emphasis. When children, teenagers, or young adults have sore throats, the nurse should encourage prompt medical attention so that a throat culture can be taken and the cause found. By means of special health education programs, high school and college students may be taught the importance of reporting *any* sore throat because some streptococcal infections do not cause serious discomfort. Parents of younger children often are unaware that illnesses apparently caused by a simple cold or a mild sore throat can be serious and may lead to rheumatic fever. The nurse should emphasize the importance of identifying the organism in any infection of the throat. A child who has a persistent sore throat that appears red and inflamed should not attend school and mingle with other children until a throat culture has been taken and the causative organism identified.

Sore throats and other upper respiratory infections caused by the group A hemolytic streptococcus usually respond to prompt and adequate treatment with penicillin or the sulfonamides. The nurse working with the child's family in the community or in the clinic should know the condition of the child and the treatment he is receiving. She should encourage parents to complete the course of treatment, which is likely to be neglected if an oral form of the drug is prescribed. When symptoms subside and the child seems better, parents may become careless and may omit the later doses of medication.

Secondary prevention of rheumatic fever is achieved largely through antistreptococcal prophylaxis. As soon as the initial attack of rheumatic fever has subsided, oral penicillin, one tablet of 100,000 or 200,000 units, taken twice daily is the treatment of choice. An alternate treatment is a long-acting, injectable penicillin, 1,200,000 units of benzathine penicillin G, intramuscularly every four weeks. If the child is sensitive to penicillin, then sulfadiazine may be given. Younger children receive 0.5 Gm. doses once daily, and older children and adults receive 1 Gm. daily. Whether or not a child has evidence of carditis, some physicians prescribe prophylactic treatment to be taken continuously for several years or longer, depending upon the child's physical condition. Careful examination of the child at periodic intervals is made to determine continuing treatment.

Although the nurse and doctor can stress to the patient that he should avoid people with colds and sore throat, this goal is often difficult to achieve within families with young children and among school-age children. Adherence to a regimen of the daily prophylactic dose of penicillin, obtaining adequate sleep and rest, eating well-balanced meals, and protection from exposure to dampness and cold will usually be the most effective method for prevention of further attacks of fever.

Taking prophylactic drugs daily after an acute attack of rheumatic fever can be very difficult for the patient. The nurse can help families to work out ways of remembering to take the medication. It is easier for everyone in the family if the patient considers taking his medication to be part of his daily personal care, as, for example, brushing his teeth. If the medication is forgotten for one or two days, the nurse should try to learn from the family the real reason why it was omitted so that it will be taken more readily in the future. She should avoid being judgmental and should realize that taking such a drug regularly can be a disturbing experience for some people. Adolescents often do not take their medication, particularly if parents remind them repeatedly and, as is sometimes the case the adolescents feel that parental wishes are not important. Often, encouragement from a nurse, such as the school nurse or a nurse in the hospital or the home who cared for an adolescent when he was ill with the fever and with whom he feels comfortable, can be much more effective than parental admonitions.

Prophylactic rheumatic fever programs have been made increasingly available with the help of the Children's Bureau of the Department of Health, Education, and Welfare. Extensive studies have been carried out by the Division for Study and Control of Heart Disease of the United States Public Health Service and by the American Heart Association.

Care of the patient. The typical picture of the acutely ill child who has had rheumatic fever and rheumatic heart disease has changed in the past decade. The very ill child with high temperature, severe joint pain and greatly dilated heart, and slow response to available treatment is now seldom seen. It is believed that improved social and economic conditions generally as well as the advent of antibiotics are responsible for this epidemiologic trend.

The treatment and care of a child with an attack of rheumatic fever is largely symptomatic. It includes good general care and understanding of the child (see pediatric texts), and care of the patient with acute joint pain (p. 921). Salicylates and bed rest are usually required. However, the length of time that the patient must remain in bed has been somewhat reduced in recent years. Occasionally the corticosteroids are given to control joint inflammation, and the child is allowed up and permitted to attend school. Usually, however, ambulation is gradual, the length of time for convalescence varies according to the individual child and the laboratory tests (primarily the blood sedimentation rate test).

Children with rheumatic fever and rheumatic heart disease are often cared for at home, and medical care is given at the doctor's office, in a hospital clinic, or in a preventive clinic of a local health department. Unless the child is seriously ill, hospitalization is not advised, providing suitable home care is available. The public health nurse often is called upon to visit the child in his home in order to help his family to plan adequate and safe care for him and to prepare him for the measures that will probably be advised to prevent future attacks. If the child is confined to bed, family members may need help in providing bedside care, including attention to good body alignment in bed and moving painful joints (Fig. 227). The most taxing time for parents and child usually comes when symptoms have decreased or disappeared but modified activity is still recommended by the doctor. Quiet yet stimulating and satisfying activities, games, and toys, help to pass the time enjoyably while avoiding exertion. When the child is allowed out of bed, supervision may be needed but has to be given with the utmost care to avoid frustration and resentment on the part of the child.

Children who have rheumatic heart disease are usually advised by the physician to lead a relatively normal, unrestricted existence in which only vigorous, competitive athletics are prohibited. The recommendations are specific for the individual patient and his particular situation, and they vary a great deal. If heart damage has been severe and permanent damage is likely, the nurse should help the child's parents to direct the child's interest toward activities that can become satisfying and rewarding and yet are not strenuous. For example, artistic interests developed from childhood might lead to skill in photography that earns recognition and a livelihood or to a variety of other satisfying occupations that are within the person's physical capacity.

Overprotection by parents is sometimes a serious problem. The nurse needs to be understanding and accepting of the parents' fears and concerns and provide sufficient time to allow discussion of them. The reason for overprotection may be very complex at times, and the nurse may need to seek consultation herself in order to understand and work through the problem with the parents. She may refer the parents to a medical social worker, if one is available, or work with the doctor in seeking psychiatric consultation.

Congenital heart disease

Congenital heart disease is discussed in detail in pediatric nursing books and will only be reviewed briefly here. Congenital heart disease occurs in about 3 of every 100 live births and accounts for about 50% of deaths caused by congenital defects in the first year of life.[51] Heart defects may be caused by heredity (defects inherent in the genes), vitamin deficiency, or the occurrence of a viral infection such as German measles in the first trimester of pregnancy. However, in the majority of cases, the cause is unknown.

The nurse should be familiar with the signs and symptoms of congenital heart disease. One of the nurse's most important contributions can be case finding. Signs and symptoms of congenital heart disease may include abnormal heart murmurs, varying degrees of cyanosis, dyspnea, generalized poor development, and clubbing of fingers and toes. The child may have no visible symptoms, such as may occur in an interatrial septal defect, and a heart murmur may be discovered during physical examination. Infants with defects such as those which occur in tetralogy of Fallot will become cyanotic soon after birth.

Congenital heart diseases usually are classified as (1) those which cause cyanosis, such as tetralogy of Fallot, transposition of the great vessels, and tricuspid atresia, and (2) those which do not cause cyanosis, such as coarctation of the aorta, aortic stenosis, patent ductus arteriosus, interatrial septal defects, interventricular septal defects, and pulmonary stenosis (Fig. 74). In *interatrial septal defects* the foramen ovale, or normal opening in the atrial septum, fails to close shortly after birth as it should, and blood returning from the lungs to the left atrium shunts over to the right atrium. An *interventricular septal defect* is an abnormal opening between the right and left ventricle through which blood from the left ventricle is shunted into the right ventricle and is recirculated through the pulmonary artery and lungs. A *patent ductus arteriosus* permits the shunting of oxygenated blood from the aorta back to the pulmonary artery. A *coarctation of the aorta* is a localized stricture just below the origin of the left subclavian artery, causing the blood pressure in the blood vessels above the constriction to become elevated and in those below the constriction to become lower than the pressure above the constriction. *Aortic stenosis* is a fusing of the commissures of the aortic valve, which obstructs the flow of blood from the left ventricle. *Pulmonary stenosis* is a narrowing of the pulmonary valve, which decreases the amount of blood flowing into the lungs. *Tetralogy of Fallot* consists of four defects: a ventricular septal defect, pulmonary stenosis, right ventricular hypertrophy, and an overriding aorta. This combination produces cyanosis, and the infant is often referred to as a "blue baby." In *transposition of the great vessels*, the aorta arises from the right ventricle instead of the left, and blood is pumped back into the circulation without having received any oxygen from the lungs. If complete congenital *atresia* (occlusion)

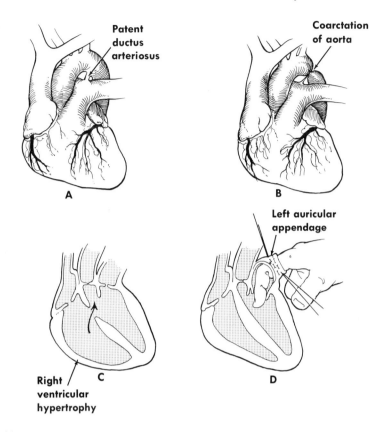

Fig. 74

Some of the more common anomalies of the heart. **A,** Communication between the aorta and the pulmonary artery, found in patients with patent ductus arteriosus. **B,** Abnormality found in coarctation of the aorta. Note the engorgement above the constriction. **C,** Abnormal opening between the right and left ventricles that exists when a ventricular septal defect is present. **D,** Technique used in a mitral commissurotomy for adhesions of the mitral valve.

of the *tricuspid valve* is present, there is no direct communication between the right atrium and the right ventricle. The right atrial blood is shunted through a foramen ovale, or an atrial defect, into the left atrium, where it is mixed with pulmonary venous blood.

Congenital heart disease no longer necessarily has an unfavorable prognosis. More accurate diagnosis and evaluation of cardiac defects is now possible by means of angiocardiograms and cardiac catheterization. In the last decade advances in anesthesiology and surgical techniques have made correction of many congenital anomalies possible, and subacute bacterial endocarditis, one of the most frequent complications, can now be arrested with penicillin or other antibiotics. The prognosis in congenital heart disease, however, varies. Patients who are treated before development of serious complications, such as retarded growth, heart muscle hypertrophy, or heart failure, have a better prognosis than if treatment is delayed. The nurse should urge parents of children with suspected anomalies of the heart to seek early medical care.

Medical treatment is preventive and supportive. The child should be protected from exposure to infections, and when they occur, he should be treated by a physician. Antibiotics usually are prescribed for infections and before and after dental therapy and surgery. Most operations attempt to repair the defect, either by closing an abnormal opening or removing or opening an abnormal obstruction. Unless the infant will not survive without surgery, as may happen when a tetralogy of Fallot is present, most surgery usually is postponed until early childhood. The operative mortality is low and the results good after most of these procedures.

Mitral stenosis

About one-half of the patients with rheumatic heart disease have mitral stenosis.[14] After repeated attacks of rheumatic fever, rheumatic nodules grow on the mitral valve at the line where the valves meet. The valves thicken and fuse together, the chordae tendineae shorten and thicken, and the valve opening narrows from 4 to 6 sq. cm. to 1 sq. cm. or less.[14] There is increased pressure in the left atrium which is reflected to the pulmonary vessels and the right ventricle, and the load on the right heart may lead to right-sided heart failure. Symptoms include dyspnea on exertion progressing to orthopnea, pulmonary edema, and hemoptysis. The patient usually becomes increasingly incapacitated, and death usually occurs between 30 and 50 years of age. Selected patients may benefit from surgery on the mitral valve (mitral commissurotomy).

Mitral commissurotomy. Mitral commissurotomy is the fracturing (breaking apart) of the stenosed leaves (commissures) of the mitral valve, which is located between the left atrium and the left ventricle. At the present time most surgeons operate on the patient who has simple mitral stenosis by the closed technique. In this operation, the thorax usually is entered through a left anterolateral incision. The fourth rib is partially resected to give adequate exposure, and then the heart is entered through the left auricular appendage. The surgeon inserts his finger through the incision into the atrium and through the mitral valve (Fig. 74). He then makes several attempts to release the leaves of the mitral valve either with his finger, with a special knife, or with a transventricular dilator.[14] At this point he will know whether or not the operation can be expected to relieve the patient's symptoms. Sometimes it is impossible to release

the stenosed valve because of excessive calcium deposits around it or because of other pathology. If any clots are found, they are flushed out to prevent their escape into the general circulation.

If the operation has been successful, there will be a decline in the pulmonary pressure, reduction of the heart size, and a gradual diminishing of the symptoms previously experienced. Many patients who have been semi-invalids are able to return to a relatively normal life. In some patients, however, the stenosis may recur after varying periods of time, and the symptoms may become worse than preoperatively. The surgeon then may attempt to relieve the stenosis by doing open heart surgery. If the valve is calcified or severely deformed, it may be replaced with an artificial ball valve. One type consists of a silicone rubber ball, a cage of stainless steel, and an outer ring of Teflon fabric.

The nursing care of the patient undergoing mitral commissurotomy is similar to that of other patients having other cardiac surgery. It is discussed in detail later in this chapter.

Chronic constrictive pericarditis

In chronic constrictive pericarditis, dense scar tissue, often impregnated with calcium deposits, forms within the pericardial space and interferes with heart action during diastole. The cause of this disease is unknown, although it is suspected that the disease is infectious in origin and that perhaps a virus may be the cause.[2] The disease is primarily one of adults; children are much less frequently affected.[2] Signs and symptoms may include all those of congestive heart failure, making it difficult for the doctor to make an accurate diagnosis.[2] Chronic constrictive pericarditis may be cured or markedly improved by *pericardial resection.*

Pericardectomy (pericardial resection, decortication of the heart). A pericardectomy is the removal of the scar tissue and pericardium that are adherent to the heart. The pericardium is separated carefully from the myocardium and removed. Almost at once, many of the patient's symptoms are relieved. A chest catheter is usually inserted for drainage postoperatively. The nursing care of patients undergoing a pericardectomy is similar to that of those having other cardiac surgery. It is discussed in detail later in this chapter.

Aortic stenosis

Aortic stenosis usually is caused by rheumatic fever. The disease attacks the valve cusps, which become stiff and calcified and obstruct blood flow. There is an elevation of left ventricular pressure and low cardiac output. Even though the obstruction may be substantial, the patient may have few clinical symptoms for some time. Some patients complain of fatigue, faintness, and angina, and roentgenograms may show a heart either of normal size or with slight enlargement of the left ventricle. Untreated aortic stenosis will contribute to, and often finally cause, congestive heart failure. Electrocardiographic changes may be the only evidence of the severity of the stenosis.

Surgery for aortic stenosis is done with the use of extracorporeal circulation, which permits full visualization of the operative area. The aortic valve may be repaired by three methods: the calcium may be removed and the fused commissures opened; the aortic valve sometimes may be reconstructed by removing one cusp and rebuilding a valve consisting of only two cusps; or part or all of the valve may be removed. When part or all of the valve is removed, artificial cusps may be stitched into normal position of the valve, or ball valves similar to those designed for the mitral valve may be used.[14] The nursing care before and after operation is the same as for patients having heart surgery for other causes.

Nursing care of the patient having cardiac surgery

The majority of the operations on the heart are being performed with full visualization (*open technique*). The heart is opened and the defect is inspected and repaired. Openings in the atrial or ventricular septa may be sutured or patched with plastic material. Valves may be opened or reconstructed, or they may be replaced with artificial cusps or ball valves. When the *closed technique* is used, the defect is not seen by the surgeon. He inserts his finger into the heart through a small incision and explores the obstructed valve with it. The surgeon may be able to open the obstructed valve with his finger, or he may have to guide a special knife or instrument into the area to release the adhesions. The closed technique is used most often to treat uncomplicated mitral stenosis. While the risks during and after surgery are greater with open heart surgery, the results generally are better than can be obtained using the closed technique. Operations such as repair of congenital defects of the heart could not be performed unless direct visualization was possible.

The open heart approach can be used only if extracorporeal circulation is maintained by means of the heart-lung apparatus (pump oxygenator). In addition, hypothermia may be used to reduce the metabolic rate, thus permitting somewhat lower flow rates with extracorporeal circulation (p. 188) and longer periods of total circulatory standstill than are tolerable at normal body temperatures.[14] Increased atmospheric pressure in special chambers is being studied for use as a supplement to either hypothermia or extracorporeal circulation. The tissues appear to become so saturated with oxygen that they withstand temporary ischemia very well. An adequate amount of oxygen can be carried dissolved in the blood, with no need for hemoglobin.[14]

Preoperative period

Before a heart operation is attempted, the patient's general health, and particularly the condition of the heart, is evaluated carefully, and he is built up to the best physical condition possible for him. He must undergo many tests, and although he probably has had previous experience in the hospital because of his heart condition, he should be given an adequate explanation of all procedures. When it has been decided that benefit can be derived from an operation, the doctor discusses the procedure with the patient and his family. He usually tells them why the operation must be done, what he hopes it will accomplish, and what will be done. If the patient is a child, the parents should explain the admission to the hospital and the operation to him as simply as possible. His age will determine the kind of explanation to be given. (See p. 172 for discussion of this preparation.)

In some instances patients or parents have

read or heard about heart operations and have come to the surgeon and asked to have the procedure done. Some men and women, faced with increasing invalidism, decide that they would like to risk an operation in the hope of being able to live more normally.

Preoperative teaching. Although the doctor has thoroughly prepared the patient for the operation and the patient has prepared himself emotionally, he is still anxious and apprehensive. Surgery on the heart carries a risk. The patient realizes that there is no substitute for the heart and that life without it is impossible. Provision should be made for him to visit with his spiritual adviser and with his family on the morning of surgery. Many patients may wish to prepare a will. The anesthetist's visit to the patient preoperatively usually gives him some reassurance.

One of the most important contributions to the care of children can be made by the nurse in her support, understanding, and teaching of the child's parents. Helping them to obtain the necessary examinations for the child and to prevent infections, and explaining necessary procedures can be tremendously saving of parents' worry and concern.

Accepting the fact that the child has a defect is sometimes the most difficult problem. Parents react in a variety of ways, but most wish to have all possible help given to the child. Helping parents to accept a "guarded" prognosis or a poor prognosis when operative procedures are recommended requires patient, careful guidance by doctor, nurse, and social worker.

The preoperative care is similar to that discussed on p. 171. Most cardiac patients are very apprehensive about the surgery, and the nurse should learn to know the patient as well as possible in order to ascertain what he should be told. For example, an explanation of chest drainage is welcomed by some patients but greatly upsets others. Preoperatively, the nurse should determine and record the amount of activity in which the patient is able to engage without becoming tired, because it will serve as a guide in determining his postoperative condition.

The doctor orders a sedative so that the patient will sleep on the preoperative night. If necessary, the medication usually can be repeated. In the morning, before the patient leaves for the operating room, the doctor usually will start an infusion. A *venesection* (cutdown) is usually done to assure a patent vein in the event of circulatory collapse. A vein in the ankle is usually used because of the proximity of the arm to the operative area. A narcotic usually is not ordered as a preoperative medication for the patient who will be undergoing cardiac surgery since it depresses respirations. Often, phenobarbital sodium, 120 mg. (2 grains), is ordered, and only 0.2 mg. ($\frac{1}{300}$ grain) of atropine sulfate is given to decrease secretions, because a larger dose might block the vagus nerve, increasing the stimuli to the sinoatrial node and causing fibrillation.

Extracorporeal circulation (heart-lung machine, pump oxygenator)

During open heart surgery the pump oxygenator is used as a temporary substitute for the patient's heart and lungs. The heart and lungs of the patient are bypassed so that the surgeon can work in a relatively bloodless field and can see the defect more clearly. Maintenance of body circulation by this artificial means also allows more time in which to correct the defect.

There are a variety of extracorporeal oxygenator systems. The most widely used are the bubble method and the screen or rotating disk types. Immediately before the operation, the machine is prepared or primed for use by filling it with 2,500 ml. (5 pints) of fresh blood that must match that of the patient. Donors are asked to report the morning of the operation to ensure freshness of the blood. Heparin is added to the blood to prevent clotting. This method may still be used, but more recently, pump oxygenators have been primed with glucose. While amounts vary, one clinic primes the unit with 16 to 20 ml. of fluid per kilogram of the patient's weight. Two-thirds of the fluid consists of 5% dextrose in water and one-third of 10% dextran 40 (Rheomacrodex) in saline solution.[18] The use of glucose leads to a significant decrease in complications and also is much less costly for the patient. Also, an oxygenator primed with glucose can be used on short notice. This is not possible with blood priming.[56]

The patient receives a general anesthetic, and an intratracheal catheter is inserted.

The surgeon then makes a bilateral thoracotomy incision, transects the sternum, and enters the pericardium. The patient receives heparin intravenously, and catheters are inserted into the superior and inferior venae cavae. By means of a Y connecting tube, these catheters are attached to the machine, and through them will pass the venous flow of blood. Another catheter is inserted into the common femoral artery and attached to the pump, and through this catheter, blood that has been oxygenated will be returned to the systemic circulation.

When all catheters are inserted and attached, the machine is set into operation, the venae cavae are occluded, and correction of the defect is undertaken. Blood is returned to the patient's body at the rate of 50 to 60 ml. per kilogram of body weight per minute to maintain the peripheral pulse at 80 to 90 per minute. A heating unit within the machine keeps the blood at body temperature. Oxygenation of blood is accomplished by means of an oxygen inlet within the machine, and carbon dioxide is removed by a chemical bath process. While the machine is in operation on a patient, heart action by electrocardiogram, brain action by electroencephalogram, and the blood pressure are monitored. These recordings allow the anesthesiologist and the surgeon to keep a constant check on the adequacy of circulation for the patient.

After the defect has been corrected, the venae cavae are unclamped, the pump is stopped, and the venous catheters are removed. Protamine sulfate is given to counteract the heparin and to restore the coagulation time of the blood to normal.

Postoperative period

Postoperative unit. Some medical centers have special units (cardiac recovery rooms) set aside to care for patients who have had cardiac surgery. Patients usually remain in these units longer than they do in regular recovery rooms.

While the patient is in the operating room, the nurse should prepare the unit for his return. It is preferable that he be in a room by himself since he will need constant observation for several days. An oxygen tent may be set up. If a mucolytic agent, such as tyloxapol (Alevaire), is to be used, appropriate apparatus for its administration should be obtained. Chest suction apparatus should be ready to attach, and a thoracentesis set, equipment for cardiac massage, and emergency stimulants should be readily available in the event that air or fluid must be withdrawn from the chest cavity or cardiac massage done as emergency measures. Infusion poles, a sphygmomanometer, and a stethoscope should also be at the bedside. Suction apparatus should be available since the patient may need to be suctioned to remove mucus. If the cardiac surgery was done while the temperature of the body was lowered (hypothermia), equipment to apply external heat or to maintain hypothermia will be needed (p. 188).

Postoperative care. The patient who has undergone heart surgery under either the closed or the open technique requires constant nursing care. The nurse must be alert for signs of hemorrhage, hypotension, fibrillation, arrhythmias, sudden chest pain, and pulmonary edema. Mortality is highest within the first forty-eight hours.

After cardiac surgery the patient is placed in an oxygen tent in Fowler's position. The doctor usually will allow him to lie on either his back or the operated side. Following thoracic surgery it is generally advisable to keep the unoperative side uppermost so that the lung on this side will be able to maintain its full expansion. When his blood pressure remains relatively stable, the patient is turned from his back to his operated side at least every two hours. The two chest catheters are attached to closed drainage and to chest suction apparatus (Fig. 132) to drain air and fluid from the pleura. The amount and color of the drainage should be checked frequently. There will be some bleeding during the first forty-eight hours, but any increased amount should be reported to the surgeon immediately. The dressings should be inspected frequently for blood. Because of the large amounts of heparin used when the pump oxygenator is used, hemorrhage is rather common. Drugs such as vitamin K and protamine sulfate are given to counteract the bleeding tendency caused by the heparin. The patient should be observed for any signs of shock, hemorrhage, spontaneous pneumothorax, mediastinal shift, cardiac arrhythmias, or congestive heart failure. Sudden hypotension with sharp pain would indicate a coronary occlusion. Blood-tinged or frothy sputum usually indicates pulmonary edema. The patient is urged to take deep breaths as soon as he awakens from anesthesia, but coughing usually is not encouraged until the blood pressure is stabilized. Following heart surgery, the patient may need constant attendance for twenty-four to seventy-two hours. If left alone, he may become extremely apprehensive, and mental stress increases the work of the heart.

The doctor may want the blood pressure reading and pulse rate taken every fifteen minutes for twenty-four hours. The frequency is decreased gradually until they are taken only twice a day. The pulse should be checked carefully for rhythm, strength, and rapidity of beat; it may be monitored. The doctor may order the apical-radial pulse rate taken since atrial fibrillation often develops about the third day in patients who have had heart surgery. The patient may be aware of palpitation. Since it may frighten him, the doctor may tell him that it can be expected. When atrial fibrillation occurs, it is controlled by medication. Depending upon the doctor's findings, digitalis or quinidine sulfate may be used, or procainamide hydrochloride (Pronestyl hydrochloride) may be given intravenously. The defibrillator or a pacemaker may be used to treat atrial fibrillation or cardiac arrest. If the patient has been on digitalis and/or mercurial diuretics preoperatively, these medications are usually resumed.

Electrocardiograms may be made continuously for the first few days. The nurse observes the readings closely and reports abnormal tracings to the doctor at once. Roentgenograms of the chest taken with a portable machine and electrocardiograms of the heart will be made daily to evaluate lung expansion and to determine heart function.

Although the patient usually is allowed clear fluids as soon as nausea subsides, supplementary intravenous fluids are given for two or three days or until he takes adequate fluids by mouth. Depending upon the postoperative cardiac condition, the doctor usually places some restriction upon the amount of fluids the patient may take. He usually is permitted to have about 1,500 to 1,800 ml. a day. The nurse, members of the auxiliary staff, and the patient should be aware of this restriction and keep accurate measurement of the fluid intake. Intravenous fluids should be administered slowly to prevent overloading the circulatory system and placing additional strain on the heart. The prescribed diet usually contains only 2 or 3 grams of salt, and this restriction is continued until all signs of congestive heart failure have disappeared, which may not be until some time after discharge from the hospital.

A self-retaining (Foley) catheter usually is inserted into the bladder; urine is collected every hour and checked for specific gravity, color, and amount. The patient should excrete 15 to 30 ml. of urine every hour. This frequent observation of his urine helps detect signs of kidney shutdown or failure, and bleeding. Disturbance of electrolyte balance with development of acidosis does occur following open heart surgery, particularly following a shunt repair. The nurse should anticipate that chemical studies of the blood will be ordered and should have the needed equipment available.

A narcotic such as meperidine hydrochloride (Demerol) may be ordered to relieve pain. Some surgeons order small doses given frequently (Demerol, 25 or 50 mg. [⅜ to ¾ grain], every two hours) since the pain is very severe and since larger doses may inhibit respirations. Pain usually persists for three or four days, caused in part by severance of the intercostal nerves. The chest catheters may also irritate the pleura and cause pain. If pain in the incision persists over a long period of time, the doctor may infiltrate the area above and below the incision with procaine. Since the pain is often made more severe by coughing, the patient may refuse to cough or take deep breaths. The pain experienced during an attempt to cough may frighten the patient so that he is afraid to try again. Therefore, coughing should be encouraged about half an hour after the narcotic is given, and whenever coughing is encouraged, the incision should be splinted manually or with a towel or drawsheet (Fig. 133). Intermittent positive-pressure respirators may be used to stimulate coughing and deep breathing. If the patient does not cough productively and if his breathing sounds moist or he has "rattles," the doctor should be notified, for he may wish to use endotracheal suction. After the chest catheters have been removed, coughing and turning usually are less difficult. There is no definite day on which the chest catheters are removed, for it depends on the amount of drainage and air present in the pleural cavity and on the reexpansion of the lungs. Usually however, they can be removed two or three days postoperatively. Antibiotics are given routinely to prevent infection.

While the patient is bedfast, the nurse should encourage him to do arm and leg exercises. They may be done passively by the nurse at first. However, as the patient becomes stronger, the doctor usually wants him to be encouraged to tighten his leg muscles, move his feet up and down, and move his arms through the full range of motion. The patient usually will not use his left arm without being urged, since motion causes pain in the operative area. To prevent a stiff, unusable shoulder, however, exercises should be gradually instituted. The nurse should supervise the exercising of the left arm and shoulder until the patient has regained full range of motion.

Many patients have profuse diaphoresis after cardiac surgery, and it may be more pronounced at night. The exact reason is not known. The patient should be kept dry and comfortable and should be reassured that it is a fairly common occurrence and that it will gradually subside. The temperature may rise markedly and remain elevated for several days. It is believed that this elevation may be due to the presence of blood within the pericardium.

Some patients experience a period of depression or even disorientation after cardiac surgery, although this reaction does not generally last very long. The patient may become very excited and fearful, or he may have hallucinations (false visual perceptions). Other patients complain of varying degrees of depression. This reaction often occurs early, and the nurse should be aware of this possibility. The cause is unknown, but it is thought that it may be caused by medication, fear, or some cerebral disturbance. Panic may develop. The family also should be prepared for this possibility. The patient needs a calm environment and much reassurance and understanding. He should be protected from anything or anyone that seems to upset him further (p. 127).

Ambulation. Mobilization of the patient depends upon the operation and the status of the heart. In general, patients who have had surgery for a coarctation of the aorta or any other surgery on the aorta are kept flat in bed for about ten days to prevent unnecessary strain on the vessel (the blood pressure is lower when the patient is flat). Some doctors do not permit the patient to be turned for several days. Before getting out of bed, the patient must gradually become accustomed to having the head of the bed elevated. When this procedure is first attempted, he may complain of dizziness and faintness. If so, he is returned to a flat position, and elevation is attempted again later. Patients who have had surgery for patent ductus arteriosus and mitral stenosis are kept in Fowler's position postoperatively and are encouraged to move their arms and legs. Unless the cardiopulmonary status is very poor, they are allowed to begin ambulation by the fifth to seventh postoperative day. Backache from lying flat on the back is common. Sometimes a hinged bed board is used as a preventive measure.

The time of ambulation for each patient depends upon his progress and condition, but it usually proceeds as follows: The first day he dangles his feet over the side of the bed for fifteen minutes in the morning and afternoon. The second day he is allowed to sit in a chair at the side of the bed for fifteen minutes in the morning and afternoon. The third day he walks around the room while he is up. The fourth day he is allowed to walk around the room and to sit in the chair for gradually increasing periods of time. By the fifth day he may walk longer distances. He should be closely supervised during ambulation, and no activity that causes fatigue, dyspnea or an increased pulse or respiratory rate should be continued. If any of these symptoms appear, he should return to bed, and the doctor should be consulted before further activity is attempted. Definite instructions are left by the doctor regarding when the patient may attempt to climb stairs. The activity should be done slowly under the supervision of a nurse. Only two or three steps should be attempted the first time, after which the number of steps is gradually increased until the patient is able to climb a flight or more, if ordered. The patient should rest two or three times while climbing one flight of stairs.

Long-term postoperative care. The patient and his family need to be told that no marked improvement will be noticed immediately after the operation—that it will be at least three to six months before the full result of the surgery can be ascertained. It is essential that all patients be given this information so that they will not be depressed by dyspnea or pain that is still present postoperatively. Sometimes, even when the patient has not benefited from surgery, he may think he feels better, and this belief should be encouraged.

In preparation for discharge from the hospital, the patient is asked to make a list of activities usually carried out at home. This list is discussed with the doctor to ascertain the activities he feels are appropriate. A woman usually will want to know if she may dust, make beds, wash dishes, and do other household chores. A man may wish to know exactly what he may do—how much he may walk, what he may do about his house and yard, and when he may report to work. Patients are usually advised to start slowly and progress gradually to more energy-consuming tasks. The doctor will want a patient to return for frequent medical follow-up examinations, at which time he will advise him regarding additional activities. The patient should not think of himself as an invalid and should be allowed to do anything that does not tire him. On the other hand, he must be restrained from attempting too much.

The family of the patient who has undergone cardiac surgery should be aware of his condition and how much he can do. Since the patient has often been an invalid preoperatively, the family may be as fearful as he is about his activity. They should understand how important it is for him to continue to see his doctor regularly and why he must continue to take his medication and remain on his diet. A public health nurse is often asked to supervise his care and activity at home.

If the patient is a child and has had congestive failure, his family will need help with medications and any diet restrictions. They should also be taught how to prepare a temperature chart, which they usually are asked to keep during the first month. After this time, danger of infection or endocarditis usually is past.

The child's parents should have ample time to review their questions and concerns, which often come out more easily during discussion of the more tangible parts of care. Most parents appreciate home visits from a nurse to be certain that what they are doing is right for their child.

Rehabilitation of the patient with cardiac disease

To help patients with diseases of the heart and circulatory system learn to live within the limits of their cardiac capacity, the nurse needs to know as much about the patient's condition as possible. She will need to know what the doctor has told the patient and his family and what limitations he has set for the patient. This information should be shared with other persons, such as the family, the social worker, the occupational therapist, the physical therapist, the public health nurse, the industrial nurse, the employer, or the schoolteacher, who may assist in the patient's rehabilitation.

It is helpful to prepare a list of the activities in which the patient usually engages at home and at work so that the doctor can check those which he considers appropriate to resume. As the patient improves, more of the activities may be added to the approved list. Such a list serves as a guide for the patient and his family, and it may help him strike a balance between too many and too few restrictions. The patient, however, must use judgment and discretion in carrying out these activities, especially the pace at which they are performed. If they cause him to be tired or out of breath, they are too strenuous. Moderation should be the guiding principle. All activities should be carried out at a slower pace, and extra rest periods should be taken. The cardiac patient should not jump out of bed, should not run or walk fast, and should avoid climbing. Walking against a high wind and exercising at a higher altitude than usual also cause additional strain on the heart.

Patients with cardiac disease should strive for equanimity. All removable burdens, such as those imposed by fatigue, obesity, infections, and emotional upsets, should be removed. It is often difficult for a patient to achieve this goal without the help of his family. Cardiac disease usually affects the lives of others as well as the life of the patient. The entire family's mode of living may have to be changed, responsibilities may need to be reapportioned, and another member of the family may even have to become the wage earner. The life of a child patient should be planned so that he is not continually frustrated by restrictions. Major adjustments cannot help but disturb the patient, especially if the patient is a mother or a father. The nurse should find opportunities to talk to the family while the patient is still in the hospital, since it is better if the family can begin to make adjustments at this time so that life will be smoother for the patient on his return home. The family members may be unaware of the changes that may be required in their lives, or if they are aware of the changes, they may need help in planning for them. They should realize that adjustments may be permanent rather than temporary. Their successful adjustment to a new way of life may have a direct effect on how long and how happily the cardiac patient will live.

The doctor will prescribe the patient's diet. On discharge from the hospital some patients will be allowed to eat a regular diet but are told to eat in moderation because large meals increase the work of the heart during digestion. If the patient is overweight, a low-caloric diet will probably be ordered. A diet low in fat may be ordered for patients with a high blood cholesterol level, since there is a possibility that it may be a factor in the development of coronary artery disease. The most common diet restriction, however, is a mild sodium-restricted diet (2,000 mg. per day) or a moderate sodium-restricted diet (600 to 1,200 mg. per day). Occasionally a strict low-sodium diet (500 mg. per day) is ordered. Both the nurse and the dietitian should work closely with the patient and the family to be sure that they understand the dietary restrictions, why they are essential, and how to prepare acceptable meals. Plans should be worked out with the homemaker so that special food will not need to be prepared for the patient. If salt is restricted, for instance, the simplest method is to cook the food for the entire family without salt, set aside the patient's portion, and season the remainder. If the patient is on restricted salt intake, he should be advised not to take medications or other substances containing salt or sodium, such as saline cathartics, sodium bicarbonate, or soft drinks containing soda water. The teaching program should be started well in advance of the patient's discharge from the hospital. Usually a public health nursing referral should be made, listing the specific problems to be checked.

Many patients with heart disease and their families can profit from regular health supervision visits by a public health nurse. If arrangements need to be made because the patient cannot climb stairs, for example, it may be helpful for the public health nurse to visit the patient's home before he is discharged. After seeing the situation, she may be able to make suggestions that will make him more comfortable and will make his care easier. If the patient happens to be a mother and housewife, minor changes, especially in the work area of the kitchen, may be possible so that she can carry out many of her housekeeping duties while seated (Fig. 75). After the patient has arrived home, problems and questions often arise with which the nurse can help. This additional help may reduce the patient's fear and the uncertainty of his family so that he will accept his restrictions more readily. If the patient cannot return to full activity, the family may need help in providing nursing care in the home. For instance, sometimes it is known that an elderly patient will be a semi-invalid. If one or more members of the family take a course in home nursing offered by the American Red Cross, it is easier for the family to give essential care. Sometimes it is possible to take the course while the patient is still hospitalized.

Provision for follow-up care should be made, and the patient should understand the importance of this care. The patient with heart disease should remain under medical supervision for the remainder of his life.

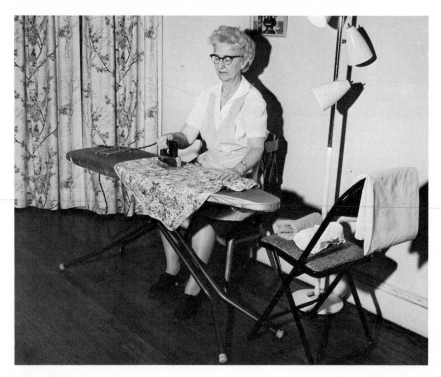

Fig. 75

The patient with cardiac disease can be helped
to make household activities easier. Note
the comfortable position and the placement
within easy reach of articles to be ironed.

In this way he may be kept in the best possible physical condition, which will cause the
least burden on his heart. He should also
avoid the danger of additional damage and
burden on the heart imposed by infections.
If possible, he should avoid colds and other
upper respiratory infections. If he does develop an infection, he should go to bed and
call a doctor. The patient with cardiac
disease will have a longer convalescence
from any illness than the normal person and
should return to full activity gradually.

When the patient with cardiac disease is
ready to return to school or work, the health
service, if one is provided, should know exactly what the patient can and cannot do.
Most patients will be allowed to return to
normal activity unless it is too strenuous or
they have marked incapacity. If the nurse in
the health service becomes aware that nor-

mal activity tires the patient, she should report this fact to her medical adviser so that
further medical follow-up can be given and
necessary adjustments made. Although many
patients may return to their former work,
some must change their type of work.

Because heart diseases do cause loss of
time at work and because the financial strain
placed on the family is great, every effort
should be made to evaluate each patient's
condition and to place him in a position
where he will be gainfully employed within
his physical limitations. Help in locating a
suitable position for the cardiac patient may
be obtained from the local branch of the
American Heart Association, from the office
of vocational rehabilitation in state employment services, and occasionally from adult
cardiac clinics in hospitals. Using the functional and therapeutic classifications set up
by the Criteria Committee of the American
Heart Association, the doctor places the patient in the appropriate categories. There
are four functional classifications and five
therapeutic classifications.

Functional classification

Class I—No limitation of physical activity
Class II—Slight limitation of physical activity

Class III—Marked limitation of physical activity

Class IV—Unable to carry on any physical activity without discomfort

Therapeutic classification

Class A—Physical activity not restricted

Class B—Ordinary physical activity need not be restricted, but patient should be advised against unusually severe or competitive efforts

Class C—Ordinary physical activity should be moderately restricted, and more strenuous habitual efforts should be discontinued

Class D—Ordinary physical activity should be markedly restricted

Class E—Complete rest, confined to bed or chair

In some communities special workshops (such as the Altro Workshops in New York City) have a demonstration and research program for cardiac patients requiring rehabilitation.

The housewife with cardiac disease should also be considered, and some rehabilitation centers and hospitals have developed programs to help her adjust to her limitations and still be able to function in her role of wife and mother. Kitchen facilities similar to those found in most homes have been provided so that she may practice work-simplification measures and plan possible adjustments in the physical setup of her own kitchen. In a booklet entitled *Heart of the Home*, prepared by the American Heart Association, work simplification is discussed and changes that can be made in the physical facilities are outlined so that the housewife with cardiac disease can manage with a minimum of effort.

Many communities now have rehabilitative help available, and no patient with heart disease should be without this type of assistance. Nurses and doctors can do much to help each patient, and this assistance may be more important than medication.

References and selected readings*

1 *Bean, Margaret A., and others: Monitoring patients through electronics, Am. J. Nursing 63:65-69, April 1963.

2 Beeson, Paul B., and McDermott, Walsh, editors: Cecil-Loeb textbook of medicine, ed. 11, Philadelphia, 1963, W. B. Saunders Co.

3 Bergersen, Betty S., and Krug, Elsie E.: Pharmacology in nursing, ed. 10, St. Louis, 1966, The C. V. Mosby Co.

4 Blake, Florence G.: Open heart surgery in children, a study of nursing care, Children's Bureau, Washington, D. C., 1964, U. S. Department of Health, Education, and Welfare.

5 *Blakeslee, Alton: How to live with heart trouble, New York, 1950, American Heart Association.

6 *Briggs, Louise Winegar, and Mortensen, J D: Nursing care of the patient with a prosthetic heart valve, Am. J. Nursing 63:66-72, Oct. 1963.

7 Cardiovascular diseases in the United States: facts and figures, New York, 1965, American Heart Association.

8 *Closed-chest method of cardiopulmonary resection, Am. J. Nursing 65:105, May 1965.

9 Coronary disease, Heart Information Center, National Heart Institute, Baltimore, 1964, U. S. Department of Health, Education, and Welfare.

10 *Crawley, Mildred: Care of the patient with myocardial infarction, Am. J. Nursing 61:68-70, Feb. 1961.

11 *Creighton, Helen, and Hufnagle, Charles A.: Aortic insufficiency and its surgical treatment, Am. J. Nursing 58:547-550, April 1958.

12 *Cross, C. Joseph: Back to work after myocardial infarction, Am. J. Nursing 62:58-61, Feb. 1962.

13 Davidsohn, Israel, and Wells, Benjamin B.: Todd-Sanford clinical diagnosis by laboratory methods, ed. 13, Philadelphia, 1962, W. B. Saunders Co.

14 Davis, Loyal, Editor: Christopher's textbook of surgery, ed. 8, Philadelphia, 1964, W. B. Saunders Co.

15 *Dean, Virginia: Measuring venous blood pressure, Am. J. Nursing 63:70-72, Oct. 1963.

16 de la Chapelle, Clarence E., and Connor, Charles A. R.: Treatment of patients after recovery from myocardial infarction, Mod. Concepts Cardiovas. Dis. 33:885-889, Nov. 1964.

17 Denham, Margaret, Abraham, Sidney, and Graves, L. M.: Nursing services outside the hospital for cardiovascular disease patients, Pub. Health Rep. 74:21-27, Jan. 1959.

18 DeWall, Richard A., Hassan, Najafi, and Roden, Thomas: A hard-shell temperature-controlling disposable blood oxygenator, J.A.M.A. 197:1065-1068, Sept. 26, 1966.

19 *Dick, Lillian S., and Grant, Marie D.: The nurse's role in rehabilitation of the child with rheumatic fever, Pub. Health Rep. 79:533-536, June 1964.

20 Douglas, Gordon W.: Rubella in pregnancy, Am. J. Nursing 66:2664-2666, Dec. 1966.

21 *Elliott, Florence C., and Winchell, Paul: Heart catheterization and angiocardiography, Am. J. Nursing 60:1418-1422, Oct. 1960.

22 Evans, John A.: Recent advances in visualization of the aorta and visceral arteries, Report of the Eighth Annual Conference on the New York Heart Association, Jan. 1962.

23 Fields, Sister Mary Lucida: The c.p.r. team in a medium-sized hospital, Am. J. Nursing 66:87-90, Jan. 1966.

24 Fletcher, Anthony P., and Sherry, Sol: Thrombolytic (fibrinolytic) therapy for coronary heart disease, Circulation 22:619-626, Oct. 1960.

25 Frank, Charles W., and others: Myocardial infarction in men, J.A.M.A. 198:1241-1245, Dec. 19, 1966.

26 Freidberg, Charles K.: Diseases of the heart, Philadelphia, 1966, W. B. Saunders Co.

---

*References preceded by an asterisk are particularly well suited for student reading.

27 Glenn, Frank, and others: The circulatory system and surgery, S. Clin. North America 41:265-496, April 1961.

28 Grace, William J., and others: Use of the permanent subcutaneous transvenous pacemaker in Adams-Stokes syndrome, Am. J. Cardiol. 18:888-891, Dec. 1966.

29 *Griep, Arthur H., and DePaul, Sister: Angina pectoris, Am. J. Nursing 65:72-75, June 1965.

30 *Grollman, Arthur: Diuretics, Am. J. Nursing 65:84-89, Jan. 1965.

31 Harrison, T. R., and others, editors: Principles of internal medicine, ed. 5, New York, 1966, Blakiston Division, McGraw-Hill Book Co.

32 *Heller, Anne F.: Nursing the patient with an artificial pacemaker, Am. J. Nursing 64:87-93, April 1964.

33 Humphries, J. O'Neal: Treatment of heart block with artificial pacemakers, Mod. Concepts Cardiovas. Dis. 33:857-862, June 1964.

34 Hypertension and hypertensive heart disease in adults, United States 1960-1962. Vital and Health Statistics, National Center for Health Statistics, series 11, no. 3, Washington, D. C., May 1966, U. S. Department of Health, Education, and Welfare.

35 *Imboden, Clarence A., Jr., and Wynn, Jane E.: Machines in perspective, the coronary care area, Am. J. Nursing 65:72-76, Feb. 1965.

36 Jenkins, Adeline C.: Successful cardiac monitoring, Nurs. Clin. North America 1:537-547, Dec. 1966.

37 Jude, James R., Kouwenhoven, William B., and Knickerbocker, G. Guy: Cardiac arrest, J.A.M.A. 178:1063-1070, Dec. 16, 1961.

38 *Kelly, Ann E., and Gensini, Goffredo G.: Coronary arteriography, Am. J. Nursing 62:86-90, Feb. 1962.

39 Kottke, Frederic J., and others: Studies of cardiac output during early phase of rehabilitation, Postgrad. Med. 23:533-544, May 1958.

40 *Leone, Lucile Petry: The attack on heart disease, cancer, and stroke. Is nursing ready? Am. J. Nursing 65:68-72, May 1965.

41 Lerner, Monroe: Mortality and morbidity in the United States as basic indices of health needs, Ann. Am. Acad. Polit. & Soc. Sc. 337:1-11, Sept. 1961.

42 Long, Janet M.: Arch aortography, Am. J. Nursing 64:97-99, Dec. 1964.

43 *MacVicar, Jean: Exercises before and after thoracic surgery, Am. J. Nursing 62:61-63, Jan. 1962.

44 Marienfeld, Carl J., and others: Rheumatic fever and rheumatic heart disease among U. S. college freshmen, 1956-1960, Pub. Health Rep. 79:789-811, Sept. 1964.

45 *Meltzer, Lawrence E.: Coronary care, electrocardiography, and the nurse, Am. J. Nursing 65:63-67, Dec. 1965.

46 Meltzer, Lawrence E., Pinneo, Rose, and Kitchell, J. Roderick: Intensive coronary care, a manual for nurses, Philadelphia, 1965, Coronary Care Unit Fund, The Presbyterian Hospital in Philadelphia.

47 Modell, Walter, and others: Handbook of cardiology for nurses, ed. 5, New York, 1966, Springer Publishing Co.

48 Modell, Walter: Drugs of choice, 1966-1967, St. Louis, 1966, The C. V. Mosby Co.

49 Moffitt, Emerson A., Sessler, Alan D., and Kirklin, John W.: Postoperative care in open heart surgery, J.A.M.A. 199:161-163, Jan. 16, 1967.

50 *Moore, Sister Mary Consilium: Nursing care of a patient with an implanted artificial pacemaker, Cardiovas. Nursing 2:19-23, Winter 1965.

51 Nelson, Waldo E.: Textbook of pediatrics, ed. 2, Philadelphia, 1964, W. B. Saunders Co.

52 *Nurse, Amy G.: But why can't I get up? Am. J. Nursing 53:172-174, Feb. 1953.

53 Nursing and summary papers, Second National Conference on Cardiovascular Diseases, Division of Nursing. Washington, D. C., 1964, U. S. Department of Health, Education, and Welfare.

54 Ochsner, John L., and Moore, Charles B.: Myocardial revascularization, S. Clin. North America 46:1525-1536, Dec. 1966.

55 Proudfit, Fairfax T., and Robinson, Corinne H.: Normal and therapeutic nutrition, ed. 12, New York, 1961, The Macmillan Co.

56 Pryor, Ray, editor: Heart disease in children, training program in cardiology, Division of Chronic Diseases, Heart Disease Control Program, Washington, D. C., Feb. 1966, U. S. Department of Health, Education, and Welfare.

57 *Rae, Nancy Mara: Caring for patients following open heart surgery, Am. J. Nursing 63:77-82, Nov. 1963.

58 *Rawlings, Maurice S.: Heart disease today, Am. J. Nursing 66:303-307, Feb. 1966.

59 Riker, William L.: Intracardiac surgery for common congenital heart lesions, S. Clin. North America 43:133-145, Feb. 1963.

60 *Ross, Jeanne: The nurse and the patient with open heart surgery, J. Nursing Ed. 1:25-29, Sept. 1962.

61 Schrogie, John J.: Cardiopulmonary resuscitation in practice, Pub. Health Rep. 81:128-132, Feb. 1966.

62 *Stamler, Jeremiah, and others: Coronary proneness and approaches to preventing heart attacks, Am. J. Nursing 66:1788-1793, Aug. 1966.

63 The heart and circulation, Second National Conference on Cardiovascular Diseases, vol. 1, parts 1 and 2, Research; vol. II, Community Service and Education, Washington, D. C., 1964, U. S. Department of Health, Education, and Welfare.

64 *Turell, David J.: The cardiac patient returns to work, Am. J. Nursing 65:115-117, Aug. 1965.

65 U. S. Department of Health, Education and Welfare, National Center for Health Statistics: Monthly vital Statistics Report, Advance Report, Final Mortality Statistics, 1964, 14:10, Jan. 14, 1966.

66 U. S. Department of Health, Education, and Welfare, Public Health Service, Communicable Disease Center: Morbidity and mortality statistics, Annual Supplement, 1964, vol. 13, Sept. 30, 1965.

67 *Varvaro, Filomena Fanelli: Teaching the patient about open heart surgery, Am. J. Nursing 65:111-115, Oct. 1965.

68 White, Paul Dudley: Heart disease, ed. 4, New York, 1951, The Macmillan Co.

69 *Wolff, Ilse S., and others: The patient with myocardial infarction, Am. J. Nursing 64:C-3—C-32, Nov. 1964.

70 *Wood, Edwin C.: Understanding the patient with heart disease, Nursing Outlook 7:90-92, Feb. 1959.

member of the family should inspect his feet periodically. In the daily, routine care of the feet, the skin and base of the nails should be gently massaged with lubricants such as lanolin or other mild creams. Alcohol is drying to the skin and is not recommended for patients with vascular disease. Each toe should be gently massaged from the distal end proximally to stimulate circulation. Powder should be used between the toes, with care being taken that it does not cake and that it is thoroughly removed at the next washing. Authorities maintain that epidermophytosis (athlete's foot), which is often a precursor of gangrene in the feet of persons with arterial insufficiency, will seldom develop if the toes and feet are kept dry at all times. Therefore, the patient who perspires profusely should powder between his toes more than once a day and should change his socks at least daily. Any kind of powder is satisfactory, although preparations containing undecylenic acid are now widely used. Small pieces of lamb's wool or cotton can be placed between the toes to absorb the perspiration.

To prevent ingrown toenails, the nails should be cut carefully at regular intervals. Before the nails are cut, the feet should be soaked in tepid water. The nails should be cut straight across and slightly rounded at the sides. They must never be cut down to the level of the tissue. Pocketknives, razor blades, or scissors should never be used. The patient should equip himself with a pair of toenail clippers. Files are usually considered safe. However, tissues can be traumatized by emery boards and files, particularly when the patient lacks normal sensation in the toes. Elderly persons with poor vision should not cut their own toenails. A member of the family should do it for them.

With daily care a toenail that has a tendency to "curl under" at the side of the toe can be trained to grow more normally, but no efforts should be made to "straighten" the nail by vigorous treatment. With the rounded end of an ordinary toothpick, a small wisp of cotton should be inserted gently under the edge of the nail. The cotton must be changed daily. Although it may be weeks before any improvement is seen, with patience and persistence most nails that tend to grow under can be made to grow more

normally unless there is aggravation by a condition such as pressure from shoes.

Medical care should be sought for blisters and for corns, calluses, and areas of thickened skin that cannot be rubbed away with a washcloth and an emery board after having been soaked. Soap poultices made of any soft soap, such as shaving cream, may be used to soften corns and calluses before rubbing is attempted. The patient with circulatory disease of any kind should be advised to seek medical advice before going to a chiropodist.

Protection from trauma and pressure. The patient should be warned to avoid injury to his feet and legs and to watch carefully for infection following trauma. He should not walk barefoot for fear of splinters causing injury. It also is dangerous for him to scratch any minor skin lesions. Many stubborn ulcers of the leg have followed the vigorous scratching of mosquito or other insect bites. Venous stasis may cause itching that can be most annoying. This itching usually follows long periods of standing and will subside if the patient rests with the feet elevated for a few minutes every hour or two. The warning not to scratch the skin is hard to heed at times. Calamine lotion is sometimes prescribed by the doctor when pruritus is troublesome. Any minor infection of the legs or the feet should be viewed as a major one by a patient with peripheral vascular disease. He should never attempt self-treatment when any signs of infection develop.

To avoid fungal infections of the feet, socks or stockings should be washed daily. If they are wool or have a tendency to shrink, they should be stretched over a dryer. Otherwise, they may constrict circulation. Sock frames can be purchased at most notion counters, or a simple, inexpensive dryer can be made from a metal coat hanger.

The patient should have at least two pairs of shoes and should wear them on alternate days, thus giving each pair a chance to air. If shoes become wet, they should be dried slowly on shoe trees to help preserve their shape. New shoes should be broken in gradually. Leather shoes are best because they give good support to the feet. Canvas, linen, or perforated nylon shoes provide ventilation, are comfortable in warm weather, and are safe if they have leather soles. Rubber-soled shoes are not advised for persons who have any kind of vascular disease since they retard evaporation and thus may contribute to the development of fungal infection. Shoes should be carefully fitted by experienced persons. They should extend about one-half inch beyond the longest toe and should be wide enough to avoid pressure anywhere on the foot and to allow fairly free movement of the toes within the shoe. The inner last of the shoe should be straight, and the longitudinal arch of the shoe should support that of the foot. Playshoes and ballet slippers, which afford little or no support are not recommended for persons with peripheral vascular disease, although there is no objection to women wearing pumps with moderately high heels. In fact, pumps are good inasmuch as the feet can be slipped

out of the shoes and the toes wiggled at intervals. However, the shoes should be roomy enough so that they can be put on again easily. The patient should be advised to shun economy when buying shoes. Ill-fitting bargain shoes may cause blisters and lead to serious and costly illness.

For sleeping hours the person with peripheral vascular disease should have light-weight covers that are loose and do not permit any pressure on the toes, which often burn and are painful. The patient who lives at home should be taught how to improvise a board at the foot of his bed to keep the weight of covers from his feet (Fig. 76). The patient who is hospitalized also should have a padded board or box at the foot of the bed. These devices are preferable to a cradle, which may hamper freedom of movement and against which the patient may accidentally strike his foot. If a cradle must be used, it should be padded and bath blankets should be placed over the cradle and tucked securely under the mattress to prevent drafts on the feet.

Rest, exercise, and posture. A careful balance of rest and exercise is necessary for

Fig. 76

The nurse instructs the patient's daughter how to improvise equipment to keep bed linen off the patient's sensitive feet.

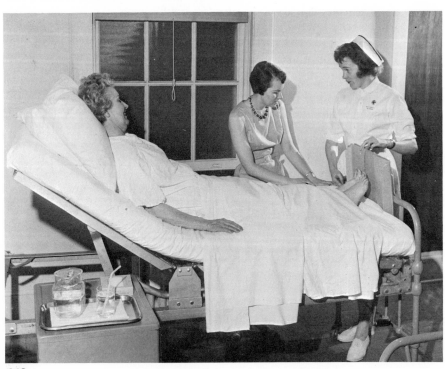

the patient with peripheral vascular disease. Exercise improves return of venous blood from the extremities to the heart, which in turn improves arterial circulation, and this is important. Too much exercise, however, increases metabolism, thereby increasing the demands placed upon the circulation to take nutrients to the tissues and to remove the products of metabolism. Complete rest may be necessary in the presence of associated medical illness such as heart disease, thrombophlebitis, or gangrene.

In regard to posture, the following is a safe guide for all patients with peripheral vascular disease (or indeed, for anyone): Do not stay in *any* position too long. This is particularly important for the elderly patient, who often has both arterial and venous disease.

Much emphasis has been placed upon elevation of the feet, and many patients believe that it will benefit them. However, it may cause damage when the patient has arterial insufficiency. The nurse must *clearly understand* the patient's condition and the doctor's orders before she attempts to give instructions in this regard. The patient with good arterial circulation but with disease such as lymphedema may safely rest for an hour or more with the feet above the level of the heart. On the other hand, the patient with arterial disease in addition to venous disease should remain in this position for only a few minutes at a time to permit venous blood to drain lest arterial flow be hindered. It is safe to assume that the flat position is best over an extended time unless the doctor has ordered otherwise.

Long periods of standing still should be avoided by persons with either venous or arterial disease, and short periods should be alternated with exercise such as rapid walking. Those who have venous disease should alternate standing and walking with elevation of the affected limbs.

The importance of posture must be stressed in the care and teaching of patients with peripheral vascular disease. The patient should sleep on a firm mattress. A soft mattress may allow enough flexion of the trunk at the hips to impede circulation to the lower extremities. It may also permit the lower limbs to be higher than the heart, which is undesirable in arterial disease. The height of a chair should be such that the knees are not bent at more than a right angle, and the depth of the seat should permit two fingers between the chair seat and the popliteal spaces. Both of these provisions will help to prevent pressure on the popliteal vessels that would obstruct arterial flow to the limbs and interfere with venous return. Furthermore, the patient should never cross his legs at the knee, since this position also causes pressure on the popliteal vessels. He should develop the habit of rotating his foot at the ankle, bending the foot up and down, and straightening the knee at intervals. Attendance at movies or other satisfying diversion can sometimes be made safe and comfortable for patients with impaired circulation by the use of these simple measures to improve circulation.

Postural exercises (Buerger-Allen). Specific exercises to empty blood vessels and to stimulate collateral circulation are sometimes prescribed for persons with arterial disease such as arteriosclerosis obliterans and thromboangiitis obliterans (Buerger's disease). These exercises are often called Buerger-Allen exercises (after the physicians who first used them). With the patient lying on his back, his legs are elevated until the feet blanch, are lowered until redness appears, and then remain flat for a few minutes. The procedure is repeated a prescribed number of times. The length of time the exercises are to be performed is varied according to the change in color of each patient's feet, but a procedure consisting of elevating the legs two or three minutes, lowering them five to ten minutes, and leaving them flat five to ten minutes is often ordered. A 45- to 90-degree angle of elevation may be ordered. If the legs are elevated at 90 degrees, the period of elevation may be shortened; for example, one to two minutes may cause blanching. A schedule of repeating the exercises five to ten times three times a day is usually prescribed.

If the nurse is asked to supervise the exercises, she should know their purpose and should not permit the feet to remain elevated after whiteness appears. If she is teaching the patient to do these exercises at home or is instructing members of his family, she must emphasize that they must watch the color of the feet while they are elevated and lower them as soon as the normal color leaves. In the hospital the overbed table covered with a pillow may be used to support the elevated limbs. At home the patient may lie on the sofa and support the elevated feet against the wall or on the arm of the sofa. A chair inverted on the bed and covered with a blanket provides a comfortable support for elevation of the feet.

Avoidance of constriction of circulation. The patient with peripheral vascular disease must not wear anything that constricts circulation. Rolled garters, knitted hose designed to stay up without garters, and girdles that cause constriction around the thighs and groin should not be worn. Some doctors also believe that tight waistbands should not be worn. Men may be advised to wear suspenders instead of belts, and women should select garter belts that do not constrict or light, full-length corsets instead of girdles. Socks that do not require garters should be worn by men. Shoelaces should be tied loosely. If edema of the feet occurs at the end of the day, the shoelaces should be loosened and relaced several times each day. Elastic shoelaces are preferred by some patients who have a moderate amount of edema of the feet or ankles.

Diet. The patient with peripheral vascular disease should avoid becoming overweight. Excess fat places an added burden on diseased arteries that already have difficulty in keeping up with tissue demands. Obesity in the patient with venous diesase increases congestion and probably lessens the effectiveness of muscles in assisting with the return flow of blood. If the patient has limited cardiac capacity in addition to vascular disease, the heart and the entire vascular system are taxed to such an extent that distribution of blood to the extremities is curtailed. Reducing diets, however, must always be under the direction of the physician. Harm can be done, particularly to the elderly patient, by rapid loss of weight, which may alter pressure within sclerosed arteries and make it possible for a clot to form, causing further depletion of the nutrient supply to tissues supplied by the arteries.

When the doctor has prescribed a reducing diet, the nurse can be of real assistance in helping to plan meals that are satisfying to the patient and yet within his caloric restrictions and financial means. The patient with peripheral vascular disease is usually advised to have a diet high in protein because it should help to prevent breakdown of tissues. If he has a lesion such as a varicose ulcer, a diet high in protein should help to promote healing. Vitamin B is important in maintaining normal health of blood vessels, and vitamin C is essential in healing and in the prevention of both internal and external hemorrhage.

It is generally recommended that patients with peripheral vascular disease take a larger amount of fluids than the normal person. As many as fifteen to twenty glasses of water or equivalent fluids are often recommended. This amount may improve the quality of the limited blood supply to the limbs by improving elimination of waste products. It is also believed that it may lessen the viscosity of the blood and thus help to prevent the formation of thrombi.

The nurse should learn about the patient's circumstances of living and their effect on his diet. For example, she should find out whether he has to climb several flights of stairs to bring groceries home. Climbing may cause severe pain in the legs because of inadequate oxygenation of the tissues. Some arrangements, therefore, must be made to assist the patient with this chore. If he lives alone, she should find out whether there is someone in his building or neighborhood who can shop for him. She may find that the young mother with a stubborn ulcer that complicated phlebitis before delivery is so harassed with feeding the baby and getting other children off to school or otherwise attended to that she neglects her own breakfast and lunch. The nurse may discover that the elderly man with arteriosclerosis develops intermittent claudication when he walks from his rooming house to the nearest restaurant, causing him to skip one or two meals each day. The assistance of the doctor and/or social worker may be needed to solve particular problems.

Drugs. In addition to medications for pain, the two important types of drugs given to patients with peripheral vascular disease are vasodilators, which dilate blood vessels, and anticoagulants, which lessen the tendency of the blood to clot. Newer drugs, which dissolve thrombi that are already formed, are now being used. These drugs show promise of great value, although their use at the present time is still experimental.

Vasodilators may be given when toxic drugs such as ergot have caused vasospasm, when arteriosclerosis has caused narrowing of the lumen of the vessel, or when a thrombus has formed in an artery and caused partial or total obstruction. If a clot is adherent to a blood vessel, an anticoagulant drug may be given with the vasodilator to prevent further clot formation. While several drugs are useful for vasodilation, the excellent vasodilatory effects of warm baths, heat to the abdomen, and hot fluids by mouth should not be overlooked.

Vasodilators. The drug *papaverine*, an alkaloid of opium, has long been known to have a relaxing effect on the smooth muscle of the blood vessels, especially if spasm occurs. It is not habit-forming. The usual dose is 30 to 60 mg. (½ to 1 grain) intramuscularly or intravenously, or 60 to 200 mg. (1 to 3½ grains) orally.[7] This drug may be used in the treatment of acute arterial occlusion associated with arteriosclerosis obliterans.

Tolazoline hydrochloride (Priscoline hydrochloride), 25 to 50 mg. (⅜ to ¾ grain), given orally three to four times a day, is an adrenergic-blocking agent (sympatholytic drug).[7] It prevents the transmission of sympathetic impulses and thus produces vasodilation. It also may be given intravenously. Some other drugs that have a similar effect and that are prescribed for vasodilation in peripheral vascular diseases are *azapetine phosphate* (Ilidar phosphate), *dibenzyl-β-chloroethylamine* (Dibenamine), and *phenoxybenzamine hydrochloride* (Dibenzyline). Toxic reactions to these drugs include palpitation, nausea and vomiting, pruritus and abnormal skin sensations, and drop in blood pressure. Toxic signs should be carefully watched for in any patient receiving these drugs and must be reported to the doctor at once. The patient who cannot tolerate one of these drugs may be able to take another without untoward reactions.

Alcohol is a very useful drug in dilating the blood vessels. The usual dosage is 30 to 60 ml. three to four times a day. The alcohol preparation often ordered is whiskey and soda, but any of the common beverages containing alcohol can be used. Some doctors order a double dose at bedtime to produce maximum effect during the hours when muscle action is not assisting with the flow of blood to the legs. *Caffeine* (contained in tea and coffee) and *theobromine* (found in chocolate) also are peripheral vasodilators, but these drugs are seldom given for their vasodilating effect. However, because they have this effect, there usually is no need to eliminate tea, coffee, and chocolate from the diet of the patient with peripheral vascular disease.

Anticoagulants. Two of the commonly used anticoagulant drugs are *heparin* and *bishydroxycoumarin* (Dicumarol), although there are many other prothrombin depressants now available.[29] These drugs are used widely in the treatment of both venous and arterial thrombosis and are used prophylactically for persons with a threatened thrombosis or threatened recurrence of conditions such as thrombophlebitis. They act therapeutically by prolonging the clotting time of the blood. They will not dissolve clots already formed but will prevent extension of a clot and inhibit formation of new ones.

Heparin is obtained from the lungs and livers of animals. It can be given only parenterally, since it is destroyed by the gastric secretions of the stomach. Its effect is almost immediate, but its action ceases after three to four hours. Heparin dosage is expressed in units or milligrams and is calculated individually for each patient; 50 mg. (5,000 units) may be given at three- to four-hour intervals, or a continuous drip of 100 to 200 mg. (10,000 to 20,000 units) in 1,000 ml. of physiologic solution of sodium chloride may be administered.[7] The average rate of flow for a continuous infusion of heparin should be about twenty to twenty-five drops per minute. When a patient is receiving this drug by infusion, the nurse must watch the rate of flow very carefully and report to the doctor if the solution stops dripping or if its rate cannot be regulated satisfactorily. This drug often is used to lower the prothrombin time until an anticoagulant, taken orally and acting more slowly, takes effect.

Dicumarol was first isolated from spoiled sweet clover after it was observed that cattle eating this food had abortions and hemorrhage. It acts by suppressing the formation of prothrombin. It takes twelve to twenty-four hours to take effect, and its action persists for twenty-four to seventy-two hours after the drug is discontinued. The usual maintenance dosage is 50 to 150 mg. per day administered by mouth.[7] Frequent determinations of the prothrombin level must be obtained and the dose regulated accordingly. Most physicians believe that the prothrombin level should be kept between 10 and 30% of normal. *Warfarin sodium* (Coumadin sodium, Prothromadin) is now widely used. Ethyl biscoumacetate (Tromexan) is another synthetic drug that has an action similar to that of Dicumarol, although it acts more quickly and its effect lasts for a shorter time.

Any anticoagulant drug requires very careful regulation as to amount and continuity of dosage, and the nurse has a responsibility in this regulation. If the dosage is too large, or if it is given in combination with acetylsalicylic acid preparations, the patient may have a hemorrhage in a vital area such as the brain. If the dosage is too small, he may have no relief from symptoms of thrombosis and may have additional thrombus formation with perhaps fatal consequences.

If bleeding results from too much heparin, *protamine sulfate,* a heparin antagonist, is given. Protamine acts almost immediately, and its effect persists for about two hours. The doctor slowly injects a 1% solution intravenously. The total amount given depends upon the amount of heparin that was given and upon the patient's symptoms. If a patient taking Dicumarol should bleed from any body orifice, such as the nose, mouth, or urinary tract, the doctor should be notified before another dose is taken. Usually the drug is discontinued, and vitamin K (menadione sodium bisulfite) or vitamin K_1 (phytonadione) is given intravenously or orally. If the hemorrhage is excessive, transfusions are given. Nursing care includes reassurance of the patient and careful observation for signs of further hemorrhage.

Anticoagulant therapy undoubtedly has prolonged the lives of many persons and enabled them to live quite satisfactorily and productively. The patient who must remain on this drug indefinitely, however, needs encouragement and sympathetic medical and nursing care. Unfortunately, the vein must be punctured at regular intervals to obtain blood for a prothrombin determination. If large doses are needed, this procedure must be done at least two to three times a week and sometimes daily. When smaller doses of anticoagulant are given over long periods, a prothrombin determination is done every one to four weeks. This experience is unpleasant for the patient, and its continuance over weeks and months may place a real restraint on the activities of the ambulatory patient. He may begin to feel trapped and hampered beyond endurance. Vacations, for example, present real problems, and even short trips must be carefully planned. In addition, although it is so important that the patient keep his appointments for prothrombin determinations, it is difficult for the physician to emphasize this fact sufficiently without the patient's realizing or suspecting that his life may be in real danger. Such a realization, of course, would cause further depression.

The patient must be taught to recognize the signs of hemorrhage and to report them immediately. He should carry an identification card stating that he takes anticoagulant drugs so that, in the event of accident, persons who give him medical care will know this fact. The identification card should also contain the name and telephone number of the physician prescribing the drug. The patient also must be told that he should not take any preparation containing acetylsalicylic acid or, in fact, any drug not prescribed by a doctor who knows that he is taking anticoagulants. If he is accustomed to taking a mild pain reliever such as aspirin periodically, he should ask his doctor to prescribe a drug that he can use. The patient should consult his doctor about drinking alcoholic beverages, too, since alcohol elevates the prothrombin time. Alcohol usually is not forbidden, but the dosage of anticoagulant is adjusted in accordance with the alcoholic intake. The intake of alcohol should be the same each day.

Proteolytic enzymes. Streptokinase-streptodornase (Varidase) and purified trypsin crystalline (Tryptar) are proteolytic enzymes that will dissolve fibrinous material and purulent accumulations, when applied to necrotic tissues after debridement. These enzymes are frequently ordered in treatment of ulcers on the legs, which may occur as a complication of peripheral vascular disease resulting from inadequate circulation. The enzyme seems to enhance the action of antibiotics and to encourage healing. The drugs are usually applied topically in the form of wet dressings or are injected into cavities.

Streptokinase and streptokinase-activated human plasma preparations (Thrombolysin lyovac) are substances that are fibrinolytic in that they can dissolve fibrin, which is an essential constituent of a thrombus. Fibrinolytic drugs are either given intravenously or injected above a thrombosed vessel. While fibrinolytic therapy holds great promise and the use of these drugs continues, studies to date seem to indicate that thrombi more than four days old are resistant to lysis and that thrombosis tends to recur after therapy is discontinued.[3,11]

Smoking. Nicotine causes spasm of the peripheral arteries. Therefore, smoking is contraindicated in all vascular diseases. Damage comes from inhaling smoke; there is no evidence that chewing tobacco or using snuff contributes to vasospasm. The relationship between arteriospasm and smoking is so definite that many doctors feel it is useless to try to treat the patient unless he gives up smoking. Smoking should be immediately discontinued in any kind of arterial vascular disease and is also contraindicated in venous disease because the arteries surrounding a thrombosed vein often develop spasms. Gangrene has even been known to follow spasm from this cause.

As ridiculous as it may seem to the non-smoker, giving up cigarettes is almost impossible for many people. The urge to smoke is almost as compelling as the urge to obtain narcotics. It is just as difficult for women as for men to stop smoking once they have become confirmed smokers. Many patients continue to smoke after they have lost a toe or a foot as a result of vascular disease although they known that the disease could be almost surely arrested if they would only stop smoking. Unfortunately there seem to be few substitutes for smoking. Candy, nuts, or raisins can be tried (if the patient is not on a reducing diet), and sometimes gum or coffee helps. Occupational therapy may help to divert the patient. Sometimes constant reminders and strict discipline do more harm than good. The need to smoke seems to be related to such a deep-seated need for gratification by this means that the nurse should be guided by the doctor in her individual approach to each patient. He should decide whether she should ignore the patient when he is smoking or whether she should reprimand him, report to his family, or take other action. Members of his family seldom seem able to help the patient to stop smoking. Often the patient will promise his family (or his doctor) that he will not smoke and then will do so surreptitiously. Reiteration of the doctor's and the nurse's faith in the patient's ability to stop smoking may yield better results than showing disapproval of his lapses. It sometimes helps if the patient can be encouraged to join a group of people who are all trying to stop smoking.[18]

Special beds. The *oscillating bed* (Sanders) may be used to improve circulation to the lower extremities. The electrically operated bed seesaws in a cycle that usually takes one to two and one-half minutes but can be regulated according to need or preference. The foot of the bed rises six inches above the horizontal and descends twelve to fifteen inches with a smooth transition from one motion to another. (See Fig. 77.) The patient should be given adequate explanation of why the bed is recommended and may need time to become adjusted to the motion. Dizziness, nausea, and headache are probably of psychic origin, but the patient is encouraged to stop the bed for a few minutes should these symptoms occur. He is given the control switch and is shown how to use it. The bed is usually stopped for meals and other necessary care, but otherwise the patient is encouraged to keep it operating both day and night. Since some patients tend to slide downward as the foot of the bed lowers, and pressure of the feet against the footboard causes pain, a padded footboard should be placed on the bed. The bed should be checked frequently by an electrician. It should work smoothly without disturbing sounds or vibration.

The *CircOlectric bed* may be used to change the patient's position at intervals and thus improve his circulation. This bed allows for more extreme changes in position than does the oscillating bed. For example, the

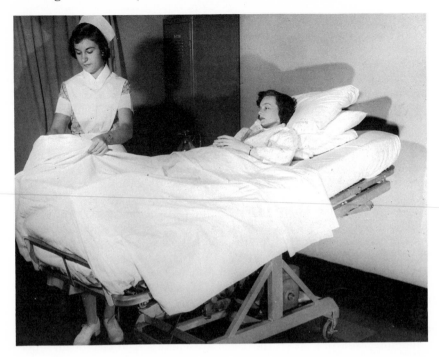

Fig. 77

The oscillating bed is used to improve
circulation. Here the student nurse
checks the temperature and color of the
affected limb. Note that a cradle is being used
to protect the feet from weight of the covers.

patient confined to bed can be placed in an
erect position if desired. The bed does not
move constantly but is changed from position to position by turning on an electric
motor. Some patients are taught to change
the tilt of the bed themselves. At first the
patient may feel quite insecure when the
bed is placed in tilted positions, and the
nurse should stay with him until he becomes
used to the position. She should also be sure
that he is secured so that he is in no danger
of falling.

Care of ulcers. Ulcers occurring in any
patient with vascular disease require meticulous care to prevent infection or to prevent further infection with new organisms.
Since local tissue resistance to infection is
lessened and the rate of healing is slowed
because of impaired circulation to the area,
a long period of healing must be antici-

pated. Wet dressings are seldom used because they cool quickly, and this cooling
may cause arteriospasm, which is harmful.
If they are ordered, they are usually used
only for short periods of time, and the nurse
must change them frequently. They may be
used to loosen crusts and facilitate drainage. Foot soaks may be used, although this
procedure cannot be sterile because it is
impossible to cleanse the entire foot sufficiently.

The patient with an ulcer on his foot usually is urged to keep off his feet, although
there is not complete agreement on the
value of this restriction. Some doctors feel
that, provided there is no direct weight-
bearing on the wound, the arterial circulation and healing are improved by a moderate
amount of moving about and by keeping
the limb in a dependent position for part
of the day at least.

Light cradles are seldom used, but occasionally the physician may feel that dry
warmth will improve healing of the ulcer.
Using extreme caution, the nurse then leaves
the wound exposed and places a cradle with
a light in it over the ulcerated part. The
bulb should never be larger than 25 watts,

374

and there should be a definite order from the doctor as to how long it should be left on and how far from the limb it should be placed. Too much heat will increase the arterial needs of the tissues and thus will be injurious.

A wide variety of drugs are used in the local treatment of ulcers in an effort to stimulate healing and prevent further infection. Castor oil and zinc oxide, nitrofurazone (Furacin), and scarlet red ointment, as well as a wide variety of bacteriostatic preparations, are often used. Streptokinase-streptodornase is applied locally. (Special treatment of ulcers occurring in conjunction with varicose veins will be described in the section in this chapter dealing specifically with that condition.)

Since many patients who have chronic ulcers of the legs and feet are not hospitalized, they must be taught how to bathe and otherwise care for themselves without contaminating the ulcer. Many elderly patients have lived with a chronic ulcer for so long that they become careless about their technique in changing soiled or loosened dressings. The patient will often benefit from a periodic visit from a public health nurse, who can reemphasize essentials of care both to the patient and to members of his family.

Tests and examinations

Several specific procedures help the physician to diagnose vascular disease and to determine the progress in treatment. Most tests are relatively simple and require no particular preparation. The patient, however, usually is in pain and fears any procedure that he believes may even temporarily increase his pain. Nervousness sometimes causes spasm of blood vessels and sensations of chilliness that may interfere with the accuracy of a test by diminishing pulsations and altering circulation. The patient should be told that the tests are painless, and the nurse should explain to him what is to be done if the doctor has not already done so. She also should see that the room is warm and, if he is going to a special room for a test, that he has sufficient clothing.

Test for intermittent claudication. Intermittent claudication is characterized by pain in the muscles caused by inadequate arterial circulation to the contracting muscles. Although this symptom usually occurs in the muscles of the lower extremities, it may occur also in the muscles of the forearm, wrists, or fingers. Except in rare instances, it is brought on only by continuous exercise and is relieved at once by resting. Knowing the amount of exercise that can be done before claudication occurs helps the doctor determine the severity of the condition and the improvement made. Unfortunately, the severity of the condition is not easy to measure. One method is to have an attendant walk with the patient to count the number of steps taken and record the time lapse before pain occurs. Sometimes mechanical devices are used. The patient stands with his foot on a pedal which he presses down, thereby lifting a weight of 6.3 kg. (13.6 pounds). This is done at the rate of 120 times per minute until the onset of pain. A normal person may continue for five to ten minutes before he has severe fatigue, whereas one with vascular disease may be able to continue only for a few seconds. While this method of testing is not entirely accurate, it is more reliable than the patient's statement of the number of city blocks he can walk before the onset of pain, since city blocks vary so much in length.

Oscillometric readings. Oscillometric readings help to determine the effectiveness of the larger arteries by measuring their pulsations. (Collateral vessels cannot be measured with an oscillometer.) An inflatable cuff is wrapped about the limb at the desired level and is connected to a delicate diaphragm that transmits arterial pressure to a needle moving across a dial that measures in units what is called the oscillometric index. The generally accepted normal oscillometric readings are given in Table 10.

Skin temperature studies. Attempts are made to record the skin temperature as a gauge to the effectiveness of the circulation to an extremity. These tests are not done too often since to be accurate they must be done in an environment with carefully controlled temperature and humidity. Normal skin temperature can be recorded by applying a thermocouple (a device for measuring skin temperature) to the skin. The temperature then is recorded on a potentiometer.

Table 10
Generally accepted normal oscillometric readings

Extremity	Oscillometric reading
Lower extremity	
Mid thigh	4 to 16
Upper third of leg	3 to 12
Above ankle	1 to 8
Foot	0.2 to 1
Upper extremity	
Upper arm	4 to 16
Elbow	3 to 12
Wrist	1 to 10
Hand	0.2 to 2

With a humidity of 40% the surface temperature of the skin usually varies from 24° to 35° C. (73° to 93° F.). Normal persons have a wider range of temperature difference in various parts of the body. For example, the forehead and the thorax are usually five to eight degrees warmer than the toes. People with arterial disease may have even greater temperature variations between the extremities and the rest of the body. The physician usually considers the skin temperature readings as only suggestive, because many factors (for example, a rise in metabolic rate) increase the temperature of the skin surface. The patient who is excited or upset by the anticipated test may have an increase in skin temperature. The test is usually done several hours after a meal since eating alters the skin temperature. Smoking also affects the accuracy of the readings.

A test for the efficiency of vasodilation in the extremities consists of immersing one of the limbs in water heated to 42° to 44° C. (107.6° to 112° F.) and then recording the skin temperature of the opposite limb. In the normal person with no vascular disease, temperature of the unimmersed limb will rise to a minimum of 34° C. (93° F.) within thirty-five minutes. A person with arterial disease may have little elevation in the skin temperature. The nurse may be asked to as-

sist with this test. An accurate bath thermometer is needed to measure the water temperature, and sufficient blankets should be used to protect the patient from chilling during and after the test.

A simpler way to test the efficiency of vasodilation in a limb is to place a hot-water bottle or heating pad on the abdomen and then manually test both extremities for elevation of skin temperature. Many doctors rely on this test since it is simple, and the hands of the experienced person are quite skillful at judging skin temperature of each limb.

Angiography. Angiography is an x-ray procedure that permits visualization of the internal anatomy of the heart and blood vessels through the intravascular injection of radiopaque contrast material. By this method, calcification and other anomalies of the arteries may be demonstrated. Calcified atherosclerotic plaques at the site of an occlusion may be visualized, and calcification can sometimes be traced throughout the entire length of an artery and can even be seen as far distally as the great toe. The information revealed by such an examination is not, of itself, evidence of arterial insufficiency, for some patients who have extensive calcification of the small arteries evidently have sufficient collateral circulation to permit good blood supply and have no symptoms of arterial insufficiency.

Radiopaque substances such as Hypaque or Renografin are injected into an artery, and serial roentgenograms are taken during the last few seconds of the injection and immediately thereafter. Usually this test is done in the x-ray department where occasionally a cutdown must be done on the vessel in order to inject the dye. When the doctor wishes to visualize the arteries of a lower extremity, the dye usually is injected into the femoral artery.

The substances used contain iodide, and the patient may have a severe reaction to the dye, with dyspnea, nausea, vomiting, numbness of the extremities, diaphoresis, and tachycardia. Any signs of a reaction should be reported at once. Occasionally a delayed reaction occurs after the patient returns to his room. Antihistaminic drugs, epinephrine (Adrenalin), and oxygen are used to combat reaction to the dye. The site of injection of the dye must be observed for signs of irritation or local thrombosis, which may occur if any of the irritating dye gets into the surrounding tissue. The area may have to be treated with massive warm packs.

The procedure is uncomfortable for the patient because, even without a reaction to the dye, he feels a flushing and burning sensation. One or more injections into deep arteries are made, and he must remain on the x-ray table for an hour or more. Afterward, he needs to be given water in generous amounts to hasten the excretion of the dye through the kidneys. He usually needs a back rub to relieve pressure areas resulting from lying on the hard table.

Capillary fragility test. A test for capillary fragility is sometimes ordered for patients with peripheral vascular disease. Since it is more often ordered for patients with suspected disease of the blood or blood-forming organs, it is described on p. 402.

Lumbar sympathetic block. Paravertebral injection of the sympathetic rami of sympathetic ganglia may be used to diagnose peripheral vascular disease. Evidence of vasodilation following the block indicates that the circulation to the limbs may be improved by subsequent injections of procaine or by sympathectomy.

With the patient in a prone or semiprone position, the doctor inserts a needle at the level of the second or third lumbar vertebra into the sympathetic tract within the spinal canal and injects 10 to 20 ml. of a 1% solution of procaine hydrochloride. If the procedure is successful, the sympathetic tracts will be blocked, causing a definite warming and drying of the skin surface of the limb on the same side as the injection. This response may be roughly measured by touch, or skin temperature studies may be done.

The patient should be told that there will be little pain associated with the test beyond the first needle prick and that there may be a sensation of tingling and warmth in the legs for several hours following the test. He should be observed carefully during and immediately following the procedure for signs of shock, which may result from the sudden shifting of so much blood into the peripheral circulation that the blood volume in the heart and vital vessels is depleted.

Arterial disease

Some arterial changes occur in almost all persons over 50 years of age, and some venous changes usually occur concurrently. For example, the elderly person suffering from arterial insufficiency often has varicosities of the veins as well. Persons who have diabetes mellitus usually develop vascular impairment more rapidly than others.

Changes in the arteries include arteriosclerosis and atherosclerosis. *Arteriosclerosis* is a hardening primarily of the middle layer of the vessel with the deposition of calcium, causing an inflexibility of the vessel and permanent narrowing of its lumen. The amount of narrowing does not always determine whether or not symptoms will occur. The occurrence of symptoms depends upon blood pressure within the vessel and the effectiveness of the collateral circulation. Arteriosclerosis affects the peripheral arteries more than the large vessels of the trunk. In *atherosclerosis,* plaques containing cholesterol, fatty acids, and other substances form in the intima, or inner wall, of the artery. Occasionally, calcium is deposited. These plaques cause distortion of the vessel and sometimes project far enough into the lumen to cause the formation of a thrombus that

377

cuts off the blood flow. Atherosclerosis affects the large vessels of the trunk more often than it does the peripheral arteries. Atheromatous changes in the arteries of the thighs and legs do occur, however, and predispose to thrombus and obstruction of the vessel lumen.

Race is not thought to affect the incidence of arteriosclerosis and atherosclerosis, although it has been reported that some Oriental groups have a lower incidence of the disease than some Occidental peoples. Nutrition, however, is thought to influence the development of arteriosclerosis and atherosclerosis, and this subject is undergoing close scientific study (p. 341). The patient should be advised to consult his physician concerning the restriction of fat in his diet, although a diet fairly high in protein and high in vitamins, with only a moderate amount of fat, is probably best for everyone.

Arteriosclerosis obliterans

Arteriosclerosis obliterans of the lower limb is an occlusive arterial disease that affects men more often than women. The media, or middle layer, of the arterial wall loses its elasticity. Atheromatous plaques form on the inner layer, or intima. As a result, the artery gradually becomes unable to transport the required amount of blood to the affected part. Symptoms appear when the blood vessels can no longer provide enough blood to supply oxygen and nutrients to the limbs and to remove the waste products of their metabolism.

Signs and symptoms. Early signs and symptoms of arteriosclerosis obliterans may include skin temperature changes, differences in color and in size of the lower limbs, and intermittent claudication. Later the patient may complain of pain in the affected part even at rest. Ulcers and gangrene may develop. Pain at rest often occurs at night, and the patient may report that it subsides with movement and particularly with walking. Very elderly patients may be awakened by excruciating cramplike pains in the muscles of the calf and the thighs that are believed to be due to lack of oxygen to the tissue (ischemia). Tingling and numbness of the toes may be mentioned by the patient, and a very common complaint is difficulty in keeping the feet and hands warm enough for comfort. Occasionally the first sign of limited circulation is necrosis following mild trauma, such as cutting the skin when trimming the nails. The disease is usually present to some extent in both limbs, although symptoms may be grossly apparent in only one. They may follow an occlusion of a fairly large artery by a thrombus. This occlusion will cause numbness, marked coldness, and a chalky-white appearance to the part of the limb supplied by the obstructed vessel.

Medical treatment and nursing care. Treatment for arteriosclerosis obliterans includes provision for general warmth, use of drugs to produce vasodilation, specific exercises to stimulate collateral circulation, carefully prescribed general exercise to maintain circulation yet not tax the arterial system, encouragement, and instruction in avoiding injury, preventing infection, and maintaining nutrition. Pain at rest may be treated by having the patient sleep with the head of the bed elevated on blocks six to ten inches in height to aid gravity in carrying arterial blood to the legs and feet. He should be advised not to walk about during the night unless he is warmly clothed and to avoid sitting with his legs over the side of the bed since he may become chilled and since right-angle knee flexion further hampers circulation. He should not rub the extremity because of the danger of trauma and of releasing an embolus into the circulation. Vigorous massage is always contraindicated in any patient with vascular disease, although gentle stroking may be permitted.

Arteriosclerosis obliterans is a chronic progressive disease for which there is no cure. Nursing care must be directed toward helping the patient to live within his limitations and encouraging him and his family to carry out medical instructions so that the disease may be held in check for an indefinite time. All nursing measures discussed earlier in this chapter under general nursing care may be necessary in caring for the patient. If the condition cannot be checked, gangrene of the extremity eventually may occur, making amputation necessary.

Thromboangiitis obliterans

Thromboangiitis obliterans (*Buerger's disease*) causes inflammation of the walls of the blood vessels, thrombus formation, and subsequent destruction of both arteries and veins. It affects men more often than women and is largely a disease of younger people, patients often being between 20 and 35 years of age when symptoms appear. Although the feet usually are first affected, vascular changes may occur in the hands and eventually throughout the entire body. The cause of inflammation is not known, but smoking definitely aggravates the condition and may even be the only cause in patients who are sensitive to inhaled smoke. As the inflammation subsides, there is partial or complete replacement of the affected blood vessels with scar tissue. The outcome of acute exacerbations, therefore, depends upon the size of the area deprived of normal blood supply and the amount of collateral circulation that can be established. Collateral vessels attempt to keep pace with the destruction, but over a period of years they usually cannot do so without treatment, and gangrene develops.

Signs and symptoms. The disease causes symptoms of inadequate oxygenation of tissues. Numbness, tingling, and vague abnormal sensations appear in the involved extremities. General chilling and exposure of the hands and feet to cold aggravate the symptoms. There may be hardened, red, and painful areas along the affected vessels, and the patient often reports that there is a burning or boring pain that is aggravated by chilling, smoking, and nervous tension. There is often edema about the areas of inflammation, and the entire limb, except where there is acute inflammation, may be cooler to the touch and whiter than normal. Cyanosis may occur when the feet are lowered.

Medical treatment and nursing care. It is often possible to arrest thromboangiitis obliterans completely and indefinitely by merely having the patient stop smoking. This restriction is considered the most important aspect of treatment. Smoking must be given up immediately, completely, and forever. Other measures are prescribed to foster circulation and to help make use of limited resources. They may include warmth, use of vasodilating drugs such as alcohol and tolazoline (Priscoline), moderate exercise, use of an oscillating bed, and instruction to prevent infection and to avoid trauma and exposure to cold. Some doctors believe that

a lumbar sympathectomy is helpful when the lower extremities are involved because it produces permanent vasodilation of the blood vessels (p. 389). In some instances the administration of typhoid vaccine to produce hyperpyrexia seems to have a beneficial effect in causing relaxation of blood vessels and improvement of circulation.

Severe pain may require narcotics, but effort is made to limit their use since there is real danger of drug addiction in young patients with a chronic disease such as thromboangiitis obliterans. The nurse can often help by emphasizing to the patient the precautions he should take to prevent the onset of acute symptoms, including pain. He should be urged not to smoke, and he should be advised to wear warm clothing, including warm gloves and footwear, in cold weather. Both of these measures prevent extensive vasoconstriction. He should be taught to avoid any injury to his feet, especially when cutting toenails. Wounds heal slowly, and gangrene may develop.

Raynaud's disease

Raynaud's disease affects young women who are usually of fairly high-strung temperament. Its cause is unknown. There is spasm of the arteries in the extremities, which lessens the blood supply. Often the hands and arms are affected before the feet. The condition may lead to coldness, numbness, cyanosis, pain, dryness and atrophy of the nails, and eventually gangrene of the ends of the fingers. The symptoms are intensified by exposure to cold and by emotional excitement. Patients often respond well to a sympathectomy in which the nerve control of blood vessels to the hands is removed, leaving the blood vessels permanently dilated. Patients in whom the condition is mild may be treated with drugs that inhibit sympathetic nervous system activity, such as Dibenamine hydrochloride. The patient is advised to avoid smoking and to keep the hands and the rest of the body warm.

Raynaud's disease is sometimes associated with scleroderma, a condition in which there is disturbance in the collagen content of the body and in which the skin becomes tightly stretched, firm, partially atrophied, and fibrosed (p. 933).

Aneurysm

An aneurysm is an abnormal enlargement of an artery at some point in its course. It may be caused by a congenital anomaly or weakness in the vessel wall, it may follow trauma, or it may be caused by a disease such as syphilis, which often attacks the aorta, or by a degenerative disease such as arteriosclerosis. By means of angiography (arteriography) and other diagnostic procedures, aneurysms in such locations as the aorta can now be clearly identified. The treatment for aneurysms usually is surgical. Treatment and care differ somewhat, depending upon the location of the aneurysm.

Aneurysm within the abdominal cavity. Aneurysms may occur anywhere in the ascending or the descending aorta or in the upper iliac arteries, which lie within the abdominal cavity. The portion of the aorta containing the aneurysm usually is resected surgically and replaced with a knitted or woven Teflon or Dacron prosthesis, carefully selected to match the vessel in size. The aorta must be clamped during the resection and insertion of the prosthesis. If the aneurysm is above the renal arteries, hypothermia and/or the heart-lung machine (pump oxygenator) may be used during the operation to provide for adequate oxygenation of vital tissues and for adequate clearance of body wastes. Hypothermia decreases the need of the tissues for oxygen and thus decreases metabolic waste products. If metabolic needs are decreased and the clamp must be in place for a short time only, the lack of circulation may be tolerated. However, if circulation must be impeded for any length of time, the blood must be shunted from the heart, through the extracorporeal circuit (heart-lung machine), to the lower aorta or the femoral artery. In other instances, before the aneurysm is resected, a temporary Teflon or Dacron prosthesis is sutured into place to shunt the blood directly from the heart or one of its main branches above the involved area to the lower aorta or femoral artery (Fig. 78). If this procedure is used, the pump-oxygenator is not necessary. Preoperative and postoperative care of the patient with an aneurysm above the renal arteries is the same as that described for the patient having heart surgery (p. 353).

If the aneurysm is below the renal ar-

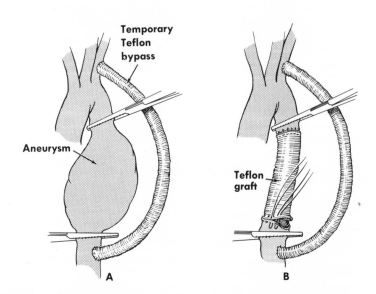

Aneurysm of the descending thoracic aorta. **A,** Temporary Teflon prosthesis has been sutured into the subclavian artery to shunt the blood around the aneurysm.
B, Aneurysm has been resected, and a permanent Teflon graft is in place.

teries, hypothermia and the heart-lung machine are not necessary because arterial flow to the lower extremities can be interrupted safely for the time needed to complete the operation. Postoperative nursing care for patients who have had this operation includes constant nursing observation for several hours and recording of blood pressure, apical-radical, posterior tibial, and dorsalis pedis pulses, and respirations every fifteen minutes until they are stabilized and then every hour for at least twenty-four hours. Skin over the dorsalis pedis pulse may be marked with ink before the operation so that its location can be easily determined postoperatively. Initial spasm may cause this pulse to be absent upon the patient's return from the operating room, but if absence of pulse continues for more than a few hours or occurs later, it may indicate a thrombosis beyond the graft and loss of arterial blood to the limb.

The patient who has had surgery for an abdominal aneurysm usually is placed flat in bed, and sharp flexion of the hip is avoided because it causes pressure on the femoral artery. Flexion of the knee is also avoided because it causes pressure on the popliteal artery. The patient can be moved gently from side to side and should dorsiflex and extend his feet at regular intervals to prevent congestion of venous blood in the lower legs. Because the incision is a long one and pain may be pronounced, the patient is able to breathe more deeply, cough productively, and move more easily if a firm abdominal binder is used and if he is instructed to support his abdomen as he coughs or moves. Often the nurse must help him. Narcotics are given fairly liberally for pain during the first few days postoperatively. Since some handling of the viscera must occur during surgery, postoperative distention is sometimes a problem. Aspiration of flatus from the stomach with a nasogastric tube may be necessary. The patient who has had an aneurysm resected must be watched for low back pain, which may indicate hemorrhage or thrombosis at the site of the graft. Pain and cramping in the legs are significant since they may indicate that a clot has formed beyond the graft and floated on to occlude an artery in the extremity. Signs of peripheral arterial occlusion

(pain, coldness, whiteness, or numbness of all or part of an extremity) must be watched for. On about the fourth postoperative day, the patient usually is permitted out of bed for a short time, and he often leaves the hospital in about two weeks.

Embolus

Emboli are blood clots floating in the circulating blood. They usually lodge at the bifurcations, or divisions, of the arteries because of the diminishing caliber of the vessels beyond these points. An embolus lodging at the bifurcation of the iliac arteries is called a *saddle embolus*. As soon as an embolus lodges, thrombi (propagated emboli) form in the involved vessel.

The signs of sudden lodging or formation of a large thrombus in an artery are dramatic. There is severe pain at the site of the thrombus formation. Fainting, nausea, vomiting, and signs of pronounced shock may appear. Almost immediately, areas supplied by the vessel may become white, cold, and blotched, and they may tingle and feel numb. Cyanosis, followed by even greater darkening and gangrene, occurs if the blood supply is completely obstructed and collateral circulation is inadequate. Vasodilating drugs are given to improve the collateral circulation, warmth is applied to the body, and a sympathetic block of the lumbar ganglia may be done in an attempt to produce vasodilation of other vessels. Heparin and Dicumarol may be given to help prevent further thrombus formation. The patient who has an acute embolic obstruction of a large artery needs constants nursing supervision. Pain is severe, and fear is pronounced.

If the patient does not respond to the medical treatment within a few hours, surgery may be performed. Surgical procedures that may be done include opening the vessel and removing the clot (*embolectomy*), removing the clot and also removing adherent substances and part of the lining of the vessel (*endarterectomy* or "reaming"), arterial resection with removal of the clot and the adherent diseased artery surrounding it with subsequent grafting, and bypassing the diseased portion of the vessel with a graft, as is sometimes done for an aneurysm. Various means are used in an endarterectomy. Recently a long catheter with a balloon has been used. It can be passed distally from a larger vessel, and the balloon can be inflated and withdrawn, bringing with it long thrombi that are filling the vessel.[10]

Embolectomy is usually the treatment of choice for aortic embolus and for an embolus of the common iliac artery. Nursing care following embolectomy is similar to that needed by the patient who has had surgery for an aneurysm. Blood pressure must be carefully recorded preoperatively so that suitable comparisons can be made postoperatively. It is important that the blood pressure not vary too much from what it was preoperatively since variation would predispose to thrombus formation. A complication that must be carefully watched for postoperatively is hemorrhage. Small arteries that may have been useless while the embolus was in the artery may not bleed freely at operation and may therefore be missed in tying bleeding vessels. They may resume normal function after the operation and cause hemorrhage.

Aneurysm of the extremity and arteriovenous fistula

Aneurysms of the arteries of the lower extremities, particularly in the popliteal area, are quite common in persons over 60 years of age who have pronounced arteriosclerosis (Fig. 79). These aneurysms often are easily palpable. Thrombi form at the site of an aneurysm, and emboli may travel to obstruct more distal portions of the artery. This type of aneurysm is sometimes confused with an *arteriovenous fistula*, which is a communication between an artery and a vein caused either by a congenital anomaly or by trauma. Both lesions produce a characteristic sound called a *bruit*. If the cause is an aneurysm, the bruit may be interspersed with the arterial pulsations, whereas the bruit caused by a fistula is often a constant soft, purring sound. Both conditions impair the supply of blood to the portion of the limb supplied by the vessel, and various signs of poor blood supply, such as atrophy, cyanosis, trophic changes, or even gangrene, may occur.

Closure of the fistula or removal of a portion of the aneurysm is the preferred treatment. If one of these measures is not possible, the vessel may be ligated unless

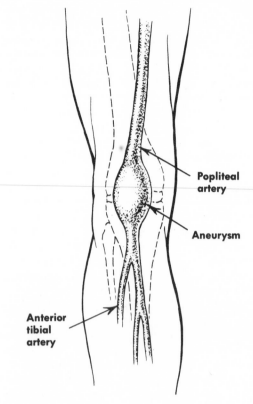

Fig. 79

Posterior view of the knee, with aneurysm of the popliteal artery. (From Newton, Kathleen, and Anderson, Helen C.: Geriatric nursing, ed. 4, St. Louis, 1966, The C. V. Mosby Co.)

ligation is incompatible with the life of tissues distal to the lesion. Arterial and plastic grafts can be used in larger blood vessels of the extremities either to replace portions of the artery that contain the aneurysm or to bypass the abnormality (Fig. 80). In addition to general postoperative care, the patient who has had this surgical procedure may be treated with any or all of the medications and other means described in this chapter to augment circulation when arterial supply is limited or when thrombosis threatens.

Venous disease

Thrombophlebitis

Thrombophlebitis is inflammation of a vein associated with clot formation. Many

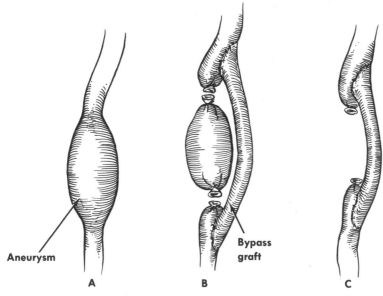

Fig. 80

Aneurysm of peripheral artery showing, **A**, aneurysm; **B**, bypass graft in place; and **C**, permanent replacement graft after resection of aneurysm.

relatively simple circumstances contribute to the development of thrombophlebitis in persons who are perhaps particularly susceptible to congestion in the venous system. For example, thrombophlebitis of superficial leg veins may follow a trip during which long hours were spent sitting in a plane or car with the knees bent sharply. Flying at high altitudes in nonpressurized cabins seems to predispose to recurrence of thrombophlebitis in persons who have a tendency toward this condition. Pregnancy is often complicated by thrombophlebitis due to interference with venous return in the lower abdomen. Thrombophlebitis may occur from inactivity following surgery, and before the days of early ambulation and emphasis on bed exercises it was a dreaded complication of surgery. Despite early ambulation, patients still develop thrombophlebitis postoperatively, and occasional deaths from subsequent emboli are reported. (For prevention of postoperative thrombophlebitis, see p. 196.) Thrombophlebitis is also caused by trauma to venous walls, with subsequent inflammation and congestion, and the irritating effects of certain drugs. Changes in blood

pressure, blood volume, and abnormal substances in the blood, such as bacteria, may also contribute to development of the condition.

Signs and symptoms. Thrombophlebitis of superficial veins is easily apparent. Upon palpation, the veins appear hard and thready and are sensitive to pressure. The entire limb may be swollen, pale, and cold, and the area along the vein may be reddened and feel warm to the touch. Deep veins in the legs may be affected, and the pain they cause when the patient dorsiflexes his foot in bed or walks is known as *Homans' sign*. Thrombophlebitis may be accompanied by reflected pain in the entire limb. Systemic reaction to the infection, which sets in rapidly in any blood vessel when free flow of blood is interrupted, may cause symptoms such as headache, malaise, and elevation of temperature. Sometimes a thrombosis in a vessel may be "silent," giving no signs or symptoms until an *embolus* is released, floats in the bloodstream, and lodges in a vital structure such as the lungs, the heart, or the brain. An embolus lodged in a vital structure may cause death within a few seconds or an overwhelming shock reaction that is followed by death or by slow recovery.

Medical treatment and nursing care. Superficial thrombophlebitis is usually treated by rest. However, physicians differ in regard to the amount of activity the patient can be allowed. Some believe that the clot is sufficiently adherent to the vein wall to make its release unlikely and that moving about helps to improve general circulation and to prevent further congestion of blood in the veins. Others believe that complete immobilization is necessary to prevent a part of the thrombus from breaking away and becoming an embolus. The patient who has thrombophlebitis of large and deep vessels, however, usually is kept quiet. He should not cough vigorously, strain at defecation, or take deep breaths, since all these activities cause a temporary rise in the blood pressure and may cause a surge of blood through the affected vessel that may dislodge a piece of the clot. Care must be taken that the patient is not frightened by these restraints, and the nurse should not hesitate to seek the doctor's help in explaining to the patient why precautions are necessary. Occasionally the doctor does a ligation of the vein above the involvement (usually at the femoral juncture) to decrease the danger of embolism, but this procedure is not possible unless there is an adequate collateral circulation. The period of immobilization depends entirely upon the response of the patient to treatment.

Continuous application of warm, moist heat may be used for both deep and superficial thrombophlebitis. Warm packs are usually ordered to cover the entire extremity and seem to have a beneficial effect, although their exact therapeutic action is not fully understood. Heating pads permanently set on "low" are best for keeping the packs at a consistently safe temperature. Many doctors prefer that the packs be applied at body temperature and that no external heat be used. They feel that packs kept at body temperature are equally beneficial and avoid the danger of releasing emboli as the caliber of the vessels changes (dilation when it is applied and constriction as it cools).

There is no medical agreement as to whether or not the limb should be elevated. Therefore, the nurse should be certain that she understands the doctor's wishes. Some physicians believe that the danger of an embolus being released is greater if the limb is elevated, whereas others believe that elevation is essential for clearing the vascular congestion and preventing further edema.

Heparin and Dicumarol are used for patients who have thrombophlebitis, and sometimes patients must remain on prophylactic doses of Dicumarol for an indefinite period to prevent recurrences of the disease. Vasodilating drugs are given to combat the arterial vessel spasm that occurs at the site of a venous thrombosis and to improve general circulation, thus increasing the rate of absorption of the thrombus.

All patients with thrombophlebitis should be observed closely for any signs of embolism, which must be reported at once. Pulmonary embolism (p. 573) is the most common type, but emboli may also lodge in the coronary vessels (p. 344) or elsewhere.

Following thrombophlebitis in a lower limb severe enough to require hospitalization or bed rest, the patient usually needs to wear an elastic stocking or elastic bandage when walking. The stocking or bandage is also often ordered for patients who have superficial thrombophlebitis, which tends to recur. After a month to six weeks, if the patient is progressing favorably, the stocking or bandage may be removed for one-half to one hour and the results noted. If there is no evidence of edema or discomfort, it may be removed for longer and longer periods until its use may be discontinued completely. Many patients wear the stockings indefinitely if their work necessitates standing for long periods of time or sitting with the knees bent. Two stockings or bandages are necessary for each affected limb so that they can be laundered as necessary.

The *elastic stocking,* preferably accurately fitted to the patient's measurements, must be obtained before the patient gets out of bed for the first time. Stockings of various lengths and sizes are stocked by many large department stores, and the measurements that must be taken can be obtained by calling the store. The most satisfactory length is one inch below the bend of the knee joint. The patient must be taught how to put on the stocking. It should be rolled on evenly before he gets out of bed in the morning. Once during the day it should be removed for a few moments and the skin very gently stroked and powdered as necessary. The stocking need not be worn during sleeping hours.

Elastic bandages may be used instead of an elastic stocking, but they are more conspicuous and are difficult to apply evenly. They may be used for short periods following surgery and are sometimes ordered for use on those occasions when the patient will be lifting heavy objects or standing still. If a bandage has been ordered for continuous use, it should be applied before the patient gets out of bed in the morning. The bandage is applied to the entire foot, usually including the heel, and extends to just below the knee or up to the groin, depending on the doctor's orders. It should be smooth and snug but must not be so tight that it interferes with circulation.

Swimming and wading in water are among the best activities for prevention of recurrences of thrombophlebitis of the lower extremities and are highly recommended for patients with other venous diseases as well. Water, which is denser than air, exerts a smooth, even pressure on the skin, and wading is especially beneficial because the greater pressure (the deeper water) surrounds the distal portion of the extremity and helps in the return flow of venous blood.

Varicose veins

Varicose veins are abnormally dilated veins occurring most often in the lower extremities and the lower trunk. In the lower limbs, the great and small saphenous veins are most often involved. At least 10% of our total population is affected by varicose veins. The highest incidence is in the third, fourth, and fifth decades of life.[21] There are several definite factors that predispose to the development of varicosities. Among them are hereditary weakness of the vein walls and prolonged standing, which places strain on the valves because muscle action is not helping to return the blood. Man's upright position further aggravates the problem, and poor posture with sagging of abdominal organs causes additional pressure. Pregnancy and abdominal tumors that cause pressure on the large veins of the lower abdomen and interfere with good venous drainage predispose to the development of varicose veins. Chronic systemic disease, such as heart disease and cirrhosis of the liver, may interfere with adequate return of blood to the heart and contribute to varicosities. Infections and trauma to the veins with resultant thrombophlebitis may lead to varicose veins, since the valves are destroyed as the acute inflammation subsides.

Signs and symptoms. Varicosities of superficial veins are often quite apparent through the skin even before they cause symptoms. They appear as darkened, tortuous, raised blood vessels that become more prominent when the patient stands and when he assumes positions that cause congestion, such as sitting with the knees crossed. Sometimes the sclerosed valves can be seen as nodular protrusions. The varicosity is more pronounced just above the valve, which has become ineffective. The patient may have pain, fatigue, feeling of heaviness in the legs, muscular cramps, and emotional reactions of discouragement and depression. Discomfort is worse during hot weather and when the patient goes to higher altitudes. It it greatly increased by prolonged standing.

The simplest test for varicose veins is known as the *Trendelenburg test.* The patient lies down with the leg raised until the vein empties completely. He then stands, and the vein is observed as it fills. A normal vein fills from below; a varicose vein fills from above, because the valve fails to retain the blood that has drained into the portion of the vessel above it.

Conservative treatment. Mild discomfort from varicose veins may be treated conservatively by advising the patient to elevate his feet for a few minutes at regular two- to three-hour intervals throughout the day, to avoid constrictions about the legs, to avoid standing for long periods of time, and to wear an elastic stocking or elastic bandage. Improvement in posture sometimes helps to prevent further development of the varicosities, and the patient may be advised by his physician to lose weight.

Ligation and stripping of veins. Surgical treatment for varicosities consists of ligation of the vein above the varicosity and removal of the varicosed vein distal to the ligation, provided, of course, that the

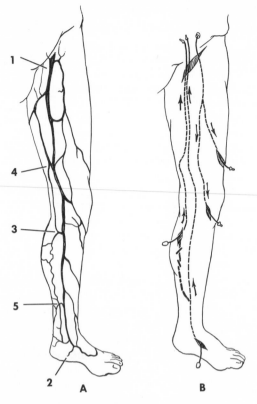

Fig. 81

A, Outline of incompetent great saphenous system, with numerals indicating main tributaries. **B,** Passing of strippers in preparation for removal of incompetent veins. (Redrawn from Allen, Edgar V., Barker, Nelson W., and Hines, Edgar A.: Peripheral vascular disease, Philadelphia, 1962, W. B. Saunders Co.)

deep veins are able to return the venous blood satisfactorily (Fig. 81). The great saphenous vein is ligated close to the femoral junction if possible, and the great and small saphenous veins are then stripped out through small incisions at the groin, above and below the knee, and at the ankle. Sterile dressings are used to cover the wounds, and an elastic bandage, extending from the foot to the groin, is applied firmly.

Ligation and stripping are usually done under general anesthesia since the procedure is very tiresome and painful. To prevent the development of thrombosis in other veins, the patient usually walks about on the day of the operation and at frequent intervals during his remaining two or three days in the hospital. Usually the foot of the bed is elevated on blocks for the first twenty-four hours to help in venous return of blood unless the patient is elderly and also has arterial insufficiency. Moving, walking, and bending are extremely difficult for the patient, and he may have more pain and discomfort following this surgical procedure than following much more serious surgery. When analgesic drugs have been ordered, they should be given for the first twenty-four to forty-eight hours.

Although the operation is considered a relatively minor one and the patient is out of bed almost at once, nursing care is important. The patient should be assisted when he walks on the first day and thereafter if he is receiving analgesic drugs. Throughout his hospitalization he should be encouraged and assisted as necessary. The elastic bandage and the dressings should be checked several times a day, since they may become loosened with walking and the wounds may be exposed. Hemorrhage from the wounds may occur and should be watched for, especially on the operative day. If bleeding does occur, the leg should be elevated, pressure should be applied over the wound, and the doctor should be notified. Since the patient has difficulty in handling himself because of the firm binding around his knees, he must be protected from accidents.

A patient who has had an operation for varicose veins should know that the condition may recur since large superficial collateral vessels may develop and in turn become varicosed. Therefore, he should take the general precautions of any patient with varicosities since the operation cures his acute symptoms but does not remove his tendency to have varicose veins. Weight reduction, posture improvement, avoidance of pressure on blood vessels, and elevation of the lower limbs should be practiced postoperatively exactly as is recommended for the patient with mild varicosities who is receiving conservative treatment only. The booklet *Varicose Veins* is useful in teaching patients who have this condition and can be obtained from the American Heart Association.

Treatment by sclerosis. Sclerosing solutions are sometimes used in the treatment of varicosities in small and early dilated tributaries of larger veins, and they may be used when for some reason varicose veins cannot be treated surgically. The solutions cause an irritation within the vein and cause a thrombus to form. As the inflammation subsides, the lumen of the vein is usually obliterated. Sodium tetradecyl sulfate (Sotradecol sodium) in a 1 to 3% solution, and sodium psylliate (Sylnasol) may be used. Both can cause allergic reactions, and an antihistaminic preparation such as dyphenhydramine hydrochloride (Benadryl) may be needed and should be readily available when this treatment is being given. If severe reaction occurs, cardiac stimulants such as caffeine sodium benzoate and oxygen may be needed.

The injection of sclerosing solutions is usually done in the clinic or in the doctor's office. The nurse must take the responsibility for seeing that emergency equipment for treating reactions is on hand and for preventing accidents to patients. Many patients are elderly, and some tend to become faint when standing for the treatment. Footstools can be equipped with side attachments and handlebars on which the patient may lean for comfort and security. The site of injection is covered with a small dressing. The patient is urged not to scratch the skin over the site of injection since scratching may lead to an infected excoriation and eventual ulceration. He also should be cautioned about bruising or otherwise traumatizing the veins, which also may lead to ulceration.

Treatment of varicose ulcers. Stasis of blood in tissues around marked varicosities, particularly when deep veins are also involved, leads to replacement of normal tissue with fibrous tissue that is firm to the touch and colored with pigment from extravasated blood cells. This condition often causes severe pruritus and general discomfort in the limb. It is called *stasis dermatitis*. Ulcers occur easily when stasis dermatitis has developed, and they are difficult to control. Ligation of varicose veins is usually necessary, since the ulcer will not heal while marked varicosities persist in the vessels above it. Besides the general measures already mentioned for any ulcers of vascular origin, treatment of *varicose ulcers* include

grafting of skin to cover the wound and the use of pressure bandages. Grafting may not be successful if the arterial supply is also affected, since poor circulation to the fibrotic tissue surrounding the ulcer causes healing to be slow. (See p. 218 for care of a graft.)

Gelatin paste bandages applied to the entire lower limb, and known as "boots," are widely used in the treatment of varicose ulcers. This dressing, or boot, provides constant even pressure that supports the superficial veins, protects the ulcer from injury and infection, and fosters healing. *Unna's paste boot* is the best known. It contains zinc oxide, glycerin, gelatin, and water, and must be melted before it is ready for application. It is applied with a brush, usually four layers of 3- or 4-inch band-

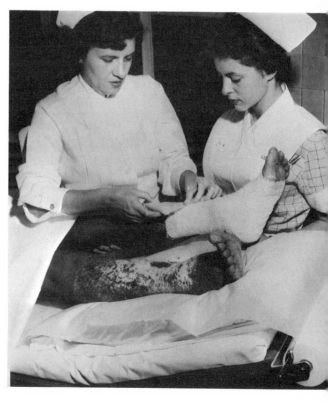

Fig. 82

The zinc oxide bandage can be applied easily to the ambulatory patient in the clinic. Note the skin discoloration around the leg ulcer.

age being alternated with layers of the paste. Many variations of this boot are now available in which the bandage comes already impregnated with the paste, sealed in a special airtight wrapping and ready for immediate use. They save time and obviate the danger of burning the patient when melted paste is used.

Before a paste bandage is applied, the patient should rest for one-half hour with the feet elevated. Hair on the legs should be shaved, and a small, dry sterile dressing should be placed over the ulcer. Adhesive tape should not be used to hold the dressing in place since it is irritating to the skin. The boot is evenly applied beginning with the instep and ending two inches below the knee (Fig. 82). It takes fifteen to twenty minutes for the paste to set. The boot is then dusted with talcum powder and may be covered with a Surgitube dressing, although a stocking or a sock may be worn directly over the boot. Boots are usually changed approximately every ten days to two weeks, depending upon the condition of the patient and the amount of drainage from the ulcer.

While caring for the patient, the nurse should learn whether or not he has been able to follow the doctor's instructions in regard to diet, rest, and exercise. She may need to refer some problems to the social worker or the doctor.

Lymphedema

Lymphedema is a swelling of soft tissue and is a result of an increase in the quantity of lymph. It occurs most often in the lower extremities, but it can occur in the arms. Lymphedema is a relatively rare condition and is seen most often in young women. It may be of unknown cause (primary), or it may be due to infection or other disease of small veins and lymph vessels. Lymphedema of the arm may be a complication of mastectomy. (It is discussed on p. 812.) Congenital underdevelopment of the lymph vessels is believed to be the cause of primary lymphedema. Symptoms often appear at the time of puberty. Lymphedema of the lower extremities begins with mild swelling on the dorsum of the foot, usually at the end of the day, which gradually extends to involve the entire limb. It is aggravated by prolonged standing, pregnancy, obesity, warm weather, and the menstrual period. Exaggerated forms of this disease are known as *elephantiasis*.

One of the greatest problems in lymphedema is the emotional reaction of patients to disfigurement. The patient often attributes difficulties encountered in working in her chosen field or social rebuffs to her disfigurement and tends to become withdrawn and depressed. The emphasis upon women's legs in our culture adds to her difficulties. One leg only may be involved, accentuating the abnormality even in fairly mild cases.

There is no cure for lymphedema, and the treatment is not too satisfactory. Therefore, the patient needs help and encouragement in learning to live with an exasperating chronic condition. Treatment is conservative, making use of basic physiologic principles to improve the lymph drainage. Since gravity helps to drain lymph from the extremities, the patient may be advised to sleep with the foot of the bed elevated four to eight inches. Very light massage in the direction of the lymph flow is recommended,[16] and the patient is advised to wear elastic stockings and to take moderate exercise regularly. Constricting clothing must not be worn, and avoiding salty or spicy foods that increase thirst and predispose to edema may be helpful. The thiazide diuretics relieve the edema in some patients.[2] Pneumatic cuffs or sleeves that help to exert a steady, gentle massage are being tried and appear to be helpful, although no spectacular results have been reported. Surgical removal of lymph nodes and vessels has been found beneficial for some patients with lymphedema due to filariasis (infection with tropical organisms that block the lymph channels). Operations also are sometimes performed to improve lymph drainage or to reduce the size of the extremity.

Special surgical procedures

Sympathectomy

Vasospasm often accompanies arterial diseases, and a sympathectomy often is done in an attempt to relieve it, although there is not full agreement as to its value. Occasionally the operation, which helps dilate the blood vessels, is done as an emergency when there is severe vasospasm from poisons such as ergot, when a limb has been frozen, or when an arterial embolism has lodged in a major vessel supplying the limb. Usually, however, before a sympathectomy is performed, the ganglia are injected with procaine to determine whether or not the treatment will be of value for the particular patient (p. 377).

A *lumbar sympathectomy* is done to dilate vessels in the lower extremity. It is accomplished by making a small incision in the lower lateral aspect of the abdomen. The peritoneal cavity is not opened, but the sympathetic ganglia supplying the lumbar region are removed and their fibers are cut. This operation may be unilateral or bilateral, depending on whether dilation of vessels is needed in both legs.

After a lumbar sympathectomy the patient should be placed on his side. Blood pressure must be taken every fifteen minutes until it is stable. Pulse rate and respiratory rate are also checked, and the patient is watched closely for signs of shock, which may result from the sudden reallocation of the blood in the dilated vessels of the lower abdomen and legs. Distention may be troublesome after a lumbar sympathectomy, and a rectal tube or rectal irrigations may be used to expel the flatus. Hourly turning should be insisted upon, and deep breathing should be encouraged. Following a lumbar sympathectomy the patient may notice a new feeling of warmth in his feet and legs. Very occasionally this warmth causes a slight discomfort and a feeling of fullness, which is relieved by wearing an elastic stocking.

To relieve vasospasm in the arms and hands, the thoracic ganglia of the sympathetic chain may be resected (*thoracic sympathectomy*). Because the ribs must be resected in this operation, nursing care is similar to that for any patient having chest surgery (p. 577). The problem of postoperative shock, which is encountered in the patient with a lumbar sympathectomy, also is present. In addition, the patient may become quite dizzy on assuming an upright position. Dizziness gradually subsides as the circulation becomes readjusted, but meantime the patient must be assisted when he is up. Elastic bandages may be ordered to prevent pooling of blood in the legs and thus lessen the circulatory problem.

Amputations

Although partial or complete amputations of either the legs or the arms may be necessary as a result of sarcoma and infections such as gas bacillus infection, the majority are necessitated by arteriosclerosis and by trauma. It is believed that amputations will increase each year because of the longer life-span and the consequent increase in the number of elderly people in whom cardiovascular disease is likely to develop, and because of an increasing number of automobile accidents.

An amputation is a serious operation that is usually done as a lifesaving measure, and it may be necessary at any age. Occasionally a deformed leg or arm is amputated because it is believed that the patient can get along better with a prosthesis than with the deformed limb. Only simple amputations of the lower limb are considered here. Selected readings pertinent to amputations of the arms[19] and to disarticulation procedures[36] are given at the end of this chapter.

Emotional reaction to amputation. Because of the severe emotional reaction to the idea of an amputation, the news that amputation is necessary is usually withheld from the patient for as long as possible. Very occasionally a patient with severe pain such as occurs in thromboangiitis obliterans may welcome an amputation. However, to most patients the thought of losing a limb is almost intolerable.

Emotional reactions of distress are normal and to be expected. In ancient times the human body with perfect symmetry was glorified, as reflected in the remarkable sculpture that remains. In some ancient cultures only the physically perfect could perform certain religious rites since it was believed that only the physically perfect should appear before God. Even though one's personal faith may emphasize beauty of the spirit rather than of the body, some feeling of rejection at marring of the body is probably felt by each of us. This feeling must be faced by the patient who must have an amputation.

Loss of the power of locomotion means loss of the power of flight, which is one of the instinctive means of self-preservation. It may be for this reason that loss of a leg depresses the patient more than loss of an arm, even though the latter is a much greater handicap. Something about the loss of power to move about at will casts a shadow on the patient's spirit that can be relieved only by the most thoughful and sensitive care. Even the patient who has suffered for a long time with a chronic disease that has hampered his freedom of motion feels the anticipated loss very keenly. Perhaps this is because there is such finality in an amputation. As long as the limb is there—imperfect though it may be—the patient usually retains the hope that normal or near-normal function will be restored. If amputation is necessary because of an accident, the suddenness of the changes in the patient's picture of himself may produce real shock.

Other emotional reactions to amputation are more tangible and more easily understood. The handicap is obvious (or at least the patient believes that it is), and he fears that he will be pitied. Young children, although they adjust to the physical limitations readily, actually may be taunted by their playmates for being different. Older children and adolescents also are handicapped in their social life and may develop serious emotional problems. To the wage earner, father, and husband, an amputation may mean that he must learn a new occupation or that he may lose his place as head of his household. To the older person, it may mean dependence upon children or upon the community.

Emotional reactions to an amputation have an enormous effect on the patient's rehabilitation. The reactions depend on the patient's emotional makeup and his response to other life crises, as well as on circumstances leading to the amputation and on the care he receives. The most perfect surgical operation and the best-fitting prosthesis are useless if the patient remains a complete invalid and a burden to himself, his family, and the community. The nurse must think of the long-range plans for the patient from the time that she learns that an amputation is necessary. It is at this time, when emotional reactions to the amputation and the idea of using a prosthesis are forming, that she can make her greatest contribu-

tion to the patient's rehabilitation by helping him to realize that his problems are not insurmountable and by watching him carefully for responses that may indicate need for care by various members of the health team.

Members of the patient's family can often be called upon for help. They are usually told of the amputation before the patient, or at the same time, so that they can help him accept the news. When the patient does know that an amputation is necessary, he often benefits from a visit from someone who has undergone the same operation and has made a full recovery. With the right mental outlook, most patients can return as functioning and useful members of society. The percentage is, of course, lower among aged persons, many of whom have other disabilities, such as cardiac disease and osteoarthritis, that slow their progress in learning to manage themselves independently.

The amputation

In amputating a limb, the surgeon endeavors to remove all diseased tissue yet leave a stump that permits satisfactory use of a prosthesis. There is not full agreement among surgeons and limb makers as to the correct levels for amputations for best use of the stump. Most agree, however, that an amputation below the knee should be in the middle third of the leg, and that thigh amputations should be in the lower third of the thigh. Each inch of bone that must be removed from the femur above the lower third decreases the function of the limb. Two and one-half inches above the knee is often considered the optimum level from the standpoint of fitting the prosthesis.

Below-the-knee amputations are best for wearing a prosthesis and permit a more natural gait than thigh amputations because knee function remains. Unfortunately, many patients with arterial disease require amputations above the knee because the poor circulation extends far up the limb.

For the best function of the limb, the stump should be long enough to permit sufficient leverage to move the artificial limb but not long enough to interfere with the movement of the joint distal to the amputation. The end of the bone should be covered with skin and subcutaneous tissue, and with muscle that is not adherent to the bone end. The stump should be healthy and firm, without creases, folds, and flabby parts. It should be painless, with no nerve endings remaining in the scar, and the scar should not fall over the weight-bearing end of the bone. The stump should have a smooth, conical contour and should be freely movable by the patient in any normal range of motion.

There are two types of amputations. One, the guillotine or circular amputation, is done when there has been serious trauma, when gas bacilli are present in the wound, or when there is moist gangrene (gangrene with infection). The blood vessels and nerves are ligated, but the wound is left open. This operation is relatively simple and quick, and can be done on patients who are quite poor operative risks. The disadvantage of this amputation is that usually another operation is necessary. Healing may take weeks or months unless a secondary, closure operation is done. Since the wound is not sutured, there also may be muscle and skin retraction, which makes the fitting of a prosthesis difficult or impossible unless the stump is operated upon again.

The flap type of amputation is by far the more satisfactory if it can be done. In this operation, a long flap of full-thickness skin is loosened from the anterior of the portion of the limb about to be amputated. Following the amputation, the end of the flap is sutured to the skin edges of the stump so that the stump is covered and the suture line is along the back of the stump. This wound usually heals completely within two weeks.

In arterial disease it has been found that, if possible, surgery should be delayed until demarcation sets in, so that healthy tissue can be more accurately identified. Otherwise, the stump may not heal because of an inadequate blood supply, and reamputation at a higher level may be necessary.

Preoperative care. If the operation is not an emergency one, the patient is told what to expect before and following the operation. The doctor explains the operation to him and usually mentions phantom limb sensation. He is also told whether it is expected that traction will be used. The nurse tells the patient that he will be turned or asked to turn and move about almost immediately following the operation, and she explains why he must be asked to lie on his abdomen. If the condition of the diseased limb permits, she may teach him to do *push-up exercises* while lying on his abdomen. Simply by using his arms to raise his chest from the bed and repeating this exercise several times at regular intervals daily, the patient can substantially improve the muscle tone and muscle strength of his arms and shoulders. He will then be able to move more easily postoperatively.

The choice of anesthetic depends upon the surgeon and the condition of the patient. General anesthesia (intravenous and inhalation) is the most frequently used. However, an amputation can be done under spinal anesthesia or with only the leg being cooled (refrigeration anesthesia), but the procedure is then very distressing to the patient since the sawing of bone can be heard despite large doses of sedation. An intravenous infusion is usually started before the patient goes to the operating room, or it is started in the operating room before surgery begins so that fluid can be given immediately if shock or hemorrhage occur.

Postoperative care. When the patient returns from the operating room or the recovery room, vital signs should be checked and signs of hemorrhage from the stump should be watched for. If there is bright red drainage, an outline of the stain should be marked on the outside of the dressing with pencil so that the rate of bleeding can be determined easily. A heavy tourniquet is always kept fastened to the foot of the bed so that it may be applied immediately if sudden, severe hemorrhage should occur. If the patient is sent to the operating room in his bed, the tourniquet should be attached to it. The nurse must know how to apply the tourniquet, and if sudden hemorrhage occurs, she does not wait for a doctor's order to use it.

Usually the stump is elevated on a plastic-covered pillow when the patient returns from the operating room, and it is left in this position for twelve to twenty-four hours to lessen edema and bleeding or serous oozing from the wound. However, the pillow must be removed after twenty-four hours at the most to prevent hip and knee contractures.

When a guillotine operation has been done, the patient usually returns to his room with traction applied to the stump to prevent retraction of skin and muscle away from the line of operation. Wide bands of adhesive tape are placed on the skin above the wound, a spreader is used, and weights are attached to provide traction. (See skin traction, p. 944.) Traction pulleys at the foot of the bed should be placed toward the center so that the patient can turn onto his abdomen. A Thomas splint sometimes is used for traction so that the patient can be moved more easily and can be out of bed without the traction's being released. (See p. 947 for care of the patient in traction.)

If the amputation is below the knee, the stump may be firmly bandaged on a padded board to prevent contracture at the knee joint. The nurse must check the padding carefully, since muscle spasm that results in pulling of the limb against the board may be so great that a pressure sore develops. If spasm seems severe, a piece of sponge rubber can sometimes be slipped between the bandaged stump end and the padded board for additional protection. Sometimes the surgeon removes the limb from the board for part of the day.

Exercises. To prevent flexion contracture of the hip, unless there is a medical order to the contrary, the patient who has had a lower-limb amputation should turn on his abdomen for a short time the day following the operation. Thereafter, he should lie on the abdomen for some time at least twice each day. Even the patient who has a limb in traction can turn on his abdomen with assistance. If the leg has been amputated below the knee, the patient can begin at once to hyperextend his thigh and leg as he lies on his abdomen. This exercise strengthens muscles in preparation for walking. If the amputation is above the knee, a medical order should be obtained before the patient hyperextends the thigh, since this exercise may cause strain on the suture line. While on his abdomen, the patient can practice the push-up exercises he started before the operation, strengthening his arm and shoulder muscles in preparation for crutch-walking.

While on his back, the patient with a recent mid-thigh amputation should be kept flat or in a low Fowler's position except for short periods of time, such as for meals. A firm trochanter roll (a sheet or bath blanket firmly rolled) should be placed along the outer side of the affected limb to prevent its outward rotation. If permitted, the patient should lie on the side of the amputation part of the time.

The patient with a below-the-knee amputation can be in a mid or high Fowler's position if he wishes, but special care must be taken to prevent flexion contraction of the knee. Usually the doctor orders the stump removed from the padded arm board or splint several times a day and has the patient sit on the edge of the bed. While sitting, he should practice extending his knee and lower limb. The nurse may be asked to press lightly against the lower limb to provide resistance.

The patient with either type of amputation should practice lifting the stump and buttocks off the bed while he is lying flat on his back. This exercise helps develop the abdominal muscles, which are necessary for stabilizing the pelvis when the patient stoops or bends.

The nurse must not become so occupied with the affected limb that she neglects the good leg and foot if the amputation involves only one limb. Supervision of regular exercises to strengthen leg muscles and care that drop foot and pronation deformities do not occur are nursing responsibilities. The patient should have a firm board or block of wood at the foot of the bed against which he can push and thereby receive essential active exercise.

When the patient is permitted out of bed, the nurse should begin to teach him self-care activities such as rising from a chair. To preserve his center of gravity and balance, the patient should keep his good leg well under him before he shifts his weight, as when rising from a chair. If a physical therapist is available, the nurse should consult him regarding exercise.

The patient who has had an amputation because of vascular disease must be reminded to take particular care of his remaining foot and leg. Exercises and other measures to keep the arterial supply as adequate as possible must be carried on while the patient is in the hospital, and he must be urged to follow his doctor's instructions carefully when he leaves the hospital.

Care of the stump. If a prosthesis is to be worn comfortably, a healthy stump is necessary. Teaching the patient how to care for his stump is a nursing responsibility that may be carried out both in the hospital and in the patient's home. The patient may be discharged from the hospital within a few weeks but may not be fitted for a prosthesis for six weeks to six months after the operation, depending on the condition of the stump.

When the wound is completely healed, the patient is taught to wash the stump daily. Most surgeons advise their patients not to soak the stump because soaking may cause maceration of the skin. The skin should be massaged gently, directing the motion toward the suture line. Alcohol or mild skin creams can be used, depending on the condition of the skin. Usually the patient is instructed to push forcefully over the bone to toughen the limb for weight-bearing. Sometimes this process is begun by placing a pillow on a footstool, chair, or high stool (depending upon the site of operation) and having the patient bear some weight on the stump while steadying himself on the bed or against the wall.

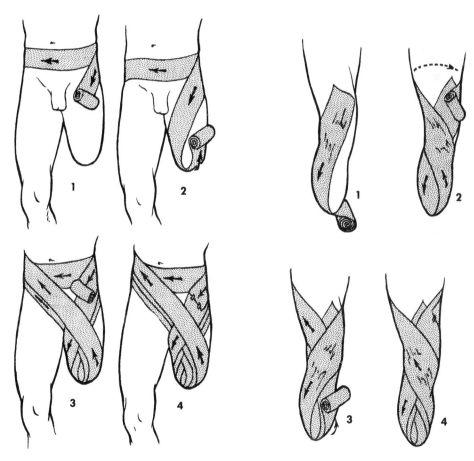

Fig. 83

The four sketches on the left side of the diagram illustrate the correct method for bandaging a mid-thigh amputation stump. Note that the bandage must be anchored around the patient's waist. The four sketches on the right side illustrate the correct method for bandaging a mid-calf amputation stump. Note that the bandage need not be anchored about the waist.

There should be no tenderness, redness, or other signs of skin irritation or abrasion at the end of the stump. The skin and underlying tissue should be firm and without flabbiness and should be without tautness over the bony end of the limb. If there is a tendency to flabbiness, the stump may be bandaged firmly both day and night. Some patients are taught to bandage the stump themselves. However, they need careful instruction and supervision. (See Fig. 83.) The bandage must not be tight enough to cause pain or numbness from hampered circulation. If it is too loose, it will defeat its purpose. If the patient is unable to apply a firm, even bandage, a member of his family may help him. The bandage should be removed and reapplied twice daily, and the skin should be washed, dried, powdered, and exposed to the air for a short time before the bandage is reapplied. The patient should have at least two bandages so that one may be washed daily; they should be layed flat to dry so as not to stretch.

When the prosthesis is used, the patient should have several pairs of stump socks of the right size. They should be made of cotton and wool and should be washed daily after use and dried over a mold to prevent shrinkage. Usually the patient wears out about one sock a month when he begins to use a prosthesis. A worn sock should not be mended because it may cause irritation to the stump. Routine care of the stump, including bathing, massage, and inspection, should be continued. If the weather is warm and the skin perspires freely, the limb should be removed from the socket, bathed, exposed to the air for a short time, and then powdered at least once during the day. The patient who works may take an extra stump sock with him so that he can change during the day in hot weather. To prevent tension on the sock as the limb is placed in the socket, a string may be attached to the end of the sock and brought through a hole that is usually left in the prosthesis below the level of the stump. The patient should be instructed to report calluses or any abnormalities on the stump to his doctor at once.

Phantom limb sensation. Phantom limb is an unpleasant complication that sometimes follows an amputation and that is difficult to treat. It is a sensation that the limb is in its normal position. The sensation may disappear if the patient looks at the stump and recalls that the limb has been amputated. *Phantom limb pain* also occurs. The patient may have the sensation, for example, that something is burning his foot, or that someone is stepping on his toes. Phantom limb pain may disappear of its own accord, or it may lessen for a time and then recur with severity. When it is really troublesome to the patient, the nerve endings may be injected with alcohol to give temporary relief. Occasionally, when pain persists, an operation is done for removal of the nerve ends that may have developed to form a tuft on a weight-bearing part of the stump. A few patients are troubled with phantom limb pain for an indefinite time following amputation, and it may interfere seriously with their rehabilitation. Reamputation is sometimes done, but even this procedure does not always bring relief since the same sensations may be experienced at the end of the new stump.

Ambulation. Teaching the patient who has had an amputation to walk with crutches, with crutches and prosthesis, and then with the prosthesis alone is a complicated task that lies within the responsibility of physical medicine. In the past, teaching the patient to walk with a prosthesis often was left to the limb maker. Although the limb maker can teach the patient a great deal about the new limb and its effective use, learning to walk well with an artificial limb requires instruction by a skilled physical therapist. It is the responsibility of nurses working with the surgeon, the social worker, the physical therapist, and other members of the professional health team to see that the patient receives continuous care, teaching, and encouragement until he is able to manage on his own.

The nurse has the responsibility to prepare every patient for *crutch-walking*, and she may have to teach the patient to use crutches if a physical therapist is not available. Therefore, every nurse should know the essentials about using crutches and something about the gaits that can be used. Preparation for the use of crutches should include exercises to strengthen the triceps, which is a muscle used to extend the elbow and is therefore most important in the satisfactory use of crutches. These exercises can be started before the operation by teaching the patient to lie on his abdomen and do the push-up exercises described on p. 391. When lying on his back, he can hold bags of sand or other weights on his palms and straighten out his elbows. In another exercise that strengthens the triceps muscles, the patient sits on the edge of the bed with his feet in a chair and, while pressing his palms against the mattress, lifts his hips off the bed. This procedure provides good exercise in extension of the elbow and helps the patient become accustomed to resting his weight on his hands. Use of an overbed trapeze bar postoperatively is helpful in that it enables the patient to handle himself much more independently than would otherwise be possible. Its use, however, strengthens primarily the biceps muscle, which is less essential in crutch-walking than is the triceps. Further preparation includes prevention of contractures and deformities that will interfere with the use of crutches and with the use of a prosthesis. Exercises to prevent hip and/or knee contractures and to maintain the muscle tone and strength in the unaffected leg are described on p. 392. Even before the stump may be healed enough to permit use of a prosthesis, the patient can learn to do a good deal to help himself (Figs. 84 and 85).

Crutches should be measured for each patient. In *method 1*, the patient lies on his back with his arms at his sides. The measurement is taken from the axilla to a point six inches out from the side of the heel. This is the length of the crutch minus three-fourths of an inch for the crutch tips. In *method 2*, the patient is measured from two inches below the level of the axilla to the base of the heel. In *method 3*, sixteen inches are subtracted from the patient's total height. Even with careful measurement, alterations may have to be made after the crutches are used. Posture, for example, may change, altering the length needed. The crutches should not cause pressure on the axillas and the patient is taught not to rest his weight on the axillary bars for more than a few minutes at a time. Pressure on the axillas causes pressure on the radial nerves which can lead to severe and sometimes permanent paralysis of the arms ("crutch paraly-

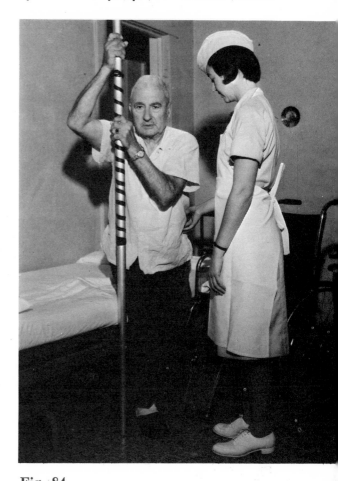

Fig. 84

Time, patience, and reassurance are needed as the elderly patient with an amputation learns to move from the bed to a wheelchair independently and safely.

sis"). The patient is taught that weight should be borne on the palms of the hands.

Before the patient attempts to walk with crutches, he should be assisted out of bed and should stand with help by the bed to get the feel of normal balance. He may then use a walker or parallel bars until he is relatively secure. At this time he should begin to practice correct standing posture, with head up, chest up, abdomen in, pelvis tilted inward, a 5-degree angle in the knee joint, and the foot straight (Fig. 86). Practice in front of a mirror is very helpful. The patient

395

(Fig. 87). The first gait that he will use is the *swing-to* or *swing-through gait* that requires no carefully guided instruction, provided the patient knows how to bear his weight and has been taught to check posture, balance, and rhythm. In this gait the amputated limb and the crutches both advance either to or beyond the level of the normal limb and are followed by the normal leg. This is a simple, fast gait that gives little leg exercise but is useful for rapid maneuvers such as are needed in crossing streets. The patient may use this gait when he begins to walk with one prosthesis, in which case both

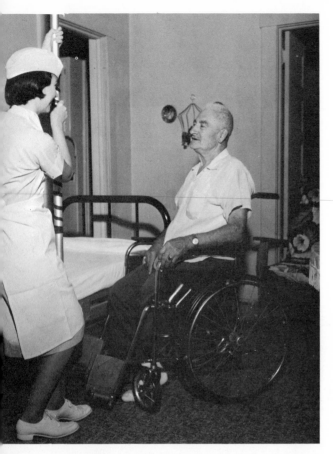

Fig. 85

The nurse demonstrates to the patient how he will proceed in moving himself from the wheelchair to his bed.

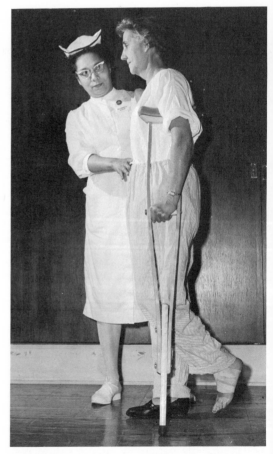

Fig. 86

In crutch-walking the patient is encouraged to maintain good posture and not to look down at her feet or the crutches.

is encouraged not to look toward his foot. Next, the patient should practice standing while supported by his crutches so that he can get the "feel" of them. The nurse should be sure that he begins at this time to bear his weight on his palms and not his axillas. Before the patient begins to try to use crutches, he should be shown the proper hand and arm position and the gait he will use. This not only helps him to understand what he must do but, if he is worried about whether the crutches will support him, it may increase his confidence.

In all crutch-walking the patient is taught to concentrate on a normal rhythmic gait

396

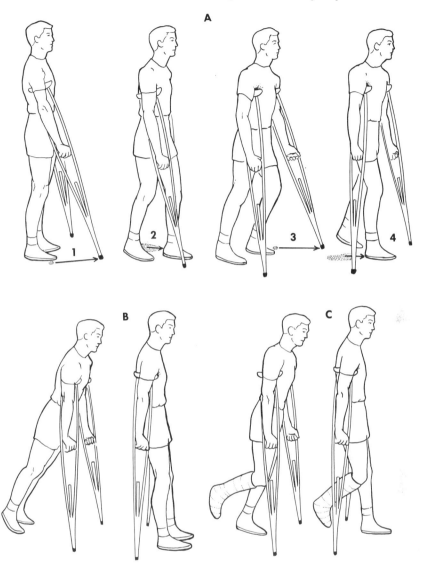

Fig. 87

A, The four-point gait. **B,** The swing-to gait. **C,** The swing-through gait.

crutches and the prosthesis move forward, followed by the normal leg.

When the patient with double amputations has been fitted with prostheses, he may be taught the *four-point gait*. This gait is taught to the count of four as follows: right crutch, left foot, left crutch, right foot. Some patients with bilateral amputations must always use this gait (which is also widely used by those with involved neuromuscular disabili-

ties and poor balance). It is a safe gait because the patient always has three points of contact with the ground at any time. Most patients progress to the *two-point gait*, in which the foot and opposite crutch move together and then the prosthesis and the opposite crutch. It is often taught to the count of two as follows: left crutch and right foot (one) and right crutch and left foot (two). The two-point gait produces a much faster gait and is easier to maintain in a rhythmic pattern than the four-point gait.

The patient with one prosthesis, may progress to one crutch and then to a cane, which should be abandoned eventually. The crutch or cane should be held in the hand on the side *opposite* the prosthesis since, as the patient normally walks, the arm on the opposite side of the body alternately swings forward. Holding the cane or crutch on the same side as the prosthesis results in an awkward, unrhythmic gait.

It is important for the nurse to know which gait the physical therapist is teaching the patient so that she may remind him if, upon leaving the physical therapy department, he reverts to a swing-to gait, for example. It is to be expected that the patient with a double amputation will learn to manage himself much more slowly than if only one limb were gone. Patients with amputations above the knee also take much longer to learn to walk and otherwise manage their movements.

The prosthesis. The doctor prescribes the type of prosthesis that is best for the patient and usually refers him to a limb maker. After the limb is made, the patient returns to the clinic, hospital department of physical medicine, doctor's office, or rehabilitation center to learn the best use of the artificial limb. The public health nurse, particularly if she is also trained in physical therapy, often gives care and supervision to the patient in his home.

The type of prosthesis is selected for the individual patient. Most prostheses are made of well-seasoned willow wood, although some are made of metal (duralumin and aluminum) and fiber materials. Metal prostheses are lighter in weight than wooden ones, but they tend to be noisy. Usually the below-the-knee prosthesis weighs about five pounds and the midthigh prosthesis about seven and one-half pounds, although the weight of the prosthesis is adapted to the size and weight of the patient and the kind of work he does.

The prosthesis has a socket, or "bucket," into which the limb fits. In the past, leather was the material most widely used, but plastic materials are now widely used since they are lighter, easier to keep clean, and odorless. The stump should fit snugly into the socket, and no more than two socks should be needed for a comfortable fit. If more are needed, the stump has shrunk and the prosthesis needs adjusting. Shrinking may continue for as long as ten years. It is usually greater after amputation of the foreleg than after amputation of the thigh. Suction cups are now quite generally used to hold the stump in the socket and obviate wearing a heavy, laced belt about the waist, although all patients with lower-limb prostheses wear some kind of waistband, and those with thigh amputations also wear a shoulder strap attachment to the waistband. The patient is advised to keep his shoulders straight and not permit the one on which the strap is worn to sag. He needs constant encouragement to use the prosthesis, particularly in the beginning, when he is adjusting to all features of the device. He should start to use the prosthesis as soon as his stump has healed.

The nurse should learn whether or not the patient is really using his prosthesis when at home. If he is not, she should learn the reason and report it to the doctor. Often she can help make the arrangements for more instruction. It is important that there be no delay, because the longer the patient puts off using the prosthesis, the less likely he is to use it satisfactorily. If crutches are used for too long, and if the patient depends on other forms of getting about, such as a wheelchair, he may have real difficulty in developing a normal rhythmic gait.

Care of the prosthesis should be reviewed with the patient. He should be taught to fasten the cuff above the stump from the bottom up, even though this method may seem more difficult at first. The cuff should be snug but not uncomfortable. If the cuff is leather, care should be taken that the stump sock is long enough to protect it from perspiration, and it should be rubbed with saddle soap at least weekly. The inside of the stump socket should be washed frequently to ensure cleanliness. Shoes should be kept in good repair and should have rubber heels. Broken shoelaces should be replaced at once. If the limb has a joint, the patient should be taught to keep this free from lint and dust, to oil the joints and locks every few weeks, and to keep screws tightened. If he feels adjustments are needed, he should return to the limb maker.

The patient should be told that his artificial limb is a tool and that it will be most useful to him when he has mastered its use. With good care it will last him three to ten years. Its value will depend on how well he can learn to balance himself, how much muscle strength he develops, and how smooth and rhythmic a gait he learns. Above all, its value will depend on his attitude toward the challenge that its use presents.

Long-term care. Most patients who have an amputation must remain under medical supervision for a long time, and it is safe to assume that any patient with an amputation needs nursing care and supervision long after the wound has healed. If possible, a public health nurse should visit the patient's home before he leaves the hospital so that she can help the family make any structural changes necessary for facilitating the patient's ambulation. If it should happen that a patient is equipped with an artificial limb but is not taught how to use it, the community nurse should initiate steps toward his rehabilitation. Occasionally the limb maker believes that the hospital clinic personnel is taking responsibility for teaching the patient to walk, and the doctor or the hospital clinic personnel believe that the limb maker is taking the responsibility. The patient may become discouraged and, after months of what appears to be a good adjustment, may lay the limb aside and return to a wheelchair or crutches. Sometimes he reports that the prosthesis is not comfortable and that he is reluctant to go back to the limb maker because of costs. If so, the nurse can help to find agencies in the community that can give appropriate assistance. It may be, however, that this statement is made by the patient to conceal a much more important and deep-seated rejection of his difficulties. This problem, of course, is much more difficult and should be reported to the doctor, who will decide what steps should be taken.

Occasionally, a patient, especially an elderly one, can use neither a prosthesis or crutches but must be confined to a wheelchair. The nurse should give special attention to the rehabilitation of this patient in an effort to make him as self-sufficient and happy as possible. Many patients can be taught to move themselves from the bed to the wheelchair, from the chair to the toilet, and even in and out of a car if bars or polecats are strategically placed. Polecats are especially useful for the patient who can pull up but not push up (Figs. 84 and 85). The patient and family often need help in arranging facilities at home, and plans should be made with the family to let the patient do useful chores such as fixing vegetables, mending, or doing small repairs. He also should be encouraged to become interested in some hobby or pastime.

There are many resources available to amputees. The National Rehabilitation Council provides financial assistance, medical aid, job-placement services, and counseling. There are many rehabilitation centers in the United States, but most of them are located in the larger cities. The division of vocational rehabilitation of the department of education in every state is, however, available to all patients. Most communities, counties, and states have voluntary programs that are designed to help the physically handicapped, including the amputee. The nurse should consult her local health department for information on the resources available to her own community. Some excellent pamphlets to use in teaching the amputee also are available: *Handbook for the Leg Amputee,** *Industrial Amputee Rehabilitation,†* and *Stump Hygiene.‡*

---

*Veterans Administration pamphlet 10-37, Washington, D. C., 1951, U. S. Government Printing Office.

†Published by Liberty Mutual Insurance Co., Boston.

‡Published by the Regents of the University of California, 1961.

References and selected readings*

1 Abramson, David I.: An approach to better circulation in the extremities, J. Am. Geriatrics Soc. 10: 605-617, July 1962.

2 Allen, Edgar V., Barker, Nelson W., and Hines, Edgar A., Jr.: Peripheral vascular diseases, ed. 3, Philadelphia, 1962, W. B. Saunders Co.

3 Anlyan, William G., and others: Fibrinolytic agents in surgical practice, J.A.M.A. 175:290-292, Jan. 28, 1961.

4 Baker, Wiley F., editor: Surgical treatment of peripheral vascular disease, New York, 1962, McGraw-Hill Book Co.

---

*References preceded by an asterisk are particularly well suited for student reading.

5 Barnes, Gilbert H.: Skin health and stump hygiene, Artificial Limbs 3:4-9, Spring 1956.

6 Beeson, Paul B., and McDermott, Walsh, editors: Cecil-Loeb textbook of medicine, ed. 11, Philadelphia, 1963, W. B. Saunders Co.

7 Bergersen, Betty S., and Krug, Elsie E.: Pharmacology in nursing, ed. 10, St. Louis, 1966, The C. V. Mosby Co.

8 Bradley, Robert L.: Amputation in the aged, J. Am. Geriatrics Soc. 8:901-902, Dec. 1960.

9 *Cannon, Jack A., and Quint, Jeanne C.: Endarterectomy and nursing the patient with endarterectomy, Am. J. Nursing 58:995-998, July 1958.

10 Chassin, Jameson L.: Improved management of acute embolism and thrombosis with an embolectomy catheter, J.A.M.A. 194:845-850, Nov. 22, 1965.

11 Cliffton, Eugene E., and others: Symposium on fibrolysin, Am. J. Cardiol. 6:367-563, Aug. 1960.

12 Crawford, E. Stanley, and others: Peripheral arteriosclerotic aneurysm, J. Am. Geriatrics Soc. 9:1-5, Jan. 1961.

13 Davis, Loyal, editor: Christopher's textbook of surgery, ed. 8, Philadelphia, 1964, W. B. Saunders Co.

14 De Bakey, Michael E., guest editor: Symposium on vascular surgery, S. Clin. North America 46:825-1071, Aug. 1966.

15 De Bakey, Michael E., and others: Basic biologic reactions to vascular grafts and prostheses, S. Clin. North America 45:477-497, April 1965.

16 Foley, William T.: The medical management of lymphedema, Mod. Concepts Cardiovas. Dis. 24:255-257, Jan. 1955.

17 Hoerner, M. Tischer: The role of lumbar sympathectomy in the treatment of obliterative peripheral vascular disease, J. Am. Geriatrics Soc. 11:781-788, Aug. 1963.

18 *James, George: A stop smoking program, Am. J. Nursing 64:122-125, June 1964.

19 *Kessler, Henry H., and Kiessling, Edward A.: The pneumatic arm prosthesis, Am. J. Nursing 65:114-117, June 1965.

20 *Knocke, Lazelle: Crutch walking, Am. J. Nursing 61:70-73, Oct. 1961.

21 *Krause G. Lynn, and Vetter, Frances C.: Varicose veins —diagnosis and treatment and nursing care, Am. J. Nursing 53:70-72, Jan. 1953.

22 Larson, Carroll B., and Gould, Marjorie L.: Calderwood's orthopedic nursing, ed. 6, St. Louis, 1965, The C. V. Mosby Co.

23 *Latham, Helen C.: Thrombophlebitis, Am. J. Nursing 63:122-126, Sept. 1963.

24 Levy, S. William: The skin problems of the lower extremity amputee, Artificial Limbs 3:20-35, Spring 1956.

25 Linton, Robert R.: Arterial occlusion and venous thrombosis, pulmonary embolism, and varicose veins, J.A.M.A. 183:191-194, 198-201, Jan. 19, 1963.

26 *Locke, Raymond K.: Foot care for diabetics, Am. J. Nursing, 63:107-110, Nov. 1963.

27 Lord, Jere W., Jr.: Cigarette smoking and peripheral atherosclerotic occlusive disease, J.A.M.A. 191:249-251, Jan. 18, 1965.

28 *Martin, Dorothy M., Case, Flossie G., and Miller, Arthur C.: Nursing care of the patient with an abdominal aortic aneurysm, Am. J. Nursing 59:60-62, Jan. 1959.

29 *Olwin, John H., and Koppel, J. L.: Anticoagulant therapy, Am. J. Nursing 64:107-110, May 1964.

30 *Sensenig, David M., and Morson, Betty J.: Buerger's disease, Am. J. Nursing 57:337-340, March 1957.

31 *Smith, Lester A.: An orthotist, prosthetist—what are they? Nursing Outlook 7:34-35, Jan. 1959.

32 Warren, Richard, and others: Surgery, Philadelphia, 1963, W. B. Saunders Co.

33 *Wesseling, Elizabeth: The adolescent facing amputation, Am. J. Nursing 65:90-94, Jan. 1965.

34 Wright, Beatrice: Physical disability: a psychological approach, New York, 1960, Harper & Row, Publishers.

35 Wright, Irving S.: The treatment of occlusive arterial disease and the treatment of thrombophlebitis, J.A.M.A. 183:186-191, 194-198, Jan. 19, 1963.

36 Young, Eleanor L., and Barnes, William A.: Hemipelvectomy, Am. J. Nursing 58:361-364, March 1958.

18

The patient with a blood dyscrasia

Study questions

1 What are the normal constituents of blood? Where are blood cells formed? How are they destroyed? What is the normal red blood cell count, hemoglobin, and hematocrit for men? For women?

2 Trace the successive processes that occur when blood clots. List the nursing responsibilities in preparing for and assisting with a blood transfusion. What observations should the nurse make while blood is being given?

3 From your understanding of physiology, explain why the patient who is anemic may have dyspnea and tachycardia.

4 Find out the price of vitamin B_{12} from your local druggist or from your hospital pharmacy. What would be the yearly expense for a patient requiring an injection of 50 μg every week?

This chapter will include only a few of the more important aspects of nursing care for patients with blood dyscrasias and diseases of the blood-forming organs. Since detailed discussion of blood transfusions and nursing problems related to the taking and giving of blood can be found in fundamentals of nursing texts, they will not be included here. (See also Chapter 3.)

Diagnostic tests and procedures

Complete blood studies. Of the many tests that may be done to help determine the patient's exact blood disease, the simplest and perhaps the most significant are the red blood cell count, hemoglobin and hematocrit determination, and the white blood cell count and smear. Platelet count and bleeding and clotting times may be ordered also. Blood for these tests is obtained from the patient's finger or earlobe. Other tests, such as prothrombin time determination, require blood from a vein. Because many patients with a blood dyscrasia have a tendency to bleed abnormally, prolonged bleeding from the puncture site or bleeding into surrounding tissues may occur. The nurse should inspect the site of venipuncture frequently to see that clotting does occur. Since frequent examinations of the blood are required to determine the pa-

401

tient's progress and are used as a guide for treatment, the patient with a blood dyscrasia should understand why they are necessary. Having blood samples taken is an unpleasant procedure, particularly when many have to be obtained.

Capillary fragility test. This simple test helps to determine the status of small capillaries that become fragile and rupture easily in certain blood disorders. If a patient has one of these disorders, what is known as the *Rumpel-Leede phenomenon* appears. A blood pressure cuff is placed on the patient's arm and inflated, and pressure about midway between systolic and diastolic pressure is maintained for fifteen minutes. When the skin is examined five minutes after removing the cuff, only one or two petechiae (small hemorrhagic spots) per square inch will normally be found. If the platelet count is low, numerous petechiae may appear. This test is painless, but it should be explained to the patient lest he become overly concerned with the results. It usually helps to tell him that every person will respond to this test with the appearance of some petechiae.

Bone marrow aspiration. A *sternal puncture*, or sternal bone marrow biopsy procedure, is done to obtain a sample of the cells active in blood cell production. It may be done when leukemia, aplastic anemia, or a number of other conditions are suspected. The biopsy is usually obtained from the sternum, but other sites, such as a vertebra or the iliac crest, may be used. Most institutions require that signed permission from the patient be obtained before this procedure is done. The procedure is upsetting to some patients, who fear that it will be painful and who dread the insertion of a needle "so near the heart" as is necessary for a sternal puncture. Actually, there is danger of puncturing the pericardium during this procedure, particularly if the sternum is abnormally thin. It is important that the patient be as relaxed and composed as possible. If he expresses extreme fear or apprehension, the nurse should report this fact to the doctor, who may then order a sedative.

For a sternal puncture the patient lies on his back, and a small pillow may be placed lengthwise under the thoracic spine to bring the sternum forward. For punctures at other sites the patient is placed in a position that gives the physician good visualization and the patient maximum comfort. The skin over the aspiration site is cleansed and prepared with an antiseptic solution, and the area is anesthetized with procaine. A few minutes are allowed for the drug to take effect on the periosteum before the sternal needle (a short, stout needle with a protecting hub to prevent its being inserted too far) is inserted and tapped gently with a small mallet until the center of the bone is entered. The stylet is then withdrawn, a dry 5 or 10 ml. syringe is attached, and a small amount (0.2 to 0.3 ml.) of material is aspirated. At this time the patient may have a feeling of mild pain or discomfort. The specimen is deposited immediately into a specimen bottle containing sodium oxalate, and several direct smears are made. The patient may have slight soreness over the puncture site for several days, but the puncture should not cause real discomfort unless pressure is exerted.

General nursing care

Chronicity of the disease. With the exception of a few conditions, such as nutritional anemia and fulminating leukemia, diseases of the blood and the blood-forming organs are chronic. Patients with these diseases are seldom cured, and knowledge of this fact colors their attitude toward treatment and may alter their efforts in carrying on from day to day. Each patient is individual in his response to knowledge that he has a chronic disease. Some patients become depressed, discouraged, and resigned to invalidism, whereas others show magnificent courage in overcoming their problems and living productively from day to day.

The nurse can help the patient by listening to him when he becomes discouraged, giving him attention and care as needed, helping him determine realistic goals, discussing the need for and encouraging him to continue medical care and treatment, maintaining a positive attitude about his progress and prognosis, and contributing to patient and family planning so that, within his limitations, he may remain a productive and contributing member of society. Individual family members may also turn to the nurse and may be in need of much the same help as the patient.

Acuity of the disease. When the patient suffers from an acute blood disease such as acute leukemia and has only a short life expectancy, the nurse's role is one of support for both the patient and the family. The family will need help in understanding the nature of the disease and in accepting the diagnosis. They will need encouragement, reassurance, and strengthening of faith in the medical care being given. Present treatment increases the length of life, controls symptoms, and may restore the patient to apparent health for periods of time. When the patient is to be at home during a remission, the nurse instructs the family in the care needed so that the patient will be protected from infection and injury but permitted to live as normally as possible. While the patient is hospitalized, the nurse should be aware of the concern of the patient's family and should try to give them necessary help by listening, observing, and answering questions. The patient is likely to be irritable, discouraged, and apprehensive. The nurse should accept his reaction and understand his need for the love and attention of his family. Volunteers can often be helpful in providing for the patient some of the attention he needs (Fig. 88).

Fatigue. Most patients with diseases of the blood and the blood-forming organs suffer from fatigue that may be almost overwhelming. The patient may go to the doctor because he is "tired of being tired." Chronic fatigue adds to discouragement and influences the patient's emotional reaction to his symptoms.

Fatigue may be caused in part by a low red blood cell count and a low hemoglobin level since insufficient oxygen is being carried to the tissues. Insufficient blood supply may cause fainting, which is fairly common among persons who have severe anemia and which may lead to serious accidents. Some patients who do not really faint complain of feeling "light-headed"; this feeling, combined with general fatigue, also predisposes to accidents. Lying flat without a pillow for frequent short periods increases arterial supply to the brain and may help to prevent the light-headedness.

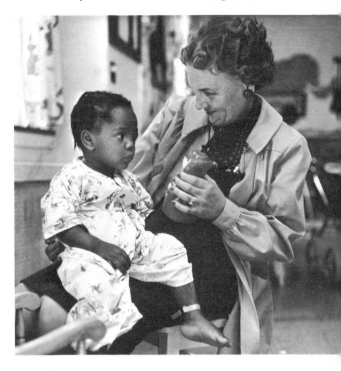

Fig. 88

The child who must have repeated hospitalizations for treatment of a blood dyscrasia benefits from a motherly interest on the part of hospital personnel. (Courtesy Muhlenberg Hospital, Plainfield, N. J.; photo by Warren R. Vroom.)

Fatigue may be lessened by specific medications and treatment such as transfusions. The nurse should question the ambulatory patient to be certain he is taking the medications as prescribed. Fatigue may decrease with better nutrition, and this fact should be emphasized to the patient. The patient should be encouraged to discuss the problem of fatigue frankly with his doctor. The ambulatory patient may feel that this complaint will appear trivial to the busy doctor and may therefore fail to mention it.

Temperature, pulse, and respirations. These three classic signs of sickness or health are particularly important when the patient has disease of the blood or the blood-forming organs. Temperature, pulse, and respirations are taken with such regularity and become so routine in hospitals that the tendency may be to regard them as not very important. This attitude is unfortunate because probably few complicated tests give clues that are as useful to the patient's progress as these simple ones give. If the temperature, pulse, and respirations are taken and recorded by auxiliary nursing personnel, the nurse has a responsibility to see that their findings are accurate and that they are correctly recorded.

Increases in pulse rate and respiratory rate are common in anemia, regardless of its cause. The heart beats faster in an effort to send the limited number of red blood cells more quickly on their way to the tissues or the lungs. The lungs work harder in response to the great need of the limited blood cells for oxygen. Increase in respiratory rate may also be a sign that a disease such as Hodgkin's disease or leukemia is causing pressure on the bronchi or the trachea, with resultant respiratory distress. Episodes of high temperature that last for several days and then disappear for several weeks, only to recur, are characteristic of Hodgkin's disease and of some forms of leukemia. Finally, increase in these vital signs may mean that the patient—whose resistance to superimposed infection is very poor—may be developing an infection of some kind.

Hemorrhage. Bleeding from various body orifices is common in persons who have blood dyscrasis. The nurse should be particularly alert for signs of bleeding from anywhere in the body. Stools should be examined at regular intervals for signs of fresh blood or for the tarry appearance characteristic of bleeding high in the gastrointestinal tract. The doctor often orders examination of stools for occult, or hidden, blood, since it is possible for patients to lose small amounts of blood regularly from the intestinal tract and to become severely anemic without frank blood or tarry stools giving any warning. Red meat is sometimes restricted for twenty-four to forty-eight hours before the stool sample is collected, and the reason for this restriction must be explained to the patient.

Urine should be noted for evidence of blood. Bright blood in the urine is usually observed by the patient, but smoky urine, caused by lesser amounts of blood, may go unnoticed.

The patient should be protected from trauma that may cause bleeding into the tissues. The ambulatory patient is cautioned to avoid bumps and similar injuries. He should not, for example, walk in the dark. If the patient is critically ill and is disoriented, his fingernails should be cut short to prevent scratching the skin, and side rails should be used to prevent falling out of bed. Tight clothing should not be worn; for example, the patient's gown should be left untied at the neck if he is inclined to be restless.

Bleeding from the mouth and gums is common in patients with blood dyscrasias. Sometimes, awareness that gums bleed excessively after brushing the teeth is the first sign to the patient that anything is wrong. Mouth care for patients with an advanced blood dyscrasia such as leukemia becomes a major nursing problem. The lips may become cracked and bleed easily, and mouth odor follows the accumulation of old blood in the mouth. The patient is often reluctant to have care given for fear that it may start fresh bleeding. Toothbrushes should never be used. The teeth and gums should be carefully swabbed with large, soft cotton applicators. Petrolatum or a similar softening cream should be applied to the lips with an applicator. A weak solution of hydrogen peroxide (1%) seems particularly effective in cleansing old blood from the mouth. Sodium perborate is sometimes used if ordered by the doctor. Carbonated beverages are sometimes a pleasant means of softening crusts of blood and exudate in the mouth. If the patient tires of sweet fluids, plain carbonated water may be tried. Zinc peroxide has been found effective for some patients. Flavored mouthwashes can be tried. Many patients like aromatic solutions such as Dobell's solution. Peppermint flavoring can also be used in solutions to cleanse the mouth. If the patient is alert and can be relied upon not to inhale the solutions, oil solutions that can be sprayed into the mouth with an atomizer help to protect bleeding or oozing surfaces. Mineral oil flavored with peppermint, oil of cloves, or menthol may make the patient's mouth feel better. The nose needs the same kind of meticulous care as the mouth. Small wicks of cotton soaked in mineral oil are usually better than nose drops because they remain longer and seldom drain into the posterior nasopharynx. These wicks are sometimes placed in the nostrils alternately, or else very small ones may be used against oozing surfaces in the nares, permitting breathing through the nostrils.

Infections. Patients with diseases involving the white blood cells are especially prone to both local and systemic infections. Staphyloccal infections are common, and a variety of other organisms are likely to attack the patient who is receiving radiation treatment, antimetabolite drugs, and steroids, and whose polymorphonuclear leukocyte response to infection is already limited by his disease.

Special care needs to be taken to prevent the exposure to infection of patients with diseases involving the tissues that form the white blood cells. Meticulous washing of the hands and strict surgical asepsis are mandatory. The environment should be kept scrupulously clean and dustless, and no person with any type of infection should be allowed in contact with the patient. Occasionally, isolation technique (reverse precautions) is ordered to protect the patient from hospital personnel and visitors (p. 61).

Since steroids and antibiotics may mask fever as a symptom of infection, the nurse needs to be particularly alert for any sign of infection such as local redness, cough, increased malaise, or anorexia. Any slight change or seemingly unimportant symptom should be called to the physician's attention.

Diet. Almost all patients with disease of the blood or the blood-forming organs should have a diet high in protein, minerals (especially iron), and vitamins. If there is gastrointestinal bleeding and if the mucous membrane of the mouth is irritated, foods containing roughage should be avoided. Hemorrhage of the gums and of mucous membrane anywhere along the gastrointestinal tract can follow the ingestion of rough food such as whole kernels of corn. Hot foods should also be avoided because the thin, irritated mucous membrane of the mouth is burned easily. Highly spiced foods are not given because they may cause irritation.

Seeing that the patient eats enough is a real nursing challenge in many instances.

The patient may be too tired or too discouraged to be interested in food, he may have a poor appetite, and he may have anorexia or even nausea from the constant presence of blood in his mouth. Companionship during meals, small, attractive servings of foods that he likes, and mouth care before meals often help to improve his appetite. The ambulatory patient or his family are often interested in suggestions for planning high-protein meals that are palatable yet within their means and for including enough vitamins yet avoiding high-roughage foods.

The patient's environment. The patient with anemia is almost always cold. Extra covers should be provided so that windows can be opened without danger of chilling. The general environment of the patient's room should be kept quiet and free from disturbance. The family of the critically or terminally ill patient should be given special consideration. If he is in a hospital, close relatives may appreciate opportunities to help in giving care. If he is at home, they may welcome assistance from the public health nurse so that they may continue to participate in care and prevent the need for hospitalization. Sometimes relatives may be overcome by their own feeling and want to avoid the sight of such things as bleeding or the patient's growing helplessness. The nurse must accept this reaction as normal for some persons.

Anemia and the anemias

Anemia is an extremely common condition in which there is an abnormal reduction in the number of circulating red blood cells and/or an abnormality of the red blood cells with a reduction of hemoglobin. Asthenia, fatigue, and pallor are the classic signs of anemia. Its main causes are loss of blood, faulty blood cell production, and excessive destruction of red blood cells.

Anemias due to excessive blood loss

Anemia resulting from frank hemorrhage such as may follow trauma, childbirth, surgery, or administration of drugs such as bishydroxycoumarin (Dicumarol) is usually apparent. It presents relatively simple medical problems provided that not too much blood is lost and the cause of hemorrhage can be corrected. The adult of average build has approximately 6,000 ml. of blood in the total circulating blood system. Usually he can lose 500 ml. without serious or lasting effects. If the loss reaches 1,000 ml. or more, serious consequences may result, and one to two months may be required for the volume to return to normal. (Care of the patient who suffers from hemorrhage is discussed on p. 91.)

The body has remarkable adaptive powers and may adjust fairly well to a marked reduction in red blood cells and hemoglobin provided the condition develops gradually. The total red cell count may even drop to almost half of its normal figure of between 4½ and 5 million per cubic milliliter of whole blood without the patient's experiencing the usual symptoms to a noticeable extent. Another example of the body's adaptive capacity is the increase in red blood cells that occurs when a person moves from a low to a high altitude (more cells are needed to carry oxygen from the rarefied atmosphere).

Chronic, unrecognized blood loss can also cause anemia. It may occur in the presence of an unsuspected gastrointestinal malignancy, a slowly bleeding peptic ulcer, or hemorrhoids that bleed without the patient's awareness. When blood loss is continuous and moderate in amount, the bone marrow may be able to keep up with the losses by increasing its production of red blood cells if enough protein and iron are supplied in food. Eventually, however, if the cause of chronic blood loss is not found and corrected, the bone marrow usually cannot keep pace with the loss, and symptoms of anemia appear.

Anemias due to defective blood production

There are several reasons for defective and inadequate red blood cell production. A diet deficient in protein and iron (raw materials from which blood cells are manufactured) and poor absorption of food from the gastrointestinal tract can lead to anemia. Lack of production of substances within the body that are essential in blood cell formation, such as the intrinsic factor

secreted by the stomach, may cause anemia. The bone marrow's capacity for manufacturing red blood cells may be depressed by toxic chemicals such as benzene and the sulfonamides, by toxins from infection, by aplasia of unknown cause, and by hyperactivity of white blood cell production, which occurs in leukemia.

Nutritional anemia. Nutritional anemia is common and may be due to lack of knowledge of the foods necessary for building normal blood cells, lack of money to purchase essential foods, or fads or notions about diet. Occasionally a nutritional anemia follows lengthy adherence to a special diet for a condition such as an allergy. To manufacture red blood cells, the body must ingest and use foods containing the essential substance (vitmain B_{12}) necessary in the manufacture of red blood cells as well as the protein and iron needed. Some foods containing these essentials are meat, eggs, yeast, and whole-grain cereals.

Nutritional anemia should be entirely preventable in a country such as ours. The nurse can help in prevention by teaching the importance of good nutrition. Emphasis should be upon the essentials of good nutrition and upon a wide selection of foods. When nutritional anemia has occurred, it is necessary for the patient to have more than the usual amounts of protein, minerals, and vitamins. Extra iron is also usually given. The simple form of ferrous sulfate usually is as effective as more elaborate trade preparations. To speed the absorption of oral preparations of iron, they are given before meals or between meals when there is little or no food in the upper digestive tract.[4] Many inorganic preparations of iron may cause irritation of the empty stomach and therefore are given after meals. The patient who is given iron should be told that the stools will be black, lest he worry about bleeding from the gastrointestinal tract. If iron is not tolerated by mouth it may be given intramuscularly. The drug is more completely absorbed by this route than when it is taken orally. An iron preparation widely used for intramuscular injection is iron-dextran (Imferon).

Pernicious anemia. Pernicious anemia was first described by Thomas Addison in London in 1849, and the term addisonian anemia is still sometimes used. In this disease a substance called the *intrinsic factor,* normally produced by the stomach mucosa, is lacking. In normal function the intrinsic factor promotes the absorption of vitamin B_{12} normally found in food (extrinsic factor). In a manner not yet fully understood, vitamin B_{12} contributes to the production of an *erythrocyte-maturing factor* that is essential to proper red blood cell formation. Without the intrinsic factor the red blood cells become abnormal. They may be large (macrocythemia), contain more hemoglobin than usual (hyperchromia), and assume peculiar shapes (poikilocytosis) and sizes (anisocytosis). A diet high in protein and iron does not correct these abnormalities, since the basic defect is not in the raw materials provided.

Pernicious anemia usually occurs after the age of 40 years. More people are affected in the temperate zones than in the far northern or southern hemispheres. In the United States the incidence is higher in the northern sections of the country, where there are many people of Nordic descent. There appears to be a hereditary influence in the development of pernicious anemia. Several members of the same family may have the disease. Many patients with pernicious anemia have characteristics in common. Many are of the Nordic race and have broad faces, blond hair that grays early, and wide-set blue eyes.

Pernicious anemia develops slowly. Fatigue is a common symptom, but it comes on so slowly that the patient seldom remembers its beginning. There may be anorexia and symptoms of poor digestion, yet little weight loss. Gastric analysis may reveal an absence of free hydrochloric acid in the stomach secretions (*achlorhydria*). The tongue becomes smooth, and the patient may notice soreness, burning, or other signs of irritation in the mouth. They may disappear, only to reappear after a few weeks or months. There is usually a characteristic waxy pallor which, as the disease progresses untreated, will turn to a light lemon yellow, with mild jaundice noticeable in the sclera. Dyspnea and palpitation also occur.

Pernicious anemia affects the nervous system. Irritability and depression are signs of the disease, and occasionally the patient even develops a psychosis that usually responds almost immediately to treatment for the anemia. As neurologic involvement develops, there may be numbness, tingling, or a burning sensation in the hands and feet. Some patients have signs of peripheral neuritis with decreased or lost sense of vibration in the feet and legs. Sense of position becomes disturbed, and eventually incoordination develops. Some patients complain of a sensation of constricting bands around the lower limbs and the trunk. It is estimated that approximately 80% of persons with pernicious anemia have some neurologic involvement by the time they seek medical care. In those with advanced disease the rectal and urinary sphincters may function poorly. Although patients with far-advanced and permanent neurologic damage are now seldom seen in the United States, some patients still have neurologic symptoms for months before they seek medical advice. When the nurse sees a patient with signs of pernicious anemia who feels that his symptoms are not serious, she should encourage him to seek medical aid at once.

There is no cure for pernicious anemia, since at the present time there is no way to help the stomach lining regain its capacity to produce the intrinsic factor. Fortunately, however, the disease can be arrested by supplying cyanocobalamin (vitaman B_{12}). Although some neurologic damage may not be completely reversible, the patient may now live out his life with no serious increase in symptoms provided he continues treatment with this drug.

The preparation of vitamin B_{12} is extremely potent, and daily intramuscular injections of as little as 1 μg will cause production of normal blood cells. Vitamin B_{12} is marketed in 5 and 10 ml. vials and in four different strengths. Each milliliter may contain 10, 15, 30, or 50 μg. An initial dose of 30 μg is given and is repeated every day or every other day for ten doses. Dosage is then usually reduced to 15 to 30 μg once or twice a week, and after a few weeks the patient can often be maintained on a dosage of 40 to 60 μg every other week. Sometimes adequate treatment is maintained with injections given as infrequently as every six months. A diet high in iron and high in protein is usually recommended.

Folic acid is now seldom used in the treatment of pernicious anemia, although it may be prescribed for certain forms of nutritional and related macrocytic anemias. For reasons not understood, folic acid enables the body to produce red blood cells of normal appearance. It does not, however, prevent the development of neurologic involvement in pernicious anemia.

Nursing care for the patient with pernicious anemia depends on the symptoms present at the time of treatment. Irritability, impatience, and apprehension should be expected and should be dealt with by showing the patient particular attention and by giving medications and other treatments on time and with as little confusion as possible. The patient may need extra warmth, special mouth care, and a carefully selected diet until severe symptoms subside. However, with present treatment the more superficial symptoms usually disappear within one or two weeks. Neurologic symptoms may be much more persistent and may even be partially irreversible despite intensive treatment with vitamin B_{12} and physical therapy. The patient may be discouraged when he finds that the neurologic symptoms do not disappear as quickly as the others. In the presence of permanent nerve damage, patience and persistence are tremendous assets to the patient in learning to manage himself effectively.

The prospect of needing intramuscular injections at weekly or biweekly intervals for the rest of one's life is not a happy one. The nurse can help the patient in his adjustment by her skill in giving injections as quickly and as painlessly as possible. She may remind him that, although injections must certainly be continued, he may need them less often when symptoms completely subside. If he must receive medication frequently, the doctor may wish the patient or a member of his family to learn to give the injections. Most patients receiving vitamin B_{12}, however, return to the doctor's office or clinic for injections, or may make arrangements through the doctor to have the public health nurse give them. The patient and his family must be taught the absolute necessity of returning regularly, since

symptoms will not reappear at once to remind them. The patient with residual neurologic involvement also needs help in learning safe and relatively simple methods of getting about without assistance. If a cane or a crutch is necessary, the patient needs to be encouraged to accept this aid.

A review should be made of the daily food intake of every patient who has pernicious anemia to be certain that he understands the essentials of a good diet. Cost may be a problem in the selection of suitable foods, particularly since vitamin B_{12} is expensive, and some of the money that the patient previously budgeted for food may be needed for its purchase. Usually the patient wiith pernicious anemia benefits from having a public health nurse visit his home to help plan low-cost, nutritious meals.

Aplastic anemia. Aplastic anemia is characterized by aplasia, depression, or cessation of activity of all blood-producing elements. There is a decrease in white blood cells (leukopenia), a decrease in platelets (thrombocytopenia), and a decrease in formation of red blood cells. The disease may be idiopathic, and it may occur in more than one child in a family. It may follow exposure to chemical agents or ingestion of certain drugs. Benzene, arsenicals, gold compounds, mustard gas, quinacrine (Atabrine), hair dyes, insecticides, streptomycin, and chloramphenicol are among the substances known to have been responsible for the development of aplastic anemia.

Symptoms of aplastic anemia may appear suddenly, but they usually develop gradually over a period of weeks and months. They include pallor, weakness, dyspnea, anorexia, headache, fever, and bleeding of the mucous membranes, often first noticed in the mouth or the nose. Treatment consists of removing causative toxic agents if they are known and of giving transfusions to raise the hemoglobin level and to supply platelets so that bleeding may be controlled. Iron, vitamin B_{12}, and high-protein foods are not effective. Antibiotics may be given to prevent and control secondary infection. The mortality rate from aplastic anemia is high, and almost all patients with the disease die. Occasionally, recovery occurs when the causative agent is found and removed. Nursing care of the patient with aplastic anemia includes all the measures mentioned in the first part of this chapter.

Anemias due to excessive destruction of red blood cells

Anemia in which there is an abnormal destruction of red blood cells is known as *hemolytic anemia.* Cells are destroyed at such a rate that the bone marrow is unable to make up the losses. Hemolytic anemia can be due to an inherited condition or to an acquired one.

Acquired hemolytic anemia can be caused by burns, snake venom, fava beans, drugs that are derivatives of benzene and toluene, certain heavy metals, or quinine. The use of incompatible blood for transfusions causes severe hemolysis of the red blood cells. Bacterial toxins from such microorganisms as the streptococcus, plasmodium, Welch's bacillus, and viruses can also cause hemolytic anemia, and marked hyperpyrexia can cause hemolysis of blood cells. Hemolytic anemia also may be caused by pathologic processes involving the spleen and causing it to destroy red blood cells excessively. The treatment for the latter is splenectomy, which will be discussed later.

An acute episode of hemolytic anemia, with rapid destruction of red blood cells, usually causes chills and fever, headache, irritability, precordial spasm, and pain. There may be abdominal pain and nausea, vomiting, and diarrhea. Urinary output may be diminished. Shock and prostration may occur, and jaundice follows the destruction of red blood cells. In chronic forms of the disease there are varying degrees of weakness, pallor, dyspnea, and palpitation. Stones may form in the biliary tract.

The prognosis of patients with acquired hemolytic anemias depends on the cause, the severity of the hemolysis, and the promptness of treatment. Treatment is directed toward eliminating the cause and maintaining renal function and fluid and electrolyte balance. The corticosteroids may be given. The anemia is usually treated by diet, but transfusions may be given. Nursing care of the patient includes all the measures discussed in the first part of this chapter.

Inherited hemolytic anemia may be due to a congenital defect resulting in formation of abnormal red blood cells. These cells are fragile and rupture easily, causing anemia and jaundice. The condition is usually chronic, but hemolytic crises similar to the acute episodes occurring in acquired hemolytic anemia do occur. These episodes frequently are precipitated by trauma, infections, or pregnancy, and therefore the patient should be instructed to seek immediate medical attention for any of these conditions. The prognosis for inherited hemolytic anemia is poorer when symptoms appear in childhood. Death usually follows a hemolytic crisis when thrombosis of a blood vessel supplying a vital area may occur.

Sickle cell anemia is one of the inherited types of hemolytic anemia. It is a chronic condition and occurs chiefly in Negroes. The disease is thought to be due to a chemical defect in the hemoglobin of the erythrocytes, and the red blood cells are characteristically shaped like sickles due to low oxygen content. This condition causes other bodily changes, including thickening of the skull bones and thinning of the long bones, with retardation of growth when it develops before full growth is attained. Other symptoms are varied and may include chronic leg ulcers, cardiac failure, and symptoms of an acute inflammation of the abdomen. Drowsiness, stupor, headaches, irritability, and convulsions can also occur. The mortality from this disease is high because there is no specific treatment. Treatment includes transfusions, sedation, oxygen, analgesics, protection from infection, and physical therapy. Frequently, packed red cells (a concentrated transfusion) are given since there is no decrease in circulating plasma in this disease.

The leukemias and lymphomas

Leukemia

Leukemia is a fatal disease of the blood-forming tissues characterized by an extensive and abnormal production of mature and immature forms of any of the white blood cells (granulocytes, lymphocytes, monocytes) that appear in the bloodstream, bone marrow, spleen, liver, and lymph nodes. Anemia is usually also present and is thought to be due to the diminished production of erythrocytes in the bone marrow as the tissue-forming abnormal leukocytes increase and spread throughout the marrow. Leukemia is a progressive malignant disease and for statistical purposes is now classified with cancer. It has increased in frequency and now accounts for about 14,000 deaths annually. The cause of leukemia is unknown. Any of the white blood cells involved may cause an acute or subacute form of the disease, with death occurring sometimes within a few weeks and usually within one year, or a chronic form, with an average course of three to five years.[3]

Treatment for both types of leukemia consists of supportive treatment such as giving blood transfusions to combat the anemia, antibiotics to treat infection, and supportive nursing. Effort is made to control the abnormal cell production, but no really satisfactory method has been found. Corticosteroids, antimetabolite drugs, and radiation treatment, including injection intravenously of radioactive substances such as phosphorus, are sometimes used. These treatments are usually used successively, with a new one being tried when objective and subjective improvement from the previous method has become minimal. (See p. 288 for the care of the patient with cancer who is receiving drug therapy.) Total body irradiation followed by bone marrow transplantation is one of the newest treatments.

Acute leukemia. Acute leukemia (whether it is lymphatic or myelocytic is often difficult to determine) usually occurs in persons under 25 years of age. Its highest incidence is in children under the age of 4. It has an abrupt onset. Symptoms include pallor, extreme fatigue, upper respiratory infection, fever, and bleeding from the mucous membrane of the mouth, nose, or other body orifices, or petechiae or ecchymoses in the skin. The total number of leukocytes of the various types is most often between 15,000 and 30,000 or less, although occasionally they may go much higher.[3] At the onset they may fall below 8,000 and may be as low as 2,000 to 3,000 per cubic milliliter or less. A severe anemia almost always develops, with the red blood cell count falling as low as 1 million per cubic milliliter, and the platelet count falling also. The lymph

nodes, spleen, and liver are usually enlarged but less so than in chronic leukemia.

The course is rapidly progressive, and while there may be a remission, death caused by hemorrhage, general debility, or infection usually occurs within a period of months.

Chronic lymphocytic leukemia. Chronic lymphocytic leukemia usually occurs in persons over 45 years of age. The onset is insidious, and the patient may complain of pallor and fatigue and may notice a painless lump in the neck, axilla, or groin. The lymph nodes, liver, and spleen are enlarged. The total white blood cell count is increased to between 30,000 and 100,000 per cubic milliliter, with 60 to 90% of these cells resembling normal small lymphocytes. The basal metabolic rate is usually increased, perhaps as a result of the increased consumption of oxygen by the leukemic cells and the accelerated rate of destruction of these cells. Abnormal bleeding usually occurs only during acute exacerbations of the disease and in the terminal phase. Average length of life after appearance of symptoms is three to five years, but some patients live eight years or more.

Chronic myelocytic leukemia. Chronic myelocytic (granulocytic and monocytic) leukemia occurs most often in persons between 35 and 45 years of age. The onset is insidious, and marked changes in the white blood cells have usually occurred before the patient has any specific complaint. Initial symptoms are usually weakness, pallor, palpitation, and dyspnea. Fever and chills often occur. There is marked enlargement of the spleen and liver, pronounced anemia, and increase in metabolic rate. Complications occur in a variety of body organs as they become infiltrated with leukocytes. An abnormal tendency to bleed occurs during acute exacerbations and immediately preceding death. The average length of life is approximately three to five years after onset of the disease.

Lymphomas

Lymphomas are tumors arising from lymphocytes or from the reticular cells of lymphatic tissues. They are considered malignant tumors and produce painless enlargement of lymph nodes throughout the body. Lymphosarcoma and Hodgkin's disease are two specific disorders classified as lymphomas. They cause about 15,000 deaths each year.

Hodgkin's disease produces painless enlargement of the lymph nodes. The first nodes to be involved usually are those in the cervical region, followed by the axillary nodes and those in the inguinal region. There is no known cause for this disease, but it is believed to be caused by an infection or a neoplastic process. Highest incidence is in young adults, and men are affected more often than women. The clinical findings vary from mild lymph node enlargement without other symptoms to generalized disease with severe symptoms including fever, excessive diaphoresis, anemia, anorexia, and weight loss. Twenty-five percent of patients with Hodgkin's disease have skin conditions such as pruritus.[13] Changes in the blood count are not significant, though leukocytosis or anemia may occur. Markedly enlarged nodes can cause severe symptoms from pressure. For example, respiration may be severely hampered by enlarged nodes in the mediastinum and neck. The average length of life is three to five years, although some patients with a benign type of disease live longer. Death is usually caused by progressive neoplastic involvement but may be due to pressure of the enlarged lymph nodes on the bronchi and mediastinum.

Since x-ray therapy appears to produce the longest remissions and the best relief of symptoms, it is thought to be the treatment of choice. Nitrogen mustard given intravenously is sometimes used as an adjunct to x-ray therapy (p. 289). Other treatment includes administration of corticosteroids, chlorambucil, antibiotics, and transfusions of whole blood or packed red cells when necessary. The aminopyrines are given for high temperature.[21]

A *lymphosarcoma* is a malignant tumor arising in the lymph nodes or mucosal lymphatic tissue. Specific complaints vary with the location of the lesion. Mediastinal and retroperitoneal lymph node enlargement may cause symptoms of pressure on adjacent organs, gastric and intestinal masses may simulate gastrointestinal carcinoma, and large, hard lymph nodes may be adherent to the skin. Fever, excessive diaphoresis, weight loss, and weakness are common. The treatment is similar to that for Hodgkin's disease. Most patients die within one or two years from this disease.

Hemorrhagic diseases

Purpura

In purpura the capillaries are exceedingly fragile, and the platelet count may or may not be reduced. There is extravasation of blood into the tissues, under the skin, and through the mucous membranes. In the skin, areas of hemorrhage may be small (petechiae) or large and "black and blue" (ecchymoses). Purpura may be secondary to other disorders or it may be idiopathic.

Secondary purpura. Secondary purpura may occur with many acute and chronic illnesses in which the bleeding and clotting times are normal. For example, dark areas of hemorrhage into the skin are characteristic of a severe, fulminating form of meningitis that swept Europe in the fourteenth century and produced the Black Death so vividly described in medical annals of that time. Some forms of purpura occur with vitamin C deficiency (scurvy), and one form of purpura, with actual abnormality in the blood, occurs with liver disease and failure to utilize vitamin K. Purpura may also occur as an allergic reaction to certain drugs such as quinine. The treatment for secondary purpura is to remove the cause if possible.

Autoimmune reactions are believed to be responsible for purpura, and they cause bleeding by increasing the permeability of the capillaries, although the platelet count is not reduced. Occasionally they appear to follow infections. *Henoch's* purpura, associated with acute abdominal symptoms, and *Schönlein's* purpura, associated with joint pains, are two syndromes that occur most often in children.[10] The bleeding from these disorders is rarely excessive, and there is no specific treatment.

Idiopathic thrombocytopenic purpura. In idiopathic thrombocytopenic purpura there is a reduction of blood platelets, the cause of which is unknown. The disease is usually seen in young people. The spleen enlarges and actively destroys platelets before their useful life is over. In response to the excessive loss, immature red blood cells (reticulocytes) appear in the bloodstream. The treatment for this condition is *splenectomy.* To lessen danger of severe hemorrhage at operation, radiation treatment to the spleen may be given to decrease its activity and to make it less vascular before surgery is attempted.

Preparation for a splenectomy is similar to that for other major abdominal surgery. Usually a transfusion is given a very short time before operation. The bleeding and clotting times are recorded, and the patient's blood is typed and crossmatched preparatory to giving additional transfusions if necessary.

Following a splenectomy the patient must be observed very carefully for signs of internal hemorrhage. As a rule he gets out of bed a day or two postoperatively to prevent thrombosis. If thrombosis does occur, its treatment is difficult because anticoagulants are considered contraindicated. Care must be taken that the patient does not bruise or otherwise injure himself when he first gets out of bed. A general diet high in iron and protein is given as soon as it can be tolerated. The patient with purpura and resultant anemia from blood loss responds very quickly to a diet high in protein and iron, together with supplementary iron.

Occasionally the patient is not cured by a splenectomy. The abdominal lymph nodes may take over the activities of the spleen, which has been removed, and may destroy platelets prematurely. If this happens, radiation therapy to the lymph nodes is sometimes given. The patient should be advised to continue under medical supervision for an indefinite time and to report any signs of bleeding to his doctor at once.

Hemophilia

Hemophilia is a hereditary hemorrhagic disease that is usually transmitted to the male by the female through a recessive sex-linked characteristic. There is one form of the disease, however, that can affect both sexes. In hemophilia the coagulation time is prolonged, and bleeding can occur at any time. The platelet count and prothrombin time, however, are normal. Hemophilia is largely a disease of children, since only one-third of patients with this condition reach the age of 30 years.

The patient with hemophilia must learn to avoid trauma of all kinds. The slightest bump will cause bruising with bleeding into tissues. Bleeding into joints is common, requiring immobilization of the affected joint. Repeated injuries cause bone destruction and deformity. The gums bleed easily, and any hemorrhage is extremely difficult to control. Care must be taken in the use of pins, nail files, scissors, and even toothbrushes. Since such care in ordinary activities is necessary, the patient and his family have serious psychologic handicaps, particularly since it is the active, growing child who is affected. Since repeated episodes of bleeding are wearing and frightening, the child may become sensitive and retiring or may attempt to defy his handicap. Social activities need to be planned to meet the patient's special needs. Minor medical problems that go almost unnoticed in the average household assume major proportions. For example, a simple tooth extraction requires hospitalization and transfusions.

Treatment consists of combating hemorrhage as it occurs by giving transfusions and by other means. Local application of fibrin foam and thrombin helps to stop external bleeding. Pressure dressings and elastic bandages may be used on joints. Giving an injection requires that particular care be taken to use a small needle, to apply pressure at the site of injection, and to inspect it for bleeding frequently for some time thereafter. The patient should have a diet high in iron. One of nature's compensations for this condition is a remarkable capacity to regenerate red blood cells when bleeding has caused their loss. The patient who has hemophilia should carry a card on his person that includes his name, his blood type, his doctor's name, and the fact that he has hemophilia, so that medical treatment will not be delayed if he should accidentally sustain injury and lose consciousness.

Polycythemia vera

In polycythemia vera there is excessive production of red blood cells, the count often being between 7 and 12 million. The hemoglobin is increased, and the patient characteristically has a reddish purple complexion, with reddening of the hands and feet. Headache, weakness, dyspnea, itching, and lacrimation may be other complaints. There may be bleeding from the skin and from the mucous membranes. This disease usually occurs in persons over 50 years of age, and the average age at death is approximately 60 years. Death is usually from thrombosis.

Phlebotomy is the main treatment and it may be necessary every six months or oftener. Radioactive phosphorus and triethylenemelamine (TEM) sometimes achieve remissions. The patient should have a diet low in iron, and the nurse can help him with the selection of foods. Other nursing care during an exacerbation consists of supportive care, with special attention to hemorrhage.

Agranulocytosis

Agranulocytosis is a disease in which production of white blood cells is depressed, and the total number of white blood cells may be reduced to between 200 and 500 per milliliter. Exposure to drugs, chemicals, and physical agents about the home can cause the disease. Sulfonamides, barbiturates, coal-tar analgesics, tripelennamine (Pyribenzamine), thiouracil, chloramphenicol, and heavy metals such as gold are examples. The nurse has a real part in the prevention of this disease. In the community she has frequent opportunity to advise against use of medications not therapeutically prescribed. In the hospital as well as in the home she must constantly be aware of the possible toxic effects of various drugs. Many times good nursing care can reduce the period of necessary treatment with drugs. Also she must be constantly alert for toxic signs of the drugs she administers.

Treatment consists of removing the offending agent. Sometimes the cause is difficult to determine, and careful history is essential. With such a low white blood cell count, precautions must be taken to control infections. The first signs of the disease may be the onset of an acute infection, with chills, fever, sore throat, and prostration. There may be enlargement of cervical lymph nodes. Infection may occur anywhere in the body. The mortality in agranulocytosis is high, although antibiotics have been found extremely helpful in controlling the infec-

tion until the cause can be found and removed. Transfusions of fresh whole blood are often given.

Infectious mononucleosis

Infectious mononucleosis is an acute disease of unknown cause. Although the theory is completely unproved, it is believed that the cause may be a virus. The disease is not new, having been described many years ago as acute "glandular fever" because of the enlargement of the lymph nodes. Infectious mononucleosis is more common in young persons, the largest number of cases occurring in those between 15 and 30 years of age. It sometimes occurs in more or less epidemic form among closely associated groups yet may also be sporadic in its appearance. Hospital personnel seem to be affected often by the disease, although this apparently higher incidence is thought to be due to better reporting. The infection is believed to be transmitted from one person to another by means of the secretions of the mouth and throat, although repeated efforts to transmit it to man in this fashion have failed. The incubation period has not been definitely established, but it is believed that it may be several weeks in length.

Signs and symptoms of infectious mononucleosis are varied. Usually it is a benign disease with a good prognosis. Malaise is a frequent early complaint, and it is often accompanied by elevation of temperature, enlargement of the lymph nodes, sore throat, headache, increased nasal secretions, aches and pains resembling those of influenza, and moderate enlargement of the liver and spleen. Jaundice, rupture of the spleen, encephalitis, and even death may occur. Diagnosis can be conclusively established by means of a test of the blood—the heterophil agglutination test. This test makes use of the fact that a certain substance that is present in the patient's blood causes clumping, or agglutination, of the washed erythrocytes (antigen) of another animal (in this case, sheep cells are used). The test is almost always positive at the end of a week of illness. Another conclusive laboratory finding is a marked increase in mononuclear leukocytes, which lends the name to the disease. At the height of the disease, the white blood cell count usually ranges between 10,000 and 20,000 cells per cubic milliliter of blood. So far, no modern antibiotic is effective in treating infectious mononucleosis, and no immunization is available.

Nursing care of the patient with infectious mononucleosis is purely symptomatic. If sore throat is severe, hot gargles may be ordered; glucose solutions often give greater relief than saline solution. Liquid and soft foods may have to constitute the patient's entire menu. An ice cap may be helpful if headache is severe. Acetylsalicylic acid is usually given for headache and generalized discomfort, and the patient is encouraged to remain in bed. If he is allowed to be up, he is advised to stay indoors and engage in little activity. The disease usually disappears within two weeks, but it may continue in a chronic form for several weeks and even months. Relapses do occur, and this fact explains the need for rest at the time of acute illness even though the patient does not feel ill and resents the time spent away from his work or regular activities.

References and selected readings*

1 American Cancer Society: 1966 cancer facts and figures, New York, 1965, American Cancer Society, Inc.

2 *Arnold, Patricia: Total-body irradiation and marrow transplantation, Am. J. Nursing 63:83-88, Feb. 1963.

3 Beeson, Paul B., and McDermott, Walsh, editors: Cecil-Loeb textbook of medicine, ed. 11, Philadelphia, 1963, W. B. Saunders Co.

4 Bergersen, Betty S., and Krug, Elsie E.: Pharmacology in nursing, ed. 10, St. Louis, 1966, The C. V. Mosby Co.

5 Cohn, Howard D.: Hemostasis and blood coagulation, Am. J. Nursing 65:116-119, Feb. 1965.

6 Crosby, William H., guest editor: Hematologic disorders, M. Clin. North America 50:1485-1720, Nov. 1966.

7 Curtin, J. A., and Marshall, B. D.: Use of antibiotics in cancer and leukemia, J. Chron. Dis. 15:713-718, July 1962.

8 Fleming, Juanita W.: The child with sickle cell disease, Am. J. Nursing 65:88-91, Sept. 1965.

9 Gruhn, John G., and Sanson, John: Mycotic infections in leukemic patients at autopsy, Cancer 16:61-73, Jan. 1963.

10 Harrison, T. R., and others, editors: Principles of internal medicine, ed. 5, New York, 1966, McGraw-Hill Book Co.

11 *Hartmann, John R., and Bolduc, Rose A.: Hemophilia: medical care and nursing care, Am. J. Nursing 56:169-174, Feb. 1956.

12 Hoaglund, Robert J.: Infectious mononucleosis, Am. J. Nursing 64:125-127, Oct. 1964.

13 *Hynes, John F., and Jansson, Eleanor B.: Hodgkin's disease, Am. J. Nursing 58:371-372, March 1958.

14 Leper, M. H.: Prophylaxis in patients receiving adrenal steroid therapy, J. Chron. Dis. 15:691-711, July 1962.

15 *Lyman, Margaret S., and Burchenal, Joseph H.: Acute leukemia, Am. J. Nursing 63:82-86, April 1963.

16 *McIntyre, Patricia Hope: Total body irradiation, Am. J. Nursing 61:62-64, Sept. 1961.

17 *McKinnie, Carol: Multiple myeloma, Am. J. Nursing 63:99-102, June 1963.

18 Molander, David W.: The malignant lymphomas, Am. J. Nursing 63:111-112, Oct. 1963.

19 *O'Kell, Richard T.: Understanding the hemophilias—A, B, and C, Am. J. Nursing 62:101-102, June 1962.

20 Onidi, Catherine: The patient with a malignant lymphoma, Am. J. Nursing 63:113-115, Oct. 1963.

21 Spear, Paul W.: The use of aminopyrine to control fever in Hodgkin's disease, J.A.M.A. 180:970-972, June 16, 1962.

22 White, Dorothy Watts: Living with hemophilia, Nursing Outlook 12:36-39, July 1964.

23 Wintrobe, Maxwell M.: Blood dyscrasias, Am. J. Nursing 60:496-500, April 1960.

*References preceded by an asterisk are particularly well suited for student reading.

19

The patient with disease of the urinary system

Study questions 1 Review the anatomy of the male and female urinary systems.
2 Review the physiology of urine formation. What are the parts of the nephron? What is the function of each part? What is the normal specific gravity of urine?
3 Review the procedure for catheterization of the urinary bladder.
4 What is the action of castor oil? Senna preparations? Licorice powder? Bisacodyl? How are each of these given?
5 What are the untoward reactions of iodide solutions given intravenously? What are the names of intravenous preparations with iodide bases that are used as radiopaque substances?
6 Review the chapter on electrolyte balance.
7 What foods are high in potassium? What are complete protein foods?
8 What are the end products of protein catabolism?
9 What is the normal nonprotein nitrogen? Blood urea nitrogen?
10 What is meant by dialysis?
11 What are the symptoms of cardiac failure? Pulmonary edema? Cerebral edema?
12 What is the action of 50% glucose? Of 50% magnesium sulfate?
13 Review procedures for measuring intake and output. What is the relation of output to intake in the normal person?
14 Review the physiology of voiding. What is the normal bladder capacity? At what point does one normally have the "urge to void"? What is retention of urine?
15 What is the normal capacity of the renal pelvis?
16 Review the signs and symptoms of hemorrhage.

17 Review the general principles of patient teaching.
18 What are the therapeutic action, the untoward results, and the method of administration of each of the following drugs: mandelic acid, methenamine (Urotropin), aluminum hydroxide gel, neostigmine bromide (Prostigmin bromide), and methantheline bromide (Banthine bromide)?
19 What is an acid-ash diet? An alkaline-ash diet?
20 How may bowel regularity be restored postoperatively? What is a paralytic ileus, and how is it treated?
21 With what large blood vessels do the renal vein and artery anastomose? At what three points are the ureters normally narrow? Which kidney is lower? What holds the kidneys in position? What is meant by the parenchyma of the kidney? By the calyxes? Is any portion of the urinary tract within the peritoneal cavity?
22 Locate the prostate in relation to the urethra, the bladder, and the rectum. Locate the external and internal bladder sphincters in women and in men.

Urology is concerned with the prevention, diagnosis, and treatment of disease of the urinary and genital systems in the male and of the urinary system in the female. However, this chapter will be concerned only with the male and female urinary systems. The male reproductive system, with

415

the exception of the obstructive lesions of the urethra, is considered in the following chapter on the reproductive system.

Whenever there is disease of any part of the urinary system, preservation or improvement of renal function is the primary objective of treatment. The reason is that the kidneys are the organs mainly responsible for maintenance of normal fluid and electrolyte balance and for the excretion of certain waste products. Without renal function, life can continue for only a few days.

The complex processes of renal function take place in the million or more nephrons located in the cortex and medulla of each kidney. The urine is excreted into the renal pelvis at a pressure of about 50 to 60 mm. Hg and passes by peristaltic action along the ureters to the collecting reservoir, the bladder, which has a lower pressure. Although the pelves, ureters, bladder, and urethra serve merely as the drainage and reservoir system, any obstruction or infection in them ultimately causes damage to the kidneys. When the pressure below the kidney becomes equal to or greater than that within the kidney, the efficiency of the system is lessened, and damage to nephrons can occur.

In 1964, disease of the kidneys and other organs of the urinary system caused 35,818 deaths in the United States.[49] Of these deaths, 13,500 were from malignancies, and the remainder were divided equally between chronic renal disease and acute urinary tract infections. In addition, 15,000 men died from hypertrophy of the prostate, a disease of the male reproductive system that causes kidney damage.

The nurse can help to reduce the amount of chronic illness and the number of deaths from disease of the urinary system by urging the person who has any symptoms of infection or obstruction of the urinary system to seek medical advice at once. Other specific ways in which she may help will be described in sections dealing with specific pathologic conditions.

The patient's emotional response to urologic disease

Fear and embarrassment are common in the patient when signs of urologic disease occur. Although most laymen have only a vague understanding of the anatomy and physiology of the urinary system, they do know that the kidneys are necessary for life. When a diagnosis of renal disease is suspected, they become frightened. Diseases that make voiding difficult not only cause discomfort but also lead to worry. Men are often fearful that disease or surgery involving the genitourinary system may decrease sexual ability. This prospect causes a man of any age to feel very much threatened. There is also a great fear of cancer. Patients with benign disease of the urinary system have been known to commit suicide because they were unable to believe the condition was nonmalignant.

The patient's embarrassment and anxiety may be expressed in a variety of ways. He may become depressed and withdrawn and may seek to delay medical diagnosis and treatment, or he may seem aggressive and perhaps even immodest. Signs of increasing anxiety should be watched for and appropriate measures taken to reduce it (Chapter 6). The patient may be too embarrassed to ask the questions that concern him most. Cultural and emotional patterns frequently inhibit discussion of the urinary and reproductive systems. Many men will be reluctant to discuss their problems with the nurse. Women may find it easier to discuss details with the nurse than with the doctor. If so, the nurse must relay information or suggest appropriate ways for the patient to discuss her problem with the doctor. Some patients may hesitate to take enough of the specialist's time to describe their problems adequately. They need to be encouraged to give full details.

The nurse should be sensitive to the patient's behavior and plan her care so that it will reduce the patient's anxiety and embarrassment. Careful explanations of the procedures to be done help to allay many fears, but for the explanations to be effective, the patient often needs some instruction in the anatomy and physiology of the genitourinary system. Simple diagrams are helpful (Fig. 89). Such instruction not only helps to overcome fear of the unknown, but it also helps to make the genitourinary system a less "unmentionable" subject because the patient learns the necessary anatomic

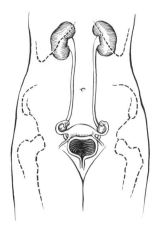

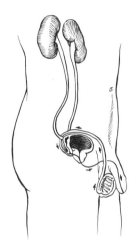

Fig. 89

The female and the male genitourinary systems and reproductive systems. The arrows indicate the route by which seminal fluid passes from the testes to the urethra.

terms with which to ask questions. Special care should always be taken to ensure the patient's privacy while he is discussing his urinary problems and undergoing examinations of the urinary system.

Making the urologic diagnosis

Since renal function is a prerequisite for life, it is fortunate that diseases in the urinary system can be diagnosed with an unusually high degree of accuracy. The urologic examination usually begins with a complete medical history and physical examination, including pelvic and rectal examinations. Thorough examination is important because urinary symptoms may be secondary to other systemic disorders. The nurse may have to interpret to the patient the need for these procedures. She may do so as she prepares him for the examinations and as she assists the doctor. Special examinations of the urinary system also are made. The necessary tests are selected carefully by the doctor. Food and fluids may have to be withheld for some tests, sedatives may be given, and catheterization or other procedures that are rather upsetting to the patient may be necessary.

Since the examinations are often done on an ambulatory basis either in a clinic or a doctor's office, the patient should be advised to bring someone with him who can be certain that he gets home safely. He or his relatives should be given printed instructions both for the preparation for examinations and for care at the conclusion of the tests. These instructions should be used as a supplement to verbal instructions, since the latter must often be given as the patient is preparing to leave the clinic and after he has had sedation. If food has been withheld, the patient should have something to eat before leaving for home.

The examinations and tests mentioned in this section are commonly done to assist in the diagnosis of many different urologic conditions. Examinations used in diagnosing specific problems will be discussed with each disorder. The preparation described is that usually given, but it may vary. For example, fluids may be withheld for only an hour before examination of infants and young children and very elderly persons to avoid electrolyte imbalance. No bowel preparation may be used on children or on patients whose ureters have been implanted into the bowel.

Examination of urine

Urinalysis. A voided urine specimen is usually examined first. About 75 to 100 ml. of urine should be voided into a clean container. Smaller quantities are acceptable for children. Urine from the first voiding of the day is preferred because it is more concentrated and abnormal constituents are less

417

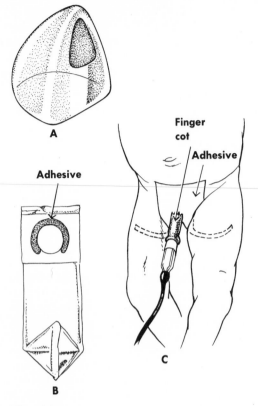

Fig. 90

Methods of collecting urine specimens from infants and small children. **A,** Birdcage feeder used for an infant girl. **B,** Plastic collecting device for boys and girls. **C,** Finger cot anchored with adhesive tape attached to drainage apparatus for collecting twenty-four-hour specimen.

likely to be missed. When a voided specimen contains abnormal constituents, a midstream, or "clean catch," specimen and perhaps a *catheterized* specimen of urine are examined. Since a catheterized specimen consists of urine that has passed through the kidneys, the ureters, and the bladder, further examination of specimens from individual kidneys may be collected by means of catheters placed through a cystoscope and into each of the ureters. This examination may locate the trouble more definitely.

A voided urine specimen is difficult to obtain from an infant or young child, and special techniques must be used. A plastic urine specimen collector treated with adhesive-

like material that adheres readily to the skin is available commercially for both boys and girls (Fig. 90). It is applied after thoroughly cleansing the area about the urinary meatus, and the open end is then attached to the drainage apparatus. A specimen of a single voiding from a male infant or a small boy can be obtained in a finger cot secured to the penis with adhesive. A single specimen can be collected from an infant girl by placing the baby on a small basin and, while holding her in an upright position, giving her a bottle. Another method is to separate the labia and place a Spicer infant urinal or a birdcage feeder over the meatus. This apparatus is secured by using two long strips of adhesive tape running from the abdomen under the buttock. Before adhesive is used on a child's skin, the skin should be painted well with tincture of benzoin to prevent irritation. Replacing the diaper prevents the child from pulling the apparatus off, but sometimes ankle and hand restraints may be needed.

Any abnormality in the specific gravity (below 1.003 or above 1.030) is usually due to inability of the renal tubules to be selective in reabsorption and excretion. For example, a marked decrease in specific gravity is found in diabetes insipidus due to a deficiency of posterior pituitary hormone, which influences renal tubular water absorption.

Multiple glass test. Occasionally it is helpful to have separate specimens from one voiding to determine if the abnormality is in the urethra, the bladder, or the prostate. The patient is asked to void about 100 ml. into the first container—the urethral "washings." Then he voids 100 ml. into a second container—the kidney and bladder "washings." If, in the male patient, prostatic "washings" are desired, the doctor gently massages the prostate immediately after the second voiding. The patient then finishes emptying the bladder, and this specimen will contain prostatic secretions.

Composite specimens. A specimen of all the urine excreted over a specific period of time often is needed. This specimen may be examined for constituents such as sugar, tubercle bacteria, and 17-ketosteroids. When urine excreted over a specified period of time is to be collected, the collection should be started at the appointed time by having the patient empty his bladder and discarding this urine. Urine from all subsequent voidings is saved, including that voided at the designated hour for closing the collection. It is important for the patient to understand that all urine must be saved; he should be instructed to void into a separate receptacle before defecation lest part of the specimen be lost.

The specimen should be kept refrigerated to prevent bacterial growth, which may alter its composition. Toluene may be added to the specimen until a film forms over the surface. This substance helps prevent bacterial growth. Sometimes formaldehyde is used as a preservative. The nurse should always check to find out how much of the specimen the laboratory needs. If only a sample is needed, the total specimen should be mixed well and a sample taken, but the total amount of urine voided in the allotted time should be recorded on the label.

If the patient is to collect the specimen at home, he should be told exactly how to collect and preserve it. He should be advised to use a jar with a tight cover and to place it in the refrigerator inside a paper bag. This will prevent contamination of food and also be more aesthetic. Advising him to return the specimen in a securely capped jar inside a paper bag may protect him from possible embarrassment.

Composite urine specimens are difficult to obtain from infants and young children. Restraints must sometimes be used. The most satisfactory method is to use the plastic material (previously described) connected to a collection bottle. For other procedures see specialized texts.[40]

When a test involves the collection of total urine output, it is important that the urine be collected from all available sources. For instance, the patient may void normally yet also have a nephrostomy tube from which urine drains. Specimens from each source should be collected in separate containers, since this may help determine the function of each kidney. Urine from a cystostomy tube and a urethral catheter may, however, be combined into one specimen because both specimens come from the bladder.

Urine culture. When infection appears to be present in the urinary system, a urine culture is often ordered. A 5 to 10 ml. specimen of urine is collected in a sterile tube under aseptic conditions. This is sent to the laboratory, where any organisms present are allowed to grow in culture media and then are identified microscopically. This information guides the doctor not only in making the diagnosis but also in ordering drug treatment.

Specimens for urine culture may be obtained either by catheterization or voiding, depending upon the doctor's wishes. The collection of a voided specimen for culture is the usual procedure because bacterial infection of the urinary tract frequently follows catheterization.

If a catheter is passed, a small amount of urine should be allowed to drain into a waste basin. Five to 10 ml. then should be collected directly into a culture tube, taking care not to touch the rim or the inside of the tube with the catheter or with the hands. The bladder should be allowed to empty completely before the catheter is removed. Cultures may also be ordered on urine taken from the renal pelves during ureteral catheterizations or when ureterostomy or nephrostomy tubes are in place. If a cotton plug is used as a stopper, the tube should be kept upright to prevent moistening the cotton and thereby contaminating the specimen.

To collect a sterile voided specimen from a woman, the nurse should first cleanse the genital area thoroughly with soap and water. Then, wearing a sterile glove, she should separate the labia so that the urinary meatus is exposed and should cleanse it as for a regular catheterization. While the nurse (or the patient, wearing a sterile glove) continues to hold the labia well separated, the patient voids. After the stream of urine has started, the nurse catches a specimen in a sterile pitcher. The specimen is then poured into a culture tube, labeled, and sent to the laboratory. This type of specimen is commonly referred to as a "clean catch" specimen.

When a urine culture is requested for a male patient, a voided specimen is usually used unless a catheter is being passed for some other reason. This is because of the danger of infecting the male reproductive tract during catheterization (p. 151). The penis should be well cleansed with a cotton

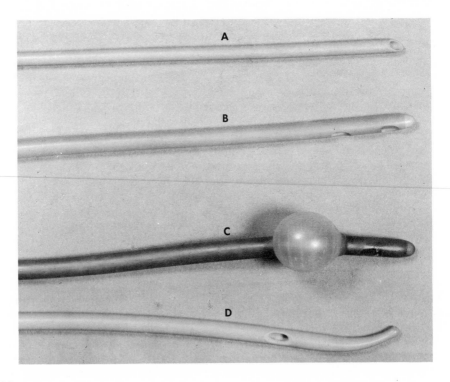

Fig. 91

Urethral catheters. **A,** Whistle-tip catheter. **B,** Many-eyed Robinson catheter. **C,** Foley catheter. **D,** Coudé catheter.

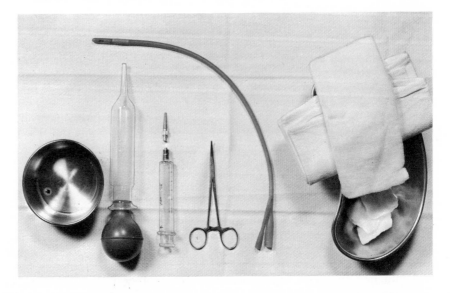

Fig. 92

Setup for inserting a Foley catheter in a male patient.

pledget saturated with a mild antiseptic such as benzalkonium chloride 1:1000; slight friction is used, and special attention should be given to the meatus. The patient is then asked to void 50 to 100 ml., which are discarded. This precaution decreases the possibility of contaminating the specimen with organisms present in the urethra. The patient then voids 10 to 15 ml. into a sterile pitcher. This urine is poured into the culture tube, labeled, and sent to the laboratory. Collection of the specimen is usually done by a male member of the nursing team or by the patient himself if he can be relied upon to use the necessary aseptic precautions.

To obtain a sterile voided specimen for culture from a child, the nurse uses the procedures for collecting a single voided specimen of urine. The local area should be cleansed especially well, and sterile collecting apparatus should be used.

Evaluating bladder function

The doctor may need to know how much urine remains in the bladder after a patient has voided. This remaining urine is known as residual urine. Normally, following voiding, the bladder contains practically no urine. If urine is retained in the bladder after voiding, it stagnates, becoming a good medium for bacterial growth. It also encourages formation of bladder stones. Sometimes a patient having difficulty with micturition may be catheterized periodically for residual urine. A decrease in the residual urine to 50 ml. or less is an indication that function is returning to normal, and catheterization usually is discontinued. The patient should empty the bladder *immediately* before catheterization. If there is a delay, additional urine will be excreted from the kidneys, giving an inaccurate result. It is best to explain the procedure to the patient and then leave him for a few moments while he voids. It is important to stress that the bladder should be completely emptied because patients with urethral obstruction often void only enough at a time to relieve pressure. With additional concentration, the patient may be able to empty his bladder almost completely. To evaluate the size and strength of the urinary stream and to estimate the difficulty that the patient has in voiding, the doctor may wish to observe the

male patient as he voids. Since this observation is more meaningful if the patient does not know that he is being watched, he may be given a basin to use rather than a urinal, and the screen or door may be left slightly ajar.

When the doctor first catheterizes a patient, various catheters should be provided. Inability to pass catheters of the usual caliber may signify stricture of the urethra. Size 14 to 20 Fr. soft rubber catheters are commonly used for women, and sizes 16 to 24 Fr. are used for men. For infants and small children, size 6, 8, or 10 Fr. may be used. (French is the scale used to graduate catheters: 1 Fr. equals ⅓ mm. in diameter.)

The doctor should be consulted before preparing the equipment for catheterization because, if he suspects much residual urine, he may use a Foley catheter, which may be left in place to provide continuous bladder drainage. If there is residual urine after the patient has been catheterized, the amount should be measured and recorded and the urine saved as a catheterized specimen to avoid having to recatheterize the patient if a sterile specimen is needed.

To avoid passing a catheter to measure residual urine, it is now fairly common practice to inject a small amount of radiopaque substance intravenously. If the dye is excreted by the kidney and passes into the bladder, it will show up on x-ray film. From a roentgenogram taken immediately after voiding, a determination of the amount of urine left in the bladder can be made. By this means, infection resulting from catheterization may be avoided. (The injection of radiopaque substance is described on p. 426.)

Evaluating renal function

If anything in the general examination or the urinalysis suggests renal damage, the doctor will probably order a number of renal function tests.

Blood chemistry tests. Since the concentration of urea in the body is regulated primarily by the rate at which the kidney excretes urea, the level of urea in the blood is a good index of renal function. When renal function is impaired, there is an elevation in the blood urea level. Either a blood urea nitrogen (BUN) test or a blood nonprotein nitrogen (NPN) test may be done. Serum creatinine levels, however, have been found to reflect renal impairment earlier and may be used in preference to, or in conjunction with, determinations of blood urea content. It is important that the patient have no food or fluid containing protein for six hours before the blood for any of these tests is obtained. Since urea and creatinine are end products of protein metabolism, only a fasting blood specimen gives an accurate index of renal function. The normal blood urea nitrogen level is 10 to 20 mg. per 100 ml.; the normal nonprotein nitrogen level is 15 to 35 mg. per 100 ml.; the normal serum creatinine level is 1 to 2 mg. per 100 ml. The nurse needs to note the blood urea and creatinine levels of patients who have renal damage. If the level is high, the patient may have impending uremia (p. 430).

When blood proteins are being lost due to faulty renal function, the albumin molecule, being smaller than the globulin fraction, is lost in larger amounts. A determination of the ratio of these two protein fractions in the blood gives an indication of the extent of the derangement and may be ordered particularly in nephrosis. The normal relationship (A/G ratio) is approximately 2:1. Since chronic disease of the kidneys causes derangement of the electrolyte system, determinations of the levels of calcium (9 to 11 mg./100 ml. of blood), phosphorus (3 to 4.5 mg./100 ml. of blood), and sodium (137 to 143 mEq./liter) may be obtained. A determination of the acid phosphatase level in the blood may be ordered, and increased levels indicate metastatic malignant involvement of the bones. The normal level varies with the method used, one method (Gutman) giving 1 to 4 units/100 ml. of blood and the other (Bodansky), 0.2 to 0.8 unit/100 ml. of blood.

Phenolsulfonphthalein test. Since phenolsulfonphthalein (a red dye) is a substance that the normal kidneys excrete completely, it is used to determine renal function. A phenolsulfonphthalein test (PSP test) may be done to estimate the amount of obstruction below the kidney that may be delaying the emptying of the renal pelves.

It is helpful for the nurse to know how this test is done in the laboratory so that she will be aware of how to prevent inaccurate results when obtaining specimens. Water is added to each specimen until it has a volume of 1,000 ml. The specimen is then alkalized because the dye is not visible in acid urine. Then the color of each specimen is compared to a standard on a colorimeter to determine the amount of dye excreted. Normally the dye will begin to appear in the bladder three to six minutes after injection, with 15 to 20% of it appearing in the first specimen and 80% being excreted within two hours. The injection of more or less than 1 ml. of dye will cause inaccuracies, because 1 ml. of phenolsulfonphthalein is the basis for the color indicator. Incomplete emptying of the renal pelves or bladder also causes inaccuracies because not all the dye excreted by the kidneys is collected. Blood in the urine and phenazopyridine hydrochloride (Pyridium), a urinary antiseptic that gives urine a red color, will also make the test inaccurate.

The test is done as follows: The patient voids, and the urine is discarded after being inspected for any red discoloration. The prescribed amount of dye is then given intravenously or intramuscularly. (Since the intravenous route gives more accurate results and is most often used, only this procedure is discussed. Specific instructions from the laboratory should be obtained for tests using the intramuscular route for administration of the dye.) Exactly 1 ml. of phenolsulfonphthalein dye is injected intravenously. Special care must be taken that the dye does not infiltrate the tissues. If it does, the test must be delayed for twenty-four hours. The patient is urged to drink several glasses of water or other fluid before the dye is injected and during the test. He may eat if he wishes. Specimens consisting of all the urine the patient can void are collected exactly fifteen minutes, thirty minutes, one hour, and two hours after the injection of the dye. Each specimen must be labeled carefully with the exact time of collection. The label on the first specimen should indicate the time the dye was injected.

Occasionally the patient is unable to void at the desired time, but urination can usually be promoted by forcing fluids. If the patient cannot void or does not appear to be emptying his bladder, the doctor should be notified. He may *very occasionally* order a catheterization done. Usually only a note of the time of voiding and of its being incomplete are made on the specimen and on the chart so that adjustments in findings can be made.

The patient who is not acutely ill can usually collect his own specimens for a phenolsulfonphthalein test if he is given a watch, properly labeled bottles, and careful instruction. The nurse must make certain that he does the test correctly and that he will send for her if he is unable to collect any one of the specimens at the appointed time.

Urea clearance test. The urea clearance test measures the efficiency of the glomerular filtration of plasma. Normally, 55 to 75 ml. of plasma are cleared of urea per minute. If an accurate result is to be obtained in the laboratory, the urine flow must be at least 2 ml. per minute. Therefore, most laboratories ask that the patient drink two glasses of water when the "discard specimen" is obtained and two more after voiding for the first urine specimen. The patient should fast until after the blood sample is taken.

The test is done as follows: The patient completely empties his bladder (the "discard specimen") and drinks the prescribed amount of water. One hour later he is asked to void again, and a blood sample is taken for blood urea nitrogen determination. All the urine at this second voiding is collected and labeled as the first specimen. The exact times at which the "discarded specimen" and this specimen were collected should be indicated. An hour later, a second urine specimen is obtained, and all the specimens, carefully identified, are sent to the laboratory. If the patient is unable to void normally and to empty his bladder completely, catheterized specimens may be ordered. If the test has been accurate, the blood urea will be elevated and the urine urea decreased in patients with poor renal function, whereas the reverse will be true if there is no disease. The two urine specimens should give comparable results.

Creatinine clearance test. A creatinine clearance test may be used instead of a urea clearance test. It, too, measures the efficiency of the glomerular filtration of plasma. A twenty-four-hour collection of urine is made, beginning and ending in the morning. At the completion of the period of urine collection, a blood sample is drawn for serum creatinine; the patient should be fasting. The normal amount of creatinine excreted in the urine in a twenty-four-hour period varies with age. A 17-year-old person will excrete approximately 1.58 grams, whereas an adult will excrete 1.2 to 1.7 grams.

Urine concentration and dilution tests. When the kidneys are damaged, the ability of the tubules to concentrate and to dilute urine is impaired. When damage is severe, the specific gravity of the urine is said to be "fixed," meaning that no matter what the fluid intake is, the specific gravity of the urine remains the same, or about 1.010 to 1.012. A fixed low specific gravity, therefore, is indicative of serious renal disease.

The ability of the kidneys to concentrate urine may be measured by several tests. The *Fishberg concentration test* is commonly used. The patient eats his usual evening meal and is instructed to take no more food or fluids until after the completion of the test the next morning. Urine specimens are collected at 6 A.M., 7 A.M., and 8 A.M. Morning specimens are collected because a normal kidney concentrates urine during the night at approximately twice the rate it does during waking hours.

The *Addis concentration test* is much more vigorous in the dehydration of the patient. It gives a more sensitive measurement, but if the patient's nonprotein nitrogen determination is high, or if he is a child under 5 years of age, it is used with caution because of the danger of precipitating a serious electrolyte imbalance. Fluids are markedly restricted for twenty-four hours. The amount allowed varies with the laboratory making the test. During the last twelve hours of the test all urine is saved.

The *Mosenthal concentration test* is a twenty-four-hour test in which neither food nor fluids are restricted. Total urinary output from 7 P.M. to 7 A.M. is saved, and then separate specimens are collected at two-hour intervals through 7 P.M.

The *Fishberg dilution test* is used to determine the ability of the kidney to dilute urine. It may be done at any time of day, but the patient should remain inactive during the test so that extra fluid and waste products are not produced by increased metabolism and fluid is not lost through perspiration or respirations. He should completely empty the bladder at the beginning of the test, and the adult should drink 1,200 ml. of fluid within one-half hour. The doctor should be consulted as to the amount to give children. Urine specimens are then collected every half hour for three hours. A person with normal hydration and normal renal function will excrete almost the entire 1,200 ml. in the three-hour period, and the urine will have a specific gravity of about 1.022. Since most patients will have difficulty in drinking 1,200 ml. of fluid in a half-hour period, it sometimes helps if water is mixed with fruit juice to make a weak fruit ade. Each specimen should include all urine voided and should be sent to the laboratory. The label on the specimen should include the exact time of each voiding.

Fig. 93

Radiorenography. Scintillation probes are in place over both kidneys. (Courtesy Veterans Administration Center, Martinsburg, W. Va.; from Abt, Arthur F., and Balkus, Vincent A.: J. Urol. **85**:95, 1961.)

Radiorenography. The radiorenogram may be used as a screening test for renal dysfunction or to study individual renal function. A radiopaque dye such as iodohippurate sodium (Hippuran) tagged with radioiodine (I^{131}) is injected intravenously. The amount used and the precautions are the same as for use of radiopaque dye for intravenous pyelography. No precautions against radioactivity need to be taken because only tracer doses are used.

As a *screening test,* voided urine specimens are collected twenty and ninety minutes after injection of the radioactive radiopaque dye and are tested with a scintillation detector or a Geiger counter for radioiodine content. Normally 75% of the radioiodine will be excreted within thirty minutes.

As a test of *individual renal function,* two methods may be used. Ureteral catheters may be inserted and urine collected from each catheter at five-minute intervals and tested. If no catheters are used, tracings are made for thirty minutes over the kidney regions using a special apparatus (gamma-ray probes, rate meters, and recorders). The probes are placed at an angle to the patient's back and are pointed directly toward each kidney. (See Fig. 93.) From these tracings

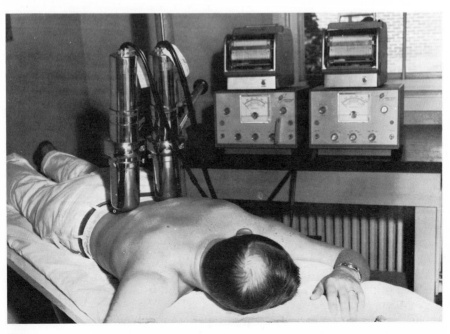

a qualitative estimate of the renal vascularity, tubular cell function, and ability of the kidney to excrete urine can be made.

Visual examination of the urinary tract

An intravenous pyelogram usually is ordered when renal or lower urinary tract disease is suspected. In this test, a roentgenogram shows the kidney shadows and the filling of the renal pelves, and it outlines the ureters and the bladder.

Before the test is scheduled, an attempt is made to learn whether or not the patient is sensitive to iodine, because the radiopaque medium that is injected intravenously contains iodine. Serious and even fatal reactions have occurred in sensitive persons. A history of allergy or of serious kidney or liver damage may also be contraindications to the use of radiopaque substances. The patient should be prepared initially for this examination by an explanation of the procedure, its purpose, and the reasons for the physical preparation. He is usually instructed to omit food and fluids from 12 o'clock the night before until after the examination is completed because a higher concentration of the radiopaque medium in the urinary tract and reduced peristalsis and the absence of gas in the intestinal tract produce a clearer roentgenogram. If the patient is an infant or a child under 7 years of age, food and fluids usually are withheld six to eight hours, but a specific order should be obtained for each child.

Since the kidneys lie retroperitoneally, it is important that the bowel be empty of gas and fecal material, which may cause shadows on the film. If the patient has received barium prior to an intravenous pyelogram, the bowel must be especially well emptied because any residual barium may obscure the kidney picture. Usually, however, this problem is prevented by carefully scheduling the tests so that those for renal function precede barium swallows, gastrointestinal series, or barium enemas. A low-residue diet may be ordered for the day before the examination, and a generous dose of a cathartic such as castor oil (30 ml.), compound senna powder (compound licorice powder, 4 Gm.), or bisacodyl (Dulcolax, 20 mg.) may be given the evening before the test. Infants and small children usually are not given any

laxative. If too much flatus is present in the bowel at the time of the roentgenogram, 8 to 10 ounces of formula may be given to the baby and a carbonated beverage to the older child, in order to stimulate peristalsis so that the flatus passes beyond the renal area. If the patient has evidence of peptic ulcers or colitis, has a colostomy or a ureterosigmoidal transplant, or is extremely debilitated, these relatively vigorous cathartics are usually not ordered. Therefore, before giving the medication, the nurse should know something about the physical condition of the patient and should bring to the doctor's attention any order for a cathartic that she believes might be contraindicated. The patient with seriously limited renal function may suffer profound electrolyte imbalance as a result of their use and of the withholding of fluids and food. Infants, young children, and occasionally elderly persons may suffer imbalance even when renal function is within normal limits.

Patients can become quite weak from drastic catharsis, and this weakness may lead to accidents. The patient who has received a cathartic should not be given sedation to induce sleep, and he should be told where to find the call light and the bathroom or bedpan. If he is elderly or debilitated, he must be urged to call for assistance to go to the bathroom.

The nurse should determine and record the effectiveness of efforts to evacuate the bowel, reporting ineffective results to the doctor. Occasionally if the cathartic has been ineffectual or if it is contraindicated for some reason, enemas or a bisacodyl suppository may be given. Enemas must be given early in the morning to allow time for excretion of the fluid absorbed during the enema and for expulsion of flatus.

For the radiogram the patient usually is placed on an x-ray table in a lithotomy position, and all the precautions discussed under placing a patient in position for a vaginal examination should be taken (p. 482). Occasionally he lies supine on a full-length x-ray table. A roentgenogram of the abdominal area (a flat plate) is taken first. It gives information as to the size, shape, and position of the kidneys and the amount of gas in the bowel, and reveals radiopaque stones anywhere along the urinary system. After this film is developed and read, the radiopaque dye is given intravenously. Sometimes, a large plastic ball is strapped firmly on the abdomen to prevent the dye from passing freely down the ureters until after the roentgenogram of the kidneys has been taken.

Several radiopaque preparations are used for intravenous pyelogram examinations. All of them contain iodine, and all may cause serious reactions in persons sensitive to the drug in this form. Diatrizoate (Hypaque) and diatrizoate methylglucamine (Renografin) are preparations widely used at the present time. The nurse never, under any circumstances, injects the substance herself. The patient should know that he may have a feeling of warmth, a flushing of the face, and a salty taste in the mouth as the doctor slowly injects the drug intravenously. These sensations usually last only a few minutes and may be relieved by taking deep breaths. The nurse should then watch for any signs of respiratory difficulty, sudden diaphoresis and clamminess, or urticaria, any of which may indicate an untoward reaction to the contrast medium. If the patient complains of numbness or tingling of any part of the body, of palpitation, or of any other unusual sensation, he must be attended constantly, and the doctor must be immediately summoned. Tripelennamine (Pyribenzamine), diphenhydramine hydrochloride (Benadryl), epinephrine (Adrenalin),

and oxygen should be available for immediate use if necessary.

Roentgenograms are usually taken seven and fifteen minutes after the drug is injected. If poor renal function is suspected, films may also be taken one and two hours later. When delayed films are necessary, the patient must either be returned to his bed or protected from discomfort on the table. If he must remain on the table, a soft bath blanket should be placed under him, and he should be assisted in changing position at fifteen-minute intervals.

Cytoscopy and retrograde pyelography. A cystoscopy is the examination of the inside of the bladder through a metal instrument called a *cystocope* (Fig. 94). The instrument is constructed with illumination, enabling the examiner to see the interior of the bladder. Newer equipment made of more flexible materials gives promise of even better visualization of the interior of the bladder in the future.[30]

A cystoscopic examination is indicated for all patients who have, or have had, hematuria because, although blood in the urine may have other causes, it is one of the earliest signs of malignant growths anywhere along the urinary system. The examination may be done as part of an intensive diagnostic study, or it may be done as an emergency diagnostic measure. By doing an immediate cystoscopy, the doctor may lo-

Fig. 94

A cystoscope inserted for examination of the bladder. **A,** Appearance of a normal ureteral orifice as seen through the cystoscope. **B,** Appearance of papillomas of the bladder as seen through the cystoscope. **C,** Appearance of a trabeculated bladder as seen through the cystoscope. Note the formation of cellules.

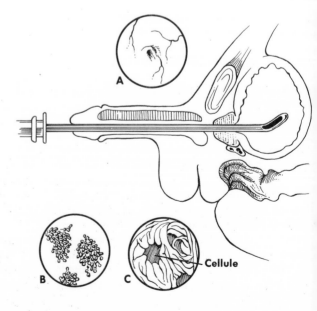

cate a point of hemorrhage in the prostate, the bladder, or the upper urinary tracts that might otherwise escape detection, because such hemorrhages frequently stop spontaneously for a time. If the examination of only the urethra and the prostate appears necessary, a shorter instrument, known as an *endoscope*, is used.

Nursing attention before and during a cystoscopic examination can contribute greatly to its success and to lessening the patient's discomfort. The patient should know what he will experience in the cystoscopy room. He may have no idea of what to expect and may be reluctant to ask the doctor. The nurse should give thorough explanations before the procedure is begun, and she should remain with the patient during the procedure, giving him reassurance and encouragement. This helps him to relax and decreases discomfort, much of which is due to contraction or spasm of the sphincters of the bladder.

Most hospitals require a signed permit before a cystoscopy, and the nurse should check to see that a permit has been signed.

Fluids are usually forced for several hours before the patient goes to the cystoscopy room, ensuring a continuous flow of urine in case urine specimens are to be collected from the kidneys. If an anesthetic is to be used, fluids may be given intravenously. Food usually is withheld from all patients because apprehension may make the patient nauseated. If the doctor expects to take roentgenograms, cathartics and enemas may be ordered as for an intravenous pyelogram. A sedative such as phenobarbital and a narcotic such as morphine or meperidine hydrochloride (Demerol) may be given about a half hour prior to the examination.

Clothing must be removed for the examination and replaced by a hospital gown and lithotomy boots. The patient is then placed in a lithotomy position on the cystoscopy table and is draped so that only the perineum is exposed. In placing the patient in position, care must be taken that pressure is not exerted upon the popliteal spaces, since pressure may cause circulatory embarrassment and lead to thrombosis in blood vessels. Because of arthritis and related disorders, some elderly patients are unable to rest comfortably in the stirrups, and it may be necessary

to use slings instead. If prolonged time on the table is necessary, the patient's legs should be removed from the stirrups at intervals and flexed and extended a few times. Extra pillows may be needed under the patient's head and shoulders.

If the patient is emotionally prepared and relatively comfortable, he should be able to relax enough so that the cystoscope can be passed with little pain, provided there is no obstruction in the urethra. Deep breathing will sometimes help the patient relax. A local anesthetic such as procaine (usually 4%) may be instilled into the urethra immediately prior to the insertion of the cystoscope. If the patient is very apprehensive or if much manipulation is anticipated, a general anesthetic may be given to avoid sudden vigorous movement during the examination, which might cause trauma to the urethra or perforation of the bladder. Chil-

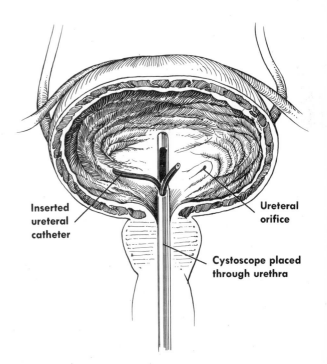

Inserted ureteral catheter

Ureteral orifice

Cystoscope placed through urethra

Fig. 95

Ureteral catheterization through the cystoscope. Note the ureteral catheter inserted into the right orifice. The left ureteral catheter is ready to be inserted.

dren are almost always given a general anesthetic for this procedure.

If the patient is not under general anesthesia, passing the instrument will be followed immediately by a strong desire to void. This is because of the pressure of the instrument against the internal sphincter and because the bladder is filled with distilled water during the examination to distend its walls and thus make visualization more effective.

When the trouble is not located in the bladder, a ureteral catheter (nylon, radiopaque, calibrated, and size 4 or 6 Fr.) is passed through the cystoscope and inserted into the ureteral opening in the bladder, up the ureter, and into the renal pelvis (Fig. 95). This procedure is known as a *ureteral catheterization* and may involve one or both of the ureters. Specimens of urine may thus be obtained directly from each kidney for microscopic examination and culture, smears for tubercle bacilli, cancer cells, and other abnormal constituents. Renal function tests of each kidney may be carried out during ureteral catheterization by injecting indigo carmine (a blue dye) or phenolsulfonphthalein (a red dye) intravenously and timing its appearance in the urine from each kidney. With normal function, the dye will appear from each side in three to six minutes. Radioiodine tests may also be done.

A sharp x-ray outline of the kidney and the ureters can be obtained by injecting 4 to 8 ml. of radiopaque substance such as Hypaque or Renografin gently up each ureteral catheter after urine specimens have been collected. While the solution is being injected, the patient who is awake may feel slight discomfort in the kidney region, but pain should not be experienced unless too much of the solution has been injected, causing overdistention of the renal pelvis. As the doctor withdraws the catheters and the cystoscope, he again injects the contrast medium (1 to 2 ml.), which fills the ureters, and then he immediately has another roentgenogram made that will show the outline of the ureters. This examination is known as *retrograde pyelography*.

Care should be taken that the patient, especially if he is elderly, does not stand or walk alone immediately afterward, since blood that has drained from the legs while he was in the lithotomy position flows back into the vessels of the feet and legs as he stands up. Accidents caused by dizziness and fainting can occur from the sudden change in distribution of blood, which reduces the blood supply to the brain. Upon returning to his hospital room or home, the patient should remain in bed for a few hours. The nurse should observe the patient's urinary output for several hours. The urine may be pink-tinged, but more extensive bleeding should be reported to the doctor. If dyes such as indigo carmine have been used, the patient should be told that the urine will be an unusual color (blue). Frequent local and systemic reactions to a cystoscopic procedure include a "full" sensation and a feeling of burning in the bladder, pain in the lower back and a sensation of chilliness. Mild analgesics such as acetylsalicylic acid and codeine sulfate may be prescribed for discomfort, but usually the greatest relief is obtained from warmth, which produces relaxation and relieves muscle tension. A heating pad or hot-water bottle may be prescribed to be applied over the bladder region or to the lower back. Warm fluids should be offered at hourly intervals for at least four hours. When the chilliness subsides, a warm tub bath may be taken. Generous amounts of fluid dilute the urine and thereby lessen irritation to the mucous membrane linings of the urinary tract.

Sharp abdominal pain should be reported to the doctor, and analgesics should be withheld until he has examined the patient because the bladder or ureters may have been perforated accidentally, causing peritonitis. Pronounced chills with marked elevation of temperature sometimes follows cystoscopic procedures. They are thought to be caused by a general systemic reaction to the foreign substances introduced, the instrumentation, and the pain. Usually these symptoms respond within a short time to extra warmth and to warm fluids by mouth, but if they persist, the doctor should be notified.

Renal angiography. The renal angiogram clearly outlines the renal blood supply. The examination is particularly indicated in cases of hypertension of suspected renal origin. It may also be used to demonstrate large renal neoplasms, abnormal renal blood vessels, and the absence of a kidney. It is sometimes used postoperatively to study the remaining renal tissue. A radiopaque dye such as Hypaque, similar to that used for intravenous pyelography, is injected intravenously or intra-arterially into large vessels not far distant from the renal vessels. The preparation of the patient is similar to that for intravenous pyelography, and the same precautions against drug reactions should be taken (p. 426).

When the contrast medium is injected intravenously, the examination may be called *intravenous abdominal aortography*. A circulation time determination is done concurrently to guide the timing of the films. The contrast medium is injected simultaneously into a large vein in each arm (see discussion on nephrotomography, p. 461). To prevent obstruction of the subclavian veins by the first ribs, the patient is asked to raise his arms and relax his shoulders during the injection. When the contrast medium is injected intra-arterially, the examination is called *aortography*. In *translumbar aortography* the aorta is punctured with a long needle inserted through the soft tissue in the lumbar region, and the contrast medium is then injected. The patient must be anesthetized. If a *femoral percutaneous aortogram* is made, a "cut-down" is made on the femoral artery. An arterial catheter is then inserted and threaded into the aorta, and the radiopaque substance is injected.

Renal failure

Renal failure, which is also referred to as *renal insufficiency* or *renal suppression,* is a serious derangement of renal function in which the kidneys are unable to carry out normal excretion of waste products and other functions essential for maintenance of fluid and electrolyte balance and therefore of life. Renal failure may be acute or chronic. When the condition progresses to the point where symptoms appear, the patient is said to have *uremia*, while the rise in the waste products in the blood is referred to as *azotemia*.

Causes of renal failure

Acute renal failure may result from acute infection of the glomeruli of the kidney, from sudden urinary tract obstruction, or from acute renal tubular necrosis (lower nephron nephrosis). It may be brought on by the ingestion of poisons such as bichloride of mercury, certain mushrooms, and carbon tetrachloride, or it may result from mismatched blood or from drugs such as the sulfonamides. It may be secondary to a decrease in the blood supply to the kidneys, as may occur in arteriosclerosis and is a fairly common complication of coronary artery disease with myocardial infarction, in which the blood pressure drops suddenly. Emboli or thrombi in renal arteries or veins may prevent flow of blood to the nephrons. There may be an insufficient blood supply passing through the kidneys due to severe dehydration, loss of blood, circulatory collapse secondary to such events as anesthesia, toxemia of pregnancy, shock resulting from internal fluid loss and unusual distribution of body fluids following burns, and severe tissue trauma.

Chronic renal failure develops from persistence of the conditions causing acute failure, in which damage to the glomeruli is irreversible so that only a very marginal or submarginal functional capacity remains. The most common causes are pyelonephritis that becomes chronic, and obstruction of long standing somewhere along the urinary tract, causing a back pressure of urine into the renal pelves and in turn a pressure on the parenchyma of the kidneys with destruction of the functioning units. Other causes include polycystic kidneys, nephrosclerosis, malignant hypertension, serum sensitivity reaction, and collagen disease. An acute infection may cause renal failure in a person whose renal function is already limited. Pregnancy may increase the workload of the kidneys enough to cause renal failure in the person who has a history of permanent damage to the kidneys and a low margin of safety in renal function.

Prognosis

The prognosis in renal failure depends upon the underlying cause. If the primary cause can be removed or corrected, as is often possible in acute renal failure, the prognosis is good. Recovery from acute glomerulonephritis with renal failure has improved remarkably in recent years. If, however, the chronic condition is irreversible and substantial permanent damage has been sustained by the glomeruli, the onset of uremia may indicate that death will occur in the relatively near future. Remissions may occur and may be prolonged by avoidance of infection, overactivity, obesity, and any other conditions that increase the work load of the damaged kidneys.

Prevention

Acute renal failure can sometimes be prevented. Federal legislation controls the distribution to the layman of drugs that may damage the kidneys. If drugs that may have an untoward effect on kidneys, such as streptomycin, are prescribed, renal function usually is evaluated periodically. Careful observation of the blood pressure should be made during and immediately after surgery, and if it is low, treatment should be instituted to prevent its falling to levels that markedly decrease the blood flow through the kidneys. Immediate restoration of fluids to patients who have sustained serious accidental blood loss also decreases the likelihood of renal damage. Patients with streptococcal infections should have medical attention, since this type of infection always precedes acute glomerulonephritis.

The removal of lesions that may obstruct the urinary tract and cause pressure on the nephrons also helps to prevent acute renal failure. Since obstruction is one of the most common causes of damage to the kidneys and of renal failure, any signs of obstruction should be reported to the doctor at once. Much renal damage is sustained because elderly men with hypertrophy of the prostate delay treatment. In children, congenital anomalies anywhere along the tract may produce obstruction with serious renal damage before symptoms occur. The nurse working in the home or in a well-baby or well-child clinic should be certain that any difficulties in voiding are reported to the physician.

In recent years pyelonephritis is being recognized as a very common condition that is responsible for much renal damage. It is believed to be the cause of over one-third of all deaths from uremia and has been found in 6 to 8% of all patients at autopsy.[19] Prevention is attempted by early treatment of infections anywhere in the body (since they may localize in the kidneys), by avoiding catheterizing any patient of either sex or any age unless it is absolutely necessary, and by careful attention to hygiene to prevent colon bacilli from entering through the urethra. Prompt changing of diapers after defecation and careful cleansing of the perineum may help to prevent pyelonephritis, which is the second most common infection of infants and more common in girls than boys. It is believed that the simple technique of cleansing from the front posteriorly after bowel evacuation may help, and the nurse should not only teach the advisability of this technique but help the woman patient confined to bed in the hospital to carry out the advised procedure. Careful sponging of the rectal area after defecation is also recommended.

Signs and symptoms

There are many signs and symptoms of renal insufficiency and impending uremia. A common symptom of acute renal failure is oliguria, or decrease in normal urinary output. Occasionally anuria, or no urinary output at all, occurs. There may be hematuria. Edema, particularly about the face, may develop in acute renal failure, and repeated examinations of the blood may show a gradual increase in the nonprotein nitrogen and creatinine content. Other signs and symptoms are similar to those in chronic uremia.

Chronic renal failure is a complex process producing profound changes that are as yet poorly understood. Accumulation of the end products of protein metabolism, such as urea nitrogen and creatinine (azotemia), always occurs. The presence of these substances in the blood, however, has not been found to be responsible for many of the signs and symptoms that appear, and many of the signs and symptoms do not respond to the usual form of treatment. For example, the patient who has twitching and other signs of tetany and is found to have a low blood calcium level, (hypocalcemia) may not respond to the administration of calcium intravenously. Some patients may have few early signs of impending uremia. Instead, symptoms of water and electrolyte imbalance may herald the disorder.

Signs and symptoms of uremia usually develop so slowly that the patient and his family may not be able to recall the time of their onset. The patient may have felt "below par" for months or years, with headaches, irritability, and mental and physical fatigue, depression, and personality change. Persistent anorexia and vague gastrointestinal symptoms are extremely frequent in early uremia and may be accompanied by long periods of hiccoughing. Halitosis is common, and diarrhea occurs occasionally. These symptoms, particularly when they occur in elderly people or in persons with a history of renal disease, indicate the need for immediate medical attention.

The patient may have nocturia, as the failing kidneys are no longer able to concentrate urine during sleeping hours. Total output of urine may be normal or even increased in quantity, yet the waste products contained therein may be below normal, resulting in a low specific gravity of the urine. Albumin may or may not be found in the urine. Occasionally the patient develops unusual thirst, and the output of urine is much above normal although edema may not occur. At other times, edema develops and is first noticed about the eyes, particularly in the morning. Later, edema develops in the lower abdomen and lower trunk, and "pitting edema" of the ankles occurs. "Pitting edema" refers to a soft fullness of subcutaneous tissue that can be depressed (pitted) with the fingertip. The indentation disappears slowly.

Pallor is usually pronounced in impending uremia and may be secondary to the anemia that always develops. Yellowish discoloration may occur in skin areas, and pruritus often develops and may be severe. These symptoms may be caused by the waste products that sometimes are deposited on the skin. In advanced uremia, these urea and salt crystals may appear as a white, powdery substance on the skin (uremic frost).

Electrolyte imbalance may lead to acidosis, with nausea, vomiting, thirst, and air hunger. Calcium metabolism is often altered, and calcium may be excreted by the failing kidney in abnormally large amounts. Its depletion may cause muscle twitching, irritability, tetany, and convulsions. Potassium retention is one of the most serious problems, since potassium intoxication causes increasing generalized weakness, cardiac failure, and pulmonary edema. Some patients

remain mentally alert for a surprisingly long time considering the extent of electrolyte imbalance, but if renal function is not restored, coma eventually occurs.

Other signs of renal failure include blurred vision, dizziness, dimness of vision, and spots before the eyes. Many times, impending uremia is detected when the patient goes to his ophthalmologist because of failing vision, and retinal hemorrhages characteristic of chronic nephritis are observed. These hemorrhages occur most often in the patient who has pronounced hypertension. Most but not all patients with uremia have hypertension. Persistent vomiting not preceded by nausea may also occur.

A fairly common accompaniment of renal failure is ulceration and bleeding of the entire gastrointestinal tract. The cause is not precisely known, although it may be related to the stubborn anemia that always occurs in chronic nephritis and in uremia. Blood may be found in the feces, and the mucous membranes of the mouth frequently bleed. It is not unusual for death to be immediately preceded by convulsions and vomiting of blood.

General treatment and nursing care in acute renal failure

There are two main objectives in the care of patients with acute renal failure. First, the primary cause is treated in an attempt to prevent further renal damage—obstructions are relieved, fluid and blood losses are replaced when there is shock, hemorrhage, or dehydration, and antidotes for poisons and injurious drugs are given when possible. Second, an effort is made to maintain the fluid and electrolyte balance as close to normal as possible and to decrease the work of the kidneys so that the injured tissues may regenerate. The following discussion is concerned only with maintaining the patient until the primary cause is removed and the kidney has had time to return to normal.

Maintaining fluid and electrolyte balance

The nurse should report early signs of renal insufficiency because early treatment for fluid and electrolyte imbalance may minimize the renal damage. Changes in the urinary output are significant. Any decrease in the urinary output below 500 ml.

a day should be reported at once, since it is known that, even if the patient fasts and goes without water, normal kidneys will excrete at least that amount of urine a day.[3] All intake by mouth and other routes and all output from the kidney and other routes, such as vomiting, must be carefully measured and recorded because this information helps the doctor determine how much fluid the patient should have. Signs of sodium and other electrolyte depletion should be reported to the doctor at once (p. 99).

When the kidneys fail to excrete an adequate amount of urine, fluids are usually limited to 800 to 1,000 ml. a day plus enough extra fluids to replace those lost through routes other than the urinary system.[3] If larger amounts of fluid are given, cardiac failure caused by excessive blood volume may occur, since the kidneys are unable to excrete the excess fluid. The salt intake varies with the individual patient and with his response to treatment. Usually no more salt is permitted than the amount that is lost daily. Large amounts of sodium retained in the body will cause retention of fluid in the tissues.[3]

Moderate amounts of complete protein foods (0.5 gram per kilogram per day) are usually ordered unless the patient develops oliguria. To decrease the work of the kidneys, it may be considered desirable to decrease protein catabolism by limiting protein foods. If oliguria occurs, food intake may be limited to carbohydrates and moderate amounts of fat. Foods high in carbohydrate, including fruit juices, may be restricted to lower the intake of potassium.

When examination of the blood shows that the potassium level is high, a *cation exchange resin* may be given either by mouth or as an enema. The cation exchange resin used most often is polystyrene sodium sulfonate (Kayexalate), administered in daily dosages of 15 to 60 Gm. by mouth, by nasogastric tube, or by enema. Cation exchange resins are inert, insoluble, synthetic substances that contain either basic or acidic groups that can combine with electrolytes in the intestinal tract, thus preventing their absorption. Their therapeutic benefit in uremia derives from their particular affinity for the potassium ion. However, they also remove sodium and calcium. The removal of

sodium may lead to acidosis (hyperchloremia). The use of cation exchange resins also may contribute to digitalis intoxication and cardiac arrhythmias, and gastric irritation, diarrhea, and fecal impaction may develop. When a resin is given by mouth, a cathartic such as citrate of magnesia and a cleansing enema or colonic irrigation are given daily to ensure the elimination of potassium from the bowel. If a resin is being given rectally, the cleansing enemas should be given several hours before the first dose of resin each day.

Intestinal catharsis may make an already weak patient weaker, so that special consideration must be given to measures that will conserve his strength. He must be given support while sitting on the bedpan, there must be provision for lengthy and undisturbed rest periods, and he must be given assistance with eating and general hygiene. Daily blood and urine specimens will be collected for determinations of sodium and potassium levels.

Since waste products are not being eliminated adequately through the kidneys, it is important that the bowels move regularly and that the skin be bathed frequently so that these routes of excretion function properly. More urea and sodium are excreted through the skin than normally, and itching may occur. The best treatment for itching is to bathe the patient with a weak vinegar solution (2 tbsp. to 1 pint of water) that dissolves the crystals on the skin.

Size of meals and time for eating should be adjusted to the individual patient. Many patients with pronounced nausea have brief periods when they can take and retain food. Ginger ale is often permissible and acceptable to the patient. It is especially helpful in alleviating the morning nausea and headaches that are characteristic of uremia. Many times, even though vomiting occurs, a meal can be tolerated about an hour later. If the patient is nauseated constantly, he may be given nothing by mouth for one to two days and receive glucose and water by intravenous infusion.

The patient who has uremia may complain of a sweet yet greasy sensation in his mouth, and his tongue may be coated. Mouth care should be given before each meal, and if the patient can tolerate hard candy, "sour balls" can be given to counteract the unpleasant sensation. They also increase the carbohydrate intake without adding potassium. Since thirst is a common complaint, fluids by mouth should be judiciously spaced throughout the twenty-four-hour period. Frequent mouth care will help to prevent drying of the mucous membranes and will add to comfort. It is especially important if the patient is vomiting or is unable to drink.

It is important to protect the patient with renal failure from infection. Any infection increases protein catabolism, increases the work load of the kidneys, and speeds the onset of uremia. Chilling must be prevented by careful ventilation of the room, with avoidance of drafts. Doctors, nurses, members of the patient's family, and others should not go near the patient if they have upper respiratory infections. Occasionally the patient is placed in a single room, and visitors are often restricted as an additional protection. Masks and gowns may be worn by staff members giving care to the patient to protect him from organisms in the hospital (reverse precautions). Careful hand washing by all personnel is mandatory. If there are surgical wounds to be cared for, special attention should be given to aseptic technique. Contamination of wounds from such sources as feces, urine, and flies should be prevented. Antibiotics often are given to prevent infection or to control spread of existing infection.

Recognition and treatment of complications

The patient must be observed carefully for signs of respiratory and cardiac complications. Hypertension usually occurs in both acute and chronic renal failure. The blood pressure may change rapidly in acute failure, and the doctor often requests that it be taken at hourly intervals. Since cardiac failure and pulmonary edema due to potassium intoxication are common complications, the nurse should be alert for tachycardia and atrial fibrillation. Cardiac insufficiency often develops and usually is treated by giving digitalis rather than by reducing the sodium intake since reduction of sodium may increase electrolyte imbalance. Mercurial diuretics are contraindicated because they may cause further renal damage and

may lead to further sodium depletion. However, mannitol may be given intravenously for its diuretic effect and has been effective in initiating diuresis in some patients with oliguria.[3] If there is edema, it is important to provide the best possible lymph and venous drainage. This goal may be accomplished by stimulating the circulation with either active or passive exercises and by elevating the edematous areas to encourage gravity drainage of lymph and venous blood. If the eyelids are puffy, the head should be elevated. In edema of the arms or legs, the parts should be supported slightly above the heart level with pillows. Edematous tissues require meticulous hygiene care and frequent change of position to help prevent pressure sores, which heal slowly and become infected easily. Usually a daily weight recording is requested. To prevent respiratory complications, the patient should be turned from side to side and encouraged to take deep breaths at two-hour intervals.

Muscle twitching anywhere in the body and convulsions are common in uremia. Persistent tremors also occur. In an attempt to prevent these problems, the doctor may ask the nurse to check for Trousseau's sign or Chvostek's sign at regular intervals, so that treatment can be started before overt symptoms appear (p. 100). If either sign is positive, the doctor is notified at once. Calcium gluconate or calcium chloride usually are kept ready to give. Sometimes hypertonic solutions similar to those used for increased intracranial pressure, such as urea in invert sugar (Urevert), may be used. However, the muscle twitching may not respond to calcium, and a barbiturate may be given intravenously, or chloral hydrate may be given by mouth or through a nasogastric tube.

If the patient continues to have generalized muscle twitching, a convulsion should be anticipated. Padded side rails should be placed on the bed and a mouth gag kept at the bedside. Even though the side rails must be padded, the bed should be placed so that the patient can see about the room. Because he is usually irritable and may become irrational, he may become upset if he feels confined. If the patient is so confused or irrational that his behavior is unpredictable, he should not be left alone. Sometimes family members can stay with him. If it is impossible to have the patient constantly attended, it is sometimes helpful to use a drawsheet restraint (with the diagonally twirled sheet placed loosely over the chest and anchored to the side rails), or a Posey belt, which will serve to remind the forgetful patient where he is and thus prevent injury if he attempts to get out of bed, may be used. Persuasion, long explanations, and arguments with the patient should be avoided since they only upset him. The nurse who has a calm voice, a calm manner, and a positive approach can usually help him. If he objects to a treatment, it is better to delay it for a short time. If he continues to resist essential treatment, however, the doctor must be notified. Loud noises and bright lights tend to increase irritability, and the number of persons entering the room, as well as frequent changes of nursing personnel, disturb the patient.

Special treatment for renal failure

The patient may be treated by *dialysis* in an attempt to provide an emergency substitution for normal renal function. Dialysis means the separation of solutes from a solvent by differential diffusion through a porous membrane placed between two solutions. Dialysis is frequently used to remove excess amounts of salicylates, barbiturates, and bromides from the bloodstream following accidental or intentional overdoses of these drugs, in a variety of other poisonings, in serious renal reaction to transfused blood, and in acute glomerulonephritis with anuria. At the present time, two methods are being used: hemodialysis by the "artificial kidney" and peritoneal dialysis.

Hemodialysis. Hemodialysis compensates for total loss of renal function, and all symptoms regress except the anemia, which does not respond to this treatment. It has proved especially useful for short-term use in acute conditions, although its usefulness is still limited by the cost, the complexity of the equipment, the need for specialized medical and nursing personnel, and sometimes the condition of the patient. Because heparin must be used, for example, the treatment is seldom done postoperatively, since hemorrhage from the wound may occur. Ambulatory patients can be treated by hemodialysis, but the inconvenience and extremely high cost limit its use for patients with chronic

uremia. Newer methods and equipment are being produced, however, that simplify the procedure and make it less expensive. Selected patients who have inadequate kidney function and yet are ambulatory are now being taught to carry out the treatment in their homes assisted by their families.[14] Peritoneal dialysis is considered to be only one-sixth to one-tenth as effective as hemodialysis, but it is much simpler to carry out and requires less elaborate facilities.

The *artificial kidney,* a complex mechanism that might be described as an external kidney, is used for hemodialysis. The patient's arterial blood is shunted into the artificial kidney. Here it circulates through special cellophane coils that resemble capillary walls in permeability and that are surrounded by a solution of approximately the same electrolyte composition as that of the normal extracellular fluid, allowing for the elimination by dialysis of moderate amounts of body waste products such as urea. The blood is then returned to the venous circulation.

For hemodialysis the patient remains in his bed and usually is taken to a special treatment room. He is weighed before and after the treatment to determine the amount of fluid loss. Several pounds may be lost from the passage of solutes and water through the membrane in the coils. Because children become dehydrated so easily, their weight may be checked throughout the procedure by placing them on special scales. Cutdowns are done on an artery and a vein (usually in the antecubital area or the wrist); plastic cannulas are inserted, and they are so constructed that they may be attached to each other under aseptic conditions at the conclusion of the treatment. The cannulas with the connecting plastic tubing provide a shunt and thus preserve the patency of the selected blood vessels for future use. A doctor or a specially prepared nurse primes the dialysis unit with two or three pints of blood. If the third pint is not used, it usually is given to the patient as a direct transfusion at the conclusion of the dialysis. When the unit is functioning properly and there are no air bubbles, the plastic catheters from the blood vessels of the patient are connected to the machine. Heparin is given at this time. Throughout the procedure, a nurse is responsible for observing the patient's general condition, state of consciousness, and vital signs. Blood pressure is checked continuously when the treatment is first started and every ten to fifteen minutes thereafter. Some drop in blood pressure is anticipated at first, and the rate of flow of blood through the unit is determined by the patient's blood pressure. For example, 50 to 100 ml. of blood per minute are permitted to flow into the machine at first. As the blood pressure stabilizes, the amount is increased to 300 to 500 ml. per minute. The patient's pulse is also carefully checked at one- to two-minute intervals at first and every ten to fifteen minutes thereafter. Any untoward signs or symptoms of reaction, such as drop in blood pressure, difficulty in breathing, complaints of pain, or lowered level of consciousness, are reported to the doctor promptly. An emer-

gency drug tray containing antihistaminic preparations and circulatory stimulants always is kept ready for immediate use.

The treatment usually is given for at least three hours. The patient may sleep during the procedure, or he may be apprehensive and restless. He may need mouth care, changing of position, and massaging of pressure areas. He may be given fluids or food, and he may need provision for normal elimination. The environment should be as quiet and unstimulating as possible under the circumstances, the patient should be kept warm and comfortable, and the room should be well ventilated. Upon completion of the treatment, the patient is returned to his room, and protamine sulfate may be given to counteract the effect of heparin. He should be watched for signs of bleeding anywhere.

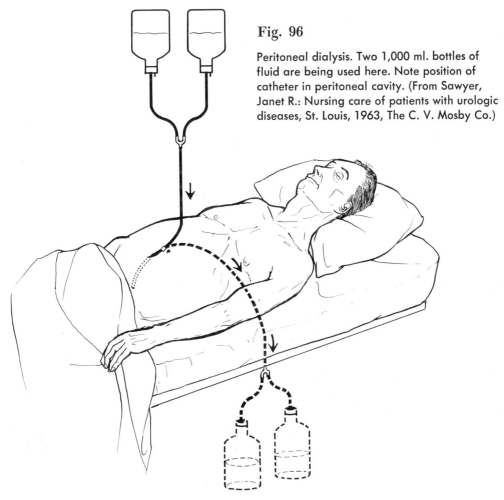

Fig. 96

Peritoneal dialysis. Two 1,000 ml. bottles of fluid are being used here. Note position of catheter in peritoneal cavity. (From Sawyer, Janet R.: Nursing care of patients with urologic diseases, St. Louis, 1963, The C. V. Mosby Co.)

If the cannulas have been removed from the artery and vein, tight dressings are applied, and they must be observed closely at frequent intervals to detect hemorrhage. Hourly checking of pulse and blood pressure may be ordered for a time if the doctor has any reason to suspect that a delayed reaction may occur.

Peritoneal dialysis. In peritoneal dialysis the dialyzing fluid is instilled into the peritoneal cavity, where the peritoneum serves as the dialyzing membrane (Fig. 96). This procedure, once it is instituted, becomes largely a nursing responsibility and may be maintained continuously for twelve to thirty-six hours.

Prior to starting the treatment, the nurse should explain it to the patient and should report any serious apprehension he has to the doctor, who may order a sedative, as in hemodialysis. The patient's weight, blood pressure, and pulse should be recorded for later comparison. After the patient has voided, the doctor anesthetizes a small area in the left lower quadrant of the abdomen with procaine hydrochloride, makes a small incision, and inserts a straight metal trocar and cannula into the peritoneal cavity (an abdominal paracentesis). The cannula is replaced by a many-eyed, semirigid nylon catheter, and the trocar is then withdrawn, leaving the catheter in the peritoneal cavity. Two liters of sterile dialyzing solution (similar to that used in the artificial kidney) warmed to body temperature are attached by tubing to the catheter and are allowed to run into the peritoneal cavity as rapidly as possible. This usually takes about ten minutes. Before the bottle is completely empty, the tube is clamped, because the remaining fluid is needed to start the siphon system for returning the flow from the peritoneal cavity. The bottle is placed on the floor, and sixty to ninety minutes later, depending on the doctor's order, the tubing is unclamped. The fluid should drain in a steady stream, emptying the cavity in about twenty minutes. If it does not, omentum probably is covering the eyes of the catheter. Applying firm pressure to the lower abdomen with both hands, moving the patient from side to side, or slightly elevating the head of the bed may remedy this problem. If these measures fail, the doctor must be called to alter the position of the catheter. If 2,000 ml. of dialyzing fluid are instilled, not less than 1,500 ml. or more than 2,500 ml. should return. If the amount varies from this, the doctor must be notified before more fluid is allowed to run into the peritoneal cavity, since dehydration or overhydration may occur.

The nurse should try to keep the patient as comfortable as possible during this tiring procedure. Although the patient must remain in a supine position, his head may be elevated slightly to prevent discomfort from pressure of the fluid against the upper abdominal organs and diaphragm. During the period between completion of drainage and restarting the procedure, he can be turned to his side for back care. The patient may have abdominal pain, especially when most of the fluid has drained out. If it is severe, the doctor may instill 2% procaine hydrochloride through the catheter. Analgesics and sedatives may be ordered to be given at intervals during the procedure.

During the first exchange, the patient's blood pressure and pulse are checked every fifteen minutes. If vital signs remain normal, they may need to be taken only every hour. However, if a hypertonic dialyzing fluid is being used or if considerably more fluid drains than is infused, fifteen-minute checks should be continued since dehydration may cause a sudden drop in the blood volume. Tachycardia, the first sign of a drop in blood volume, should be reported to the doctor at once. Any signs of overhydration, such as bounding pulse, increased blood pressure, or dyspnea, should also be reported.

It is important to keep an accurate record of all intake and output during the procedure. The patient is allowed to eat and drink, and there may be fluid loss from urine or other routes. Overall fluid balance should be checked after each exchange. The body weight is checked at least every twenty-four hours; 0.5 to 1% of the total body weight should be lost each day to prevent overhydration. Blood chemistry studies such as nonprotein nitrogen, serum potassium, and sodium tests are ordered to be carried out at frequent intervals.

At the termination of the period of peritoneal dialysis, the catheter is removed by the doctor, and a dry, sterile dressing, heavy enough to absorb any further drainage, is applied over the incision. This dressing should be changed as necessary, using aseptic technique. The incision usually seals over in a day or two. The patient should be observed for any signs of peritonitis such as fever, abdominal pain, or a tender, rigid abdomen.

The patient convalescing following acute renal failure

If the patient can be maintained during the crucial period of acute renal failure, diuresis will usually occur during the second week of renal failure, and function will gradually return to normal over a period of weeks. As recovery occurs, the fluid intake is increased to equal the output. It is important to watch for signs of dehydration due to sodium depletion and for signs of sodium retention (edema) during this period because the sodium-water balance may be unstable. Until renal function returns to normal, a high-caloric, low-protein diet, with plenty of fluids, should be continued and only moderate activity allowed.

Since a period of convalescence is necessary following acute renal failure, arrangements may need to be made for care in a nursing home or in a convalescent home.

General treatment and nursing care in chronic renal failure

In chronic renal failure (*chronic uremia*) the treatment is designed to maintain physiology as close to normal as possible in order to keep the patient relatively comfortable for as long as he lives. Much of the treatment and nursing care is similar to that for acute uremia. Therefore, only variations in this care will be discussed.

Provided that the urinary output does not decrease or edema does not increase, fluids are forced in chronic renal failure since the kidney has a lessened ability to concentrate solids and more fluid is needed to excrete wastes. If there is edema, however, fluids must be restricted. An accurate record of the intake and output should be kept, and fluids should be forced only to the point at which a positive balance of intake and output is maintained.

Since the patient usually has severe an-orexia, many physicians feel that he should have any food that appeals to him, although an attempt is made to give him a well-balanced diet. Salt should not be used in excess, but neither is it limited by these doctors unless there is edema. Some doctors, however, believe that the diet should be low in salt and low in protein since these restrictions may lessen strain on the limited kidney reserve. Salt substitutes containing potassium are contraindicated for patients with renal disease because the kidneys are often unable to eliminate potassium normally. Vinegar, lemon, brown sugar, minced parsley, mint, rum, cloves, cinnamon, and salt-free tomato juice are a few suggested flavorings that may make unsalted foods more palatable. Often the patient can tolerate fruit juices and carbonated beverages when other foods are rejected, and foods prepared in his own home may be more acceptable to him than hospital meals. Relatives may be permitted to bring foods to the very ill patient in the hospital provided that they are able to do so and know what seasonings must be avoided. If the gastrointestinal tract becomes ulcerated, bland foods and fluids may have to be given.

Mouth care is extremely important since mouth sores, once developed, are almost impossible to cure. Mineral oil is an acceptable protective lubricant for the alert patient. A water-soluble lubricant with a vegetable base, such as K-Y lubricating jelly, is preferable for the stuporous patient. Hydrogen peroxide is helpful in removing caked blood from the mouth and the nose.

The patient should be kept active and occupied within the limits of his strength for as long as possible. Since he usually has failing vision, safety measures similar to those needed for patients with eye conditions should be employed. The patient may enjoy being read to or listening to the radio. If he cannot see, his mail should be read to him, and he should be kept informed of headlines in the daily papers so that he is able to maintain contact with the world around him. Although vision is poor, he may be able to feed himself for some time. The nurse or a member of the patient's family should tactfully indicate the foods being served and their placement on the tray. Later the patient may need to be fed by others, and ultimately tube feeding may be required.

Severe anemia, which is common in chronic uremia and contributes to the patient's general weakness, is usually treated by blood transfusions. Hematinic drugs appear to be of little value.[3] If blood cells are hemolyzing, corticosteroids may be given. Acidosis is usually not treated unless hyperventilation causes the patient distress. If the patient can tolerate oral medications, he often is given aluminum hydroxide, which decreases the absorption of phosphates in the gastrointestinal tract and helps alleviate symptoms of acidosis. The phosphates, rather than being absorbed into the blood, combine with the aluminum to form aluminum phosphate, which is eliminated through the bowel. Sodium bicarbonate may also be given by mouth to combat acidosis. When oral medications cannot be tolerated, intravenous solutions such as ⅙ molar lactate may be given.[3]

The patient with chronic renal failure easily contracts systemic infection. Preventive nursing measures are the same as for the patient with acute renal failure. Other complications of chronic uremia are the same as those described in the discussion on acute renal failure, but the treatment is never so vigorous. Tetany, convulsions, cardiac failure, and pulmonary edema are managed in the same way, but dialysis is rarely used. If there is edema, it is important to provide the best possible lymph and venous drainage, as described on p. 433.

Giving emotional support to the family is probably one of the most important duties of the nurse who is caring for a patient with either acute or chronic uremia. The patient requires many treatments that may alarm the family even more than they do the patient. A brief, simple explanation of the reasons for procedures may prevent anxiety, which often is transmitted from the family to the patient. If the family wishes to participate in care, there is much that they can do to help maintain a pleasant, safe, calm environment for the patient. However, they must understand the need for the proper environment and must be helped to plan appropriately. Often both the patient and the family appreciate visits from their spiritual adviser. The nurse, by her interest and attitudes during this period, can do a great deal to help the family accept the patient's ultimate death if it is inevitable. When the patient becomes comatose, additional care will be required. (See p. 162 for care of the unconscious patient.)

The patient with disease directly impairing renal function

Nephritis

Nephritis, or Bright's disease, is a general term sometimes used to describe noninfectious inflammatory and degenerative diseases affecting the nephrons of the kidney. Under this classification are such diseases as acute glomerulonephritis and subacute and chronic glomerulonephritis.

Acute glomerulonephritis. Acute glomerulonephritis directly affecting the glomeruli and their function is a disease seen usually in children and young adults. It occurs twice as often in male as in female patients. Although the cause is unknown, the patient with this disease usually gives a history of a recent upper respiratory infection, such as tonsillitis, laryngitis, sinusitis, common cold, or grippe, or has recently recovered from scarlet fever or chickenpox. Hemolytic streptococci either have been the causative organisms or have caused complications, although the organisms are not present in the kidneys when glomerulonephritis occurs.

Because of the association between acute glomerulonephritis and streptococcal infections, early treatment of the latter with antibiotics seems advisable as a prophylactic measure. Potential foci of infection, such as diseased tonsils, may be removed after the acute infection has subsided.

The onset of acute glomerulonephritis may be either sudden or insidious. The patient may not present a classic picture with all the common symptoms but may have only one or two of the common symptoms.

If the onset is insidious, the patient may complain of weakness, pallor, and anorexia, followed by hematuria, puffiness of the face (especially about the eyes), headache, and decreased urine volume. Hypertension may be present. Nausea, vomiting, a low-grade fever, and nocturia are common. If the disease is of the acute, or fulminating, type, the patient suddenly develops generalized edema, blurring of vision, marked hypertension, and nitrogen retention. The condition may rapidly progress to uremia and result in death.

Laboratory findings in glomerulonephritis vary widely, but albumin, casts, and red and white blood cells are almost always present in the urine. The blood urea nitrogen level is usually only slightly elevated. The specific gravity of the urine may be high because of the reduced filtration rate in the glomeruli, the continuing normal reabsorptive function of the distal tubules, and the retention of fluid in the tissues.

Treatment of acute glomerulonephritis consists of supportive measures. Bed rest is usually prescribed. The room should be kept at a constant temperature to avoid the patient's becoming chilled. If he is in a cool room or is ambulatory, warm pajamas and bedsocks should be used for additional warmth. Exposure to upper respiratory infections should be avoided, since even a mild infection such as the common cold may reactivate the renal disease. Since the period of bed rest may be long and the patient does not usually feel ill, the nurse needs to help him understand why bed rest is necessary. She should make arrangements to keep him occupied and relatively content during waking hours. The patient is allowed to begin progressive ambulation when the blood sedimentation rate and the blood pressure have returned to normal levels. If ambulation causes any increase in albuminuria or hematuria, the patient must return to bed rest. This setback may cause the patient to become discouraged, depressed, and hostile to treatment. He should be encouraged to discuss his feelings, and it should be explained to him that return to complete bed rest is not an unusual occurrence.

Diet restrictions depend on the symptoms. Effort usually is made to give the kidneys rest by reducing the intake of protein, the end products of which must be eliminated by the kidneys. If there is edema, salt may be restricted. If there is anuria or oliguria, fluids, protein, and potassium are restricted, and carbohydrate is forced in the same manner as for the patient with lower nephron nephrosis. As improvement occurs, a low-protein diet (50 to 60 grams of protein daily) is usually ordered. It should consist mainly of complete protein foods, which should be divided equally among the three usual meals to ensure their maximum utilization. If this diet is tolerated and improvement continues, a normal diet is often ordered.[3]

The nurse should be alert for signs of complications such as cardiac failure, pulmonary edema, or increased intracranial pressure, which may develop if the glomerular damage is not quickly repaired. Since cerebral edema may develop within a few hours, the patient with any elevation of blood pressure should have his blood pressure and pulse checked at least twice a day and preferably every four hours.

Acute glomerulonephritis is usually self-limiting, with complete recovery occurring within a few days to a year. Only about 5% of patients with this condition die, and the deaths are usually due to complications.[3] A few patients with acute glomerulonephritis may develop the chronic form of the disease. However, the severity of the symptoms, provided death from complications can be prevented, seem to have little relationship to the prognosis. A patient with a rather mild case of acute glomerulonephritis may develop chronic glomerulonephritis, whereas the patient who is acutely ill and has severe hypertension may recover completely and have no recurrences.[3]

Subacute and latent glomerulonephritis. When complete recovery from acute glomerulonephritis has not occurred in six to eight weeks, the disease is termed subacute. In this stage, recurrent streptococcal infections often produce acute exacerbations. If symptoms continue up to or beyond a year, the disease is termed chronic. When no symptoms are present but albumin and cylindrical casts continue to be present in the urine, the term latent nephritis is used.

During the subacute and latent stages of nephritis, the patient may continue his normal activities. He should, however, avoid fatigue. The rules of good general health should be stressed in an effort to prevent exacerbation of the nephritis. Upper respiratory infections should be prevented, if possible, and all infections deserve early medical attention. Diet is not restricted, but fluid intake should be kept high. Since the patient usually feels well, he often must be convinced of the need to follow the prescribed regimen and to return for routine medical follow-up. Examinations are usually done at least annually and may include renal function tests and studies of the blood to determine the status of the disease. If symptoms recur at any time, the patient should be advised to seek immediate medical attention even though he may have been thoroughly examined only a short time previously.

Chronic glomerulonephritis. Although chronic glomerulonephritis may follow the acute disease, the majority of patients with this disease give no history of acute glomerulonephritis. The name actually is a misnomer in that there is no real infection in most instances. Various symptoms of failing renal function, none of which are usually severe, may bring the patient to the doctor. He may notice the slow onset of dependent edema that comes and goes. He may complain of headache, especially in the morning. It is usually associated with hypertension. Hypertension may also cause dyspnea upon exertion. Blurred vision may lead the patient to consult an ophthalmologist, who may be the first to suspect chronic nephritis because there are changes in the retinas of the eyes. Nocturia is a common complaint since the kidneys are unable to concentrate urine efficiently and must work overtime and eliminate more fluid to excrete sufficient waste products. Occasionally chronic nephritis is discovered during a routine physical examination because of the presence of albuminuria, or it may be discovered by the school nurse, who observes marked visual change and lassitude in a student. Weakness, lassitude, and weight loss are common but nonspecific symptoms of chronic nephritis.

Early in the disease, urinalysis shows the presence of albumin, cylindrical casts, and blood in microscopic amounts. At this stage, renal function tests may be normal, but the ability of the kidneys to concentrate urine will gradually decrease as the glomeruli become fibrotic. Finally, when only a few glomeruli are left to function, the tubules begin to degenerate. Reabsorption and excretion decrease, there is less albuminuria, cylindruria, and hematuria, and the specific gravity becomes "fixed." At this time the nonprotein nitrogen level in the blood increases.

With any exacerbation of hematuria, hypertension, and edema, however, the patient is put to bed, and the treatment is similar to that for acute glomerulonephritis. If sleeplessness, irritability, and headache become distressing, sedatives are ordered. Chloral hydrate and bromides are usually the most effective. The patient should be urged to take rest periods during the day and avoid excessive emotional and physical exertion. Obese patients usually are placed on reducing diets. The treatment is basically that described for hypertension associated with cardiac disease (p. 338).

Patients with chronic glomerulonephritis who become pregnant seem to be susceptible to toxemia and to spontaneous abortion. Some patients have no difficulties during pregnancy, but others may develop a severe toxemia and must have labor induced prematurely. The patient who has had nephritis of any kind must be urged to see a physician if she plans to become pregnant, to report at once if pregnancy occurs, and to follow the physician's instructions carefully during pregnancy.

The course of chronic glomerulonephritis is unpredictable, but it ultimately terminates in death. Some patients with rather marked decrease in renal function and hypertension may be able to lead a normal life for years, whereas others with identical symptoms may progress quickly to uremia and death. As chronic glomerulonephritis continues into the later stages, the complications are the same as those described for chronic uremia.

It is wise to encourage the family of the patient whose condition seems to be deteriorating rapidly to begin to make arrangements for terminal care. The social worker in the hospital or in the public health agency can often help the family make suitable plans.

Kidney transplants are being done more and more frequently in an effort to prolong the lives of patients with chronic renal failure. As of March, 1964, 342 of these transplants had been done, and 121 of the patients were still alive; 23 had lived six to twelve months, and 3 had lived over three years.[27] The biggest problem in this method

440

of treatment, in addition to the technical difficulty of the operation on a chronically ill patient and the problems of securing a suitable donor kidney at the right time, is the tendency of the body to reject the grafted kidney, which, like all tissues from another person (homografts), acts as a foreign body. Drugs such as azathloprine (Imuran), 6-mercaptopurine, actinomycin C, and prednisone are given in an attempt to ensure the continued life of the graft, and at this writing there is hope that before very long a means will be found to overcome the body's response of rejecting grafted tissue from other persons. Kidneys may be transplanted into the groin or into a relatively normal location within the body cavity. (See current periodicals for details.[27]) If the patient has two very poorly functioning kidneys, sometimes the poorer one is replaced. The most involved kidney may be removed, depending upon whether or not it is infected or is in some way more of a detriment to the patient than no kidney in that location, upon the condition of the other kidney, upon the chances of the grafted kidney's surviving, and upon other circumstances.

The nephrotic syndrome

The term nephrotic syndrome designates a condition or a group of conditions that involve the glomeruli of the kidney and that produce the characteristic manifestations: severe generalized edema, which is particularly noticeable around the eyes and the abdomen, pronounced albuminuria and hypoproteinemia, and usually hyperlipemia (increase of lipids in the blood). The cause of this syndrome is unknown, but it is believed that some pathology develops that alters the capacity of the glomeruli to retain protein. In adults, particularly, the nephrotic syndrome resembles chronic glomerulonephritis and may develop into chronic nephritis with nephrotic characteristics. Some patients with nephrotic syndrome may develop uremia, while others recover spontaneously.

Nephrosis is now considered part of the nephrotic syndrome in most classifications of diseases of the kidney. This condition occurs most often in children, and before ACTH and the adrenocorticosteroids were available, it was an extremely difficult condition to treat and had a fairly high mortality rate. Now, with the aid of these hormones, the prognosis usually is good.

Medical treatment of the nephrotic syndrome in children consists of giving ACTH or the adrenocorticosteroid hormones and limiting salt intake to that found in natural foods. A diet high in protein usually is prescribed to compensate for the losses in the urine. Often the diet ordered contains 1 gram of protein daily per kilogram of body weight plus an amount equivalent to the protein lost in the urine. Total urine output for each twenty-four-hour period may need to be collected and sent to the laboratory to determine total protein losses. Transfusions may be given if anemia is pronounced and in an effort to raise the protein level in the blood and thereby lessen the edema. Dextran blood volume expanders are also used for this purpose. The patient with this condition needs particular attention paid to the prevention of infection, since the edematous tissues are susceptible to trauma and infection and the body defenses are impaired by the hypoproteinemia. If renal damage has occurred beyond that which alters the ability of the glomeruli to retain protein, then all the medical and nursing measures described in the care of patients with acute or chronic glomerulonephritis or uremia may be necessary.

Renal hypertension

Hypertension may be neurogenic or renal in origin. Renal hypertension is known to result from a primary lesion of the renal blood vessels, from pyelonephritis and glomerulonephritis, from congenital anomalies of the urinary tract that obstruct the kidneys, and from other obstructive lesions of the urinary tract. If hypertension, regardless of the origin, continues unchecked over a period of time, the renal arterioles, as well as arterioles elsewhere in the body, become sclerosed and cause the blood supply to the kidneys to gradually decrease. This is known as *nephrosclerosis*.

The care of the patient treated medically is similar to that of the patient with hypertensive cardiac disease (p. 338) and the patient with chronic glomerulonephritis. Effort is made, by giving drugs such as products of rauwolfia, to lower the blood pressure, since continuing hypertension leads invariably to cerebral vascular accident, cardiac failure, or uremia.

Pyelonephritis

An inflammation of the renal pelvis is known as *pyelitis*. This condition rarely exists alone. The infection most often has invaded the parenchyma of the kidney, causing an *acute pyelonephritis*. This condition progresses to chronic pyelonephritis involving the renal pelves and the glomeruli. Chronic pyelonephritis was found to be present in 6 to 8% of all autopsies in several series, although death was due to a variety of causes, and probably it accounts for over one-third of all patients dying of uremia.[19] When the condition develops from the lower parts of the tract upward, the causative organism is most often *Escherichia coli*. The streptococcus is sometimes the causative organism and more often so when the condition follows a blood-borne infection involving primarily the parenchyma and upper calyxes of the renal pelvis. (For ways in which the nurse may help to prevent this very common and very serious condition, see p. 430.) Pyelonephritis is exceedingly common during pregnancy and indeed may be the first sign to a woman that she is pregnant. It probably is due to the physiologic stasis of urine in the upper urinary system caused by the developing fetus, although it is more common in the first trimester of pregnancy than later. Pyelonephritis may be due to obstruction anywhere along the urinary tract and develops often in men who have prostatic hypertrophy, which interferes with free passage of urine.

The usual symptoms of pyelonephritis are fever, malaise, tenderness of the costovertebral angle, pyuria, and leukocytosis. The onset is often heralded by a chill. Pyelonephritis may be preceded by cystitis, which may cause fever, malaise, pyuria, frequency, and pain on micturition.

If the patient with acute pyelonephritis is treated promptly with antibiotics, fluids, rest, and drainage of urine (if necessary), the prognosis usually is good. If treatment is inadequate, acute pyelonephritis progresses to *chronic pyelonephritis*. Patients with chronic pyelonephritis have repeated exacerbations. Each attack causes further renal damage, and the patient may eventually succumb to renal failure.

General care of the patient receiving treatment for obstruction of the urinary tract

The patient with urologic disease presents many unique nursing problems. For medical treatment to be effective, the nurse needs a clear understanding of the principles and techniques she should use in providing for the patient's nursing needs. Many patients hospitalized because of urologic conditions are in the geriatric age group. Prostatic hypertrophy, a disease of aging men, is one of the most common problems treated by the urologist. Because most of these elderly patients will have one or more other chronic diseases in addition to the acute urologic condition, the nurse should be alert for exacerbations of such common chronic ailments as cardiac decompensation, diabetes mellitus, emphysema, and arthritis.

Maintenance of fluid intake and urinary output

The maintenance of an adequate urinary output and of an adequate fluid intake might be considered a specific urologic nursing measure, since obstruction and infection of the urinary system are the most common disorders treated by the urologist. Usually both conditions are present, and the treatment is based primarily upon removal of the obstruction. Often urinary drainage must be diverted, at least temporarily, by placing a catheter into the urinary system above the obstruction to allow for maximum drainage. If the obstruction cannot be corrected medically, surgical removal will be required. Occasionally a permanent means of diverting urinary drainage must be provided.

Urethral catheterization. A *coudé* catheter, which is a soft, red rubber, *curve-tipped* catheter, is often used for catheterizations, and it is usually the catheter of choice for men patients, because it is easily inserted into the curved male urethra. A *whistle-tip* catheter or a *many-eyed* Robinson catheter may also be used. If a catheter is to be left indwelling for drainage, a Foley or a Foley type of catheter usually is used (Fig. 91). (See p. 421 for correct size of catheters to use.) The nurse should review catheterization procedures in texts on fundamentals of nursing or in a specialized text on urologic nursing. If the nurse, in carrying out an order for catheterization, finds it difficult to pass the catheter, the procedure should be discontinued and the doctor notified. Traumatic catheterization predisposes to urinary tract infection, and it is possible to perforate the urethra or bladder. It is not unusual to be unable to pass a standard catheter in patients with urethral disorders. Catheterization requiring the use of special equipment such as catheter directors, filiform catheters, or sounds are not nursing procedures. Moreover, the nurse should *never* catheterize a patient in the early postoperative period following urethral or bladder surgery.

When the doctor is to catherize a woman, the nurse should prepare the equipment and drape the patient for the procedure. She should remain with the patient and should encourage her to take deep breaths, which will relax the sphincter muscles of the bladder and make the procedure less uncomfortable. When a man is to be catheterized, the nurse should place a protective pad under the thighs and cover the patient with a draw sheet or bath blanket from the chest to the knees. After the patient and the equipment are ready (a culture tube and a sterile specimen bottle should always be available because the doctor often decides that a specimen is needed), the nurse leaves the male patient alone with the doctor. She returns when the procedure is finished to see that the patient is comfortable and to take care of the specimen and the equipment.

If a self-retaining catheter with an inflatable balloon (*Foley, Gilbert*) is to be inserted, the doctor will need a bulb syringe, a basin, and irrigating solution, such as sterile physiologic solution of sodium chloride, in order to irrigate the catheter to determine if it is correctly placed. A syringe (5 to 30 ml., depending upon the size of the balloon) with a catheter adapter or a needle, depending upon the type of catheter, is needed to inflate the balloon (Fig. 92). Black silk should be available to tie off the inflation tube of a Foley catheter because a metal clamp may be accidentally released and may cause irritation or pressure on surrounding tissues. Self-sealing catheters, which require no clamp, are now available. If a retention catheter is to be left in place, the nurse should ask the doctor the type of

Fig. 97

A to **C**, Catheters used to drain the renal pelvis: **A**, ureteral catheter; **B**, Malecot, or batwing, catheter; **C**, Pezzer, or mushroom, catheter. **D**, Stylet used to insert Malecot and Pezzer catheters.

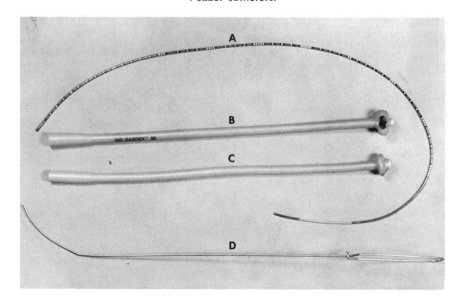

drainage he plans to use and should have the equipment ready to be connected as soon as the catheterization is completed.

Maintaining urinary drainage with a catheter

The nurse should know *why a catheter has been inserted and what cavity it is draining.*

Types of catheters and their anchorage. If the ureter is obstructed or partially obstructed, a catheter must be placed directly into the renal pelvis to assure adequate drainage. If there is complete obstruction of the ureter, a *nephrostomy tube,* usually a Pezzer (mushroom) or Malecot (batwing) catheter (Fig. 97), may be inserted through the substance of the kidney into the renal pelvis, from a surgical wound made laterally and posteriorly in the kidney region. A *pyelostomy tube* is placed directly into the pelvis—it is not passed through the cortex and the medulla. The kidney may also be drained by a *ureterostomy tube* (a whistle-tip or a many-eyed Robinson catheter), which is

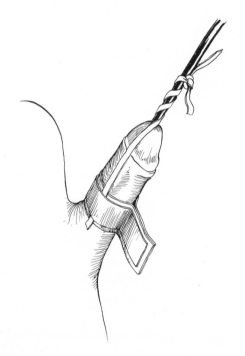

Fig. 98

A method of securing a straight catheter used as an indwelling catheter in a male patient.

passed through an incision made in the upper outer quadrant of the abdomen into a surgical opening in the ureter above the obstruction. The catheter is passed up the ureter to the renal pelvis. The renal pelvis may be drained by a *ureteral catheter,* which is passed by means of a cystoscope to the bladder and up the ureter to the renal pelvis (Fig. 95). Ureteral catheters inserted through a cystoscope may be left in place even though the cystoscope is withdrawn. This procedure is frequently done prior to gynecologic or extensive lower colon surgery, in which there may be danger of accidentally injuring an unrecognized ureter. A ureteral catheter may also be left in place to provide better drainage of the renal pelvis in certain conditions, such as when a stone is lodged in the ureter. If the patient has two functioning kidneys but only one is being drained by a ureteral catheter, there will also be a collection of urine in the bladder. The output from each kidney—that obtained from the ureteral catheter and that coming directly from the bladder—should be recorded separately.

If there is obstruction below the bladder, constant drainage is necessary to preserve renal function because the back pressure produced by inadequate emptying of the urinary system will ultimately damage the nephrons. The most common means of draining the bladder is through a *urethral catheter.* Usually a self-retaining type such as a Foley or a Gilbert catheter is used. Sometimes a coudé, a many-eyed Robinson, or a filiform catheter will be used as an indwelling catheter for male patients since a straight catheter can be adequately anchored to the penis (Fig. 98). The method of anchoring is as follows: (1) cut two strips of adhesive tape 1½ by 4 inches; (2) cut two pieces of twill tape 12 inches long; (3) shave the penis and apply tincture of benzoin to the mid-shaft; (4) apply one strip of the 1½ by 4 inch adhesive tape, bringing the edges together beyond the penis (this permits easy removal and allows for expansion in case of penile erection); (5) place one end of each piece of twill tape over the adhesive tape on either side of the penis and apply the second strip of adhesive to hold the tapes in place; (6) wind the two pieces of twill tape in alternate directions around the catheter and tie them securely near its tip.

When the urethra is completely obstructed or when there is danger of infection of the male genital system because of extended urethral intubation, *cystostomy drainage* may be necessary. A catheter (usually a Malecot or a Pezzer) is placed into the bladder through a suprapubic incision. Sometimes postoperatively the bladder will be drained by both a cystostomy tube and a urethral catheter. If so, each catheter will not necessarily drain equal amounts, but both should be kept open, and the total output should be measured and should be adequate.

It is important that catheters be adequately anchored to prevent accidental dislodgment. Self-retaining urethral catheters rarely need further anchoring. Cystostomy, nephrostomy, and ureterostomy tubes should have two points of anchorage to prevent their being dislodged. The openings made for the insertion of these tubes are essentially fistulas that rapidly decrease in size upon removal of the catheter, and even a half hour after removal it is often impossible to reinsert a catheter of the same size. If the catheter is inserted during an operation, it usually is sutured in place. In that case, only the two-flap adhesive anchorage is necessary. (See procedure on p. 444.) If the tube is not sutured in place, a piece of adhesive tape should be placed around the catheter, leaving a tab to pin to the dressing. When the patient has no dressing, the catheter can be gently curved (taking care not to kink it) and attached to the abdomen at two points by two-flap adhesive anchorage.

Checking catheters. Catheters must be checked frequently. Since the purpose of using a catheter in any patient with disease of the urinary system is to provide better urinary drainage, catheters should never be left clamped nor be allowed to become completely or partially plugged. A catheter that is directly draining a kidney must *never* be clamped for even a very short period of time because the normal pelvis has a capacity of only 5 to 8 ml. Also, in case of accidental removal, catheters should be reinserted promptly.

To check a catheter for patency, disconnect the drainage tubing at the catheter and allow the urine in the tubing to drain. Then reconnect the catheter to the tubing and hold the connector at a slight elevation so that the urine will be draining against gravity (running uphill) to fill the connector. If, under these conditions, urine appears in the connector within a minute or two, the catheter is draining adequately. If there is little drainage, one should make sure that the patient is not dehydrated. Drainage often will start within half an hour after

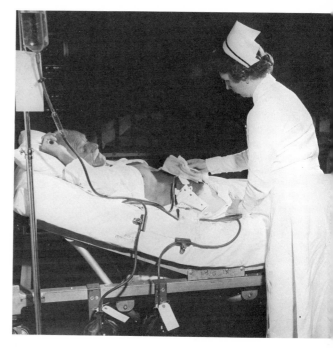

Fig. 99

The nurse is checking the drainage from the suprapubic tube and the Foley catheter. Note that she checks the glass connection proximal to the catheters. This setup is for continuous irrigation of the bladder. The card for recording the amount of irrigating fluid used is readily available on the pole. The drainage bottles are labeled according to which contains urine draining from the suprapubic tube and which contains urine draining from the urethral catheter. Note that the drainage tubing has no loops between the mattress and the drainage bottles.

the patient is given two or three glasses of water. The drainage system, starting with the drainage bottle and working back to the catheter, should be systematically checked to be sure that it is not obstructed at any point. A catheter or the drainage tubing may be blocked by a blood clot or a plug of mucus that sometimes may be dislodged by gently "milking" the tubing. If drainage remains poor, the catheter should be irrigated. The doctor often leaves an order to irrigate the catheter if necessary. If there is no order, or if irrigation is not successful, the doctor should be called. No catheter should be allowed to drain inadequately for more than an hour.

The color of urinary drainage should be checked and recorded. An accurate check of the color can be made only at the connector next to the catheter, since the urine in the drainage bottle is a collection of several hours (Fig. 99). One should be alert for any evidence of hemorrhage, report it immediately, and take added precautions to prevent stoppage of the catheter drainage by kinking of the catheter or by other means. If there is any hematuria, the nurse should watch carefully for further bleeding. Clots can form in fifteen to twenty minutes, and it may be necessary to aspirate them or to change the catheter. Purulent and dirty-appearing urine suggests infection; cloudy urine suggests albuminuria; smoky urine suggests hemoglobinuria. Certain foods and drugs may also cause color and odor changes in urine. The consumption of large servings of beets may cause the urine to be red temporarily. Phenazopyridine hydrochloride (Pyridium), a urinary antiseptic, also turns the urine red. Asparagus may cause the urine to appear cloudy and to smell musty. Mucous shreds and small pieces of tissue may also appear in urine.

While the catheter is being checked, the surrounding skin should be inspected for dryness and cleanliness. Occasionally, following a traumatic urethral intubation, there may be marked edema of the foreskin. This should be reported to the doctor immediately. It usually is treated by sitz baths or by cold applications to the penis. Inspection of the catheter and genital area will be less upsetting to the patient if it is done in a matter-of-fact, efficient manner and without undue exposure. He should be told why the inspection is being made. If there is a man on the nursing team, it is usually preferable that he cleanse the genital area of the male patient.

The drainage system

Proper maintenance of the drainage system to which a catheter is connected is an essential nursing function. Catheters usually are attached to *straight drainage* and allowed to drain by gravity. To drain a closed cavity by gravity, air must be accessible in the drainage system. Since there is less danger of infection and there is better drainage when the tubing is not immersed in the urine drained, it is preferable to use a drainage system in which the tube is attached to a bottle cap that has an air outlet (Fig. 100, *B*) or to a plastic bag similarly equipped. This system of drainage also decreases odor. With the infections, either this system is often used, or the catheter may be clamped and then opened periodically for drainage.

To provide complete drainage of a cavity by gravity, the receptacle must be lower than the cavity to be drained, and the tubing must run directly from the level of the cavity to the drainage receptacle, with no loops of tubing below the level of the drainage bottle. Clipping the tubing to the bed and coiling the excess length on the bed help to prevent any interference with the flow of urine.

If thick-walled latex tubing is used, obstruction of drainage due to kinking can be reduced. Care should be taken not to obstruct the lumen when attaching the drainage tubing to the bed. A large paper clamp is convenient to use and is unlikely to squeeze or kink the tubing (Fig. 99). To prevent clamping off of tubes by the weight of a patient lying on them and also to lessen the danger of pressure and injury to the skin, it is best to run drainage tubing over the thigh. However, if this position causes kinking, the tubing should be run under the knee or directly to the foot of the bed, where it will not be under any body part. Special care must be taken that nephrostomy and ureterostomy tubes are not kinked when the patient is on his side.

The lumens of the connectors and the

tubing should be comparable in size to the lumen of the catheter. The inner bore for any tube draining urine should be at least 8 mm. in diameter. Improperly cleansed catheters, connectors, or drainage tubing may cause partial obstruction of their lumens.

To keep catheters and drainage systems in good condition, immediately after use they should be soaked in cold water to which a detergent such as Solvental has been added. Next, warm water and soap should be forced through the lumens with a syringe. Then 5% acetic acid (full-strength white vinegar) should be forced through in order to dissolve urate crystals, followed by hydrogen peroxide to remove any old blood. The glass connectors can be cleansed easily with a small tube brush, and benzene or ether can be used to remove adhesive from the outside of the tubes. After a final thorough rinsing in cold water, the catheters and tubing are ready for sterilization.

When a white sediment begins to encrust a connector, or when tubing rubbed between the fingers feels "sandy," the equipment should be changed. Usually the catheter will also need changing at this time. Ordinarily, tubing will need to be changed only once a week. If the bottles are cleansed and boiled daily, however, there will be less odor. Disposable calibrated plastic drainage bags are now available commercially.

The use of an "up bottle" (a small drainage receptacle that can be attached to the gown or to the thigh) provides for a system of straight drainage for the ambulatory patient. If there is to be complete drainage of the intubated cavity while the patient is out of bed, this system must be used. A flat 8-ounce bottle attached to the gown with tape and a safety pin works satisfactorily as an "up bottle"; plastic leg urinals now on the market are also useful (Figs. 32 and 102). Patients should be cautioned not to fasten the "up bottle" so high that the catheter or tubing is kinked or must drain against gravity. "Up bottles" and leg urinals do not provide adequate drainage for the patient who is in bed because no gravity is provided.

Catheter irrigation. If adequate fluids are being given and if there is no hematuria with clots, it is unusual for a catheter to need irrigation. The safest and most effective means of irrigating the urinary system is by "internal irrigation" (fluids by mouth or parenterally).

When tubes are irrigated, one should realize that the purpose of the procedure is to maintain patency of the tube and to prevent obstruction, not to lavage the organ that the tube drains. Vigorous irrigation of the kidney and bladder will almost certainly damage these structures and spread infection, resulting in pain, hematuria, chills, fever, and even abscess formation. Gentleness is mandatory. All equipment must be sterile, and the greatest care must be taken not to introduce infection during the procedure. Sterile normal saline solution is usually used to irrigate catheters because it is isotonic and because its clarity makes observation of the return flow easy.

If a catheter is to be irrigated, one needs to consider the size of the cavity into which the fluid is being instilled. The renal pelvis should never be irrigated with more than 8 to 10 ml. of fluid. The fluid should be instilled gently and allowed to drain back by gravity. Most patients will tolerate 75 to 100 ml. of fluid in the bladder, but one should never use more fluid than a patient can tolerate without pain. Irrigations are carried out until the returns are clear. If fluid flows in readily but fails to return, there probably is a clot acting as a valve over the eye of the catheter. In this situation, do not continue to add fluid but try to dislodge the clot by "milking" the tubing. If this is unsuccessful, the doctor should be called. He may use a suction syringe to evacuate the clots. (The Toomey syringe is the type often used.) A nurse should not use a suction syringe because the mucous membrane lining of the bladder can be damaged if too much pressure is exerted.

If the urethral catheter needs frequent irrigation, it may be practical to set up *intermittent irrigation,* which is simply an adaptation of the method of irrigation in which a syringe and a basin of solution are used. The reservoir flasks holds the irrigating solution, and the tubing from the flask to the catheter allows the solution to flow through the catheter upon release of the inflow clamp, provided that the drainage tubing has been clamped (Fig. 100). This

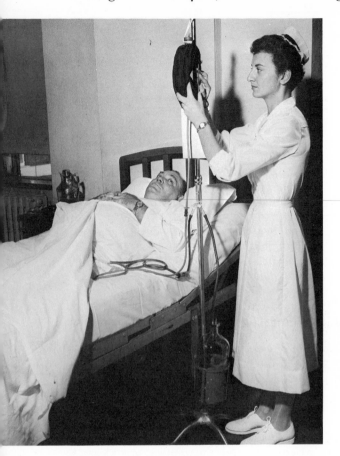

A

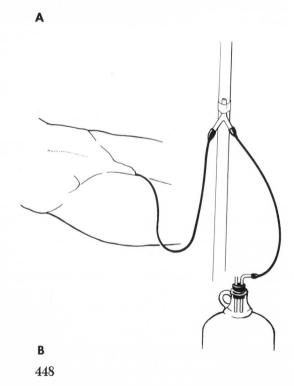

B

Fig. 100

A, The nurse is checking the amount of fluid left in a Kelly flask. Note the setup for intermittent irrigation and that the catheter is attached to high decompression drainage by means of the Y tube attached to the standard. The Kelly flask is covered because silver nitrate solution, which turns black if exposed to light, is being used. **B,** Placement of the Y connecting tube on the standard as it is used to decompress the bladder.

method obviates the danger of contamination and breakage of an irrigation set left at the bedside. It also makes using a new set for each irrigation unnecessary.

If intermittent irrigation is used, an accurate record of the amount of fluid used for irrigating must be kept because the solution returns into the drainage bottle. The amount of irrigating fluid used must be subtracted from the total drainage each time the drainage bottle is emptied so that the urinary output may be accurately recorded. This method of irrigation is not safe for kidney irrigations because the inflow cannot be regulated carefully enough to allow only 8 to 10 ml. of fluid to be instilled at a time.

If the catheter provides for both inflow of irrigating fluid and outflow of drainage, such as a three-way Foley catheter does, or if the patient has both a cystostomy tube and a urethral catheter in place, the doctor may order *constant irrigation*. The equipment is identical to that used for intermittent irrigation except that a dripometer is placed below the Kelly flask (Fig. 99). The rate of the drip may be increased or decreased as necessary to keep the catheter draining well. When using this method, it is also necessary to provide accurate recording of urinary output, for the drainage will be made up of both urine and irrigating solution. Sometimes irrigation with 5% glucose in water is ordered because some absorption takes place when an irrigation is constant, and the doctor may not wish sodium chloride to be absorbed.

Care of a patient
after removal of a catheter

The nurse needs to be aware of the urinary output of patients from whom catheters have been removed. The man with an enlarged prostate or the patient who has recently had a catheter removed may be asked to record the *time* and *amount* of each voiding for several days. The nurse should teach the patient how to record this information. If the patient is confined to bed, the nurse may do the recording herself. She should always note the amount of urine voided at least every four to eight hours and report inadequate output to the doctor.

For a few hours after a catheter is removed, the patient may have some dribbling because the sphincters of the bladder have been dilated. Dribbling usually can be controlled if the patient is taught to do perineal exercises (p. 156). Continued dribbling should be reported to the doctor since it may indicate that a bladder sphincter muscle has been damaged. It is important to find out if the incontinence is complete (constant dribbling) or if it is only "on urgency" because such information guides planning for the patient's rehabilitation. Another pertinent observation is whether the patient is incontinent in all positions (lying, sitting, or standing). If the major problem is muscle weakness, he will probably have the least difficulty with control when in a prone position and the most while walking. A patient who is having difficulty regaining normal urinary control should limit his fluids after 6 P.M. so that sleep will not be disturbed unduly.

No patient who has an adequate fluid intake should go longer than six to eight hours without voiding. If the patient has a small bladder capacity, such as may be present after a bladder resection, it is expected that he will void more frequently. It is not unusual for such a patient to need the catheter replaced since it is impossible to know how much edema is present around the bladder neck until after the catheter has been removed.

The color and consistency of the urine should be noted. Some patients develop a cystitis (inflammation of the bladder) that is caused by incomplete emptying of the bladder. The urine may appear cloudy or even purulent. It is not unusual for some hematuria to occur from eight to fourteen days after urologic surgery, especially if bleeding has been controlled during surgery by fulguration (electric desiccation), which is followed by a period of sloughing in which the dead tissue breaks away from the healing wound. If hemorrhage occurs, the doctor should be informed because it is sometimes necessary to use some kind of hemostasis to prevent serious secondary hemorrhage.

The relationship of fluid intake
to urinary output

The nurse not only must keep a careful record of the patient's total fluid intake and urinary output but also must study the the record critically in relation to the expected ratio of intake to output. A well-hydrated person who is not losing fluid by other routes will normally excrete amounts of urine almost equal to his fluid intake. Any marked decrease in this ratio is indicative of renal failure (suppression). However, one should be certain that decreased output is not caused by retention of urine in the bladder.

Unless the patient's cardiac or renal status contraindicates forcing fluids, all adult patients with urologic disorders should drink between 2,500 and 3,000 ml. of fluid a day. Young children should be given slightly more fluid than the normal amount (p. 92). Not only does an increased amount of fluids serve to irrigate the urinary system, but it also prevents waste materials from passing through the system in concentrated form, predisposing to the formation of calculi. This advice should not be given only during the acute stage of the illness but should also be included in the health-teaching plan.

Care of the patient
requiring urologic surgery

Emotional support. The basic needs of patients requiring urologic surgery are the same as those of any other surgical patient. However, since urologic surgery may necessitate mutilation of normal anatomy, the patient may have to adjust to the problem of "being different," such as having to adjust to a new route of urine excretion. The

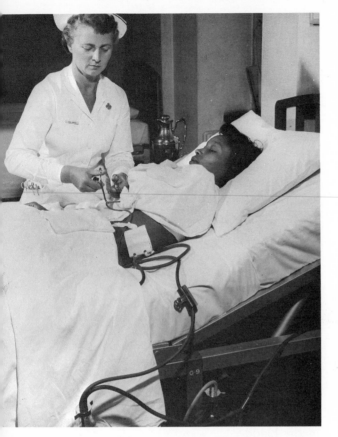

A

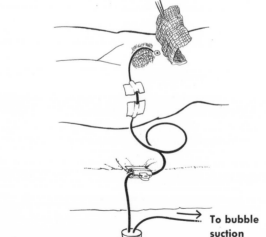

B

Fig. 101

A, The nurse is incorporating a sterile catheter attached to "bubble" suction drainage into a gauze dressing. This apparatus will collect urine draining from a ureterolithotomy incision. **B,** Note that the catheter is anchored to the skin with two flaps of adhesive tape, that the drainage tubing is attached to the bedclothes with a clamp, and that the excess tubing is coiled on the mattress.

To bubble suction

male patient may be made sterile, impotent, or both by some operative procedures. If a radical operative procedure is contemplated, the doctor usually discusses the implications in detail with the patient and his family. Many doctors feel that the patient should make the final decision to undergo such an operation. While attempting to reach a decision, the patient often is very depressed. If he accepts surgery, he usually has a second period of depression at the time active rehabilitation begins.

During these stages there is little that the nurse can do except to give moral support by providing for privacy, allowing extra family visits if they seem to help the patient, caring for his physical needs, and answering or channeling to appropriate persons the questions raised by either the patient or his family. The patient also is often helped by talking with his spiritual adviser, with understanding members of the family, and with patients who have made good adjustments following similar surgical procedures. The nurse should be alert for changes in mood or behavior that might indicate the need for psychiatric guidance.

Hemorrhage. Hemorrhage may follow such operative procedures as transurethral prostatectomy, suprapubic prostatectomy, nephrolithotomy (complete kidney split), and nephrectomy. If drainage tubes are used, the bleeding may be visible. After surgery involving the urinary system, urine is usually dark red or pink, but it should not be bright red or viscid or contain clots. The wounds often normally drain copious amounts of light red urine, but bright red blood on dressings indicates hemorrhage. Following surgery on the kidney, the nurse should look along the posterior edge of the dressing for blood draining over the sacral area. If the patient has a suprapubic incision, blood may be noted along the side of the dressing and in the inguinal region. The classic symptoms of hemorrhage, including pallor, skin clamminess, and apprehension will usually be present. The blood pressure drops and the pulse becomes rapid and thready. Since many patients with urologic disease have hypertension, the blood pressure may be relatively high but still represent a marked drop for the individual. If hemorrhage occurs, the doctor should be called at once. If the bleeding is external, a pressure dressing should be applied over the incision while awaiting the doctor's arrival. If the patient is lying in a pool of blood, the nurse should slip some absorbent material under him until after the doctor has examined him. His bed should then be changed if he can be moved at all. The patient should be protected from the sight of blood on his bedding or in the tubing and bottle.

Dressing materials and material for intravenous therapy should be at the bedside. If the patient has a catheter in place, materials for irrigation should be prepared. In addition, a suction syringe, several liter bottles of sterile physiologic saline solution, and several large waste basins should be available. The patient should be placed flat in bed, or the physician may order him to be placed in the position used for shock, with the lower extremities raised above the level of the heart.

Dressings. Since urine drains from many urologic incisions for several days and sometimes much longer, the nurse working with a urologic patient is more likely to have an order to change postoperative dressings as necessary than is the case when she cares for other surgical patients. Montgomery straps are often used to hold these dressings in place. It is not necessary nor is it good practice to allow dressings to become saturated with urine. Not only is the patient made very uncomfortable, but frequently he is also unable to rest, the skin becomes irritated, and there is an unpleasant odor.

There are many ways to prevent the patient from lying in wet dressings, and the nurse should ask the doctor for an order to use appropriate procedures. If the wound must be kept sterile, incorporate a small, sterile, many-eyed Robinson catheter inside a sterile 4-inch by 8-inch dressing and place it with the eyes directly over the drainage site. Fasten the catheter and gauze in place with a strip of adhesive tape, and attach the end of the catheter to a suction apparatus (Fig. 101). This method not only keeps the patient dry but it also permits the amount of drainage to be recorded. The patient may be out of bed but only within range of the suction.

Any suction used to drain closed cavities and affecting the mucous membrane or the skin surface should be limited to a specific, constant negative pressure; 5 cm. (2 inches) of negative pressure are often ordered. Suction may be used directly from the source if an electric pump on which the amount of negative pressure exerted can be regulated (Gomco or Stedman pump) is used. Tubing from the pump is attached to one arm of a drainage-bottle cap, and the catheter tubing is attached to the other arm.

When the amount of suction cannot be regulated at the source, methods to decrease it must be used. It can be decreased by placing a bottle containing water between the source of suction and the drainage apparatus. A glass tube with one end open to the air is inserted through a cork and immersed a specific number of inches under water placed in one bottle, the "water" bottle. The depth of immersion determines the amount of suction; for 5 cm. (2 inches) of negative pressure, the end of the tube must be under 2 inches of water. Since the water bubbles when the apparatus works smoothly, this method is called *"bubble" suction.*

Tubing from the source of suction may be connected to the drainage system by one of two methods:

Method 1. Using a three-holed cork in the water bottle, attach tubing from the source of suction to a glass connector inserted in one hole. Attach one end of a piece of tubing to a second connector and the other end to one arm of the drainage-bottle cap. The long glass tube regulating the suction and open to the air is in the third

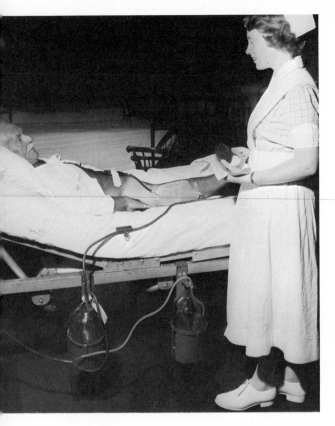

Fig. 102

The nurse has just removed the suction cup from a draining suprapubic wound and has placed a drainer attached to a plastic leg bag over the fistula. The patient is now ready to get up. Note that the suction cup was connected to "bubble" suction drainage.

hole. The other arm of the drainage-bottle cap is attached to the drainage tubing. This setup is similar to that depicted for chest drainage in Fig. 132 except that the drainage tube is not immersed in water.

Method 2. Tubing should run from the source of suction to one arm of a Y connector. Tubing from a second arm of the Y connector is attached to a glass connector inserted into one hole of a two-holed water-bottle cork. The long glass tube open to the air is inserted through the other hole. Tubing from the third arm of the Y connector it attached to one arm of the drainage-bottle cap. The drainage tubing is attached to

452

the other arm of the drainage-bottle cap (Fig. 101).

Suprapubic wounds may sometimes be kept dry by the use of a piece of equipment known as a *suction cup* (Fig. 102). A suction cup can be used only after the sutures have been removed. Before applying it, protect the skin around the area with tincture of benzoin and then place the cup so that the drainage spout is uppermost over the fistula. Be careful not to cover the air outlet in the top of the cup, since the increased suction that is produced may cause the skin under the cup to blister. Securely fasten the cup in place by a wide strip of adhesive tape, Montgomery straps pulled snugly together, or skin cement applied to the edges of the cup. Attach the cup to "bubble" suction. If the patient is to be out of bed or if gravity drainage is needed, a drainer cup may be substituted for the suction cup. It differs from the suction cup in that it has no collecting tube around the inner edge and will cause blistering of the skin if attached to suction drainage. It must be used only with gravity drainage. (See Fig. 102.)

If the urethral catheter is still in place and if there is leakage from the suprapubic wound, the catheter should be checked to ensure that it is draining and is properly placed. The urethral catheter should provide for draining of urine, and the suprapubic wound should be dry.

Another method sometimes used to drain urine from an abnormal opening is the application of a large-sized ureterostomy cup over the fistula, attaching it to straight drainage.

Disposable *plastic ileostomy bags* may be secured over the fistula with skin paste. Since the opening in these bags can be cut to the appropriate size, the skin can be completely protected from urine. The bag may be emptied as necessary, and no dressings are required. This method often works well following ureterolithotomy when the drain is still in place.

In still another method, a 12-inch square of rubber dam is used. An opening large enough to fit around the draining wound is cut in the center, and the rubber dam is pasted to the skin area immediately surrounding the fistula. Dressings are then placed over the drainage site, with the rubber dam folded over them in envelope style. (See Fig. 103.) Montgomery straps will be needed to hold such a dressing in place. If this method is used, dressings still require frequent changing. Although the patient may be dry externally, the urinary drainage lies in a pool over the incision. Unless the dressings are frequently changed, the wound will become infected from organisms growing in the stagnant urine. Patients can usually be taught to change their own dressings when necessary.

None of the methods described works well with every patient. The nurse must study the type of wound, the placement of the incision, and the contour of the surrounding tissue to determine the most satisfactory method for the particular patient.

Frequently, in changing a urologic dressing, a catheter must also be irrigated. If the wound opens into the same cavity drained by the catheter, the same sterile field may be used for the irrigation and the dressing. Each kidney and the bladder are considered separate cavities, and care must be taken not to cause cross-contamination. Irrigation should be done before redressing the wound since some fluid may seep out through the incision.

Planning home care for the patient with urinary drainage

In some urologic conditions, patients will be discharged from the hospital with a catheter still in place in the bladder or in one of the kidneys. It may be only a temporary measure (preparatory to surgery or for a short period postoperatively), or it may be permanent. The doctor usually wants the patient or a member of his family to be taught to care for the catheter. If an ileal conduit operation has been done, the patient must learn to care for the stoma and the equipment used. This care is smiliar to that needed when an ileostomy has been done (p. 667). *The nurse in the hospital should plan the teaching program* so that the patient, under supervision and using his own equipment, will be able to assume complete care of himself before discharge.

Care at home may require additional adjustment, however. Although the nurse in the hospital may suggest types of equipment

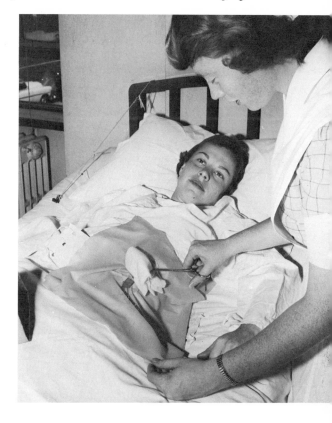

Fig. 103

The student nurse is changing the dressing over a drain that is inserted into a ureterolithotomy wound. Rubber dam has been pasted to the skin around the drain so that urine will not run over the skin.

that can be used, a visit to the home prior to the patient's discharge will give the family and the public health nurse the opportunity to gather and make ready for use the necessary equipment. The public health nurse should visit the patient and his family at regular intervals until they are comfortable with the arrangement for care. (For details of instructions given to patients having catheters in use indefinitely, see specialized texts.[40])

Obstruction and infection of the urinary system

Obstruction and infection of the urinary tract are common causes of renal failure.

453

Rarely is one condition seen without the other. If obstruction is the primary problem, residual urine will form, and it is a good culture medium for bacterial growth. If infection is the primary condition, it frequently causes edema and inflammation, resulting in scarring, which leads to obstruction.

Whenever obstruction occurs at any point along the urinary system, the tubal system above the obstruction becomes dilated. No matter what has caused the obstruction and/or the infection, the symptoms are the same.

Hydronephrosis

Obstruction of the upper urinary tract eventually causes hydronephrosis, or dilatation of the renal pelvis. Common symptoms of hydronephrosis are pain, nausea, vomiting, local tenderness, spasm of the abdominal muscles, and a mass in the kidney region. The patient may, however, have no symptoms. The pain is caused by the stretching of tissues and by hyperperistalsis. Since the amount of pain is proportionate to the rate of stretching, a slowly developing hydronephrosis may cause only a dull flank pain, whereas a sudden blockage of the ureter, such as may occur from a stone, causes a severe stabbing (colicky) pain in the flank or abdomen. The pain may radiate to the genitalia and thigh and is caused by the increased peristaltic action of the smooth muscle of the ureter in an effort to dislodge the obstruction and force urine past it. Narcotics, such as morphine and meperidine, and antispasmodic drugs, such as propantheline bromide (Pro-Banthine) and belladonna preparations, are usually used to relieve severe colicky pain.

The nausea and vomiting frequently associated with acute ureteral obstruction are caused by a reflex reaction to the pain and will usually be relieved as soon as pain is relieved. A markedly dilated kidney, however, may press on the stomach, causing continued gastrointestinal symptoms. If the renal function has been seriously impaired, nausea and vomiting may be symptoms of impending uremia.

When the upper urinary tract becomes infected, symptoms of pyelonephritis appear. If the infected kidney is completely obstructed, no pus or bacteria may be found in the bladder urine.

When obstruction occurs, the treatment consists of reestablishing adequate drainage from the urinary system. This may be temporarily accomplished by placing a catheter above the point of obstruction. Sometimes surgery must be performed to insert a catheter (for example, nephrostomy). Later, definitive treatment is dependent upon the cause. The infection is treated with antibiotics, chemotherapy, fluids, and rest. Urinary antiseptics such as methenamine (Urotropin) and methenamine mandelate may also be given. For these drugs to be effective, the urine must be acid in reaction. Sodium biphosphate (sodium acid phosphate) or enteric-coated ammonium chloride may be ordered. Ammonium mandelate, which is antiseptic and also tends to make the urine acid in reaction, is also used.

The patient is frequently acutely ill, but if he has severe colic, he may not be able to remain in bed until the pain has been relieved. It is not unusual to see a patient with acute renal colic walking the floor, "doubled-up" and vomiting. After narcotics

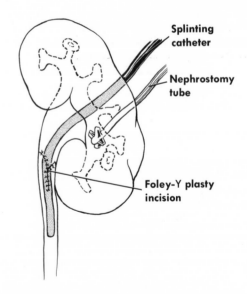

Fig. 104

Placement of a splinting catheter after repair of a ureteropelvic stricture. Note the use of a nephrostomy tube for drainage of urine during healing of the anastomosis.

have been given, such a patient must be protected from injury due to dizziness. As the pain eases, the patient can usually be made relatively comfortable in bed. As soon as the nausea subsides, large amounts of fluids should be urged.

Kidney infections

Blood-borne infections of the kidney occasionally cause a perinephritic abscess or a renal carbuncle. The *perinephritic abscess* forms in the soft tissue of the kidney. A *renal carbuncle* is a localized abscess of the cortex of the kidney. The patient may have symptoms of obstruction dependent upon the location of the abscess, but he frequently has fever, chills, flank tenderness, malaise, and leukocytosis.

Treatment usually consists of the administration of antibiotics, fluids, and rest, but incision and drainage may be required. Following incision and drainage, nursing care will be the same as that for any patient having renal surgery, but the wound drainage usually will be purulent (p. 203). If the causative organism is staphylococcus, the patient is placed on isolation.

Ureteral constriction

Hydronephrosis may be caused by constriction of the ureteral lumen. The constriction may be due to trauma but is often caused by a congenital anomaly. Often symptoms may not appear for years. The constriction, however, finally increases and causes an acute obstruction. In a child or adult with undiagnosed recurrent attacks of acute pyelonephritis, the possibility of a congenital lesion is always considered.

A plastic repair of the ureter must be done to relieve ureteral strictures. A flank or suprapubic incision is made, depending on the location of the stricture. If a ureteropelvic stricture has been repaired, the patient usually will return from the operating room with a nephrostomy tube in place and a splinting catheter in the ureter (Fig. 104), which prevents a new stricture from forming as the ureter heals. Some urologists do not use catheters because they believe they cause irritation and predispose to new strictures. The patient will require the routine care given any patient having renal surgery plus the special considerations mentioned here.

The splinting catheter is usually a small catheter that extends into the ureter to a point below the anastomosis. It is brought out through the wound beside the nephrostomy tube. No drainage should come through this catheter. If it does, it is likely that the nephrostomy tube is partially blocked or that the splinting catheter has slipped into the renal pelvis. The splinting catheter is incorporated into the dressing, not attached to drainage, and it usually is not removed until two or three weeks postoperatively.

The nephrostomy tube may be left in place for several months. Many patients go home with it and return later for its removal. Before it is removed, evidence of ureteral patency is desirable. The evidence may be obtained by several methods. The patient may be taken to the x-ray department and radiopaque dye run by gravity into the nephrostomy tube. If the ureter is patent, the dye will pass through it into the bladder, and the roentgenograms will give evidence of the size of the lumen.

A *burette test* may be ordered to test the patency of the nephrostomy tube. In this test the nephrostomy tube is attached to a calibrated burette, placed so that the center is at kidney level, and filled with a solution of methylene blue dye to a level equal to renal pressure. This procedure is done by the doctor. The patient remains flat in bed during this test, which may last from four to twenty-four hours. A burette reading is taken every hour. Notation should be made of the activity of the patient at the time of the reading, since any activity that causes increased intra-abdominal pressure, such as turning, coughing, and straining, will give an elevated reading. If the ureter is patent and the patient is quiet, the reading will not fluctuate from the original reading by more than 2.5 to 5 cm. (1 to 2 inches). If the ureter is still obstructed, the urine will become stagnant in the renal pelvis, causing increased pressure. The burette readings will progressively increase, and the urine will be forced out through the top of the burette. If pressure increases, the test should be immediately discontinued and the nephrostomy tube reattached to straight drainage equipment. Otherwise, infection is likely to occur. Before the nephrostomy tube is finally removed, it is usually clamped for a day or two. If fever or back pain occurs, the catheter will be reattached to drainage apparatus.

If the stricture is at the ureterovesical juncture, the surgery is done through a suprapubic incision. The ureter is partially resected as it enters the bladder and then reimplanted into the bladder a short distance from the original site. The splinting catheter may then be brought out through the urethra or through the ureterostomy onto the abdominal wall. This catheter is used for drainage and as a splint. The patient may or may not have a cystostomy incision with urinary drainage through a cystostomy tube.

If the strictures are bilateral, as is often true in patients with congenital lesions, bilateral nephrostomies are performed, and later the ureters are resected and replaced by a graft, such as a piece of ileum, or are partially resected and reimplanted into the bladder.

Nephroptosis

Since the kidneys are not anchored in place by ligaments but are kept in normal position by blood vessels, the fatty pads surrounding them, and the pressure of the abdominal organs, they may drop slightly under certain circumstances, such as when a patient has lost a considerable amount of weight. This is known as nephroptosis, commonly called "dropped kidney" or "floating kidney" by the layman. The right kidney, which normally is lower than the left, is most frequently affected. The liver, a very large organ, lies directly above the right kidney.

Nephroptosis rarely causes severe symptoms. The patient may have a "dragging ache" in the flank that is usually relieved by bed rest. Occasionally the doctor suggests that the patient sleep in the Trendelenburg position. He may elevate his bed at home by placing 6-inch blocks under the foot of the bed. If higher elevation is desired, the footboard can be placed on the seat of a sturdy straight chair. A *kidney belt* may be ordered to help keep the kidneys in normal position. It should be applied before arising in the morning and fastened from the bottom up. A high-caloric diet may be ordered if the condition follows weight loss, because additional weight helps to restore the fatty pads around the kidneys.

Conservative treatment is usually effective, but occasionally the kidney drops enough to cause the ureter to become kinked, impairing the flow of urine. In such cases, *nephropexy* is done. In this procedure, the kidney is sutured to the adjacent structures in order to straighten the ureter and provide adequate drainage of the renal pelvis. The patient is usually kept either flat in bed or in the Trendelenburg position for two weeks to prevent tension on the sutures. The nursing care is similar to that given any patient undergoing surgery of the kidney.

Renal calculi

Renal calculi can develop at any age. Although the cause is not completely understood, it is known that the problem is essentially one of crystallization around a microprotein matrix, which may be pus, blood, devitalized tissue, crystals, tumors, or a foreign body such as a catheter. Stasis of urine is known to predispose to formation of some stones (phosphatic), especially if there is associated infection that makes the urine markedly alkaline.

Patients with fractures or other bedridden patients who cannot move about freely are prone to develop renal calculi. This probably is due to the excessive amount of calcium released from the bones in patients who remain in bed without normal activity and to stasis of urine in the lower calyxes of the kidneys when the erect posture is not assumed. To prevent the formation of renal calculi, patients usually are mobilized early or at least turned from side to side in bed every one to two hours. If a patient cannot walk, the doctor may order him placed in a wheelchair or, if necessary, on a tilt table (board) twice a day for an hour or two or in a CircOlectric bed. If his legs are immobilized, he should be encouraged to exercise his arms. Using a trapeze also helps to prevent formation of renal calculi.

Hyperparathyroidism and gout are metabolic diseases that result in hyperexcretion of calcium and uric acid, respectively. These substances are excreted through the kidneys and may form stones.

Since recurrence of renal calculi is common, not only must the immediate problem be treated, but the reason for stone formation must also be discovered, if possible, and treated. Therefore, intensive diagnostic studies may be done after the removal of stones.

The patient usually seeks medical care because of symptoms of obstruction and/or infection. He may have gross hematuria due to trauma from the jagged stone, although hematuria from stones is more often microscopic. Sometimes he complains of frequency and urgency—symptoms of cystitis. The bladder infection is probably a direct extension of an infection behind the stone. Any or all of these symptoms may occur. Often a stone is "silent," causing no symptoms for years. This is true especially of large renal stones.

Diagnostic procedures. The diagnosis of calculi is made from the history and by intravenous pyelography. Sometimes a cystoscopic examination is done, and a ureteral catheter with wax applied to the tip may be passed. This procedure is done if there is any suspicion that the defect in the ureter is a tumor rather than a stone. A stone may scratch the wax.

If it is impossible to pass a catheter beyond the stone, so that a retrograde pyelogram is necessary, a perforated bulb tip may be placed on the ureteral catheter to block the ureter, and the pressure thus created forces some of the dye beyond the stone. This procedure is known as *Woodruff pyelography.*

Stones are usually sent for laboratory study to determine their composition. The results serve as a guide in further search for the cause and in determining suitable prophylactic treatment.

Twenty-four hour urine specimens may be analyzed for their chemical content. Tests to determine blood uric acid levels are done if gout is suspected. Tests for calcium and phosphorus blood levels and the *Sulkowitch test,* to determine the calcium content of the urine (a single urine specimen), may be ordered if hyperparathyroidism is suspected. A parathyroid screening test may be done. Infections and obstructive lesions are looked for (p. 453).

Medical and nursing care. Most renal calculi pass out through the urethra spontaneously. All patients with relatively small stones therefore should have the urine strained.

Urine can be strained easily by placing two opened 4-inch by 8-inch gauze sponges over a funnel. The urine from each voiding should be strained, and one needs to watch closely for the stone, because it may be no bigger than the head of a pin, and the patient may not realize it has passed. Stones larger than 0.5 cm. in diameter are rarely passed.

If there is no infection and if there is not a complete obstruction, the stone may be left in the ureter for several weeks. The patient is usually allowed to continue work, and the stone is closely observed by x-ray examination. A person who is up and about is more likely to pass a stone than is a person who is in bed. Therefore, the patient should be urged to move about actively. Fluids should be taken freely.

Patients frequently have two or three attacks of acute pain (renal colic) before the stone passes. This is probably because the stone gets lodged at a narrow point in the ureter, causing temporary obstruction. The ureters are normally narrower at the ureteropelvic and ureterovesical junctions and at the point where they pass over the iliac crest into the pelvis. If the stone is to pass along the ureter by peristaltic action, the patient must expect some pain. He should determine his tolerance to pain and anticipate when he needs medication to prevent colic. Drugs used include morphine sulfate and meperidine hydrochloride (Demerol) for direct pain, and atropine, methantheline bromide (Banthine), and propantheline bromide (Pro-Banthine) to depress the smooth muscles of the ureter and lessen pain from spasm.

If the stone fails to pass, one or two ureteral catheters may be passed through a cystoscope up the ureter and left in place for twenty-four hours. The catheters dilate the ureter, and when they are removed, the stone may pass into the bladder.

If the patient shows signs of infection, an attempt is made to pass a ureteral catheter past the stone into the renal pelvis. If such an attempt is successful, the catheter is left as a drain, since pyelonephritis will quickly follow if adequate urinary drainage is not reestablished.

The very narrow ureteral catheters may be most effectively attached to drainage

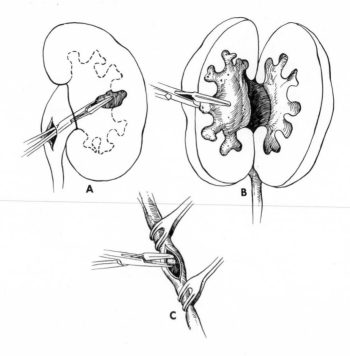

Fig. 105

Location and methods of removing renal calculi from the upper urinary tract. **A,** A pyelolithotomy, the removal of stone through the renal pelvis. **B,** A nephrolithotomy, the removal of a staghorn calculus from the renal parenchyma (kidney split). **C,** A ureterolithotomy, the removal of stone from the ureter.

equipment without encroaching on the catheter lumen by punching a small hole in the rubber top of a medicine dropper and threading the catheter through it. To make the hole, use a large, red-hot needle or pin. Hot metal permanently perforates rubber. The medicine dropper top is then attached to the glass connector of the drainage tubing. If there is a catheter in each ureter, consult the doctor to determine which is right and which is left. Label the catheters with adhesive tape. Check ureteral catheters frequently to see that they are draining. If the urine is purulent, the catheters may become obstructed. If there is no order for irrigation or if patency cannot be reestablished by irrigation, the doctor should be notified at once. Patients with ureteral catheters should be kept in bed and in a low Fowler's position to prevent pull on the catheters and their possible dislodgment.

If the stone has passed to the lower third

of the ureter, it can sometimes be removed by *manipulation*. Special catheters with corkscrew tips, expanding baskets, and loops are passed through the cystoscope, and an attempt is made to "snare" the stone. This procedure is done under anesthesia, and the patient knows that if the manipulation is unsuccessful, he may have surgery immediately. The aftercare of a patient on whom manipulation has been carried out is the same as that following cystoscopy. Any signs suggestive of peritonitis or a decreased urinary output should be carefully watched for, since the ureter occasionally is perforated during manipulation.

The operation for removal of a stone from the ureter is a *ureterolithotomy*. A roentgenogram is taken immediately preceding surgery, since the stone may have moved, and it is desirable to make the incision into the ureter directly over the stone. If the stone is in the lower third of the ureter, a rectus incision is made. If it is in the upper two-thirds, a flank approach is used. If the patient has a ureteral stricture that causes stones to form, a plastic operation to relieve the stricture may be done as part of the operation.

Removal of a stone through or from the renal pelvis is known as a *pyelolithotomy*. Removal of a stone through the parenchyma is a *nephrolithotomy*. (See Fig. 105.) Occasionally the kidney may have to be split from end to end (a kidney split) to remove the stone. Patients in whom such a split is done may have severe hemorrhage following surgery.

Nursing the patient who has ureteral surgery. The patient who has had a ureterolithotomy through a rectus incision needs the routine postoperative care given any patient who has had abdominal surgery. The incision, however, will drain large amounts of urine for two or three weeks postoperatively because the ureter usually is not closed with sutures for fear that closure will cause strictures to form. A tissue drain is placed proximal to the ureteral incision and may be left in place for a week or more. (For special nursing measures that should be used to care for the draining urinary fistula, see p. 451.) Occasionally a ureteral catheter will be left in place for several days.

If the ureter has been approached through a flank incision, nursing care includes the general care given any patient with renal surgery and care of the urinary fistula.

Nursing the patient with a flank (kidney) incision. Whenever there has been a flank incision, there are special nursing responsibilities. Because the incision is directly below the diaphragm, deep breathing is painful and the patient is reluctant to take deep breaths or to move about. He tends to splint his chest and, therefore, is likely to develop atelectasis or other respiratory complications. He needs adequate medication for pain. Usually he will need a narcotic every four hours for twenty-four to forty-eight hours after surgery. After this time, medication may be slowly tapered off. After the patient has been given enough medication to relieve pain and mechanical support has been given to the incision, he should be encouraged to expand the rib cage fully and to cough at least every two hours. He should turn from side to side while he is in bed, and he should be encouraged to get up as soon as permitted. Most patients will be more comfortable turning themselves. After renal surgery the patient can turn to either side unless he has a nephrostomy tube inserted. Even then, he can be tilted to the affected side, with pillows placed at his back for support. It must be ascertained that the tube is not kinked and that there is no traction upon it.

Following surgery on the kidney, most patients have some abdominal distention, which may be due in part to pressure on the stomach and intestinal tract during surgery. Patients who have had renal colic prior to surgery frequently develop paralytic ileus postoperatively. This condition may be related to the reflex gastrointestinal symptoms caused by the pain. Because of the problem of abdominal distention following renal surgery, the patient is often given no food or fluids by mouth for twenty-four to forty-eight hours postoperatively. A nasogastric tube may be passed prophylactically. Fluids by mouth should be started slowly, and the nurse should watch for signs of distention. It is preferable to give warm fluids. Iced fluids, citrus fruit juice, and milk tend to cause flatus and gastric distress in some patients and usually are not given. By the fourth postoperative day most patients tolerate a regular diet. Fluids are usually forced to 3,000 ml. a day, and the doctor may believe it desirable for the patient to continue to take this amount of fluids throughout his life.

If distention occurs, a rectal tube and heating pad may be ordered. Neostigmine (Prostigmin) and carminative enemas may also be ordered. If neostigmine is given, a rectal tube usually is inserted for twenty minutes after its administration. In addition, the patient should be helped to turn frequently, since turning encourages the gas to pass along the bowel.

Hemorrhage may complicate renal surgery. It occurs more often when the highly vascular parenchyma of the kidney has been incised. (See p. 450 for a discussion of hemorrhage in urologic surgery.) The bleeding may occur on the day of surgery, or it may occur eight to twelve days postoperatively, during the period when tissue sloughing normally occurs in healing. Because of the possibility of hemorrhage, some doctors put the patient who has had extensive surgery of the parenchyma back to bed for three or four days after the eighth postoperative day. The nurse should observe the patient closely during this period for any signs of hemorrhage.

Following renal surgery, the patient frequently will have a nephrostomy or a pyelostomy tube inserted. He may have a moderate amount of urinary drainage on his dressing, but if the catheter drains adequately, this diminishes steadily.

Prophylaxis and home care. Since urinary calculi are likely to recur or to develop following surgery on the kidney, patients should understand the importance of following prescribed prophylactic measures. A patient who has had any renal pathology should drink fluids freely for the remainder of his life. It is unwise for him to consume large amounts of high-calcium foods, although adequate nutrition should be maintained. Because toxins from infections are eliminated through the kidneys, and because infections may localize in the urinary tract and produce an alkalinity of the urine, he should avoid upper respiratory infections and any other infections. If he develops an infection, he should force fluids, take extra rest, and seek medical attention at the first sign of complications. He should return to his doctor for examination as recommended.

Special medications and diets designed to eliminate conditions conducive to the formation of stones may be prescribed. Phosphatic calculi comprise about 21% of all calculi and develop in alkaline urine.[13] Their prevention depends upon keeping the urine acid and preventing infection. Enteric-coated ammonium chloride is often used to assure acidity of the urine.

The Shorr regimen has given beneficial results in the prevention of phosphatic calculi. A diet containing only 1,300 mg. of phosphorus daily is prescribed, and 40 ml. of aluminum hydroxide gel are taken after meals and at bedtime. The aluminum combines with the excess phosphorus, causing it to be excreted through the bowel instead of through the kidney, thus decreasing the possibility of stone formation. Patients who must have a catheter in use for long periods of time may be placed on this regimen prophylactically.

Aluminum hydroxide gel tends to constipate some persons. Usually this tendency can be counteracted by eating additional raw fruits and vegetables or drinking a glass of prune juice each morning. If not, a mild cathartic such as psyllium seed (Metamucil) may be prescribed. Patients should be advised not to take mineral oil routinely because it may decrease absorption of vitamin A. Since the patient usually discontinues the regimen because of constipation, the nurse should anticipate this and tell him that bowel regularity can often be maintained by drinking plenty of fluids, eating fresh fruits and vegetables, which will add bulk to the diet, and defecating at a regular time each day.

Calcium oxalate crystallization accounts for over 50% of all urinary tract calculi.[13] These calculi occur in acid urine and in the absence of infection, obstruction, or hyperthyroidism. Attempts are made to prevent recurrences by prescribing a diet high in phosphorus. Sodium or potassium phosphate, to be taken by mouth in dosages of 1 to 3 Gm. daily, may also be prescribed.

Sometimes stones are found to contain both oxalates and phosphates. The diet and drug therapy prescribed for these patients is highly individualized.

Cysts and tumors of the kidney

Masses in the kidney may represent cysts or tumors. Either may eventually result in obstruction.

A *solitary cyst of the kidney* may usually be differentiated from a tumor by intravenous or retrograde pyelography. The solitary cyst may be aspirated with a needle because it often occurs in the renal cortex. However, it usually is explored surgically because it occasionally contains malignant cells. Fluid from a cyst is usually sent for cytologic examination. If there is no evidence of carcinoma, the renal capsule covering the cyst is removed (*decapsulation*).

Polycystic disease is a familial disease characterized by multiple cysts of both kidneys. The cysts press on the parenchyma and cause death from renal failure. There is no specific treatment, and the patient usually dies at a fairly early age.

Tumors of the kidney are usually malignant. They grow insidiously, producing no symptoms for a long time, and finally the patient seeks medical care because of hematuria, dragging back pain, or weight loss. Unfortunately, the hematuria is often intermittent, lessening the patient's concern and causing procrastination in seeking medical care. Any patient with hematuria should have a complete urologic examination, since it is only by immediate investigation of the first signs of hematuria that there is any hope of cure.

Wilms' tumor is an embryonal type of highly malignant growth occurring in children (usually under 7 years of age). It metastasizes early. A mass in the abdomen may be the first sign, and later, hematuria and anemia may occur. The treatment is nephrectomy and radiation treatment if there is no evidence of metastasis.

Tumors of the renal parenchyma, often called *hypernephromas,* are the most common tumors of the kidney. They rarely occur before the age of 30 years. A small tumor in the parenchyma may not be apparent in a routine pyelogram. Therefore, special techniques that gives pictures of sections of the kidney may be used. *Tomography, laminography, planigraphy, stratigraphy,* and *body section radiography* are plain roentgenograms of a section of the body taken with a rotating x-ray tube. No physical preparation of the patient is needed. A *nephrotomogram* is a tomogram taken after intravenous injection of a radiopaque dye. The patient is placed on an x-ray table, and a circulation time study (p. 314) is done to guide the timing of serial roentgenograms about to be taken. A radiopaque dye such as sodium acetrizoate (Pyelokon R), with dehydrocholic acid (Decholin) added, is then given intravenously. The patient is instructed to indicate the moment that he tastes the Decholin, and the films are then taken. Physical preparation of the patient is the same as that for intravenous pyelography. He should be instructed to expect the same sensations when the dye is given, and he should be observed for the same drug reactions. Since the regulation of the time interval is dependent upon the patient's cooperation, the nurse should explain the procedure carefully so that the patient will understand his role.

If a series of "metastatic" roentgenograms show no signs of metastasis, and if there is good function of the unaffected kidney, the diseased kidney is removed. This operation is called a *nephrectomy* and may be done through a lumbar (flank), retroperitoneal, or thoracic approach.

The nursing care following nephrectomy is similar to that of any patient who has had renal surgery. The patient usually has less distention than patients who have had a nephrolithotomy or other operation performed on the kidney. There should be only a minimal amount of serosanguineous drainage on the dressing. Since the renal vessels, which are normally short, are often involved in the tumor mass, they may be difficult to ligate at operation. Therefore, the patient should be carefully observed for signs of internal hemorrhage. If a suture should slip from a renal vessel, death from exsanguination may occur quickly. Blood is usually kept available for immediate emergency use, and the doctor may request that an emergency hemostatic tray be kept at the bedside. The patient also should be observed closely for symptoms of spontaneous pneumothorax (p. 574) since the pleura may be accidentally perforated during the operation. If the thoracic approach is used, a catheter will be inserted into the thoracic cavity, and the nursing care of the patient will be similar to that described on p. 577.

Following surgery for a malignant tumor that is radiosensitive, the patient is usually given a course of x-ray therapy. He will not necessarily be hospitalized during this time. Radiation also may be used over the metastatic sites as palliative treatment for the patient with an inoperable tumor.

Benign prostatic hypertrophy

Benign prostatic hypertrophy (prostatism), the cause of which is unknown, is a common urologic disease. The prostate is an encapsulated gland weighing about 25 grams. It encircles the urethra directly below the bladder, and as it hypertrophies, it impinges upon the bladder outlet.

More than half of all men over 50 years of age have some symptoms of prostatic enlargement. Although the patient's main complaint is inability to void, destruction of renal function is the most serious conse-

461

quence of this disease. The patient first notices that the urinary stream is smaller and more difficult to start as the urethra becomes partially obstructed by the adenomatous growth. As time goes on he may develop frequency, urgency, and burning on urination. These are symptoms of cystitis, caused by prolonged incomplete emptying of the bladder. Stagnant urine is held in trabeculae or cellules formed by sagging of the atonic mucous membrane between overworked hypertrophied muscle bands in the bladder (Fig. 94). The patient complains of increasing frequency as the bladder fails to empty completely at each voiding and, therefore, refills more quickly to the amount that causes the urge to void (usually 250 to 500 ml.). Nocturia is used as a good index of frequency since it is not normal to awaken frequently to void.

The earlier treatment is instituted, the greater the likelihood of an uncomplicated course. Therefore, if any of the problems just mentioned come to the nurse's attention, she should recommend immediate urologic examination in the hope that treatment can be given before renal damage occurs.

Management of acute retention. It is not uncommon for men with prostatic disease to be admitted to the hospital with acute retention of urine (inability to void). This condition occurs especially after drinking alcoholic beverages and after being exposed to cold. If the patient has acute retention, a urethral catheter will be inserted. When the residual urine is more than 1,000 to 1,500 ml., the catheter may be connected to a decompression drainage apparatus, since sudden emptying of an overdistended bladder may cause loss of bladder muscle tone.

Decompression drainage is an arrangement which encourages bladder muscles to maintain their tone since the urine must flow against gravity and the bladder does not empty completely. If the mechanical pressure caused by a markedly distended bladder is suddenly released from the large abdominal vessels and bladder mucosal capillaries, the patient may faint or develop hematuria. As blood rushes to fill the vessels, the blood supply to the brain is momentarily depleted, causing dizziness and faintness. The hematuria is caused by the rupture

of some of the capillaries in the mucosa of the bladder.

The decompression may be high (5 to 8 inches above bladder level), medium (3 to 5 inches above bladder level), or low (at bladder level). A Y tube is attached to a standard at the desired level. The tubing from the catheter is connected to one arm of the Y, and the tubing to the drainage bottle is connected to another arm. The third arm of the Y tube is left open as an air outlet. (See Fig. 100.) Since changing the position of the bed, such as raising the bed to a high Fowler's position for meals, changes the bladder level of the patient, the Y tube must be adjusted accordingly.

The catheter will usually be attached to the high decompression drainage apparatus first and the level then lowered an inch at a time (usually every hour) until low decompression is reached. It may then be attached to straight drainage equipment.

Preoperative preparation (medical and nursing). The treatment for prostatic enlargement is surgery. Some patients require catheter drainage prior to prostatic surgery. The results of the examinations with radiopaque media and of renal function tests are used to determine the need. If a catheter is inserted, it should be connected to drainage at all times since the purpose is to provide an empty bladder, which in turn provides for more complete emptying of the renal pelves. Some patients will have so much renal damage that a cystostomy tube is inserted, and they are sent home with the inserted tube for several months until renal function can be restored to a satisfactory level and prostatic surgery can be performed. If no catheter is used, the patient should measure and record the time and amount of each voiding for twenty-four to forty-eight hours. Such a record gives a fairly accurate picture of the severity of his difficulties.

The usual diagnostic procedures are a blood urea nitrogen test or a blood nonprotein nitrogen test, intravenous pyelography (excretory urography), cystoscopy, and occasionally, urethrography. (A *urethrogram* is a roentgenogram of the urethra. There is no special preparation. A jellylike radiopaque substance is injected into the urethra, and a roentgenogram is taken.) A

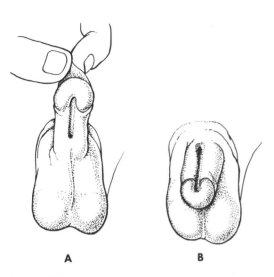

Fig. 108

A, Hypospadias. **B,** Epispadias.

During his convalescence he should take the same precautions previously suggested for patients who have had other types of prostatectomy operations.

The adenomatous tissue of the prostate can also be enucleated through a perineal incision. This procedure is called *perineal prostatectomy*. The incision is made between the scrotum and the rectum. The posterior capsule of the prostate is incised, and the adenoma is removed.

Preoperative and postoperative care following perineal prostatectomy is similar to that given a patient having a radical perineal prostatectomy (p. 522). The patient, however, will not be impotent, and he is no more likely to have urinary incontinence after a simple perineal prostatectomy than after any type of uncomplicated prostatectomy. Convalescent care is the same as for patients who have had other types of prostatectomies.

Bladder diverticula and bladder calculi

A *diverticulum of the bladder* is a large herniated sac of bladder mucosa that has sagged between the hypertrophied muscle fibers. Diverticula are usually seen in men and are often secondary to chronic prostatic obstruction. Since the diverticulum holds stagnant urine, infection often occurs, and calculi may form. Diverticula are excised surgically, and the bladder wall is repaired. The care is the same as that for a patient having a bladder resection.

Bladder stones may be removed through a suprapubic incision, or they may be crushed with a lithotrite (stone crusher) that is passed transurethrally. This procedure is known as a *litholapaxy*. Prior to this procedure a continuous irrigation of the bladder with a solution such as magnesium and sodium citrate (G solution) may be ordered to soften the calculi.

Following bladder stone removal, the bladder may be irrigated (intermittently or constantly) with an acid solution such as magnesium and sodium citrate (G solution) to counteract the alkalinity caused by the infection and to help wash out the remaining particles of stone. If there has been a suprapubic incision, the care of the incision is similar to that following a suprapubic prostatectomy.

Congenital anomalies of the bladder and the urethra

Exstrophy of the bladder and epispadias are developmental anomalies that often occur together (Fig. 108). They result from failure of the midline to close adequately during fetal development and may vary a great deal in their extent. *Exstrophy of the bladder* may consist of only a small fistula leading to the surface on the lower abdominal wall and draining urine, or it may be so extensive that most of the interior of the bladder is visible or is partially everted on the outer abdominal wall. Usually the sphincter muscles of the urethra are faulty, and other anomalies, such as undescended testicles, may be present. *Epispadias* is a failure of closure of the midline on the dorsal surface of the penis. *Hypospadias* is failure of normal closure of the midline on the ventral surface of the penis and may extend from the glans to the perineum. Hypospadias is almost always accompanied by *chordee*, a ventral curvature of the penis caused by abnormal fibrous tissue beneath the shaft of the penis distal to the urethral opening, and most easily noted when penile erection occurs. Both epispadias and hypospadias can

467

usually be noted when the newborn infant is examined closely, even if the defect is only slight. Usually a defect that appears only minimal causes a urinary stream that is far from normal.

Operations for exstrophy of the bladder may include attempts to reconstruct the sphincter muscles of the urethra and to close the ectopic bladder opening. The surgery done depends upon the degree of abnormality. Infection and bladder calculi are frequent if closure cannot be done and normal function cannot be restored soon after birth. Nephrostomies may be done prior to reconstructive surgery, and if satisfactory repair cannot be made, permanent diversion of urinary drainage may be necessary by means of a ureteroileostomy (ileal conduit) (Fig. 109) or other means.

The treatment for epispadias and hypospadias is surgical reconstruction of the urethra. Usually a cystostomy is done prior to surgery to ensure adequate urinary drainage. A problem postoperatively is incontinence, which may be treated with postoperative exercises. Treatment may consist of several operations in stages, so that hospitalization may be prolonged or have to be repeated. As growth occurs, scar tissue may fail to be absorbed sufficiently, and distortions may occur or interference with urinary flow may develop. For these reasons the doctor usually wishes to see the child at regular intervals for years. The nurse should impress upon the child's family the importance of keeping medical appointments as advised and to report any difficulty the child may develop in voiding at once. (For further details in the care of the patient having surgical treatment for these conditions, see specialized nursing texts.[40]

Cystitis

Cystitis is an inflammation of the lining of the bladder. It is often secondary to infection or obstruction elsewhere in the urinary tract. As a primary condition, it is seen more frequently in women than in men and is usually associated with a nonspecific urethritis. It is sometimes caused by vaginal trauma and contamination of the urethra with organisms in the vagina and rectum. A urine culture, however, may yield no growth of organisms. Frequency, urgency, and severe burning on urination are the usual symptoms, but hematuria may occur.

Because cystitis may precede or accompany pyelonephritis, which is a serious disease (p. 442), the person who has any signs of cystitis should seek medical care without delay. Treatment includes antibiotics, chemotherapy, and fluids. Hot sitz baths give relief, and tincture of hyoscyamus, an antispasmodic drug, and potassium citrate, a urinary alkalizer, may be prescribed. Irrigation of the bladder with a mild antiseptic solution such as potassium permanganate 1:8,000 or acetic acid 1:3,000 may be ordered, and is often followed by instilling a 5% solution of mild silver protein (Argyrol). Cystitis frequently becomes chronic and is than extremely difficult to cure. A wide variety of treatments may be tried. The urethra may be dilated to open the ducts of the periurethral glands and to allow them to drain. Dilation is followed by the instillation of an antiseptic solution such as silver nitrate 1:1,000 to 1:10,000. Cortisone may be given systemically for its anti-inflammatory action. Partial cystectomy, irrigation, and even psychotherapy may be tried. Improvement of general health and the eradication of vaginal infection may help. Unless fluids are contraindicated by other disorders, the patient should drink generous amounts of fluid in order to dilute the urine and relieve the discomfort.

Tuberculosis of the urinary system

Although painless gross hematuria often is the initial symptom of renal tuberculosis, other symptoms of cystitis, such as frequency and pain upon micturition, may be the first complaint. Urinalysis may reveal a pyogenic infection, which is secondary to tuberculosis and often is recurrent. When infection of the bladder continues to recur, a search for tubercle bacilli usually is made. Twenty-four-hour or single urine specimens are sent to the laboratory for detection of tubercle bacilli by culture or guinea pig inoculation. Single urine specimens should be the first-voided morning specimen since more organisms are likely to be present in a concentrated specimen. Pyelograms are taken and often show "ragged" calyxes, which are indicative of renal tuberculosis.

A history of pulmonary tuberculosis or

close contact with someone with tuberculosis is usually revealed in the history of the patient with tuberculosis of the urinary system. The pulmonary lesion, however, may have been minimal and never diagnosed. The organisms reach the kidneys through the bloodstream, but there may be no symptoms until several years after healing of the original lesion. The disease is usually seen in patients between 20 and 40 years of age and is more common in men than in women.

If the disease is unilateral but far advanced, a nephrectomy usually is done. Preceding the operation, the patient is given short courses of antitubercular drug therapy in various combinations. Following surgery, drug therapy is continued, sometimes for as long as two years. If the disease is bilateral, or unilateral and early, an extensive course (eight months to one year) of antituberculosis drug therapy is given. (See p. 555 for medical treatment of pulmonary tuberculosis.) The urine is examined at regular intervals.

The nurse should take time to explain and answer questions about the disease, its communicability, and the probable rehabilitation course. If a pulmonary lesion is not active, the patient with tuberculosis of the urinary system may not have to be isolated. Patients may worry about giving tuberculosis to others or fear that they can never safely have sexual intercourse again. The patient should not have sexual intercourse while there are tubercle bacilli in the urine because it is possible to spread the disease to other persons by this means. Patients are taught to wash their hands thoroughly with soap and water after any contact with urine or the genitalia. If there is a draining wound or lesion, soiled dressings should be wrapped in paper and disposed of immediately. Linen contaminated with urine or drainage should be boiled for twenty minutes and then washed.

Tumors of the urinary bladder

Hematuria should always be investigated. Although it occurs in nonmalignant urinary tract diseases, painless hematuria is the first symptom in the majority of tumors of the bladder. It is usually intermittent, and patients may therefore fail to seek treatment.

Cystitis may be the first symptom of a bladder tumor since the tumor may act as a foreign body in the bladder. Renal failure due to obstruction of the ureters sometimes is the reason the patient seeks medical care. Vesicovaginal fistulas may occur before other symptoms develop. The last two conditions indicate a poor prognosis, because usually the tumor has infiltrated widely.

Medical treatment and nursing care. Most bladder tumors start as *benign papillomas* or as *leukoplakia.* Although these conditions may be successfully treated by early fulguration, a new tumor may appear five or more years later. Any patient who has had a papilloma removed should have a cystoscopic examination every six months because further symptoms may not appear until a new papilloma has become a far-advanced tumor. Repeated cystoscopies may seem unacceptable to patients who dread them. The necessity for frequent examination should be fully explained by the doctor and the explanation reinforced by the nurse. Emphasis can be placed on how fortunate the patient is to know about his disease so that early treatment, the only successful treatment of bladder tumors, can be instituted if necessary. If he had never had symptoms from the papilloma, cancer might have been far advanced prior to diagnosis.

Carcinoma of the bladder is diagnosed by cystoscopy and biopsy. The treatment is dependent upon the size of the lesion and the depth of the tissue involvement. Small tumors with minimal tissue layer involvement may be adequately treated with *transurethral fulguration* or excision. The patient may or may not have a Foley catheter inserted after surgery. The urine may be pink-tinged, but gross bleeding is unusual. Burning on urination may be relieved by forcing fluids and applying heat over the bladder region by means of a heating pad or a sitz bath. The patient is discharged within a few days after surgery.

If a cancerous lesion of the bladder is small and superficial, *radioisotopes* contained in a balloon of a Foley catheter may be inserted into the bladder. The catheter is attached to drainage, and all urine must be saved and sent to the radioisotope department for monitoring prior to disposal. Severe cystitis and proctitis usually result from this

469

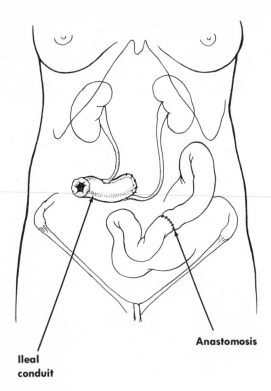

Ileal conduit

Anastomosis

Fig. 109

Ileal conduit.

treatment, and the patient may be very uncomfortable for several days or weeks. Forcing fluids gives some relief from the symptoms, and urinary antiseptics and antispasmodic drugs are usually ordered. A low-residue diet and mineral oil may be ordered to keep the stools soft and lessen rectal discomfort.

Sometimes radioactive substances such as *radon seeds* are implanted around the base of a tumor. This usually is done through a cystotomy but may also be done transurethrally through a cystoscope. If a cystotomy has been done, the patient may have a cystostomy tube inserted, but more often a urethral catheter will be used, and the cystotomy incision will be completely closed. (See p. 280 for precautions that should be taken when radiation treatment is used.) Radiation treatment usually causes a rather severe cystitis, which is treated by giving sedatives, antispasmodic drugs, fluids, and heat locally.

External radiation of tumors of the bladder with x-rays or cobalt teletherapy is rarely done except as a palliative treatment for inoperable cancer. Unless the urinary stream has been diverted prior to radiation, contraction of the bladder and serious cystitis often occur. If a urinary diversion procedure has been done, however, radiation of the bladder may decrease bleeding from the tumor and relieve pain.

Chemotherapy using purine antagonist drugs such as 5-fluorouracil occasionally may be used to treat tumors of the bladder that have metastasized. The drugs may be given either orally or intravenously. (See p. 288 for dosages and for nursing care necessary when these drugs are given.)

Surgical procedures. If the tumor involves the dome of the bladder, a segmental resection of the bladder may be done. Over half of the bladder may be resected, and although the patient may have a capacity of no more than 60 ml. immediately postoperatively, the elastic tissue of the bladder will regenerate so that the patient is able to retain from 200 to 400 ml. of urine within several months.

The decreased size of the bladder, however, is of major importance in the postoperative period. The patient will return from surgery with catheters draining the bladder both from a cystostomy opening and from the urethra. This is to obviate the possibility of obstruction of drainage, since it would take only a very short time for the bladder to become distended and there would be danger of disrupting the suture line on the bladder. One or both of the catheters may be drained by "bubble" suction. Since the bladder capacity is markedly limited, the catheters usually cause severe bladder spasm. Usually the urethral catheter is not removed until three weeks postoperatively. Sometimes, if the cystostomy wound is not completely healed, the urethral catheter will have to be left in place longer.

As soon as the urethral catheter is removed, the patient becomes acutely aware of the small capacity of the bladder. He usually will need to void at least every twenty minutes. He needs to be reassured that the bladder capacity will gradually increase. Meanwhile, he should be urged to force fluids to 3,000 ml., but he should be advised to space the fluids so that time spent in the bathroom is not an inconvenience. He should thus take large quantities of fluids at one time, limit fluids for several hours before he plans to go out, and take no fluids after 6 P.M.

Cystectomy. A cystectomy, or complete removal of the bladder, usually is done only when the disease seems curable. Complete removal of the bladder requires permanent urinary diversion. This may be accomplished by various methods. The ureters may be transplanted into the intact bowel *(uretero-intestinal anastomosis).* A sigmoidal colostomy may be performed to divert the fecal stream, and the ureters may then be transplanted into the lower bowel *(anal bladder).* A section of the ileum may be resected with its blood supply and closed at one end. The other end of the section is brought to the skin as an ileostomy and the ureters are transplanted into it. This procedure, which is called an *ileobladder* or *ileal conduit,* is used most often at the present time. (See Fig. 109.) The ureters may be brought directly onto the abdomen (ureterostomies), although this procedure is seldom done. A new procedure, *colocystoplasty,* has been used also. A portion of sigmoid is resected and fashioned into a bladder. The urethra and ureters are anastomosed to it in an anatomic position that is as nearly normal as possible. After healing, there is relatively normal physiologic bladder function. Whether or not this procedure is feasible depends partly upon the extent of the cystectomy.

The patient whose ureters are transplanted into the normally functioning bowel is usually socially acceptable, but hydronephrosis and renal infection frequently occur. The kidneys may empty poorly because the rectum normally has a higher pressure than the bladder due to fecal contents and peristalsis. As the ureters and renal pelves dilate, bacterial organisms easily start an infection. The intestinal tract also has absorptive powers, and waste products in the urine may be reabsorbed, upsetting the electrolyte balance of the body. This has been found to be a serious disadvantage of anastomosis of the ureters to the bowel.

Recently, many urologists have come to feel that transplantation of the ureters into

an ileobladder is the diversional procedure of choice since the patient seems able in most cases to cope with an ileostomy bag used for drainage, and the problem of reabsorption of substances from the urine through the segment of ileum does not seem to present serious problems.

Immediately after the cystectomy the patient is usually acutely ill. Since not only the bladder but also large amounts of surrounding tissue are removed (the male patient also has a radical perineal prostatectomy), the patient may have a circulatory disturbance. This may be surgical shock, thrombosis, or cardiac decompensation. There is a long vertical or transverse abdominal incision, and there may be a perineal incision. The patient may be given nothing by mouth for several days, and a nasogastric tube may be inserted. The nursing care is the same as that given any patient after major abdominal surgery plus the routine care for a perineal wound and the care of the diverted urinary drainage.

Nursing the patient with an ileal conduit. The most common method of urinary diversion is via the ileobladder. The nurse who encounters other, newer procedures should refer to recent periodicals.[5,20,45,50]

Preoperatively the patient who is to have an ileal conduit constructed is given a bowel preparation (usually cathartics, enemas, one of the sulfonamides such as sulfathalidine, or neomycin, and a clear-liquid diet) for three days. If surgery is delayed for any reason, the doctor should be consulted before continuing the regimen longer since vitamin B and K deficiencies may result, and sometimes fungus infections occur. Fluids, vitamins, and glucose may be given intravenously to supplement the diet.

Following an ileal conduit procedure, the patient usually returns from the operating room with a catheter inserted through the ileostomy opening to provide for urinary drainage. Since the ileum secretes mucus, the catheter usually needs to be irrigated gently every two to four hours. Sometimes no catheter is used, and an ileostomy bag (usually a plastic one) is secured over the opening to collect drainage. Regardless of what method is used, the nurse must watch carefully for, and report at once, any signs, such as lower abdominal pain or decreased urinary output, that indicate distention of the isolated segment of ileum with urine, since distention may cause the suture line to rupture, or it may cause back pressure on the kidneys. The collection bag should be emptied frequently so that it cannot contribute to back pressure and stop drainage. Special ileal conduit bags that can be attached to drainage apparatus are available, and they are preferable to a regular ileostomy bag. Swelling about the stoma may also prevent emptying of the conduit. Swelling about the ureteroileal anastomoses or pressure of distended organs against the conduit may prevent drainage from the ureters.

Symptoms of peritonitis (fever, abdominal pain) should be watched for carefully and reported at once. After this type of surgery, the intestinal anastomosis may leak fecal material, or the ileal conduit may leak urine into the peritoneal cavity. If leakage occurs, an emergency operation is done to repair the weakened area.

The patient usually has a nasogastric or intestinal tube inserted for several days after an ileal conduit procedure to prevent distention of the bowel with resultant pressure on the intestinal anastomosis. (Details of care relating to the intestinal anastomosis are discussed on p. 680.)

The doctor usually changes the ileostomy bag and dilates the stoma daily for several days postoperatively. This procedure then may become a nursing responsibility, and later it is taught to the patient. In dilating the ileal stoma, a finger cot should be slipped onto the finger to be inserted, and the finger cot should be well lubricated with water-soluble jelly. The finger is inserted gently through the opening and into the conduit. This procedure may have to be done daily at first, but later, once a week usually suffices. In doing this procedure and in teaching the patient, the nurse should stress proper aseptic technique so that organisms are not introduced into the conduit. Washing of hands is imperative before any care is given. When a bag is being used for drainage, the doctor periodically inserts a catheter into the conduit to determine how much residual urine is in it. If there is a large amount of residual urine, permanent catheter drainage may have to be used, or the patient may be taught to insert a catheter several times a day to drain the ileal conduit.

A temporary ileal conduit bag is used for about six weeks or until the stoma has shrunk to its permanent size. The stoma should then be measured carefully, and a pattern of the exact size of the opening needed should be made. The cuff of the bag should exert no pressure on the stoma, and no skin surface should be exposed. Using the pattern, a surgical supply house will provide permanent bags. Usually at least two bags are ordered so that they can be cleaned and aired alternately.

Ileal conduit bags are applied by a method similar to that used for ileostomy bags (p. 668). Since the skin must be dry, it is easier to apply the bag when the patient has had nothing to drink for three or four hours. Placing a cotton ball over the ileal opening while the skin is prepared helps to prevent urine from draining onto it. Care of the skin and the equipment are the same as for the patient who has an ileostomy. Care should be taken that clothing does not constrict the bag. Depending upon the placement of the ileostomy opening, it may be preferable for men to wear suspenders rather than a belt, and a girdle or support with an opening cut out over the bag should be worn.

A written procedure that includes a list of equipment and where to procure it, the steps of routine care, and management of problems that frequently are encountered is helpful for the patient learning to care for his own ileal conduit.

The ileal conduit is placed in such a way that it should not act as a reservoir but only as a passageway from the ureter to the outside. Therefore, patients with ileal conduits should have less difficulty with electrolyte imbalance than those in whom the bowel serves as a reservoir. Some problems do occur, however, and the patient should be advised to report signs of renal failure or electrolyte imbalance such as nausea, vomiting, diarrhea, or lethargy to the doctor.

Nursing patients with other types of urinary diversion. Patients who in the past have had other types of urinary diversional procedures may be admitted to the hospital or be seen by the nurse in the home. Therefore, she must know how to cope with the problems presented by these patients.

After *ureterointestinal anastomosis*, the bowel adjusts to being a reservoir for urine. The stool will be soft, but the patient will be able to tell when he needs to void and when he needs to defecate. He will be able to retain about 200 ml. of urine. If the patient is incontinent or has symptoms of renal failure or electrolyte imbalance, a large rectal tube (28 Fr. attached to drainage) is left in the rectum. It often is secured in the gluteal fold with a double-flap adhesive tape anchorage. Ethyl aminobenzoate ointment may be used to lubricate the tube because of its local anesthetic effect. The urinary output should be carefully measured and recorded. The tube must be removed for the patient to defecate and then be reinserted.

Even if rectal tube drainage is not used during the day, patients with ureterointestinal anastomoses often are advised to insert a tube each night. When the tube is out, the patient should be urged to void every four hours to minimize the reabsorption of waste products and to improve emptying of the renal pelves. Any nausea, vomiting, diarrhea, or lethargy should be reported to the doctor. These symptoms are suggestive of electrolyte imbalance, and alkalizing or acidifying drugs may be prescribed. The patient should not be given enemas, rectal suppositories such as bisacodyl, or strong cathartics such as castor oil or licorice powder because the increased peristalsis in the lower bowel may force contaminated urine up the ureters. Small doses of milk of magnesia may be ordered if a cathartic is necessary. The patient usually is encouraged to eat a regular diet and to drink approximately 3,000 ml. of fluid daily.

When an anal bladder has been constructed, urinary output is cared for in a manner similar to that used by the patient with ureterointestinal anastomoses. Fecal discharge, however, is through a colostomy. (See p. 682 for care of the patient who has a colostomy.)

When the patient has cutaneous ureterostomies, the urine is drained either through ureterostomy cups or ureteral catheters inserted into the renal pelves. Catheters inserted into ureterostomies are cared for in a manner similar to that for any catheter draining the renal pelvis. *Ureterostomy cups* (Singer cups) are applied to the skin with skin paste or double-sized adhesive disks and may require changing only every two or three days. Patients are taught to care for these cups themselves, but the nurse should know correct procedure so that she may assist them as necessary. Because few patients now use this method, it will not be described fully here. (For the details of the procedure, consult specialized texts.[40])

If the patient wearing a cup complains of back pain, the cup should be removed at once and the doctor notified unless, on removing it, the ureter drains. If it does, the drainage apparatus should be checked carefully for blockage before reapplying the cup. Catheters may need to be inserted to provide drainage. Each time the cup is removed, the patient should take a warm bath. If this is not possible, the skin around the ureterostomy opening should be washed thoroughly and a warm compress placed over it for about fifteen minutes. If the skin is irritated, a heat lamp (60-watt bulb placed 2 feet away from the abdomen) should be used for twenty minutes. The cup should be reapplied since the cement and the pressure exerted by the cup have healing properties. A ureteral catheter sometimes may have to be inserted until the skin heals. If the stoma swells, provision of an air outlet by inserting a No. 20 hypodermic needle with the hub uppermost into the tubing close to the cup may help. If the cup irritates the stoma, a plastic postoperative ileostomy appliance should be used until the swelling subsides (p. 668).

Trauma to the urinary tract

The urinary tract may be seriously damaged by external trauma. If the pelvis has been fractured, one should observe the patient for any signs of a perforated bladder or urethra. There may be no urinary output, the urine may be bloody, or there may be symptoms of peritonitis. When the lower urinary tract is injured, provision must be made for urinary drainage at once. A cystostomy frequently is performed. Reparative surgery is undertaken when the patient's condition warrants it.

The kidney may be contused, torn, or completely ruptured by an external blow. Since spontaneous healing may occur, the patient is observed closely, and surgical intervention is usually necessary only if the kidney has been ruptured or if severe hemorrhage follows.

References and selected readings*

1 Ball, Thomas L.: Gynecologic surgery and urology, ed. 2, St. Louis, 1963, The C. V. Mosby Co.

2 Barry, Kevin G., and Malloy, John P.: Oliguric renal failure, J.A.M.A. 179:510-513, Feb. 17, 1962.

3 Beeson, Paul B., and McDermott, Walsh, editors: Cecil-Loeb textbook of medicine, ed. 11, Philadelphia, 1963, W. B. Saunders Co.

4 Bell, Alexander H., and Shanahan, Douglas A.: The management of undescended testicle, S. Clin. North America 64:1571-1582, Dec. 1964.

5 Berman, Henry I.: Urinary diversion in treatment of carcinoma of the bladder, S. Clin. North America 45:1495-1508, Dec. 1965.

6 Boyd, Julian D., and Murdock, Harold R., Jr.: Urinary excretion of radiohippuran as a measure of renal function, J. Urol. 86:294-295, Sept. 1961.

7 Campbell, Meredith F., editor: Urology, ed. 2, vols. 1-3, Philadelphia, 1963, W. B. Saunders Co.

8 *Ceccarelli, Frank E., and Smith, Perry C.: Studies on fluid and electrolyte alterations during transurethral prostatectomy, J. Urol. 86:434-441, Oct. 1961.

9 Charghi, Ali, and others: A method of urinary diversion by anastomosis of the ureters into a sigmoid pouch, J. Urol. 94:376-379, Oct. 1965.

10 Cox, Clair E., and Hinman, Frank, Jr.: Incidence of bacteriuria with indwelling catheters in normal bladders, J.A.M.A. 178:919-921, Dec. 2, 1961.

11 *Creevy, C. Donald, and Tollefson, Dorothy M.: Ileac diversion of the urine and nursing care of the patient with an ileac diversion of the urine, Am. J. Nursing 59:530-536, April 1959.

12 *Davis, Joseph E.: Drugs for urologic disorders, Am. J. Nursing 65:107-112, Aug. 1965.

13 Elliot, James S.: Urinary calculus disease, S. Clin. North America 45:1393-1404, Dec. 1965.

14 Fellows, Barbara: Hemodialysis at home and adapting to long-term hemodialysis, Am. J. Nursing 66:1775-1781, Aug. 1966.

15 *Fellows, Barbara: The role of the nurse in a chronic dialysis unit, Nurs. Clin. North America 1:577-586, Dec. 1966.

16 Fraser, Sir Kenneth: Hypospadias, S. Clin. North America 64:1551-1570, Dec. 1964.

17 Goodman, Louis S., and Gilman, Alfred, editors: The pharmacological basis of therapeutics, ed. 3, New York, 1965, The Macmillan Co.

18 Greenhill, J. P., editor: Obstetrics, ed. 13, Philadelphia, 1965, W. B. Saunders Co.

19 Harrison, T. R., and others, editors: Principles of internal medicine, ed. 5, New York, 1966, McGraw-Hill Book Co.

20 Hradec, Eduard A.: Bladder substitution, indications and results in 114 operations, J. Urol. 94:406-417, Oct. 1965.

21 Hunt, James C., and others: Diseases of the kidney, M. Clin. North America 50:925-1186, July 1966.

22 *Kasselman, Mary Jo.: Nursing care of the patient with benign prostatic hypertrophy, Am. J. Nursing 66:1026-1030, May 1966.

23 *Kelly, Ann E., and Gensini, Goffredo G.: Renal arteriography, Am. J. Nursing 64:97-99, Feb. 1964.

24 *Leadbetter, Guy W., and Leadbetter, Wyland F.: Indications and techniques for renovascular surgery on hypertensive patients, J. Urol. 85:105-114, Feb. 1961.

25 LeBlanc, Gilbert A., and Richardson, J. Francis: Elimination of catheters, tubes and packs in suprapubic prostatectomy, J. Urol. 86:431-433, Oct. 1961.

26 *Lombardo, Louis J., Jr., Heyman, Arnold M., and Barnes, Roger W.: Injuries of the urinary tract due to external trauma, J.A.M.A. 172:1618-1622, April 2, 1960.

27 Longmire, William P., Jr.: A current survey of clinical experience in tissue and organ transplantation, S. Clin. North America 45:407-421, April 1965.

28 Lubash, Glenn D.: Acute renal failure, Hosp. Med. 1:14-18, April 1965.

29 Mackinnon, Harold A.: Urinary drainage: the problem of asepsis, Am. J. Nursing 65:112, Aug. 1965.

30 Marshall, Victor F.: Fiber optics in urology, J. Urol. 91:110-114, Jan. 1964.

31 *Merrill, Arthur J.: Nutrition in chronic renal failure, J.A.M.A. 173:905-911, June 25, 1960.

32 *Mohammed, Mary R. B.: Urinalysis, Am. J. Nursing 64:87-89, June 1964.

33 Morris, George C., Jr., DeBakey, Michael E., and Cooley, Denton A.: Surgical treatment of renal failure of renovascular origin, J.A.M.A. 182:609-612, Nov. 10, 1962.

34 *Mossholder, Irene B.: When the patient has a radical retropubic prostatectomy, Am. J. Nursing 62:101-104, July 1962.

35 Mueller, C. Barber: The mechanism of acute renal failure after injury and transfusion reaction and its prevention by solute diuresis, S. Clin. North America 45:499-508, April 1965.

36 *Murphy, John J., and Schoenberg, Harry W.: Urologic aspects. In Cowdry, E. V., editor: The care of the geriatric patient, ed. 2, St. Louis, 1963, The C. V. Mosby Co.

37 Newton, Kathleen, and Anderson, Helen C.: Geriatric nursing, ed. 4, St. Louis, 1966, The C. V. Mosby Co.

38 *Nursing Division, Memorial Center: Home care for the patient after urologic surgery, New York, 1954, Memorial Center for Cancer and Allied Diseases.

39 *Santora, Delores: Preventing hospital-acquired urinary infection, Am. J. Nursing 66:790-794, April 1966.

*References preceded by an asterisk are particularly well suited for student reading.

40 *Sawyer, Janet R.: Nursing care of patients with urologic diseases, St. Louis, 1963, The C. V. Mosby Co.

41 *Schlegel, J. U.: Pyelonephritis, J. Urol. 86:12-16, July 1961.

42 Schreiner, George E.: Toxic nephropathy, J.A.M.A. 191:849-850, March 8, 1965.

43 *Sharp, Robert F.: Hydronephrosis: development of present concept of management, J. Urol. 85:206-210, March 1961.

44 *Shebelski, Dorothy I.: Nursing patients who have renal homotransplants, Am. J. Nursing 66:2425-2428, Nov. 1966.

45 Sister M. Agnes Clare Frenay: A dynamic approach to the ileal conduit patient, Am. J. Nursing 64:80-84, Jan. 1964.

46 *Spence, Harry M., and Littlepage, Sylvia: Genitourinary injuries and nursing care, Am. J. Nursing 55:970-974, Aug. 1955.

47 Stewart, B. H., and others: Differential function studies in renal hypertension: indications and techniques, J. Urol. 94:7-14, July 1965.

48 Twiss, Mary R., and Maxwell, Morton H.: Peritoneal dialysis, Am. J. Nursing 59:1560-1563, Nov. 1959.

49 U. S. Department of Health, Education, and Welfare: Morbidity and mortality, annual supplement, 1964, Sept. 30, 1965.

50 *Walsh, Michael Adrian, Ebner, Marion, and Casey, Joseph William: Neo-bladder, Am. J. Nursing 63:107-110, April 1963.

51 Winter, Chester C., Roehm, Marilyn M., and Watson, Harriet Grant: Urinary calculi—medical and surgical management and nursing care, Am. J. Nursing 63:72-76, July 1963.

20

The patient with disease of the reproductive system

Study questions

1 Review the anatomy of the male and female reproductive systems.

2 Review the menstrual cycle. During which period does ovulation occur? What is the relationship of estrogen and progesterone to the cycle?

3 Review the methods of draping a patient for a pelvic examination and of assisting the physician with this examination.

4 What physical, hormonal, and psychologic changes occur at puberty in girls? In boys?

5 List the male hormones. What physiologic changes do they stimulate? List the female hormones. What physiologic changes do they stimulate?

6 Review the following basic nursing procedures: catheterization, insertion of retention catheters, use of T binder and methods of securing perineal dressings, measurement of drainage and care of drainage equipment, use of cold applications.

7 What are the main purposes of a douche? Review the procedure. What solutions are most often used?

8 What are the purposes of using heat lamps and sitz baths? What is the physiologic principle for these therapeutic actions? Review both procedures.

Diseases of the reproductive systems, especially cancer, take a high toll of human life. In addition, many other pathologic conditions can occur, and many of them go untreated for long periods of time. The nurse has a responsibility to assist in general health education, to direct patients to good medical care, and to understand the treatment available and the nursing care needed when disease has developed.

Health education

Many people, especially women, turn to nurses with questions and problems related to the reproductive system. The nurse should, therefore, have a sound knowledge of the normal system and its function. She should also be able to recognize deviations from normality so that she may guide the patient to medical care when it is needed. She will need to use great skill in helping people to talk about these problems, for many people hesitate to express themselves freely. The nurse with an understanding and accepting attitude can provide an atmosphere that makes it easier for people to discuss their problems.

Preparation for puberty

Sex education. The nurse is in a position not only to answer parents' questions regarding themselves but also to advise them of the importance of sex education for their children and of how and what to teach. Often parents want to teach their children, but they do not know how to proceed. They should themselves understand the anatomy and physiology of the reproductive system. Sex education is usually simple for parents who are prepared to give frank answers as the child grows and asks questions. For young children, lengthy explanations are not necessary. The child needs only direct answers to his specific questions.

In addition to individual teaching of parents, the nurse can assist with sex education by working through groups. The school nurse and the public health nurse are most likely to have this opportunity, but in the smaller community any nurse who expresses interest may be called upon by civic groups. The nurse may participate in parent-teacher programs and, by using drawings, filmstrips and films, explain normal reproductive processes. Church groups may give some instruction, and other groups, such as the Girl Scouts, may include some instruction in courses in personal hygiene. By planning with parents the course content to be taught to their children, many difficulties and misunderstandings are avoided, and often the parents learn facts that they need to know before they can contribute to their children's understanding of sex. The school nurse may help teachers in physical education to cover content in this area and may assist with, or herself teach, courses in hygiene for children at various age levels. Some schools are now adding discussion periods on sex education for teen-agers.

The nurse should evaluate critically articles in daily papers and popular magazines so that she may guide parents in the use of the information they offer. Often she can be helpful in suggesting books that the parents may read in anticipation of their children's questions or that they may make available to their children. There are many pamphlets and books on sex education, but only a few can be mentioned here. Most state departments of health supply useful material. *How to Tell Your Child About Sex** is helpful to parents in answering typical questions. *The Gift of Life*[†] is an excellent booklet to put into the hands of children. *A Girl Grows Up*[‡] is highly recommended for teen-age girls. *Attaining Manhood*[§] is good for the adolescent boy. *The Adolescent Years*[‖] is written for parents. Three books[¶] on reproduction that are written for various age levels are as follows: *The Story of Life,* for boys and girls about 10 years old; *How Life Goes On and On,* for high school girls; and *The Age of Romance,* for college girls. *The Wonder of Life,*[**] by a pediatrician and a teacher, explains sex and reproduction frankly for the preadolescent boy and girl. Especially recommended for Roman Catholics is *Parents, Children and the Facts of Life.*[††]

Menstruation. Many women ask questions regarding menstruation. Their understanding may have been limited by no instruction except that passed to them by friends or by misinformation given to them by their parents who were unfamiliar with physiologic functions. On the other hand, the nurse may find women who know about the entire menstrual cycle but have difficulty in accepting it as a normal periodic process.

Instruction concerning menstruation should precede its onset, usually referred to as the menarche. Menstruation is a normal process and should be treated as such. The "period" or the "monthly period" are sensible and accurate terms to use. The psycho-

---

*Hymes, James L.: Public Affairs Pamphlet, No. 149, New York, 1949, Public Affairs Committee, Inc.

†Prepared by the New York State Office of Public Health Education, Albany, 1951, New York State Department of Health.

‡Fedder, Ruth: ed. 3, New York, 1967, McGraw-Hill Book Co.

§Corner, George: ed. 2, New York, 1952, Harper & Row, Publishers.

‖Wettenberg, William W.: New York, 1955, Harcourt, Brace & Co.

¶Published by the American Medical Association, Chicago, Ill.

**Levine, Milton I., and Seligman, Jean H.: New York, 1940, Simon & Schuster, Inc.

††Sattler, Henry V.: Garden City, New York, 1956, Image Books.

logic implications of "being sick" and "having the curse" are poor. The girl should know how menstrual flow comes about, what its purpose is, and any special care that she should give herself during this time. She will probably have little discomfort if she has adequate rest, maintains good posture, eats a balanced diet, and participates in regular, moderate exercise. There may be slight discomfort in the lower back, legs, and pelvis, particularly on the day of the onset, and a slight tendency to fatigue. Some adolescent girls are concerned about circles that appear under their eyes during menstruation and that they fear are obvious; additional rest will usually control this problem. Girls should know that breast changes may occur either preceding the period or at various times throughout the monthly cycle; in some instances, rather marked tenderness and enlargement of the breasts occur. Mild mood swings also occur in the normal menstrual period and should be understood and accepted, but excessive allowances should not be made for them.

Normally there is a loss of from 30 to 180 ml. of menstrual fluid during the period, which usually lasts from three to five days. One-half to three-fourths of the fluid is blood and the remainder is mucus, fragments of endometrial cells, and desquamated vaginal epithelium.[34] The average woman probably needs approximately a dozen napkins for the entire period. Tampons can be used unless a tight hymenal ring makes their insertion and removal uncomfortable. They should be changed frequently during the height of flow. If the string should break and the tampon cannot be removed, a doctor should be consulted at once.

There is considerable individual variation in speed of onset, in duration, and in regularity of menstrual flow. Some irregularity is usual in the first few months and may continue for a few years or even indefinitely in some women. The pattern of the menstrual cycle may be upset by such things as changes in climate, changes in working hours, emotional trauma, and acute or chronic illness. Any of these factors may alter the total life pattern temporarily and produce change in the nerve centers in the hypothalamus. This upset causes a change in the rate and timing of the secretion of the pituitary hormones,

which probably maintain the normal menstrual cycle. An early menstrual period or absence of the period is not significant if it occurs only one month, but if either condition continues, a gynecologist should be consulted. Girls should be advised to report any marked change in amount of duration of flow as well as marked irregularity.

Clots should be reported since normally the menstrual fluid does not clot unless retained in the vagina for a prolonged period of time. It is believed that the endometrium produces an unknown lytic or anticoagulant agent that prevents clotting in the uterus. There is no alteration in the coagulability of the blood during menstruation.[34] A recent study[18] shows a relatively high incidence of marked discomfort during menstruation by young girls and the large consumption of a variety of medications by them. They should be encouraged to treat minor discomforts with rest, warmth, and small amounts of acetylsalicylic acid and to avoid the use of patent medicines and other unprescribed remedies.

During menstruation a bath should be taken at least once daily. Although a warm tub bath often allays any slight pelvic discomfort, showers are preferable during this period from the esthetic standpoint. It is well to avoid cold baths and showers, particularly if there is a tendency to discomfort. Many women, however, use tampons and go swimming during their period with no ill effects.

Regarding marriage

It is advisable for engaged couples to have complete physical examinations prior to marriage, including a serologic test for syphilis (now compulsory in all except five states). Women should have a pelvic examination. At this time a tight hymenal ring, which could make intercourse difficult, can be dilated or incised, provided this procedure is psychologically and culturally acceptable to both the woman and her prospective husband.

Prior to marriage the couple should talk freely with their doctor, with their religious adviser, and particularly with each other concerning the physical, psychologic, and religious implications of sex. It is important that cultural differences be considered, and any questions or differences regarding intercourse and size and spacing of the prospective family should be discussed at this time. *Married Love,*[*] *Marriage Manual,*[†] and *Sex Life in Marriage*[‡] are books often suggested for reading either shortly prior to or immediately following marriage. Roman Catholic engaged couples are encouraged to read *Beginning Your Marriage*[§] and *The Catholic Marriage Manual.*[‖]

Married women often ask nurses about intercourse. Tremendous variation exists in the sexual activity of married couples. With adequate knowledge, patience, and understanding, a husband and wife can usually work out a plan that is satisfactory to both. Frequency of intercourse may vary from one or more times a day to once a month or less. The frequency normally drops considerably after the first year or two of marriage.

From 25 to 50% of married couples have some difficulty in intercourse because of emotional maladjustment. This often is due to worry or guilt feelings related to the sexual act or to inability to meet cultural standards for satisfactory intercourse. This may result in frigidity in women and impotence in men. The couple should be urged to discuss these problems frankly with their doctor and spiritual adviser since reassurance and additional sexual education may relieve the situation. A few persons may need psychiatric treatment.

Married couples should understand the menstrual cycle and should know the times during the cycle when fertilization is most likely to occur. For most normal women who have a regular cycle of twenty-eight days, the period of ovulation falls between the fourteenth and sixteenth day after the beginning of the previous menstrual period. If couples have a reasonable cause for

using the rhythm method of family planning, physicians usually instruct them to avoid intercourse three days before and three days after ovulation. However, ovulation may not be regular, and fertilization has been known to occur on any day of the monthly cycle.

Absence of menstruation (*amenorrhea*) in the recently married woman who is having intercourse regularly usually indicates pregnancy. Regardless of the cause of amenorrhea, medical advice should be sought at once.

Some women may have a slight vaginal discharge following intercourse. If it is irritating, a douche with plain water or with a tablespoon of white vinegar to a quart of water may be taken from one to three hours after intercourse. For marked discharge not alleviated by this means, medical advice should be sought. Normally, douches are not needed for cleanliness, and it is inadvisable to take a douche routinely. However, some normal women have a troublesome odor, especially in warm weather and following the menstrual period, which can be relieved by an occasional douche with warm water or vinegar in water.

The reproductive system in later life

The *climacteric,* or "change of life," is frequently misunderstood by both men and women. The nurse should provide a patient with factual information to help allay fears and to give supportive encouragement if he or she has actually reached this time of life. The climacteric begins in women with the end of the active childbearing period, which is usually between 44 and 49 years of age. If it occurs before 42 or if menstruation continues after 50 years of age, the patient may be normal, but medical consultation is recommended because disease may be the cause. Every woman after the climacteric, as well as before, should be examined by a gynecologist at least once each year. The climacteric, which usually lasts from one year to eighteen months, is a period in which there is a gradual decline in ovarian function. It leads to the cessation of menstruation, or the *menopause.* During this time the interval between menstrual periods becomes increasingly longer or irregular, and the flow usually decreases in amount. Many women go

---

[*]Stopes, Marie C.: ed 24, New York, 1939, G. P. Putnam's Sons.

[†]Stone, Hannah M., and Stone, Abraham: New York, 1952, Simon & Schuster, Inc.

[‡]Butterfield, O. M.: New York, 1962, Emerson Books, Inc.

[§]Cana Conference of Chicago, Chicago, 1957, Distributed by Delaney Publications, Oak Park, Ill.

[‖]Kelly, George A.: New York, 1958, Random House, Inc.

through this interval of life with little awareness of its occurrence.

Approximately 10% of all women have pronounced symptoms of the climacteric. Vasomotor reactions producing hot flashes and excessive perspiration may occur and are caused by lack of stimulating hormones to or in the ovaries. Headaches, nervousness, heart palpitation, and sleeplessness may occur, and depression and other emotional reactions, such as feelings of futility or uselessness, may appear. Unfortunately, the climacteric often comes at the very time when children are moving away from home and emancipating themselves. This fact in itself may make the woman feel that the better part of her life is over. Keeping busy, developing new interests, and recognizing her emotional reactions as an expected adjustment to a new hormonal environment help the woman to maintain a normal outlook. Most women's symptoms are relieved by a sedative such as phenobarbital or one of the ataractic (tranquilizing) drugs. Female hormones (primarily estrogen) are prescribed widely during the climacteric to combat marked depression and relieve many of the other annoying symptoms. Usually they are prescribed to be taken for twenty-one days and omitted for seven days each month, but this schedule may be adjusted to the menstrual cycle of the particular patient. If the patient has a history of cancer of the reproductive system, including the breast, hormones are never given because it is believed that their use may stimulate growth of cancer cells that may remain in the body. There seems to be no evidence, however, that the use of estrogens contributes to the development of primary cancer. Some studies have indicated that there may be less primary cancer among women who have taken these hormones and also a lower incidence of coronary artery disease. Since the administration of small doses of estrogenic hormones helps to preserve normal vaginal mucosa and delay the involutional changes involving the secondary sexual characteristics, many doctors now believe that their use in small amounts should be continued indefinitely.

Men may also have a climacteric. However, it is usually less severe than in women and occurs at a much older age, or it may never occur. At this time men also suffer from feelings of depression and uselessness as the sexual drive diminishes. They, too, frequently have vasomotor instability. These changes may tempt some men to be promiscuous in an effort to prove to themselves that the aging process has not affected their virility.[5]

It is an erroneous assumption that sexual activity must end with the climacteric. The frequency simply is decreased. Many women have a capacity to enjoy normal intercourse up to 65 years of age and beyond. This may be true even when the actual cessation of menstruation has occurred at a relatively early age. Men, too, often continue a fairly active sexual life after many signs of normal aging, such as hypertrophy of the prostate, have developed.

Women may have pain with intercourse (dyspareunia) after the menopause because of shrinkage or adhesions of the vaginal canal due to tissue atrophy. This condition occasionally is treated surgically by a plastic repair of the vagina, but usually estrogenic hormones are given. Treatment is determined by the physician after reviewing the wishes and living pattern of the patient. A low-grade vaginal infection may also follow atrophy of the cells lining the vagina. It sometimes responds to vinegar-and-water douches, but if it continues, estrogen hormones may be prescribed. The older woman with such an infection should be advised to bathe frequently in a tub of warm water and to soak for fifteen to twenty minutes at each bath.

With the onset of the climacteric, the predisposition to cancer of the sex organs, which are at this time undergoing involutional changes, seems to increase for both sexes. After the age of 35 years, every woman, married or single, should have a yearly pelvic examination, including a cytologic smear of cervical secretions, since regular examination is the best way to diagnose early cancer of the female reproductive system. Women who have had children are more prone to cancer of the cervix than single women, but cancer of any part of the reproductive system is quite common in all women. Since cancer of the cervix has an unusually good prognosis if diagnosed and treated early, any delay in diagnosis by failure to have regular examinations is deplorable.

After the age of 40 years, the prostate gland also becomes unusually prone to carcinoma. Every man over 40 years of age should have a yearly rectal examination, since by this simple means many carcinomas of the prostate may be diagnosed early enough for treatment to be satisfactory.

Examination of the reproductive tract

Both men and women often put off medical examinations of the reproductive system, since this type of examination arouses intense emotional reactions in both sexes. Fear, embarrassment, and cultural background play an important part in this emotional distress. In our culture, people frequently are afraid that their anxieties concerning carcinoma, venereal disease, sterility, or the climacteric will be verified. Many people are embarrassed to discuss problems concerning their sexual life, such as inability to perform in the culturally accepted pattern during intercourse. Many are embarrassed by the necessary exposure of the external genitalia during the medical examination. A person may also be fearful that some condition will be discovered that will require surgery which will result in sterility. The nurse who is sensitive to the many thoughts and fears that may trouble the patient will be better prepared to help him accept the necessary medical examination.

It often reassures patients to know that medical information will be given only to the doctor and that this information goes no farther. They should know that complete, frank answers to the doctor's questions will help considerably in determining the cause of any difficulty and in planning suitable treatment. Patients should be encouraged to discuss with the doctor any other related problems that may be of concern to them but about which the doctor may fail to ask specifically. The woman should be prepared for the questions she will be asked. If she is told that before the doctor examines her he will probably ask her all about her monthly periods and about her pregnancies and deliveries, she is given a chance to think through her answers

under less pressure and thus can give more accurate information.

It is necessary to explain to the patient the procedures that will be performed during the examination, what he or she will be expected to do, and what the doctor will do. For example, any likelihood of a cramping discomfort (which will occur if *anything* is introduced into the cervical canal), should be explained to the patient. A calm, thoughtful, interested, yet matter-of-fact manner often helps put patients at ease. The nurse should appraise each patient and adjust her approach accordingly. Some patients, particularly girls who are very fearful, may need either a much more personalized or, perhaps, a more detached approach. It is important for a woman to know that the nurse will be present during the examination and for a man to know that, after the nurse has made the necessary preparations for his examination, he will be left alone with the doctor.

Examination and diagnostic measures used for female patients

Pelvic examination. The pelvic examination is relatively simple. However, if the patient is extremely upset and unable to relax sufficiently for satisfactory palpation, or if any undue pain is anticipated, it may occasionally be done under anesthesia. An anesthetic usually is necessary if a complete examination of a young girl must be done.

The following equipment is needed:

Several speculums (various sizes)
Rubber or plastic gloves (correct size for the doctor) and talcum powder
Lubricating jelly (water soluble, vegetable base)
Applicators
Cotton balls

In addition the physician may request the following:

Uterine tenaculum forceps
Sponge forceps
Biopsy forceps
Cautery unit with cautery tips

Good light is important for a pelvic examination. Probably the best lighting is obtained with a head mirror. Gooseneck lights also are used frequently.

The patient should void immediately prior to the examination since an empty bladder makes palpation easier, eliminates any possible distortion of the position of the pelvic organs caused by a full bladder, and obviates the danger of incontinence during the examination. The urine specimen should be saved.

Ambulatory patients should always be told what clothing must be removed, since panties or girdles interfere with the examination, waste time, and cause unnecessary embarrassment to both the patient and the doctor.

The woman should know that the examination may be somewhat uncomfortable. It should not be painful unless disease makes it so. She can help most in making the examination effective and brief by relaxing as completely as possible. Breathing through the mouth often helps to relax the abdominal muscles. She should be assured that her modesty will be maintained. While on the table she will be draped, the door will be kept closed, and the nurse will be present during the entire procedure.

Several positions may be used (Fig. 110). The doctor will indicate the one in which he wishes the patient placed. The nurse should check to see that the patient does not have arthritis or any other condition that may limit position or movement and will interfere with her assuming the desired position. Some positions, such as the knee-chest position, are uncomfortable and embarrassing for patients of almost any age or physical condition. As the nurse places the patient in the position desired, she should explain why the position is necessary for an adequate examination.

1. *Dorsal recumbent position (also known as lithotomy position) (Fig. 110).* The lower leaf of the examining table should be dropped before the patient gets onto the table, since dropping it may be frightening to her after her feet have been placed in the stirrups. There should be a footstool handy, and the patient should be guided to step on the stool, turn, sit down on the edge of the table, and then lie back. It is better to place both legs in the stirrups at the same time. Gentleness is essential in order to prevent muscle strain, particularly if the patient is anesthetized. Metal stirrups are the most satisfactory. However, if they are being used, the patient should wear her shoes because the heels help to hold the feet in the stirrups.

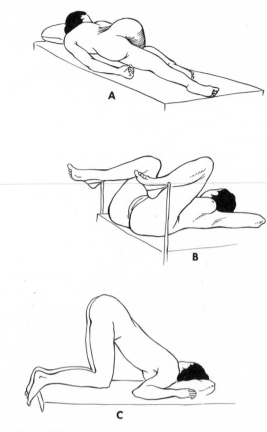

Fig. 110

The various positions that can be assumed for examination of the rectum and the vagina. **A**, Sims' (lateral) position; note position of the left arm and right leg. **B**, Lithotomy position; note position of the buttocks on the edge of the examining table and support of feet. **C**, Knee-chest (genupectoral) position; note placement of the shoulders and head.

Care must be taken to see that there is no pressure on the legs when sling stirrups are used, since nerve damage can occur. The buttocks need to be moved down so that they are even with the end of the table. The nurse should see that the pillow under the head is pulled down at the same time to assure comfort for the patient. The patient is then draped in such a manner that only the perineum is exposed. The triangular drape is most often used since it provides a flap that can be brought down for protection if a few moments should intervene between draping and examination.

If this examination must be done in bed, the patient is placed across the bed with her feet resting on the seats of two straight chairs. This method can be used in the home if necessary.

2. *Sims' position (used also for rectal examination) (Fig. 110).* For this position the patient is placed on her left side, with her left arm and hand placed behind her. The left thigh should be only slightly flexed, and the right knee should be flexed sharply upon the abdomen. She should be draped so as to expose only the perineum.

3. *Knee-chest position (Fig. 110).* After dropping the lower end of the examining table, have the patient get on her hands and knees on the table. The buttocks will be uppermost, and the thighs should be sharply flexed on the trunk. The patient's head should be turned to one side and should rest on the table. The arms should be flexed and resting well forward (often above the patient's head), and the knees should be apart. The feet should extend over the lower edge of the table to prevent pressure on the toes. Drape so as to expose only the perineum. If this examination must be done in bed, place the patient crosswise on the bed.

The pelvic examination consists first of inspection of the external genitalia for signs of inflammation, bleeding, discharge, swelling, erosions, or other local skin changes. If the patient is a virgin, a very small speculum may be used, or examination with the speculum may be omitted. Using the speculum, the doctor examines the vaginal walls and can actually see the cervix, thus making it possible to note any unusual signs, such as alteration in the normal size or color, tears, erosion, or bleeding. The nurse should see that the light is adjusted so that the vaginal canal and cervix are well illuminated. If no other light is available, the nurse may hold a flashlight to provide suitable lighting. A digital examination then follows; for this the doctor will need gloves and lubricating jelly. Placing one or two fingers in the vagina, he palpates the abdomen with his other hand. He concludes with a rectal examination, using one finger. (See Fig. 111.) By digital examination he can usually detect abnormalities in the placement, contour, motility, and tissue

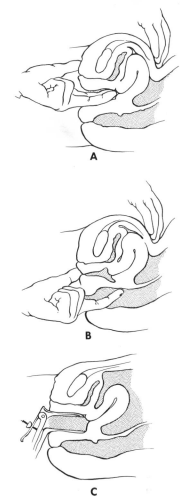

Fig. 111

Methods of pelvic examination. **A,** Digital examination of the vagina with abdominal palpation to determine size and position of uterus. **B,** Digital rectal examination with abdominal palpation. **C,** Examination of the vagina and cervix using a bivalve vaginal speculum.

consistency of the base of the bladder and the uterus and its adjacent structures, including the ovaries, the fallopian tubes, and the rectum.

Responsibilities of the nurse during the examination include being present during the entire procedure for the protection of both the patient and the doctor, encouraging the patient to relax, and assisting the doctor as necessary. Additional equipment that may be needed should be available in the room so that she will not have to leave the patient unattended. This equipment will depend upon the doctor and the patient, but may often include materials for taking and preserving smears for cytologic study, packing for use following biopsy, and tampons.

Following the examination, the nurse should quickly remove any lubricating jelly or discharge that may be on the genitalia and should assist the patient from the table, taking both legs out of the stirrups simultaneously. In elderly patients, unnatural positions, such as knee-chest and lithotomy, may alter the normal circulation of blood sufficiently to cause faintness. Extreme care must be taken not to leave an elderly patient sitting on the table. With the aid of a footstool, the nurse should assist her from the table and help her to a chair where she may wish to rest for a moment before beginning to dress. If necessary, the nurse may help the patient to dress, and during this time or later she may explain any statements made by the doctor that are not clear to the patient. She tells the patient that after she is dressed the doctor will wish to talk to her again.

Equipment should be rinsed with cold water, washed well with soap and water, rinsed, and sterilized. The linen or other protective covering on the table should be changed. Often a protective waterproof square covered with a treatment towel or paper towel or napkin is placed under the buttocks to prevent cross contamination of the linen. The protective square must be thoroughly washed with soap and water if it has become moistened.

After the patient has completed her interview with the doctor, the nurse is responsible for follow-up teaching as necessary. She may further explain information or orders given by the doctor, such as the technique of douching, provide general health education, discuss the time and importance of her next appointment, and explain any referrals to a special department or doctor.

Schiller's test. This test is based on the knowledge that abnormal cells do not take iodine stain in the same way as normal ones.

A solution of iodine is injected onto the cervix. Early cancerous lesions and also benign lesions, such as areas of cervicitis, may show up as glistening areas of a lighter color than surrounding tissue, and this simple test helps the doctor decide whether or not other diagnostic procedures should be done. Since iodine stains clothing, the patient usually is advised to wear a pad for several hours after the test.

Cytologic test for cancer (Papanicolaou smear test). This test is based on the simple fact that tumor cells, as well as normal cells, of such structures as the fallopian tubes, the uterus, and the vagina exfoliate and pass into the cervical and vaginal secretions. When these secretions are aspirated and smears made, lesions of the cervix and of the lining of the fallopian tubes and the uterus may be detected in their early stages. Malignant lesions in the ovaries and in the outer structures, such as the outer layers of the uterus, do not, of course, exfoliate cells that are available for study in this manner.

In diagnosing cancer of the uterus, the smear test has been found to be 89% accurate for cancer of the cervix in situ, and 96% accurate when invasion of surrounding tissues has occurred.[24] The test is extremely valuable in leading the doctor to suspect cancer of the cervix while there is yet no visible or palpable evidence of tumor growth. Cancer of the cervix, one of the most common forms of cancer in women, may thus be treated much earlier than was previously possible, and the rate of cure is relatively high. The patient should understand, however, that the smear test is not necessarily conclusive and that biopsy or even operation may be necessary to verify the diagnosis. It is also used to screen patients needing further examination as well as to measure the effectiveness of radiation and surgical treatment. Many patients are familiar with the vaginal smear test from descriptions given in popular magazines. It is not painful, and some patients are taught to take smears themselves daily, especially when the doctor is interested in determining the pattern of endometrial growth in women with sterility problems or in those having estrogen therapy (Fig. 112).

Experimentation is now under way in having women take their own smears, which are then mailed for study. Although these tests may be less informative than when done by a physician, who also takes a smear from the cervix, they may prove to a most valuable early screening procedure. At present far too few women are having this test done regularly. It is hoped that the home test will prove to be practical and that it will eliminate some of the reasons, such as inconvenience and cost, that prevent many women from having periodic testing done by their physician.[54]

Smears for cytologic study may be taken from the vagina or, under sterile precautions, from within the cervix. The test is not done if profuse bleeding has occurred or if catheterization or curettage has been done within two weeks of the examination. The test will not be accurate if the patient has taken a douche within two hours of the examination, since the significant cells may have been washed away.

If the equipment must be sterilized with moist sterilization and if it is needed for use before it has thoroughly dried, it should be rinsed in equal parts of 95% alcohol and ether to hasten drying.

The equipment needed for taking a vaginal cytologic smear includes a vaginal pipette with a rubber bulb, an applicator for obtaining secretions from the external mouth of the cervix, a spatula for scraping around the cervix in order to obtain cells loosened but not yet exfoliated, slides, a widemouthed bottle containing equal parts of 95% alcohol and ether, and appropriate labels and laboratory slips.

With the patient in lithotomy position, the doctor takes the smears before he begins the vaginal examination. Dry, clean, unlubricated equipment is used, and the label on the slide is checked to be sure that it contains the name of the patient, the date, and the source of the specimen. After air is expressed from the bulb of the vaginal pipette, the pipette is inserted with an upward and backward motion so that the specimen will be obtained from the posterior fornix, which is most likely to contain cells from the fallopian tubes, the cervix, and the vagina. A specimen of the secretion is aspirated, and the pipette is withdrawn. The secretion is then expressed thinly and evenly on the prepared slide, and the slide is placed in the solution

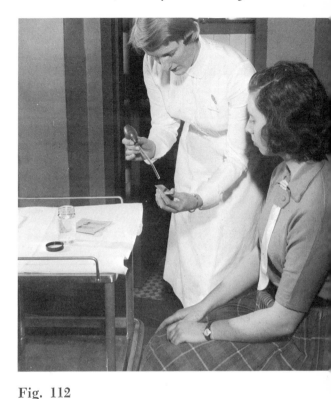

Fig. 112

The nurse shows the patient how to fix the slide after taking a vaginal smear; a necessary procedure if the patient must make daily smears at home.

of ether and alcohol, or five drops of a commercially available fixative (Cyto-Dry-Fix) are added to the wet smear. The secretion must not be permitted to become dry, since the cells will be distorted in appearance if drying occurs. Patients who take their own smears often do the aspiration while standing with one foot on a low stool or chair.

Obtaining an endocervical smear is a sterile procedure that is done only by the doctor. The preparation is the same as for a vaginal smear except that a sterile metal cannula with a bulb or syringe attached is needed. The patient having this test will have some discomfort due to the dilation of the cervical canal, but there should be no real pain. There may be some cramping pain from uterine contractions after the procedure. Usually heat applied to the lower

485

abdomen and the administration of acetyl-salicylic acid will give relief.

Tests for pregnancy. In addition to physical signs such as softening of the cervix (Hegar's sign), there are several tests for pregnancy. They are based on the knowledge that chorionic gonadotropin is produced by the pituitary gland in sufficient amounts after one month of pregnancy to affect gonads of experimental animals. Urine of the patient is injected into rabbits, mice, frogs, toads, or rats. The urine specimen should be the first voided in the morning, since this urine is likely to be more concentrated. Two tests commonly used are the *Friedman test* and the *Aschheim-Zondek test.*

In the Friedman test some of the patient's urine is injected into a nonpregnant female rabbit; corpora lutea or corpora hemorrhagica in the ovaries occurring twenty-four hours after injection of the urine indicates a positive reaction. In the Aschheim-Zondek test the patient's urine is injected into immature mice, the ovaries of which are examined 100 hours later; again, maturation of the ovaries occurs if the test is positive. A quicker test is done by injecting the patient's urine into a male frog. Tests of the frog's urine are taken at thirty-minute intervals for three hours, and presence of spermatozoa in the frog's urine is a positive test. Newer tests are now being done that utilize antigen factors in the pregnant woman's urine. In men the Aschheim-Zondek test is used to diagnose a type of testicular tumor in which chorionic gonadotropin is present in the urine.

Culdoscopy and related procedures. A culdoscopy is an examination in which the doctor attempts to see the cause of disease in the pelvis by inserting an instrument (culdoscope) through the posterior fornix into the cul-de-sac of Douglas (Fig. 113). A tubal pregnancy, for example, can sometimes be observed by this means. Usually the patient is hospitalized for the procedure, which is done in the operating room under sterile conditions and with the patient under anesthesia. Occasionally sedation and only local anesthesia are used. *Peritoneoscopy* and *laparoscopy* are similar procedures through which pelvic structures may be observed by approaching from above rather than through the vagina. Air may be injected and roentgenograms taken to outline pelvic structures more fully, and a radiopaque, aqueous medium may be injected into the uterus and

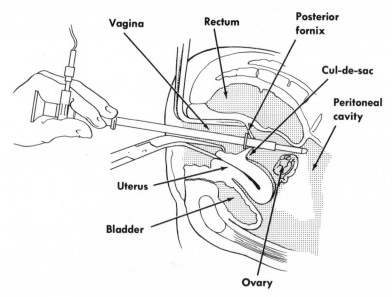

Fig. 113

With the patient in the knee-chest position, the culdoscope is inserted through the posterior fornix of the vagina into the cul-de-sac of Douglas. Note that the ovaries can be seen.

the fallopian tubes (p. 492). Following these procedures, air in the abdominal cavity may cause discomfort similar to that following the Rubin test for patency of the fallopian tubes.

After procedures in which air enters the abdominal cavity, the patient is placed in a face-lying position with a pillow under the abdomen. Occasionally a tight abdominal binder and pressure on the abdomen are prescribed.[33] The knee-chest position should be avoided for several days since the unhealed wound may permit air to enter the abdominal cavity. The patient should not take a douche or have sexual intercourse for a week. Hemorrhage occurs very occasionally. Since infection could develop, the patient should be observed for signs of infection, such as elevation of temperature and pain or discomfort in the lower abdomen.

A *culdocentesis* is a procedure in which a needle is inserted through the posterior fornix of the vagina into the cul-de-sac of Douglas for the purpose of removing, for study, pus or other abnormal fluids that may be present. Usually this procedure is done in the doctor's office and does not require hospitalization. Surgical aseptic precautions are used so that infection will not be introduced into the pelvis.

Cervical biopsy and cautery. Sometimes the doctor wishes to send a piece of cervical tissue to the laboratory for pathologic examination. The biopsy procedure will usually be scheduled for a week after the end of the menstrual period, since the cervix is more vascular immediately before and after menstruation. The patient should know what is to be done and why. She should know that there may be momentary discomfort, but that no actual pain will be felt because the cervix does not contain pain fibers. If a cautery is to be used to treat erosion, to remove small polyps from the mouth of the cervix, or for other reasons, she should be told that a small, lubricated sheet of lead will be placed against the skin under the lumbar area as a safety device for grounding electrical charges and that there will be slight bleeding which will be controlled by a tampon or packing that will be inserted by the doctor. The odor of burning tissue when a cautery is used nauseates some patients. They should be told that the

odor may be noticed but that it actually is insignificant and that the procedure usually is over quickly.

In addition to the equipment needed for a pelvic examination, the nurse should have the following items available:

Biopsy forceps
Uterine tenaculum forceps
Specimen bottle containing 10% formalin or, if specimen can be delivered to pathology laboratory immediately following procedure, wet saline sponge and waxed paper may be used (specimens should be labeled with patient's name, date, source of specimen, and doctor's name)
Cautery unit and cautery tips
Gauze packing or tampon

Following the procedure, the nurse should be certain that the patient understands the doctor's instructions. Sometimes the main points are written out for her. Instructions will vary, but they usually include the following:

1. Rest more than usual for the next twenty-four hours. Avoid lifting and marked exertion.

2. Leave the tampon or packing in place as long as the doctor advises (usually eight to twenty-four hours).

3. Report to the hospital or doctor's office if bleeding is excessive. (Usually more than occurs during a normal menses is considered excessive.)

4. Do not use an internal douche or have sexual relations until the next visit to the doctor unless he has given you specific instructions as to when intercourse can be safely resumed.

5. If cauterization has been done, an unpleasant discharge, caused by sloughing of cells destroyed, may appear four to five days following the treatment. A warm bath several times each day will help this condition, which should not last more than a few days.

The doctor may suggest a douche if there is a vaginal discharge. Usually vinegar (2 tbsp. of white vinegar to 2 quarts of water) is ordered. The nurse should make sure that the patient knows how to take a douche. The temperature should be 40° C. (105° F.) unless otherwise ordered. Most doctors prefer that patients take the douche while lying in the bathtub rather than while sitting on the toilet seat (Fig. 114). A douche pan may be

Fig. 114

A vaginal douche should be taken while lying in the bathtub. A douche pan may be placed under the patient in the tub if desired.

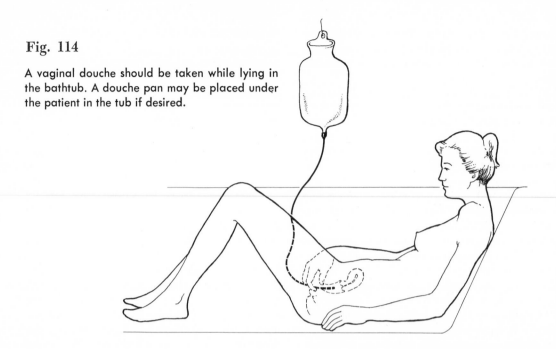

placed in the tub if so desired. A bath should be taken first to lessen the chance of contamination. The douche tip should be inserted upward and backward and moved about to prevent fluid from being forced into the mouth of the cervix and to ensure flushing of the posterior fornix. If a medicated or hot douche is to be taken, the labia should be held together for a few moments to allow the vagina to fill up and thus benefit all areas. Douches prescribed to provide local heat should be continued for about a half hour. Petroleum jelly may be used to prevent burning the sensitive tissues of the labia. Following douching, the tub should be well cleaned with soap and warm water.

Dilation and curettage. Dilation of the cervix and curettage (scraping) of the endometrial lining of the uterus are minor surgical procedures usually done at the same time either to diagnose disease of the uterus or to correct excessive and prolonged bleeding. Occasionally dilation of the cervix alone is done to treat dysmenorrhea or to treat sterility caused by stricture or stenosis of the cervical canal. Since the procedure is carried out under general anesthesia, the patient needs physical and emotional preparation and care similar to that given any

patient undergoing general anesthesia. In addition, the patient should be told preoperatively that the pubic and perineal area will be shaved if this will be done. Some doctors now believe that shaving is not necessary and that the discomfort during regrowth of pubic hair can be avoided.[44] She should know that a nurse will be present with her during the entire procedure, and that she will not be exposed any more than during a pelvic examination. Sometimes the perineal shave and entire preparation is done in the operating room after the patient has been put to sleep and placed in the lithotomy position. If this procedure is followed, the patient should know what is planned. Otherwise she may worry because the preparation is not done in her room or be upset when she awakens from anesthesia to find that it has been done. As in all surgery involving the perineum and lower abdomen, the lower bowel and bladder must be empty so that they will not interfere with the operation or be damaged.

At the conclusion of the operation, packing is placed in the cervical canal and vagina, and a sterile pad is placed over the perineum. When the patient returns to her room, the nurse should check the pad for any excessive bleeding every fifteen minutes for two hours and then every one to two hours for eight hours. Usually the pad is only slightly stained. Any excessive bleeding should be reported to the doctor. For the comfort of the patient, the pad should be anchored with a sanitary belt and changed as necessary. Sterile perineal pads are used until the packing is removed, usually within twenty-four hours after operation.

The packing in the cervical canal may cause cramps similar to moderately severe menstrual cramps, since a dilated cervical canal stimulates uterine contractions. Usually codeine sulfate and acetylsalicylic acid are ordered to relieve cramps and are given every four hours for the first twenty-four to forty-eight hours as necessary. Any really severe abdominal pain that is not relieved by analgesics should be reported at once. A very uncommon but serious complication of curettage is accidental perforation of the uterus during the procedure, with resultant peritonitis.

Voiding may be difficult following a dilation and curettage because of the pressure of the packing against the urethra or because of local trauma and irritation from the procedure. Usually, however, the patient is permitted to be up almost as soon as she reacts from the anesthetic, and she can void if permitted to use the bathroom. Any packing that extends beyond the vagina should be kept dry during voiding if possible, and the patient should be instructed to protect the vaginal orifice from fecal contamination by cleansing with a backward motion.

Patients often go home the day after a dilation and curettage. They can resume most of their normal daily activities, increasing to normal activity in about a week. Vigorous exercise such as horseback riding, tennis, and dancing are usually advised against, since these activities may tend to increase pelvic congestion. The patient should abstain from sexual intercourse until her return visit to the doctor, at which time he will advise her as to when intercourse may safely be resumed. The menstrual cycle usually is not upset by a dilation and curettage, but a vaginal discharge may appear during the healing period. The doctor may prescribe a vinegar-and-water douche for this (p. 487).

Examination of the female infant and the young girl. At birth the infant girl should be examined for evidence of any abnormalities of the external genitalia. *Gynatresia* (imperforate hymen) is a relatively minor abnormality that can usually be noted at an early age. It should be corrected before the onset of the menses. The nurse in the hospital and the public health nurse should observe the newborn girl and should be certain that the infant's mother knows what is normal. Some mothers actually do not know what the external genitalia of a small girl should look like. Diagrams and pictures often help to clarify points for them. Infants born to women who have taken the hormone progesterone to maintain their pregnancy should be observed particularly carefully because large doses of this hormone causes abnormalities of various kinds. Some of the changes produced by this hormone are reversible with puberty. Without alarming the mother, the nurse should urge that any abnormality noted be brought to the physician's attention.

Unless there are definite indications making examination necessary, detailed examination of the internal genital system usually is not done until after puberty. When examination is necessary it may be done under general anesthesia. A urethroscope may be used to visualize the cervix when a speculum cannot be used. Atresia of the vagina, absence of the vagina or the uterus (agenesis), double vagina, double uterus, or anomalies of the ovaries are some of the abnormalities that may be found.

Examination and diagnostic measures used for male patients

Examination of the male genitalia. Physical examination of the reproductive system in the male patient consists of careful inspection and palpation of the scrotum, noting skin lesions, differences in size and contour of the scrotum, and any evidence of swelling. Transillumination of the scrotum is done to detect absence of testicles and any unusual density of the structures contained within the scrotal sac. By means of a rectal examination, the doctor can detect enlargement and general consistency of the prostate gland (Fig. 115) and any nodules in the adjacent tissues. The penis, foreskin, and meatus are inspected for signs of le-

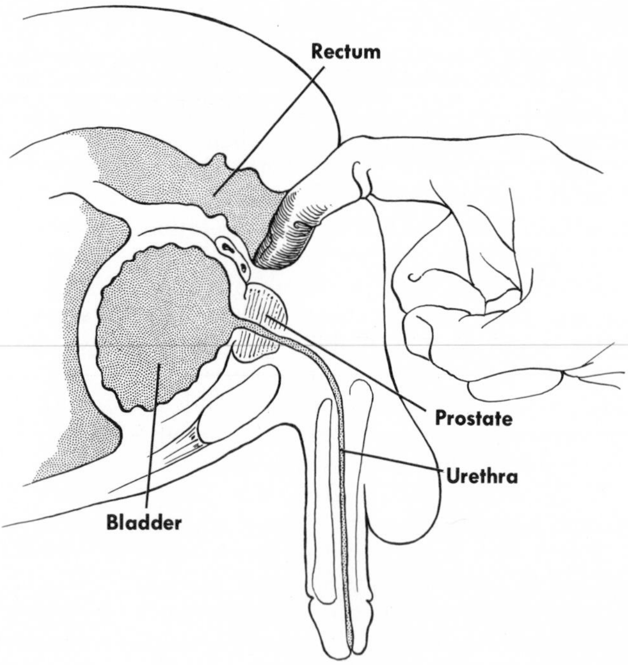

Fig. 115

Digital examination via the rectum to determine the size and consistency of the prostate gland. Note location of the gland in relation to other structures.

Rectum

Prostate

Urethra

Bladder

sions or other abnormalities. By means of cystoscopic examination the doctor can detect prostatic encroachment on the urethra and observe the condition of the urethral and bladder mucosa. This procedure is not a part of routine examination, however. X-ray visualization and catheterization of the seminal vesicles to obtain specimens are also sometimes done.

The nurse should see that the patient is draped and that he understands what the doctor will do and what will be expected of him, such as giving a specimen of urine and breathing deeply to make palpation easier for the doctor. He should not empty his bladder immediately before examination because the doctor may, by watching him void, be able to identify signs of possible urethral obstruction. Necessary equipment is prepared, and the nurse then leaves the patient alone with the doctor.

After the examination, the male patient may have questions to ask the nurse. If he is to have special examinations or treatments later, the nurse is responsible for explaining the preparation and the procedure to him. (See p. 426 for preparation for cystoscopic procedures and aftercare.)

Prostatic smears. If cancer or tuberculosis of the prostate is suspected, a prostatic smear may be desired. The doctor first massages the prostate via the rectum. The next voided urine specimen is collected in an appropriate container (a sterile bottle for acid-fast [tubercle] bacilli; a bottle containing alcohol, 95%, for Papanicolaou or cytologic examination) and sent to the laboratory.

Testicular and prostatic biopsies. Testicular and prostatic biopsies may be obtained either by aspiration of cells through a needle or by obtaining a specimen of tissue through a surgical incision. Both of these procedures are carried out under sterile conditions using local or general anesthesia. If a general anesthetic is to be used, the preoperative and postoperative care is similar to that given any surgical patient. The incision used to obtain a testicular biopsy is a small one in the scrotum, usually about 1 inch in length. The only dressing is usually a sterile 4-inch by 8-inch gauze sponge inside a firm scrotal support. The patient may go home the evening of the operation, returning to have the sutures removed or to be prepared for further treatment if the biopsy shows that it is necessary.

To obtain a prostatic biopsy, a small incision is made in the perineum between the anus and the scrotum. The dressing is usually held in place by a two-tailed binder. The patient must be instructed to be careful not to contaminate the incision while cleansing himself following defecation. If the incision is accidentally contaminated, the area should be carefully cleansed. Irrigation of the perineum by pouring sterile water over it or by washing with sterile sponges and benzalkonium chloride (Zephiran) is sometimes ordered following defecation. A heat lamp with a 60-watt bulb placed 12 inches from the perineum is often used two or three times a day to encourage healing. The patient must be in a position in which the scrotum is elevated so that the heat strikes the incision. The best method is to allow the scrotum to rest on a wide piece of adhesive tape extending from thigh to thigh. Occasionally an exaggerated Sims' position gives satisfactory wound exposure. When the sutures have been removed, sitz baths are used instead of the lamp treatment, and they add a great deal to the general comfort of the patient. Usually following a prostatic biopsy the patient remains in the hospital until the laboratory findings are reported. A patient who has had a needle, or aspiration, biopsy will not usually require hospitalization and has no dressings.

Frequently patients, both men and women, show signs of anxiety and depression following diagnostic procedures that necessitate waiting for pathologic reports. The nurse should reassure them by emphasizing their intelligence in seeking medical advice and, without undue discussion, should let them know that results of the examination will be available soon.

Evaluation of infertility problems

The problem of infertility among married couples is of major medical and social concern. It has been estimated that one out of every six to ten couples in the United States is unwillingly childless. It was many years before the husband was considered as a possible cause of sterility, but it is now known that almost as many men as women are responsible for barren marriages and that many times both husband and wife are responsible. Thus, both should be urged to seek medical attention. Sterility problems always deserve medical consultation to correct deficiencies and to clarify the problem.

Evaluation of male fertility. Some doctors prefer to carry out a complete examination of the husband first, as it is more easily accomplished. Following a thorough physical examination, the first special test will be *multiple semen examinations* to determine the presence, number, maturity, and motility of the sperm. The husband should bring a specimen of semen to the doctor immediately after emission because sperm cells quickly deteriorate. The date of the last emission and the time of this specimen should be recorded. The absence of sperm in the semen may indicate a stricture somewhere along the vas deferens or absence of sperm production. A normal sperm count is approximately 60 million per milliliter of semen, at least 75% of which have normal motility and are normal in shape. A sperm count below 20 million per milliliter of semen and a motility rate of under 40% with over 25% of misshapen forms are known to lower the chance of fertilization of an ovum.

A *biopsy of the testicle* will show sperm production if the absence of sperm in the semen (azoospermia) is due to stricture of the tubal systems beyond the testes. Occasionally strictures may be repaired by a plastic surgery procedure (vasoepididymal or vasovasal anastomosis), but the results are often poor. Bilateral cryptorchism, or undescended testicles, even though corrected, may be the cause of sterility because of failure of the testicles to develop their sperm-producing function. This is particularly true if the correction is not done before puberty. Men sometimes will have no further sperm production following orchitis as a complication of mumps or following x-ray exposure of the testicles. A lack of vitamins A and E in the diet may also cause some atrophy of the spermatogenic tissue.

When the husband is completely aspermatic, conception is impossible, and the couple should consider adoption of children if they really want a family. If the sperm count and the motility rate of the sperm cells are low, the doctor usually prescribes thyroid extract and vitamins, and treats any low-grade infections. Testosterone may be prescribed. It is important for the patient to eat a well-balanced diet, to maintain normal weight, to obtain adequate rest, and to participate in moderate exercise (preferably outdoors). The doctor will suggest that the couple have frequent intercourse during the fertile period (fourteen to sixteen days after the beginning of the menstrual period). Several days of continence should be practiced just prior to this period. If these methods are unsuccessful, the injection of several drops of the husband's semen into the upper portion of the cervical canal may produce a pregnancy.

Evaluation of female fertility. The wife should also have a thorough physical examination, including a pelvic examination. In addition, a systematic check is made of each organ that might affect the reproductive system and of each gland influencing it (Fig. 169).

In order for the ovum to be fertilized, the vagina, cervix, and uterus must be completely patent and have mucosal secretions that are not hostile to the sperm. Normally semen is alkaline in reaction, cervical secretions are alkaline, and vaginal secretions are acid. The Huhner test and vaginal and endometrial smears give necessary information about the secretions.

In the *Huhner test* the doctor aspirates cervical secretions within one hour after intercourse and examines them for the presence and viability of the sperm cells. The woman should be instructed not to void, douche, or bathe between intercourse and the examination. She should use a perineal pad and go immediately to the doctor's office. If the sperm are being killed by the secretions, vaginal smears are examined, and an appropriate antibiotic may be given to change the flora in the woman's vagina and cervix, timing its administration so that the secretions are most favorable to the sperm at the time of ovulation. If the secretions are too acid or too alkaline, medicated douches may be ordered. A douche using sodium bicarbonate (1 tbsp. to 1 quart of water) taken just before intercourse has been found to increase the motility of the sperm cells in many cases.[59] If the sperm cells do not reach the uterus, dilation of the cervix may be tried.

The ovary must be producing ova, estrogen, and progesterone for an ovum to be fertilized and implanted and retained in the uterus. *Endometrial biopsy* and *vaginal smears* taken premenstrually give some of this information, but a *complete endocrine work-up* may also be indicated. Urine studies to determine the amount of gonadotropin in the urine are used to study function of the pituitary gland. Hypothyroidism or general health that is below par may prevent an otherwise normal woman from conceiving. (See p. 731 for studies done.) Thyroid hormones sometimes are given, and vitamins C and E and extra rest may also be prescribed.

If the wife has an irregular menstrual cycle, it is important that she keep a temperature chart for several months to help the doctor determine her exact period of ovulation. The temperature will usually be lower at ovulation (the time at which conception most likely will take place) and then will rise abruptly as the corpus luteum begins to produce progesterone. It will drop to a lower level again a day or two before the start of the menstrual period. The temperature should be taken rectally before arising each morning. The temperature chart should be interpreted by the doctor since there may be individual variations.

If the ovum is to reach the uterus, the fallopian tubes must be mechanically patent and not in spasm. The *Rubin test* will provide the doctor with information concerning patency of the tubes. In this test the patient is prepared as for a pelvic examination, and then compressed air or carbon dioxide is forced into the uterus under sterile conditions. If the fallopian tubes are open, the doctor will be able to hear free air in the peritoneum on auscultation. The patient will feel pain under the scapula on the same side as the patent tube. If considerable pressure is required to force air into the tubes, there may be spasticity or partial stricture. Roentgenograms of the uterus and fallopian tubes (*hysterograms*) may be taken by forcing a sterile, aqueous, radiopaque substance through the uterus into the tubes. This examination is usually not carried out more than seven days after the end of the menstrual period, since ovulation may be taking place.

The patient should prepare for these tests

by taking a laxative the night before the examination and an enema or a bisacodyl suppository in the morning so that distention of the bowel will not obstruct the fallopian tubes and so that the roentgenograms will not be distorted by gas shadows in the intestine. Soluble phenobarbital and an analgesic are usually given since there will be some discomfort during and after this examination. Low abdominal pain, cramps, nausea, vomiting, and faintness occur occasionally. After the examination is over, the patient usually has "gas pains"; they may be relieved by lying on the abdomen, with the head lower than the feet, for one or two hours, since this position allows the gas to rise into the lower pelvis. Since the x-ray medium may stain the patient's clothing, she should wear a perineal pad for several hours, or the doctor may insert a tampon and give instructions as to when it should be removed.

Tubal strictures may be the result of acute or chronic infections involving the fallopian tubes. Although they sometimes can be repaired by plastic surgery, the results are successful in only a few instances. Tubal insufflation is often therapeutic in itself, opening the fallopian tube(s) enough to allow the free passage of the fertilized ovum into the uterus.

A displaced uterus may occasionally be the only known cause of the infertility. Treatment usually consists of pelvic exercises, such as the knee-chest position, the "monkey trot," or other exercises as described in specialized tests, and/or the use of a pessary.

The couple should not be disappointed if, even with medical treatment, pregnancy does not occur immediately, since many normal couples must wait many months and even years before pregnancy occurs. Pregnancy has been known to occur after years of childless marriage, perhaps because the couple begin to accept the situation and thus become more relaxed. Often no physical cause for sterility can be found in either the husband or the wife. Many couples will benefit simply from reassurance of normality. Others may need marriage counseling or psychiatric help to gain insight into psychologic and emotional problems that may be preventing conception.

Nursing related to disease of the female reproductive system

Advances in medical science have made it possible to treat effectively many diseases of the female reproductive system, but for optimum benefit from treatment an early diagnosis is essential. As the layman becomes better informed about normal reproductive functions throughout life, he or she should be able to recognize and report symptoms indicative of early disease. Since the nurse is often the first member of the health team consulted about symptoms related to the reproductive system, she needs to know those for which she may safely suggest conservative hygienic measures and those for which she should guide the patient to seek medical advice. If disease is found, she may also play an important part in helping the patient accept the prescribed treatment as well as in providing nursing care that is coordinated with the efforts of other disciplines to return the patient to a normal productive life.

Common gynecologic disorders

Abnormal menses

Dysmenorrhea. Pain with menstruation is known as dysmenorrhea. Although studies and estimates vary enormously (from 3 to 47%),[34] it is generally believed that at least one-third of all women suffer from dysmenorrhea in varying degrees. Studies in industry have shown dysmenorrhea to be one of the most important causes of absenteeism among working women, resulting in loss of two or more days a month for many employees. Present wide use of the antiovulatory drugs has compounded problems in analyzing and in treating this condition.[4]

The nurse frequently is asked for practical suggestions to relieve dysmenorrhea. Since dysmenorrhea occurs more frequently in individuals who have poor posture, take little exercise, and have poor eating habits, the nurse should encourage good general health practices. In helping with the immediate problem she should determine if the period is in any way abnormal. If it is not, she can suggest rest in bed for an hour or two and application of heat to the lower abdomen. She should advise against repeated use of large amounts of analgesics such as acetylsalicylic acid, which is widely used by the laity without medical prescription. Reading something interesting while resting may bring faster relief. A person who is busy, either mentally or physically, doing something she enjoys is less likely to notice discomfort. These measures will suffice in most instances, but anyone with further difficulty or consistent dysmenorrhea should be urged to seek medical attention. There are many causes that are not obvious, and curative treatment can be given only when the cause of the difficulty is known.

When the patient visits the doctor, a pelvic examination is usually performed, and health practices are analyzed. Congestion of blood in the pelvic cavity or intrapelvic pressure resulting from constipation, a full bladder, or a tumor often causes menstrual pain. Frequently no definite cause can be determined, and the patient may again be urged to try such health measures as securing adequate rest, improving posture, participating in moderate exercise, eating a nonconstipating diet, and taking warm, rather than cool, baths during the menstrual period. The nurse who by her own attitude shows that she considers menstruation to be a normal function and who augments the patient's understanding of normal sexual functions by giving explanations whenever possible may help some women make a better adjustment to the menstrual cycle.

If premenstrual fluid retention causes slight swelling of the abdomen and ankles, limiting salt and fluids during the week prior to the onset of menstruation may help. Tenderness of the breasts, either immediately preceding the onset of menstruation or at any other time during the cycle, headache, and pronounced mood swings are due to hormonal influences. The patient in whom these difficulties are marked should consult a gynecologist, since they may be due to hormonal dysfunction or other causes. For marked fluid retention the doctor may order a low-sodium diet.

Although displacement of the uterus may cause dysmenorrhea, many women with known displacements have no difficulty. Some patients with displacement complain of chronic backache, pelvic pressure, easy fatigue, and leukorrhea in addition to painful menstruation.

Common kinds of displacement are *anteflexion, retroflexion, and retroversion* of the uterus caused by congenitally weak uterine ligaments, adhesions following infections or surgery in the pelvic region, or the strain of pregnancy on the ligaments. A space-filling lesion in this region or even a full bladder or rectum may also displace the uterus enough to cause symptoms. Normally the body of the uterus flexes forward at a 45-degree angle at the cervix. In retroflexion this angle is increased. In anteflexion it is decreased. In retroversion the whole uterus is tipped backward. (See Fig. 116.)

If the displacement is not due to some coexistent pelvic disease, various pelvic exercises may be recommended by the doctor in an attempt to return the uterus to a normal position. These exercises, employing the principles of gravity, stretch or strengthen the uterine ligaments. Some exercises used are knee-chest exercises, the monkey trot, lying on the abdomen two hours a day, and premenstrual exercises.[45] Corrective exercises for poor posture may also be prescribed.

In doing *knee-chest exercises,* the patient is instructed to assume a knee-chest position (Fig. 110) and to separate the labia to allow air to enter the vagina, since this helps to produce normal position of the uterus. This position should be maintained for five minutes two or three times a day.

In doing the *monkey trot,* the patient is instructed to walk about on her hands and feet, keeping the knees straight. This should be done for five minutes two or three times a day.

Premenstrual exercises as described in specialized texts are believed by some doctors to be helpful in selected patients with dysmenorrhea. Other gynecologists believe that equally good results are obtained by attention to posture and general exercise to improve muscle tone throughout the body.

The nurse may be responsible for teaching the patient how to do prescribed exercises. The patient should begin exercising gradually; for example, knee-chest position

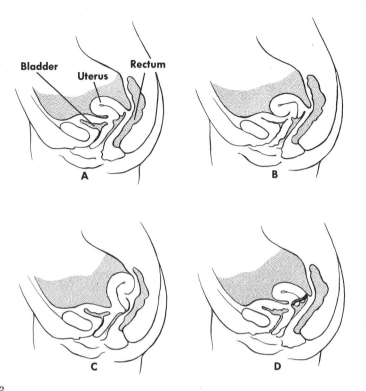

Fig. 116

Normal and abnormal positions of the uterus. **A,** Normal anatomic position of the
uterus in relation to adjacent structures. **B,** Anterior displacement of the uterus.
C, Retroversion, or backward displacement of the uterus. **D,** Normal anatomic position
of the uterus maintained by use of a rubber S-shaped pessary.

should be maintained only one minute the
first time, two minutes the second time,
with gradual progression up to five minutes.
Results from a program of exercising will
not be noticed immediately. The patient
should be told this and should be encouraged to exercise regularly over a period of
months. Performance of exercises should be
reviewed each time the nurse sees the
patient.

If the uterus can be manually returned to
a normal position, a *Smith-Hodges pessary*
may be inserted for a trial period to learn
whether malposition causes the dysmenorrhea (Fig. 116). The pessary is an appliance
introduced into the vagina for the purpose
of supporting the uterus in a normal position. Sometimes, after the removal of the
pessary, the uterus will remain in normal
position. If, after about a six-month trial,

the uterus still returns to its displaced position upon removal of the pessary, and if the
pessary has relieved the symptoms, the ligaments may be shortened surgically through
an abdominal incision. While the pessary is
in use, the patient usually is instructed to
take a daily cleansing douche with warm tap
water to remove extra vaginal secretions
caused by its use. The pessary is usually
changed every three to six weeks. If it is left
in place indefinitely, it may cause erosion of
the cervix and become adherent to the
mucosa.

A stricture of the cervical canal may cause
dysmenorrhea. If so, dilation of the cervical
canal may relieve the discomfort. Dysmenorrhea may be due to endocrine disorders,
but extensive diagnostic tests of hormone
function are done only when there seems to
be no other possible cause. In some instances

psychiatric therapy may be needed to attempt to relieve symptoms. The nurse may be helpful in making this treatment acceptable to the patient.

If dysmenorrhea is incapacitating and unrelieved by conservative therapy, a *presacral neurectomy* may be performed. In this procedure the pain (sensory) fibers from the uterus are interrupted surgically through an abdominal incision. If a pregnant woman has had this operation, she will not feel uterine contractions during labor, and contractions must be palpated carefully to prevent precipitate birth of the baby.

Amenorrhea. Amenorrhea is the absence of menstruation. Before the seriousness of this symptom can be ascertained, one needs to know if there has ever been menstruation and if there has been any recent change in the normal life pattern or in the general state of health of the patient. It is not unusual for a woman to miss one period, especially if she is adjusting to a change in her life pattern. If menses continue to be absent, however, medical consultation should be advised.

The most common cause of amenorrhea, aside from the menopause, is pregnancy. Some women, however, continue to menstruate during the first months of pregnancy. Menses are also usually absent at least until six weeks after delivery of the baby, and sometimes throughout the period of lactation. If a girl is over 14 years of age and has not started to menstruate, she should be examined by a gynecologist to rule out a congenital deformity such as imperforate hymen or absence of the vagina, uterus, or ovaries. If there is no apparent cause for the failure to menstruate regularly, endocrine studies may be done. Sometimes thyroid and ovarian hormones need to be supplemented. Nutritional anemia, wasting chronic illness such as tuberculosis, and psychogenic factors such as fear of pregnancy or desire for pregnancy may cause amenorrhea. A certain type of ovarian tumor (arrhenoblastoma) also causes amenorrhea.

Abnormal menstruation. Abnormal bleeding from the vagina requires immediate medical attention. There are two types: *menorrhagia,* or prolonged profuse menstrual flow during the regular period, and *metrorrhagia,* or bleeding between periods.

Metrorrhagia may be only a slight spotting to be significant.

Menorrhagia in an adolescent girl may be due to a blood dyscrasia or to an endocrine disturbance. This is called *functional bleeding.* Menorrhagia in adult women is likely to be a symptom of an ovarian tumor, a uterine myoma, or pelvic inflammatory disease.

Metrorrhagia may be a symptom of many disorders, including benign or malignant uterine tumors; pelvic inflammatory disease; abnormal conditions of pregnancy such as a threatened abortion, ectopic pregnancy, or hydatid mole; blood dyscrasias; senile vaginitis; and bleeding at ovulation caused by the withdrawal of estrogen. The wide use of combined ovarian hormones such as norethindrone to suppress ovulation sometimes causes bleeding at irregular times. If there is no delay in seeking medical examination, metrorrhagia should not cause undue anxiety since its cause may not be serious. However, the cause, not the symptom, must be treated, and the nurse has a responsibility to help disseminate this information to all women. Early diagnosis and treatment increase the possibility of cure even when the cause is a malignancy.

Vaginal infection

Many women complain of *leukorrhea,* a white vaginal discharge. It is normal to have a slight white vaginal discharge the month prior to the menarche and then monthly around the period of ovulation and just prior to the onset of menstruation. Ordinarily the vagina is protected from infection by its acid secretion and by the presence of Döderlein's bacilli. Occasionally, if the invading organisms, such as the colon bacillus, are very numerous, or if the resistance of the person is lowered by malnutrition, aging, disease, or emotional disturbances, a *vaginitis* may develop. Profuse discharge, yellow discharge, and mucoid discharge are abnormal and are signs of vaginitis, inflammation, or infection. Urethritis usually occurs simultaneously because the mucous membranes of the vagina and urethra are contiguous. The discharge may be irritating and cause redness, edema, burning, and itching. The burning and pruritus may be aggravated by voiding and by defecation.

496

Medicated vaginal jellies and vaginal suppositories are frequently prescribed for patients with vaginitis. The nurse will need to instruct the patient in the procedures for their use. Vaginal jelly is dispensed in a tube to which is attached an applicator. The applicator is inserted into the vagina in a manner similar to the way a pipette is inserted when obtaining a vaginal smear. The medication is then expressed into the vagina and the applicator is withdrawn. A vaginal suppository may be inserted directly into the vagina. It is dissolved by body heat, and the medication may be absorbed through the vaginal mucosa.

Simple vaginitis. Simple vaginitis is caused by contamination of the vagina with organisms from the rectum such as *Escherichia coli* or with other common pyogenic organisms such as staphylococci and streptococci. The organisms are usually introduced from outside sources such as clothing or a douche nozzle. Simple vaginitis is treated with warm douches of a weak acid solution such as vinegar (1 tbsp. to 1 quart of water). This solution increases the acidity of the bacterial environment within the vagina. To help control the infection, beta-lactose, a sugar that stimulates the growth of Döderlein's bacilli, may be prescribed as a vaginal suppository, and sulfonamide cream may be prescribed as an intravaginal application. The sulfonamide cream should be applied after douching. Sitz baths, taken two or three times a day to help relieve local irritation, and thorough gentle cleansing of the perineum with water after voiding and defecating are recommended.

Trichomonas vaginitis. Trichomonas vaginitis is one of the most common forms of vaginal infection and is often found in combination with other infecting organisms. A protozoan called the *Trichomonas vaginalis* is probably the causative agent. Symptoms include a persistent irritating discharge. The disease is diagnosed by examining a drop of vaginal secretion microscopically. When this test is to be made, a dry speculum should be offered the doctor. The slide should be dry and warm, and as soon as the drop of vaginal secretion is placed on the slide, a drop or two of normal saline solution should be added.

A relatively new synthetic drug, metronidazole (Flagyl) is proving to be remarkably effective in treatment of trichomonas vaginitis. Treatment consists of 250 mg. (5 grains) tablets taken by mouth two to three times a day for ten days. Specific local treatment consists of the local use of suppositories, powders, or jellies containing antibiotic drugs, sulfonamides, or carbarsone, which is an arsenical preparation effective against protozoans. Warm vinegar-in-water douches may also be prescribed. Sunshine, rest, good nutrition, and treatment of any focal infections may help to improve the patient's general resistance.

Trichomonads sometimes attack the cervix, bladder, or rectum. If the cervix is involved, the infected portion may need to be surgically removed (conization of the cervix). When the bladder is infected, instillations of mild silver protein (Argyrol) or sulfonamide solutions are used, and carbarsone suppositories may be used to clear up persistent rectal involvement. Trichomonas vaginitis often resists treatment and may persist for months and years despite extensive treatment. It is discouraging and distressing to the patient. If she is to be encouraged to continue the treatment and not "shop around" in her effort to be cured, she needs to be treated with much patience and understanding.

Monilial vaginitis. Monilial vaginitis is a fungus infection commonly seen in patients with uncontrolled diabetes mellitus because the fungi thrive on sugar. A white membrane appears in the vagina, and there is a very irritating, watery discharge mixed with white cheesy particles. If the infection is due to untreated diabetes mellitus, it usually responds to better control of the blood sugar level. Local treatment consists of painting the vagina three times weekly with aqueous gentian violet, 5%, and the nightly instillation of caprylic compound (Naprylate). Douches should not be taken during the period of treatment. Since gentian violet stains clothing, a perineal pad should be provided for the patient who has been treated with this drug. Monilial infection is sometimes resistant to treatment and tends to recur just when it is believed that treatment has been successful. Total recovery may be aided by attention to the improvement of general health.

Senile vaginitis. Senile vaginitis (atrophic) is cause by the invasion of the thin, atrophied, postmenopausal vaginal mucosa by pyogenic bacteria. The main symptom is an irritating vaginal discharge which is sometimes accompanied by pruritus and burning. The treatment is the same as that for simple vaginitis. Estrogenic hormones, given by mouth or applied locally as ointment, will help to restore the epithelium to normal and are used widely.

Perineal pruritus

Perineal pruritus, or excessive itching of the perineum, is a very common and very aggravating affliction that may be due to a variety of causes. It may be due to senile changes in the skin of the perineum, vitamin A deficiency, or the irritation from a chronic vaginal discharge or from the high sugar content of urine in persons with uncontrolled diabetes mellitus. Pediculosis pubis, allergies, cancer of the vulva, scabies, and superficial skin infections such as *tinea cruris* (a fungal infection) may be the cause. Sometimes the cause of the itching cannot be found. The pruritus is made worse by scratching and rubbing; edema, redness, excoriation of the skin, and infection may complicate the original condition.

Perineal pruritus is treated by correcting the aggravating cause if it can be found. Because perineal pruritus, like pruritus in any location of the body, is increased by nervous tension, small doses of sedatives such as phenobarbital or chloral hydrate may be given when symptoms are severe. Frequent bathing, sitz baths, and soothing lotions such as calamine lotion are helpful. The patient is urged not to scratch or further irritate the condition, and to avoid fecal contamination by careful cleansing from the front backward following defecation. Hyrocortisone ointment has been found to be extremely effective in controlling perineal pruritus and is now widely used.

Cervicitis

Cervical erosion is the mildest form of cervicitis. A small, reddened, irritated area appears about the external mouth of the cervix. It occurs in both married and single women, and the cause is obscure. Inflammation of the cervix may be due to an acute pyogenic infection such as sometimes follows abortion and childbirth, or it may be due to lodging of the gonococcus in a cervical erosion or laceration. This is known as *acute cervicitis*. If inadequately treated, it may become chronic.

In some instances the erosion may be diagnosed as *congenital* erosion. The erosion appears similar to acute cervicitis, but distinction is made because it occurs in girls before puberty and in virgins, in which case trauma and infection from external sources do not appear to be related to the cause.

In untreated cervicitis, the local tissues are constantly irritated, and there is some evidence that this irritation predisposes to cancer. Since leukorrhea, the only symptom of cervicitis, does not appear unless there is severe irritation, the presence of unrecognized cervicitis must be determined by pelvic examination, including visualization of the cervix. If the practice of returning to the doctor for a careful examination six weeks after the birth of every baby were adhered to, much chronic cervicitis could be prevented. The cervix is frequently lacerated as it stretches and thins out to allow the baby to pass through the birth canal, and the torn surfaces do not always heal properly. At the examination made six weeks following delivery, improperly healed lacterations of the cervix can be cauterized so that the everted portion of the mucosa is turned back into the cervical canal. This minor procedure can be done in the doctor's office or the clinic, and it will prevent chronic inflammation. Cervical erosions are often discovered during routine pelvic examinations. A biopsy is taken, and the erosion is then cauterized with silver nitrate.

Acute cervicitis can usually be adequately treated with hot douches and the local application of antibiotics. Antibiotics also may be given both orally and parenterally.

In chronic cervicitis the infection has extended deeper into the tissues, and the patient must be hospitalized for at least one day for *conization* of the cervix. This is the removal of a cone-shaped portion of the cervix containing the infected tissue. The nursing care is the same as that required after a dilation and curettage. In addition, hemorrhage, which may occur from the operative site, is treated by such means as packing the vagina, raising the foot of the bed, and keeping the patient absolutely quiet for several hours. Very occasionally the patient must be returned to the operating room for resuturing or cauterization of the site of hemorrhage. Untreated chronic cervical infections eventually may extend into the uterine cavity and into the pelvic cavity, causing endometritis (inflammation of the uterine lining) and pelvic inflammatory disease.

Bartholinitis

The Bartholin glands, located at the base of the labia majora and secreting a lubricating mucus through an opening between the labia minora and the hymen, may become infected with a variety of organisms, including the gonococcus, staphylococcus, streptococcus, or *Escherichia coli*. With infection the duct from the gland may become obstructed, and severe redness, edema, and tenderness ensue, making even walking difficult. Sometimes the abscess that forms ruptures spontaneously, but surgical incision for drainage is often required. Usually the patient with this condition is treated on an ambulatory basis. Before rupture of the abscess, hot sitz baths and/or local heat in the form of compresses is prescribed. Antibiotics are given systemically, and a gauze packing may be inserted at the time of incision. Careful instruction in perineal care is needed to avoid further contamination after defecation.

Occasionally the acute inflammation subsides, leaving fibrotic or scar tissue. When this occurs, the gland develops a cystic dilation or a *Bartholin's cyst*. The cyst may vary in size from a few centimeters in diameter to the size of a hen's egg. The cyst is mobile and is not tender. If it grows to be of sufficient size to cause difficulty in walking or during intercourse or if it shows signs of inflammation, it may be excised surgically.

Pelvic inflammatory disease

Pelvic inflammatory disease is an inflammatory process within the pelvic cavity that may involve the fallopian tubes, the ovaries, pelvic peritoneum, pelvic veins, or pelvic connective tissue. Inflammation of the fallopian tube is known as *salpingitis*, and inflammation of the ovary is known as *oophoritis*.

Pelvic inflammatory disease frequently is a complication of acute infectious processes such as gonorrhea, puerperal infection, and tuberculosis. The rupture of any adjacent structure may spill organisms into the pelvic cavity, producing secondary inflammation; for example, when the appendix perforates, pelvic peritonitis usually follows. Prevention or early and adequate treatment of the original infection should decrease the incidence of this problem.

Pathogenic organisms such as gonococci and staphylococci are usually introduced from the outside and pass up the cervical canal into the uterus. They seem to cause little trouble in the uterus but pass into the pelvis either through thrombosed uterine veins, through the lymphatics of the uterine wall, or by way of the fallopian tubes. Here they cause an inflammation. Before the discovery of penicillin, the gonococcus was the most common organism causing pelvic inflammatory disease. This organism typically invades the pelvis through the fallopian tubes. Pus forms in the tubes, and adhesions develop so that sterility often follows. Tubercle bacilli usually are carried to the location of inflammation by the blood and from the lungs. Although a generalized peritonitis can occur, the infection usually is localized in the lower abdomen, causing abscess formation and adhesions of the pelvic viscera. An abscess of the cul-de-sac of Douglas is common. In this location the abscess may rupture spontaneously into the vagina or may require surgical incision through the vagina for drainage.

Signs and symptoms of pelvic inflammatory disease may include severe abdominal and pelvic pain, malaise, nausea and vomiting, and elevation of temperature, with leukocytosis. Often there is a foul-smelling, purulent vaginal discharge. The patient is usually hospitalized and placed on bed rest in a mid-Fowler's position to provide dependent drainage so that abscesses will not form high in the abdomen, where they might rupture and cause generalized peritonitis. The sulfonamide and antibiotic drugs are almost always given. Heat applied to the abdomen, either a hot-water bottle or an electric heating pad, or a hot vaginal douche to be taken twice a day may be ordered. Heat improves circulation to the involved parts, and thereby allays the discomfort caused by stasis of blood and enhances the effectiveness of the body's natural defenses—leukocytes. If there is a vaginal discharge, tampons should not be used, since the drainage may be coming from the vaginal wall and a tampon would obstruct it. If the patient is hospitalized, the nurse should instruct her and ancillary personnel to report any change in the amount, appearance, or odor of vaginal discharge. If the patient is ambulatory, she should be advised to watch for these changes and told that she should not have sexual intercourse during the acute stage of the disease.

Pelvic inflammatory disease becomes chronic unless it is quite vigorously treated at its onset. Chronic pelvic discomfort, disturbances of menstruation, constipation, and periodic exacerbation of acute symptoms sometimes occur. Occasionally the patient may be considered neurotic because of the repeated and nonspecific nature of her complaints. The most serious of the complications of pelvic inflammatory disease is *sterility,* which is caused by scar tissue that closes the fallopian tubes. Strictures of the salpinges may cause an *ectopic pregnancy,* since the fertilized egg may not be able to reach the uterus even though the smaller sperm has been able to pass the stricture and produce conception. Adhesions form as a result of chronic inflammation, and the ovaries, fallopian tubes, and uterus may have to be completely removed.

Puerperal infection

Puerperal infection is a uterine infection following interruption of pregnancy or a normal delivery. It usually is caused by streptococci, and the usual route of infection is through the vagina and the cervical canal. With improved obstetric care, puerperal infection now occurs most frequently in women who have had criminally induced abortions. Puerperal infections may occur, however, if the membranes have been ruptured for several days before delivery, if the removal of the placenta has been incomplete, or if clots or edema prevent normal drainage from the uterus following delivery. When the baby is delivered at home, or elsewhere where it is impossible to use aseptic technique, there is increased danger of infection. If contamination has occurred, or if any symptoms of infection appear after

a delivery, antibiotics are given. If pieces of the placenta have been retained, a dilation and curettage of the uterus will be performed because the retained tissue not only causes continued bleeding but also serves as a culture medium for organisms. Uterine cramps, continued vaginal bleeding, or scanty normal uterine drainage *(lochia)* following delivery should be noted and reported so that appropriate treatment may be started if necessary.

Tuberculosis

Tuberculosis of the female reproductive system most frequently involves the fallopian tubes but may also involve the uterus, ovaries, and pelvic peritoneum. It is secondary to a lesion in the lungs. The tubercle bacilli reach the pelvis through the bloodstream but rarely cause symptoms in the pelvis until eight to ten years following occurrence of the primary lesion. Often the pulmonary lesion was minimal and was never diagnosed.

The symptoms are those of acute pelvic inflammatory disease plus (sometimes) the general malaise, weight loss, afternoon temperature elevation, and night sweats that are typical symptoms of tuberculosis. Since the lung lesion is usually inactive, isolation is not necessary. The precautions used for patients with tuberculosis of the urinary system should be followed since the vaginal discharge may contain live tubercle bacilli (p. 469).

The treatment is that given for pulmonary tuberculosis—rest and antituberculosis drug therapy. Sexual intercourse is prohibited. If treatment is ineffectual, the affected pelvic structures may be removed surgically.

Abortions

An abortion is the expulsion of, or removal of, a fetus before it is viable, or before twenty-eight weeks of fetal life. The term miscarriage is used by the laity to indicate spontaneous abortion without human interference and is used occasionally by the medical profession to indicate a pregnancy lost in the second trimester (late abortion). The term abortion is commonly used if the fetus weighs under 1,000 grams. The infant weighing more than that amount is usually viable, and the term *premature labor* is used. It is estimated that 10 to 20% of all conceptions results in abortion. Over one-half of these abortions occur because of some abnormality in the fetus and result from Nature's effort to terminate the development of an imperfect infant.[58]

There are several kinds of abortions. A *threatened abortion* is one in which there is a bloody vaginal discharge and sometimes uterine contractions. In this condition the cervix does not dilate, and immediate bed rest and conservative treatment can often prevent abortion. An *inevitable abortion* is one that occurs despite conservative treatment of early signs. A *complete abortion* is one in which the fetus and all the surrounding tissues are passed, whereas in an *incomplete abortion* some of the products of conception remain in the uterus. A *missed abortion* is one in which the fetus dies (usually early in pregnancy) but is not expelled for as long as two months thereafter.

A *spontaneous abortion* is one that occurs naturally with no known specific cause. It may be due to intrinsic factors, such as a defective ovum or sperm or an improperly placed placenta, or it may be due to extrinsic factors, such as hormonal imbalance or chronic debilitating disease such as tuberculosis. *Habitual abortion* is the repeated abortion of successive pregnancies with no known cause. Many kinds of treatment, such as bed rest during the entire pregnancy, thyroid extract, stilbestrol and progesterone in an attempt to prevent sloughing of the endometrium, and psychotherapy, have been tried. None are really satisfactory, although hormones appear to have helped in some instances.

A *therapeutic abortion* is one performed by a physician when serious maternal disease threatens the mother's life. Usually more than one physician is called in for consultation before decisions is reached to perform this procedure. The patient's husband is always consulted before a therapeutic abortion is considered, and often the spiritual adviser must also be consulted. For details of the convictions of certain religious groups on this subject, the nurse should consult special references. The Roman Catholic viewpoint, for example, is available in material on medical ethics.

A *criminal abortion* is the illegal destruction of the products of conception by the patient or by others. Figures on the frequency of this procedure vary and cannot be accurate since most criminal abortions are performed secretly. It is roughly estimated, however, that at least 1 million such operations are performed annually.[59] Criminal abortions are responsible for a large number of maternal deaths each year since they are almost always performed by unskilled persons. A rough estimate is that 10,500 deaths occur annually.[59] Infections often follow criminal abortions and still cause many deaths each year. Some women die because they hesitate to seek competent medical care when complications of a criminal abortion occur. Some fatalities have been caused by the ingestion of huge doses of drugs in an effort to induce abortion. Others have been due to trauma, such as perforation of the uterus by crude instruments in unskilled hands. The nurse is often in a situation in which she can stress to women that there is no safe way to induce an abortion and that there are no drugs that can be taken to safely dislodge a fetus normally implanted in the uterus. If asked for information on birth control, the nurse can suggest that the patient consult her physician.

The nurse can often encourage the patient to continue with her pregnancy. If the patient is unmarried, she should direct her to agencies especially equipped to help her. Many of our larger cities, for example, have local branches of the Florence Crittenton League, which serves unmarried mothers. The Salvation Army maintains facilities for care of pregnant women in many cities. Local health departments or their equivalents are usually able to provide information about available resources. The nurse must, in all instances, avoid planning with the unmarried pregnant woman for the disposition of her unborn child. She should refer such a matter to the doctor and to reliable social agencies.

The patient who enters the hospital with a history of *threatened, partial,* or *complete abortion* is put on bed rest. Antibiotics are usually ordered to combat infection. The patient's temperature should be taken carefully and recorded. Pain in the abdomen should be reported at once. If abortion is inevitable or if partial expulsion of the products of conception has occurred before the patient was admitted, drugs such as neostigmine (Prostigmin) and ergot may be given to stimulate the uterus to expel its remaining contents. The patient should not go to the bathroom but should use a bedpan. Auxiliary nursing personnel should be instructed to save all bedpan contents since pieces of placental tissue and even a fetus may be passed unknowingly by the patient while she is having a bowel movement. If a fetus is over 5 months, papers recording a stillbirth should be filed with the Bureau of Vital Statistics.

Surgical treatment. If tissue is retained following an abortion, a procedure known as *evacuation of retained secundae* (ERS) must be performed. This is similar to a dilation and curettage, and the preoperative and postoperative nursing care is the same.

General nursing care. The patient who has had an abortion needs understanding and thoughtful nursing care. Regardless of the cause of the abortion or the circumstances surrounding it, the patient usually has a severe emotional reaction. She may, for example, have lost the fetus after years of attempting to become pregnant, or she may have experienced another of a series of abortions when she desperately wants a child and is approaching the age limit for future pregnancies. If so, it is not unusual for the patient to cry, and she should be made to feel that this is normal and to be expected. If the patient wishes to talk, this may decrease her depression. Sometimes it is at this time that the patient may want information about adoption.

The patient who has had a criminal abortion may experience a feeling of relief from knowing that she is no longer pregnant, but she almost invariably suffers from guilt and often from grief as a result of the death of the fetus and of a realization of her life situation that led to abortion. The patient who has had an illegal abortion presents a difficult nursing and medical care problem because she seldom gives the doctor a correct story of her condition and the treatment she has received. Occasionally the nurse who is particularly skillful in gaining the patient's confidence may get information that is helpful to the doctor. The patient also may talk about her feelings if the nurse gives the impression that she has time and is willing to listen and if her attitude suggests that she will not judge the patient. The nurse may then be able to plan with the patient for ways to get the help she needs through a social worker, a spiritual adviser, or other sources.

Ectopic pregnancy

An ectopic pregnancy is one in which the fertilized ovum becomes embedded outside the body of the uterus. Since it is almost always located in the fallopian tube, the term *tubal pregnancy* is often used.

This condition occurs most often in women who have a narrowed fallopian tube due either to inflammation or to a congenital stricture. The sperm may be small enough to pass through the stricture, but the larger fertilized ovum may be unable to do so. It may then attach itself to the tubal wall and develop into an embryo. As the embryo grows, the fallopian tube stretches and finally ruptures. This rupture usually occurs within the first six weeks of pregnancy. The patient experiences a sudden severe pain on one side of the abdomen and has a history of amenorrhea and often of suspected pregnancy. She may go into shock quickly after the onset of pain because of massive hemorrhage into the peritoneal cavity.

Emergency treatment for shock and hemorrhage is given. Early treatment of a ruptured ectopic pregnancy is imperative to prevent death from hemorrhage. Immediately upon diagnosis the patient is prepared for a salpingectomy. If there has been prolonged bleeding preoperatively, the postoperative course may be complicated by peritonitis since the blood in the abdomen becomes infected with organisms.

The nursing care combines the aspects of emergency treatment of a patient who has sustained a severe hemorrhage, general care of a patient who has had major abdominal surgery and who may have peritonitis, and care of a woman whose pregnancy has been terminated prematurely. The patient needs reassurance regarding future pregnancies. She needs to understand that since ova are produced from alternate ovaries, she still has a good chance to become pregnant and have a normal baby.

Hydatidiform mole

A hydatidiform mole is a tumor mass of fetal cells in the uterus that masquerades as a pregnancy. The cause is unknown, although a defective ovum is assumed to be involved. The uterus rapidly increases in size, and the ovaries also increase in size because of enlargement of the ovarian follicles. The hormonal balance is upset and usually causes uterine bleeding. Hydatidiform mole is usually a benign condition and is relieved by curettage of the uterus to remove the abnormal growth. If all tissue is not removed, however, there is some suspicion that cancer may develop either in the uterus or elsewhere in the body because the cells may get into the bloodstream. Since some spontaneous abortions actually may be the expulsion of hydatidiform moles, all aborted tissue should be sent for pathologic examination. Women who have hydatidiform moles are followed medically with periodic Aschheim-Zondek tests. If cancer develops, this test will become positive.

Uterine displacement due to relaxation of the pelvic musculature

Downward displacement of the uterus is caused by a relaxation of the muscles of the pelvic floor. It usually results from unrepaired lacerations due to childbirth. With better obstetric care, use of episiotomies to prevent tearing of the pelvic muscles, and immediate repair of all tears, fewer women should require vaginal wall repairs late in life than is now the case. Perineal exercises practiced following delivery help to prevent relaxation. Apparently relaxation may also be caused by a congenital weakness of the muscles of the pelvis because it occurs occasionally in women who have had no children.

As the uterus begins to drop, the vaginal walls become relaxed, and a fold of vaginal mucosa may protrude outside the vaginal orifice. This is known as a *colpocele*. With the relaxation of the vaginal walls, the bladder may herniate into the vagina (a *cystocele*), or the rectal wall may herniate into the vagina (a *rectocele*). (See Fig. 117.) Both conditions may occur simultaneously.

A sign of relaxation of the pelvic muscu-lature is a dragging pain in the back and in the pelvis. It is made worse by standing on the feet or by walking. The patient who has a cystocele may complain of urinary incontinence accompanying activity that increases intra-abdominal pressure, such as coughing, laughing, walking, or lifting (stress incontinence). The cystocele may become so pronounced that, in order for the patient to void, the bladder must be pushed back into place by holding the finger against the anterior vaginal wall. If the patient has a rectocele, she may complain of constipation and resultant hemorrhoids.

Older women may have suffered from these conditions for years and yet may not have sought medical attention. They may remember that their mothers had a similar condition and think that it is to be expected in women who have borne children. Since they are not incapacitated, some decide not to spend money to have reparative surgery that they know is available. Some delay seeking treatment because they dread surgery. However, untreated displacements of the uterus may cause complications such as cervical ulceration and infection, cystitis, and hemorrhoids.

Vaginal repair. Cystoceles and rectoceles are treated by plastic operations designed to tighten the vaginal wall. The operation is done through the vagina. The repair for a cystocele is called an *anterior colporrhaphy;* that for a rectocele, a *posterior colporrhaphy.* Old tears of the pelvic floor, usually caused by childbearing, may also be repaired. Such repair is called a *perineorrhaphy.*

The patient should have routine preoperative preparation, and a cleansing douche is frequently ordered the morning of surgery. When surgery involving the vagina is done, postoperative nursing care includes prevention of pressure on the vaginal suture line and prevention of wound infection. Perineal dressings are seldom used. *Perineal care* is given at least twice a day and after each defecation. Sterile cotton balls moistened with benzalkonium chloride, bichloride of mercury, or normal saline solution may be used, or the patient may be placed on a douche pan and the solution poured over the perineum. Cleansing is always done away from the vagina toward the rectum so that

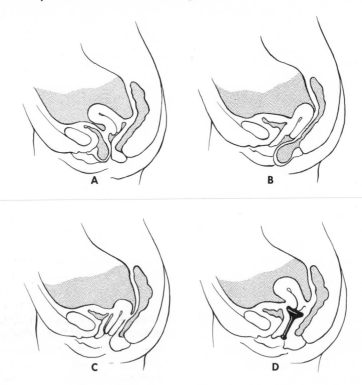

Fig. 117

Abnormalities of the vagina. **A,** Cystocele—downward displacement of the bladder toward the vaginal orifice. **B,** Rectocele—pouching of the rectum into the posterior wall of the vagina. **C,** Prolapse of uterus into vaginal canal. **D,** Stem pessary in place to maintain normal anatomic position of the uterus.

fecal contamination is avoided. A heat lamp may be used for one hour two or three times a day to encourage healing of the perineum. The heat lamp should be used after perineal care to help dry the area and thereby prevent sloughing of tissue. If the patient complains of perineal discomfort, an ice pack applied locally helps to reduce swelling and gives relief. A plastic bag, filled with ice, firmly tied and covered, makes an adaptable pack. When sutures have been removed, sitz baths are usually ordered. Beginning on the tenth postoperative day, most doctors prescribe a daily vaginal douche with normal saline solution. Occasionally douches are ordered during the immediate postoperative period. Sterile equipment and sterile solution should then be used. The douche nozzle should be very gently inserted and very carefully rotated.

After discharge the patient who has had a vaginal repair should continue to take a daily douche and a daily tub bath. The doctor also usually orders mineral oil to be taken each night. When she returns to the clinic or to the doctor's office, she is told when to discontinue the douches and the mineral oil. The doctor also tells her when it is safe for her to resume sexual intercourse. Patients who have had vaginal repair procedures, like other patients having gynecologic surgery, need to avoid jarring activities and heavy lifting for at least six weeks postoperatively.

If a posterior colporrhaphy is scheduled, a cathartic may be given approximately twenty-four hours before surgery, and several enemas usually are given preoperatively to help assure an empty bowel at the time of surgery and immediately thereafter. Up to twenty-four hours preoperatively the patient may be permitted only clear liquids by mouth to further reduce bowel contents. Postoperatively the patient may be kept flat in bed or in a low Fowler's position to prevent increased intra-abdominal pressure or strain on the wound. Special attention must be given to exercise for the patient's legs, to having her turn frequently, and to having her cough deeply. For five days, only liquids are permitted by mouth, and camphorated tincture of opium (paregoric) is also given to inhibit bowel function. At the end of this time mineral oil is given each night, and an oil retention enema is given the morning after the first laxative is given. Only a soft rectal tube and small amounts of oil (200 ml.) should be used. The nurse should discourage straining to produce a bowel movement. Enemas for relieving flatus and for cleansing the bowel usually are not given until at least a week postoperatively.

After an anterior colporrhaphy an indwelling catheter is usually left in the bladder for about four days. The catheter should keep the bladder completely empty. If a catheter is not used and if the patient is taking sufficient fluids, voiding should be checked at least every four hours. No more than 150 ml. of urine should be allowed to accumulate in the bladder. It is usually very difficult to catheterize a patient following a vaginal repair since the urethral orifice may be distorted and edematous. Having the patient take deep breaths may help in locating the orifice because it dilates slightly with each breath. A soft rubber catheter should be used. The patient is usually allowed out of bed immediately after surgery. A regular diet is given, and mineral oil is taken each night to lessen need to strain on defecation.

Sometimes a vaginal plastic procedure does not relieve the *stress incontinence* caused by a cystocele and by general relaxation of the pelvic floor. When this happens, the ligaments about the bladder neck may be shortened in such a way that the bladder drops less easily into the vagina. The degree of incontinence may be tested by filling the bladder to various levels with sterile normal saline solution, and then having the patient cough or strain while standing. If the incontinence is marked, the patient may be placed in a lithotomy position while the doctor fills the bladder with normal saline solution and supports the bladder neck with a finger or with a clamp in the vagina to test the effectiveness of the bladder with this support. If the patient can cough and strain down without being incontinent, she is considered a good candidate for the operation. The surgery is done through a suprapubic incision, and it is usually combined with further vaginal repair. A urethral catheter is inserted, and the nursing care is similar to that following a vaginal repair. If the catheter does not drain freely or if the patient without a catheter does not void within four to six hours, the doctor should be notified. Pressure from a full bladder may disrupt the repair.

Prolapse of the uterus. Prolapse of the uterus, or *procidentia uteri,* is a marked downward displacement of the uterus. The severity of the displacement is designated as first, second, or third degree. In a first-degree prolapse the cervix is still within the vagina. In a second-degree prolapse the cervix protrudes from the vaginal orifice. In a third-degree prolapse the entire uterus, suspended by its stretched ligaments, hangs below the vaginal orifice. In both second-degree and third-degree prolapses, the cervix becomes irritated from clothing, the circulation becomes impaired, and ulceration often follows.

The usual treatment for a uterine prolapse is hysterectomy. This procedure may sometimes be done by the vaginal route. If any operation is contraindicated because of the age or general condition of the patient, a *Gellhorn* or *stem pessary* may be inserted to hold the uterus up in the pelvis (Fig. 117). A string should be attached to the pessary, and after its insertion the patient pins the string to her underclothing. This type of pessary occasionally becomes displaced and might cause the patient embarrassment.

Fistulas

Fistulas can occur in several locations (Fig. 118). They may occur when a malignant lesion has spread or when radiation treatment has been used for a malignancy,

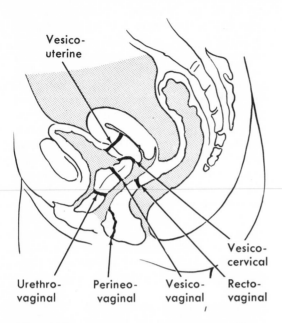

Vesico-
uterine

Urethro-
vaginal

Perineo-
vaginal

Vesico-
vaginal

Vesico-
cervical

Recto-
vaginal

Fig. 118

Types of fistulas that may develop in the vagina and uterus.

or they may be caused by trauma at operation.

Ureterovaginal fistulas complicate gynecologic treatment rather frequently. In treating cancer of the uterus, either by radiation or surgery, or occasionally when a hysterectomy is done, the blood supply to the ureter may be impaired or other damage may occur. The ureteral wall sloughs, and a fistula opens from the ureter to the vagina. This causes a constant drip or urine through the vagina. A ureterovaginal fistula usually heals spontaneously after a period of time. If it does not, repair procedures may be attempted, and occasionally an ileobladder must be made (p. 471).

Vesicovaginal fistulas, or fistulas between the bladder and the vagina, and *urethrovaginal fistulas,* between the urethra and the vagina, may follow radiation of the cervix, gynecologic surgery, or trauma during delivery. It is impossible to perform surgery to repair the fistula until the inflammation and induration have subsided. This may take three to four months. A suprapubic incision is made into the bladder, the fistula tract is dissected out, and the defect is closed by primary closure or by using a graft from the bladder or adjacent mucosal wall.

Postoperatively the patient usually has both a suprapubic tube and a urethral catheter inserted to drain the bladder. These tubes are sometimes attached to a "bubble" suction drainage apparatus in order to assure that the bladder is kept empty. Bladder drainage is maintained for about three weeks or until the wound is completely healed. The catheters should not be irrigated unless it is absolutely necessary, and only very gentle pressure should be used when irrigating them. Signs of urinary drainage from the vagina should be noted. There is normally a small amount of serosanguineous drainage from the vagina for a few days postoperatively. Vaginal douches may be ordered and should be given gently and with very little pressure from the fluid. The patient is kept on bed rest for several days, and then she is usually allowed to sit at the side of the bed. She will need to remain in her room and beside her bed if "bubble" suction is being used. Such confinement is tiring since she is not acutely uncomfortable. Visitors, television, radio, reading materials, and a variety of occupational therapy activities may help her to pass the time satisfactorily.

The results of repair operations for fistulas are not always successful. The patient must sometimes have several operations, and each successive hospitalization increases her anxiety about the outcome of surgery and lessens her ability to accept the discomforts and inconveniences entailed. All possible nursing measures should be taken to prevent infection and to be certain that free drainage of urine is assured. Obstruction of drainage tubes may place pressure against the newly repaired vesicovaginal wall and cause healing tissue to break down, resulting in return of the fistula.

Rectovaginal fistulas are less common than vesicovaginal fistulas. The constant escape of flatus and fecal material through the vagina is particularly distressing to the patient, especially so because rectovaginal fistulas are quite resistant to satisfactory surgical treatment They may be due to the same causes as vesicovaginal fistulas.

Surgical repair is usually done through the rectum. It may not be satisfactory, and operations may have to be repeated. The nursing care is similar to that needed by patients following surgery for other types of rectal fistulas (p. 693). In addition, the patient will need sympathetic understanding and encouragement since the emotional reactions are much more severe.

If there is dribbling of fecal material into the vagina, it may be temporarily lessened by giving a high enema, and the patient who is at home is encouraged to do this procedure before going out. After surgery, of course, enemas are never permitted until healing is complete. They may be given while the patient is awaiting operation. A soft rubber catheter should be used and should be directed carefully on the side of the rectum opposite the fistula. The catheter must go beyond the fistulous opening, or else the fluid will return through the vagina and no benefit will be derived from the treatment. While a constipating diet will temporarily prevent fecal material from going into the vagina, it eventually will cause pressure and may aggravate the condition and increase the size of the fistula. The patient, therefore, is advised against restricting diet and fluids in an effort to control bowel action.

Most patients with vesicovaginal and rectovaginal fistulas tend to become withdrawn. Occasionally, however, a patient becomes immune to the odors, and this presents a serious problem to her family. It puts a strain on family relationships at a time when the patient is desperately in need of approval and acceptance. Often it is better for the doctor or nurse to bring the problem to the patient's attention than to have it mentioned by a member of the family, but the nurse should consult the doctor before discussing this matter with the patient. The nurse can then help the patient to devise means of caring for herself so that she can be assured that she is free of odor. Chlorine solution (for example, 1 tsp. of chlorine household bleach to 1 quart of water) makes a satisfactory deodorizing douche, and this solution is also excellent for external perineal irrigation. Sitz baths and thorough cleansing of the surrounding skin with mild soap and water are helpful. Deodorizing powders such as sodium borate can be used. Care is time-

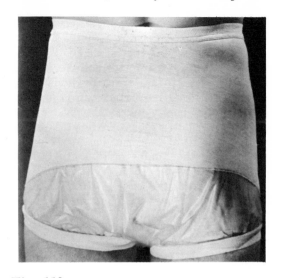

Fig. 119

Pants with plastic reinforcement of the crotch. They usually give adequate protection to the woman with stress incontinence. (Courtesy Ferguson Manufacturing Co., Grand Rapids, Mich.)

consuming and must be repeated at regular intervals to ensure cleanliness. Protective pants can be worn. Some large department stores now stock plastic pants for women that button at the side to avoid bulkiness (Fig. 119). A protective apron worn backward under other clothing or a petticoat with a posterior lining of plastic waterproof material also protects the patient from embarrassment of soiling clothing or furniture when she is seated.

The patient needs encouragement from the medical and nursing staff, and she needs assurance that they understand her problem. When fistulas persist, married couples have special problems that require patience and understanding. Husband and wife should be encouraged to plan together a recreational and activity schedule that will help to minimize tensions until normal sexual relations can be resumed.

Tumors

Among women in the United States, malignant tumors of the reproductive system (exclusive of the breast) rank as the second cause of death from malignant disease and

507

will account for approximately 23,550 deaths in 1966 by present estimates.[2] In the last ten years there has been an almost 25% decrease in deaths from cancer of the uterus, due in large part to wider use of the Papanicolaou test for detection of cancer of the uterus in its early stages. However, it is estimated that in 1966 approximately 9,000 women will die of cancer of the cervix, 4,000 of cancer of the fundus uteri; and 9,000 of cancer of the ovaries.[2]

Cancer of the cervix. The most common cancer of the female reproductive system is cancer of the cervix, which is three to six times more common than cancer of the fundus of the uterus. Cancer of the cervix most often occurs in women who are between 30 and 50 years of age and who have had children. The incidence is also higher in married than in single women regardless of whether or not they have had children. It is believed that 75 to 90% of all women with this condition could be saved by early and adequate treatment.[2] When the cancer is localized (in situ) and has not spread to surrounding tissues at the time of treatment, the rate of cure is almost 100%, whereas the five-year survival rate is only 50% when invasion of other tissues has occurred at the time of treatment.[24] In 1929, the Cancer Committee of the League of Nations developed for statistical study an international classification for cancer of the cervix. This classification originally ranged from Stages I to IV. However, since the discovery of the Papanicolaou smear technique, Stage 0 has been added (Table 11).

Probably one of the greatest responsibilities of the nurse is to encourage every woman over 35 years of age to have a yearly pelvic examination, including a Papanicolaou smear test, and to be aware of the warning signs of cancer of the cervix. If there is early diagnosis, the prognosis is excellent because the preclinical stage (Stage 0) of cancer frequently exists five to ten years before the visible Stage I lesion appears. In the early stages the symptoms are a slight watery vaginal discharge, lengthening of the menstrual period, or occasional spotting of blood between periods. Spotting is often noticed following intercourse, after taking a douche, after defecating, or after heavy lifting.

If treatment is not instituted, the disease will advance progressively, with the vaginal discharge becoming dark, bloody, and foul smelling due to infection and necrosis of tissue. Bladder or rectal symptoms such as fistulas or symptoms of pressure may appear. As lymph glands anterior to the sacrum become involved, back and leg pains occur from pressure on the nerves. Emaciation, anemia, and irregular fever, secondary to the local infection and tissue necrosis, may then follow. The woman with untreated cancer of the cervix has a life expectancy of from two to four years following the appearance of the cervical lesion.

Cancer of the fundus uteri. It is believed that 30 to 40% of all postmenopausal bleeding is due to cancer of the body of the uterus.[1] If the irregular vaginal bleeding is heeded and medical attention sought,

Table 11

Cancer of the cervix

Stage	0	I	II	III	IV
Involvement	Confined within epithelium of cervix	Completely confined to cervix	Extends outside cervix but does not involve pelvic wall or lower third of uterus	Involves pelvic wall and lower third of vagina	Extends beyond Stage III; involves (1) bladder or (2) rectum or (3) metastatic spread

there is a good chance of cure because malignant tumors of the body of the uterus grow slowly and metastases occur late. Since these tumors often arise from a polyp, anyone who has *uterine polyps* or who has had polyps removed from the uterus should have periodic pelvic examinations.

Cancer of the fundus may be treated by panhysterectomy or by irradiation therapy (intrauterine radiation and deep x-ray therapy to the pelvis). Often intrauterine irradiation is used preoperatively to shrink the tumor and to decrease the amount of local infection so that the operation will be safer and more easily performed. Since tumors of the fundus of the uterus occur later in life, the surgical course is frequently complicated by other conditions commonly seen in geriatric patients, such as hypertension, diabetes mellitus, poor circulation, and malnutrition.

Fibroid tumors of the uterus. Approximately one-half of women who are over 50 years of age develop myomas or fibroid tumors of the uterus. These benign tumors are more prevalent in Negro women and in women who have not had children. They are benign lesions and very rarely become malignant. With the advent of the menapause they tend to disappear spontaneously because their growth is stimulated by ovarian hormones.

Menorrhagia is the most common symptom of myomas. If the tumor is very large, it may cause pelvic circulatory congestion and may press on surrounding viscera. The patient may complain of low abdominal pressure, backache, constipation, or dysmenorrhea. If a ureter is compressed by the tumor, there may be signs and symptoms of ureteral obstruction. Sometimes the pedicle on which a myoma is growing becomes twisted, causing severe pain. Large tumors growing into the opening of the fallopian tubes may cause sterility, those in the body of the uterus may cause spontaneous abortions, and those near the cervical opening may make the delivery of a baby difficult and may contribute to hemorrhage postpartally.

The treatment of fibroid tumors depends upon the symptoms and the age of the patient and upon whether she wants more children and how near she is to the menopause. If the symptoms are not severe, the patient may simply need close medical supervision. If the tumor is near the outer wall of the uterus, a *myomectomy* (surgical removal of the tumor) may be performed. This operation leaves the muscle walls of the uterus relatively intact. If there is severe bleeding or obstruction, a *hysterectomy* (surgical removal of the uterus) is usually necessary. Occasionally, if surgery is contraindicated or if the patient is approaching the menopause, x-ray therapy or radiation is used to reduce the size of the tumor and to stop vaginal bleeding.

Cancer of the ovary. Cancer of the ovary appears to be increasing in the United States, and so far it has defied all attempts at early diagnosis. Over one-half of all patients having this condition are inoperable when the disease is discovered, and the five-year survival rate is only 15 to 20%.[55] Most gynecologists believe that the only hope for the patient lies in early and vigorous treatment of ovarian cysts, which may be precursors of malignant disease. They believe that all patients suspected of having tumors of the ovary should have an exploratory abdominal operation, because malignant tumors of the ovary usually give no symptoms until local metastasis occurs and there is ascites from increased pressure within the portal system, edema of the legs from pressure on veins passing through the pelvic cavity, or pain in the back or the legs from pressure on nerves, or until there are symptoms of distant metastasis. The silent onset and growth of ovarian tumors almost surely doom the patient in whom diagnosis is not made prior to onset of symptoms. The only effective means of assuring early diagnosis is a pelvic examination every six months, including careful ovarian palpation, and surgical exploration of any questionable ovarian growth. If possible, the ovary and the tumor are completely removed at operation. If the tumor is malignant, the operation often is followed by deep x-ray therapy. Chemotherapy has prolonged the lives of some patients; nitrogen mustard and TEM are drugs often used, and the alkylating agent chlorambucil has been found to produce a favorable response in approximately 25% of all patients.[58] (For the nursing care of patients receiving these drugs see p. 288.)

Benign tumors of the ovary. Benign tumors of the ovary may cause changes in the secondary sex characteristics. One type produces marked feminizing characteristics, precocious menstruation, resumption of menstruation after the menopause, or prolongation of the menopause. Another type causes development of male characteristics, such as voice changes, male distribution of hair on the face and body, flattening of the breasts, and cessation of menstruation. Symptoms can be relieved by surgical removal of the tumor.

Ovarian cysts. The most common ovarian growth is a cyst of the graafian follicle or corpus luteum. This usually reabsorbs spontaneously. There are, however, other types of ovarian cysts arising from various types of tissue. Some are partly solid, such as the *dermoid cyst*, which may contain skin, hair, teeth, and bone. Others grow very large and cause distortion of the abdomen. Ovarian cysts are surgically removed. This usually includes an *oophorectomy* (removal of the ovary).

Sometimes an ovarian cyst twists on the pedicle that carries its blood supply, causing sudden, sharp pain and shock. An emergency oophorectomy is done since without blood supply the tissues rapidly become necrotic.

Endometriosis

Endometriosis is a condition in which endometrial cells that normally line the uterus are seeded throughout the pelvis and occasionally extend to as distant a location as the umbilicus (Fig. 120). The disease appears to be increasing, although the increased incidence may be due to better diagnosis and recognition of the condition. It is not known how endometriosis first develops. Theories include congenital presence of endometrial cells out of their normal location, their transfer by means of blood vessels or the lymphatic system, and reflux of menstrual fluid containing endometrial cells up the fallopian tubes and into the pelvic cavity. None of these theories has been proved. With each menstrual period the endometrial cells are stimulated by the ovarian hormones and bleed into the surrounding areas, causing an inflammation. Subsequent adhesions may be so severe that pelvic organs may become fused together, and occa-

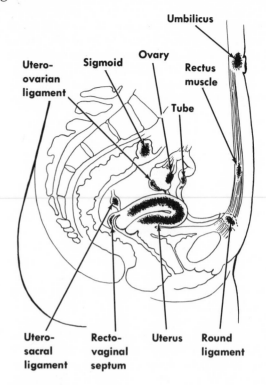

Fig. 120

Sites of endometrial implants.

sionally causes a stricture of the bowel or interference with bladder function. Encased blood may lead to palpable tumor masses, which often occur on the ovary and are known as *chocolate cysts*. Occasionally these cysts may rupture and spread endometrial cells still farther throughout the pelvis.

Usually endometriosis progresses very gradually and does not produce symptoms until the patient is in her thirties or forties. Occasionally, however, symptoms appear when the patient is in her teens. The characteristic symptom of endometriosis is pain and general discomfort accompanying menstruation that becomes progressively worse and that was not present at the onset of the menses. This one characteristic feature should alert the nurse to urge that the patient see a gynecologist at once. Many women with severe pain related to menstruation have been judged to be neurotic when in reality they were suffering from endometriosis. Other symptoms of endometriosis are a feeling of fullness in the lower abdomen, dyspareunia, and general poor health. Sometimes the disease is far advanced and yet has caused no symptoms at all.

Although a great deal of study of endometriosis is under way at present, its response to treatment is still variable and poorly understood. For this reason treatment is highly individualized. If the woman is young and wants to have children, the treatment for endometriosis is usually as conservative as possible. Pregnancy is beneficial because menstruation ceases during this time. If a young married woman has endometriosis, the couple usually is advised to have their family without delay because fertility rate is low and sterility due to adhesions may occur, and because surgery that would prevent a pregnancy may have to be done within a reasonable period of time. Nursing the infant is also recommended because it delays the onset of menstruation following delivery. The antiovulatory drugs are now widely used in the treatment of endometriosis and are given in large doses (usually up to four times the dosage given when used only to suppress ovulation). This dosage produces a situation known as a pseudopregnancy and causes the errant endometrial cells to be temporarily quiescent. Norethynodrel (Enovid), for example, in dosages up to 40 mg. daily may be given for extended periods. The disadvantages of this treatment are that irregular bleeding may occur and that the symptoms of early pregnancy, including nausea, vomiting, depression, and fatigue, may be troublesome. It is not believed that they should be given indefinitely. Androgens are also given occasionally, but their masculinizing effects limit their usefulness.

When the involvement is severe and does not respond to hormonal treatment, surgery may be necessary. A *panhysterectomy* (removal of the uterus with the cervix, the fallopian tubes, and the ovaries) may be done. Removal of the ovaries prevents further bleeding of endometrial implants that cannot be removed, and it has been found that removal of the uterus alone has lead to prolonged regression of the implants in some instances.[53] If the patient is in the premenopausal time of life and the ovaries must be removed, she may be given very small amounts of estrogen to preserve secondary sexual characteristics and permit more normal living. The menopause stops the progress of this condition.

Disease of the vulva

Cancer of the vulva is seen most often in women over 60 years of age who have *chronic leukoplakia of the vulva*. The skin appears white and thickened, itches, and is easily fissured. If leukoplakia in women approaching 60 years of age does not respond to more conservative treatment, some doctors recommend a *vulvectomy*, or surgical excision of the vulva, to prevent the development of cancer. If cancer is already present, the treatment is also vulvectomy. However, in addition, *bilateral inguinal node dissection* may be done, and deep x-ray therapy may be used. Patients with cancer of the vulva are often poor operative risks because of concurrent medical conditions related to age.

Kraurosis vulvae. Another condition seen in older women, kraurosis vulvae, causes a shrinking of the skin of the vulva. The skin is shiny and thin and itches severely. Kraurosis vulvae is not a precancerous condition, but it sometimes requires surgery because adhesions may interfere with voiding and with sexual intercourse. Cortisone ointment is often helpful. Occasionally female hormones are given, and local injections of alcohol may be tried to relieve the pruritus.

Nursing the patient having a vulvectomy and inguinal node dissection

The patient having a vulvectomy has some special nursing needs in addition to routine preoperative and postoperative care. Preoperatively she is given enemas, and postoperatively she is given a low-residue diet. These measures obviate the need for straining to defecate and help prevent contamination of the vulval wound. A Foley catheter usually is used to provide urinary drainage. When the catheter is removed, the patient may be unable to void due to difficulty in relaxing the perineum. Sitz baths may help. If the inguinal nodes have been dissected, a heat lamp may be directed to the groins. After all the sutures are removed, hot sitz baths may be substituted for the heat lamp. Large amounts of tissue are removed from the vulva and the groins during the operation, and the sutures are usually quite taut, leading to severe discomfort. The patient will usually need analgesic medication at frequent intervals during the two or three weeks before sutures can be removed. Following an inguinal node dissection, pillows need to be arranged to prevent undue pulling on the taut inguinal sutures when the patient moves. If the patient is lying on her side, she will be more comfortable if her upper leg is supported by a pillow. If she is lying on her back, a low Fowler's position puts less tension on the sutures. Wound hemorrhage is a possible complication.

The vulval wound is frequently left exposed, but if a dressing is used, it should be held in place with a T binder. The wound is cleansed twice a day with solutions such as hydrogen peroxide, normal saline solution, benzalkonium chloride, pHisoHex, or other antiseptic solutions. Following this, a heat lamp is used to dry the area. The heat also improves local circulation, thus stimulating healing.

The wounds following a vulvectomy or an inguinal node dissection also heal slowly, and the patient may become quite discouraged. Diversional occupations and socializing with other patients may help to keep the patient from thinking too much about herself and help her to pass the time. Privacy should be assured, and women should be encouraged to express their feelings concerning this disfiguring surgery. Some women feel that their femininity has been irreparably damaged or that the disfigurement may end their sexual life. Actually, by the time the patient is discharged, the wounds are usually healed, and the convalescence will be similar to that following any surgical procedure. Sexual intercourse, for the married patient, can usually be resumed.

Nursing the patient receiving radiation therapy

Internal radiation is used to treat cancer of the cervix and cancer of the body of the uterus because of the accessibility of these body parts and because of their generally favorable response to this form of treatment. The radioactive materials most often used are radium and cobalt (Co^{60}) or iridium (Ir^{192}), which have been made radioactive by artificial means. (For discus-

sion of radiation treatment and the general nursing care and precautions involved, see p. 278.)

It is important that all normal tissues remain in their natural position and do not come nearer to the radioactive substance than is anticipated and than is provided for by the protective materials used. The patient is usually given a cleansing enema before the treatment starts and is given a low-residue diet to prevent distention of the bowel, and a catheter may be inserted to prevent distention of the bladder. Gauze packing is usually inserted into the vagina to push both the rectum and the bladder away from the area being irradiated. Enemas are not given during the treatment. To prevent any displacement of the radioactive substance, the patient is kept flat in bed and is allowed to turn only from side to side. A roentgenogram is taken after the radioactive substance is inserted to determine its exact location.

The colpostat and tandem incorporating radioactive cobalt and intrauterine applicators or needles containing radium or radioactive iridium are most often used (Fig. 121). The amount of radioactive substance used and the number of hours it is left in place are determined by the amount of radiation needed to kill the less resistant cancer cells without damaging normal cells. Radioactive materials used for internal treatment must be removed at exactly the indicated time, and the nurse is often responsible for reminding the doctor to do this. If possible, the time of insertion should be planned so that removal will be at a convenient hour; for example, not in the middle of the night or during visiting hours.

Since the presence of *anything* in the cervix stimulates uterine contractions, the patient who has a colpostat or intrauterine applicator in place may have severe uterine contractions as a result of dilation of the cervix. The patient should know that they will occur. Often a narcotic is given at regular intervals while the applicator is in place. There will be foul-smelling vaginal discharge from destruction of cells. Good perineal care is essential, and it must be remembered that since the patient must lie on her back, she will need assistance. A deodorizer is helpful.

Patients may develop radiation sickness,

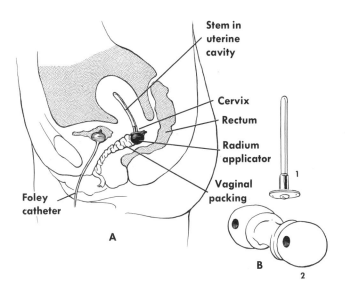

Fig. 121

A, Radium applicator in place in the uterus. Note the Foley catheter to decompress the bladder and that vaginal packing is used. **B, 1,** Intrauterine applicator; **2,** colpostat.

with nausea, vomiting, diarrhea, malaise, and fever. This probably is a systemic reaction to the breakdown and reabsorption of cell proteins. (See p. 283 for discussion of care.) Local reaction may include cystitis and proctitis. Camphorated tincture of opium (paregoric) helps relieve the diarrhea. If it is severe, a cornstarch enema (1 tbsp. of cornstarch to 250 ml. of lukewarm water) may be ordered. Oil retention enemas are also sometimes given. The patient is urged to drink at least 3,000 ml. of fluid a day to help relieve any irritation of the urinary system.

Since the woman who is receiving radiation treatment usually either knows or suspects the diagnosis, she is likely to be depressed. The nurse should plan to spend some time talking with her but should remain at the distance that is safe (see p. 280). She should explain to the patient that this precaution is necessary because nurses are in frequent contact with radioactive material. Close members of the family should be encouraged to visit when it is considered safe for them to do so (p. 284).

Following the removal of the radioactive agent, the catheter is removed, a cleansing enema is given, and the patient is allowed out of bed. Vaginal discharge will continue for some time, and the patient may need to take douches for as long as the odor and vaginal discharge persist. Usually douches are ordered twice a day. The patient who is returning home needs detailed instruction in how to give herself douches and what solutions to use. Some vaginal bleeding may occur for one to three months after irradiation of the cervix or the body of the uterus. The patient who is at home should report persistent rectal irritation to the doctor. Emollient enemas may be prescribed to be taken at home. The patient is usually discharged from the hospital within a day or two after the applicators are removed but may return for another course of radiation.

Complications to watch for following radiation of the uterus are vesicovaginal fistulas, rectovaginal fistulas, ureterovaginal fistulas, cystitis, phlebitis, and hemorrhage. Each is due to irritation and destruction of adjacent tissue either by the radiation or by extension of the disease process. The patient is urged to report even minor symptoms or complaints to her doctor.

If the patient is treated by x-ray therapy for a lesion of the reproductive system, the care is the same as that given a patient receiving this treatment elsewhere in the body (p. 281). However, one important point should be emphasized: the patient should always void immediately before the treatment to prevent damage to the bladder.

Nursing the patient who must have all or part of the female reproductive system removed

Surgery such as a bilateral oophorectomy or a hysterectomy upsets most women emotionally. All women worry about the effect it will have on their femininity and wonder about possible changes in secondary sex characteristics. Young women may feel bitterly disappointed because they can no longer have children. Some women worry about gaining weight, although weight gain is more often due to overeating than to hormonal changes. It is true that the childbearing function will be terminated, but usually the vagina is intact so that several weeks following surgery married women can resume normal sexual intercourse.

Older patients are usually less upset by the prospects of surgery of this kind than are those who have not reached the menopause. Postoperatively, however, almost all patients feel weepy and depressed for several days. This apparently is due to a change in hormonal balance and to psychologic reaction. The patient often is unable to explain why she is depressed and crying. During this period, she needs understanding and sympathetic care since she may appear somewhat unreasonable at times. Families need to be helped to accept these unusual responses calmly, and a husband may need to reassure the patient repeatedly of his love and affection.

Hysterectomy. If a hysterectomy is to be performed, the preoperative physical preparation is the same as that for any other abdominal surgery, except that the perineum is completely shaved. A vaginal douche may be given. Postoperatively the patient has an abdominal dressing and wears a perineal pad. If a vaginal hysterectomy is performed, there will be no abdominal incision, but sterile perineal pads will need changing frequently. The dressings should be observed for any sign of bleeding every fifteen minutes for two hours and then at least every hour for eight hours. There is normally a moderate amount of serosanguineous drainage. The perineal pad should be held in place with a T binder, and some doctors prefer that a snug scultetus binder be applied to the abdomen, especially if there has been a *radical hysterectomy* (removal of the ovaries, tubes, uterus with the cervix, and parametrial tissue) and extensive node dissection. (See Fig. 122.)

Following a hysterectomy, especially one in which there has been extensive node and parametrial resection, the bladder may be temporarily atonic as a result of nerve trauma, and a Foley catheter is used to maintain constant drainage of the bladder. If no catheter is used and if the patient is unable to void within eight hours, she is usually catheterized. The catheter (if used) is removed on the third or fourth postoperative day, and the patient may be catheterized if abnormal residual urine is suspected.

Abdominal distention may complicate a hysterectomy. It is caused by nerve damage, by handling of the viscera during operation or by sudden release of pressure on the intestines such as occurs on removal of a large myoma. Some doctors insert a nasogastric tube prophylactically following surgery, and most doctors restrict food and fluids by mouth for twenty-four to forty-eight hours. There is usually an order for a rectal tube and for a heating pad to the abdomen to be used as necessary. If the surgery has been extensive, a soft rectal tube should be selected to prevent trauma to the bowel. A carminative enema is usually given on the second or third day postoperatively. When peristalsis returns, the patient is started slowly on fluids and food.

There may be interference with circulation during hysterectomy, and thrombophlebitis of the vessels of the pelvis and upper thigh is a rather common complication. The patient should never rest with the knees bent or with the thighs sharply flexed. The knee gatch should not be used, and the bed should not be raised at the head to more than a mid-Fowler's position. The patient should exercise her feet and legs every hour, and she should move about in bed, turning from

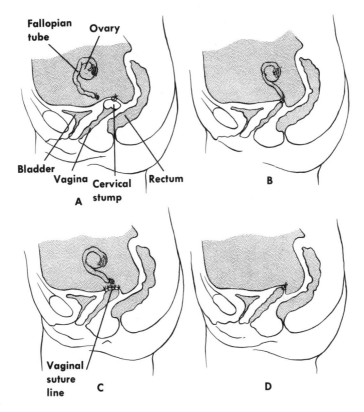

Fig. 122

A, Cross section of a subtotal hysterectomy. Note that the cervical stump, fallopian tubes, and ovaries remain. **B,** Cross section of a total hysterectomy. Note that the fallopian tubes and ovaries remain. **C,** Cross section of a vaginal hysterectomy. Note that the fallopian tubes and ovaries remain. **D,** Cross section of a panhysterectomy. Note that the uterus, fallopian tubes, and ovaries are completely removed.

her side to her back and to a partial face-lying position. A pillow can be used to support the abdominal wound. The head of the bed should be put completely flat for a short time every two hours. These precautions help prevent stasis of blood in the pelvic vessels. If the patient has varicosities, the doctor may order elevation of the legs for a few minutes every two or three hours to permit blood to drain from the legs. Ace bandages may be ordered to be applied from the toes to the groin. They should be reapplied twice a day to assure a snug, even pressure. The patient often is permitted out of bed the day following the operation. Other nursing care is the same as that following

any abdominal surgery. Special attention should be given to any complaint of low back pain or to lessened urinary output since it is possible that a ureter could have been accidentally ligated. Very occasionally, the ureter, the bladder, or the rectum is traumatized.

The patient should know what surgery has been done, what changes in herself she should expect, and what care she needs when she leaves the hospital. If a *total hysterectomy* has been done, she will not menstruate. A *subtotal hysterectomy*, however, permits menses to continue, since a portion of the uterus with its endometrial lining is left. She should not have sexual intercourse until told

515

by the doctor that it may be safely resumed. Most patients are more comfortable if they wear a girdle. Heavy lifting should be avoided for about two months. Activities such as riding over rough roads, walking swiftly, and dancing tend to cause congestion of blood in the pelvis and should be avoided for several months. Physical activity that does not cause strain, such as swimming, may be engaged in since it is helpful both for the physical and mental well-being of the patient.

Unilateral salpingectomy and oophorectomy. The patient who has a unilateral salpingectomy (removal of one fallopian tube) or a unilateral oophorectomy (removal of one ovary) usually requires postoperative nursing care similar to that given any patient having abdominal surgery. If the surgery is done to remove a large ovarian cyst, however, the patient may have considerable abdominal distention due to the sudden release of pressure on the intestines. The care is similar to that given for distention following a hysterectomy. If the surgery is done to remove a tumor which has caused changes in sex characteristics, the patient is usually quite sensitive and needs much understanding and encouragement from the nurse. She may shun others prior to surgery, and it is wise to let her have privacy if she so desires. She may be reassured that following surgery the abnormal sexual changes will gradually disappear. If the patient seems to withdraw from contact with others, the nurse should spend extra time with her provided she seems receptive to the nurse's interest.

Bilateral oophorectomy and radiation of the ovaries. The patient who has a bilateral oophorectomy or radiation treatment of the ovaries has specific problems. Although immediate preoperative and postoperative nursing needs are no different from those of the patient with other abdominal surgery, she will have an emotional reaction to being sterile that will need consideration. The extent of this reaction depends upon her age, whether or not she already has or wants children, and her emotional makeup. She also will have symptoms of the climacteric. When the menopause is artificially induced, the symptoms are often more severe than in the normal climacteric. Therefore, at least a portion of an ovary is left unless this is detrimental to the patient's prognosis. Estrogens relieve the symptoms and may be given to most patients unless surgery has been done for a malignancy. A bilateral oophorectomy may have been done primarily to remove the hormonal supply. This procedure is now used quite frequently in conjunction with radical mastectomy for cancer of the breast. The period of adjustment after a bilateral oophorectomy is long and is often trying not only for the patient but also for her family.

Pelvic exenteration. In a pelvic exenteration all reproductive organs and adjacent tissues are removed. Nursing care includes the care given the patient having a hysterectomy, the care given the patient having an abdominal perineal resection of the bowel, and the care given the patient having an ileobladder with transplantation of the ureters. Since this operation includes a radical hysterectomy, pelvic node dissection, cystectomy, vaginectomy, and a rectal resection, it requires unusual physical, social, and emotional adjustments on the part of the patient. Since it has not been found to help patients with cancer of the uterus more than less extensive operations and radiation treatment, it is not widely done at this time.

The patient who has had a pelvic exenteration will have both urine and feces passing from the body through openings in the abdominal wall. She cannot contemplate having children, cannot have sexual intercourse, and will have symptoms of the menopause. Until she is able to accept her situation realistically, her rehabilitation will progress very slowly. This acceptance cannot be forced upon the patient, but she must be encouraged gradually to resume self-care. She will undoubtedly have recurring periods of depression and discouragement. She should be helped to express her feelings and be given ample time and consideration by the nurse in order to do so. The family should understand what the surgery will entail, and they too, need encouragement. Acceptance of the situation by the patient's husband is a very important factor in giving her the reassurance and courage necessary to face her future, and he, too, may need to talk about his feelings with the nurse or others.

Nursing the patient with incurable disease of the female reproductive system

The patient with incurable disease of the female reproductive system frequently has a lingering terminal illness. Most carcinomas of the female reproductive system do not metastasize to vital areas such as the liver. By direct spread they eventually cause death from carcinomatosis and from kidney failure that results from obstruction of both ureters by the tumor.

The nursing care is the same as for any patient with a terminal cancer elsewhere (p. 290), but there are some special measures that help to make the patient more comfortable. Frequent changes of position help relieve abdominal and pelvic pressure, and alternate hot and cold applications to the abdomen may bring some relief from pain. Often the use of these measures and the prescription of mild analgesics such as acetylsalicylic acid keep the patient comfortable for an indeterminate time and delay the need for narcotics. Most physicians believe that the patient should be kept relatively comfortable by the use of drugs to relieve pain. Now that synthetic narcotics are available, there is less danger of the patient's developing addiction or tolerance to drugs since it is possible to change from one to another. A chordotomy is sometimes done to relieve severe pain (p. 916).

As cells die and are expelled, vaginal discharge may be profuse and have a foul odor. This is upsetting to the patient, her family, and her friends. The most effective means of decreasing the odor is to give the patient perineal care every four hours and to give a cleansing douche at least twice daily. Copious amounts of water shouuld be used. Solutions containing chlorine are useful in destroying odors, and aromatic trade preparations added to the water may make the patient feel cleaner and more acceptable.

Meticulous care must be given to the skin since the patient is usually emaciated and may develop pitting edema. If the patient has ascites, she may rest better if the head of the bed is elevated.

Nursing related to disease of the male reproductive system

The nurse must be particularly aware of the reactions and feelings of male patients who have disease of the reproductive system. She should not hesitate to ask the

Fig. 123

A, Bougie for urethral dilation. **B**, Filiform. Note the long, fine, flexible tip. **C**, Metal sound for urethral dilation.

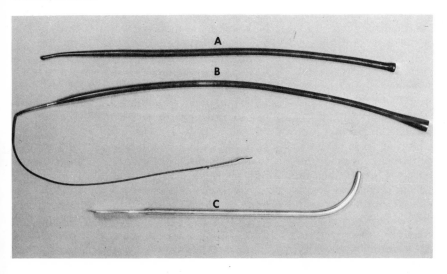

doctor to discuss with the patient any problems that can best be handled by him.

Infections

Nonspecific pyogenic organisms, as well as specific organisms such as gonococci and tubercle bacilli, may cause stubborn infections of the male reproductive system. Urethritis, prostatitis, seminal vesiculitis, and epididymitis are the most common infections. Infecting organisms may reach the genital organs by direct spread through the urethra or they may be borne by blood or lymph.

Because urethral infection spreads so readily to the genital organs, men should not be catheterized unless it is absolutely necessary. Every means should be used to help them void normally. They are often allowed to stand to void even when they are to be on bed rest otherwise. Because of the length and curvature of the male urethra, some trauma to the urethral mucosa is likely to accompany catheterization or the passage of instruments such as a cystoscope. The distal part of the urethra is not sterile, and trauma makes the area susceptible to attack from the bacteria present. Fluids should be given liberally following passage of instruments through the urethra.

Nonspecific urethritis. Nonspecific urethritis is an inflammation of the urethra caused by such organisms as staphylococci, *Escherichia coli, Pseudomonas,* and streptococci. Although the symptoms and complications are essentially the same as those of gonorrheal urethritis, this infection is rarely caused by sexual contact. The patient complains of urgency, frequency, and burning on urination. There may be a purulent urethral discharge. (See p. 529 for discussion of gonorrheal urethritis.)

Treatment of nonspecific urethritis consists of antibiotics and chemotherapy, hot sitz baths, and increased fluid intake. To drain periurethral glands, the urethra may be dilated with sounds (Fig. 123). Dilation is followed by the instillation of a mild antiseptic such as 1:10,000 silver nitrate solution. Physical rest, improvement of general health, and decreased sexual activity are usually suggested. Nonspecific urethritis is difficult to cure and may become a chronic problem that ultimately results in chronic prostatitis.

Prostatitis. The patient with prostatitis usually has acute symptoms of urinary obstruction. He suddenly has difficulty in voiding, perineal tenderness and pain, and elevation of temperature. There may be hematuria. Treatment is usually conservative, consisting of antibiotics and chemotherapy, forcing fluids, physical rest, and local application of heat by sitz baths and/or low rectal irrigations.

Before having a rectal irrigation, the patient should have a cleansing enema. Then, by means of a Y connector on the rectal tube, tap water is allowed to flow alternately in and out of the rectum. The use of 2,000 ml. of water 46° C. (115° F.) and the insertion of the tube only three to four inches into the rectum will concentrate heat in the area of the prostate gland.

Prompt treatment of prostatitis may obviate the need for an indwelling catheter by preventing edema of the prostate and resultant obstruction of the urethra. Occasionally *prostatic abscesses* complicate the clinical course and may have to be drained surgically. Recurrent episodes of acute prostatitis may cause fibrotic tissue to form, and a prostatectomy may be necessary to relieve the resultant obstruction (p. 463).

Epididymitis. Epididymitis, one of the most common infections of the male reproductive system, may be caused by any pyogenic organism, but it frequently is a complication of gonorrhea or of tuberculosis of the urinary system. The patient complains of severe tenderness, pain, and swelling of the scrotum, which is hot to the touch. His temperature may be markedly elevated, and he has general malaise. He often walks with a characteristic "duck waddle" in an attempt to protect the affected part. This walk may first disclose difficulty in the patient who is too embarrassed to describe his trouble.

The patient with epididymitis is usually put to bed and the scrotum elevated either on towel rolls or with adhesive strapping (Fig. 125). Ice is used to help reduce the swelling and to relieve the pain and discomfort. Heat is usually contraindicated because the normal temperature of the scrotal contents is below normal body temperature, and excessive exposure to heat may cause destruction of sperm cells. If an ice cap is used, it should be placed under the scrotum and should be removed for short intervals every hour to prevent ice burns. Antibiotic therapy is given. At least three quarts of fluid should be taken daily. When the patient is allowed out of bed, he should wear a scrotal support.

Patients with *tuberculous epididymitis* are placed on a tuberculosis regimen (p. 555). If a drainage fistula (scrotal fistula) develops, contamination of others with the drainage must be prevented.

Since bilateral epididymitis usually causes sterility, special attention is given to the prevention of this infection. Untreated epididymitis leads rather rapidly to necrosis of testicular tissue and septicemia. When bladder drainage over a long period of time is necessary, a cystotomy is done so that a urethral catheter is avoided. An older patient who must have surgery of the prostate such as a transurethral resection, that will require leaving a urethral catheter in place for a long time may be advised to have a *bilateral vasectomy* to prevent any infection from descending via the vas deferens to the epididymis. Often the operation is done prior to any cystoscopic examination. Since bilateral vasectomy causes sterility, it is seldom done on young men. Permission must be granted by the patient. The vasectomies are done through two very small incisions in the scrotum or in the groins. Local anesthesia is used. Postoperatively the patient should still be watched for symptoms of epididymitis, since the organisms may have invaded the epididymis prior to the vasectomy.

Paraphimosis. Paraphimosis is a condition in which the prepuce is retracted over the glans and forms a constriction that is sometimes impossible to reduce as edema develops in the glans (Fig. 124). Cool compresses are applied to the penis and it is elevated for a short time before gentle attempt is made to reduce the prepuce. If this measure fails, emergency surgery must be done. A dorsal slit is made in the prepuce to prevent necrosis of the glans due to impairment of its blood supply. A circumcision usually is done later to prevent recurrences.

Circumcision, or surgical excision of the prepuce, is widely recommended for all male infants. The reasons are that it makes cleansing of the area so much simpler and that cancer of the glans penis is almost un-

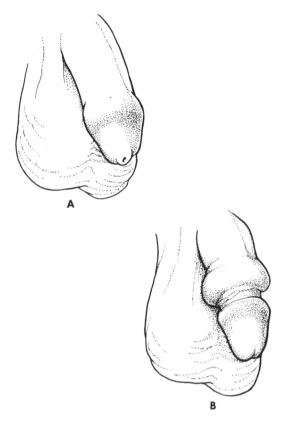

Fig. 124

A, Phimosis. Note pinpoint opening of foreskin. **B,** Paraphimosis. Note foreskin is retracted but has become a constricting band around penis.

known among men who were circumcised soon after birth. If the operation is done a few days after birth, no general anesthetic is needed. Some patients, even if they need anesthesia, are not hospitalized for more than a few hours for this operation. The wound is covered with gauze generously impregnated with petroleum jelly. Bleeding usually is controlled by applying a pressure dressing that may be bulky and that sometimes must be removed before the patient can void. It should be removed cautiously and replaced after voiding with a petroleum jelly dressing. If the patient goes home, he or his mother, if the patient is a child, is taught to change the dressing at each voiding for a few days and to try, if possible, to avoid fecal contamination of the area. Instruction is also given to be alert for signs of bleeding. If severe bleeding occurs, a firm dressing should be applied to the penis and the patient should go at once to the doctor's office or the hospital emergency room. Very occasionally, if bleeding persists, it is necessary to resuture the wound. Frequently an estrogen preparation is prescribed for adult patients for several days after surgery to prevent penile erections, which are painful.

Orchitis. An infection of the testicle is known as orchitis. It may be caused by pyogenic bacteria, the gonococcus, or the tubercle bacillus, or it may be a complication of mumps contracted after puberty. Although the latter occurs in a relatively small percentage of the cases, if bilateral it usually causes sterility. Any boy after puberty or man who is exposed to mumps usually is given gamma globulin immediately unless he has already had the disease. If there is any doubt, globulin usually is given. Although it may not prevent mumps, the disease is likely to be less severe with less likelihood of complications.

The symptoms and the treatment of orchitis are the same as those of epididymitis. Stilbestrol, which inhibits normal function, cortisone, and antibiotics may be given. Sometimes the tunica albuginea must be excised surgically to improve circulation to the testicle.

Scrotal and testicular enlargement

Immediate medical attention should be sought for any swelling of the scrotum or the testicles within it. Scrotal enlargements should be diagnosed—not treated symptomatically with suspensories, which give relief and encourage procrastination.

Hydrocele. A hydrocele is a benign, painless collection of fluid within the tunica vaginalis that leads to swelling of the scrotum. It occurs fairly often in infant boys as well as in adults. The cause is usually unknown. Occasionally hydrocele is treated by aspirating the fluid and injecting a sclerosing drug such as urea hydrochloride into the scrotal sac, but excision of the tunica vaginalis (hydrocelectomy) is the preferred treatment. Postoperatively a pressure dressing is applied on the scrotum, which is elevated (Fig. 125). The patient should be observed carefully for any symptoms of hemorrhage. Bleeding may

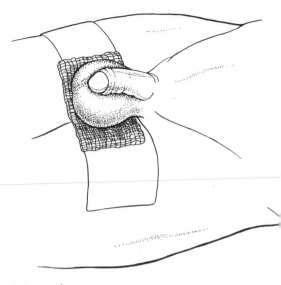

Fig. 125

Bellevue bridge.

not be external. The patient needs a scrotal support when he is up and about and may still require one after he is discharged from the hospital. He should have two scrotal suspensories since they should be washed each day. Immediately after operation or following an infection, most patients require an extra large suspensory or perhaps an athletic support (jockstrap).

Testicular neoplasm. Cancer of the testicle is usually painless, but it may be accompanied by an aching or dragging sensation in the groin and by swelling of the testicle. The swelling is frequently first discovered by the patient following trauma, but it usually is not caused by the trauma. Testicular swelling should always make one suspicious of neoplasm of the testicle. This condition is usually seen in men between 25 and 35 years of age, and it accounts for about 3% of all malignant tumors of the male reproductive system.[19]

An *undescended testicle* is much more likely to become malignant than one that is in the scrotum at birth or descends shortly thereafter. This is an important reason for encouraging parents to consent to surgical intervention to bring down a testicle of a young boy. This does not eliminate the possibility of a neoplasm, but the testicle is located in a position where it may be examined carefully and regularly.

Men with suspicious testicular swelling are asked to collect a first-voided morning urine specimen. This is sent for an Aschheim-Zondek test, the same test used to detect pregnancy in women. One type of testicular tumor, the one with the poorest prognosis, gives a positive Aschheim-Zondek reaction. For all types of testicular tumors, the testicle is removed surgically (orchiectomy) and the adjacent area is explored for metastatic node involvement. Metastasis often has occurred before the initial lesion is discovered.

The patient with cancer of the testicle is usually given a course of radiation therapy, and a *radical node dissection* may be done. This dissection may be unilateral or bilateral.

Following a radical node dissection, there is danger of hemorrhage. Active movement may be contraindicated since nodes may have been resected from around many large abdominal vessels, but gentle passive turning and leg and arm movement are essential to prevent postoperative pneumonia and thrombosis. Deep breathing should be encouraged at hourly intervals. A turning sheet and a chest support are usually helpful. The patient is extremely uncomfortable and needs frequent and large doses of narcotics and sedative drugs.

When a radical node dissection is done, the patient may be placed in a Trendelenburg position for two weeks to allow the kidney to become fixed in place, since frequently all the fatty tissue supporting it must be removed. The patient may need to be fed and bathed during this period. He may have difficulty voiding in this position. For defecation, permission from the doctor may have to be obtained to lower the foot of the bed. Occupational and diversional therapy should be provided. Since many patients find it impossible even to read in the Trendelenburg position, they may appreciate being read to, having the use of books that can be projected on the ceiling, or having access to "talking books" used by blind persons.

Since radiation therapy often is begun the day after surgery, the patient may develop radiation sickness during his hospital stay or during continued treatment as an outpatient. Hormones and chemotherapy are not effective in slowing the progress of cancer in this organ.

Patients and their families are extremely upset by the diagnosis of neoplasm of the testicle. The doctor frequently is quite frank with the family and with the patient because he believes the man needs to be able to make necessary arrangements to provide for his family. The patient's prognosis may be measured in only months or in several years. Some patients are openly depressed. Others may seem to be taking the news too well. The nurse should listen carefully to both the patient and his family and sometimes suggest that help be obtained from others, such as the social worker or the spiritual adviser. (For further discussion, see p. 277.)

Spermatocele. A spermatocele is a nontender cystic mass containing sperm. It is attached to the epididymis. Since the lesion is benign and usually there are few symptoms, excision is rarely necessary. If the patient is uncomfortable, he is usually advised to wear a scrotal support to prevent undue discomfort until after he has a family. Large masses may then be excised.

Varicocele. A varicocele is a dilation of the spermatic vein and is commonly seen on the left side only, probably because the left spermatic vein is much longer than the right. A varicocele on the right side only is suggestive of an abdominal tumor. The use of a scrotal support is usually all that is necessary to relieve any dragging sensation, but the spermatic vein may be ligated.

Torsion of the testicle. Torsion of the testicle or kinking of the spermatic artery causes severe pain, tenderness, and swelling of the testicle. It often follows activity that puts a sudden pull on the cremasteric muscle such as may occur from jumping into cold water. Operative intervention may be indicated and must be done within a few hours because interruption of blood supply to the testicle causes necrosis of the organ.

Cancer of the prostate gland

On autopsy examination, from 15 to 20% of all men past 55 years of age have been found to have microscopic carcinoma of the prostate gland. Although many of these men did not have clinical symptoms, it is known

521

that the incidence of clinical cancer of the prostate gland increases with increasing age. It is believed that probably 25% of men in the seventh and eighth decades of life have cancer of the prostate gland.[21]

Cancer of the prostate gland is most often diagnosed when the patient seeks medical advice because of symptoms of urethral obstruction or because of sciatica (low back, hip, and leg pain). The pain is caused by metastasis of the cancer to the bones. This form of cancer frequently occurs concurrently with benign prostatic hypertrophy that causes the urethral obstruction. However, the cancer itself may be so far advanced as to cause obstruction.

Most carcinomas of the prostate gland are adjacent to the rectal wall and can be detected by rectal examination before symptoms appear. Since cancer of the prostate gland that causes obstruction of the urethra or back and leg pains may be too far advanced for curative treatment, one can readily understand the need for men past 40 years of age to have routine rectal examinations. It is usually the lesions that are detected prior to symptoms that can be cured. A biopsy of any suspicious mass is taken.

An elevated acid phosphatase in the blood serum suggests cancer of the prostate gland, but since the acid phosphatase produced by prostatic cancer is not absorbed by the blood until the lesion has extended beyond the prostatic capsule, it is not a useful technique for early diagnosis.

In patients in whom a diagnosis is made prior to local extension of the cancer or distant metastasis, a *radical resection of the prostate gland* usually is curative. The entire prostate gland, including the capsule and the adjacent tissue, is removed. The remaining urethra is then anastomosed to the bladder neck. Since the internal and external sphincters of the bladder lie in close approximation to the prostate gland, it is not unusual for the patient to have urinary incontinence following this type of surgery. He also will be both impotent and sterile. The perineal approach is most often used, but the procedure may be accomplished by the retropubic route (Fig. 107).

If the patient is to have a perineal approach in surgery, he is given a bowel preparation, which includes enemas, cathartics,

and phthalylsulfathiazole (Sulfathalidine) or neomycin preoperatively and only clear fluids the day before surgery to prevent fecal contamination of the operative site. Postoperatively he may be permitted nothing by mouth, clear liquids, or a low-residue diet until wound healing is well advanced. He may also be given camphorated tincture of opium to inhibit bowel action. If the retropubic approach is used, the preoperative care is similar to that of any patient having major surgery.

Regardless of the surgical approach, the patient returns from surgery with a urethral catheter inserted. A large amount of urinary drainage on the dressing for a number of hours is not unusual. It should decrease rapidly, however. There should not be the amount of bleeding that follows other prostatic surgery and, since the catheter is not being used for hemostasis, the patient usually has little bladder spasm. The catheter is used both for urinary drainage and as a splint for the urethral anastomosis. Therefore, care should be taken that it does not become dislodged or blocked. The catheter is usually left in the bladder for two or three weeks.

The care of the perineal wound is the same as that following a perineal biopsy except that healing is usually slower. If there has been a retropubic surgical approach, the wound and possible wound complications are the same as for a simple retropubic prostatectomy (p. 466).

Since perineal surgery causes relaxation of the perineal musculature, the patient may suddenly have fecal incontinence. It is disturbing to the patient and sometimes can be avoided by starting perineal exercises within a day or two after surgery. Control of the rectal sphincter usually returns readily. Perineal exercises should be continued even after rectal sphincter control returns since they also strengthen the bladder sphincters, and unless the bladder sphincters have been permanently damaged, the patient will regain urinary control more readily on removal of the catheter. (See p. 156 for perineal exercises.)

The patient with carcinoma of the prostate gland is often very depressed after surgery, because he suddenly realizes the implications of being impotent and perhaps permanently incontinent. He usually has been told by the doctor before the operation that these consequences are possible, but he may not have fully comprehended their meaning. He needs to be encouraged, and provision should be made to keep him dry so that he will feel able to be up and to socialize with others without fear of having obvious incontinence. (See p. 158 for ways to manage incontinence.) Until the doctor has ascertained that return of urinary sphincter control is unlikely, a method that gives only partial protection, such as the use of a bathing cap, is preferable since the patient is more likely to attempt to regain voluntary control.

When cancer of the prostate gland is inoperable, or when signs of metastasis occur following surgery, medical treatment is given. Relief from conservative treatment is quite dramatic in many patients and may last for ten years or more in some instances. Usually the response is quite good for about a year and then the patient's condition begins to deteriorate.

The Huggins treatment may be used for inoperable cancer of the prostate gland to cause atrophy of the local lesion, control metastases, and relieve pain. It is based on the elimination of androgens by removal of the testicles and/or the giving of estrogenic hormones. The estrogen given is usually stilbestrol, 5 mg. ($\frac{1}{12}$ grain) a day for one to two weeks. The dosage is then reduced to 1 mg. $\frac{1}{60}$ grain) a day. This measure frequently will relieve the pain. Stilbestrol causes engorgement and tenderness of the male breasts. It may also cause nausea. Severe side effects should be reported to the doctor so that the dosage or type of estrogenic preparation may be adjusted. If a large tumor does not diminish in size with this treatment, some of the prostate gland may be resected to relieve obstruction. This procedure is most often done transurethrally (p. 463).

When symptoms begin to recur, or if the patient is very uncomfortable and needs immediate relief when the diagnosis of cancer is first made, a *bilateral orchiectomy (castration)* may be done. This operative procedure is technically minor and is often done under local anesthesia, but it may cause the patient considerable psychologic distress. The patient's permission for sterilization must be obtained. If he is married, he is usually urged to discuss the operation with his wife. This surgery eliminates the testicular source of male hormones and seems to cause regression or at least slows the cancer growth. Very occasionally, a hypophysectomy may be done to further reduce hormonal stimulation.

Lesions of the external genitalia

Any lesion of the external genitalia requires medical attention, and no ulcer of the genitalia should be treated by the patient before seeing the doctor lest the diagnosis be obscured. Although lesions are present in a wide variety of conditions, they should always be considered infectious until proved otherwise, since each of the venereal diseases, with the exception of gonorrhea, produces a genital lesion or ulceration. These lesions will be discussed in the section to follow, which deals with the venereal diseases.

Cancer of the penis. Cancer of the penis is far less common than formerly but it still accounts for almost 3% of all cancers in males. Apparently it could be eliminated completely since carcinoma practically never develops in men who have been circumcised as infants. Usually the patient is over 50 years of age, but the condition has developed in men in their twenties. Most often the glans is the site of the initial malignant lesion.

Treatment for carcinoma of the penis is surgery with partial or total amputation of the penis. Removal of adjacent tissues and inguinal lymph nodes may be necessary, and this treatment may be followed by radiation therapy. Occasionally radiation therapy is used before surgery is done. Radiation therapy may be given externally, or needles, seeds, or plaques containing radioactive substances may be used. The physical nursing care is similar to that needed by women who have had a vulvectomy with inguinal node dissection (p. 511). Since the treatment causes such serious changes in a man's total life, the emotional reactions are profound, and very specialized care is needed. For further discussion of the treatment and the nursing care involved, see specialized nursing texts.[50]

Venereal disease

Syphilis and gonorrhea are communicable diseases that affect the reproductive tract primarily. Since the incidence of these diseases is increasing, it is important for the nurse to understand their epidemiology—how they are spread and how they can be controlled.

Syphilis

Development and diagnosis of the disease

Syphilis is caused by the spirochete, *Treponema pallidum*, a delicate spiral-shaped organism that is between a protozoan and a bacterium in form. The spirochete is destroyed by soap and water and by drying and can live only a few hours outside a warm environment such as that provided by the human body. It is transmitted from person to person largely through direct contact and less often by transfer from the mother's blood to that of the unborn child. Live spirochetes can also be transmitted through blood transfusions, although they die after refrigeration for more than three hours.

Syphilis is diagnosed by the observation of live treponemes in the material obtained from an early syphilitic lesion and by tests on blood and spinal fluid when the disease is well established. Blood and spinal fluid tests are of two kinds, but the underlying principle of both is the fact that an antibody-like substance, *reagin*, is present in the blood of the infected person. This reagin reacts with certain prepared cells of animal tissue that are termed *antigens*. If a precipitate is obtained, the test is termed a *flocculation test*, an example of which is the *Mazzini test*. If all complement in the serum is bound by the test, so that none is left to combine with other antibody substances, it is known as a *complement-fixation test*, an example of which is the *Wassermann test*. These tests have a variety of names, having been named after the men who modified and improved them. False positive reactions in the serologic tests occur fairly often, particularly after recent infections or immunization, or in the presence of early collagen disease. A new test, the *treponema-fixation test*, or *Nelson test*, is proving valuable in ruling out false positives in the serologic test for syphilis (often abbreviated S.T.S.).

Syphilis differs from most infectious diseases in its slow progress, its tendency toward chronicity, and its invasion of a large number of organs and body systems. Eventually about one-fourth of those persons infected are crippled or die if the disease remains untreated.[5] The disease is described in stages. *Early syphilis* includes the time during which the initial lesion, or *chancre*, develops at the site of exposure and the time of early spread of the disease throughout the body, when a rash and other secondary lesions may develop and disappear only to reappear at intervals for as long as two years. *Early latent syphilis* refers to the interval of two to four years when body defenses have not yet been fully mobilized and infectious exacerbations may occur. *Late latent syphilis* designates the disease after four years of infection, when reappearance of infectious lesions is unlikely.

Persons who are untreated usually transmit the disease to others through sexual contact during the first three years of infection, although in rare instances it appears that lesions in latent syphilis may also be infectious. It is uncertain how long spirochetes can be carried in the seminal fluid, but there seems to be evidence that untreated persons have transmitted the disease during sexual intercourse as long as ten years after infection. There is no evidence that an infection in the father can in any way affect an unborn child when the mother is not infected. Spirochetes may pass through the placental barrier to the fetal bloodstream at or after the fourth month of fetal life. This transfer occurs in approximately one-half of the instances in which treatment is not given to the expectant mother with active syphilis. Active syphilitic infection in the fetus leads to its death in many instances and to malformations of various kinds, such as saddle nose and interstitial keratitis of the eyes, in many of the infants born alive.

Syphilis is almost always acquired through sexual contact. The spirochetes pass through minute breaks in the mucous membrane and skin, where they begin to multiply within an hour. Within three days the organisms have entered the bloodstream, and at the end of the incubation period of about three weeks (ten days to ten weeks), the initial lesion, or chancre, appears. This lesion, a painless indurated ulcer, is usually found on the genital area but may appear on the lip, in the mouth, or on the nipple. It may develop on the wall of the vagina, on the cervix, or within the male urethra, where it will not be observed by the patient. Adjacent lymph nodes are almost always somewhat tender and enlarged, but these symptoms, together with malaise and headache, may not be recognized as more than a minor indisposition if the chancre is not evident.

While the chancre is present, the serologic blood test is negative because insufficient reagin has been produced to render it positive. The chancre is, however, teaming with live spirochetes, and fluid obtained from the lesion will reveal them easily under a dark-field microscope. It is unfortunate if the patient is given penicillin before this test is done because this antibiotic causes disappearance of the spirochetes within twenty-four hours, and the opportunity to make a definite diagnosis by observation of the living organisms is thus lost. Diagnosis must then be made by means of the serologic test, which must be delayed for a few weeks until sufficient reagin is produced and which is subject to the hazards of false negative reactions, which will cloud the laboratory picture. The patient may then remain inadequately treated and develop complications of latent syphilis.

If not treated, the chancre heals within three to eight weeks. The *secondary* manifestations usually occur immediately after the healing of the chancre, or about six weeks after the initial infection, although they may be delayed for as long as six months and may never appear as a distinct stage. A *rash* resembling that of almost any dermatitis may appear. *Mucous patches* (condyloma lata) may be present in the mouth and on the mucous membrane of the genital area and the perianal skin. These signs may be accompanied by headache, malaise, and sore throat. *Acute iritis* and *retinitis* sometimes occur as secondary metastatic manifestations of the disease, and occasionally there is patchy *loss of hair* (alopecia areata). The disease is highly infectious during the time

when secondary manifestations are present. Lesions on the skin and mucous membrane contain large numbers of spirochetes that are readily transmitted to others; organisms are in the seminal fluid and in the milk of lactating mothers. The serologic test will be positive. The secondary manifestations of early syphilis usually disappear after a few weeks even without treatment, although they have a tendency to recur at intervals.

The late stage of syphilis is divided into late latent (asymptomatic) syphilis and late symptomatic syphilis. About 80% of infected persons are in the late latent group.[40] These individuals are usually discovered to have the disease through routine serologic tests. If undiscovered, they usually live their normal life-span and die of some other cause. The remaining 20%, however, have late symptomatic syphilis and are less fortunate unless treatment is given. The spirochetes attack internal organs by the development of cellular deposits, or *gummas*. The brain, spinal cord, heart, lungs, liver, or bones may be attacked by the organism, and serious damage can result. Gummas seldom contain live spirochetes but are disturbing because they tend to break down and form ulcers or abscesses, which eventually heal spontaneously even when no treatment is given. In the late stage the disease is seldom infectious since the spirochetes have retreated to inaccessible places in the body as body defenses have been further mobilized.

During the chronic stage of syphilis, the heart and blood vessels are often affected. Lesions may develop in the heart muscle or valves, and aneurysms may occur in the large blood vessels, particularly in the aorta. Damage may occur to the central nervous system, causing optic atrophy, tabes dorsalis, and general paresis (p. 885). There may be some racial differences in either vascular or central nervous system diseases, although both complications may occur in either the white or the Negro race. The chronic manifestations may occur as early as a year or two after the initial infection, they may be delayed until as many as twenty years have elapsed, or they may never occur at all.

Treatment

Hospitalization is seldom necessary for persons who have contracted syphilis. The disease is usually treated in the doctor's office, in the hospital clinic or in community clinics, or in homes of patients by doctors and public health nurses. The year 1943 was a revolutionary one in the treatment of syphilis. Before that time the treatment had been tedious and had required weekly injections of arsenicals and other "heavy metal" drugs for twelve to eighteen months and sometimes longer. In 1943 it was shown that penicillin was remarkably effective in treating early infectious and early latent syphilis. The ideal dosage and distribution of dosage have not been conclusively established, but 2,400,000 to 6,000,000 units of penicillin are given in a period of one to three weeks, depending upon the stage of the disease. This dosage is believed to effect a cure in 80% of all patients with early syphilis.

Patients in whom diagnosis is made and treatment started in the early chancre stage never experience the signs and symptoms described for untreated syphilis. It is established almost beyond doubt that biologic cure can be effected by adequate treatment in the early stages of the disease. This means that all living spirochetes within the body are destroyed. Results of treatment have been difficult to analyze because reinfection is possible and is rather frequent in persons treated for early infectious syphilis. Whether or not reinfection is possible in late latent syphilis and whether or not the disease is completely eradicated in this stage have not been determined. The blood and spinal fluid may remain negative for a long time and then become positive even when reinfection has not occurred, although this occurrence is exceedingly rare. Possibly the organisms are harbored somewhere in the body and released at intervals under certain conditions not yet understood.

Incidence, prevalence,
social significance, and control

Syphilis is probably as old as civilization, although the country of its origin is debatable and uncertain. Hand in hand with civilization, it has gone to new lands and taken a heavy toll on peoples whose natural defenses were low. There is evidence that some host resistance is transmitted through generations, since the disease is not so virulent in Western countries as it was centuries ago.

There is, however, no natural immunity to syphilitic infections, and no way to produce an artificial immunity has been found. One infection by the spirochete does not produce an immunity to recurrent disease upon further exposure.

Syphilis has no respect for class or person. The prevalence is higher in the Negro than in the white population, but this is thought to be due to social rather than biologic causes. The disease is more common in men than in women, probably because of greater exposure. The incidence and prevalence of syphilis are increased by war and by frontier migration, both of which take young people away from their homes and lead to increased promiscuity. Since the disease is so often spread by casual sexual encounters, it increases in any situation in which promiscuity is common as, for example, in social and cultural groups in which mores do not require rigid adherence to monogamy and in adolescent groups in unfavorable home and community environments.

With the advent of penicillin in 1943 and the establishment of rapid treatment centers, great strides were made in the control of syphilis. Over the next ten years the very optimistic view developed that syphilis would soon disappear completely. With the closing of rapid treatment centers in 1953, the individual physician and hospital clinics were relied upon to treat infected patients on an ambulatory basis. State and local health departments were to maintain the services of case finding, contact tracing, referral, and treatment for persons unable to pay for private care. A national average of approximately 6,500 cases was maintained until 1958. From 1958 to 1961 reports showed infectious syphilis morbidity rates to have tripled, increasing from 6,600 cases in 1958 to 18,700 in 1961.[40] Since then, further increases have occurred. In 1963 the reported deaths from syphilis were 2,666, and in 1964 114,314 cases were reported.[40]

There are several reasons for the increased incidence of syphilis. Federal funds for venereal disease control measures were decreased. It was assumed that state and local health departments would take over responsibility. These departments, however, began to make budgetary cuts and reduced the numbers of personnel assigned to this work.

Health workers themselves transferred to other fields, believing the disease was well under control. Treatment of patients rested with the individual's voluntary efforts. Medical and nursing schools gave less attention to teaching the diagnosis and treatment of syphilis while efforts in the field of chronic and degenerative diseases overshadowed the needs of what appeared to be a waning problem.

The single factor probably contributing the most to the increase of syphilis has been the general letdown in morals and behavior. Sexual promiscuity, particularly in the younger age groups, has increased, and primarily the large urban areas have been involved in this increase.[40]

Syphilis is not simply an infectious disease caused by spirochetes that responds quickly to the administration of penicillin. It is caused by a social and emotional unhealthiness as well as by spirochetes. Therefore, it has not responded well to methods of mass control that have been effective in other communicable diseases such as typhoid. The disease thrives among emotionally immature persons in poor environments. Incidence is high among young people from broken homes who seek affection, acceptance, love, and security in unsound sexual relationships. These young people attempt to justify or "prove" themselves or try to achieve acceptance by promiscuous sexual behavior. Its incidence is also high among sexual deviates, who are often lonely and out of the common stream of human contacts.

The public's attitude toward syphilis is a major obstacle in its control. Often the immediate assumption is that anyone who has the disease has been guilty of moral wrongdoing. The average person thinks of the method of exposure and not of the complex social and emotional climate that made the disease possible. Actually, syphilis may be contracted congenitally or by an innocent married partner. Fear of detection leads many persons to fail to report symptoms. Lack of education is another obstacle to control. Many young people do not know the symptoms and do not know the dangers of failure to receive treatment. Complete ignorance of the fact that a person under treatment is not infectious leads employers to dismiss workers without reason. This situa-tion seriously militates against efforts to have patients remain under treatment, since many of them are reluctant to ask for time off for treatment lest the nature of their medical problem be discovered.

Several practices in this country help in the detection and control of syphilis. Forty-five states now require that a serologic test for syphilis be made before a marriage license is issued. In some states the law requires that physicians order serologic tests for syphilis for all pregnant women under their care. All approved hospitals and almost all recognized physicians order a serologic test for all antenatal patients and for all persons who give blood for transfusion. Most hospitals require a serologic test for syphilis for all patients admitted for care, and these tests reveal a significant number of persons with the disease. Industrial health services usually incorporate multiphasic screening tests, which almost always include the serologic test for syphilis.

The nurse's role

The nurse's responsibilities include assisting in programs for the prevention of the disease, case finding, assisting with education and treatment of infected persons, interviewing patients for contacts (persons who have been exposed sexually to the patient and who may have the disease also), helping to secure medical care for contacts if necessary, and giving nursing care to patients who have not had adequate treatment and are in advanced stages of the disease.

Before the nurse can be effective in working with patients with syphilis, she must face her own emotional reactions squarely. The patient is often young, fearful of pain, and unaccustomed to his surroundings in the clinic or the doctor's office. Above all, he fears that his family and friends will learn of his predicament and that they will think less of him because of it. He must be certain that information he divulges will be kept in strict confidence, and he should be treated as a patient who has a medical problem and not as one who has sinned. In all contacts with patients who have syphilis, regardless of the circumstances that may unfold, the nurse must refrain from passing moral judgment. The nurse who is successful in working with these patients is the one who can create an atmosphere in which the patient feels free to discuss all aspects of the problem. This need not mean that the nurse accept the patient's standard of conduct for herself but that she show sincere professional concern. She is interested in whether or not the patient is under treatment and in teaching him why he should remain under medical care. Other concerns are who the contacts are, how they may be brought under treatment if necessary, and how the situation may be improved so that events such as those encountered are less likely to recur.

The patient should know that syphilis is a reportable disease and that he, as well as the persons he names as contacts (if they are shown to have the disease), must be reported to the department of health. He should know that numbers instead of names are used in public places such as clinic waiting rooms so that there is little danger of others learning the nature of his disease unless he chooses to tell them. He should recognize the importance of reporting at intervals for checkups as recommended by his doctor, because a few persons either are resistant to the drugs or have only slight resistance to the disease. Serologic tests, made at intervals as specified by the doctor, reveal whether or not a relapse of active infection has occurred.

The nurse should not only reexamine her own attitude toward the disease but should also make use of every opportunity to change the attitude of the public. Group meetings of citizens or patients, association with her less-informed colleagues, and face-to-face relationships with patients all afford opportunities. All young people should know about the disease. In educational programs conducted in venereal disease clinics, patients themselves have stated that they wished they had known more about syphilis at an earlier age. Since good family relationships are so important in preventing syphilis, the nurse should try to help parents to solve their own problems and to prepare their children to be good members of the family and of the community. Premarital counseling, including sex education, is important in the prevention of syphilis. The *Social Hygiene News*,* a

---

*Published by the American Social Hygiene Association.

monthly publication, is helpful in keeping the nurse informed in the field of venereal disease. The dangers of reinfection by spirochetes should be stressed in all health teaching. The effectiveness of penicillin in treatment of syphilis has produced mixed results. It has been a boon in making treatment easier, cheaper, safer, and more convenient and in rendering the patient noninfectious much more quickly than with any other treatment. On the other hand, according to some authorities, treatment has become so simple that patients tend to take the disease too lightly, to believe that they are immune to reinfection, or to believe that they need not worry about reinfection since they can again be easily cured. The incidence of reinfection in patients treated early is quite high, again demonstrating that not only must the spirochete be killed but also that the causes of promiscuity must be controlled if the disease is to disappear. The nurse should participate in community activities designed to improve the environment for young people. For example, better recreational opportunities for teen-agers tend to lessen sexual promiscuity and thus aid in the prevention of syphilis.

Contact investigation. The nurse often interviews the patient and reviews with him his understanding of the disease. Her success in obtaining the names of contacts and in securing the patient's confidence and cooperation in treatment depends largely on her objectivity, her sincerity, and her discretion. With the appropriate outlook and attitude, she is often surprisingly successful in obtaining information that is difficult for the patient to impart to anyone. If the nurse is to win the patient's confidence, she must make him feel that she is concerned about the disease and what it is doing to him as a person and to his associates. The patient should be given the opportunity to inform his contacts of the urgency to seek medical care voluntarily. Many situations in contact investigation become exceedingly complex and difficult (in the case, for instance, of a married patient who has contracted the disease extramaritally). Although the real burden of contact investigation in many clinics rests with the nurse, she may occasionally refer a patient to the social worker, to a community agency, back to his doctor, or to his spiritual adviser, depending upon the particular circumstances.

In contact investigation it is necessary to identify and bring under medical supervision all sexual contacts of the past three months if the patient has a primary lesion, all contacts for the past six months if secondary manifestations are evident, and all contacts for the past year if the patient is in the stage of latent syphilis. In late latent syphilis effort is made to determine the contacts at the time the disease was probably acquired, since such persons may also be suffering from latent syphilis that should be treated in the hope of preventing cardiovascular, neurologic, and other late complications. In latent and congenital syphilis all members of the immediate family should be considered. It is not always necessary to examine the children of the patient, since the likelihood of congenital syphilis may already have been ruled out by routine blood tests done premaritally, upon induction to the armed services, or at the time of a hospital admission. Because the problem of syphilis is such a personal one, most clinics designate one nurse to receive phone calls, make appointments, and provide further information requested by the patient's contacts. This nurse's extension number is also given to the patient for distribution to his contacts in the event he notifies them first. Form letters and individual letters are sent out to patients who fail to report to the clinic as arranged. Telegrams have been effectively used by some clinics and health departments. In the event that contacts fail to report or patients with infectious disease fail to report for follow-up, law requires that the names be submitted to the local health department, which assumes the legal responsibility for the control of communicable disease.

Chronic disease. The nursing care of patients with chronic organic pathology from syphilis is similar to nursing in other conditions except that it is given within the framework of the patient's and his family's guilt feelings about the original cause of his trouble. *Gastric* crisis is one late manifestation that is most distressing to the patient. He has severe abdominal pain and nausea and vomiting. The pathology is in the nervous system, not in the stomach. *Optic atrophy* is sometimes treated by fever therapy, usually induced by giving a foreign protein such as milk intramuscularly or by placing the patient in a fever cabinet. *General paresis* occurs when there has been extensive and permanent damage to the brain. Patients with this condition occupy a large number of beds in mental hospitals throughout the country. Fever therapy and the new drugs, such as chlorpromazine, are of some benefit in controlling violent behavior, but far more important than any kind of treatment is prevention of the original infection and early and complete treatment when it occurs.

Gonorrhea

Gonorrhea is a venereal disease that has been prevalent since ancient times. In the United States it is estimated that 1 million new reportable cases occur each year. It is said that gonorrhea is the most underreported disease of mankind.[40] Many persons are infected several times during their lives since one attack does not confer immunity.

The initial symptom of gonorrhea is burning on urination, occurring usually forty-eight hours after exposure. This symptom is followed by a thick yellowish green discharge from the urethra in men and women and from the vagina in women. Women may also complain of redness and tenderness of the labia and of the vaginal and urethral orifices. Pain on walking and on sitting is common. Diagnosis is made from the history of exposure by sexual contact and by identification of the gonococcus organism in the discharge.

The treatment of gonorrhea consists of the administration of 300,000 units of penicillin daily for three or four days as soon as diagnosis has been made. If the organism is resistant to penicillin, one of the other broad-spectrum antibiotics is used. Usually cultures are taken from the urethra or the vagina daily, and the antibiotic is given until three negative cultures have been obtained. Since organisms can be harbored and cause reinfection, cultures are often taken weekly for three months. If the cultures are negative over this period of time, the patient is considered cured. If treatment with penicillin is begun within a day or two of the onset of symptoms, patients rarely develop the complications, such as epididymitis and salpingitis, that were common before the antibiotics were discovered.

In women the organism may lodge in Skene's glands, on either side of the urethral meatus, or in Bartholin's glands, in the vulvovaginal region. It may then be necessary to dilate the urethra with sounds to facilitate drainage from areas where the organisms have become lodged. The formation of a *Bartholin's gland abscess,* which must be incised and drained, is not unusual in patients who have delayed seeking medical attention (p. 499). It is important that the disease be treated successfully before the onset of the woman patient's next menstrual period because at this time the infection may ascend through the uterus to the fallopian tubes, which may lead to pelvic inflammatory disease and salpingitis with subsequent sterility.

In men the gonococcus may be harbored in the glans penis, causing a *balanitis* which may require surgical drainage and circumcision when the inflammation has subsided. Circumcision of male babies definitely decreases the possibility of local infection of the penis. Infection may travel up the reproductive and urinary tracts, causing urethral strictures, prostatitis, seminal vesiculitis, and epididymitis. The long, tortuous path of the epididymis becomes bound down with adhesions, and the lumen of the duct becomes closed by strictures, resulting in sterility. If urethral strictures occur, the patient has difficulty in voiding and may require periodic dilation of the urethra with sounds. Occasionally an external or internal urethrotomy or a plastic repair of the urethra is necessary.

The doctor emphasizes to the patient that sexual contact must be strictly avoided. Sexual stimulation should also be avoided, since it may produce congestion of blood in the area and increase the discomfort.

Patients with acute gonorrhea are rarely hospitalized. The nurse, however, is responsible for teaching the patient in the hospital clinic, in the doctor's office, or in the home. The patient must be taught to care for himself and to protect himself and others. Anything that comes in contact with discharge, such as bedclothes, washcloths, towels, and underclothing, must be used only by the patient, must be separated from other linen, and must be washed well with soap and hot water. The gonococcus, although it thrives in dark, moist, protected parts of the body, does not long survive sunshine, exposure, drying, and soap and water. The patient should wash his hands thoroughly each time he goes to the bathroom or otherwise contaminates his hands. Women patients usually wear a protective pad. They should not use tampons, which may obstruct free flow of drainage. Men patients occasionally wear an athletic support to protect their clothing.

The greatest care must be taken to protect the eyes from infection. The mucous membrane of the eyes is particularly susceptible, and before the use of penicillin and the sulfonamide drugs, gonorrheal ophthalmia was the cause of much blindness, particularly to newborn infants who were exposed to infection during birth. The patient must be cautioned to wash his hands thoroughly before washing his face and to wash his face under running water.

Very young girls are extremely susceptible to gonorrheal infection of the vagina. They should never be permitted to share the same bed with persons who have the disease and must be carefully protected from exposure when members of their family have gonorrhea.

The patient with gonorrhea should drink large amounts of fluid. This measure helps to "wash out" the organisms and decreases irritation of concentrated urine on the inflamed tissues of the meatus and surrounding area. Hot douches may be ordered for their cleansing effect and to stimulate circulation and therefore stimulate healing. In giving a douche, the nurse usually wears gloves, but the patient, giving her own, should be instructed to rely on careful handling of equipment and thorough washing of her hands. Sitz baths or warm tub baths twice a day or more often may also be ordered for their stimulating effect. The tub should be thoroughly cleansed with hot water and soap and, if at all possible, should not be used by the rest of the family.

The patient must understand the importance of keeping his appointments for medical care. Unfortunately, gonorrhea occurs more commonly in persons who are not always responsible in their conduct. One of the difficulties in the management of this disease is due to its common occurrence among certain groups of people who almost take it for granted. Contracting the disease may even be considered a sign of manhood. The serious results of failure to secure treatment are not too well understood, and the startling success in treatment of gonorrhea by giving penicillin has resulted in overconfidence of patients, particularly since resistance of the organism to penicillin now occurs quite frequently. Some persons have become careless about reporting a fresh exposure since they are so certain of cure when symptoms become troublesome for them. Complications sometimes develop while they are delaying treatment or are ignoring instructions to return to the doctor.

Lesions of the external genitalia

Chancroid. Chancroid is a venereal disease seen in both men and women and is caused by *Ducrey's bacillus.* It is characterized by a raised lesion on the external genitalia one to five days after the contact. This lesion becomes a pustule and then develops into a painful ulcer, with extensive local inflammation and spread. It is treated locally with sulfathiazole powder and systemically with chloramphenicol or chlortetracycline.

Lymphogranuloma venereum (lymphogranuloma inguinale). Lymphogranuloma venereum is a venereal disease caused by an agent intermediate between a virus and a rickettsia carried via the lymph stream. It is believed at this time that a bacterial organism may also be involved in the development of the disease. It is diagnosed by a positive *Frei test* (blood test). At any time from six to sixty days after contact the inguinal nodes in men and the perirectal nodes in women become very swollen and tender, and sometimes ulcerate. These nodes are known as *buboes.* Rectal strictures and fistulas and urethral strictures develop, and superficial painless ulceration may occur also. There may be complete destruction of the bladder or bowel sphincter muscles, with resultant incontinence. If there is interference with lymph channels, elephantiasis, a hard lymphatic swelling of the lower trunk and legs, that completely distorts their size and shape, may also develop and may make walking about impossible. Until the advent of chlortetracycline, which has proved quite effective in treatment, the treatment was unsatisfactory. Some patients also respond to the sulfonamide drugs.

References and selected readings*

1 American Cancer Society, Inc.: A cancer source book for nurses, New York, 1963, American Cancer Society, Inc.

2 American Cancer Society, Inc.: 1966 cancer facts and figures, New York, 1965, American Cancer Society, Inc.

3 Ball, Thomas L.: Gynecologic surgery and urology, ed. 2, St. Louis, 1963, The C. V. Mosby Co.

4 Beacham, Daniel Winston, and Beacham, Woodward Davis: Crossen's synopsis of gynecology, ed. 6, St. Louis, 1963, The C. V. Mosby Co.

5 Beeson, Paul B., and McDermott, Walsh, editors: Cecil-Loeb textbook of medicine, ed. 11, Philadelphia, 1963, W. B. Saunders Co.

6 *Behrman, S. J.: Management of infertility, Am. J. Nursing 66:552-555, March 1966.

7 *Brown, William J.: Venereal disease control, Am. J. Nursing 61:94-96, April 1961.

8 *Bruehl, Frances Sabina, and Lesh, Ruth Ellis: The nurse in the gynecologist's office, Am. J. Nursing 55:187-192, Feb. 1955.

9 *Busse, Geraldine: Promiscuity and venereal disease, Nursing Outlook 4:223-225, April 1956.

10 Campbell, Meredith F., editor: Urology, vols. 1 and 2, Philadelphia, 1963, W. B. Saunders Co.

11 *Cianfrani, Theodore, and Conway, Mary Kate: Ectopic pregnancy, Am. J. Nursing 63:93-95, April 1963.

12 *Clark, Charles Walter: When patients ask you about sex, Am. J. Nursing 53:73-76, Jan. 1953.

13 Copenhaver, Edward H., and Iliya, Fawzi A.: Treatment of urinary stress incontinence—a current appraisal, S. Clin. North America 45:765-773, June 1965.

14 *Cromwell, Gertrude E.: The teenager and venereal disease, Am. J. Nursing 59:1738-1739, Dec. 1959.

15 Davidsohn, Israel, and Wells, Benjamin B.: Todd-Sanford clinical diagnosis by laboratory methods, ed. 13, Philadelphia, 1962, W. B. Saunders Co.

16 *Deschin, Celia S.: VD and the adolescent personality; Taylor, Susan Daggett: Clinic for adolescents with venereal disease, Am. J. Nursing 63:58-66, Nov. 1963.

17 *Eichner, Eduard: Progestins, Am. J. Nursing 65:78-81, Sept. 1965.

18 *Fay, Audrey B.: Dysmenorrhea, Am. J. Nursing 63:77-79, Feb. 1963.

19 Fletcher, E. Colby: Essential urology, ed. 4, Baltimore, 1961, The Williams & Wilkins Co.

*References preceded by an asterisk are particularly well suited for student reading.

20 *Funnell, Joseph W., and Roof, Betsy: Before and after hysterectomy, Am. J. Nursing 64:120-122, Oct. 1964.

21 Garvey, Fred K.: Disease of the genitourinary organs in the male and the urinary organs in the female. In Johnson, Wingate M., editor: The older patient, New York, 1960, Paul B. Hoeber, Inc.

22 Glynn, Robert: Vaginal pH and the effect of douching, Obst. & Gynec. 20:369-372, Sept. 1962.

23 Golub, Leib J.: New exercises for dysmenorrhea, Am. J. Obst. & Gynec. 78:152-155, July 1959.

24 Graham, John B., Sotto, Luciano S., Jr., and Paloucek, Frank P.: Carcinoma of the cervix, Philadelphia, 1962, W. B. Saunders Co.

25 Greenhill, J. P., editor: Office gynecology, ed. 8, Chicago, 1965, The Year Book Medical Publishers, Inc.

26 Greenhill, J. P., editor: The yearbook of obstetrics and gynecology, 1965-1966, Chicago, 1965, The Year Book Medical Publishers, Inc.

27 Harrison, T. R., and others, editors: Principles of internal medicine, ed. 5, New York, 1966, McGraw-Hill Book Co.

28 *Harvard, B. Marvin: Ureteral injuries in routine pelvic surgery, M. Clin. North America 43:1713-1729, Nov. 1959.

29 *Hodgkinson, C. Paul, and Hodari, A. A.: Trocar suprapubic cystostomy for postoperative bladder drainage in the female, Am. J. Obst. & Gynec. 96:773-783, Nov. 15, 1966.

30 *Hofmeister, Frederick J., Reik, Robert P., and Anderson, Nancy Jane: Vulvectomy—surgical treatment and nursing care, Am. J. Nursing 60:666-668, May 1960.

31 Hresachyshyn, M. M.: A critical review of chemotherapy in the treatment of ovarian carcinoma, Clin. Obst. & Gynec. 4:885-890, Sept. 1961.

32 Huffman, John William: Gynecology and obstetrics, Philadelphia, 1962, W. B. Saunders Co.

33 *Iorio, Josephine: Culdoscopy: nursing care, Nursing Outlook 12:35, Sept. 1964.

34 Israel, S. Leon: Mazer and Israel's diagnosis and treatment of menstrual disorders and sterility, ed. 4, New York, 1959, Paul B. Hoeber, Inc.

35 Kasselman, Mary Jo: Nursing care of the patient with benign prostatic hypertrophy, Am. J. Nursing 66:1026-1030, May 1966.

36 Kelso, Joseph W., and Funnel, Joseph W.: Management of gynecologic-urologic complications, Am. J. Obst. & Gynec. 79:856-865, May 1960.

37 *Lammert, Albert C.: The menopause—a physiologic process, Am. J. Nursing 62:56-57, Feb. 1962.

38 Lee, Raymond A., Welch, John S., and Spraitz, Anton F.: Use of posterior culdotomy in pelvic operation, Am. J. Obst. & Gynec. 95:777-780, July 15, 1966.

39 Lefson, Eleanor, Lentz, Josephine, and Gilbertson, Evelyn: Contact interviews and the nurse interviewer, Nursing Outlook 10:728-730, Nov. 1962.

40 *Lentz, John William, and Hall, Madelyn N.: Venereal disease control in the twentieth century, Nursing Outlook 10:722-726, Nov. 1962.

41 *Lewis, George C., Jr., and others: Cancer in situ of the cervix, Am. J. Nursing 64:72-86, April 1964.

42 *Manfredonia, Genevieve: Radiation therapy for cancer of the cervix, Am. J. Nursing 59:513-515, April 1959.

43 Marshall, Minna H., and Caillouette, James C.: Septic abortion, Am. J. Nursing 66:1042-1048, May 1966.

44 *McGowan, Larry: New ideas about patient care before and after vaginal surgery, Am. J. Nursing 64:73-75, Feb. 1964.

45 *Menaker, Jerome S.: When menstruation is painful, Am. J. Nursing 62:94-96, Sept. 1962.

46 *Miller, Norman F., and Avery, Hazel: Gynecology and gynecologic nursing, ed. 5, Philadelphia, 1965, W. B. Saunders Co.

47 *Mossholder, Irene B.: When the patient has a radical retropubic prostatectomy, Am. J. Nursing 62:101-104, July 1962.

48 *Novak, Edmund R.: Benign ovarian tumors, Am. J. Nursing 64:104-109, Nov. 1964.

49 Novak, Edmund R., Jones, Georgeanna Segar, and Jones, Howard W.: Novak's textbook of gynecology, ed. 7, Baltimore, 1965, The Williams & Wilkins Co.

50 *Sawyer, Janet: Nursing care of patients with urologic diseases, St. Louis, 1963, The C. V. Mosby Co.

51 Schima, Marilyn E.: Starting sex instruction for sixth grade boys, Am. J. Nursing 62:75-76, Sept. 1962.

52 *Scott, Roger B.: Common problems in geriatric gynecology, Am. J. Nursing 58:1275-1277, Sept. 1958.

53 Sheets, Joseph L., Symmonds, Richard E., and Banner, Edward A.: Conservative surgical management of endometriosis, Obst. & Gynec. 23:625-628, April 1964.

54 *Stewart, Muriel J.: Testing home tests for cervical cancer, Am. J. Nursing 65:75-76, Dec. 1965.

55 Stone, Martin L., and Weingold, Allan B.: Cancer of the ovary, Hosp. Med. 1:33-38, Sept. 1965.

56 Sturgis, Somers H.: Treatment of ovarian insufficiency, Am. J. Nursing 64:113-116, Jan. 1964.

57 Taylor, E. Stewart: Beck's obstetrical practice, ed. 8, Baltimore, 1966, The Williams & Wilkins Co.

58 Taylor, E. Stewart: Essentials of gynecology, ed. 3, Philadelphia, 1965, Lea & Febiger.

59 *TeLinde, Richard W.: Operative gynecology, ed. 3, Philadelphia, 1962, J. B. Lippincott Co.

60 Titchener, James L., and others: Problem of delay in seeking surgical care, J.A.M.A. 160:1187-1193, April 7, 1956.

61 Top, Franklin H.: Communicable and infectious diseases, ed. 5, St. Louis, 1964, The C. V. Mosby Co.

62 U. S. Department of Health, Education, and Welfare: Morbidity and mortality, annual supplement, 1964, Sept. 30, 1965.

63 *Valk, William L., and Foret, John D.: The problem of vesicovaginal and ureterovaginal fistulas, M. Clin. North America 43:1769-1777, Nov. 1959.

64 World almanac and book of facts for 1965, New York, 1965, New York World-Telegram & The Sun.

65 Youmans, John B., and others: Symposium on syphilis and other venereal diseases, M. Clin. North America 48:571-814, May 1964.

21

The patient
with
pulmonary disease

Study questions

1 Review the anatomy and physiology of the lungs and diaphragm. How does lack of function in the diaphragm affect respiration?
2 Which muscles can be used as accessory muscles in breathing? What is meant by residual air?
3 Explain the exchange of oxygen and carbon dioxide in normal respiration. What is the normal respiratory rate? What is the normal carbon dioxide level in the bloodstream? How does carbon dioxide content affect respiration and general body function? What is meant by the hypoxic stimulus to the respiratory center?
4 Review the drugs that facilitate the raising of sputum.
5 How many diseases can you name that begin with symptoms of the common cold?

There are numerous diseases that may affect the respiratory system. They include both acute (short-term) and chronic (long-term) diseases, and some are communicable. The most significant pulmonary diseases are those that are chronic. According to the National Health Survey reports for July, 1963, to June, 1965, approximately 30 million people in the United States had asthma, chronic bronchitis, or other chronic respiratory conditions, including emphysema.[18] Because many acute and chronic pulmonary diseases are preventable, at least to some extent, the nurse should know what causes them to develop and how they are spread, as well as the care needed by the patient when the disease is far advanced.

Since most diseases of the respiratory tract are not reportable, the full extent of both acute and chronic illness is difficult to estimate. However, known facts about disability caused by chronic respiratory diseases indicate clearly that they are a serious health problem and cause tremendous loss in the nation's productivity. Disability benefits as reported by the Social Security Administration show that emphysema is the second most frequent single condition for which disability claims are made. The annual payment of disability benefits for emphysema alone is estimated at 80 million dollars.

The objectives of health education in relation to pulmonary diseases are the same as for other diseases. Prevention, early diagnosis, prompt and often continued treatment, limitation of disability, and rehabilitation should be emphasized for all persons. Early symptoms of respiratory diseases are probably those most often ignored by the general population. Perhaps this is because, with the exception of influenza and some types of pneumonia such as that caused by Friedländer's bacillus, respiratory diseases often develop slowly and progress without the individual's awareness. Nurses should encourage individuals and families to get proper medical attention if they have symptoms such as cough, difficulty in breathing, production of sputum, shortness of breath, and nose and throat irritation that does not subside within two weeks. These symptoms are suggestive of respiratory disease and should be investigated.

With increased study and new knowledge about the respiratory diseases, the methods of treating patients with these diseases is changing rapidly. The American Thoracic Society, the medical section of the National Tuberculosis Association, publishes a journal* that is an excellent source of current information on all acute and chronic respiratory diseases. The National Tuberculosis Association also publishes the *Bulletin*, many booklets and pamphlets, and newsletters that are useful to nurses in education of the public and in teaching patients.

Diagnostic examinations and related nursing care

X-ray examination of the chest

X-ray examination is probably familiar to most patients and the general public. Roentgenography has had very wide use as a screening test, and as a diagnostic measure. When chest disease is suspected, a roentgenogram is almost always ordered to help identify the disease and to visualize its effects and the extent of the disease process. Various types of roentgenograms may be ordered. For survey purposes a *microfilm* may

---

*American Review of Respiratory Diseases, published by the National Tuberculosis Association, New York, N. Y.

be used. If this small plate indicates any abnormality, a large plate is made. A large x-ray plate may be called an AP (anteroposterior view). *Lateral* views may be ordered. *Stereoscopic* roentgenograms may be made because they give a three-dimensional (depth) view. When carcinoma is suspected, *tomography* may be ordered. A tomogram is a roentgenogram of a layer of tissue at any depth. A series of tomograms are made in such a way as to give depth views of various sections of the lung.

If the patient is acutely ill, a portable x-ray machine may be brought to his bedside, and the nurse assists the patient into correct position and protects him from exposure. If oxygen is being used, it must be discontinued because of the danger of its igniting. The x-ray plate is covered and then placed flat on the bed. If the patient can sit up, the plate is put in place, he leans back on it, and the bed is lowered as far as can be tolerated. If he is unable to sit up, he is turned on his side, the plate is correctly placed on the bed, and he is rolled onto it.

If the patient is ambulatory or well enough to be moved, he is taken to the x-ray department in a wheelchair or on a stretcher for the procedure. He must always be accompanied, and the nurse should be certain that he is wearing an open-backed gown and has removed or will remove from his person or his gown all metal above the waist, since metal restricts the passage of the x-rays and will cause a shadow on the film. Care should be taken that such articles are not misplaced or lost.

Fluoroscopic examination

Frequently the physician will do a fluoroscopic examination of the patient's chest prior to taking the roentgenogram. Fluoroscopy helps the doctor to evaluate pulmonary function. He can observe what muscles are being used, estimate the adequacy of ventilation and the uniformity of the distribution of air, and often locate the sites of pulmonary diseases. Air trapped in the lungs is easily seen under the fluoroscope. The contours and action of the diaphragm can be observed as well as rib movement, width of interspaces, and size and contour of the heart.

Whether fluoroscopic examination is done

in the doctor's office or in the hospital, the patient must go to a room where the fluoroscope is installed. He may need assistance in rising to a sitting position or in remaining still during the examination. If he is in a wheelchair, he is assisted to a stool in front of the machine. The doctor wears an apron and gloves containing lead to protect him from the x-rays, and he uses plastic goggles to aid his adaptation to the dark. Fluoroscopic examination is done with the lights off, and the doctor operates the machine with a foot pedal. The patient needs a careful explanation of the procedure and should be told that he will be in darkness, and that he may be asked to hold his breath for a few seconds during the examination. He should be assured that there will be no pain.

Examination of sputum

Examinations of sputum are usually required when chest disease is suspected. The mucous membrane of the respiratory tract responds to inflammation by an increased flow of secretions that often contain the offending organisms. Microscopic examination of a *smear of the sputum* often gives useful information in diagnosis. A *culture of the sputum* may be ordered also. Suitable growth media are inoculated with the sputum. Growth on media of the same organism as that identified on microscopic smears will help confirm a diagnosis. The sputum may be examined for carcinoma cells by using the Papanicolaou technique. It may also be examined grossly for color, consistency, and special constituents. Clear mucoid "currant jelly" sputum is indicative of possible carcinoma of the lung. Purulent blood-streaked sputum has long been considered suggestive of tuberculosis. Thick tenacious sputum containing casts of bronchioles is often found in asthmatic bronchitis.

Tests to be done on sputum should be explained to the patient so that he will understand the need for obtaining a suitable specimen. He should be instructed to collect only sputum that has come from deep in the chest. When instructed inadequately, patients often expectorate saliva rather than sputum. They are likely to exhaust themselves unnecessarily by shallow, frequent coughing that yields no sputum suitable for study and that affords them little relief from

discomfort. The first sputum raised in the morning is usually the most productive of organisms. During the night, secretions accumulate in the bronchi, and only a few deep coughs will bring them to the back of the throat. If the patient does not know this fact, upon awakening he may almost unconsciously cough, clear his throat, and swallow or expectorate before attempting to procure a specimen.

The patient should be supplied with a widemouthed bottle or jar and instructed to expectorate directly into the bottle. Since the sight of sputum is often objectionable to the patient, and particularly to persons about him, the outside of the container should be covered with paper or other suitable covering. To prevent the possibility of contamination of the air with organisms in the sputum, a screw-top or tight-fitting lid should be kept over the top of the container. Usually 4 ml. of sputum are sufficient for necessary laboratory tests and examinations. Occasionally, however, all sputum collected over a period of twenty-four to thirty-six hours is needed. If there is any delay in sending the specimen to the laboratory, it should be placed in the refrigerator.

Sputum collection using saline inhalation. Inhalation of a heated saline solution is being used to help patients raise sputum for specimens. A 10% solution of saline in distilled water is placed in a heated nebulizer, and a fine spray is produced by attaching the nebulizer to compressed air or oxygen. When inhaled, the heated vapor condenses on the surface of the tracheobronchial mucosa and stimulates production of secretions.

Patients who have difficulty raising sputum for specimens can learn this procedure readily. The patient needs careful instruction in coughing deeply before starting the inhalation. He should be seated in front of the nebulizer before starting preparations for inhalation. He should be taught to take about four deep breaths. The first two times he should inhale deeply and expel the air slowly. The third time he should inhale deeply and forcefully blow the air out through his mouth. The fourth time, he should inhale quickly and cough. As he finishes the preparatory breathing and cough, he should place his mouth over the mouthpiece of the nebulizer and inhale. Inhalation of the vapor should be repeated for a few minutes or until coughing is stimulated. Some patients begin to cough after the first inhalation. The patient should have a supply of tissues in his hand to cover the cough and should expectorate the sputum into the collection container.

The patient should be asked to rest for a few seconds between periods of inhaling and coughing so that he does not become overtired. If the patient complains of lightheadedness or dizziness, he should be encouraged to sit quietly and to breathe normally for a few minutes. If he complains of nausea, the inhalations should not be continued. The patient usually feels nauseated for only a few minutes, and it may be associated with factors other than the inhalation. The advantage of this method of raising sputum is that the patient can do the procedure at any time of the day and needs no special preparation. Many hospitals and outpatient facilities are now using this method in preference to gastric lavage.

If the patient has suspected tuberculosis and specimens are being collected for screening purposes, the hospital or outpatient personnel should use some precautions. The room should be well ventilated so that there are frequent changes of air. If the patient is known to have sputum positive for tubercle bacilli, the extra precaution of wearing a mask may be taken. Special ultraviolet lights may be installed to rid the rising circulating air of infectious droplets. They are installed high enough to protect the patient and the personnel from direct exposure to the light.

Gastric washings. A gastric aspiration may occasionally be done to collect sputum. Since most patients swallow sputum when coughing in the morning and during sleep, an examination of gastric contents may reveal causative organisms. Breakfast is withheld for gastric aspiration. (The procedure for passing the nasogastric tube is the same as that discussed on p. 637.) Once the tube is passed, a large syringe is attached to the end, and by gentle suction a specimen of stomach contents is withdrawn. The specimen is placed in a covered bottle, and the tube is withdrawn. The specimen is examined microscopically on slides, and culture media are inoculated as is done with other sputum samples. For the patient the disad-

vantages of this method of sputum collection are the discomforts of going without food and the passage of the nasogastric tube.

Pulmonary function tests

Pulmonary function tests are done to assess lung function, to rule out nonorganic types of dyspnea such as that caused by psychoneurotic disorders, and to differentiate diseases of the lungs. They also may be used to evaluate the disability caused by diseases of the lungs. Localized disease of the lung such as carcinoma, tuberculosis, or lung abscess may have little effect on pulmonary function, whereas generalized disease such as emphysema or fibrosis may produce a significant alteration of pulmonary function.

The physiologic tests of pulmonary function are of two general kinds. One tests the bellows action of the chest and lungs for movement of air in and out of the alveoli (ventilation) and the distribution of inspired gas to the alveoli. The second is concerned with the *diffusion* of a gas across the alveolar capillary membrane to and from the blood *perfusing* the pulmonary capillaries of the lungs. The nurse should be familiar with the tests that are more commonly used so that she can explain them to the patient and tell him how he may help to achieve successful tests.

Measurement of pulmonary volumes and capacities. To determine the functional capacity of the lungs, vital capacity, timed vital capacity, tidal volume, and residual volume tests may be ordered. A *tidal volume test* measures the gas inspired and expired with each normal breath. A *vital capacity test* measures the maximal amount of air that can be exhaled after maximal inhalation. The vital capacity can be timed for 0.5 second to 3 seconds, and by reviewing the tracings, the physician can determine if there is delayed expiration. A *residual volume test* measures the gas remaining in the lungs at the end of a normal expiration. The *total lung capacity* is the sum of the vital capacity and the residual volume. On the basis of these few simple tests the physician begins to differentiate the type of pulmonary functional impairment the patient may have. There are numerous tests and techniques of studying pulmonary function that have been developed, and they may be found in specialized texts.

The patient is usually instructed how to participate in the tests by the physician or the technician in the testing laboratory. For all these tests the patient is asked to breathe only through his mouth. A recording device and a spirometer are used. When the patient breathes through the mouthpiece and connecting tube, the action of the spirometer is recorded on a revolving drum. A noseclip is usually used so that the patient cannot breathe through his nose. Although a noseclip may seem like a small, harmless piece of equipment, the patient often becomes apprehensive about it. He should be allowed time to adjust to the clip. Fear of cutting off the air supply, particularly when a person has a breathing limitation, may cause anxiety. Nurses can allay some of the patient's apprehension by giving him clear and confident explanations.

Bronchospirometry. Bronchospirometry measures both the ventilatory efficiency and the oxygen-absorptive function of the lungs. It gives an accurate determination of the degree of respiratory impairment. For this test a double-lumen catheter may be introduced into the trachea (see discussion of bronchogram for care of the patient, p. 538). A noseclip is used, and air is inhaled or exhaled through the tracheal catheter, which is attached to a device that measures both the amount of air inhaled and the amount of air exhaled. Samples of arterial blood are taken to determine the arterial oxygen and carbon dioxide tensions. This test is usually done in a special laboratory.

The patient may have many pulmonary function tests performed in the cardiopulmonary laboratory in the same day. He may become exhausted not only because of his chest condition and breathing difficulties but as a result of having to lie still so long, listening to the staff give each other directions, being exposed to noise and lights, and being under so much tension. The nurse should try to make him as comfortable as possible. Personal hygiene needs should be taken care of immediately to make him physically more comfortable.

Bronchography and bronchoscopy

Examinations by bronchography and bronchoscopy are somewhat complicated diagnostic procedures that may be ordered. Both procedures are unpleasant and uncomfortable for the patient. A thorough explanation of what will happen and what will be expected of him during these examinations can do much to allay his anxiety. Since instruments are passed through the mouth and pharynx, making the patient apprehensive about being able to breathe, he should practice breathing in and out through the nose with the mouth open. He can also practice consciously relaxing the shoulders and hands while lying on his back. Clenching the fists causes the neck muscles to tense, interfering with the procedure. If the patient is to have a bronchoscopic examination, he should know that the room lights will be off, that his eyes will be covered, and that a mask and gloves will be used by the doctor and his assistants.

A *bronchogram* enables the doctor to visualize the bronchial tree by x-ray film after the introduction of a radiopaque liquid such as Dionosil. To lessen the number of bacteria introduced from the mouth into the bronchi, the patient should pay particular attention to oral hygiene on the night before and on the morning of the procedure. No food or fluids are allowed for eight hours preceding the examination. Since, if the smaller bronchi contain secretions, the radiopaque liquid will not reach them, postural drainage may be ordered for the morning the bronchogram is made. Usually the patient remains in postural-drainage position for about fifteen minutes, and he should breathe deeply and cough. Mouth care should follow. The patient should be asked about any loose or capped teeth or dental bridges. Dental prostheses should be removed, and loose teeth should be brought to the doctor's attention.

Approximately one hour before the injection of the radiopaque substance, the patient is given a mild sedative such as Seconal to relax him and to counteract the effect of the tetracaine (Pontocaine) or cocaine used for local anesthesia. Usually 0.5% Pontocaine or cocaine is used. The doctor anesthetizes the pharynx, larynx, and major bronchi immediately before the radiopaque substance is introduced. The patient should be told that the local anesthetic will taste bitter and that he should not swallow it but expectorate into the emesis basin or tissues

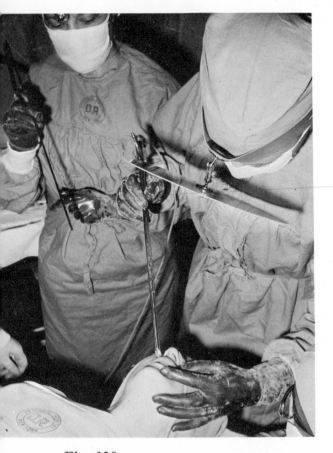

Fig. 126

Patient having a bronchoscopy. Note position
of head and neck. The nurse is prepared
to aspirate after the bronchoscope is passed.
(From Horowicz, Clara: Am. J. Nursing **63**:107,
May 1963.)

provided. When the gag reflex disappears,
a metal laryngeal cannula is passed into the
trachea, and then a catheter is passed
through the nose into the cannula and into
the trachea. The radiopaque substance is
then introduced, and the patient is tilted into
various positions to distribute it to the
bronchi and bronchioles. A series of roentgenograms is then taken. Following this
procedure, postural drainage is usually ordered to help remove the radiopaque substance from the lungs. No permanent damage results, however, if some of it remains
for an indefinite period. Food and fluid

should be withheld until the gag reflex
returns, which can be tested by gently
tickling the posterior pharynx with a cotton
swab.

A *bronchoscopic examination* is performed
by passing a bronchoscope into the trachea
and bronchi (Fig. 126). Preparation of the
patient for a bronchoscopic examination is
similar to that for bronchography except
that postural drainage is less often ordered.
In addition to a spray anesthetic, cocaine
may be applied locally by holding small cotton pledgets soaked in solution in the posterior fossa of the pharynx. If the patient is
very apprehensive or if a sponge biopsy
(abrasion of the lesion with a sponge) is to
be done or a tissue biopsy obtained, intravenous anesthesia may be used. The bronchoscope is a long, slender, hollow instrument through which light can be reflected
and visual examination of the trachea and
major bronchi with their branchings can be
made. Bronchoscopy may be done to remove a foreign body, to facilitate free air
passage by removal of mucus plugs with suction, to obtain a biopsy and samples of secretions for examination, and to observe the air
passages for signs of disease.

Following bronchoscopy, the patient is
given no food or fluids until the gag reflex returns. Some doctors prefer that the
patient lie flat after this procedure, while
others prefer a semi-Fowler's position. Unless intravenous anesthesia is used, the patient is awake and conscious although
rather drowsy from the sedation. Rather
than attempt to swallow saliva, he should
lie on his side and let mucus from the mouth
flow into disposable tissues or a small emesis
basin conveniently placed. He should be
urged to lie quietly and not try to talk,
cough, or clear his throat since these activities only increase the secretions and the desire to clear the throat. A pencil and a piece
of paper should be at the bedside so that he
can write if he needs to communicate. He
should have his call light within easy reach,
and he should be instructed to signal for the
nurse if he feels uncomfortable. Occasionally, severe laryngeal edema follows this
procedure causing respiratory embarrassment and perhaps even necessitating a
tracheotomy.

The patient may be hoarse and have a

sore throat for several days following a bronchoscopy. Warm fluids by mouth may relieve the soreness, and sometimes warm gargles are ordered. If the discomfort is severe, acetylsalicylic acid, 0.3 Gm. (5 grains), may be dissolved in the mouth and then swallowed. Inhalation of warm, moist steam may also be prescribed.

If a biopsy is taken during bronchoscopy, the patient is kept under close surveillance until clotting occurs—usually five to seven minutes. His sputum should be observed carefully for a few hours after the procedure for signs of hemorrhage. The patient should not smoke for several hours because smoking may cause coughing and start bleeding. Although normally the sputum may be streaked with blood for a few days after a biopsy has been taken, any more pronounced bleeding must be reported at once to the doctor.

Acute respiratory diseases

Viral infections

Viral infection is exceedingly prevalent. There are now over seventy viruses recognizable in man, and many of them cause respiratory disease.[29] Some diseases may be caused by one virus, or different viruses may cause the same symptoms.

If specific signs are not evident, the clinical illness is termed a common cold, viral infection, fever of unknown origin, acute respiratory illness, or the grippe. The most common specific respiratory illnesses caused by the various viruses are epidemic pleurodynia (Bornholm's disease), acute laryngotracheobronchitis, viral pneumonia, and influenza. Most adults have developed antibodies for the more common viruses, and most viral infections are relatively mild. However, they are frequently complicated by secondary bacterial infections. When new strains of the Asian flu virus develop, severe epidemics may ensue, and many people may die from secondary infections such as pneumonia.

The common cold

Few persons escape having a "cold." The general population averages three colds per person each year.[4] The frequency of their occurrence, the numbers of people affected, the resulting economic loss, and the possibility that a cold may lead to more serious disease are reasons why colds merit serious attention.

Since persons with colds are rarely hospitalized, the nurse will encounter them at work, in public places, or in their homes. It is important for her to note the symptoms at the onset of the cold. Many other more serious diseases begin with a cold or with symptoms resembling those of the common cold. Because a cold is considered a minor but bothersome condition and because the patient has possibly had many colds, he, rather than a physician, makes the diagnosis. Helping persons to realize the importance of an illness that may appear slight but that may have serious consequences is an integral part of nursing.

The common cold is caused by a filtrable virus, and it is spread rapidly, easily, and directly by droplet infection. Symptoms of a cold usually appear suddenly, and the infection may be full-blown within forty-eight hours. The acute inflammation usually begins in the pharynx, and there is a sensation of dryness or soreness of the throat. This is followed by nasal congestion with a thin, watery, profuse discharge and frequent sneezing. The eyes may water, the voice may become husky, breathing may be obstructed, and sense of smell and taste may diminish. Often a cough develops, and it may become productive of sputum.

The patient with a cold may have various complaints. At times he may feel lethargic and have vague, aching pains in the back and limbs. Most adults are afebrile, but those with a tendency toward developing complications, such as persons with chronic illness and low resistance, may have a temperature elevation. The course of the cold is variable, but ordinarily it lasts from seven to fourteen days. It is difficult to determine when the cold ends and when complications appear. Laryngitis and tracheitis may be part of the cold. Tracheobronchitis is a complication usually due to secondary bacterial infection. Acute sinusitis and otitis media may follow the common cold.

Prevention. There is no known way to prevent the common cold, and there is no specific treatment. However, there are measures that help to prevent the development of a cold, complications, and transfer to other persons. Attention to good general hygiene, with plenty of rest, and adequate diet, and sufficient exercise and fresh air presumably help to maintain resistance to colds. The nurse should teach that the patient can go through the usual course of a common cold without difficulty if he obtains enough rest.

The nurse should emphasize to the patient with a cold the importance of avoiding spread of his cold. Crowded places, such as the theater, should be avoided by persons with colds. The patient should particularly avoid coming into contact with and therefore exposing infants and young children, persons who have chronic chest disease such as bronchiectasis, those who have recently had an anesthetic, and elderly people. He should remember to cover his nose and mouth when sneezing, coughing, and clearing his throat. Frequent washing of hands, covering of coughs and sneezes, and careful disposal of waste tissues are protective health measures that are advisable for everyone in everyday life, but they become increasingly important when known respiratory infection exists. Since the common cold is a communicable disease, the principles of protection of oneself, as well as the ways in which a cold can be transferred to others, should be remembered.

Treatment. All treatment of colds is directed toward relief of symptoms and control of complications. If the patient has an elevated temperature and complains of headache and muscular aching, he should seek the advice of a physician. Acetylsalicylic acid may be prescribed for mild aches and discomfort. Salicylates, however, do not influence the course of the common cold and lack specific action in this disorder.

If the patient has *nasal congestion,* the physician may recommend nose drops. Ephedrine, 0.5 to 2% aqueous solution, with isotonic sodium chloride solution is used frequently. (See p. 588 for method of administration.) This medication shrinks swollen nasal tissues and allows for the free passage of air. Many physicians advise against the use of nose drops, maintaining that constriction of blood supply to the tissues lowers resistance. In general, oily solutions are not recommended because of the danger of the inhalation of oil droplets, which might cause lipid pneumonia. Nasal sprays containing antihistamine may be ordered. They should be given with the patient sitting upright. The nurse should emphasize to patients and their families the importance of using only prescribed solutions and only those that are fresh. Nose drops should be prescribed by a doctor, and only the specified amount should be used; excessive use may only aggravate symptoms. Many persons prefer a medicated nasal inhaler since it can be carried easily in a pocket and is more pleasant to use. Benzedrex containing propylhexedrine is an example of one that is widely used. Propylhexedrine is a volatile drug with minimum stimulating effect on the central nervous system.[5] Soft disposable paper tissues or old, soft cotton handkerchiefs should be used to help prevent dryness, redness, and irritation about the nose. Some dryness can be prevented by treating the skin early in the cold with mild soothing creams, such as cold cream.

The *dryness, cough,* and *"tickling sensation"* in the throat so often associated with a cold can be relieved in a variety of ways. There are many cough drops and lozenges on the market. Lozenges relieve irritation and are pleasant to use. Patients should be advised not to use them just before dozing off to sleep since they may be accidentally aspirated into the trachea during sleep. A mixture of honey and lemon may be preferred to cough medications by some patients. This mixture increases mucus secretions and thereby softens exudate and facilitates its expectoration. It also relieves the dryness that predisposes to coughing. Some people report that undiluted lemon or orange juice is helpful. A section of the fruit with the rind may be placed at the bedside for easy accessibility during the night. Hot fluids often relieve coughing. The patient may be advised to keep a small vacuum bottle of hot water or other liquid at the bedside. If cough medication has been taken, it should not be followed by water because the effect will be dissipated. Patients should keep prescribed cough medications within reach to avoid chilling from getting out of bed during the night. If the cough associated with a common cold persists or does not yield to the simple home remedies mentioned or to specific medication that may have been ordered, the patient should be urged to report to his doctor.

Pneumonia

Pneumonia can occur in any season, but it is most common during the winter and early spring. Persons of any age are susceptible. However, those with lowered resistance are most often affected. The use of anesthetics and of large doses of morphine may be contributing causes since they slow reflex action of the epiglottis, permitting aspiration of infected secretions from the upper respiratory tract. Chilling and exposure may permit organisms already present to become active. Alcoholics are particularly susceptible to pneumonia because of general malnutrition, frequent exposure to cold, and poor general health practices. Elderly persons are susceptible to pneumonia because of the slowing of reflex action of the epiglottis and because of limited expansion of the rib cage and poor aeration of the lungs. Organisms such as pneumococci in the nasopharyngeal secretions may be carried to the distant bronchioles and to the alveoli, where they may cause an acute inflammation. Accumulation of fluid in the alveoli caused by such conditions as cardiac failure, viral infection of the lungs, trauma to the thorax, or pulmonary stasis resulting from prolonged bed rest in the same position provides an ideal medium for the growth of bacteria. Pneumonia is also a communicable respiratory illness, and it may be spread directly from person to person by droplet infection. The pneumococcus causes 95% of all primary pneumonia of bacterial origin.[4] Other bacterial causes of the disease are Friedländer's bacillus, tubercle bacillus, and streptococcus.

The *staphylococcus organism* is being seen more often than previously as a cause of pneumonia particularly among debilitated hospitalized patients with such illnesses as collagen disease, leukemia, and chronic liver disease. The sudden or insidious onset of marked elevation of temperature, increase in pulse and respiration rate, and aching pain and dry cough in the debilitated hospital patient are evidences that staphylococcal pneumonia may be developing.[25] The incidence is higher among patients who have been receiving antibiotic treatment.[25]

Prevention. Pneumonia can often be prevented in susceptible patients by careful nursing care. Preoperative and postoperative patients, those receiving heavy sedation for any reason, alcoholics, elderly patients, chronically ill patients, those with gross limitation of movement, and those with difficulty in swallowing need frequent mouth care to help reduce the number of bacteria in the mouth. Frequent turning or help in changing position will lessen the possibility of stasis. Prompt suctioning of secretions in patients who cannot cough and expectorate secretions forcibly will reduce the chances of aspiration and accumulation of fluid in the lungs. These patients will need special attention when they are being given medication, food, or drink by mouth. An apprehensive patient with swallowing difficulties needs time to learn to swallow with expiration. He needs constant encouragement in his efforts to relax and continue his efforts to swallow safely.

Staphylococcal pneumonia in the hospitalized patient may sometimes be prevented by employing at least partial medical isolation technique or asepsis. The debilitated patient should, ideally, never be placed on the same unit as any patient suffering from a staphylococcal infection of any kind. Wearing an isolation gown over the uniform when giving direct care to the patient gives a little protection and is sometimes the practice. The utmost care should be taken by the nurse to wash her hands thoroughly before doing anything for the patient and after caring for any other patient.

Medical treatment and nursing care. The patient with pneumonia has a temperature elevation and may have shaking chills and a cough. Thick, purulent sputum is common in staphylococcal pneumonia. Increased temperature and pulse are indications that body defenses are mobilized into action, and additional strain on the body will be detrimental. Bed rest is a "must." The nurse can help to assure adequate rest for the patient by helping him with personal hygiene, keeping the environment generally quiet, allaying

541

fears and apprehension, and arranging for regular rest periods during the day. If the disease is severe, the patient should move only enough to maintain good general circulation. Sometimes passive exercises are prescribed by the doctor. The patient should be told that he must not try to help. Otherwise he may feel impelled to move when he does not have energy to expend in this way.

When the temperature is elevated, both fluids and salt are lost. Fluids are encouraged and additional salt may be given either in food or in intravenous fluids. If the patient is nauseated or otherwise unable to take sufficient fluids by mouth, infusions may be given. If the patient's temperature becomes extremely high, hypothermia may be used (p. 188).

Since the treatment and prognosis of pneumonia depend upon the causative organism, the sputum is examined for type of organism, and cultures are grown. A sputum specimen for examination should be obtained *before* administration of the drug is started, and it is a nursing responsibility to help obtain this specimen as quickly as possible.

Pneumonia is now classified according to the offending organism rather than the anatomic location (lobar or bronchial), as was previously the practice. The type of organism determines the drug or drugs that are given. Medications must be carefully given as ordered to ensure that the amount necessary to combat the infection is present in the bloodstream. The patient should be observed carefully for any untoward reaction to the drug he is receiving, and such a reaction should be reported to the doctor at once.

If antimicrobial therapy can be instituted promptly, the temperature drops markedly in twenty-four hours, the pulse rate may become normal, and the patient may feel generally much better. When the temperature falls, the patient usually perspires profusely. He should be kept warm and protected from drafts. Clothing that becomes damp with perspiration should be changed at once. The patient should be observed closely for "pseudocrisis." In this condition the temperature falls but the pulse remains elevated and the patient's general condi-

tion does not improve. The lowered temperature indicates failure of the body's resources to meet the threat of bacterial infection in an adequate way.

Because of high temperature, dehydration, and mouth breathing, the patient needs frequent mouth care. Maintenance of cleanliness of the mouth may also inhibit extension of infection to the ears. Herpetic blisters about the mouth are common and are a source of much discomfort to the patient. Tincture of benzoin can be applied, and sometimes camphor ice is beneficial. Cold cream can be used to soften the crusted areas. If the nostrils are dry or are crusted with exudate, swabs moistened with water or hydrogen peroxide can be used, and cold cream can be applied to the external nares.

Chest pain in pneumonia is caused by inflammation of the pleura and usually is confined to the affected side. Involvement of the pleura and empyema often complicate staphylococcal pneumonia.[4,25] Pain may be severe and stabbing in nature and may be exaggerated by coughing and by deep breathing. Respirations are often described as "grunting." Close observation of the chest may show that there is limitation of movement of the affected side. The patient may use accessory muscles to aid in breathing instead of expanding the lower chest fully. The patient with severe chest pain usually needs help and encouragement in changing his position at intervals. Lying on the affected side may relieve the pain since this position helps to splint the painful side of the chest. Raising the head of the bed will often make it easier for the patient to breathe, but he may need pillows to support the arms, since otherwise the weight of the arms dropping forward puts a strain on the shoulder girdle and increases fatigue. Oxygen is often used for the patient who has severe chest pain and difficulty in breathing adequately since the higher concentration of oxygen makes deep breathing less necessary for obtaining an adequate supply of oxygen. (For care of the patient receiving oxygen, see texts on fundamentals of nursing.) Occasionally pain is severe enough to require regional block of the intercostal nerves (p. 185). If narcotics are used, codeine is usually the drug prescribed since it is less likely to inhibit productive coughing than the stronger narcotic drugs.

Severe cough and blood-tinged, or "rusty," sputum are characteristic of pneumonia. The patient must be encouraged and helped to cough deeply to produce sputum from the lungs and not expend needed energy in raising secretions from the upper trachea and posterior pharynx only. The nurse can help the patient to cough without too much pain by giving prescribed medications and by helping to splint the chest as the patient coughs.

In severe pneumonia, peristaltic action may be decreased. The nurse should report failure to have a bowel movement and any distention, rigidity, or tenderness in the upper abdominal quadrant, since these conditions are signs of paralytic ileus (p. 207). If peristalsis becomes suppressed or absent, there is respiratory distress due to elevation of the diaphragm by the accumulation of gas and fluid in the gastrointestinal tract, and vomiting may occur. Enemas are seldom given because they will be retained unless siphoned back, and they may increase distention and discomfort. Bisacodyl suppositories may be effective. Insertion of a rectal tube or the administration of neostigmine (Prostigmin) may help to relieve distention. A nasogastric tube may be inserted and intravenous fluids containing electrolytes given, since electrolyte imbalance will be made worse by continuous removal of stomach secretions, and potassium loss may contribute to the development of paralytic ileus. Peristalsis seems to be encouraged by exercise. If the patient's condition permits, sitting up in bed or even walking a little often helps. Eating solid food also appears to prevent the occurrence of paralytic ileus in some instances. For this reason, if patients are able to take this kind of nourishment, some physicians order solid food for those who are quite ill. However, the patient who has had paralytic ileus or in whom the condition has threatened should not be given foods that are gas forming.

Prevention of complications. With the advent of antibiotics and better diagnostic measures such as x-ray procedures, complications during or following pneumonia are rare in otherwise normal persons. Atelectasis, delayed resolution, lung abscess, pleural effusion, empyema, pericarditis, meningitis, and relapse are complications that were quite common in the past. Strict adherence to the prescribed medical treatment, careful accurate observation, and sufficient time for convalescence now ensure the average patient a smooth recovery from pneumonia. However, pneumonia and influenza still rank sixth as a cause of death in the United States. Aged persons and those with chronic illness are likely to have a relatively long course of convalescence from pneumonia, and there is a great possibility of their developing complications. Recently there has been an increase in the incidence of staphylococcal pneumonia subsequent to influenza. Consolidation of lung tissue, pleural effusion, and empyema frequently occur soon after the onset of this type of pneumonia and may cause death.

Acute bronchitis

Bronchitis can be acute or chronic. Acute bronchitis is an inflammation of the bronchi and sometimes the trachea (tracheobronchitis). It is often caused by an extension of an upper respiratory tract infection such as the common cold and is, therefore, communicable. It also may be caused by physical or chemical agents such as dust, smoke, or volatile fumes, and since 9,500 communities in the United States have an air pollution problem, bronchitis is an increasing public health problem.[46]

The patient with acute bronchitis usually complains of chilliness, malaise, muscular aches, headaches, a dry, scratchy throat, hoarseness, and a cough. The temperature may be elevated. The patient may be confined to bed at home or in the hospital. In either case, exposure to others should be kept to a minimum.

Early in the disease the patient's main complaints are the dry, irritating cough and the feeling of tightness and soreness in the chest that follows coughing. The patient may obtain relief by the same means as those described for the common cold. Mustard plasters over the anterior chest may help to counteract local soreness (see texts on fundamentals of nursing). Cough may be relieved by cough mixtures or aerosol drugs. Humidifying the air eases breathing and lessens irritation. Tincture of benzoin, menthol, or oil of eucalyptus may be ordered for the steam vaporizor for its soothing and aromatic effect. As the disease progresses, secretions usually increase. Congestion and dryness of the bronchial mucous membrane are then relieved.

The treatment of acute tracheobronchitis is usually conservative in an attempt to prevent extension of infection to the smaller bronchi, the bronchioles, and the alveoli of the lungs. The patient usually is kept on bed rest and should avoid prolonged activity of any type. He should be protected from drafts, and he should take from 3,000 to 4,000 ml. of fluid daily. A simple bland diet is usually most easily eaten. Often antibiotics are given if the patient has an elevation of temperature.

Most patients need a period of convalescence following an attack of acute bronchitis. Patients usually complain of weakness and fatigability. The nurse should caution the patient to guard against overexertion, including return to work without medical approval. He should be encouraged to take extra rest, to eat a well-balanced diet, and to avoid conditions that might expose him to further infection or predispose him to possible relapse.

Chronic respiratory diseases

Tuberculosis

Tuberculosis has affected man from the earliest times. It has even had periods of relative acceptance. It has been considered fashionable, disgraceful, and mysterious. Today, more than ever, there is need for better interpretation and for clearer understanding of the disease. It is still looked upon by many as being associated with uncleanliness and with careless living. Many families hesitate to admit that tuberculosis has attacked one of their members. Fear of the disease is one of the greatest barriers to control and treatment. This fear exists among health workers as well as patients, their families, and the general public. Although attempts are made constantly to learn more about how tuberculosis affects the body, there is still much about the disease that is controversial and poorly understood. If nurses clearly understand what is known

about the disease, they can do a great deal to help assure eradication of barriers to effective control and treatment.

Tuberculosis trends

Since the discovery of the antituberculosis drugs and successful treatment of tuberculosis with chemotherapy, the mortality rate for tuberculosis has declined steadily. The United States death rate from tuberculosis for 1964 was 4.3 per 100,000 population, an all-time low.[18] Recently an increased number of persons have been discovered to have newly active disease. From 1953 to 1960 both the mortality and the morbidity rates declined, but in 1963 there was an increase in the number of new cases.

Examination of the statistics for 1963 shows that one-third of all new active cases reported were among the nonwhite population. There were a greater number of cases reported among children under 15 years of age, with the greatest increase being among children 5 to 14 years of age. Among nonwhite men and women and white women over 45 years of age, there was a marked increase in the disease. (See Fig. 127.)

The standstill and reversal of the trend in the number of persons with newly active disease were attributed partly to better reporting but also to the fact that efforts toward prevention and control had been relaxed. Many persons believed that tuberculosis was truly disappearing in this country because such effective treatment for the disease was available. However, availability of effective treatment does not ensure actual treatment for every patient.

As of 1964, the number of persons with newly active tuberculosis declined again, and the provisional figures for 1965 show further decrease. The 1964 figures showed that the new active case rate among men was double that for women. The nonwhite population had an incidence of over three and one-half times as high as that for the white population, but almost half of all the new active cases occurred among white men. The highest incidence was among persons 45 to 64 years of age and among those 65 years and over (Table 12).

In the United States there are over 60,000 persons discovered to have newly active disease each year, and 10,000 of these are persons with reactivation of the disease. The

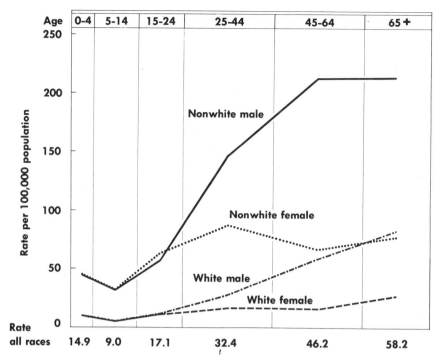

Fig. 127

New active tuberculosis case rates by age, race, and sex in the United States, 1963. (From Reported tuberculosis data, 1965 edition, U. S. Department of Health, Education, and Welfare.)

total number of persons with active tuberculosis is estimated to be 110,000; 250,000 persons have inactive disease, and another 250,000 persons have had contact with someone who has active disease.[60] Thus, 610,000 Americans need attention because of tuberculosis, and an unknown number have the disease without knowing it. The number of deaths and the incidence of new disease are higher in the large cities than in towns and rural areas.

It is believed that eradication of tuberculosis in the United States is possible by intensifying all aspects of the control program. Improved case finding, treatment of active disease, careful medical follow-up of persons who have inactive disease, prevention of relapses in those with inactive disease, determination of the extent of infection and disease in contacts, careful follow-up of those suspected of having disease, and prophylactic treatment for all persons at risk of having the disease are part of a comprehensive control program.

Prevention of tuberculosis infection would decrease the reservoir of people capable of transmitting the disease. Even if all new exposure to infection could be stopped now, there would still be a chance of many persons' developing tuberculosis in the future. In the year 2000, 8 million people infected in 1960 will still be living, in addition to those infected after 1960.

Prevention and control of tuberculosis

Identification and treatment of persons with active pulmonary tuberculosis should be given the highest priority in treatment. If treated with proper antituberculosis drugs, most persons with active tuberculosis will become noninfectious in two to four months.

Examination and follow-up of each of the *contacts*, or persons who have associated with the patient, will add further to the prevention of spread of the disease. There are at

Table 12

New active tuberculosis case rates and death rates per 100,000 population, by age, in 1964*

	Age (years)					
	0-4	**5-14**	**15-24**	**25-44**	**45-64**	**65 and over**
New case rate	13.7	8.5	15.6	30.6	42.7	53.3
Death rate	0.4	0.1	0.4	2.4	8.3	21.0

*From Tuberculosis facts in the United States, New York, 1966, Epidemiology and Statistics Division, National Tuberculosis Association.

least five contacts for each new active case reported annually.[18] Since these persons may have become infected, it is particularly important that they be followed medically during the first year after this exposure to a person with active disease. It has been estimated that nineteen persons per thousand contacts will develop the disease, and about half this number will develop the disease in the first year.

Tuberculin testing of the contacts will indicate presence of infection (p. 549). A chest roentgenogram and a general physical examination will show any signs of clinical pulmonary tuberculosis. Findings on a chest roentgenogram suggestive of disease and a positive tuberculin test identify those persons who are *suspect*. All persons suspected of having the disease need repeated chest x-ray and physical examinations to be certain that active disease is not present.

In addition to these control measures, persons who are at special risk of developing tuberculosis should be given attention. If they are infected with the tubercle bacillus, persons with diabetes mellitus and silicosis and those who have had gastric resection are prone to develop the disease. Infants, preschool children, adolescents, and young adults have a higher susceptibility to tuberculosis than other age groups. Every effort should be made to find the susceptible persons and to follow them medically to prevent their developing active disease.

Sex, race, and socioeconomic conditions should be considered in the tuberculosis con-

trol program. Older white men seem to be very susceptible to the disease. Crowded living conditions with poor ventilation and poor standards of nutrition contribute to the incidence of tuberculosis.

In 1963 the Surgeon General of the United States, disappointed with reports of the higher incidence of tuberculosis, appointed a task force to study the problem. This group's report, entitled *The Future of Tuberculosis Control, a Report to the Surgeon General,** was published at the close of 1963.

One of the recommendations made by the task force was that all children who enter school for the first time should receive a tuberculin test. The number of children in the community who react to tuberculin testing because they have been infected with the tubercle bacillus is an indication of the extent of exposure within the community. Tracing and testing the contacts and associates of children about to enter school who have positive reactions is comparatively easy to do because children at this age have a limited number of known associates. The child's infection can be traced to close family members, other relatives, neighbors and their children, and possibly baby-sitters and domestic workers. In addition, the task force recommended testing all schoolteachers and other school employees. When infection and

---

*This report is obtainable from the Superintendent of Documents, U. S. Government Printing Office, and should be read by all nurses.

disease is discovered among schoolchildren, school bus drivers or teachers may be the source.

The United States Public Health Service has made a renewed effort to intensify tuberculosis control. To date, seventy-one special projects in thirty-seven states, the District of Columbia, and Puerto Rico are under way. These projects provide services to nonhospitalized patients, to persons with active disease, and to those whose disease has been inactive less than five years. They also provide examinations and prophylactic treatment for contacts of recently diagnosed cases. Many projects are emphasizing reduction of infection by identifying persons who might infect children and conducting tuberculin testing of schoolchildren and school employees.

Prophylactic treatment is offered to persons who have recently converted from a negative tuberculin test to a positive test. Prophylactic treatment consists of taking isoniazid tablets daily for one year. Any child under the age of 3 years discovered to have a positive test is considered a recent converter, and in fact may have tuberculosis because of his high susceptibility. Prophylactic treatment also is given to children with positive tests, to young adults, and to persons with high susceptibility to the disease, as mentioned earlier in this chapter.

The National Tuberculosis Association has been working steadily through its constituent and local organizations to disseminate information about the disease, offering chest x-ray examination programs, and setting up tuberculin testing programs with health departments.

The local organizations help to evaluate problems of tuberculosis in the community and find out what methods of control are being used. After collecting the necessary information, the local association passes it along to members of the community by means of exhibits, posters, talks, the press, films, and television. Local organizations work closely with hospitals, departments of health and of welfare, and local physicians. They also give guidance to families and patients.

Vaccination

Efforts continue in search of a more satisfactory tuberculosis vaccine. Presently, BCG (Bacille Calmette Guérin) vaccine is in use in some parts of the United States and in many countries throughout the world. This vaccine contains avirulent tubercle bacilli. They are alive, but through many generations of growth in artificial media (attenuation) they have lost their ability to produce disease. The vaccine should be given only by persons who have had careful instruction in the proper technique. A multiple-puncture disk is used, as shown in Fig. 128. When there is a positive reaction to skin-testing with tuberculin, when acute infectious disease is present, or when there is any skin disease, BCG vaccine is not given. Possible complications following vaccination are local ulcers, which occur in a relatively high percentage of persons vaccinated and abscesses or suppuration of lymph nodes, which occur in a small percentage.

In countries where living conditions are such that transmission of the disease is to be expected, BCG vaccine is given early in life and then repeated after twelve to fifteen years. The intradermal method is used to administer the vaccine so that a uniform controlled dose can be given.

Large-scale vaccination in the United States is unnecessary, but selected groups who are tuberculin negative and who are very susceptible to tuberculosis are being given BCG vaccine in the belief that it may offer some protection. Migrant workers, persons in crowded urban areas, and those in continual contact with infectious persons at home, inmates, patients, and employees in institutions such as mental hospitals, prisons, and old-age homes are among those to whom BCG vaccine is likely to be given. (See p. 548 for method used.)

Infection and disease

Tuberculosis is caused by a bacillus, the *Mycobacterium tuberculosis*, or tubercle bacillus—a gram-positive and acid-fast organism. Microscopic study of a slide prepared from the positive sputum of a patient with active disease reveals the organisms quite readily. The tubercle bacillus is able to survive outside its host particularly when it is embedded in sputum or pus, but growth outside the host requires very special conditions. Carefully prepared cultures on the most favorable media grow quite slowly. Mycobacteria other than *Mycobacterium*

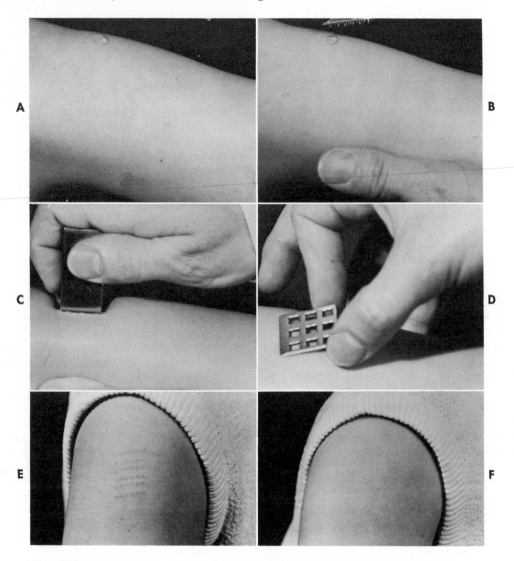

Fig. 128

Vaccination with BCG. **A**, A drop of BCG vaccine is placed on the arm. **B**, The drop of vaccine is spread by tapping with the wide end of a metal disk. **C**, The points of the metal disk are pressed through vaccine to penetrate the skin. **D**, The vaccine is redistributed by a tapping motion. **E**, The site of vaccination after thirteen days. **F**, The site of vaccination after ninety days; note absence of scar. (Courtesy Research Foundation, Chicago, Ill.)

tuberculosis have been identified and studied. (See p. 557 for their description.)

Infection occurs when the tubercle bacilli are inhaled into the alveoli of the lungs. This first reaction depends upon the allergic state of the person, the size of the dose, and the virulence of the organisms. Inflammation occurs within the alveoli (parenchyma) of the lungs, and natural body defenses attempt to counteract the infection. Lymph nodes in the hilar region of the lung may be involved as they filter drainage from the infected site.

The inflammatory process and cellular reaction produce a small, firm, white nodule called the *primary tubercle*. The center of the nodule contains tubercle bacilli. Cells gather around the center, and usually the outer portion becomes fibrosed. Thus, blood vessels are compressed, nutrition of the tubercle is interfered with, and necrosis occurs at the center. The area becomes walled off by fibrotic tissue around the outside, and the center gradually becomes soft and cheesy in consistency. This latter process is known as *caseation*. This material may become calcified (lime deposits), or it may liquefy. The first infection is usually successfully overcome, and the calcified nodule is known as the *Ghon tubercle*. The evidence on x-ray film of the calcified lymph nodes and *Ghon tubercle* is sometimes referred to as the *primary complex*.

Persons who have been exposed to the organism become sensitized to the tubercle bacillus, and this sensitivity can be confirmed by skin testing with tuberculin. Sensitization, once developed, remains throughout life. Evidence that tubercle bacilli have been taken into the body does not mean that one has tuberculosis. It is important for nurses to remember this fact and to explain it to persons who are having a tuberculin test.

Tuberculosis infection is unlike other infections. Usually, other infections disappear completely when overcome by the body's defenses and leave no living organisms and generally no signs of the infection. However, a person who has been infected with tubercle bacilli harbors the organisms for the remainder of life. The tubercle bacilli remain in the lungs in a dormant, walled-off, or so-called resting stage. Under either single or combined physical or emotional stress, these bacilli may become active and begin to multiply. If body defenses are low, active tuberculosis may develop. Most persons who have active tuberculosis developed it in this manner.

Diagnosis and course of the disease

Tuberculin skin testing. Tuberculin skin testing provides evidence of whether the individual tested has been infected by tubercle bacilli. A negative tuberculin skin test usually rules out disease and past infection. A positive test indicates that infection has occurred.

Two substances are used in tuberculin skin testing: OT (old tuberculin), which is prepared from dead tubercle bacilli and contains their related impurities, and PPD (purified protein derivative), which is a highly purified product containing protein from the tubercle bacilli in a dry, stable form. PPD is made up in the desired dilution from tablets immediately before use. OT comes in liquid form, having been prepared in various dilutions each week during the culture of the living organism.

The tuberculin test that gives the most accurate results is the *Mantoux test*, or intracutaneous injection of either PPD or OT. A tuberculin syringe and a short (½ inch), sharp, 24-gauge to 26-gauge needle are used. With the skin (usually the inner forearm is used) held taut, the injection of an exact amount of the PPD or OT is made into the superficial layers, and it produces a sharply raised white wheal. Weak dilutions are used first. If the reaction is negative, stronger dilutions are used. This precaution prevents severe local reactions that might occur in highly sensitive individuals if the higher dilutions were used initially. If old tuberculin is used, tests are begun with a dilution of 1:10,000 or 0.001 mg. of OT. If this test is negative, successive tests with 1:1,000, 1:100, and 1:10 dilutions are made. If PPD is used, the first strength contains 0.00002 mg. of tuberculoprotein, and the second strength contains 0.005 mg. The most frequently used strength of PPD is an intermediate strength of 0.0001 mg. per dose, or 5 tuberculin units (5 Tu). Each injection dose is 0.1 ml. For broad screening and case finding purposes, a single test of intermediate strength is recommended. Interpretations of the tests are made after forty-eight to seventy-two hours. A positive reaction may begin after twelve to twenty-four hours with an area of redness and a central area of induration, but it reaches its peak in forty-eight hours. The area of induration (not the erythema) indicates how positive the test is. Induration should be examined in a good light and palpated gently. Tuberculin reactions should always be measured and recorded in millimeters as the largest diameter of the induration. When successive dilutions are being used, it is advisable to have tests read by the same person since individual variation in interpretation cannot be prevented. If the test is negative, there may be no visible reaction or there may be only slight redness with no induration.

The *Sterneedle tuberculin test* is a modification of the British Heaf test in which a multiple skin puncture is made. A special applicator that holds a sterile, six-needle cartridge is used. The forearm is cleansed with acetone and the cartridge tip is dipped into concentrated tuberculin PPD solution. The tip is placed on the forearm and rotated 90 degrees to spread the solution. The needle points are then released by pressing the plunger of the applicator. Reactions are read three to seven days following the test. A positive reaction shows induration of at least four puncture sites.

Another multiple-puncture tuberculin test is the *Tine test*. The Tine test unit consists of four stainless steel points, each 2 mm. long, attached to a plastic holder. The points of the tines are precoated with old tuberculin. The forearm is cleansed with acetone, and the tines are pressed against the skin so that four puncture sites and a circular depression on the skin are visible. The results are noted forty-eight hours after application and are positive if there is 2 mm. or more of induration at any one puncture site.

One of the most important steps in tuberculin testing is the accurate measurement of reaction. Recent studies have shown that persons with larger-sized reactions—10 mm. or more—are at greater risk of developing tuberculosis than are persons with smaller reactions. Any reaction of 5 mm. or more is considered a positive test, but persons with 10 mm. or more of induration are given priority in follow-up examinations.

Other diagnostic tests. Results of roentgenograms and sputum examinations will either rule out the possibility or confirm a diagnosis of tuberculosis. Both tests have been described (pp. 534-535). Blood-streaked sputum in the absence of pronounced coughing may be the first indication to the patient that anything is wrong. Pathologic changes may have occurred in the lungs, but sputum examination may not show tubercle bacilli. However, if the nodules produced in the parenchyma of the lung become soft in the center, then caseated and liquefied, the lique-

fied material may break through and empty into the bronchi and be raised as sputum. Cavities in the lung may appear on x-ray film and may be present in more than one lobe of the lung.

Tuberculosis diagnosis and classification. Tuberculosis is diagnosed and classified according to the extent of the disease in the lung (minimal, moderately advanced, far advanced), the status of clinical activity (active, quiescent, inactive, activity undetermined), the bacteriologic findings (sputum positive or negative), the therapeutic status (previous chemotherapy or surgical procedures), and the exercise status (amount of exercise prescribed). It is important for the nurse to understand fully the patient's complete diagnosis and classification in order to help carry out prescribed treatment and follow-up that may prevent a possible reactivation of inactive disease or transmission of the disease to others. Details of diagnosis and classification are available in special references.[14]

Preventing transmission of infection and disease

Pulmonary tuberculosis is spread either directly or indirectly from one individual to another, usually by the inhalation of tubercle bacilli. Despite the fact that many people inhale tubercle bacilli during the course of their lives, the majority overcome the infection, and active clinical tuberculosis does not develop. The defensive forces of the body overcome the first bacterial invasion. Tuberculosis does not often follow the swallowing of tubercle bacilli, but one can be indirectly exposed by putting contaminated fingers or utensils in the mouth.

The best way for the nurse to protect others from active pulmonary tuberculosis is by helping the tuberculosis patient to understand how the disease is transmitted and how he can prevent bacilli from reaching the surrounding atmosphere and in turn infecting those who breathe the air. The nurse should teach the patient to cover his mouth and nose when clearing his throat, sneezing, or coughing. He should use disposable tissues whenever possible and should discard them in the toilet or collect them in a paper bag that subsequently can be burned. The patient should wash his hands after handling any sputum or receptacle containing sputum.

The most effective way to kill the tubercle bacillus in moist sputum is by burning. All tissues and disposable receptacles for the collection of sputum should be burned. Direct sunlight destroys the bacillus in from one to two hours. Five minutes at boiling temperature and thirty minutes at pasteurizing temperature, 61.7° C. (143° F.), kill the bacillus. Autoclaving also destroys the bacillus. Disposable articles may be used if desired.

Studies have shown that tubercle bacilli reach the air about the patient by forceful expulsion of air from the lungs, as in sneezing or coughing.[58] Droplets within the exhaled spray vary in size; the larger ones fall rapidly and settle. Droplets expelled into the air begin to lose moisture by evaporation, and the smaller the droplet the more quickly it dries. Many small droplets, therefore, dry in the air, and the remaining tiny solid particle is called a droplet nucleus. The nuclei are much smaller and lighter than droplets and are carried easily by air currents.

Tubercle bacilli are 0.5 to 1.5 microns in size. For comparison, a red blood cell is 6 to 8 microns, a particle of dust averages 200 microns, and a droplet is 10 to 90 microns in size. Only those particles that are 5 microns or less in size can possibly enter the alveoli of the lungs. Any larger-sized droplet or dust particle is trapped in the upper respiratory tract and expelled by ciliary motion and/or coughing. Thus, only droplet nuclei containing tubercle bacilli are capable of causing infection.

The natural movement of air in a room carries droplet nuclei along, and if windows are kept open or air is circulated mechanically, changes of air dilute the contaminated air below the level where infection can take place. If the patient who has positive sputum has been taught to cover coughs and sneezes, air contamination in his room is even lower.

Tubercle bacilli in droplet nuclei are highly susceptible to sterilization by sunlight. Ultraviolet light also kills tubercle bacilli in droplet nuclei. Lights installed in air ducts through which room air passes or mounted high on side walls of the room are effective.

It is important that the nurse understand how tubercle bacilli are transmitted through the air so that she can teach the patient how to protect others and also to allay fears that family members and others may have about contracting the disease. The patient who is taking antituberculosis drugs is the least likely to transmit the infection even if the organisms are resistant to treatment. The most infectious patient is one who has thin, watery sputum that contains the tubercle bacilli. When caring for the patient with active disease and positive sputum, the nurse has no need to wear a mask and gown. Droplet nuclei that come to rest on walls, floors, or clothing cannot be inhaled. Masks are of little value since droplet nuclei can pass through them and in many instances are breathed in around the edges of ill-fittting masks. One newer type of mask, the Ultra-Filter, has been proved quite effective as a filter. If the patient is so ill that he is unable to cover his cough or if he is incapable or unwilling to do so, the nurse should wear an effective mask when she is near the patient.

Since many patients with active tuberculosis are cared for in their own homes, the nurse should help patients and their families to understand the communicability of tuberculosis and the precautions that must be taken. Family members and friends may be frightened at the thought of contact with the patient and with articles he has touched. On the other hand, they often point to long, intimate contact they have had with the patient without developing the disease. Careful observation of the family will help the nurse determine how many and what kind of explanations are needed regarding spread of infection. If the family is overly cautious in handling the patient's personal articles, the nurse may need to advise against discarding articles that are costly to replace. In contrast, if the family is too casual in regard to spread of the disease, the nurse should urge more caution in care of sputum and in exposure to the patient's cough. If possible, the patient should occupy a room alone, but if he is allowed to stay at home, he usually does not need to be strictly isolated from the rest of the family. Careful planning with the family often helps to ensure that he will not infect others yet can be located so that he and his family can be as happy as possible under such circumstances. The susceptibility of babies and very small children must be emphasized in all teaching of the patient and of his family.

Nursing care

Acceptance of the disease. Acceptance of a diagnosis of tuberculosis and of its many implications for the future is difficult for anyone. The patient and/or his family should be referred to a public health nurse immediately after the diagnosis of tuberculosis is made since she can help him make arrangements for hospitalization, give initial explanations, and begin essential teaching. It is important that any problems that might interfere with acceptance of the disease be identified early since the earlier efforts are made to solve them, the less difficult they may be to overcome.

Real acceptance of the disease, however, may come only after months of illness and after steady help and support from the family, the doctor, the social worker, and the nurse. The acceptance of facts and realities varies according to each patient's basic personality and his lifelong pattern of behavior in stress situations. The nurse should realize that for some time after the diagnosis is made and treatment started the patient's true self may not be evident. At first the patient may seem to accept everything, and then, little by little, his behavior may reveal that he has not accepted the disease at all. For example, the patient may be pleasant and agreeable, accept suggestions readily, and follow recommended medical treatment carefully for the first month or two. But when the third or fourth month is reached, he may begin to complain about numerous little things, he may object to taking medications, and he may make occasional critical remarks. The length of time necessary for "cure" is often the most difficult problem for the patient to face. Particularly is this true if time must be spent in a hospital away from his family, job, and usual way of life.

Some patients do not have the capacity ever to accept the disease, and they may experience frustration and despair at the changes in their lives that it entails. The patient may completely "block out" all thoughts of the disease and continue as if nothing had really happened. This is likely to be true of patients who refuse care. Other patients may welcome the long period of rest and the lessening of life's responsibilities. However, as recovery progresses and they must once again face adjustment to normal life, they may experience fear and anxiety. Since the treatment of tuberculosis extends over a long period of time, periodic reevaluation and follow-up are necessary. Conferences among staff members caring for the patient provide an excellent opportunity for all persons to discuss their observations and interpretations.

There is a high incidence of alcoholism among patients with tuberculosis, probably because of the increased possibility of alcoholics coming into contact with tubercle bacilli during drinking bouts and because of their decreased resistance to infection. Many of these patients have been committed to the hospital for care by legal action after refusal to obtain treatment although their disease is a threat to the health of their family and the community. They present the dual problem of the patient with alcoholism (p. 132) and the patient with tuberculosis who cannot accept his disease.

Increasing attention needs to be given to patients who refuse treatment and thus stand in the way of eradication of tuberculosis. The nurse often is the member of the medical team called upon to work with these patients. Patience and understanding as well as flexibility in trying new approaches are essential in working with them. Although the patient needs explanations as to the need for treatment and time to make his own decisions regarding means of obtaining it, delaying tactics should be discouraged by setting limits. Avoidance of questions that permit categorical refusal is wise. It is often helpful to discover the person for whose judgment the patient has the greatest respect and to seek his help in encouraging treatment. This person may be the doctor, a clergyman, a family member, or a close friend. Patients who have completed treatment for tuberculosis and are well again often are helpful in answering specific questions the patient may have and may thus relieve many of his anxieties. Appropriate measures to alleviate financial and social problems impeding hospitalization of the patient should be instituted as soon as possible. Every effort should be made to make the patient feel there is sincere concern for his and his family's welfare. In spite of all efforts, some patients will not consent to treatment. Sometimes, if they become suddenly worse, they may then be receptive to treatment, and the opportunity to work with them and help them at this time should not be missed.

Acceptance of tuberculosis as a disease by the nurse is closely related to her ability to know and to help the patient with tuberculosis. The nurse who has a fear of tuberculosis may show it in her behavior. Most patients with tuberculosis are extremely sensitive to ways in which various health workers approach them. If the nurse is obvious about precautions in giving care, she may cause the patient to feel rejected. Her touch when giving physical care, or even when placing articles such as food trays within reach, may be clues to him as to her acceptance of him with his disease. Nurses may be fearful of the disease for various reasons. If the nurse is conscious of her fear, discussion with a more experienced person may help her to learn more about the disease, to accept it better, and therefore to alter her own feelings and reactions.

The majority of patients with tuberculosis are able to assume responsibility for most of their own care. Proper rest, good nutrition, prescribed drugs, prescribed activity, and attention to good body alignment are essential. The nurse's major responsibility is to help the patient learn what he should do and why, and to give encouragement and supervision in the simple but essential elements of good care. Group teaching often is a very productive method of instructing both patients and family members since they often learn from each other and give each other emotional support (Fig. 129).

Today, many patients with tuberculosis are not hospitalized or are hospitalized for much shorter periods of time than in the past. Since the newer drugs are more effective in controlling the communicability of the disease, some physicians feel that it is safe and better for the patient to remain at home and either visit the doctor's office or

Fig. 129

Some of the best opportunities for teaching occur during discussions with small groups of patients. General health principles, as well as understanding of disease, can be discussed. Here the nurse is discussing the selection of well-balanced meals.

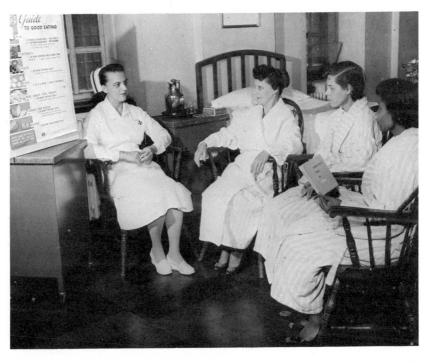

a clinic for his medication and have a public health nurse make regular visits.

Provision for rest. Rest must be mental as well as physical and therefore presents a challenge to the nurse and to all other persons responsible for the patient's care. Learning why mental rest is impossible for the patient is sometimes difficult, but continued friendly interest usually leads to understanding. Loneliness, need for privacy, financial worries, and concern for loved ones are only a few of the many problems that may be interfering with rest.

It is often extremely difficult for the average patient with tuberculosis who feels well and looks well to remain on limited activity for even short periods of time.

Activity. Activities are progressively increased as the patient's physical condition improves. With the use of antituberculosis drugs, activity can usually be advanced more rapidly than previously, but specific doctor's orders for each increase in activity must be obtained.

If the patient is being treated at home, a definite schedule of activities must be arranged. Upon visiting a patient at home, the nurse may find that he is doing more than is advisable or recommended. It is particularly difficult for many persons to conform to a routine of restricted activity if they remain at home. If patients have had a period of hospitalization first, it is more likely that a daily program will have been planned with them, and carrying it out at home is less difficult.

Patients at home who have not had the advantage of working closely with a medical and nursing staff may find themselves adding activities one by one with little awareness that they are doing so. For example, a housewife may feel well and, seeing work to be done, may be tempted to do more than is advisable. She may add new activities daily with little realization that she is doing so.

Men who have been used to regular working hours may feel guilty about being home during those hours. Since they are temporarily unable to support their families, they may feel that they must help with chores about the house, and they argue that some of these duties are light and will do them no harm. It is important that members

of the family clearly understand the patient's rest and activity schedule so that they can help him to carry out the doctor's orders.

If the patient must remain hospitalized for a period of time, members of the staff or the patient's family are his only contacts with the outside. Thus, in conversation, many patients rely on the nurse to learn about the latest movies, various shows, community activities, prices in stores, and the like.

Small day-by-day routine tasks and activities should be planned. The patient should be encouraged to maintain interest in his appearance and in his grooming. Manicures, shampoos, and hair styling can and should be done. Any patient who has a long-term confining illness may value his smallest possessions in a way quite different from the person who is well and participating actively in life. Personal belongings tend to collect, and the patient needs help in sorting and arranging them.

Ordinary small routine activities that every well person takes for granted can be very important to the patient on limited activity. If an organized occupational therapy department is available, the patient is encouraged to engage in activities appropriate to his prescribed program. The interest of others in his projects adds to his enjoyment. Patients may enjoy telling the nurse about their projects or even teaching her some of the skills involved. When occupational therapy service is not available, the nurse can teach some simple skills to patients or arrange for them to take responsibility for small jobs such as distributing mail and taking orders for papers. Some patients who are allowed activity enjoy doing these and similar jobs.

Diet. Food and meal schedules can present many problems in the care of patients with tuberculosis. Adequate nutrition is essential to increase or to maintain natural body resistance and to help in the repair of damaged lung tissue. Some patients may have lost weight, and they may lack appetite. If the patient is hospitalized, members of his family can help by occasionally preparing food and bringing it to the patient. It may replace the regular hospital meal, or it may be used as a supplement to the meal. The patient's appetite is sometimes improved by serving food he particularly enjoys. A weekly record of weight is often requested since, when other outlets for their interest are restricted, some patients may be too preoccupied with food, and they may gain weight. Occasionally patients with tuberculosis are overweight, and reasonable dieting may be ordered. The nurse may then need to help make low-caloric foods attractive and satisfying.

Chemotherapy. Whether the patient with tuberculosis is being treated at home or in the hospital, the same drugs are given. Streptomycin, para-aminosalicylic acid (PAS), and isoniazid (INH) are the drugs in common use. These three drugs are considered to be the "first-line," or primary, medications in the treatment of tuberculosis. If they prove to be ineffective or if the patient develops resistant tubercle bacilli, the "second-line," or secondary, drugs are used. These drugs are cycloserine (Seromycin), pyrazinoic acid amide (Pyrazinamide), viomycin (Viocin), kanamycin (Kantrex), and ethionamide (Trecator).

Previously untreated pulmonary tuberculosis can nearly always be controlled bacteriologically with drugs alone. Most failures of drug therapy are due to either errors in choice of drug or the failure of the patient to take the drugs regularly as prescribed.[4] Choices of drugs are made with the objective of both effective treatment of disease and minimizing the development of drug resistance.

Susceptibility testing. Prescriptions for antituberculosis drugs are made according to the susceptibility of the organisms isolated from the patient's sputum to the three primary drugs, isoniazid, para-aminosalicylic acid, and streptomycin. Susceptibility testing indicates the effectiveness of a specific drug in inhibiting the growth of the organism or the organism's resistance to the drug. The doctor may start the patient on drugs to which it is anticipated the bacilli will be susceptible until testing can be done.

Testing is done by growing cultures of the organisms in special media. The culture plate is divided into sections so that the organisms, if present in the patient's sputum, can grow on one section. Each of the other three sections contains a medium plus one of the three primary drugs. Thus, if the or-

ganisms multiply on the plain medium but do not appear on the medium with the drug, those organisms are susceptible to the drugs. The testing usually takes about three weeks, which is about half the time formerly required to grow cultures of tubercle bacilli.

Although it is the physician's responsibility to make susceptibility tests, the nurse should understand the basis upon which drugs are prescribed and help the patient understand the various changes in drugs that may be prescribed for him and why he may be receiving drugs that are different from those received by other patients.

Delay of drug resistance is achieved by giving at least two drugs in combination. As tubercle bacilli multiply in the lungs, the strains of organisms develop mutants (organisms that are new and different from their parent organisms), and these developing strains may be resistant to one of the drugs but not the other. Thus, the presence of a second drug to which the organism is still susceptible in the bloodstream inhibits the growth of the new strain.

Drugs frequently used. Isoniazid and PAS are by far the most common combination given. The daily dose of isoniazid for an adult is usually 5 mg. per kilogram of body weight (about 300 mg. daily) given orally in three doses. Higher doses are given to some patients who have severe or acute disease. The daily dose of PAS in adults is 12 Gm. orally (200 mg. per kilogram of body weight), usually in three divided doses and taken following meals.

PAS commonly causes gastrointestinal symptoms, especially early in treatment. Some physicians reduce the dosage temporarily to 4 to 6 Gm. daily and then increase the dosage when the intolerance to the drug has subsided. Nausea, vomiting, and poor appetite are the usual symptoms. Taking the pills following meals or with milk helps most patients. Some who receive PAS in powder form prefer to have the medication mixed in a glass of milk, which produces a consistency similar to that of a milkshake. Other signs of intolerance to the drug are skin rash, fever, headache, malaise, and sore throat. The nurse should observe the patient closely during the first six weeks of therapy for signs of hypersensitivity so that the dosage can be reduced if necessary.

555

Isoniazid causes little toxicity. Occasionally, however, symmetrical peripheral neuritis may develop, particularly in patients who are malnourished or who are receiving large doses of the drug. To prevent neuritis, the physician usually orders pyridoxine, 50 to 100 mg. daily. Occasionally isoniazid may effect memory and the ability to concentrate, and rarely it may cause psychosis.

Streptomycin is often given as part of an initial program of treatment. It is given daily for six to twelve weeks or more, depending upon the patient's response, in 1 Gm. doses, intramuscularly. Smaller doses may be prescribed for elderly patients or for patients who have hearing impairment or renal damage. The most important untoward reaction to streptomycin is vestibular damage with resulting dizziness and staggering. Skin rash, itching, and fever can occur. Although renal damage is uncommon, the doctor usually orders urinalyses and blood urea nitrogen determinations at periodic intervals. (For chemotherapy programs and toxicities of the secondary drugs, see pharmacology texts.)

Patients' problems with chemotherapy. It is imperative that the patient who has tuberculosis take the prescribed medication regularly and without interruption. Since the patient must take drugs daily usually for at least two years, he may become discouraged and stop taking the drugs. If symptoms of intolerance to the drug such as those produced by PAS occur, he may simply stop taking the one drug and continue with the other. The patient may feel quite well, work regularly, yet must continue the therapy. Because he feels well and has been able to increase his activity, he may be tempted to discontinue the drugs altogether or perhaps take the one drug that bothers him the least. He may forget to take one dose occasionally, but usually this causes no ill effect. If forgetfulness becomes habitual, however, it may be an indication that he is becoming lax about following treatment. The nurse should help all patients to develop a daily routine for taking the drugs. For those who have difficulty, drug calendars or diaries may help.

Some patients stop taking drugs and then restart them. Because they may feel guilty about this interruption in therapy, they do not tell the doctor or nurse, and it may not be evident until susceptibility tests are done that show that drug resistance has developed. The nurse can help by allowing time for patients to talk about themselves, their families, and their treatment. This may be done when the patient visits a health department clinic to receive his new supply of drugs, when he comes for his periodic medical examination, or when the nurse visits him in his home. Patients may be asked to collect a urine specimen periodically for examination. The urinalysis may give some indication of how consistently the drugs are being taken. The best indication, of course, is the progress of the patient. If he improves, therapy is effective and the medications probably have been taken as prescribed.

Continuing care and follow-up. It is extremely important that each patient who has or who has had active tuberculosis continue with medical care throughout his lifetime. Tuberculosis is a chronic, communicable disease in which relapses may occur. Studies show that most relapses occur within the first five years after the disease has become inactive, and may occur within two years.[11] Unless patients continue with medical care and periodic examinations, they may be completely unaware that the disease has become active again. If it has, they may do harm to themselves and may expose others.

Rehabilitation. Careful planning for the time when the hospitalized patient will return home should start as soon as possible. His care at home should be reviewed with the members of his family. They should be urged to have a public health nurse visit their home to help them arrange for continued care. The public health nurse may continue the teaching begun in the hospital, and she should be advised of any problems that have been detected during hospitalization and the progress made in solving them.

The patient may have viewed his future with uncertainty for so long that he finds it difficult to express an interest in his future. The social worker is often helpful to him in making plans for the future as well as in taking care of immediate social and economic problems. The doctor may feel that the patient will need to return to a different type of work. If so, assistance in vocational rehabilitation is available to many patients and may include vocational retraining or counseling and guidance regarding future work. If the nurse, in the absence of a social worker, must be responsible for determining the eligibility of the patient for this help, she can obtain guidance from the local tuberculosis association and the state health department. Plans for return to work often are considered after the patient has been at home for some time, and the public health nurse or nurse in the clinic may need to initiate action.

Surgical treatment for tuberculosis

When medical treatment has failed to check and heal the disease process, surgical treatment for tuberculosis may be necessary. Surgical treatment for tuberculosis includes pneumonectomy, lobectomy, partial lobe resection, and wedge resection. Usually parts of the lungs with active disease are resected, and as much lung tissue as possible is preserved. The nursing care and descriptions of operative procedures are explained later in this chapter in the section on thoracic surgery (p. 575).

Extrapulmonary tuberculosis

Tuberculosis may attack other parts of the body besides the lungs, such as the larynx, the gastrointestinal tract, lymph nodes, skin, skeletal system, nervous system, and urinary and reproductive systems.

Tuberculous meningitis. The onset of symptoms of tuberculous meningitis usually is sudden. The patient has marked constipation, an elevation of temperature, chills, headache, convulsions, and sometimes loss of consciousness. If untreated, this disease causes death, but with the use of antituberculosis drugs, it is usually controllable. A twelve-month course of medical treatment is necessary, however, and the nurse must help to make the patient and his family realize that it is absolutely necessary. Streptomycin, isoniazid, and PAS are all given concurrently.

Signs of sensitivity to drugs or toxic reactions must be watched for particularly carefully, as with any other type of tuberculosis.

Skeletal tuberculosis. Since the advent of antituberculosis drugs, better case finding methods, pasteurization of milk, and tuberculin testing of cattle, skeletal tuberculosis is growing less common. It is most common in children, but adults also are sometimes affected. Although tubercle bacilli may attack any bone or joint in the body, the spine, hips, and knees are most often involved. Deformities occur as a result of bone destruction. Tuberculosis of the spine is now rare in the United States. The "hunchback" deformity it causes can still be seen in some people, particularly in those who have come from countries where standards for pasteurization of milk and tuberculin testing of cattle were not rigid. (For nursing care of patients having tuberculosis of the spine, see specialized texts on orthopedic nursing.)

Unclassified mycobacteria

Pulmonary disease that is indistinguishable from tuberculosis can be produced by a number of species of mycobacteria other than *Mycobacterium tuberculosis*. Four groups have been identified thus far. Groups I and III have been studied extensively. They are chronic in nature, produce cavities in the lungs, and frequently are associated with emphysema. Laboratory tests and skin sensitization tests are used to identify the organisms. However, some patients may be diagnosed as having tuberculosis until tested. For more details about these diseases, see references at the end of this chapter and statements from the American Thoracic Society.*

CHRONIC OBSTRUCTIVE LUNG DISEASE (ASTHMA, CHRONIC BRONCHITIS, PULMONARY EMPHYSEMA)

The common characteristic of asthma, chronic bronchitis, and pulmonary emphysema is that chronic obstruction of the lung airways develops and makes breathing difficult. These conditions may have developed suddenly but usually have developed gradually over a long period of time. Often the patient cannot recall the time of onset of trouble in breathing. A chronic or recurring productive cough usually is the first symptom, but many people ignore it. If symptoms are minimal, many persons continue in their usual way until symptoms become severe. By this time, emphysematous changes have occurred in the alveoli and are irreversible.

---

*American Review of Respiratory Diseases 87:459-462, March 1963.

Chronic obstructive lung disease has increased spectacularly in recent years. Death rates, particularly for men, have risen sharply. In 1950 the death rate for men with emphysema was approximately 1.5 per 100,-000 population, and in 1963 it had risen to approximately 14.5 per 100,000 population. Increased consumption of cigarettes, the increasing age of the population, and greater accuracy in reporting the primary cause of death have contributed to this rise.

Although causes of most chronic obstructive lung diseases are unknown, many factors have been shown to be related to their development. The Surgeon General's Advisory Committee, in its report on smoking and health, listed cigarette smoking as the most important cause of chronic bronchitis. It also stated that a relationship exists between pulmonary emphysema and cigarette smoking. Bronchopulmonary infections have not been shown to cause obstructive lung disease, but if anatomic and physiologic abnormalities are present, these infections may hasten the development of severe, destructive lung disease. Air pollution contributes to the occurrence of these chronic diseases, and certain occupations, involving exposure to dusts, fumes, molds, and fungi, are known to damage the lungs. Allergenic factors may also contribute to the development of chronic lung disease.

Chronic bronchitis

Chronic bronchitis is most prevalent among men over 35 years of age who are heavy cigarette smokers, although the disease does occur in nonsmokers as well. Hypersecretion of mucus occurs, and both bronchi and bronchioles are affected. The patient coughs to rid the air passages of these secretions, and repeated coughing and secondary irritation from smoke or other irritating inhalants increase the irritation and inflammation. Repeated irritation and coughing cause loss of cilia, aggravating the condition.

Relief of symptoms can be achieved to some extent by avoiding the irritants that increase the irritation. Nurses can learn from the patient and his family some of the circumstances that initiate the persistent cough and increase it. A medication such as potassium iodide or a mucolytic enzyme, used in a hand nebulizer, may be ordered to thin secretions. Other measures that may make these persons more comfortable will be described later. The most important action the nurse can take is to assist persons with symptoms to obtain medical care and thus perhaps prevent more serious lung disease.

Asthma

Children often have asthma, and men and women in every age, race, and occupational group contract asthma. Most people who have asthma seem to inherit a tendency to be sensitive (allergic) to various substances (p. 74). For most persons, asthma comes and goes in "attacks."

Persons who have asthmatic attacks usually seek medical care because attacks are both incapacitating and frightening. If allergens are discovered as the offending substance, injections to desensitize the person may be given. (See p. 76 for techniques in desensitization.)

After asthma has become established in the patient, other factors besides the antigens to which he was originally sensitive may precipitate an acute attack. Emotional stress, changes in temperature and humidity, irritating fumes and smoke, strong odors, and physical exertion have been known to precipitate attacks. The patient must often make an attempt to lessen emotional stress and to control physical exertion since these factors are less amenable to management than are specific excitants such as drugs or foods. If the underlying cause of the allergy is obscure or if it is resistant to treatment, the recognition and control of secondary factors may be the main approach to treatment.

Nursing care. There is perhaps no disease in which knowing the patient well is more important than in asthma. Since sensitivity tests can be done with only a very small fraction of the substances with which the patient is in contact, the doctor usually makes the diagnosis on the basis of a careful history. Knowing how the patient lives, how he spends his leisure time, what he eats, what type of work he does, his social contacts, and many other circumstances may give useful clues as to the cause of his trouble. Although the allergist urges patients to report seemingly trivial and insignificant details, they often hesitate to do so since they are used to reporting only physical changes within themselves. If the nurse is alert, she can often be of real help to the doctor in learning the cause of the allergic reaction. In conversation with the patient, for example, she may learn that a relative had just visited and brought a pet with her.

The nurse may make observations regarding emotional stresses that appear to aggravate the patient's condition. Careful observation of his relationships with members of his family may give clues to sources of emotional stress. Some patients remain in the hospital during an acute episode and return home relieved of serious symptoms. However, unless his circumstances can be improved, family relationships and general socioeconomic conditions that cause stress may send the patient back to the hospital with another attack.

Patients with chronic bronchial asthma may gain a sense of security while in the hospital and may be reluctant to return home. Asthmatic attacks can be precipitated by plans for discharge, and the patient's stay may thus be prolonged. Patients with severe emotional insecurity may find help in psychotherapy.

Signs and symptoms. Asthmatic attacks often occur at night. The person awakens with a feeling of choking. He can neither get enough air into his lungs nor can he breathe air out satisfactorily. The bronchioles react with swelling of the mucosa, muscle spasm (bronchospasm), and increased amount of thick secretions. The patient's breathing has a characteristic wheezing sound as he attempts to draw air through the constricted and obstructed airways. Cyanosis may develop. When an attack starts, the patient should sit upright. He should be given something on which to lean forward, such as an overbed table. Since, during an acute attack, the patient uses the accessory muscles of respiration in his effort to get enough air, leaning forward helps him to use them more effectively. Since his only concern during an acute attack is breathing, he must be protected from falling and from other injury. He should be given medication for relief of the attack as soon as possible, and he should be constantly attended until acute symptoms subside. The attack usually ends with the patient coughing up large quantities of thick, tenacious sputum. He may become completely exhausted from increased physical effort, and he should rest quietly after the attack. He usually perspires profusely, and he may need change of clothing and special protection from chilling. Most attacks subside in one-half to one hour, although asthmatic attacks following infection may continue for days or weeks.

Patients who are severely affected with asthma and who have attacks that are difficult to control with the usual medications may develop *status asthmaticus.* In this case the symptoms of an acute attack continue. The patient is acutely ill. When he is admitted to the hospital, he needs emergency treatment. Prolonged attacks cause exhaustion, and death from heart failure may occur. Oxygen is administered by mask, and positive pressure may be used intermittently. In extreme cases, when the air passages appear seriously obstructed, a mixture of helium and oxygen may be given by endotracheal tube or by mask. Helium has a high rate of diffusion and a lighter molecular weight than oxygen, so that it can be inhaled with less effort. During an acute attack, the alveoli progressively distend as in emphysema, and actually acute emphysema exists. Unless relaxation of the bronchioles can be accomplished, insufficient oxygen passes through the alveolar membrane into the bloodstream, and the patient becomes progressively more cyanotic. The patient needs constant observation, and he should have everything done for him. Repeated attacks of status asthmaticus may cause irreversible emphysema, resulting in a permanent decrease in total breathing capacity.

Some patients have *chronic mild asthma.* Symptoms are not noticeable when the patient is at rest. However, after exertion such as laughing, singing, vigorous exercise, or emotional excitement, the patient develops dyspnea and wheezing. These attacks are controlled with medications, and patients usually can continue their usual mode of living with few modifications and no serious lung changes. They are not hospitalized, but they sometimes come to outpatient clinics for medical supervision.

Treatment. The treatment of asthma is directed toward symptomatic relief of attacks, the control of specific causative factors, and the general care for maintenance of optimum health. The chief aim of various medications is to afford the patient immediate and progressive bronchial relaxation. A drug often given to control mild attacks is *epinephrine* (Adrenalin), which relaxes smooth muscles in the respiratory tract and counteracts the bronchial constriction that occurs during attacks. Epinephrine, 0.2 to 1 mg. (1/300 to 1/60 grain) in a 1:1,000 solution, is given subcutaneously or intramuscularly and may be repeated every five to ten minutes for two or three doses. Frequent repeated doses can be avoided by giving epinephrine in oil, 0.4 to 3 mg. (1/150 to 1/20 grain) of a 1:500 solution, intramuscularly every six to twelve hours. This provides slower systemic absorption and prolongs the effect. Some patients who have frequent mild attacks are taught to give their own injections, or a member of the family may be taught to give the injections.

Patients with chronic bronchial asthma are maintained at home on active drug therapy and return to the doctor's office or the clinic for periodic supervision. Many patients take *ephedrine sulfate*, 25 mg. (⅜ grain), by mouth every four hours during the day. Ephedrine sulfate, like epinephrine, relaxes hypertonic muscles. The stimulating effects of ephedrine sulfate can be lessened by combining ephedrine with a mild sedative such as phenobarbital, 15 mg. (¼ grain), taken by mouth several times a day. *Theophylline ethylenediamine* (aminophylline) may be given during acute attacks. The dosage is 0.25 to 0.5 Gm. (3¾ to 7½ grains) intravenously or intramuscularly. Aminophylline suppositories, 0.5 Gm. (7½ grains), can also be given rectally every eight to twelve hours. Tablets are available that combine theophylline, ephedrine, and phenobarbital. They are taken four times a day when attacks are frequent or for prophylaxis. Each tablet contains theophylline, 130 mg., ephedrine hydrochloride, 24 mg., and phenobarbital, 8 mg. Many patients are treated with other drugs to dilate the bronchi. These drugs are given by inhalation. The patient who is ambulatory will need instruction in the use of a nebulizer. *Isoproterenol hydro-chloride* (Isuprel), 0.5 ml. of 1:200 solution, is often used.

Hand nebulizers may be of the glass container type with a small opening through which air is pumped with a hand rubber bulb, producing a spray of medication that is inhaled into the lungs. Several types of nebulizers are available that make use of a plastic holder and a cartridge containing the medication. The latter has some advantage in that, with only slight pressure of the finger on the cartridge, a measured dose of a very fine spray is ejected. The main points to be taught to the patient, regardless of the type of nebulizer used, is to exhale first as completely as possible, to place the open end of the nebulizer into his mouth, and after beginning to inhale deeply, to direct the aerosolized medication toward the back of the throat, and finish taking the deep breath. He should hold his breath for as long as possible and then should exhale slowly, pursing his lips. The latter helps to create increased pressure in the airways and carries the medication farther into the bronchioles and alveoli.

Expectorants such as *potassium iodide* or *ammonium chloride* may be given to help loosen thick bronchial secretions. The dosage of potassium iodide is usually 0.3 Gm. (5 grains) by mouth three times a day after meals. Sedatives help to keep the patient quiet and to provide for better rest. However, they are used with caution to avoid depressing respiratory function and to avoid the danger of addiction. If a narcotic is needed, *meperidine hydrochloride* (Demerol), 50 mg. (¾ grain), given intramuscularly every four hours, is used in preference to morphine. *Barbiturates* such as phenobarbital, 30 mg. (½ grain), by mouth every four hours during the day and pentobarbital, 100 mg. (1½ grains), by mouth at night help to give the patient steady sedation. *Codeine*, 15 mg. (¼ grain), or *elixir of terpin hydrate with codeine*, 5 ml. (1 dram) every four hours, helps to control excessive coughing, thus permitting more rest. In asthma following infection, various antibiotics are used, depending on the organism involved. Adrenocorticosteroids are sometimes used for patients with severe asthma that does not respond favorably to other drug therapy.

Pulmonary emphysema

Approximately 75% of the individuals with emphysema have chronic bronchitis. Pulmonary emphysema usually follows repeated respiratory infections that cause changes in the bronchial walls and in the alveoli. Low-grade infection and inadequate drainage of exudate result in mechanical stretching and thickening of the walls of the bronchioles. Asthma, which causes the bronchial mucosa to become edematous with subsequent obstruction of air passages, also leads to emphysema. Emphysema may follow distention of the lungs that may occur as the lung expands to fill space in the pleural cavity following surgery such as the removal of a lung. Occasionally this same reaction occurs after destruction of a portion of the lung from disease such as tuberculosis or silicosis. Many elderly patients have emphysema as one of several diseases. Accurate statistics on the incidence of chronic pulmonary emphysema are not available, although it is said to be the most common chronic disease of the lungs, and the incidence is believed to be increasing. Medical research is presently directed toward studies to determine what relationship, if any, may exist between substances inhaled in breathing and this disease.

Chronic emphysema develops in middle or later life and is more common among men than women. Fairly early signs include severe "smoker's cough" upon awakening and a visible tightening of the neck muscles as the patient makes an almost conscious attempt to take a full breath of air. The nurse should urge any person who has these signs to stop smoking if he does smoke and to visit his doctor, because the condition if developing, may be delayed in its progress by early treatment. As the disease progresses, the patient develops increasing dyspnea on exertion and chronic fatigue until most of his available energy is spent in getting enough air.

In efforts to increase breathing comfort, the patient with emphysema uses the upper intercostal muscles. Full use of the diaphragm is diminished, and eventually the diaphragm flattens in a fixed position. Thus expiration is prolonged and difficult, with the patient literally having to squeeze air from his lungs. Patients sometimes make a blowing sound through the mouth in an effort to force exhalation. The abdomen often protrudes because of loss of muscle tone, and the chest becomes barrel-shaped because of elevation of the rib cage. After a long period of diminished alveolar function, the patient's breathing under ordinary activity becomes jerky or spasmodic. With exertion, expiration is further impaired. The carbon dioxide level in the blood may increase due to the diminished supply of oxygen and to changes in exchange of oxygen and carbon dioxide across the alveolar membrane. Breaths are taken until the oxygen level of the blood rises and then may cease until it again falls to a level that reflexly triggers inspiration.

If the patient is in danger of developing acute pulmonary insufficiency *(carbon dioxide narcosis),* he may be placed in a respirator or given assistance in breathing by a volume cycle type of intermittent positive-pressure breathing (IPPB) machine. This improves the exchange of air since it supplements the respiratory muscle action and provides for exchange of air in the absence of central nervous system stimulation. Oxygen is given cautiously and at a low liter flow until the carbon dioxide level is lowered and the physiologic stimulus for breathing is restored. Because narcotic drugs such as morphine tend to depress respirations and may contribute to the development of carbon dioxide narcosis, they are seldom ordered.

Polycythemia may result as a compensatory mechanism for carrying more oxygen in the bloodstream, and *cor pulmonale* (a marked rise in the pressure in the pulmonary artery to accelerate blood flow through the lungs and maintain circulation) is a frequent complication of pulmonary emphysema. It is treated by increased attempts to improve ventilation, but it may eventually cause right heart failure (p. 318).

Treatment. Complete cessation of smoking is advised by the physician, and many physicians consider this to be the most important part of treatment.

Inhalation of medications. Inhalations of bronchodilating drugs may be very effective in assisting patients to obtain better ventilation of the lungs. Isoproterenol (Isuprel) 1:200 and racemic epinephrine hydrochloride (Vaponephrine) are examples of drugs commonly used. Usually four to eight drops are used, and they usually are diluted. With the force of compressed air or oxygen, a fine spray is produced and can be inhaled easily. Powdered drugs (aerosols) may also be used. These drugs may be administered four times a day. Diluents, detergents, and mucolytic agents such as sodium ethasulfate (Tergemist), distilled water, and tyloxapol (Alevaire) may be given to help liquefy and thin secretions. Antibiotics also may be administered by aerosol. Choice of the latter will depend upon the organisms involved. These medications are administered effectively in nebulizers attached to compressed air or oxygen or electric motor airpumps. Nebulization may also be used in combination with positive-pressure breathing treatments.

The nebulizer may be connected by rubber tubing to a tank of compressed air, or a low concentration of oxygen may be used. Midway in the rubber tubing connection, a glass Y tube or a slightly bent glass tube with a tiny opening on one side is inserted. The air is turned on after the desired medication has been placed in the nebulizer. Usually 4 to 6 liters of gas per minute are sufficient. The nurse should test the kind and amount of spray briefly by placing a finger over the open end of the Y tube. If a fine spray cannot be seen or felt on the hand, the equipment is not working properly. Most patients learn to use the nebulizer themselves. The patient needs to learn how to breathe and when to close off the opening with his finger. The opening in the glass tube or the open end of the Y tube should be closed on inhalation and left open on exhalation. The principles of breathing with the use of the nebulizer are the same as with the use of a hand bulb. If the patient has dyspnea, he may wish to take several normal breaths before repeating a cycle of deep inspirations with the nebulizer.

Intermittent positive-pressure breathing. Intermittent positive-pressure breathing (IPPB) therapy is prescribed by the physician as an aid to pulmonary ventilation. It increases the tidal volume, improves distribution of inhaled gas, increases arterial oxygen saturation, facilitates the elimination of carbon dioxide, and assists in regulating respiratory acid-base levels. The pressure range ordered usually ranges from 12 to 20 cm. H_2O, with 20 cm. being the desirable level. Patients may be started at lower levels until they become accustomed to the treatment. Patients usually receive three or four treatments of twenty minutes each daily. This number may be decreased as the patient improves and particularly if the patient is expected to use this treatment at home.

Gas mixtures used may be oxygen with air dilution, 40% oxygen and 60% helium, or compressed air. A humidifier should be used to counteract the drying effect of the gas.

IPPB machines are basically of two types. Many varieties are manufactured. One type employs a pressure cycle and the patient has control; the other has a volume cycle over which the patient has no control. The first is helpful to increase alveolar ventilation, to make coughing more effective, and to reduce the effort of breathing. The second type is used for patients whose ventilatory efforts no longer can produce a satisfactory tidal volume because of muscular exhaustion or because of central nervous system depression (carbon dioxide narcosis). This type of machine has largely supplanted the tank type of respirator (p. 853).

Breathing exercises. Breathing exercises are helpful to some patients with emphysema. Some institutions offer breathing improvement clinics. Patients exercise together in groups and find this arrangement stimulating as well as beneficial. Since many of the patients are elderly and may not be able to notice an immediate improvement in their breathing, they need encouragement to maintain interest and effort in learning the exercises and in practicing them faithfully. The chief aim of exercises is to increase the force of exhalation largely by increasing motion of the diaphragm. If the patient can lie flat, he should lie on his back, with the knees bent, and take in a deep breath while letting his abdomen rise. In exhaling, he should contract the abdominal muscles as he forces the air out. Placing the hands on the abdomen while doing this exercise helps the patient to concentrate on breathing with the abdominal muscles. If he must be in a sitting position, the same exercise can be done. In addition, he should let his body relax completely while breathing out and should lean forward, allowing the arms to hang loose. Other simple exercises to increase forceful expiration are conscious forceful blowing out of air, hissing through the teeth, blowing into paper bags, blowing a pencil along a table top, and blowing into balloons. (For further details see reference at the end of this chapter.[23])

Care at home. Unless there is an acute attack of dyspnea caused by overexertion, or unless an acute infection in the lungs occurs, patients with emphysema remain at home. The nurse should help the patient and his family to plan so that he may live a fairly satisfactory life within the limitations of his disease. The effectiveness of treatment prescribed has been found to depend a good deal, at times, upon the patient's understanding of his illness. Daily schedules may need rearrangement so that activities are not too intensive or engaged in all at one time. For example, almost all patients with emphysema have a severe bout of coughing upon arising as secretions that have accumulated during the night are raised; a period of rest should be planned following this. If the patient goes to work, he may have to arise earlier than usual to allow time for rest after the exertion of coughing. Since sudden exertion taxes the respiratory system and usually precipitates more coughing, the patient's morning schedule should be planned so that he can arise, dress slowly, and eat breakfast in a leisurely manner. Means of getting to work and the daily work schedule may also need modifications to provide a fairly leisurely pace with rest periods at intervals.

GENERAL NURSING CARE IN RESPIRATORY DISEASE

Difficulties in breathing. The patient with respiratory disease may have very slight or severe difficulty in breathing. There may be obstruction to the free passage of air through the bronchi and/or damage to lung tissues. The patient may have both of these difficulties. If so, more effort is required for breathing, and the patient is more aware of breathing. This is tiring and unpleasant. With increased difficulty in getting air, most patients become apprehensive and even panicky. A nurse who understands this can be a

great comfort to the patient. The presence of another person often helps the patient to control fear and eases his efforts in breathing.

Position. The most comfortable position for more relaxed breathing is a semiupright or upright sitting position. In these positions the lungs and respiratory muscles are not cramped and thus are not working against resistance. A pillow placed lengthwise at the patient's back will support him and will keep the thorax thrust slightly forward, allowing freer use of the diaphragm and therefore deeper breathing. For patients who must be upright, the overbed table with a pillow on top can be used as a support and a resting place for the head and arms. If the patient has marked breathing difficulty and is not sufficiently alert or is very alert and fearful, side rails should be used for additional security. The patient may also use them to pull himself up into a higher sitting position. If the patient is at home and has a chronic problem, he may prefer to sit up in a large chair that supports him well and to lean toward a smaller chair placed in front of him. This chair should be blocked to prevent it from slipping.

Since the diaphragm becomes flattened and less active, some patients find breathing is helped by wearing an elasticized abdominal support. The support is often made of material similar to that used in elasticized girdles. Men may need to be persuaded to wear this kind of support but, upon trial, learn how much the support adds to comfort and accept it quite readily. Pressure from the girdle must be from below the umbilicus upward, so that the flattened diaphragm is forced up into the thorax.

Ventilation

Proper ventilation and temperature of the room will help the patient to breathe more easily. Irritants such as smoke should be excluded. Patients may have preferences as to room temperature and amount of fresh air, and the nurse should respect these preferences. In general, most patients breathe more easily if the air is cool. Occasionally an oxygen tent is used for its air-cooling effect. An air-conditioned room may make breathing easier.

For patients with nose, throat, and bronchial irritation, warm, moist air produced by a *vaporizer* may be beneficial. A vaporizer can be used to humidify the air throughout the room, or it can be put in close proximity to the patient so that he can inhale the steam as it is released. The large electrically operated vaporizers used in hospitals serve to moisten the air in the entire room. Water flowing from a gallon-sized jar is heated to form steam that is then directed out through a long, flexible spout. Inhalations of plain steam or of an aromatic medication such as tincture of benzoin or menthol are often ordered.

If the patient is at home, the nurse can help him and his family to improvise equipment for inhalations and for proper humidity. An empty coffee can or a shallow pie tin can be filled with water and placed on an electric plate in the patient's room to increase humidity. If the inhalation is to be directed, an ordinary steam kettle or a kettle with a longer improvised paper spout may be used. The paper needs to be changed frequently. A few drops of menthol or oil of eucalyptus can be put into the water. Benzoin will cause corrosion in the kettle, which is exceedingly difficult to remove. The kettle and electric plate should be placed a safe distance from the patient's face so that he can breathe the medicated steam, yet not be burned by accidentally tipping the kettle or by touching the hot plate. After the twenty-five to thirty minute treatment, equipment should be removed from the bedside.

Small electric vaporizers can be purchased at most local drug stores. They usually consist of a pint-sized or larger jar with a heating element extending into the jar. The jar should be filled with ordinary tap water and a pinch of salt added to hasten heating. The top of the jar holds a small, removable perforated cup, to which is attached a small metal spout. Cotton saturated with medication is placed inside the cup, and the small metal spout is fitted over the cup. As the water boils, the medicated steam is directed out through the small spout. Jars for the set are usually replaceable and inexpensive.

If breathing is so difficult that the patient cannot get enough oxygen from the air, it may be necessary to give additional oxygen. Dyspnea and cyanosis are not always present, and increased pulse rate may be the first detectable sign of oxygen shortage. The nurse, therefore, should check the patient's pulse rate carefully as well as his color and the character and the rate of respirations. Oxygen may be administered by tent, by nasal catheter, or by mask. The method used depends on the patient, his need, and the concentration of oxygen necessary. If oxygen is not readily available, increasing the amount of fresh air may help. The nurse should be familiar with operation of the various devices used to administer oxygen and should check frequently to note whether they are operating properly. (For details of nursing care of patients receiving oxygen, see texts on fundamentals of nursing.)

When the patient is having difficulty in the exchange of inspired and expired air, oxygen or sometimes compressed air may be given under *positive pressure*. Intermittent positive-pressure breathing machines such as the Bennett respirator are most often used. These are discussed in the section dealing with emphysema. In an emergency, mouth-to-mouth breathing may be used (p. 241).

Continued uncorrected difficulty in breathing may cause an excess of carbon dioxide or a deficiency of carbon dioxide in the bloodstream. The former is due to incomplete exhalation and causes acidosis. The latter is due to hyperventilation and causes respiratory alkalosis (p. 101). If the patient's greatest difficulty is exhalation and if inspiration becomes slower and deeper, there is danger of carbon dioxide narcosis, and oxygen should *not* be given, since a low oxygen level in the blood may be the only stimulus for respiration. The nurse must notify the doctor at once if this occurs.

Coughing

Two of the most troublesome symptoms of respiratory disease are the increase in mucous secretions as a result of inflamed mucous membranes and the stimulation of coughing due to irritation of the respiratory tract. If coughing is productive, the patient should be encouraged to cough in order to keep air passages clear and allow sufficient oxygen to reach the alveoli. Changing the patient's position will help to prevent pooling of secretions in the lungs and will stimulate coughing. The patient should be instructed to breathe as deeply as possible to loosen secretions and to stimulate productive coughing. For an effective cough, the patient should take a deep inspiration, contract the diaphragm and intercostal muscles, and exhale forcefully. Any sputum raised should always be expectorated, not swallowed. If he cannot cough forcefully enough to raise sputum and if his respirations are very shallow or sound very moist, he is often given a medication to thin the secretions. The medication may be given as a nebulizer treatment so that it is applied topically to the respiratory passages.

Many patients with obvious, noisy respirations caused by accumulated sputum hesitate to cough because they fear that coughing will cause pain. The nurse can assist these patients by placing her hands on the front and back of the chest to give support as the patient coughs (Fig. 133). A towel placed around the chest and held snugly as the patient coughs may also be used.

Although coughing is a physiologic protective reflex, constant nonproductive coughing and hacking can lead to exhaustion. Medications, therefore, are often prescribed for coughing. The type prescribed depends on the nature of the cough and the secretions. The purposes of various cough medications are to increase secretions, to decrease secretions, to thin secretions so that they can be raised and expectorated more easily, or to depress the cough reflex.

Sedative expectorants increase secretions, protect irritated membranes, and lessen the amount of coughing. Increased secretions may result in a productive cough and make paroxysms of coughing less frequent. For this purpose, ammonium chloride in wild cherry or orange syrup is often ordered, and other mixtures such as iodide solutions or ipecac syrup are sometimes used. Detergent drugs, such as Tergemist and Alevaire, and normal saline solution have been found to be effective in thinning secretions. The mucolytic enzymes, trypsin (Tryptar) and pancreatic dornase (Dornavac), are useful if the secretions are purulent. Stimulating expectorants, such as terpin hydrate, diminish secretions and promote repair and healing of the mucous membrane.

When the main objective of treatment is to suppress coughing, drugs depressing the cough center in the medulla are ordered. Codeine is frequently used and may be added to elixir of terpin hydrate, but there is danger of addiction in its prolonged use. Recently some new nonnarcotic drugs with actions similar to codeine have been prescribed widely. Among them are dextromethorphan (Romilar hydrobromide) and noscapine (Nectadon).

When respiratory difficulty is severe, secretions are present, but coughing is unproductive, intratracheal suctioning and occasionally bronchoscopy are necessary. By means of bronchoscopy, mucous plugs may be loosened or removed and intratracheal suctioning made more effective. Equipment for emergency bronchoscopy may be kept in the patient's room. When this procedure is ordered the nurse must see that electrical outlets are adequate and that the necessary equipment is assembled in one place and ready for immediate use. (See p. 538 for care of the patient during bronchoscopy.)

Postural drainage. Postural drainage may be used to assist the patient who has difficulty in raising sputum. By means of gravity, secretions flow into the bronchi and trachea and into the back of the throat and can be raised and expectorated more easily. A position providing gravity drainage of the lungs can be achieved in several ways, and the procedure selected usually depends on the age of the patient and his general condition, as well as the lobe or lobes of the lungs where secretions have accumulated. The young patient may tolerate farther lowering of the head than an elderly patient, whose vascular system adapts less quickly to change of position. A severely debilitated patient may need a modified procedure because of the danger of an accident. To accomplish postural drainage, the patient may lie across the bed on his abdomen, with his head and chest extending over the edge of the bed. A chair or a high stool can be placed on the side of the bed so that he can support himself in this jackknife position. A small basin or widemouthed cup can be placed on the chair, which should be protected with newspaper.

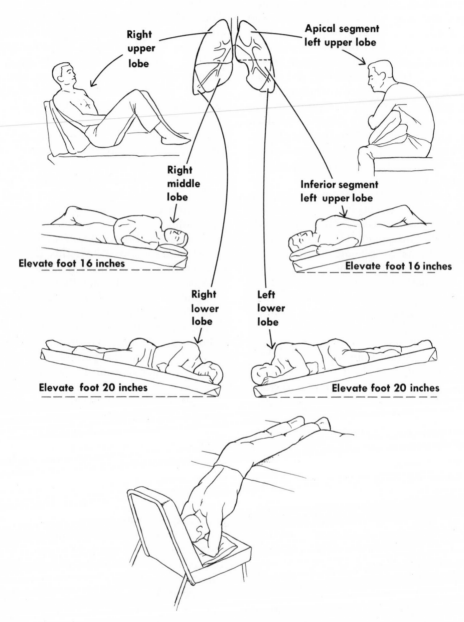

Fig. 130

Postural drainage requires that the patient assume various positions to facilitate the flow of secretions from various portions of the lung into the bronchi, trachea, and throat so that they can be raised and expectorated more easily. Drawing shows the correct position to drain various portions of the lung. At the bottom of the drawing is illustrated a frequently ordered and less specific position, in which the patient lies across the bed, with his arms resting on a pillow on a chair.

A Gatch bed can be used for postural drainage. Most patients prefer this method because it provides more support and therefore is less taxing than being suspended over the side of the bed. The knee-gatch is raised as high as possible, and the patient lies over the bend in the bed foundation so that his head and chest are dependent. To provide something firm on which the patient can rest his arms and hands for more security and to provide a place for the sputum container, a board can be placed flat across the lower part of the bed frame in the space between the springs and the mattress.

Postural drainage achieved merely by putting blocks under the casters at the foot of the bed sometimes produces excellent results. The footboard of the bed may also be supported on the seat of a firm chair to provide a position in which the head is lowered. Tilt boards (special tables that can be raised or lowered to any angle) or Stryker frames are sometimes used, but many doctors prefer raising the foot of the bed since this entails much less exertion for the patient.

The nurse should know the part of the lung affected and should help the patient assume a position that is best for draining that portion (Fig. 130). For example, if the right middle lobe of the lung is affected, drainage will be accomplished best by way of the right middle bronchus. The patient should lie on his back with his body turned at approximately a 45-degree angle. The angle can be maintained by pillow supports placed under the right side from the shoulders to the hips. The foot of the bed should then be raised about twelve inches. This position can be maintained fairly comfortably by most patients for half an hour at a time. On the other hand, if the lower posterior area of the lung is affected, the jackknife position already described is most effective.

Patients having postural drainage of any kind are encouraged to breathe deeply and to cough forcefully to help dislodge thick sputum and exudate that is pooled in distended bronchioles, particularly after inactivity. Any medication to thin secretions, dilate the bronchioles, or stimulate expectoration should be given fifteen to twenty minutes before postural drainage is started. The patient may find that he can raise sputum upon resuming an upright position even though no drainage appeared while he was lying with his head and chest lowered.

Since some patients complain of dizziness when assuming position for postural drainage, the nurse should stay with the patient during the first few times, and she should report any persistent dizziness or unusual discomfort to the doctor. Postural drainage may be contraindicated in some patients because of heart disease, hypertension, or age. However, most patients can be taught to assume the position for postural drainage and can proceed without help. Often patients with a chronic problem need to be taught to do this independently so that they can continue at home. The position usually is maintained for ten minutes at first, and the period of time is gradually lengthened to fifteen or twenty or even thirty minutes as the patient becomes accustomed to the sometimes almost "upside-down" position. At first, elderly patients usually are able to tolerate the unusual position only for a few minutes. They need more assistance than most other patients during the procedure and immediately thereafter. They should be assisted to a normal position in bed and requested to lie flat for a few minutes before sitting up or getting out of bed. This helps to prevent dizziness and reduces danger of accidents.

The patient may feel nauseated because of the odor and taste of sputum. Therefore, the procedure should be timed so that it comes at least forty-five minutes to an hour before meals. A short rest period following the treatment often improves the appetite. The patient needs mouth care following postural drainage. Aromatic mouthwashes should be available for frequent use by any patient who is expectorating sputum freely.

Care of sputum. Since the causative organisms may not be known early in the respiratory disease, the nurse should use caution in the disposal of sputum and should instruct the patient to protect others. The patient who is coughing or clearing his throat forcefully should be instructed to cover his mouth and nose with several thicknesses of disposable tissues to prevent possible spread of infectious organisms. The nurse should be calm and matter-of-fact in doing this so that the patient does not feel that he is dangerous to others or that he has some dread disease.

Used tissues should be folded carefully and placed in a paper bag or flushed directly down the toilet. If a bag is used, it should be closed and preferably burned. Used tissues should be collected from the bedfast patient at frequent intervals, and whoever handles the bags should wash his hands thoroughly to avoid transfer of infection to others.

If the patient has a copious amount of sputum, he may be instructed in the use of a sputum cup. Waxed paper cups with lids may be used. In some hospitals the waxed paper cups are placed in metal containers. At least once daily, the inner cup should be discarded and a fresh one provided. The metal containers frequently become contaminated with sputum and therefore should be washed and boiled often. Some hospitals have a schedule for boiling them daily.

If the patient cannot care for and dispose of his own sputum, he must have assistance. Tissues may be placed in the patient's hand, and a paper bag may be placed on each side of the bed so that he does not have to turn to dispose of the soiled tissues. The bedfast patient who handles his own sputum should be offered soap and water with which to wash his hands before meals.

Appetite and nutrition

The odor and taste in the mouth caused by frequent raising of sputum may seriously affect appetite and may impair nutrition. Provision should be made for oral hygiene before meals, washing of hands should be encouraged, and sputum cups or other evidence of sputum should be removed before meals are served. Some patients find that a strong, clear, well-seasoned broth helps to make the mouth feel fresher and improves appetite for the rest of the meal. Other patients report that beginning a meal with acid fluids, such as grapefruit or tomato juice, improves acceptance of other food. The nurse should report food preferences to the dietitian.

Frequently, patients with breathing difficulties tolerate regular full meals poorly. Smaller and more frequent meals are taken with greater comfort, and thus nutrition is maintained. Gas-forming foods should be avoided. Taking fluids frequently also helps to keep mucous secretions thin. The patient should try to take fluids every few hours. This measure will also help to counteract constipation and thereby lessen straining and exertion.

Rest

Adequate rest is important in combating respiratory disease. During respiratory illness, however, normal sleep may be interrupted for a number of reasons. The patient may be plagued with frequent coughing, and breathing may be difficult. Airways may become blocked with secretions, and the patient may be awakened by the resultant increased difficulty in breathing.

The nurse should be alert for signs of what irritates the patient, precipitates cough, and therefore prevents rest. For example, excessive talking, smoking, or laughing, or sitting in a draft or in a dry, overheated room may predispose to coughing. Cough medications given before the hour of sleep and when rest is disturbed by coughing are often helpful. However, when the patient has noisy breathing and it is obvious that secretions are present in the respiratory tract, he should be encouraged to cough deeply and to expectorate until the airway is free of obstruction before medication is given. A suitable position in bed and changes in position also help the patient to rest more quietly. Room temperature and ventilation should be kept at what the patient feels is best for him.

Prevention of new infection

Patients with any type of respiratory disease should protect themselves against exposure to new infection. They should avoid outdoor exertion in cold weather and extremes of cold or humidity. If they must go out in cold, damp weather, warm clothing should be worn. If the clothing gets wet, it should be changed immediately. Smoking should be discouraged. Undue emotional stress may also lessen the patient's resistance and increase susceptibility to additional infection.

OTHER CHRONIC LUNG DISEASES
Bronchiectasis

Bronchiectasis means dilation of the bronchus or bronchi. When infection attacks the bronchial lining, inflammation occurs and an exudate forms. The progressive accumulation of secretions mechanically distends the bronchioles. With repeated infection, the bronchioles become permanently distended and appear saccular and cylindrical in shape. Their expulsive force is diminished, and they may remain filled with exudate. Only forceful coughing and postural drainage will empty them. Bronchiectasis may involve any part of the lung parenchyma, but it usually occurs in the dependent portions or lobules. The disease begins in young people, many patients showing symptoms by the age of 20 years. The initial contributing factor is a congenital weakness in the structure of the alveoli so that elasticity is not normal. Bronchiectasis may occur without previous pulmonary disease, but it usually follows such diseases as bronchopneumonia, lung abscess, tuberculosis, or asthma.

Symptoms of bronchiectasis vary with the severity of the condition. The patient may complain of fatigue, weakness, and loss of weight. Appetite can be affected by the fetid sputum. The condition may be develop so gradually that the patient is often unable to tell when symptoms first began. Clubbing of the fingers is common, as it is in other chronic respiratory disease. The patient's chief complaint in bronchiectasis is severe coughing (brought on by changing position) that is productive of large amounts of sputum and causes dyspnea. The patient may have a paroxysm of coughing when he gets up in the morning and again when he lies down.

Treatment of bronchiectasis is not very satisfactory. Surgical removal of a portion of the lung is the only cure (p. 576). Therefore, patients who have bronchiectasis that involves both lungs are not amenable to surgical cure and do not have a good prognosis. The life expectancy usually is considered to be no more than twenty years. Many patients develop cardiac complications resulting from the extra strain on the heart caused by inability of the lungs to oxygenate the blood adequately.

Postural drainage at least twice a day helps to remove secretions and thus helps to prevent coughing. (See previous discussion, p. 565). During severe episodes of coughing, the patient should not be left alone, since a large plug of thick secretion may block a large bronchiole and cause severe dyspnea and cyanosis. Occasionally, a bronchoscopy may be done to remove the plug of mucus or to break adhesions that may be interfering with postural drainage by blocking passage to the main bronchi. Antibiotics may be used in the treatment of bronchiectasis. Although these drugs do not cure the condition, they may prevent further infection and are often used prior to surgery, both by parenteral and inhalation routes. If the involvement of the lung is widespread, oxygen may be used. Nursing care should stress good general hygiene, which may contribute to relief of symptoms. Adequate diet, rest, exercise, and diversional activity are important, and avoiding superimposed infections such as colds should be emphasized. Frequent mouth care is essential, and cleansing the mouth with an aromatic solution before meals often makes food more acceptable.

Pulmonary fibrosis

Pulmonary fibrosis is extensive scarring of lung tissue with areas of calcification. It often develops in persons whose work involves inhalation of dusts such as coal, marble, or iron over long periods of time. When it is caused by stone or marble dust, it is known as *silicosis*. Pulmonary fibrosis also occurs with collagen diseases such as scleroderma, polyarteritis nodosa, and systemic lupus erythematosus. It may complicate histoplasmosis and tuberculosis in which there has been extensive bilateral involvement.

The patient with pulmonary fibrosis has respiratory embarrassment because of limited usable lung tissue. Cardiac complications may follow since heart action must be increased to make up for respiratory impairment. There is no cure and no specific treatment for pulmonary fibrosis. Breathing exercises may be prescribed in an effort to preserve, for as long as possible, the elasticity of lung tissue. The patient is cautioned to avoid strenuous exercise that will tax the respiratory and cardiac systems and, above all, to guard against exposure to upper respiratory infection.

In recent years adrenocortical steroids have been used in the treatment of pulmonary fibrosis. They appear to improve the condition especially when it follows or accompanies collagen disease. (For problems associated with the administration of these steroids, see p. 63.)

Histoplasmosis

Histoplasmosis is a fungus disease that affects the lungs. Now that more has been learned about the disease, it is recognized that the incidence is quite high in the United States. It is most prevalent in the rural sections of the central states, but its incidence is also high in the mid-Atlantic states. It is estimated that one in four of the farm population has been exposed to the disease. It is not communicable from man to man. Organisms are transmitted to man by inhaling spores that thrive in moist, dark, protected soil. The disease masquerades as either influenza or chronic tuberculosis with cavities. It is diagnosed by the presence of nodular infiltrations found on roentgenography and a skin reaction to the intradermal injection of histoplasmin. This test is done by a method similar to the Heaf test for tuberculosis. An indurated area of 5 mm. or more appearing at the site of injection within forty-eight hours is considered a positive reaction.

Histoplasmosis responds to treatment with an antibiotic drug, *amphotericin B*. Since it must be given intravenously and causes toxic reactions, such as gastrointestinal symptoms, headache and cough, the patient is hospitalized and observed closely during treatment. The infusion containing the drug is given over a five-hour or six-hour period. It is administered every other day for about eight weeks. Acetylsalicylic acid and promethazine hydrochloride, an antiemetic antihistamine, are often given a half hour before the infusion is started and repeated as necessary. Hydrocortisone may be given to reduce the side effects. A blood urea nitrogen test or nonprotein nitrogen determination is usually taken every two or three days during treatment because the drug may cause kidney damage. Any symptoms of potassium deficiency (p. 99) or anemia (p. 405) should be reported to the doctor at once. The general nursing care is similar to that for the patient with noninfectious tuberculosis.

Nurses working in areas where this disease is prevalent have an important role in helping to locate sources of infection and in teaching the public to prevent inhalation of potentially infected material. Since the disease can be fatal and children appear to be particularly susceptible, the nurse should point out potential danger to rural families when it is known that the soil is contaminated.

OTHER CHEST CONDITIONS
Lung abscess

A lung abscess is an area of localized suppuration within the lung. It usually is caused by bacteria that reach the lung through aspiration. The infected material lodges in the small bronchi and produces inflammation. Partial obstruction of the bronchus results in the retention of secretions beyond the obstruction and the eventual necrosis of tissue. Before the advent of antibiotics and specific chemotherapy, lung abscess was a fairly frequent complication following pneumonia. When a lung abscess forms, various organisms are found. Lung abscess may follow bronchial obstruction caused by a tumor, a foreign body, or a stenosis of the bronchus. Children particularly may aspirate foreign material, such as a peanut, and a lung abscess results. Metastatic spread of cancer cells to the lung parenchyma may also cause an abscess, and occasionally the infection appears to have been borne by the bloodstream. In recent years the incidence of lung abscess due to infection has decreased, and secondary lung abscess following bronchogenic carcinoma has increased.

Symptoms of lung abscess include cough, elevation of temperature, loss of appetite, malaise, and, if the condition is of long standing, clubbing of the fingers. Unless the abcess is walled off, so that there is no access to the bronchi, the patient usually raises sputum. There may be hemoptysis, and often the patient raises dark brown, or "chocolate-colored," sputum that contains both blood and pus.

The patient's course in lung abscess is influenced by the cause of the abscess and by the kind of drainage that can be established. If the purulent material drains easily, the patient may respond well to postural drainage, antibiotic therapy, and good general supportive care. Small adhesions that may be interfering with drainage into the bronchi may be broken by means of a bronchoscopic procedure. Today, surgical treatment to establish drainage has become increasingly less necessary. Chemical debridement is accomplished by nebulizer administration of crys-

:alline trypsin (Tryptar). Trypsin, 125 mg., s dissolved in water, 2 ml., and inhaled daily as a spray for five to ten days. Antibiotics also are given systemically. Special care needs to be given to be sure the patient is in a position for postural drainage that will drain the affected portion of the lung. (See discussion of postural drainage, p. 565.) If Tryptar is being given, the postural drainage should follow its administration to enhance drainage. Productive coughing must always be encouraged after a nebulizer treatment, and sputum should never be swallowed. Frequent mouth care is exceedingly important and should always be given before meals.

Medical treatment cannot cause a walled-off abscess to disappear, and surgery may be necessary. If surgery is done, the portion of lung containing the abscess is removed. If the abscess is due to carcinoma, the surgery may be much more extensive.

Empyema

Empyema means pus within a body cavity. It usually applies to the pleural cavity. Empyema occurs as a result of, or in association with, other respiratory disease, such as pneumonia, lung abscess, tuberculosis, and fungus infections of the lung, and also following thoracic surgery or chest trauma. It is now occurring fairly often as a complication of staphylococcal pneumonia. The patient with any kind of lung infection or chest injury should be observed closely for signs of empyema, which include cough, dyspnea, unilateral chest pain, elevation of temperature, malaise, poor appetite, and unequal chest expansion. The condition may develop several weeks after an apparently minor respiratory infection. The diagnosis can usually be made from the signs and symptoms and the medical history, but it is confirmed by a roentgenogram of the chest and examination of the lungs under a fluoroscope. Sometimes a thoracentesis is done to confirm the diagnosis of fluid in the pleural space, to obtain a culture of the organisms, and to relieve the patient's respiratory symptoms. (For details of equipment needed for this treatment, see texts on fundamentals of nursing.)

If a *thoracentesis* is to be done, the procedure should be explained to the patient. It is important that he be instructed not to move when the needle is inserted lest damage to the lung or pleura occur. Usually procaine is used to eliminate pain at the site of insertion of the needle. However, when the pleura is entered, a sensation of pain or pressure may occur. The patient should be in a sitting position, and he should be made as comfortable as possible. Sometimes leaning forward over an overbed table that is well padded with pillows is satisfactory, since the table can be raised to support the arms and shoulders and keep them slightly elevated. Raising the arms and shoulders elevates the ribs and makes it easier for the doctor to carry out the procedure. If the patient is extremely ill, apprehensive, or debilitated, two nurses must assist with this procedure. One attends and observes the patient and the other assists the doctor. The patient's respiratory rate should be taken several times during the procedure, and he must be watched for any changes in color and breathing, and for excessive diaphoresis. The needle and syringe should be carefully checked to see that they fit snugly since no air should be permitted to enter the pleural cavity. After the fluid is withdrawn into a 20 or 50 ml. syringe, it should be placed in a proper container and carefully labeled for microscopic examination and for culture. Following a thoracentesis the patient is watched for signs of coughing or raising blood, since these signs might indicate that the lung was traumatized inadvertently.

After diagnosis and determination of the organisms within the pleural space, treatment is begun. The patient is given the antibiotic that is specific for the infecting organism. Subsequent thoracenteses usually will be performed to determine the activity of remaining organisms. The primary aim of treatment is to clear the infection, eliminate fluid, and promote expansion of the lung. When organisms disappear and only a small amount of fluid remains, the lung will expand to its normal size. This usually takes a few months.

During the period of intensive chemotherapy and while he has definite symptoms, the patient is kept on bed rest. He is usually more comfortable lying on his affected side since this position helps to splint the chest and thus to lessen pain. A firm mattress also lessens discomfort. If he has dyspnea, the head of the bed may need to be elevated to facilitate lung expansion. The doctor may not want the patient to turn to the unaffected side because this may increase the danger of spreading the infection and also may further the danger of mediastinal shift. Medication such as codeine to suppress cough and relieve pain may be ordered. Changes in pulse rate, color, and rate of respiration are most important since sudden changes may indicate mediastinal shift, with subsequent pressure on the normally functioning lung.

Mobility is encouraged during convalescence, and the nurse should allow the patient opportunity to help himself in his own daily personal care. She should encourage use of the extremities on the affected side since the patient may feel activity will cause renewed pain or regression of the disease. When the infection is controlled and the pleural space is obliterated, the arm can be used for stretching and reaching without harm. During convalescence exercises to lessen the chances of postural deformity should be done by the patient and are usually ordered by the physician.[40]

Since the discovery of the antibiotics and specific chemotherapeutic agents, surgery is seldom necessary in the treatment of empyema. Occasionally, when infection persists, adhesions form, and areas become walled off, it may be necessary to resort to surgical drainage. A surgical incision may be made into the chest and a thoracotomy tube (catheter) inserted at the lower level of the infected cavity. The catheter is attached to water-seal drainage or suction and left in position until the drainage subsides. (See nursing care of the patient with chest drainage, p. 577.) If the pleura has firmly adhered to the chest wall so that there is little danger of the occurrence of a pneumothorax, Penrose drains may be placed in the incision in a manner similar to that used for any infected wound. The care is then that of any infected, draining wound. The patient should be observed carefully, however, for any signs of pneumothorax.

Carcinoma

During the last thirty years there has been a startling increase in the incidence of carcinoma of the lung. There were 49,187 deaths from malignancies of the respiratory

tract in 1964.[66] The American Cancer Society estimated that there were 55,000 new cases of carcinoma of the lung in 1965 and 50,000 deaths in 1965.[2a] It is now the most common form of cancer among men, leading all other respiratory system disease as the cause of death among white men. Carcinoma of the lung is six times as frequent among men as women. Most people who develop the disease are over 45 years of age. Some of the factors believed to be involved in this increase in incidence of carcinoma of the lung include more accurate diagnosis and a tendency to name the lung as the primary site.

The cause of carcinoma of the lung is unknown, but it is believed that chronic irritation contributes to its development. Special occupations in which workers are exposed to radioactive substances or to certain chemicals are felt to be of significance in the production of carcinoma of the lung. History of heavy smoking is common, and it is almost certain that it is a factor contributing to the disease. Statistical studies show that ten times as many people who smoke die of cancer of the lung than those who do not smoke. Studies show, too, that the more a person smokes the greater the risk of developing lung cancer. Laboratory studies have shown that the tar in cigarette smoke contains a number of agents that will produce cancer in animals, and other studies show that cigarette smoke weakens the natural defenses of the lungs.[57] Air heavily polluted with smoke, the exhaust from automobiles, and other industrial fumes probably is a contributing factor as well.

Prevention is the best protection against carcinoma of the lung because early detection of the disease is most difficult, and at the present time only about one patient in twenty is "cured" (living at the end of five years).[57] From available research data it seems evident that curtailing smoking is a primary preventive measure. The nurse should be active in teaching the dangers in smoking and should herself set a good example to others in this regard. It is especially important that teen-agers be given specific facts concerning the dangers involved in cigarette smoking because they are not likely to be habitual smokers at that age. People who are already habitual smokers should also be urged to stop smoking, even though it may be very difficult for them to do so. Since it is also highly possible that air pollution affects the lungs and may predispose to the development of carcinoma, the nurse should also encourage and actively support community programs to decrease the amount of air pollution.

Carcinoma of the lungs may be either metastatic or primary. Metastatic tumors may follow malignancy anywhere in the body. Metastasis from the prostate, uterus, thyroid, larynx, breast, and suprarenal gland is common. Metastasis to the lung may be discovered before the primary lesion is known, and sometimes the location of the primary lesion is not determined during the patient's life.

Since most new growths in the lungs arise from the bronchi, the term *bronchogenic carcinoma* is widely used. The growth of new cells produces bronchial narrowing, and eventually a cough and dyspnea develop. The symptoms produced by the new growth depend upon its size and location. If the growth is small and is located in the main bronchus, there may be a cough. On the other hand, if the growth is in a small bronchus in the periphery of the lung, it may grow to a considerable size before producing symptoms. Very often there are no early signs of the disease. Close observation of patients and investigation of small, seemingly unimportant symptoms can be important in early case finding. Attention should be given to persistent cough. Shortness of breath, unexplained fever, and loss of weight may be warning signs.

Time is very important in the treatment of lung cancer. If carcinoma is detected while it is still confined to a local area, immediate surgery, with removal of all or part of a lung (lobectomy or pneumonectomy), may be successful. The nursing care of the patient following surgery of the lung is discussed later in this chapter.

Radiation therapy may be used in the control of the growth of cancer of the lung when it is not possible to remove all the growth surgically. If the disease is allowed to go untreated, life expectancy is probably lessened.

Radioactive gold (Au[198]) is sometimes left in the pleural cavity following surgery to help destroy any malignant cells that may remain in surrounding tissue or lymph nodes. It is also used in the treatment of pleural effusion (fluid exuded into the pleural cavity from the surface of the lungs and producing symptoms similar to those seen in empyema), which rather often complicates far-advanced carcinoma of the lung. The radioactive gold may also be given through a thoracentesis. (See p. 278 for care of patients receiving x-ray therapy or radioactive substances.)

Metastasis occurs to the mediastinal lymph nodes, to the walls of the esophagus, to the pericardium and heart, and to the opposite lung or to the cervical lymph nodes. If the patient has advanced carcinoma of the lung, marked dyspnea, with wheezing, weakness, loss of weight and of appetite, cough, and pain are the usual symptoms. All supportive nursing measures should be used to make the patient as comfortable as possible. (See p. 290 for details.)

Efforts to detect malignant lesions of the lung early while curative treatment may be possible must be continued. The nurse should urge all persons, particularly men over 40 years of age, to have an x-ray examination of the chest periodically in addition to a yearly physical examination. As a result of various public education media, many people have become more conscious of early signs of pulmonary cancer, but there is still a great need for them to learn about diagnostic tests that are available, including x-ray examinations, bronchoscopic examinations, and cytologic studies of sputum. The nurse should know of available cancer detection clinics in her community and should assist patients to secure proper medical supervision.

Pulmonary embolism and pulmonary infarction

Pulmonary embolism is the lodgment of a clot or other foreign matter in a pulmonary arterial vessel, and pulmonary infarction is the hemorrhagic necrosis of a part of the lung parenchyma due to interruption of its blood supply, usually as a result of embolism.[4]

The embolism usually comes from a thrombosed vein in the pelvis or the lower extremities. It may cause symptoms before any signs of venous thrombosis appear at its place of origin.

The size of the pulmonary artery in which the clot lodges determines the severity of symptoms and the prognosis. If the embolus is sufficiently large, immediate death may occur before any symptoms are reported by the patient. If it is less severe, the patient may complain of sudden sharp upper abdominal or thoracic pain, be dyspneic, cough violently, and have hemoptysis; shock may develop rapidly. If the embolus is a small one and the area of infarction is small, the symptoms are much milder. The patient may have cough, pain in the chest, slight hemoptysis, and elevation of temperature with increase of leukocyte count in the blood. An area of dullness can be detected by the doctor upon listening to the patient's chest sounds.

If the patient survives a severe pulmonary infarction, he needs immediate medical attention. While awaiting the doctor he should be kept in bed and as quiet as possible. A high Fowler's position usually helps breathing. The subsequent medical and nursing care are similar to that needed by the patient who has an acute myocardial infarction (p. 344). If the infarction is a mild one, the treatment is more conservative and resembles that provided for the patient with pneumonia. In either case an immediate attempt is made to locate the original source of the embolus and to treat the thrombosis.

The development of techniques to provide extracorporeal circulation (p. 354) has made it possible to remove emboli from the pulmonary arteries—a major step forward, since pulmonary emboli cause many deaths. At present this surgery is done quite rarely and, of course, it is possible only when the patient survives the initial infarction. The nursing care following pulmonary artery surgery combines that needed after any operation on major blood vessels (p. 381) and the postoperative care of patients having thoracic surgery, as well as the care of the patient being treated medically for pulmonary embolism.

The best treatment for pulmonary embolism is prevention. Prevention of thrombophlebitis in patients undergoing surgery is discussed on p. 197. The nurse must remember, too, that thrombosis can occur easily in the patient who is being treated only for a medical condition. This is particularly true when the patient is elderly and has chronic vascular and cardiac disease. The *very same* nursing measures that are employed to prevent development of thrombophlebitis in surgical patients must be used.

Pneumothorax

Pneumothorax is a condition in which there is air in the pleural cavity between the lung and the chest wall (Fig. 131). It usually results from the rupture of an emphysematous bleb on the surface of the lung, but it may also follow severe bouts of coughing in persons who suffer from a chronic chest disease such as asthma. It occurs when wounds have penetrated the chest wall and perforated the pleura. Rather frequently it occurs as a single or recurrent episode in otherwise healthy young people. Air in the pleural space reduces normal negative intrapleural pressure and causes the heart and mediastinum to shift toward the unaffected side. Loss of negative pressure on the affected side prevents expansion of the lung, and the mediastinal shift hampers activity of the lung on the unaffected side so that severe dyspnea develops.

A *spontaneous pneumothorax* occurs without warning. The patient has a sudden sharp pain in the chest, accompanied by dyspnea, anxiety, increased diaphoresis, weak and rapid pulse, fall in blood pressure, and cessation of normal chest movement on the affected side. When a spontaneous pneumothorax is suspected, a doctor should be summoned immediately. The patient should not be left alone. He should be reassured and urged to be quiet and not to exert himself. Oxygen and equipment for a thoracentesis should be assembled at once. Air is immediately aspirated from the affected pleural space, and the level of pressure is brought to normal if possible. If air continues to flow into the pleural space, continuous drainage of air with closed-chest drainage equipment is necessary. If the cause of the condition is trauma, treatment is to seal the chest wound and then to aspirate air from the pleural space.

The patient who has had a spontaneous pneumothorax is usually most comfortable in a sitting position. Physical activity is kept at a minimum for at least twenty-four hours. The patient is asked to remain as quiet as possible and to avoid stretching, reaching, or moving suddenly. He should breathe normally and not hold his breath. His pulse rate and respirations must be checked frequently. Roentgenograms are always ordered to determine the amount of air in the pleural cavity and the amount of collapse of the lung, as well as the degree of mediastinal shift. When roentgenograms are taken, the patient needs help to prevent overexertion.

When air no longer is expelled from the pleural cavity through the underwater suction drainage system, the patient's symptoms have subsided, and the lung has completely reexpanded, the patient is allowed out of bed. He may be advised to avoid strenuous exertion, which increases rate and depth of respirations for a time, but usually he may return to relatively normal activity rather

quickly. If there are frequently recurring episodes, the portion containing the defect may be resected from the lung and the parietal pleura abraded to produce an adhesion to the faulty lung area.

Thoracic surgery

Many of the conditions and diseases described in the previous sections of this chapter are either entirely or partially corrected by a surgical procedure. Intelligent nursing care of patients undergoing thoracic surgery depends upon knowledge of the anatomy and physiology of the chest, of the surgery performed, and of procedures and practices that assist the patient to recover from the operation. When endotracheal anesthesia became possible, surgery of the chest was given a great impetus. Before that time it had not been possible, except in the rarest of cir-

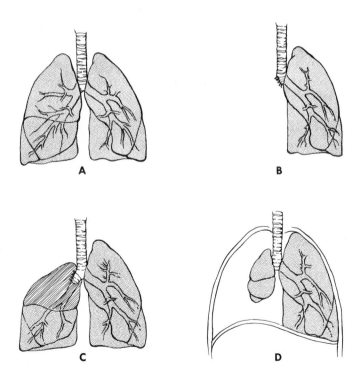

Fig. 131

A, Normal expanded lungs. **B,** Surgical absence of the right lung following a pneumonectomy. **C,** Surgical absence of the right upper lobe following a lobectomy. **D,** Complete collapse of the right lung (atelectasis) due to air in the pleural cavity (pneumothorax).

cumstances, to operate upon the lung without causing collapse of the good lung and death. By means of endotracheal anesthesia, it is possible to keep the good lung expanded and functioning even when it is subjected to atmospheric pressure. Endotracheal anesthesia is used for surgery involving the lungs and for most chest surgery in which the pleural space is entered.

Operative procedures

Lobectomy. A lobectomy, the removal of a lobe of the lung, is the most common of all lung operations (Fig. 131). It may be done for conditions such as bronchiectasis, cysts of the lung, lung abscess, benign lung tumors, and tuberculosis. A *thoracotomy incision* is made into the chest, and one or two ribs usually are resected. When the pleura is entered and the lung is exposed to atmospheric pressure, it collapses. The main bronchus to the lobe is resected, closed, and carefully covered with pleura to prevent the leakage of air. The affected lobe is then removed, the pleura is closed, and the other lobes are reexpanded with oxygen by the anesthesiologist. Drainage catheters are usually inserted through short incisions above and below the resected lobe. The upper catheter provides for removal of air, and the lower catheter permits drainage of fluid.

Pneumonectomy. A pneumonectomy, or removal of an entire lung, may be done for conditions such as cancer, lung abscess, bronchiectasis, and tuberculosis (Fig. 131). This procedure carries a greater risk than lobectomy. Although the operative procedure is technically simpler than a lobectomy, the nature of the disease and the extent of lung involvement may make surgery difficult and may make the patient a poorer operative risk. The phrenic nerve is crushed to allow the diaphragm to rise on the affected side and help obliterate the cavity left by removal of the lung. The incision usually is closed without drainage tubes. The cavity left by the removal of the lung is smaller than might be expected because of the elevation of the diaphragm on the operative side and because of the slight shifting of the mediastinum. The normal negative pressure found in the chest draws fluid into the cavity from the surrounding tissues. This fluid becomes incorporated with red and white blood cells,

and eventually a cheesy material forms and fills the space, preventing the other lung and the heart from shifting toward the affected side.

Partial resection of the lung. Partial resection or removal of a diseased part of a lobe of the lung is usually done to excise a localized bronchiectasis, a lung abscess, an emphysematous bleb, or a localized tuberculous cavity that fails to heal by other methods of treatment. The success of this procedure depends on the determination of the exact part of the lobe involved. After the bronchioles have been ligated, the anesthesiologist fills the lung with oxygen to demonstrate the collapsed area. The diseased part of the lobe is removed. Drainage catheters are inserted, and the incision is then closed.

Thoracoplasty. An extrapleural thoracoplasty, or extensive rib resection, is done primarily for tuberculosis. When the ribs are removed, the chest wall becomes depressed and the underlying lung collapses, thus obliterating the cavity. When more than three or four ribs are to be removed, the operation is done in two stages; the first three ribs are removed in the first operation, and portions of the next four are removed in the second operation. Since the operation causes a deformity of the chest wall, it usually is done only when the patient is too ill to undergo a lobectomy. This surgical procedure also may be done after a pneumonectomy to decrease the size of the space to be obliterated.

Decortication. Decortication is the removal of a thick membrane that may form over the lung following empyema. This membrane constricts the lung and prevents it from expanding fully. The operation is done through a thoracotomy incision. Usually a rib is resected and the membrane surgically removed from the lung. A catheter usually is placed in the chest cavity and attached to a closed drainage system.

Exploratory thoracotomy. An exploratory thoracotomy is an operation done to confirm a suspected diagnosis of lung or chest disease. Intratracheal anesthesia is used, and a surgical opening into the thorax is made. If cancer is suspected, a biopsy is taken, and if there has been bleeding into the pleural cavity, the lung is examined in order to locate the bleeding point. If possible, the bleeding is controlled. This operation may be done following traumatic injury in which there has been damage to the lungs or the pleura.

Nursing care of the patient who has chest surgery

Preoperative care. If the patient who is to have chest surgery has an understanding of what is expected of him preoperatively and postoperatively, he will be less apprehensive and better able to help himself. A full explanation of all tests that will be made helps him to accept the preoperative preparation.

In preparation for chest surgery, the patient usually has a bronchoscopic examination, gastric aspirations, roentgenograms of the chest including tomograms, and sputum examinations. He may be asked to do postural drainage several times a day and to take various medications. If he is hospitalized, drugs such as racemic epinephrine hydrochloride (Vaponefrin) may be given by nebulizer. Tests and treatments often are done on an outpatient basis either in a clinic or in a doctor's office. Because the patient will not be under close supervision, it is important that the clinic nurse or office nurse makes sure that the patient understands all directions and that he is able to carry out necessary procedures. Close members of his family may be called upon to help. When it is advisable that the patient be hospitalized for the preoperative examinations and preparation, instructions should still be given.

The operation is discussed with both the patient and his family. The preoperative nursing care is similar to that discussed on p. 170. The patient should understand that he may receive oxygen postoperatively either by mask, catheter, or tent because this practice is routine for patients undergoing chest surgery. He should know that he will be turned and asked to cough every two hours postoperatively to help bring up secretions from the lungs and prevent complications.

The nurse should instruct the patient how to cough (p. 196). Patients who practice coughing preoperatively usually will cough more effectively postoperatively. Exercises to preserve symmetrical body alignment, full range of motion of the shoulder, and maximum pulmonary function are usually started during the preoperative period and continued postoperatively. In some hospitals the physical therapist instructs the patient. The nurse, however, must provide follow-up instructions and is responsible for seeing that the patient carries out the instructions properly. Many times the nurse must take the responsibility for teaching the exercises. If so, she should find out the exercises the doctor feels should be used and, if possible, should obtain assistance from a physical therapist in how best to provide each specific exercise. Articles in current nursing periodicals are helpful.[40]

If a catheter is to be used for drainage of the chest, the patient can be told that it will be used to drain fluid that normally accumulates after a chest operation. He should also be told to expect to have pain for some time postoperatively because intercostal nerves are severed, but he should be told that medication can be given for this pain and that he must not let it prevent him from coughing. If he has pain on breathing deeply, he should not hesitate to ask whether medication can be given. The patient should also know that the doctor may start an infusion in a vein in the leg before he goes to the operating room. The skin is often incised and a polyethylene tube inserted into the vein to obviate the danger of infiltration of the fluid and of collapse of the vein in the event of shock.

Chest drainage. When there is a possibility that there may be leakage of air, fluid, or blood into the chest cavity from the lung, chest wall, or any other thoracic organs or tissues that have been operated upon, a means of escape must be provided for such fluid or air to prevent impaired breathing and to prevent mediastinal shift. Catheters (drainage tubes) placed in the chest usually are placed above and below the resected area. The upper catheter allows air to escape. The lower catheter allows fluid to drain. When the patient breathes out, he pushes the air and fluid from the chest cavity into the catheters, and then gravity forces them down into the drainage bottle. By coughing and breathing deeply, the patient forces the fluid out, and the lung can then expand more fully.

The catheters are attached to a *closed*

drainage system (underwater drainage) that prevents outside fluid or air from entering the chest cavity and causing collapse of the lung. Closed drainage is accomplished by attaching the catheter from the chest to a tube that is submerged under sterile water in a drainage bottle. If the drainage bottle is below the level of the bed, the normal negative pressure created in the pleural cavity will not be great enough to draw water up the tube on inspiration. However, sterile tubing, drainage bottles, and water should always be used lest, through some accident, the fluid is drawn back into the chest cavity.

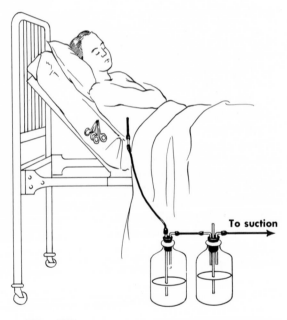

To suction

Fig. 132

Chest catheter in place. The chest catheter is attached to a closed drainage system. Note that the glass tube in the drainage bottle connected to the tubing of the chest catheter is below the level of the water. The bottle to the right of the drainage bottle regulates the amount of suction transmitted to the drainage bottle, the chest catheter, and the pleural cavity. The two clamps attached to the bed are available for use when the tubing is disconnected. If two catheters are used, a Y connecting tube may be used, or both catheters may be connected to separate bottles and then attached to the control bottles.

If the patient is not able to cough or if the drainage is such that respiration is not enough to force the fluid out through the drainage tube, suction may be attached to the catheter (Fig. 132). Many chest suction machines with regulators are available commercially. However, the usual type of suction machine or wall suction may create more suction than is desired, and a control bottle may be placed between the drainage bottle and the suction machine to regulate the amount of suction being exerted. By placing a specific amount of water in a control bottle, having an airtight system, and placing a glass tube in such a way that one end is exposed to the air and the other end is in the water, the amount of suction can be controlled. The amount of suction is regulated by the number of centimeters the tube open to the air is submerged under the water (generally 4 to 10 cm.). If the glass tube is submerged 8 cm. (3 inches), 8 cm. of negative pressure (suction) are exerted to draw fluid from the chest.

Chest drainage is adjusted by the doctor, who determines how much sterile water should be in the bottles and how far below the water level the glass tube in the control bottle should be. A mark is often placed at the initial water level and the bottle calibrated so that it is not necessary to empty it to determine if drainage is flowing steadily. The actual drainage from the chest cavity is determined by subtracting the amount of water initially placed in the drainage bottle from the total amount of drainage at the time of emptying. The doctor may be responsible for measuring the drainage in the bottle and for refilling the bottle with sterile water as necessary. In many institutions, however, measuring and refilling are nursing functions, in which case the nurse must be certain that the tube from the chest is clamped off close to the chest wall before the stopper is removed from the bottle. Care must be taken to measure drainage accurately, to use aseptic technique in handling and sterilizing the equipment, and to carry out this procedure as quickly as possible. Sometimes extra sterile bottles and tubing are available so that used equipment can be replaced immediately. The bottle should be filled with sterile water to the prescribed level and the system made airtight before the tube from the chest is unclamped. The tube should be reattached to drainage as soon as possible, however, lest fluid congeal in the tube or expansion of the lung be delayed.

In caring for the patient who has a chest catheter attached to a closed drainage system, the nurse should check the equipment frequently to be sure that the system is airtight and that drainage is not obstructed by kinks, blood clots in the tubing, or other causes. When the patient is lying on his operated side, the tube should be protected from kinking or from pressure by placing towels on either side of it to make a trough or by having the patient lie with a rubber ring under the operated area. Two clamps should be kept at the bedside. If the drainage or suction system seems to be working improperly or if the drainage bottle is broken or cracked, both clamps should be placed immediately on the catheter close to the wound dressing. The drainage bottles should never be raised above the level of the bed, since this will permit the fluid to drain back into the chest cavity. The glass tube in the drainage bottle must *always* be under water, the rubber tubing should be attached snugly to the glass connecting tubes, and the bottle stoppers should fit tightly to prevent air from leaking into the system. If the catheter is patent, the water will rise and fall in the glass tube in the collection bottle on inspiration and expiration. If the tubing becomes blocked or if the lung has reexpanded, the water will remain at one level. If the nurse notices that the fluid in the tubing does not rise or fall with breathing, the doctor must be immediately notified since he must determine the cause. A clogged tube with drainage dammed up behind it may cause the heart and the great vessels to shift positions and cause respiratory and circulatory distress. When shifting occurs, the patient is said to have a *mediastinal shift*. The pulse becomes very rapid and "fluttery," and signs of shock will soon appear. Mediastinal shift is a serious complication and must be watched for after any type of chest surgery. It also may occur after the injection of air in collapse therapy or following trauma to the chest. A thoracentesis may be done as an emergency measure to draw air or fluid out of the pleural cavity on the affected side

and thereby lessen its pressure upon the mediastinum.

A roentgenogram is taken with portable equipment within a few days. If it shows the lung to be fully expanded and reveals no fluid level, the chest catheters are removed. When the catheters come out, the intercostal muscles contract, thereby closing the openings and preventing the entrance of air into the chest cavity. As an additional precaution, petroleum jelly gauze is applied immediately over the openings and is covered and taped securely with adhesive tape. The small openings heal quickly.

Postoperative care. When the patient returns from the operating room, vital signs should be checked, oxygen administered as ordered, and the chest tube attached to a closed drainage system. The patient should be watched for signs of shock or hemorrhage. The dressings must be observed for drainage. A moderate amount of serosanguineous drainage is expected for the first day. There will be some bleeding through the chest catheter during the first forty-eight hours, but the amount should not be excessive and should be observed closely. Dyspnea, cyanosis, or sudden sharp pain in the chest should be reported at once. These are signs of *spontaneous pneumothorax*. If this condition is not treated promptly by aspiration of air or fluid by means of a thoracentesis, a mediastinal shift may occur. When the patient has reacted from anesthesia, he should be placed in a semi-Fowler's position to facilitate breathing. Since a firm bed lessens pain, a hinged fracture board should be put under the mattress prior to surgery.

The patient should be turned at least every two hours. Many doctors believe that the patient should lie on his operated side most of the time since this position lessens pain, permits better expansion of the unaffected lung, facilitates drainage, and helps to prevent spread of any possible infection to the mediastinum and the unaffected lung. Some surgeons believe that the patient should be turned on alternate sides and will specifically order this measure.

The patient is encouraged to cough. Coughing is made easier for the patient by splinting the wound with the hands or by having the patient sit up in bed and splint-

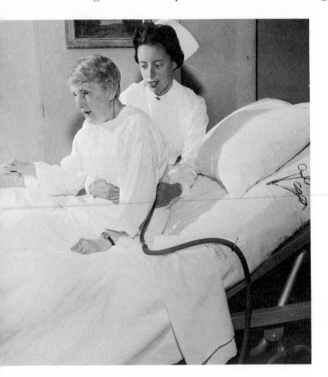

Fig. 133

The nurse is splinting the chest by applying pressure; this lessens muscle pull and pain as the patient coughs.

nacious, and thus it can be more easily expectorated. A physiologic solution of sodium chloride may be given through the oxygen tent, by nebulizer, or with an intermittent positive-pressure breathing machine to help liquefy mucus. After an inhalation, the patient should be encouraged to cough and bring up as much sputum as possible. Steam inhalations and inhalations of drugs such as isoproterenol hydrochloride (Isuprel) or racemic epinephrine hydrochloride (Vaponefrin) also may be used.

Exercise is started early (sometimes on the day of operation) to prevent the shoulder and arm on the affected side from becoming stiff, with subsequent loss of full range of motion. The patient has a natural tendency to protect his operated side, but overprotection can quickly cause stiffness, atrophy of muscles, and an awkward posture. A full-length mirror helps the ambulatory patient to check his own posture. Passive exercise may be given for a few days after surgery. The preoperative program for active arm and shoulder exercises should then be initiated and supervised by the physical therapist or the nurse. The patient needs encouragement to do exercises since he fears that they will increase pain. Exercises can be planned for a suitable interval after analgesic medication has been given. Active movement of the arm through full range of motion should be done two to three times a day within a few days. It must be remembered that the patient cannot do exercises to ensure complete range of motion of the shoulder unless he is upright or lies on his abdomen. Exercises such as elevating the scapula and clavicle, "hunching the shoulders," bringing the scapulas as close together as possible, and hyperextending the arm can be done only in these positions. Since lying on the abdomen may not be possible at first, these exercises should be done when the patient is sitting on the edge of the bed or when he is standing.

The patient who has had extensive chest surgery usually requires a long convalescence. He may feel weak and tired for a long time. This is especially true if much of the lung has been removed and vital capacity is reduced. He is likely to complain of pain in the incision for weeks after the operation. If it is really severe, the doctor may infiltrate the nerves in the area with procaine. Some

ing the chest with a towel or a drawsheet (Fig. 133). To make it easier for him to sit up, the nurse may place a pull rope at the foot of the bed to assist him in rising and in remaining upright for short periods.

Morphine or meperidine hydrochloride (Demerol) is usually ordered for pain. Medication for pain should be given as needed and may be required frequently during the first few postoperative days. The patient is extremely uncomfortable and will not be able to cough or turn unless he has relief from pain. In some instances the dosage of the drug is decreased so that it may be given oftener and yet not depress respirations. The tube in the chest causes pain, and the patient may attempt rapid, shallow breathing to splint the lower chest and avoid motion of the catheter.

The patient is encouraged to take fluids postoperatively, and he can progress to a general diet as soon as it is tolerated. Forcing fluids helps to keep the mucus less te-

patients complain of a feeling of numbness in the area of the incision. However, feeling will eventually return, and the patient is reassured by knowing this. The pain and numbness are caused by the interruption of intercostal nerves.

If the operation is for tuberculosis, the precautions used for any patient with active tuberculosis should be followed, since although the diseased area is removed, tubercle bacilli may still be in the respiratory tract. Since walled-off organisms may be released at operation, isolation precautions may be ordered for the patient whose sputum has been negative preoperatively. Both he and his family should know why isolation is necessary. The first few days postoperatively the patient generally is too ill to be expected to do such things as "cover his cough." The responsibility for carrying out good technique should rest with the nurse during this time. Usually the nurse wears a mask and gown that are discarded for laundering after removal.

Special care following a pneumonectomy. The nursing care of a patient following a pneumonectomy is essentially the same as that for patients having other kinds of pulmonary surgery except that the drainage catheter is not used. Patients who have had a lung removed have a markedly lowered vital capacity, and exercise and activity should be limited to that which can be done without dyspnea. Since the body must be given time to adjust to getting along with only one lung, the patient's return to work may be delayed. If the diagnosis is cancer, radiation therapy is usually given, and it may be started before the patient leaves the hospital. (See p. 278 for further discussion of nursing care for patients receiving radiation therapy.) The patient who has had a pneumonectomy for cancer is urged to report to his doctor at once if he has hoarseness, dyspnea, pain on swallowing, or localized chest pain, since these difficulties may be signs of metastasis.

Special care following a thoracoplasty. After a thoracoplasty, early movement of the arm and shoulder is exceedingly important, since several ribs have been removed and there is a tendency for a deformity to develop that may involve the entire shoulder girdle on both sides of the body. Position in bed and postural exercises to prevent drooping of the shoulder on the unaffected side should be emphasized. Scoliosis can easily develop in persons who have had a thoracoplasty without sufficient attention to posture postoperatively. A physical therapist may be able to give helpful suggestions regarding exercises that may be carried out while the patient is in the hospital. When patients return home, most of them need extra supervision either by a physical therapist or by a public health nurse who is experienced in orthopedic nursing.

Chest trauma

Fracture of the ribs. The fourth, fifth, sixth, seventh, and eighth ribs are most commonly fractured. Fractures of the ribs are caused by blows, crushing injuries, or strain caused by severe coughing or sneezing spells. If the rib is splintered or the fracture displaced, sharp fragments may penetrate the pleura and the lung. Patients with questionable rib fractures should have a roentgenogram of the chest made and should be observed carefully for signs of pneumothorax or hemothorax.

The patient with a rib fracture complains of pain at the site of the injury which increases on inspiration. The area is very tender to the touch, and the patient splints his chest and takes shallow breaths. Unless the lung has been penetrated, the usual treatment for rib fracture is strapping the chest with adhesive tape from the affected side to the unaffected side or applying a circular strapping, using an Ace bandage. A chest binder also may be used. If adhesive tape is used, the skin may be shaved and painted with tincture of benzoin to prevent blistering and other irritation. When the pain is severe and is not relieved by strapping and analgesic medications, the doctor may do a regional nerve block. This procedure consists of infiltrating the intercostal spaces above and below the fractured rib with procaine, 1%. If the lung has been penetrated, the patient may raise bright red sputum. If this occurs, an exploratory thoracotomy is usually done.

The patient who has a fractured rib is usually more comfortable in a semi-Fowler's position. After the chest is strapped, he should be encouraged to take as many deep breaths as possible. Since pain may prevent him from breathing easily enough to sleep, provision should be made for him to have medication. Because the patient with a rib fracture is often treated in the doctor's office or in the emergency room of a hospital and then discharged, his family should also be instructed about his position for comfort, medications to take, and the need for deep breathing. If the patient has difficulty breathing or develops sudden, sharp chest pain, he should call the doctor or return at once to the hospital emergency room.

Penetrating wounds of the chest. When a knife, bullet, or other foreign object has entered the chest, the major problem is not injury to the chest wall but injury to structures within the chest cavity. Penetration of the lung can cause leakage of air from the lung into the pleural cavity (pneumothorax). Blood may also leak into the pleural cavity (hemothorax). As the air or fluid accumulates in the pleural cavity, it builds up positive pressure, which causes the lung to collapse and may even cause a mediastinal shift, thus compressing the opposite lung and the heart. The patient then has serious difficulty in breathing and may go into shock. His pulse may become weak and rapid and his skin cold and clammy, and his blood pressure falls rapidly.

Emergency treatment must be instituted to remove the air or blood from the pleural cavity before death from cardiac or respiratory failure occurs. An emergency thoracentesis is done, and a catheter may be inserted and attached to a closed drainage sytem. When the patient's condition permits, the chest is opened and the injury is repaired or a section of the lung is removed.

If an open wound of the chest has been sustained, it should be covered immediately to prevent air from entering the pleural cavity and causing a pneumothorax. Several thicknesses of material may be used, and these are anchored with wide adhesive tape, or the wound edges may be taped tightly together. If an object such as a knife is still in the wound, it must never be removed until a doctor arrives. Its presence may prevent the entry of air into the pleural cavity, and its removal may cause further damage. The patient who has sustained a penetrating wound of the chest should be placed in an upright position and taken to a doctor immediately.

References and selected readings*

1 A statement of the American Thoracic Society: Chemotherapy of pulmonary tuberculosis in adults: the choice of drugs in relation to drug susceptibility, Am, Rev. Res. Dis. 92:508-512, Sept. 1965.

2 *Ahlstrom, Pearl: Raising sputum specimens, Am. J. Nursing 65:109-110, March 1965.

2a American Cancer Society, Inc., 1966 cancer facts and figures, New York, 1965, American Cancer Society, Inc.

3 *Andrews, Neil C., and MacVicar, Jean: Resection for pulmonary tuberculosis and the patient with a pulmonary resection, Am. J. Nursing 59:962-970, July 1959.

4 Beeson, Paul R., and McDermott, Walsh, Editors: Cecil-Loeb textbook of medicine, ed. 11, Philadelphia, 1963, W. B. Saunders Co.

5 Bergersen, Betty S., and Krug, Elsie E.: Pharmacology in nursing, ed. 10, St. Louis, 1966, The C. V. Mosby Co.

6 Blake, Mary: Probe of 38 Oregon tuberculosis relapse patients in 1963, NLN exchange no. 73, New York, 1965, National League for Nursing.

7 Blomquist, Edward T.: Program aimed at eradication of tuberculosis, Pub. Health Rep. 78:897-905, Oct. 1963.

8 *Burgess, Alex M.: A comparison of common methods of oxygen therapy for bed patients, Am. J. Nursing 65:96-99, Dec. 1965.

9 Chronic obstructive lung disease, a manual for physicians, Portland, 1965, Oregon Thoracic Society.

10 Closed drainage of the chest, a programmed course for nurses, Public Health Service publication no. 1337, Washington, D. C., 1965, U. S. Department of Health, Education, and Welfare.

11 Comstock, George W.: Untreated inactive pulmonary tuberculosis—risk of reactivation, Pub. Health Rep. 77:461-470, June 1962.

12 *Creighton, Helen, and Coulter, William Wallace, Jr.: The whys of a pulmonary function test, Am. J. Nursing 60:1771-1774, Dec. 1960.

13 Davis, Loyal, editor: Christopher's textbook of surgery, ed. 8, Philadelphia, 1964, W. B. Saunders Co.

14 Diagnostic standards and classication of tuberculosis, New York, 1961, National Tuberculosis Association.

15 *Drummond, Eleanor E.: The respiratory disease campaign—nursing actions, Am. J. Nursing 63:98-101, March 1963.

16 Dubois, René J., editor: Bacterial and mycotic infections of man, ed. 3, Philadelphia, 1958, J. B. Lippincott Co.

17 *Elwood, Evelyn: The battle of breathlessness in nursing care of the disoriented patient, no. 13, New York, 1963, American Nurse's Association.

18 Facts about selected respiratory conditions in the United States, New York, 1966, National Tuberculosis Association.

19 *Feldmann, Floyd: How to use the tuberculin test, Am. J. Nursing 59:856-859, June 1959.

20 *Frenay, Sister Mary Agnes Clare: Drugs in tuberculosis control, Am. J. Nursing 61:82-85, April 1961.

*References preceded by an asterisk are particularly well suited for student reading.

21 *Furcolow, Michael L., and Rakich, Jennie H.: Histoplasmosis and nursing aspects of histoplasmosis, Am. J. Nursing **59**:79-83, Jan. 1959.

22 Guide for follow-up of tuberculosis, New York, 1963, American Public Health Association.

23 *Haas, Albert: Essentials of living with pulmonary emphysema, a guide for patients and their families, patient publication no. 4, New York, 1963, The Institute of Physical Medicine and Rehabilitation.

24 Hadley, Florence, and Bordicks, Katherine J.: Respiratory difficulty: causes and care, Am. J. Nursing **62**:64-67, Oct. 1962.

25 Harrison, T. R., and others, editors: Principles of internal medicine, ed. 5, New York, 1966, McGraw-Hill Book Co.

26 *Hebert, William M., and Schlesinger, Eva M.: Crushing injuries of the chest and nursing the patient with a crushed chest, Am. J. Nursing **59**:678-684, May 1959.

27 *Heimlich, Henry J.: Postoperative care in thoracic surgery, Springfield, Ill., 1962, Charles C Thomas, Publisher.

28 *Horowicz, Clara: Bronchoscopy as an outpatient procedure, Am. J. Nursing **63**:106-107, May 1963.

29 *Huebner, Robert J.: Seventy newly recognized viruses in man, Pub. Health Rep. **74**:6-12, Jan. 1959.

30 *Hueper, Wilhelm C.: Lung cancer, air pollutants as a cause, Am. J. Nursing **61**:64, 66-68, April 1961.

31 *Introduction to respiratory diseases, New York, 1964, National Tuberculosis Association.

32 *James, George: A "stop-smoking" program, Am. J. Nursing **64**:122-125, June 1964.

33 Jenkins, Daniel E.: Current status of the atypical mycobacteria, Clin. Notes Res. Dis. **4**:3-12, Fall 1965.

34 Johnson, Karl M.: Some newly discovered respiratory viruses, Am. J. Nursing **63**:67-69, Nov. 1963.

35 *Kelley, Winfield O., and Poole, Hazel: Skeletal tuberculosis and nursing the patient with skeletal tuberculosis, Am. J. Nursing **57**:332-336, March 1957.

36 *Kressler, Alta: Teaching patients with tuberculosis, Am. J. Nursing **59**:1116-1118, Aug. 1959.

37 *Kurihara, Marie: Postural drainage, clapping and vibrating, Am. J. Nursing **65**:76-79, Nov. 1965.

38 Lefkowitz, Lewis B., Jr.: The common cold syndrome, Am. J. Nursing **63**:70-74, Dec. 1963.

39 Lichtenstein, M. R.: The current status of tuberculosis, World-Wide Abst. Gen. Med. **7**:8-18, Nov.-Dec. 1964.

40 *MacVicar, Jean: Exercises before and after thoracic surgery, Am. J. Nursing **62**:61-63, Jan. 1962.

41 *Malinoski, Victoria F.: Air pollution research, Am. J. Nursing **62**:64-67, Jan. 1962.

42 Manual of intermittent positive-pressure therapy, Los Angeles, 1965, The Hospital of the Good Samaritan Medical Center.

43 McFarland, J. Wayne: Lifeline for ex-smokers, Nursing Outlook **12**:50-52, July 1964.

44 McGrath, Dorothy, and Kruger, Betty K.: Chest suction using mercury instead of water, Am. J. Nursing **62**:72-73, June 1962.

45 Miller, William F., and others: Severe respiratory depression, J.A.M.A. **180**:905-911, June 16, 1962.

46 National Conference on Air Pollution, Pub. Health Rep. **74**:409-427, May 1959.

47 Pace, William R.: Pulmonary physiology in clinical practice, Philadelphia, 1965, F. A. Davis Co.

48 Reported tuberculosis data, Public Health Service publication no. 638, Washington, D. C., 1965, U. S. Department of Health, Education, and Welfare.

49 *Richie, Jeanne: The tuberculosis patient who refuses care, Nursing Outlook **8**:621-623, Nov. 1960.

50 *Riley, Richard L.: Air-borne infections, Am. J. Nursing **60**:1246-1248, Sept. 1960.

51 Riley, Richard L.: Protective measures; reasonable or ritualistic? Nursing Outlook **7**:38-39, Jan. 1959.

52 Riley, Richard L., and O'Grady, Francis: Airborne infection, New York, 1961, The Macmillan Co.

53 *Rodman, Theodore: Management of tracheobronchial secretions, Am. J. Nursing **66**:2474-2477, Nov. 1966.

54 *Safer ways in nursing to protect against airborne infections, New York, 1962, National Tuberculosis Association.

55 Saltman, Jules: Emphysema—when the breath of life falters, Public Affairs Pamphlet no. 326, New York, 1962, Public Affairs Pamphlets.

56 *Schwartz, William S.: Management of common pulmonary diseases, J.A.M.A. **181**:134-141, July 14, 1962.

57 Shall I smoke? New York, 1960, American Cancer Society, Inc.

58 *South, Jean: Tuberculosis handbook for public health nurses, ed. 4, New York, 1965, National Tuberculosis Association.

59 *Stephan, Phyllis Jean: Nebulization under intermittent positive pressure, Am. J. Nursing **57**:1158-1160, Sept. 1957.

60 *Task Force on Tuberculosis Control: The future of tuberculosis control, a report to the Surgeon General, Public Health Service publication no. 1119, Washington, D. C., U. S. Department of Health, Education, and Welfare.

61 Tuberculosis facts in the United States, New York, 1966, National Tuberculosis Association.

62 Vaughan, Victor C., III: The place of drug therapy in childhood asthma, Am. J. Nursing **66**:1049-1052, May 1966.

63 Weaver, Barbara, and Williams, Elsie L.: Teaching the tuberculosis patient, Am. J. Nursing **63**:80-82, Dec. 1963.

64 Williams, M. Henry, Jr., and Robinson, Faulkner: Pulmonary emphysema and nursing care of the patient with pulmonary emphysema, Am. J. Nursing **63**:88-96, Sept. 1963.

65 Wolcott, M. W., and Murphy, J. D.: The changing picture of lung abscess therapy, Dis. Chest **32**:62-69, July 1957.

66 World almanac and book of facts, 1965, vol. 80 (edited by Harry Hansen), New York, 1965, New York World-Telegram & The Sun.

67 World Health Organization Expert Committee on Tuberculosis, eighth report, no. 290, Geneva, Switzerland, 1964, WHO Technical Report Series.

22

The patient with ear, nose, or throat disease

The purpose of this chapter is to give the nurse an understanding of the causes of ear, nose, and throat diseases and the sequence of complications so that she is better able to teach health and prevention of disease. The close link between minor infections of the ears, nose, and throat and more serious disease makes prompt care of these conditions most important, and therefore every nurse should be concerned with prevention of these common infections.

Diagnostic procedures, treatments, and nursing care of patients with specific diseases of the ear, nose, and throat are discussed only briefly. For more detailed information concerning specialized care, refer to the references preceded by an asterisk at the end of this chapter and to other periodicals and special publications on this subject.

Common diagnostic procedures

Visual examinations. The mucus membrane lining the antra of the nares is examined easily by using a nasal speculum, a head mirror, and a standing light. The light should be bright and should be placed about nine inches to the right of, and slightly behind, the patient's head. The room should be darkened. The speculum stretches the nasal vestibule so that the light reflected from the head mirror can shine into all parts of the nose. A cotton-tipped applicator may be needed to remove secretions or to take a culture. A vasoconstrictor such as epinephrine (Adrenalin) may be applied to shrink the mucous membrane and give a better exposure. The throat often is examined superficially with a tongue depressor and flashlight. For a more extensive examination of the posterior nares and the throat, a nasopharyngeal mirror, a head mirror, a tongue depressor, and a light are used. To prevent its becoming foggy and failing to reflect, the nasopharyngeal mirror is warmed with hot water or an alcohol lamp before use. Because this examination may make the patient gag, he should be instructed to breathe through his mouth while the mirror is being directed toward his pharynx.

The larynx may be examined by an indirect or direct method. For an *indirect laryngoscopy,* the patient sits in a chair with his head tilted back and is asked to stick out his tongue. The physician then grasps it with a gauze sponge and pulls it forward and downward. A warmed laryngeal mirror is introduced into the back of the throat until the larynx is visualized. It is examined at rest and during attempts to speak (phonation). If the gag reflex is very sensitive, the pharyngeal wall may be sprayed with a light, topical anesthetic, such as 2% cocaine. A *direct laryngoscopy* is performed on children, on adults who are unable to cooperate for an indirect examination, and on all patients with suspicious lesions of the larynx. A sedative such as phenobarbital sodium is given an hour before the examination, which usually is performed under local anesthesia for which a drug such as 10% cocaine is used. If general anesthesia is used, atropine also will be given. For direct laryngoscopy, the patient is placed in a reclining position, with his head, manually supported by a doctor or nurse, extending over the edge of the table. The laryngoscope, a hollow, metal tube with a handle at the proximal end and a light at the distal end is introduced by a doctor through the mouth into the hypopharynx, elevating the epiglottis, and making the interior of the larynx easily visible. Benign surgical procedures, such as a biopsy or the removal of a small benign tumor, may be performed through this instrument.

After a laryngoscopy under local anesthesia, the patient should not eat or drink anything until the gag reflex returns, usually after about four hours. The gag reflex can be tested by "tickling" the throat with a tongue blade or applicator. After the gag reflex returns, the patient should try first to drink water since, if it is accidentally aspirated into the trachea or lungs, it is the fluid least likely to cause an untoward reaction.

The normal frontal and maxillary sinuses can be visualized by illuminating them in a dark room with a specially shaped, lighted bulb or a lighted transillumination tip. This examination is referred to as *transillumination.* If disease is present, the light will not penetrate the sinuses, or it will reveal fluid levels indicative of obstruction to drainage of the sinuses. Roentgenograms of the sinuses may be ordered to help establish the diagnosis of sinusitis. No physical preparation is necessary. No contrast medium is used, since the normal sinus is filled with air which itself casts a shadow in contrast to surrounding structures.

The ears may be examined with an aural speculum and with reflected light supplied by a head mirror. The ear canal often has to be cleansed of cerumen, desquamated epithelium, and other accumulations with a cotton-tipped applicator or a cerumen spoon before the eardrum can be seen. An *otoscope* with its magnifying lens usually is used to supplement the examination with the speculum, particularly for the examination of small children. Young children who have difficulty remaining still may have to be restrained for examination of the ears, nose, or throat.

Audiometric testing. The ability to hear pure tones (simple sound waves) and to discriminate speech can be tested with an electric audiometer. The chart of the hearing curve is called an *audiogram* (Fig. 134). Only the weakest intensities (pressure exerted by sound) that can be heard by the patient at each frequency are recorded on the audiogram. Intensity of sound is measured in decibels (considered the unit of hearing) and is defined as the least intensity of sound at which pure tone can be heard. Speech that is comfortably loud ranges in intensity from approximately 40 to 65 deci-

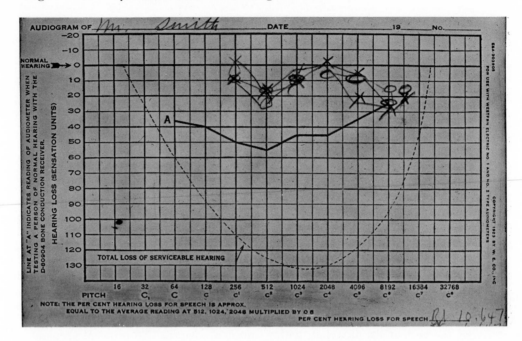

AUDIOGRAM OF *Mr. Smith* DATE_____ 19____ No.____

Fig. 134

An audiogram. (From Parkinson, Roy H.: Eye, ear, nose, and throat manual for nurses, ed. 8, St. Louis, 1959, The C. V. Mosby Co.)

bels. The term frequency refers to the number of sound waves emanating from a source per second, and is expressed in cycles per second (cps). A child or young adult can usually hear frequencies from about 20 to 20,000 cps. Hearing is most sensitive in the frequencies from 500 to 4,000 cps, the range in which most important speech sounds occur. The information gathered by audiometry helps the doctor determine if a hearing loss is present, what frequencies are affected, and whether the disease causing the hearing loss is in the middle ear, the inner ear, or is due to nerve damage.

For the best results, audiometry must be performed in a soundproof room. Group examinations, such as are done in schools, are helpful only in discovering children who need individual examination (Fig. 135). To test the intensity of sound by air conduction, the patient wears earphones and is instructed to signal with his finger when he hears the tone and when he no longer hears it. The higher frequencies are tested first, and the operator alternately increases and decreases

the intensity of sound until he finds the dial setting at which the person being tested can just perceive sound. When the patient's air conduction audiogram is above the 30-decibel level at 500, 1,000, and 2,000 cps, he usually has adequate hearing for ordinary social and economic contacts.[3] To test the ability to hear vibrations transmitted by bone conduction, a bone oscillator, which produces mechanical vibrations of the skull, is held against the head. The recording is done in the same way as for air conduction. To test how well a patient can hear and understand speech, the examiner introduces words into the earphones, and the patient is tested for his speech reception threshold (ability to hear words correctly 50% of the time), discrimination (how well the test words are understood), most comfortable loudness level, and the threshold of discomfort.

Hearing may be tested by other methods that may be used in conjunction with audiometry. Tuning forks are useful for determining rapidly the lower and upper tone limits within the speech range. The forks

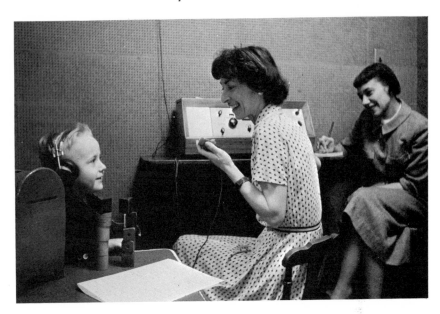

Fig. 135

Testing of a child's hearing with an audiometer. Note the soundproof walls. The child's mother is observing. (Courtesy New York League for the Hard of Hearing, New York, N. Y.)

also help differentiate between conductive and nerve hearing impairment, two types of hearing impairment that are discussed on p. 612. Tests with the tuning forks are known as the Weber, the Rinne, and the Schwabach tests. Other methods include having the patient tell when he hears a watch ticking or someone whispering behind him.

Until a child is 5 or 6 years of age, he is difficult to test by conventional methods because of lack of motivation, short attention span, and limited motor coordination. Therefore, special procedures that require only simple responses and that are interesting to the child are used. Most communities have screening programs to test the hearing of schoolchildren in order to detect any hearing impairment that might interfere with learning. Some communities also have these programs for the preschool child.

Insufflation. Insufflation of the eustachian tubes may be done either to test their patency or to force them open mechanically. A simple insufflation procedure is to have the patient compress his nose with his thumb and forefinger and swallow (*Valsalva* procedure). If he can feel the passage of air up the eustachian tube to the middle ear, or if the doctor, looking through the otoscope, can see the eardrum move outward as the patient swallows, the tube is patent. An-

other method is to force air into the nostril as the patient swallows water. A Politzer bag (a specially constructed rubber bag equipped with a nasal tip) is inserted into one nostril and the other nostril is compressed by the doctor's fingers. As the patient swallows a sip of water, pressure is applied on the bag, forcing air into the nasopharynx and the eustachian tubes. The physician, listening through a rubber tube connecting his ear with the patient's ear, can hear if air passes into the middle ear.

Air may also be forced into the eustachian tubes by means of a catheter inserted through the nose into the nasopharyngeal opening of the tubes. Finding the opening may be a tedious and uncomfortable procedure for the patient. To make the procedure easier, a weak solution of cocaine (1%) may be applied to the mucous membrane to desensitize it as the catheter is maneuvered into place. When the catheter passes into the orifice, the Politzer bag is attached to the catheter and air is instilled as the physician listens to its passage through tubing attached to his ear and the patient's. If passage of air into the tube cannot be heard, it may be due to stenosis or to anatomical irregularities of the eustachian tubes. This procedure is not done when there is an acute infection because of the danger of trauma to the eustachian tube and introduction of new infection to the middle ear.

Infections of the nose and sinuses

Infections of the nose, throat, and sinuses are among the most frequent complications of the common cold. The nurse, therefore, should be aware of the signs of these infections and of their complications.

The patient with rhinitis

Acute rhinitis. Simple, acute rhinitis *(coryza)* is an inflammatory condition of the mucous membranes of the nose and accessory sinuses caused by a filtrable virus (common cold). It affects almost everyone at some time in his life and occurs most often in the cold, winter months. It is generally believed that the infecting agent is present in the nose and sinuses at all times and that fatigue and chilling are among many factors influencing susceptibility. The patient usually complains of dryness of the nose, eyes, and soft palate, general malaise, chilliness, and headache. These systems are followed in twelve to twenty-four hours by obstruction to nasal breathing due to swelling of the mucous membrane and a profuse, watery nasal discharge. Sneezing, tearing of the eyes, and nasal irritation also occur, and the postnasal discharge may cause pharyngitis, laryngitis, or bronchitis. Infants and young children are particularly susceptible to this infection, which may spread to the middle ear and cause an otitis media. They should be isolated from persons with colds, and if they develop a cold, they should be observed carefully for symptoms suggesting otitis media. If a high temperature occurs, or if the child becomes restless, rolls about in bed, or pulls at his ear, medical attention should be sought.

Most people with colds do not go to their physician unless symptoms persist or make them very uncomfortable. Medical treatment, if sought usually consists of rest, fluids, moist inhalations, and the intranasal use of astringent solutions such as ephedrine sulfate, 1%, racephedrine hydrochloride, 0.25 to 3%, phenylephrine hydrochloride (Neo-Synephrine hydrochloride), 0.25 to 1%, or naphazoline hydrochloride (Privine), 0.1%. These drugs are applied locally and relieve the nasal congestion by constricting the capillaries and diminishing hyperemia. They may be ordered to be used every four hours for several days. However, with continued use, they lose their effectiveness. Mild antiseptics such as mild silver protein (Argyrol), 10%, may be ordered. Some of these medications may be obtained without a prescription, but since they may contain drugs that produce tension, restlessness, and palpitation of the heart, the advice of a physician should be asked before using them. Aqueous solutions are preferable to solutions with oil bases since they are more easily absorbed and, if they are aspirated into the lungs, are less likely to cause lipoid pneumonia. Any of the various antihistaminic drugs may be ordered to alleviate symptoms such as sneezing and tearing of the eyes. Since these drugs usually cause drowsiness, they should not be used when driving a car or working near moving machinery.

Since people usually instill their own nose drops or administer their own nasal sprays or inhalators, they should be taught the correct method. No more than three drops or three sprays of solution should be instilled into each nostril at one time unless more medication is specifically prescribed. To administer nose drops a person should sit in a chair and tip his head well backward, lie down with the head extending over the edge of the bed, or lie down and place a large pillow under the shoulders so that the head is tipped backward. He should remain in this position for five minutes after the drops are instilled to allow the solution to reach the posterior nares. If, after ten minutes, he still has marked congestion, another drop or two of the solution may be used. The mucous membrane of the anterior nares by this time should have become constricted so that the solution may reach the posterior nares more easily. Some physicians feel that the instillation of nose drops is too upsetting for children and order nasal decongestants such as pseudoephedrine, 30 mg. (½ grain), by mouth every three or four hours and steam inhalations. A small syringe with a glass nozzle may be used to aspirate the mucous discharge from the nose of infants to clear the nose so that they can breathe and be able to take their feedings. To administer a nasal spray or use an inhalator, the person sits upright with his head tilted slightly backward. The atomizer is placed at the entrance of the nostril and, while occluding the opposite nostril with finger pressure, squeezed. The inhalator is placed in the nostril, and after occluding the opposite nostril, the person inhales. Occluding the opposite nostril prevents the entrance of air and thus allows the medication to be forced high up into the nasal cavity.

If the nasal discharge persists for more than about a week, or if the patient develops an elevation of temperature, he should be urged to visit his doctor. People who have recurrent colds should seek medical attention because nasal deformity such as enlarged turbinated bones or a deviated septum and chronic sinusitis may cause the repeated attacks. Repeated colds eventually may lead to chronic rhinitis. (For further discussion of the common cold, see p. 539.)

Chronic rhinitis. Chronic rhinitis is a chronic inflammation of the mucous membrane of the nose caused by repeated, acute infections or an allergy. Nasal obstruction accompanied by a feeling of stuffiness and pressure in the nose is the chief complaint. A nasal discharge is always present and may be serous, mucopurulent, or purulent, depending upon the amount of secondary infection present. Polyp formation may occur, and the turbinates may enlarge as a result of the chronic irritation. Complaints of frontal headache, vertigo, and sneezing are common.

Antibiotics may be used to treat the infection. After the offending allergens have been identified, they should be avoided by the patient. Antihistamines are helpful in alleviating symptoms. The polyps or the hyperplastic tissues may require surgical removal (polypectomy, turbinectomy).

Nasal irrigations may be used in the treatment of chronic rhinitis, and the nurse may be asked to assist with them. The details of this procedure are described in texts on fundamentals of nursing. Care should be taken

that both nostrils are open and that the pressure exerted is no greater than that produced when an irrigating can is held 30 to 37.5 cm. (12 to 15 inches) above the level of the nose.[23] Greater pressure increases the danger of forcing infected material into the sinuses or the middle ear. The patient should breathe through his mouth during the procedure, and the irrigating tip should be removed from the nostril if he must sneeze or cough. The position of choice for the irrigation is one in which the patient sits upright with the chin bent forward so that the eustachian tubes will be above the stream of solution. The patient should not blow his nose for one-half hour after the procedure in order to avoid forcing residual irrigating fluid through the eustachian tubes into the middle ears. This procedure is dangerous if performed on a child who is crying or struggling to avoid the procedure.

The patient with sinusitis

Acute sinusitis. Acute sinusitis is an inflammation of one or more of the sinuses. It usually follows acute rhinitis or other respiratory diseases, such as pneumonia or influenza, and is caused by infection extending through the nasal openings into the sinuses. Abscessed teeth or tooth extraction occasionally causes an acute maxillary sinusitis. Streptococci, staphylococci, or the pneumococcus bacilli usually are the infecting organisms. Sinusitis also may be an allergic reaction.

The patient with acute sinusitis often complains of a constant, severe headache and of pain over the infected sinuses. Maxillary sinusitis may cause pain under the eyes, whereas frontal sinusitis often causes pain over the eyebrows. The patient may have the sensation of "pain in the bone" upon even slight pressure over the affected sinus. Pain from the ethmoid and sphenoid sinuses usually is referred and is felt at the top of the head. Occasionally there may be noticeable swelling over the maxillary or frontal sinuses or there may be orbital edema. The patient may have nausea, purulent discharge from the nose if the duct is not closed, obstruction to nasal breathing, fever, and general malaise. Fever usually is proportional to the amount of obstruction present and the virulence of the infection. If the sinus is completely obstructed, the temperature may be as high as 40° C. (104° F.). The throat may be sore from irritation caused by post-nasal drainage. Complications of severe untreated sinusitis include osteomyelitis in the adjacent bone, an abscess that may involve the brain, venous sinus thrombosis, and septicemia.

Objectives in the care of patients with acute sinusitis are to establish drainage of the sinuses and to control the infection. Sulfonamides and antibiotics are given for their specific action upon the causative organisms. Drugs such as phenylephrine hydrochloride (Neo-Synephrine hydrochloride), 0.25%, and ephedrine sulfate, 0.25 to 3%, which constrict the blood vessels and thus reduce hyperemia and improve drainage, may be given as nose drops or by inhalation. Antibiotics and mucolytic agents such as Alevaire or plain normal saline solution may be given by inhalation.

If medication is being given by atomizer or nebulizer, the adapter should be placed in one nostril and the other nostril closed. The patient then should be instructed to breathe through his nose with the mouth closed. Medication is then forced by air pressure (created with a hand bulb) through a small opening in the atomizer. Such pressure breaks the large droplets of fluid into a fine mist. If a nebulizer is used, the solution is usually forced through the apparatus by a current of oxygen or compressed air (p. 562).

Acetylsalicylic acid usually relieves the pain from sinusitis, but occasionally codeine or even morphine sulfate or meperidine (Demerol) may be necessary. Heat over the sinuses also gives some relief from pain. Hot wet dressings or a heat lamp may be ordered. Moist steam in the room may help to facilitate drainage. Humidity of 40 to 50% will add to the patient's comfort, and the room temperature should be kept constant since room temperature changes aggravate sinusitis. Drainage of the maxillary sinuses by the use of gravity may be accomplished by having the patient lie on his abdomen with his head extended over the side of the bed.

If conservative measures do not cure an acute sinus infection, the doctor may irrigate the maxillary and frontal sinuses with normal saline solution by inserting a trocar and cannula through the openings of the sinuses. Following irrigation, a sulfonamide or antibiotic solution may be instilled into the sinuses. The maxillary sinuses are the ones most often treated in this way. If it is impossible to insert the trocar and cannula through the normal opening, the nasal mucosa may be anesthetized with cocaine and the antrum (maxillary sinus) perforated with a trocar and cannula. This procedure is known as an *antrum puncture.* The nurse should explain it to the patient and should urge him to breathe through the mouth during the procedure. She should remain with him while the treatment is given, since, although it is not actually painful, it causes a sensation of pressure and may produce dizziness and nausea.

Since early treatment of acute sinusitis is much more successful than treatment after the condition becomes chronic, patients with symptoms of acute sinusitis should be urged to seek medical attention at once. Chronic sinusitis is difficult to cure and may lead to further complications such as ear infections and bronchiectasis.

Chronic sinusitis. In chronic sinusitis the mucous membrane lining a sinus becomes thickened from prolonged or repeated irritation and infection. The patient usually has a chronic purulent nasal discharge, a chronic cough caused by a postnasal drip, and a chronic dull sinus headache that is present upon awakening and usually subsides during the day because the varied positions and movement of the head help the sinus to drain. There also may be loss of the ability to smell.

The treatment of chronic sinusitis may be surgical. Removal of nasal deformities such as a deviated nasal septum, hypertrophied turbinated bones, or nasal polyps that are obstructing the sinus openings may give relief. Sinus irrigations may be done to ensure better drainage. If the condition is caused by an allergy, it responds to general treatment of the allergy.

The person with chronic sinusitis should avoid chilling, and cold, damp atmospheres. Change to a warm, dry climate, though helpful to some people, should not be thought of as necessarily helpful for all patients. The patient is advised not to smoke, because smoking further irritates the damaged mucous membranes. Air-conditioning often causes discomfort, particularly if the outside air is warm and moist. The person with chronic sinusitis often sleeps poorly and lacks pep and vigor in his living and in his work. Persistent postnasal discharge is believed to contribute, as the person grows older, to bronchiectasis, a chronic lung disease.

Operations on the sinuses. If the patient has recurrent attacks of sinusitis, it may be necessary to provide better drainage by permanently enlarging the sinus openings or by making a new opening and removing diseased mucous membrane. Surgery usually is done during the subacute stage of infection. An opening into the maxillary sinus may be made through the nostril (antrotomy) or through the mouth under the upper lip (*Caldwell-Luc* operation). The Caldwell-Luc operation is not performed on children because they may have unerupted teeth near the site of the incision. While the ethmoid, frontal, and sphenoid sinuses can be approached through the nose, operations through an incision made in the upper half of the eyebrow and extending downward along the side of the nose provide better visualization for the surgeon and are considered safer. (See Fig. 136 for location of the sinuses.) Surgery through the nostril is usually done under local anesthesia.

Nursing care of the patient undergoing a sinus operation. To prevent the swallowing or aspiration of bloody drainage from the nose and throat, postoperatively the patient who has had a general anesthetic should be turned well to the side. Upon recovery from the anesthesia or following local anesthesia, the patient may be in a mid-Fowler's position, which will help to decrease edema at the operative site and promote drainage. Ice compresses are usually applied over the nose or an ice bag is placed directly over the maxillary or frontal sinuses. The ice constricts blood vessels, decreasing oozing and edema, and relieves pain. The patient should be watched carefully for hemorrhage. Repeated swallowing by the unconscious patient may indicate hemorrhage.

Gauze packing is usually inserted into the nares and usually remains there for forty-eight hours. Consequently the patient breathes through his mouth. His lips and mouth become dry and need frequent care. Aromatic solutions are refreshing, and cold cream helps to prevent dryness of the lips. Steam inhalations often are ordered. The patient should be reminded not to blow his nose, since this procedure may cause trauma to the operative site and bleeding.

If a Caldwell-Luc procedure has been performed, the patient usually is given only liquids for at least twenty-four hours and a soft diet for three or four days. Fluids should be given liberally to all patients following surgery of the sinuses. If there is an oral incision, mouth care should be given before meals to improve the appetite and after eating to decrease the danger of infection.

Fever or complaints of tenderness or pain over the involved sinus should be reported to the doctor since they may indicate postoperative infection or inadequate drainage. Antibiotics may be given prophylactically. For a week or two postoperatively, there may be

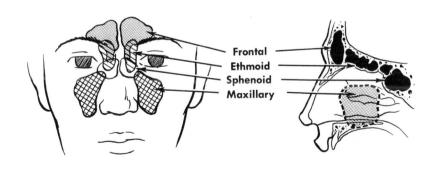

Fig. 136

The location of the sinuses.

Frontal
Ethmoid
Sphenoid
Maxillary

swelling of the area or a black eye. Numbness of the upper lip and upper teeth may be present for several months after a Caldwell-Luc operation.

The patient with nasal obstruction

Nasal polyps. Nasal polyps are grapelike growths of mucous membrane and loose connective tissue. They may be caused by irritation to mucous membranes of the nose or sinuses from an allergy or by chronic sinusitis. Since they may obstruct breathing or may bleed, nasal polyps are removed. They are excised through the nose by a snare or biting forceps (a polypectomy).

Deviated septum. The septum, which is normally thin and straight, may be deviated from the midline and protrude more to one side of the nasal passage than the other. It may cause a nasal obstruction that increases when infection or allergic reaction occurs. If the obstruction is marked, harsh breathing will result. There may be a postnasal drip, or the mucosa may become dry so that crusts form. This deformity of the septum is common in older children and adults. It may be congenital but usually is the result of an injury. Persons who break their noses often fail to have them set, sometimes not realizing that a bone is broken. The nurse should encourage persons with trauma to the nose to seek medical attention since, if not treated, a broken nose can lead to chronic sinusitis and chronic rhinitis, even though it may cause no immediate problem.

If the deformity causes nasal obstruction, a *submucous resection* may be performed. After a local anesthetic has been administered, an internal incision is made on one side of the nasal septum from top to bottom. The mucous membrane is elevated away from the bone, the obstructive parts of the cartilage and bone are removed, and the mucous membrane is sutured back into place. Plastic reconstruction may be necessary if a large part of the septum must be removed. Packing is placed in both nostrils to prevent bleeding and to splint the operative area.

Hypertrophy of the turbinates. If the turbinates hypertrophy and cause nasal obstruction, they may be shrunk by the use of a cautery blade inserted into the middle turbinate or by an injection of a sclerosing solution such as sodium morrhuate, 5%. The bone of the inferior turbinate sometimes is removed through a submucous resection. Because the mucous membrane covering the turbinates are not injured or removed during these procedures, they continue to serve as a protective lining and to warm inspired air.

Nursing care of the patient undergoing nasal surgery. Most nasal surgery on adults is done under local anesthesia. The patient, however, should not be given anything by mouth for six hours preoperatively, since he may become nauseated during the operation. Usually he receives a sedative and a narcotic preoperatively. Children require a general anesthetic and may be given a drug such as atropine.

Packing, either gauze or a tampon, is usually placed in the nose at the conclusion of the operation. If a tampon is used, the string attached to it should be securely fastened with adhesive tape to the face so that the tampon will not slip back into the throat. Should the tampon slip into the throat, the patient may have respiratory difficulty, and the nurse may have to grasp the tampon with a forceps and pull it forward through the mouth. Gauze packing occasionally extrudes from the posterior nares into the throat. If extrusion is slight yet bothersome, it should be reported to the doctor, and sedatives, if ordered, can be given. If it is obstructing breathing, the doctor is notified immediately. The packing is pulled forward through the mouth with forceps and replaced.

Following nasal surgery there is danger of hemorrhage. Blood may be evident on the external dressing that is applied under the nose, or the patient may expectorate or vomit bright red blood. The back of the throat should be examined to see if blood is running down into it. The patient's pulse may be rapid, or he may swallow repeatedly. Some oozing on the dressing is expected, but if it becomes pronounced or if any other symptoms appear, the doctor should be notified, and material for repacking the nose should be prepared. This material consists of a hemostatic tray containing nasal tampons, gauze packing, a few small gauze sponges, a small rubber catheter (used for inserting a postnasal plug), a packing forceps, tongue blades, and scissors. A head mirror, a good light, epinephrine (Adrenalin) 1:1,000 or some other vasoconstrictor, applicators, and a nasal speculum should be available.

If the dressing under the nose becomes soiled, it may be changed as necessary. This is very important from an esthetic standpoint. Sedation and encouragement are necessary because of general discomfort and apprehension caused by having the nasal passages packed and having to breathe through the mouth. The patient can be reminded that it will soon be removed. Frequent mouth care should be given, and fluids should be given freely. Postnasal drip, the presence of old blood in the mouth, and the loss of the ability to smell lessen the patient's appetite. Because it is difficult to eat while the nose is packed, most patients prefer a liquid diet until the packing is removed (twenty-four to forty-eight hours postoperatively), but they may have whatever food is tolerated.

After the nasal packing has been removed, the patient is asked not to blow his nose for forty-eight hours because blowing may start bleeding. Fever should be reported to the doctor because it may be due to infection. Since the patient has swallowed blood, the doctor may order a mild cathartic such as milk of magnesia to hasten the expulsion of material from the gastrointestinal tract. It is normal for the stools to be tarry for a day or two.

Following nasal surgery the patient frequently has discoloration about the eyes and should be prepared for it. To decrease local edema, he is kept in a mid-Fowler's position. Ice compresses usually are used over the nose for twenty-four hours to lessen discoloration, bleeding, and discomfort. If a bowl of ice cubes and three or four wet 4-inch by 4-inch gauze sponges are left within easy reach at the bedside, the patient may apply the ice compresses.

Similar care is given the patient who has a plastic procedure on the nasal septum. Such a patient should know that the cosmetic result of the operation cannot be evaluated for several weeks. Otherwise he may be disappointed. A protective dressing of adhesive tape or a plastic or metal mold usually is placed over the nose after a plastic procedure on the nasal septum and also after a reduction of a fractured nasal septum. If the patient has a fractured nose, however, the doctor usually removes the protective dressing daily to manually mold the broken parts. Firm healing develops about the tenth day. If a splint is used, the nurse should watch the skin about it to make sure that no pressure areas develop.

Complications of rhinitis and sinusitis

Epistaxis. Epistaxis, or nosebleed, may be caused by local irritation of the mucous membranes due to chronic infections or lack of humidity in the air that is breathed, violent sneezing or nose blowing, or trauma to the nose resulting in damage to or rupture of the superficial blood vessels. General or systemic causes may be hypertension and arterial blood vessel changes, blood dyscrasias such as leukemia, or a deficiency of vitamin K or vitamin C. In adulthood, nosebleeds are more common in men than in women. They are most frequent in early childhood and puberty. Patients who have frequent nosebleeds need a complete medical examination to determine the cause.

Most nosebleeds come from the tiny blood vessels in the anterior part of the nasal septum. This bleeding usually can be controlled at least temporarily by compressing the soft tissues of the nose against the septum with a finger. Firm pressure should be maintained for five to ten minutes, and it may be necessary for as long as a half hour. Ice compresses may be applied over the nose. If these measures do not control bleeding, the help of a doctor should be sought. The anterior nares may be packed with gauze saturated in Adrenalin 1:1,000. The exact bleeding spot may then be cauterized with a silver nitrate stick or an electric cautery. Hemostatic agents such as topical thrombin or an oxidized pack such as Gelfoam may be used. If the Gelfoam pack is applied, it usually is left in place until it dissolves in approximately four days.

Bleeding from the posterior part of the nasal septum is more common in the elderly person and is more likely to be severe. If the bleeding point cannot be seen and treated as described above, a postnasal pack may be inserted. Because this procedure is extremely painful, sometimes causing faintness, patients usually are admitted to the hospital. The pack is left in place two or three days and then removed very gently. If the bleeding has been severe, a transfusion may be necessary. Carbazochrome (Adrenosem) may be helpful in severe cases of epistaxis due to blood dyscrasias. Vitamin K may be administered when a deficiency of prothrombin is suspected, and vitamin C may be given if increased capillary fragility is the cause of bleeding. To prevent recurrent hemorrhage, the patient should be warned not to blow his nose vigorously.

Nosebleeds may cause real and severe apprehension since bleeding may be profuse, not only dripping from the nose but also flowing into the throat. The patient should be kept quiet, and stained clothing should be removed. If he remains in an upright position with the head forward, less blood drains into the throat. A basin and tissues should be provided for expectorated blood, and the patient should be urged not to swallow blood because it may cause nausea and vomiting.

Infections of the external tissues about the nose. The skin about the external nose is easily irritated during acute attacks of rhinitis or sinusitis. Furunculosis and cellulitis (inflammation of connective tissue) occasionally develop. (See p. 780 for discussion and treatment of furunculosis.) Infections about the nose are extremely dangerous since the venous supply from this area drains directly into the cerebral venous sinuses. Septicemia, therefore, may occur easily. No pimple or lesion in the area should ever be squeezed or "picked"; hot packs may be used. If any infection in or about the nose persists or shows even the slightest tendency to spread or increase in severity, medical aid should be sought.

Infections of the throat

Acute pharyngitis

Acute pharyngitis is an inflammation of the pharynx caused by hemolytic streptococci, staphylococci, or other bacteria or filtrable viruses. A severe form of this condition often is referred to as "strep throat" because of the frequency of streptococci as the causative organisms. Dryness of the throat is a common complaint. The throat appears red, and soreness may range from slight scratchiness to severe pain with difficulty in

swallowing. A hacking cough may be present. Children often develop a very high fever, while adults may have only a mild elevation of temperature. Symptoms usually precede or occur simultaneously with the onset of acute rhinitis or acute sinusitis. Pharyngitis can occur after the tonsils have been removed since the remaining mucous membranes can become infected.

Acute pharyngitis usually is relieved by hot saline throat gargles. An ice collar may make the patient feel more comfortable. The doctor may prescribe acetylsalicylic acid by mouth, as a gargle, or as Aspergum. Lozenges containing a mild anesthetic may help relieve the local soreness. Moist inhalations may help relieve the dryness of the throat. A liquid diet usually is more easily swallowed, and a generous amount of fluid is encouraged. If the temperature is elevated, the patient should remain in bed, and even if he is ambulatory and has no fever, he should have extra rest. Occasionally sulfonamide drugs or antibiotics are used to treat severe infections or are prescribed prophylactically to prevent superimposed infection, particularly in persons who have other disease such as rheumatic heart disease.

Acute follicular tonsillitis

Acute follicular tonsillitis is an acute inflammation of the tonsils and of their crypts. It usually is caused by the streptococcus bacillus. It is more likely to occur when the patient's resistance is low, and is very common in children. The onset is almost always sudden, and the symptoms include sore throat, pain on swallowing, fever, chills, general muscle aching, and malaise. In children, the temperature may rise suddenly to 40.5° C. (105° F.). These symptoms often last for two or three days. The pharynx and the tonsils appear red, and the peritonsillar tissues are swollen. Sometimes a yellowish exudate drains from crypts in the tonsils. A throat culture usually is taken to identify the offending organism.

The patient with acute tonsillitis should remain in bed and take generous amounts of fluids by mouth. Hot saline throat irrigations are usually ordered, and a sulfonamide preparation or antibiotics are usually given. Acetylsalicylic acid and sometimes codeine sulfate may be ordered for pain and discomfort. An ice collar may be applied to the neck, and if the temperature is over 39° C. (102° F.), an alcohol sponge bath may be given. Until the temperature subsides and the sore throat improves, a bland diet is given. After the temperature returns to normal, the patient should be kept in bed for forty-eight hours, since heart and kidney damage, chorea, and pneumonia are rather common complications of tonsillitis. Most doctors feel that patients who have recurrent attacks of tonsillitis should have a tonsillectomy. This procedure is usually done from four to six weeks after an acute attack has subsided.

Since the patient with acute tonsillitis is usually cared for at home, the nurse should help in teaching the general public the care that is needed. The office nurse, the clinic nurse, the nurse in industry, the school nurse, and the public health nurse have many opportunities to do this teaching.

Peritonsillar abscess

A peritonsillar abscess, or *quinsy*, is an uncommon, local complication of acute follicular tonsillitis in which the infection extends from the tonsil to form an abscess in the surrounding tissues. The swelling on the involved side displaces the uvula, resulting in difficulty in swallowing, talking, and opening the mouth. In some cases, saliva may drool from the patient's mouth, and he may be unable to swallow at all. Pain is severe and may extend to the ear on the affected side. If antibiotics to which the offending organism is sensitive are given early, the infection subsides. If an abscess forms, incision and drainage are necessary. During the operation, the patient's head usually is lowered and suction applied as soon as the incision is made. This prevents the patient from aspirating the drainage. Hot saline irrigations, an ice collar, or narcotics may help to relieve discomfort. If acute follicular tonsillitis is treated adequately, peritonsillar abscess is unlikely to occur.

Chronic enlargement of the tonsils and adenoids

Tonsils and adenoids are lymphoid structures located in the oropharynx and the nasopharynx. They reach their full size in childhood and atrophy during puberty. When the adenoids enlarge, usually as a result of chronic infections but sometimes for no known reason, they cause nasal obstruction. The person breathes through his mouth, may have a dull facial expression, and may have reduced appetite since the blocked nasopharynx may interfere with swallowing. In children, the enlarged adenoids may block the openings to the eustachian tubes in the nasopharynx, predisposing to middle ear infections and hearing impairment. Hypertrophy of the tonsil does not usually block the oropharynx but may affect speech and swallowing and cause mouth breathing.

Tonsillectomy and adenoidectomy. The tonsils and adenoids are removed when the adenoids become enlarged and cause obstructive symptoms, when they are chronically infected, or when the patient has repeated attacks of tonsillitis. Chronic infections of these structures usually do not respond to antibiotics, and they may become foci of infection, spreading organisms to other parts of the body, such as the heart. If a child's tonsils must be removed, the adenoids, even if they are not infected or enlarged, usually are removed too as a prophylactic measure. If possible, the removal of the tonsils is postponed until the child is about six years of age, but obstructing adenoids may be removed earlier.

The patient who is to have a tonsillectomy and adenoidectomy usually is admitted to the hospital on the morning of the operation. Children should be prepared carefully for the experience (p. 172). The complete examination is done in the doctor's office, but the general physical condition, urine, blood count, and bleeding and clotting times are rechecked before surgery. The operation will be postponed if there are signs of fever, upper respiratory disease, or other conditions that would complicate the induction of anesthesia or the postoperative course. The operation is performed on children under general anesthesia. In adults, the tonsillectomy may be done under either general or local anesthesia. In the operating room, after the tonsils are removed, pressure is applied to stop superficial bleeding. Occasionally, bleeding vessels are tied off with sutures or an electrocoagulation current is used.

Postoperatively, the patient who has had a tonsillectomy may have a small amount of

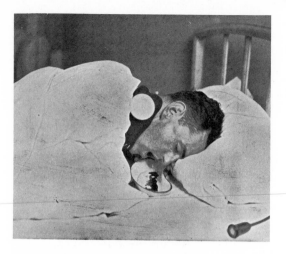

Fig. 137

This patient has just returned from the operating room after having a tonsillectomy. Note the pillow under the chest and the support of the head so that there is free drainage from the mouth. (From Parkinson, Roy H.: Eye, ear, nose, and throat manual for nurses, ed. 8, St. Louis, 1959, The C. V. Mosby Co.)

dark, bloody drainage from the operative area and may vomit blood that he has swallowed. Until he has reacted fully from the anesthesia, he should be propped on his side or placed on his abdomen with a pillow under his chest and an emesis basin under his mouth (Fig. 137). When the patient is awake, he is permitted to sit up in a mid-Fowler's position. Sometimes an ice collar is applied about the throat to make the patient more comfortable and possibly to lessen the chance of hemorrhage. Young children usually resist the application of an ice collar, and therefore it is not used.

Following a tonsillectomy or an adenoidectomy, the patient should be watched carefully for signs of hemorrhage. He is urged repeatedly as he is awakening and thereafter not to cough or attempt to clear his throat since these actions may initiate bleeding. Efforts should be made to prevent the small child from crying lustily. If he has fully responded from anesthesia, he may be rocked. If the patient swallows frequently, hemorrhage should be suspected, and the

throat should be inspected since any signs of hemorrhage must be reported to the doctor at once. Vomitus containing bright red blood should be reported at once, and the specimen should be saved for the surgeon's inspection. It is especially important to watch the patient who is asleep for signs of hemorrhage, since he may swallow blood and lose a very large amount without any external evidence of bleeding. The pulse rate should be taken every fifteen minutes for the first hour and every half hour for several hours thereafter.

The doctor may be able to control minor postoperative bleeding by applying a sponge soaked in a solution of epinephrine to the site. The patient who is bleeding excessively often is taken to the operating room for surgical treatment to stop the hemorrhage. This may be done by ligating or by cauterizing the bleeding vessel. If sutures must be used, the patient will have more pain and discomfort than he would have following a simple tonsillectomy. He may be unable to take solid food until the sutures have been absorbed.

After a tonsillectomy, the patient usually is kept in bed for twenty-four hours. When vomiting has ceased, fluids and bland nourishment are offered. While the patient usually will only take small amounts because of pain, he should be urged to take large swallows because they hurt less and because more fluid can thus be taken. Drinking through a straw is not advisable because of the danger of physical trauma and because the suction on the throat may cause bleeding. Ice-cold fluids are most acceptable and are given frequently. Ice cream usually is well tolerated, and ginger ale, cold milk, and cold custard usually are offered next, followed by cream soups and bland juices such as pear juice. The morning after surgery the patient is usually offered such foods as refined cereal and soft-cooked or poached eggs. When he goes home, he is advised to avoid citrus fruit juices, hot fluids, rough foods such as raw vegetables and crackers, and highly seasoned foods for at least a week because they irritate the operative area.

If the patient is old enough to chew gum and not swallow it, he usually is given Aspergum before meals and at bedtime to relieve the pain in the throat and ears and to help keep the throat muscles supple. Pain in the ear is a common complaint postoperatively. Acetylsalicylic acid by mouth may be given for this pain. Some doctors suggest that older children and adults gargle gently after the first postoperative day. The gargle solution is prepared by dissolving 0.3 Gm. (5 grains) of acetylsalicylic acid and ½ tsp. of sodium bicarbonate in half a glass of water. Some of this fluid may be swallowed without harm.

Most patients are discharged from the hospital the day after surgery, but some are permitted to return home the night of the operation. If so, the child's parents should be instructed to watch for bleeding and to report it to the doctor at once. The child is usually kept in bed for two or three days and indoors for a week. Adult patients may be up and about as soon as they return home but may be advised to remain indoors for three days. Usually the patient is told to avoid exposure to the sun, vigorous exercise, and coughing, sneezing, clearing of the throat, and vigorous blowing of the nose since these actions may cause bleeding. If bleeding occurs at any time, the patient should contact the doctor. The tough, yellow, fibrous membrane that forms over the operative site begins to break away between the fourth and eighth postoperative days, and hemorrhage may occur. The separation of the membrane accounts for the throat's being more painful at this time. Pink granulation tissue soon becomes apparent, and by the end of the third postoperative week the area is covered with mucous membrane of normal appearance.

The adult patient or the parents of the young patient should be given specific instructions for home care. Most hospitals and most laryngologists have these instructions written out. Acceptable foods and fluids should be outlined. The diet can be increased as tolerated. The patient should continue to drink plenty of fluids (2,000 to 3,000 ml. daily) to help relieve the objectionable mouth odor common after any oral surgery. If the patient does not have a bowel movement after a day or two, a mild cathartic is usually ordered. Parents should be told that the stool may be dark or black for a day or two because blood has been swallowed at operation. A temperature of 37.7° to 38.5° C. (99° to 101° F.) may be expected for the first two or three days, and discomfort in the ears should also be expected. Persistence of temperature elevation or of discomfort in the ears, however, should be reported to the doctor. The patient usually returns to the hospital clinic or to the doctor's office for a follow-up examination about one week after the operation.

The nurse may need to help some mothers plan ways to amuse the sick child. He should be allowed to play in his bed but should take a short rest in the midmorning and midafternoon. Most children like to be read to, to color, to do puzzles, and to watch selected television programs. A sick child's interest span is short, however, and one must be prepared to have various pastimes ready. Visits from other children should be restricted for the first week since they may bring upper respiratory infection to the patient.

Laryngitis

Simple acute laryngitis. Simple acute laryngitis is an inflammation of the mucous membrane lining the larynx, accompanied by edema of the vocal cords. It may be caused by a cold, sudden changes in temperature, or irritating fumes. The symptoms vary from a slight huskiness to a complete loss of voice. The patient's throat may be sore and scratchy, and he often has a cough. Laryngitis usually requires only symptomatic treatment. The patient is advised to stay indoors in an even temperature and to avoid talking for several days or weeks, depending on the severity of the inflammation. Steam inhalations with aromatic vapors such as tincture of benzoin, oil of pine, and menthol may be soothing. Cough syrups or home remedies for cough such as those suggested on p. 540 may be tried. Smoking or being where others are smoking should be avoided.

Acute laryngitis may cause acute respiratory distress and prostration in children under 5 years of age. Because the larynx of the infant and young child is relatively small and is susceptible to spasm when irritated or infected, it becomes partially or totally obstructed more easily. After exposure to cold air, or as a result of an upper respiratory infection, the child may develop a hoarse, barking cough and an inspiratory stridor (a form of *croup*). He may become restless, the muscles about the clavicle may be visibly retracted as they attempt to help the patient get more air, and the child's nostrils may flare. The child may sit up and grasp his throat as he tries to breathe. He may be completely well before and after the attack, which may last one-half to three hours. The doctor may order warm, moist inhalations and the administration of 2 ml. of ipecac to induce vomiting and reduce the laryngeal spasm. The child will be less frightened if he is held or if someone remains with him during the attack. A sedative may be ordered. If the condition becomes worse despite conservative treatment, a tracheotomy may be necessary.

Chronic laryngitis. Some people who use their voices excessively, who smoke a great deal, or who work continuously where there are irritating fumes develop a chronic laryngitis. Hoarseness usually is worse in the morning and in the evening. There may be a dry, harsh cough and a persistent need to clear the throat. Treatment may consist of removal of irritants, voice rest, correction of faulty voice habits, steam inhalations, and cough medications. The doctor may order spraying of the throat with an astringent antiseptic solution such as hexylresorcinol (S. T. 37). To do this procedure properly, the patient must use a spray tip that turns down at the end so that the medication reaches the vocal cords and is not dissipated in the posterior pharynx. He should place the spray tip in the back of the throat with the bent portion behind the tongue. He should then take one or two deep breaths and on inhalation spray the medication. This procedure may cause temporary coughing and gagging. Many medications used as throat sprays are now sold in plastic squeeze bottles with tube and spray tip attached.

Tracheotomy and tracheostomy

A *tracheotomy* is an operation in which an artificial opening is made in the trachea to allow the patient who has obstruction above this area to breathe. It also may be performed to provide a way for aspirating secretions from the trachea or bronchi of the unconscious or paralyzed patient who cannot cough. It may be done as an emergency measure or it may be done prophylactically when severe edema of the larynx and throat are anticipated. If the opening is permanent (for example, following removal of the larynx), the term tracheostomy (tracheal stoma) is used. These operations may be done on patients of all ages. The preoperative care is similar to that required when a tracheotomy is done.

The patient who has had a tracheotomy is apprehensive and is often fearful of choking. Discussion of postoperative routines with the patient before the tracheotomy is performed helps the patient to know what to expect, and knowing what to do may help to alleviate his fear. Every patient and his family should know that he will be attended constantly until he has learned to care for himself safely, and they should be told that he will be unable to speak. The patient should be taught how to communicate with others by writing on a pad or a slate. Placing a bell in the unit often reassures him, since it makes him feel that he can attract attention as necessary.

After the opening into the trachea is made (Fig. 138), a silver, nylon, or plastic tube is inserted to keep the tracheostomy patent. Gauze tapes, attached to either side of the tube, are tied securely behind the neck to prevent the tube from becoming dislodged by coughing or other exertion, since, if it is removed, the opening will close except in tracheostomies of long standing. Tubes are available in sizes No. 2-0 to No. 8. No. 2-0 may be used for the premature or newborn infant, while No. 6 is used most often for adults. The tracheostomy tube consists of two parts—the outer cannula, which is secured with the gauze tape and is removed only by the surgeon, and the inner cannula, which is removed at regular intervals for cleaning. The silver tracheostomy tube has a lock that must be opened to remove the inner cannula.

The operative wound may be sealed with a plastic spray, or a small dressing may be placed around the tracheostomy tube. Although drainage should be minimal, the wound should be inspected frequently for bleeding during the immediate postoperative period. The dressings may be changed as they become moistened with drainage or mucus. A single layer of gauze often is placed over the opening of the tube to prevent powder, crumbs, or other substances

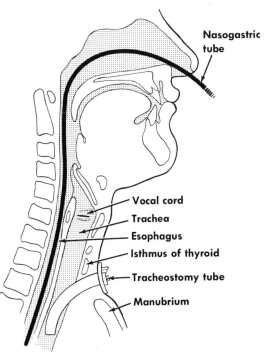

Fig. 138

Position of a tracheostomy tube and a nasogastric tube, if used.

from being aspirated into it. To prevent dry air from irritating the trachea and causing crusts to form, moisture usually is added to the air either by a humidifier or by moistening the gauze placed over the tracheostomy tube. Elbow restraints occasionally may be used to prevent infants from removing the tube or putting objects into it.

Maintaining a patent airway. One of the nurse's main responsibilities is to see that tracheostomy remains patent so that the patient has a free exchange of air. The patient is placed in a mid-Fowler's position for comfort and to make breathing easier. The patient should be attended constantly for twenty-four to forty-eight hours because of the possibility of respiratory embarrassment from blockage of the tube by secretions and because he is fearful of not being able to breathe and becomes restless when left alone. Oxygen may be administered, and Alevaire or Tergemist may be used to help liquefy mucous secretions so that they will

be easier to cough up or to remove by suction. Later, potassium iodide or ammonium chloride may be given orally for this purpose. Analgesics and sedatives are ordered to be given judiciously so as not to cause respiratory depression. If the patient is having any respiratory distress, the tube should be suctioned. If mucus is blocking the inner cannula and cannot be removed by suction, the inner cannula should be removed to open the airway. When the mucus is thick, the inner cannula should be cleaned, sterilized, and replaced at once because the outer tube may also become blocked. If, despite these measures, the patient becomes cyanotic, the doctor should be summoned at once. To remove secretions, the nurse must sometimes suction the tube every five minutes during the first few hours. The patient who is able to cough up secretions probably will require suction less frequently. The amount of mucous secretions subsides gradually, and the patient may go for several hours without the need for suctioning. However, even if secretions are minimal, the patient will be apprehensive and needs constant attendance.

Suctioning the tracheostomy tube. In preparation for suctioning the tube, the nurse should wash her hands and use a sterile catheter (No. 8 or 10 for children and No. 16 or 18 for adults) attached with a glass Y tube to a suction machine. The Y tube permits fingertip control of suction and prevents the buildup of pressure within the catheter (Fig. 42). The tip of the catheter is moistened with sterile saline solution and inserted into the tracheostomy tube, with the Y valve open to prevent traumatizing the mucous membranes. Some surgeons wish the suctioning catheter inserted only about 4 inches, lest the trachea be traumatized; others believe that it should be inserted as far as it will go easily in order to stimulate coughing. The nurse turns the patient's head to the right and tilts his chest to the left to aspirate his left main bronchus. The head is turned to the left and the chest tilted to the right to aspirate the right main bronchus. When the lowest point of permitted suctioning is reached, the open end of the Y tube is occluded and the secretions are aspirated as the tube is rotated 360 degrees and withdrawn slowly. If the patient coughs, the catheter should be removed because its presence obstructs the trachea and the patient must exert extra pressure to cough around it. As coughing occurs, the nurse or the patient should have tissues ready to receive the mucus since it may be ejected with force. The patient may cough more readily if the tracheostomy tube is held in place, since he may be afraid that it will come out with vigorous coughing. If the mucus is tenacious and difficult to remove, the doctor may order a few drops of sterile saline solution instilled into the tube before suctioning is done. Each time suctioning is done, the procedure should be continued until no further secretions return. Some patients are taught to suction their own tracheostomy. They need a mirror to see to do this procedure.

Fig. 139

This 82-year-old man cares for his own tracheostomy tube. He is about to clean the inner tube with a small tube brush. (From Newton, Kathleen, and Anderson, Helen C.: Geriatric nursing, ed. 4, St. Louis, 1966, The C. V. Mosby Co.)

After each suctioning, the catheter is rinsed in a solution, such as sterile saline solution, and then kept at the bedside, wrapped in a sterile towel or placed in a container of solution such as benzalkonium chloride. Extra sterile catheters should be available in case the one in use becomes contaminated. When suctioning of the nose or mouth is also necessary, separate catheters and solutions must be provided to avoid introducing pathogens normally found in the nose and throat into the lower respiratory tract. The same machine may be used. Disposable catheters may be used and discarded after each use.

Care of the patient having a tracheotomy. Every three hours, or more often if mucus collects and partially obstructs the lumen, the inner cannula of a tracheostomy tube is removed and cleaned. Cold water, soap, pipe cleaners, and a small test tube brush are used for cleaning. Hot water is not used because it increases the coagulation of the mucus, making the mucus difficult to remove. The tube may be soaked in a solution of half-strength hydrogen peroxide to soften the congealed secretions. The tube should be in-

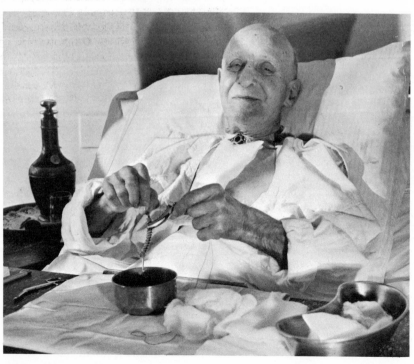

spected to see if the mucus has been removed. Gauze may be threaded through it to remove excess secretions and solution. After being cleaned, the tube is boiled for five minutes and then cooled. Before the inner tube is reinserted, suction should be used to remove secretions that may have accumulated in the lumen of the outer tube. If the patient is to be discharged with the tube in place, he is taught to care for it and to change it himself (Fig. 139). He may begin to do this within a few days of the operation, and often he is happier being able to care for himself.

The doctor may change the outer tube every twenty-four hours. The tapes holding the outer tube can be replaced as necessary, but a second nurse should always be present when this procedure is done. One nurse places one hand firmly behind the patient's neck and, with the other, holds the tube in place by supporting the T portion of the tube with her fingers. The second nurse then adjusts the knot or changes the ties.

If the outer tube should come out for any reason, the passageway for air is immediately obstructed. A tracheal dilator or a curved hemostat and a pair of scissors with which to cut the tape if the tube is only partially out should be conveniently placed in the patient's room. The nurse should use the dilator to maintain an open airway while she signals for assistance. (See Fig. 140.) An extra outer tube that is sterile and the correct size for the patient should always be kept in the room. The parts of the plastic tracheostomy tubes are interchangeable, but the silver ones must be matched. Many hospitals require that an emergency tracheotomy set be on the unit at all times. Likelihood of serious interference with breathing if the outer tube comes out becomes less as the wound heals. However, most ambulatory patients are advised to carry a small pair of scissors and a hemostat with them and are told how to use these instruments in an emergency.

Fig. 140

Material that should be kept at the bedside of a patient who has had a tracheotomy.
A, Scissors to cut the tape if the tube becomes blocked and needs to be removed immediately. **B,** Obturator used in insertion of a tracheostomy tube. **C,** Outer portion of a tracheostomy tube with tapes for tying around the neck. **D,** Inner portion of a tracheostomy tube. **E,** Tracheostomy dilator used to keep the trachea open if the tracheostomy tube becomes blocked and must be removed.

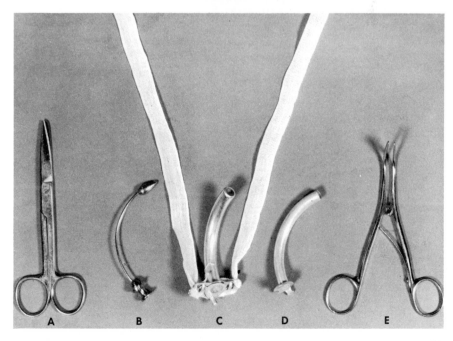

The patient who has had a simple tracheotomy may have fluids a few hours after the operation. He needs encouragement in his first efforts to swallow since he is fearful that food and fluids will go the wrong way. This is not a serious danger, although the patient may cough when he first attempts to drink fluids. The suction machine must be available and ready for immediate use at all times. Fluids are usually given parenterally during the first twenty-four hours. By the second postoperative day, the patient can drink readily and can eat most foods. However, foods that may be somewhat difficult to swallow, such as mashed potatoes, are usually avoided for a few days.

Mouth care is especially important. The patient often has marked halitosis following this operation and may be sensitive about it. He should be encouraged to drink large amounts of water because this measure will contribute to good mouth hygiene and will help to thin mucous secretions.

The patient usually is advised to avoid talking until the tracheotomy opening is occluded for increasing periods prior to removing the tube completely. Therefore, a pad and pencil should be readily available to him. With the doctor's permission, patients who must have the tube left open for extended periods can be taught to cover it momentarily with a finger while they speak.

Use of the tube is discontinued gradually. Usually it is first partially closed with a rubber cork, and if the patient can breathe adequately, the tube may then be completely corked for a day before it is removed. When the tube is removed, the skin edges are pulled together with strips of adhesive tape. After a few days, the wound is healed and air no longer escapes through it.

Patients who go home with the tracheostomy tube still in place must be provided with necessary supplies or with instructions as to where to secure them and with knowledge of how to care for themselves. They should have suction equipment. Suction machines can be rented for home use or obtained in many communities through the local chapter of the American Cancer Society. Suction can be provided by attaching a suction hose to a water faucet. Many hardware stores carry the necessary equipment. The amount of suction is controlled by the stream of water.

Cancer of the larynx

If treated early, cancer of the larynx is one of the most curable of all malignancies. It comprises about 5% of all malignant lesions, and approximately 6,000 persons in the United States have this disease.[4] Cancer of the larynx limited to the vocal cords grows slowly because of the scarcity of lymph vessels in the area. Elsewhere in the larynx, such as the epiglottis, lymph vessels are abundant, and cancer of these tissues often spreads rapidly and metastasizes early to the deep lymph nodes of the neck. Hoarseness is an early symptom of cancer of the vocal cords. If treatment is given when this first sign (due to the tumor's preventing complete approximation of the vocal cords) appears, a cure usually is possible. Signs of metastases of cancer in other parts of the larynx include a sensation of a lump in the throat, pain in the Adam's apple that radiates to the ear, dyspnea, dysphagia, enlarged cervical nodes, and cough.

Cancer of the larynx is ten times more common in men than in women, and it occurs most often in persons past 60 years of age. There seems to be some relationship between cancer of the larynx and heavy smoking, chronic laryngitis, vocal abuse, and family predisposition to cancer. Any person who becomes progressively hoarse or is hoarse for longer than two weeks should be urged to seek medical attention at once. The diagnosis of cancer of the larynx is made from the history, from visual examination of the larynx with a laryngoscope, and from a biopsy and microscopic study of the lesion.

Partial laryngectomy. If the tumor has not involved the muscles and if the motility of the cord is normal, a partial laryngectomy may effect a cure in early carcinoma of the vocal cords. The most common technique is to make an opening into the larynx through the thyroid cartilage *(laryngofissure)* and remove the involved cord and tumor. As healing takes place, scar tissue fills the defect where the diseased cord was removed and becomes a vibrating surface within the larynx. This tissue permits husky but acceptable speech. A tracheostomy tube is inserted at the time of operation but is removed when edema in the surrounding tissues subsides. For forty-eight hours postoperatively, food may be supplied intravenously or by a nasogastric tube. The patient may then take fluids by mouth. Other care is similar to that given the patient having a tracheotomy for other reasons. The patient who has had a partial laryngectomy usually is not on absolute voice rest but is not permitted to use his voice until the doctor gives specific approval (usually three days postoperatively). He should then only whisper until healing is complete, after which time he usually adjusts quite readily to his relatively minor limitation of speech.

Total laryngectomy. When cancer of the larynx is advanced, a total laryngectomy may be performed. This procedure includes removal of the epiglottis, thyroid cartilage, hyoid bone, cricoid cartilage, and two or three rings of the trachea. The pharyngeal opening is closed, the anterior wall of the esophagus is reinforced, and the remaining trachea is brought out to the neck wound and sutured to the skin. It forms a permanent opening *(tracheostomy)* through which the patient breathes. He no longer breathes through his nose or mouth, and he no longer has a laryngeal voice. A radical neck dissection also may be done to remove metastases to surrounding tissues and lymph nodes. In certain selected cases radiation therapy may be used instead of surgery.

The patient who is to have a laryngectomy is told by the doctor that he will breathe through a special opening made in his neck and that he no longer will have normal speech. He is often depressed by this news, which threatens his economic, social, and emotional status, as well as his life. It is helpful for the patient to be visited by another patient who has made a good recovery from laryngectomy and who has undergone rehabilitation successfully. No one else can give the patient the reassurance that he can regain speech as well as a fellow patient. Many large cities have a "Lost Cord Club" or a "New Voice Club," and the members are willing to visit hospitalized patients. Information regarding these clubs may be obtained by writing to the International Association of Laryngectomies.* Local speech rehabilitation centers may be available to supply instructive films and other resources. The local chapter of the American Cancer

---

*American Cancer Society, Inc., 521 W. 57th Street, New York, N. Y. 10019.

Society and the local health department also have information available. If possible, the family, too, should learn about the method of esophageal speech that the patient will learn to use.

The preoperative and postoperative care of the patient is essentially the same as that described for tracheotomy. Some patients may not have a tube in the tracheostomy after the operation because the sutures keep the stoma open and because their surgeons believe that there is less tissue reaction and a better stoma if no tube is used. Other patients will return with a laryngeal tube, which is somewhat larger than the tracheostomy tube, in the opening. It will remain there until the wound is healed and a permanent fistula has formed, usually in two or three weeks. Frequent suctioning is necessary in the early postoperative period to keep the trachea free of secretions.

If a radical neck dissection has also been performed, the patient may have a pressure dressing applied that may interfere with respirations. The patient is more comfortable and can breathe better if he is placed in a mid-Fowler's position. If drains have been inserted in the wound, drainage may be noted on the dressing soon after the operation. A catheter may be inserted into the wound and attached to suction. The dressing then may be small or absent, and the drainage from the wound should be minimal (p. 625).

A nasogastric tube may be inserted for the instillation of food and fluids at regular intervals (Fig. 138). The use of the tube to give food is thought to minimize contamination of the pharyngeal and esophageal suture lines and to prevent fluid from leaking through these wounds into the trachea before healing occurs. Some surgeons feel that, with modern suturing and drainage techniques, tube feedings are not necessary, and they permit the patient to take food and fluid by mouth after the second postoperative day. If the nasogastric tube is used, it is removed as soon as the patient can swallow safely. The patient then needs careful attention in his first attempts to swallow. He may feel that he is choking, and may have severe coughing that is frightening and painful. It is extremely important that the nurse be present when swallowing is first attempted and that she be prepared to suction the trachea and bronchi at once if aspiration does occur. Only water should be given until the patient has become accustomed to swallowing.

The patient who has a tracheostomy must take some special precautions. He must not go swimming and must be careful while bathing or taking a shower that water is not aspirated through the opening into the lungs. He is advised to wear a scarf or a shirt with a closed collar that covers the opening yet is of porous material. This material substitutes for some of the functions normally assumed by the nasal passages, such as the warming of air and the screening of dust and other irritating substances.

Speech rehabilitation may be started as soon as the tracheostomy tube has been removed. Information regarding learning alaryngeal speech may be obtained by writing to the American Speech and Hearing Association* or to the International Association of Laryngectomies. Most patients learn esophageal speech faster if they go to a special speech clinic. Speech centers such as the National Hospital for Speech Disorders in New York City and the Cleveland Hearing and Speech Center are located in various communities. Although the patient may need to go to a nearby city for this instruction, he usually must remain away from home for only one or two weeks. If his emotional outlook is good, his ability to learn esophageal speech is remarkable. About 75% of patients who have their larynx removed master some sort of intelligible speech in two or three weeks, some in two to six lessons. The average patient can return to work one or two months after leaving the hospital.

To learn esophageal speech, the patient must first practice burping. This provides the moving column of air needed for sound, while folds of tissue at the opening of the esophagus act as the vibrating surface. The patient must learn to coordinate his articulation with the esophageal vocalization made possible by aspirating air into the esophagus. His new voice sounds are natural although somewhat hoarse. The qualities of speech provided by the use of the nasopharynx are still present, however. The patient may have

digestive difficulty during the time he is learning to speak. This difficulty is due to the swallowing of air as he practices, to the unusual strain on abdominal muscles, and to nervous tension. The patient should be told that digestive difficulty may occur and that it should not be a cause for alarm. It abates with proficiency in speaking.

If the patient is unable to learn esophageal speech in sixty to ninety days after surgery, an artificial speech aid such as a battery-powered and battery-operated vibrator may be prescribed for him. Various mechanical devices are available, and the newer ones permit a more natural type of speech, providing pitch inflections and volume control. The local chapter of the American Cancer Society may help the patient to obtain a speech aid at a reduced rate. It costs approximately twenty-five dollars.

Diseases of the ear

General nursing in diseases of the ear

A few simple rules should be borne in mind by the nurse when doing treatments on the patient with ear disease. It is important to avoid further infection by washing hands thoroughly before doing any treatment and by seeing that all equipment and material used are sterile. Trauma must be avoided. Hard articles such as a glass medicine dropper, a hairpin, or a toothpick or match should never be inserted into the ear lest the eardrum be perforated accidentally. The auditory canal must never be obstructed by a medicine dropper, irrigating tip, wick, or anything else, since obstruction may produce pressure beyond the obstructing object and damage the eardrum. The nurse should never insert any object beyond where she can see easily and she should instruct the patient who cares for himself to be equally careful in placing anything in the ear canal.

A good practice in doing any treatment for the ear canal is to have an adjustable light, such as a standing gooseneck light, that does not need to be held. The nurse should be able to see exactly what she is doing, and her hands should be free to hold the ear for good visualization and to do the treatment. For best visualization of the ear canal and of the drum, the outer ear is held

---

*1001 Connecticut Avenue, N.W., Washington, D. C. 20036.

down and out in an infant or small child and up and back in an adult.

Ears that are draining are often treated by using dry wipes. Sterile applicators may be used, and often they are prepared on the unit, since commercial ones often are hard and ineffectual. *Wicks* (single pieces of gauze picked up at the center, twisted, and then sterilized) may be inserted gently into the ear canal by the doctor or the nurse to serve as drains to encourage passage of exudate. The loose end extends outside the ear canal. A wick saturated with a medicated solution may be used both as a drain and for local compress effect. A wick also may be inserted after ear drops have been given to distribute and help retain the medication in the ear canal. It must be changed often and never allowed to become hardened with exudate because this may interfere with the flow of drainage.

Irrigations may be ordered in disease of the auditory canal, and they often are used when wax (cerumen) has become impacted in the auditory canal. However, they are seldom used if the eardrum is ruptured, for fear of introducing further infection into the middle ear. When an irrigation is ordered, the irrigation solution should be no warmer than 38° C. (100° F.). The ear is easily stimulated by temperatures that are above or below body temperature, and they may cause vertigo. The patient should sit with the head tilted slightly forward and toward the affected side, holding the emesis basin directly below the ear. The irrigation also may be done with the patient lying down while the nurse sits in a chair. Air should be expelled from the bulb syringe prior to instilling solution, and the tip of the syringe should be directed either toward the roof or toward the floor of the canal but not straight inward. The canal should not be completely obstructed by the syringe since this would keep solution from flowing back and would cause pressure against the eardrum. To assure complete drainage of the irrigation fluid, the nurse should have the patient lie on the affected side for several minutes. The external ear should then be dried thoroughly to prevent excoriation of the skin.

If the patient is to irrigate his ear at home, the nurse should teach him how to do it correctly. By sitting at a wash basin, the patient may manage alone, but it may be better to have the treatment done by a responsible and informed family member. The public health nurse may give this instruction in the patient's home.

Ear drops should be at room temperature because vertigo may result from the stimulation of the ear by high or low temperatures. The patient should lie on his side with the affected ear uppermost. The external ear should be cleansed with a sponge and the canal straightened with one hand, while three or four drops of the prescribed medication are instilled into the ear with a medicine dropper. After the drops are inserted, the patient should remain on the nonaffected side for about five minutes so that the medication will have a chance to reach all of the ear canal. The external ear should be dried thoroughly to prevent skin irritation.

The external ear

External otitis. The external ear may be affected by acute and chronic forms of such conditions as eczematous dermatitis, diffuse dermatitis, fungus, and bacterial infections. These conditions may be associated with systemic diseases, with diseases of the skin of the adjacent face, neck, and scalp, or with diseases of the middle ear. They may be caused by trauma or be the result of a primary invasion of organisms. Any symptoms of redness, scaling, itching, swelling, watery discharge, or crusting should be referred to the otologist since, if these diseases are not treated, chronic changes may result, causing thickening of the skin and stenosis of the external canal.

Local treatment may include application of medicated ointments or powders, compresses to provide heat, soften crusts, or supply medication, and cool applications to lessen inflammation and relieve discomfort. Burow's solution (aluminum acetate solution) often is used for its astringent action, which has a cooling and soothing effect. Antibiotic preparations, such as those containing bacitracin, neomycin, and polymyxin, and the corticosteroids may be prescribed to be applied locally.

When compresses are used, the pillow should be protected, and a loose gauze plug should be placed in the outer ear canal. This plug can either be moistened with solution if the outer ear canal also is involved or be used dry to prevent spread of the infection to the inner part of the canal. Compresses of single-thickness gauze fit the contours of the outer ear best. They should be quite moist yet not dripping. Ice caps are too heavy to use on the exquisitely sensitive external ear. To apply cold, a light application can be made by placing about two cupfuls of crushed ice in a small sealed plastic bag.

Furunculosis of the external auditory canal. Furuncles or boils usually are confined to the external auditory meatus and most often are caused by the *Staphylococcus aureus* or *albus.* They cause severe pain because there is little expansile tissue in the area, and as they enlarge the skin becomes taut and is under great pressure. The swelling may occlude the auditory canal, causing temporary deafness. The administration of antibiotics systemically may resolve the condition, an incision and drainage may be necessary, or wicks treated with antibiotics or drugs such as Burow's solution may be inserted. Acetylsalicylic acid, codeine, or hot compresses may be given to relieve discomfort. When drainage occurs, pain usually subsides.

Impacted cerumen. A certain amount of cerumen in the ear canal is normal, and persons who have no wax have itching and scaling in the ear canal. Occasionally, when the cerumen becomes impacted and causes pain or temporary deafness, it must be removed by the doctor. He may ask the patient to instill several drops of warm sweet oil or hydrogen peroxide into the auditory canal for several days to soften the wax. It can then usually be removed by irrigation with a metal Pomeroy syringe or with a cerumen spoon. Since there is danger of perforating the eardrum, this treatment should be done by a doctor or by a nurse specialist.

Foreign bodies in the ear. Children and mentally disturbed adults occasionally insert foreign bodies such as beans, peas, paper, erasers, crayons, chalk, or buttons into their ears. These articles should be removed by a doctor because there is danger of traumatizing the canal wall, eardrum, or middle ear while probing for them. Insects may get into the ear. Their movements cause pain and noise. A few drops of mineral oil, alcohol, or ether instilled into the ear will either kill or anesthetize the insect. It may then be removed with a forceps or washed out.

The internal ear

Serous otitis media. Serous *(catarrhal)* otitis media is a condition in which sterile serum is present in the middle ear and interferes with hearing. Normally, the nasopharyngeal end of the eustachian tubes opens periodically to permit the passage of air up into the middle ear as swallowing or yawning occurs. This air helps to maintain the pressure within the middle ear equal to that of the external ear. When the opening of the eustachian tube is blocked by nasopharyngeal infections or enlarged adenoids, or when its lumen is swollen by allergic reactions, air cannot enter. The remaining air eventually is absorbed by the mucous membrane lining, and a negative pressure is created that draws fluid from the surrounding tissues into the middle ear. A sudden change in atmospheric pressure, such as that which occurs in flying, can also produce this condition. Ascending from a high atmospheric pressure to a low atmospheric pressure moves air from the middle ear out through the eustachian tube, but as a person descends, air may be unable to pass through the eustachian tube back into the middle ear. Gum chewing or swallowing helps to open the tube, thus permitting air to enter the middle ear.

Serous otitis media may be acute or chronic. It may last for a few days or persist for years. The patient may complain of a sense of fullness or blockage in the ear, hearing loss, a low-pitched tinnitus, and an earache. The eardrum usually appears retracted upon examination. The condition resolves as the cause of the eustachian obstruction is removed. Gentle inflation of the eustachian tube may bring relief. Aspiration of the fluid with a needle or through a myringotomy incision may be necessary in some instances. A polyethylene or Teflon tube sometimes is inserted through an opening in the eardrum to equalize pressure and to speed the absorption of the fluid.

Early and adequate treatment of nasopharyngeal infections and allergic conditions can usually prevent chronic serous otitis media from developing. Since this disease is a cause of conduction deafness in children, the nurse should urge mothers of children who complain of persistent earache to seek medical advice. Any person who complains of tinnitus or who seems to have loss of hearing should be advised to seek medical attention promptly.

Acute purulent otitis media. Acute purulent otitis media is an acute inflammatory process in the middle ear. It is common in infants because their eustachian tubes are short and straight, and thus almost any infection in the nasopharynx has direct access to the middle ear. This disease most often follows the common cold or tonsillitis but may complicate measles or scarlet fever. It may also be caused by the forcing of contaminated water into the middle ear through the eustachian tube while swimming and by blowing the nose improperly. People should be urged to avoid swimming in uninspected pools and in stagnant water, and they should be taught to blow the nose gently, lest infected material be forced into the middle ear. The offending organism usually is the streptococcus or the staphylococcus, which reaches the middle ear by way of the eustachian tube. In children under 6 years of age, however, the offending organism more often is the pneumococcus or the *Haemophilus influenzae.*

The infection usually begins with local engorgement of the blood vessels, which causes swelling of the mucous membrane lining of the eustachian tubes, middle ear, and mastoid cells. As the inflammatory condition progresses, a serous exudate develops in the middle ear and becomes serosanguineous and, later, mucopurulent. The pressure of the exudate may cause the eardrum to rupture. The fluid may drain into the external auditory canal or it may be forced back into the mastoid cells.

In the early stages, the patient complains of a sensation of fullness in the ear. As the infection progresses, the eardrum bulges and the pain becomes severe and throbbing. The pain may cause the child to tug on his ear, or the infant may roll his head from side to side, cry constantly, and refuse to eat. There may be decreased hearing in the affected ear, tinnitus, and fever, which in the child may range as high as 40° to 41.1° C. (104° to 106° F.).

Since antibiotics have been used to treat acute tonsillitis, pharyngitis, rhinitis, and sinusitis, otitis media is no longer a common complication of these conditions. When otitis media does develop, antibiotics are given at once, and the infection usually subsides before acute, painful symptoms occur. Treatment also may include bed rest, the administration of acetylsalicylic acid or codeine for pain, the instillation of warm ear drops such as Auralgan (antipyrine and benzocaine in glycerine) to relieve discomfort, the application of dry heat such as a hot-water bottle, and the forcing of fluids. Usually otitis media is treated on an ambulatory basis, and parents of the infant or young child need careful instruction in his care.

A *myringotomy* (incision into the eardrum) may be performed to permit the fluid that has collected in the middle ear to drain. The procedure usually is performed in the doctor's office or in the clinic. If necessary, a short-acting anesthetic such as nitrous oxide or a topical anesthetic such as ethyl chloride may be used. A single incision is made in the eardrum, and the fluid may be aspirated and cultures taken. It is extremely important that free drainage continue so that it does not cause pressure against the mastoid cells. Cotton may be placed loosely in the outer ear to collect drainage. It should be replaced when it becomes moist, in order to lessen the danger of secondary infection. Dry wipes may be used to remove excess drainage. Petrolatum may be placed around the outer ear to prevent it from becoming excoriated from the drainage. Parents and patients should know that the discharge may be infectious and that the hands should be washed after changing cotton plugs or cleaning the ear. Elbow restraints may be necessary to keep the young child from touching his ear and the drainage. Antibiotics usually are continued for several days after the discharge has stopped. If the patient has a rise in temperature, complains of headache, or becomes drowsy, irritable, or disoriented, the doctor must be notified at once. These signs may indicate that the eardrum needs to be reopened, that mastoid cells are involved, or that a brain abscess or meningitis is developing. A myringotomy incision usually heals completely and does not affect hearing.

Acute mastoiditis. An acute infection of the middle ear usually is accompanied by some inflammatory reaction in the mucosa of the adjacent mastoid process. If the middle ear infection is not treated early or adequately, or if the infection is particularly virulent, acute mastoiditis may occur. The streptococcus, pneumococcus, staphylococcus, or *Haemophilus influenzae* bacillus may be the causative organism. The inflammatory reaction proceeds from edema of the tissues to the formation of exudate and pus that fill the mastoid cells. Pressure on the blood supply causes necrosis to develop and an abscess to form. There may be pain in the ear, mastoid tenderness, fever, headache, and a profuse discharge from the affected ear.

Treatment consists of the use of antibiotics, bed rest, ear drops, medication for pain, and forcing of fluids. If an abscess forms or if the symptoms persist or become worse and cause an elevation of temperature, vertigo, or facial paralysis, surgery is performed. Through an incision in front of or behind the ear, the necrotic mastoid cells are removed, a small rubber drain is inserted, and the wound is closed *(simple mastoidectomy)*. The middle ear is left intact, and hearing is not affected.

Preoperative preparation for a simple mastoidectomy is similar to the routine preoperative care given any patient. If the earache is severe, an ice bag may be used, and acetylsalicylic acid or codeine sulfate may be ordered.

Postoperatively a tight, bulky dressing is applied that provides some hemostasis (Fig. 141). The dressing may be reinforced as necessary, but it is not changed by the nurse. The doctor usually changes it daily. There may be a small amount of serosanguineous drainage apparent on the dressing, but signs of bright blood on outer dressings should be reported at once. If the tissues around the dressing become edematous, the doctor should be notified because the dressing may need to be loosened. Any signs of facial paralysis, such as inability to smile or to wrinkle the forehead, should be reported. Headache, vomiting, stiff neck, dizziness, irritability, or disorientation may forewarn of

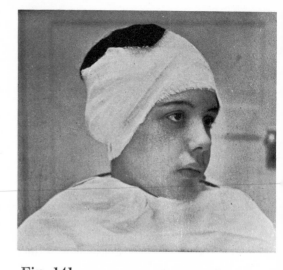

Fig. 141

A mastoid dressing. (From Parkinson, Roy H.: Eye, ear, nose, and throat manual for nurses, ed. 8, St. Louis, 1959, The C. V. Mosby Co.)

a septic thrombosis of the lateral sinus in the brain, meningitis, or brain abscess. A chronic purulent otitis media also occasionally follows this operation, necessitating more radical mastoid surgery.

The patient usually is allowed out of bed within twenty-four to forty-eight hours. Fluids are forced throughout the postoperative course. The nurse should use the postoperative period to teach good health practices. The patient may be prone to future hearing difficulties and should be told that help is available if they occur.

Chronic purulent otitis media. Chronic purulent otitis media is characterized by chronic purulent discharge from the middle ear. It is a sequela to acute otitis media and involves both the middle ear and the mastoid cells. The mastoid bone cells become thickened, and polyps may develop from the mucous membrane of the middle ear. The patient's main complaint may be deafness, occasional pain, or dizziness. If chronic purulent otitis media is permitted to progress unchecked, meningitis, brain abscess, or facial paralysis may eventually occur because the infection gradually erodes the surrounding bone.

Another complication of chronic purulent otitis media is *cholesteatoma.* It occurs when the eardrum has been ruptured and the ear has drained for some time. Skin cells from the ear canal grow into the middle ear, where their normal excrescences combine with mucus and purulent exudate to form a mass that becomes firm and erodes the tissue surrounding it. This mass must be removed surgically.

The best treatment for chronic purulent otitis media is prevention by early treatment of the acute disease. If the chronic condition does occur, it should be treated as soon as it is recognized. The treatment is a *radical mastoidectomy* or a *modified radical mastoidectomy.* An incision is made either behind the ear or directly in front of it, and the mastoid cells are completely removed, converting the middle ear and the mastoid space into one cavity. If the hammer and anvil bones have not already been eroded, they and the remaining tympanic membrane also are removed. The radical mastoid cavity may be allowed to gradually reline with epithelium, or a graft of skin or muscle may be applied. Packing is placed into the wound to keep the graft in position, to hold the external meatus open, and to provide hemostasis. The packing is removed gradually through the external ear. The ungrafted radical mastoid cavity usually is healed two to three months after the operation. Hearing may be permanently lost in the ear, although many people, even after a radical mastoidectomy, have enough hearing left to manage without a hearing aid.[23]

Fortunately, a radical mastoidectomy is required much less often now that antibiotic drugs are used to treat acute infections. With continued attacks of acute infection, however, some organisms may become resistant to certain antibiotics, and treatment may become a problem.

Nursing care for the patient with a radical mastoidectomy is similar to that given the patient having a simple mastoidectomy.

Myringoplasty and tympanoplasty. When chronic perforations of the eardrum cause conductive hearing loss, a *myringoplasty* may be performed. The opening in the eardrum is surgically enlarged, and a piece of skin, vein, or fascia, large enough to fit the opening, is sutured over it. Gelfoam or clotted blood may be used to fill the middle ear space to support the graft, and packing is placed outside, in the external ear, to help keep the graft in position. If the graft takes, a large degree of tympanic function will return.

Other parts of the middle ear also require reconstructive surgery, and the procedures are known collectively as *tympanoplasty.* They may include removal of any scar tissue that interferes with the function of the ossicles, replacement of diseased ossicles with plastic or metal prostheses, and reconstruction of the eardrum. These procedures usually are not performed on children because they are highly susceptible to infections that reach the middle ear by way of the eustachian tubes, and therefore the graft is likely to become infected.

Labyrinthitis. Labyrinthitis is an infection of the inner ear (the labyrinth) and usually is a complication of chronic middle ear infection. The inner ear helps maintain equilibrium, and infections there, in addition to producing loss of hearing, disturb the function of the semicircular canals, causing severe vertigo, nausea, vomiting, and nystagmus (abnormal jerking movements of the eyes).

The patient who has labyrinthitis is kept in bed and given massive doses of antibiotics. If vomiting persists, fluids must be given parenterally. However, fluids by mouth usually are retained if they are taken in small amounts and if the patient lies with his head perfectly still. Since the patient is quite dizzy, side rails should be placed on the bed to prevent him from falling. An operation such as a radical mastoidectomy is sometimes done to remove the source of the infection. His other nursing care is similar to that for the patient with Ménière's syndrome.

Ménière's syndrome. The cause of Ménière's syndrome is unknown. There is hypertension of the endolymphatic fluid circulation in the cochlea due to increased production of endolymph or to decreased absorption of it. Atrophy of the hearing mechanism eventually occurs. The patient is incapacitated by severe attacks of vertigo, sometimes to the extent that he is unable to cross a room without falling. He describes a sensation of dizziness, severe tinnitus (ringing in the ears), and a feeling that the room is spinning about him. During an attack, any sudden motion of the head or eyes tends to precipitate nausea and vomiting. The patient may appear withdrawn and irritable as well as acutely ill. Attacks may occur at intervals of weeks or months. They may disappear without treatment or they may continue until the patient is completely deaf in the affected ear. When the eighth nerve (acoustic) dies, symptoms cease.

Diagnosis is made from the patient's history and from the results of a caloric test made to differentiate this disease from an acoustic neurinoma. The *caloric test* consists of dripping cold water into the ear. This procedure causes a normal patient to become dizzy, and it precipitates a severe attack in one who has Ménière's syndrome. Patients with acoustic neurinomas have no reaction to this test.

There are many types of treatment, and they all may be prescribed for the patient during the course of this disease. In order to reduce the hypertension, fluid intake may be limited and diuretic drugs such as chlorothiazide (Diuril) may be ordered. If the sodium ion is thought to be a factor in the production of fluid, a salt-free or low-salt diet may be prescribed. Vasodilating drugs such as nicotinic acid often are used. Dimenhydrinate (Dramamine) may be given to control nausea, vomiting, and dizziness. If the medical therapy does not control the disease and the patient is incapacitated by the vertigo, surgical removal of the membranous labyrinth may performed, resulting in disappearance of the vertigo and loss of hearing in that ear.

Since sudden movement or jarring aggravates the vertigo, the patient usually prefers to move at his own rate and to take care of himself. If one stands directly in front of him when talking, so that he does not have to turn his head or his eyes, he will experience less dizziness. Although movement increases the symptoms, the patient should be encouraged to move about in bed occasionally and to permit gentle back care to preserve good skin tone. Lying quietly on the unaffected side with eyes turned toward the direction of the affected ear sometimes is recommended to relieve an acute attack. The patient should not try to read, and bright glaring lights should be avoided. Side rails should be on the bed at all times, and the patient should not attempt to get up and walk without assistance lest he injure himself. Because it is usually very difficult to get the patient with Ménière's syndrome to take food or fluids, efforts should be made to obtain something that he will eat or drink.

Otosclerosis. Otosclerosis is a progressive condition in which the normal bone of the inner ear is replaced by abnormal osseous tissue. The new growth of bone forms about the oval window and then about the stapes and blocks its movement so that it is unable to vibrate effectively in response to sound pressure. The other ossicles also may be involved in this process. The cause of otosclerosis is not known, but it tends to run in families, and it is more common in women than in men. In some women, pregnancy may be a precipitating factor. According to one source, a focus of otosclerotic bone can be found in one out of eight middle-aged adult white females and one out of fifteen adult white males examined.[21] The hearing loss is gradual and usually becomes noticeable some time between puberty and 30 year of age. Usually both ears are affected one more than the other, and tinnitus is a troublesome symptom. The treatment for hearing loss due to otosclerosis is a stapedectomy.

Stapedectomy. After a local anesthetic has been administered, an incision is made deep in the ear canal close to the eardrum so that the drum can be turned back and the middle ear exposed. Working through an electric microscope, the surgeon frees and removes the stapes and the attached footplate, leaving an opening in the oval window. The patient can usually hear as soon as this step is completed. The opening is closed with a vein graft, a plug of fat, or Gelfoam, which the body eventually replaces with mucous membrane cells. A plastic tube, a steel wire, or a Teflon piston is inserted to replace the stapes, and is attached at one end to the incus and at the other to the graft or plug to transmit sound to the inner ear. (See Fig. 142.)

The patient usually is kept in bed for forty-eight hours, and he remains flat for the first twenty-four hours, with the operative ear

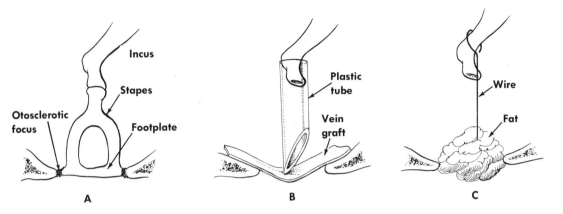

Fig. 142

Two methods of performing a stapedectomy. **A,** Stapes immobilized by otosclerosis. **B,** Replacement of stapes with a plastic tube and closure of the opening in the oval window with a vein graft. **C,** Replacement of stapes with a fine wire and sealing of the opening in the oval window with a ball of fat removed from the earlobe. The wire and fat apparently cause no reaction.

always kept uppermost. If postoperative pain occurs, it usually is relieved by codeine sulfate, 60 mg., or meperidine hydrochloride, 100 mg. Postoperative trauma and edema may cause vertigo for a few days. Drama-mine, 50 mg., is given every six hours to relieve it. The patient should be cautioned against rapid turning since it may cause vertigo. To prevent falls, side rails should be on the bed and the patient should have supervision and assistance when getting out of bed and walking. Antibiotics usually are given to help prevent postoperative infection, and the patient is instructed not to blow his nose for a week to prevent air and organisms from being forced up the eustachian tube. Sneezing should also be avoided, but if a sneeze appears imminent, the patient is advised to open his mouth wide and to sneeze as lightly as possible. He should not lift heavy objects or bend over until such activity is approved by the surgeon. He usually is advised not to wash his hair for two weeks and not to get water into his ear for six weeks. The patient may be discouraged because hearing may be less than he had experienced in the operating room or be less than he had expected. However, the packing in in the ear and postoperative edema

may cause some of this loss, and the full effects of the operation cannot be evaluated in the immediate postoperative period. The usual hospital stay is four or five days. The packing usually is removed in the doctor's office or in the clinic about the sixth day, and most patients are allowed to return to work in two weeks. During the first week the patient may be advised to wear cotton in the ear when outdoors. He should avoid exposure to persons with colds, which might be acquired and lead to middle ear infections. Flying should be avoided for six months after the operation.

Hearing loss

It is estimated that more than 12 million adults and 3 million children in the United States have some kind of hearing defect. Four million of these persons are seriously handicapped, and about 760,000 are totally deaf.[9] For psychologic reasons, hearing loss, hearing defect, or impairment of hearing are the terms used to describe the patient's handicap.

Most hearing difficulties begin in childhood. With adequate treatment of upper-respiratory infections, treatment of aching and draining ears, and care to avoid foreign objects in the ears, hearing loss often can be prevented. The nurse should be alert to every opportunity for health teaching concerning the conservation of hearing. Screening programs in the communities for detecting children with possible hearing losses are helpful in limiting the handicap by getting the child to the doctor. The nurse in industry can help prevent deafness due to noise of high intensity by teaching the employees why they should wear their earplugs. The person who seems to be inattentive or who has a strained facial expression, particularly when conversing or listening to others, may be hard of hearing. Persons with faulty articulation in speech may be deaf. Their faulty articulation may result from not being able to hear themselves speak. The person who habitually fails to respond when spoken to or who makes mistakes in carrying out directions should be encouraged to have his hearing tested. The repetition of "What did you say?" or "uh huh" with a quizzical expression is often a symptom of hearing loss. Persons with marked hearing loss frequently tend to withdraw from others in an attempt to conceal their difficulty.

Hearing is one of man's primary means of communication and helps keep him in touch with reality and his environment. Every effort should be made to develop, protect, and preserve it. As hearing diminishes, the impact of not understanding others and of not being understood may make the person withdraw from social situations, and he may become anxious and insecure. His fear of inadequacy and inferiority may make him suspicious and depressed. When hearing is completely gone, the individual may find his silent world almost intolerable. Loneliness and isolation eventually may lead to disorientation or the lack of desire to live. The nurse can help find and direct the person with a hearing loss and his family to the appropriate agencies for assistance. There may be ways of improving his hearing through medical or surgical therapy. If the loss is irreversible, aural rehabilitation may make it possible for him to understand and communicate with others again so that he can lead a useful, meaningful life. Unfortunately, many persons who have a hearing loss are in the older age group and usually also have some loss of vision, making rehabilitation more difficult.

Types of hearing loss. Hearing loss is classified in several ways. Any interference with the conduction of sound impulses through the external auditory canal, the eardrum, or the middle ear produces a conductive type of hearing loss. The inner ear is not involved, and sound directed to it will be heard clearly. Conductive hearing loss may be due to impacted cerumen or a foreign body in the external auditory canal, a thickening, retracting, scarring, or perforation of the eardrum, pathologic changes in the middle ear that prevent movement of one or more of the ossicles, or a fixing of the stapes due to otosclerosis. At the present time, it is only the conductive type of hearing loss that can be treated effectively.

Sensorineural hearing loss results from disease in the inner ear or its neural pathways. Some of the causes include arteriosclerosis, infectious diseases such as mumps, measles, and meningitis, toxicity to drugs such as quinine, dihydrostreptomycin, or neomycin, neurinoma of the eighth cranial nerve, blows to the head or the ears, and degeneration of the organ of Corti due to exposure to noise of high intensity. Treatment usually is not effective for sensorineural loss because the damage has been done by the time the patient goes to the doctor and the process is irreversible. In many cases sensorineural hearing loss can be prevented by such measures as avoiding toxic drugs, controlling noise in industry and wearing ear protection when exposed to loud noises, and early and adequote treatment of middle ear infections such as otitis media and of systemic diseases such as measles so that the disease does not involve the inner ear. Many persons have hearing losses caused by a combination of the two main types of difficulty.

Rehabilitation. The purpose of rehabilitation of persons with a hearing loss is to reestablish and maintain oral communication by means of hearing aids, maximum application of any remaining hearing ability, and increased use of the other senses. The patient may be fitted with and taught to use a hearing aid. He is taught how to use his remaining hearing ability more effectively by developing his listening skills to improve the hearing he has left and to compensate for what he has lost. Speech reading is taught to supplement the hearing function, and includes lipreading and the study of facial ex-

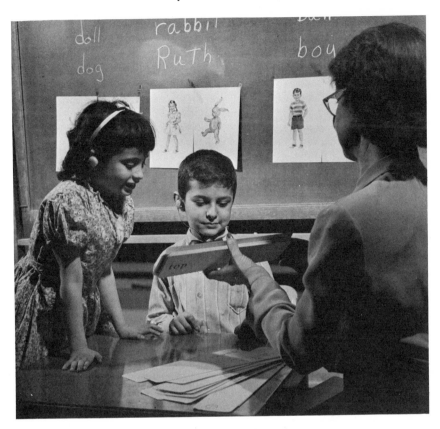

Fig. 143

Children with hearing difficulties practice reading preparatory to joining classes for children with normal hearing. Note the hearing aids. (Courtesy New York League for the Hard of Hearing, New York, N. Y.)

pressions, gestures, and body movements used in speech. Speech training is given to develop, conserve, or correct speech. The patient's acceptance of the fact that he has a hearing loss, his desire to seek help, his use of the facilities available, together with high motivation, perseverance, and patience, contribute to the success of a program of rehabilitation.

Services for persons with a hearing loss may be offered by audiology clinics sponsored by universities, hospitals, community programs, local or state departments of health and education, or the Veterans Administration. The national organizations are available to give information and counseling.*

*American Federation of the Physically Handicapped, Inc., 1370 National Press Building, Washington, D. C. 20004; American Hearing Society, 919 18th Street, N.W., Washington, D. C. 20006; American Speech and Hearing Association, 1001 Connecticut Avenue, N.W., Washington, D. C. 20036; National Association of the Deaf, c/o Byron B. Burnes, 2495 Stattuck Avenue, Berkeley, Calif. 94700.

In working with the patient who has difficulty hearing, the nurse should be aware of certain considerations and should teach them to others who are in contact with people who have a hearing loss. Speak in a normal voice, and tell the patient when he speaks too loudly that it is not necessary to do so. This will help him to regain his normal modulation. Always talk directly to a deaf patient, making sure that the light is on your face. This helps him to lip-read. Speak clearly, but do not accentuate words. If the patient does not seem to understand what is said, express it differently. Some words are difficult to "see" in lip-reading. Do not smoke or cover the mouth while speaking to a person with limited hearing. If he wears a hearing aid, wait until he adjusts it before speaking. Do not avoid conversation with a person who has a hearing loss. It has been said that to live in a silent world is much more devastating than to live in darkness, and persons with hearing loss appear, by and large, to have more emotional difficulties than those who are blind.

Habilitation is necessary for the child who is born deaf or becomes deaf in early childhood, because he has never acquired language and speech. He is educable, but his education requires more time. The child who has never heard speech it unable to imitate it. He should start attending a special nursery school at the age of 3 or 4 years, since a period of about three years is required for

a child to learn sufficient language to begin the first grade (Fig. 143). He may then attend classes with children who have normal hearing or go to a public or private school for deaf children.

Hearing aids. Hearing aids are instruments used to increase the sound reaching the ear of the person with a hearing loss. They do not improve the ability to hear, but they make the sound louder. Hearing aids usually are prescribed when the patient has difficulty in understanding speech in his occupation or in everyday conversations. A loss in the better ear averaging more than 30 decibels in the speech range of 500 to 2,000 cps indicates the need for a hearing aid. Patients with a conductive hearing loss benefit most from wearing a hearing aid because their loss usually is in the low and middle frequencies, for which most good hearing aids can compensate. They will not hear as well as they did with normal hearing, but they will be able to hear speech in the frequencies at which most ordinary conversations occur (50 to 60 decibels at 300 to 3,500 cps). Because patients with sensorineural loss usually have a hearing loss in the higher frequencies, an intolerance for loud speech and noise, and difficulty in understanding what is being said, they may find the amplification by the hearing aid annoying and impractical for them. Elderly people often have difficulty adjusting to the use of the hearing aid, partially because their hearing loss usually is of sensorineural origin. Their problems also may be due to a lack of patience, of concentration, or of the mental energy needed to learn to use a hearing aid. Small children with a hearing loss may be fitted with a hearing aid before they begin to crawl and will learn to use it at all times.

The hearing aid usually consists of a microphone used to receive spoken speech and environmental sounds and to convert them into electrical signals, an amplifier to strengthen electrical signals, a receiver to convert electrical signals back to sound, and a battery to supply the electrical power. A variety of hearing aids are available. They may be worn on the body (Fig. 144), built into the temple bow of eyeglasses, or worn as individual units behind the ear or in the ear canal. Hearing aids are not custom-built, and only minor adjustments can be made

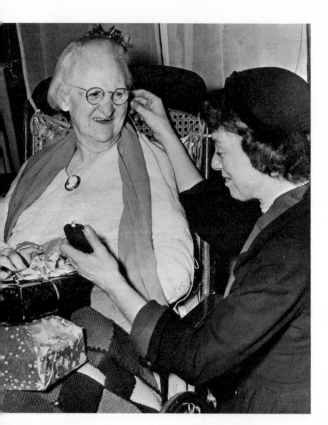

Fig. 144

A nurse from New York League for the Hard of Hearing assists an elderly patient to adjust her hearing aid. (Courtesy New York League for the Hard of Hearing, New York, N. Y.)

for individual patients. The cost of a single unit is between $85 and $350; binaural aids are much more expensive. Upkeep cost varies between $30 and $100 per year, depending upon the repairs needed and the number of batteries used.

The patient should also be instructed in the care of his hearing aid. The ear mold or plug may be washed daily in mild soap and water, with a pipe cleaner used to cleanse the cannula. It should be thoroughly dried before being reconnected to the receiver. The transmitter of a hearing aid worn on the body should be worn so that the microphone faces the speaker, and it should not be covered by heavy clothing. Men often wear it in their shirt or upper coat pocket. Women may fit it into a special pocket sewed on the outside of their underclothing. Children often wear it in a fabric harness placed over their undergarments. The person who uses a hearing aid should carry an extra battery and cord at all times.

References and selected readings*

1 Armstrong, Inez L., and Browder, Jane J.: The nursing care of children, ed. 2, Philadelphia, 1964, F. A. Davis Co.

2 Beeson, Paul B., and McDermott, Walsh, editors: Cecil-Loeb textbook of medicine, ed. 11, Philadelphia, 1963, W. B. Saunders Co.

3 Boies, Lawrence R., Hilger, Jerome A., and Priest, Robert E.: Fundamentals of otolaryngology, ed. 4, Philadelphia, 1964, W. B. Saunders Co.

4 Davis, Loyal, editor: Christopher's textbook of surgery, ed. 8, Philadelphia, 1964, W. B. Saunders Co.

5 Fuerst, Elinor V., and Wolff, LuVerne: Fundamentals of nursing, ed. 3, Philadelphia, 1964, J. B. Lippincott Co.

6 *Gardner, Warren H.: Adjustment problems of laryngectomized women, Arch. Otolaryng. 83:31-42, Jan. 1966.

7 Gellis, Sydney S., and Kagan, Benjamin M.: Current pediatric therapy, 1966-1967, Philadelphia, 1966, W. B. Saunders Co.

8 Gilmore, Stuart I.: Rehabilitation after laryngectomy, Am. J. Nursing 61:87-89, Jan. 1961.

9 Havener, William H., Saunders, William H., and Bergersen, Betty S.: Nursing care in eye, ear, nose, and throat disorders, St. Louis, 1964, The C. V. Mosby Co.

10 Hoenig, Leah: A hearing program for schoolchildren, Am. J. Nursing 63:85-87, May 1963.

11 Klotz, Robert E., and Robinson, Mildred: Hard-of-hearing patients have special problems, Am. J. Nursing 63:88-89, May 1963.

12 Marlow, Dorothy R., and Sellew, Gladys: Textbook of pediatric nursing, ed. 2, Philadelphia, 1965, W. B. Saunders Co.

13 Monteiro, Lois: The patient had difficulty communicating, Am. J. Nursing 62:78-81, Jan. 1962.

14 Nelson, Waldo E.: Textbook of pediatrics, ed. 8, Philadelphia, 1964, W. B. Saunders Co.

15 O'Neill, John J.: The hard of hearing, Englewood Cliffs, N. J., 1965, Prentice-Hall, Inc.

16 *Quimby, Margaret Ann: Care of patients with labyrinthine dysfunction, Am. J. Nursing 60:1780-1781, Dec. 1960.

17 *Ronnei, Eleanor C.: Hearing aids, Am. J. Nursing 63:90-93, May 1963.

18 *Riley, Edward C.: Preventing deafness from industrial noise, Am. J. Nursing 63:80-84, May 1963.

19 Robinson, Mendell: A four-year study of the stainless steel stapes, Arch. Otolaryng. 82:217-235, Sept. 1965.

20 Ryan, Robert E., Thornell, William C., and von Leden, Hans: Synopsis of ear, nose, and throat diseases, ed. 2, St. Louis, 1963, The C. V. Mosby Co.

21 Shambaugh, George E., Jr.: Surgery of the ear, Philadelphia, 1959, W. B. Saunders Co.

22 Sheehy, James L.: Ossicular problems in tympanoplasty, Arch. Otolaryng. 81:115-122, Feb. 1965.

23 Shepard, Mary Estelle: Nursing care of patients with eye, ear, nose, and throat disorders, New York, 1958, The Macmillan Co.

24 Sykes, Eleanor M.: No time for silence, Am. J. Nursing 66:1040-1041, May 1966.

25 *Totman, Laurence E., and Lehman, Roger H.: Tracheostomy care, Am. J. Nursing 64:96-98, March 1964.

26 Yanagisawa, Eiji, and Kirchner, John A.: The cuffed tracheotomy tube, Arch. Otolaryng. 79:80-87, Jan. 1964.

*References preceded by an asterisk are particularly well suited for student reading.

23

The patient with disease of the teeth and mouth

Study questions

1 Review the anatomy of the teeth, jaws, and mouth. How are the teeth formed? To what is the tongue attached?
2 What main purpose is achieved by chewing food? What enzyme is present in saliva and what is its function?
3 Review the location and function of the thoracic duct.
4 From your notes on fundamentals of nursing, review the measures that can be used to control unpleasant odors in the mouth.

This chapter will consider prevention of and nursing care in diseases of the teeth, and infections, tumors, and trauma involving the mouth and closely related structures. In all these conditions prevention is much more important than treatment and attempted cure after disease has become well established.

The mouth has special emotional significance for every individual, perhaps because it is associated in infancy with food, sucking, warmth, love, and security. It continues to be associated throughout life with survival through the intake of food and with pleasurable sensations related to love and companionship, acceptance and belonging. Therefore, severe emotional reactions frequently occur when treatment involving the mouth is necessary. The patient may refuse to visit his dentist, may go into complete panic when the jaws must be wired and normal eating is impossible, and may refuse to accept the fact that a lesion in the mouth is any threat to his health. An understanding of what may be some of the patient's unspoken and often unrealized fears will enable the nurse to give him better care. Patience in explaining tests and treatments often helps. Sometimes merely taking time to explain to the patient how he may be fed following a mouth operation may make the difference between his acceptance or rejection of the procedure. Sometimes the patient needs time to accept the need for referral to a doctor or dentist and to accept the suggested treatment.

Diseases of teeth and closely related structures

General prevention. Teaching the prevention of disease of the teeth and related structures is an important health education responsibility of nurses. Responsibilities vary according to the needs of patients or groups of patients. They include providing public information about overall preventive health measures such as the fluoride treatment of water, proper daily care of teeth and gums to preserve their health, care related to satisfactory use of artificial dentures, diet, general mouth hygiene including regular visits to the dentist, and alertness to the possible significance of lesions anywhere in the mouth.

No organized teaching plan is necessary, and no unit of time need be specifically set aside for dental health education. The nurse must have at her command certain facts to use throughout her day's work. Almost every patient needs to learn about care of the teeth and mouth, whether he is admitted to the hospital with an acute illness or confined to his home because of a heart condition, an infection of his foot, or any other cause.

Nurses will probably be asked about some common misconceptions, and they should know the answers.[13] For example, there is no evidence that any general systemic disease is caused by decayed teeth. There is no evidence that calcium is removed from the mother's teeth during pregnancy and lactation regardless of how deficient in calcium her diet may be. There is, however, abundant evidence that a diet adequate in calcium, phosphorus, and other essential elements during pregnancy contributes to good tooth formation in the growing fetus and that a diet rich in these substances is essential during the years of life when the permanent teeth are being formed. Calcium is deposited in the buds of the permanent teeth almost immediately after birth. A high-calcium diet after teeth have erupted

probably has no effect whatever on their preservation, but local action of other foods such as carbohydrates is of tremendous importance.[14]

General care of the teeth. The nurse is frequently asked about the kind of toothbrush to use and about general care of the teeth. The important points to emphasize are a proper brush, correct method of brushing, and correct time of brushing (after eating).

There is general agreement among dental authorities that toothbrushes should be small enough to reach all tooth surfaces. Usually two or three rows of bristles are recommended, depending on how much space exists between the cheek and the outer tooth surface. Bristles should be straight across the brushing surface, since tufts of bristles may traumatize the gums. Bristles should be firm but not hard. While nylon bristles dry quickly and are durable, natural bristles are preferred because they are less abrasive. Every person should have two toothbrushes and should use them alternately, permitting each brush to dry thoroughly between uses; this helps to prevent bacterial growth and to keep the brush firmer. The electric-powered toothbrush is easy to use and safe to operate. Its use may encourage children to brush their teeth more often and may help incapacitated persons to clean their teeth more thoroughly.[18] The individual, detachable brushes make it convenient for use in a family or hospital unit.

Brushing the teeth should remove debris from between the teeth, stimulate the gums, and yet not traumatize the delicate gingival papillae between the teeth (Fig. 145). Because the oral mucosa of the child is thin and easily injured, brushing of the teeth usually is not started before the third year. The child should be taken to the dentist at the age of 3 years and every six months thereafter. Many people brush their teeth by passing the bristles quickly across the lateral surfaces of the teeth. This method damages the enamel, does not clean between the teeth, and may injure the gums. The brush should be placed along the gum line with bristles toward the roots of the teeth. Then the bristles should be brought down over the gum and teeth with a gentle sweep, always using a downward or upward motion. Cross-

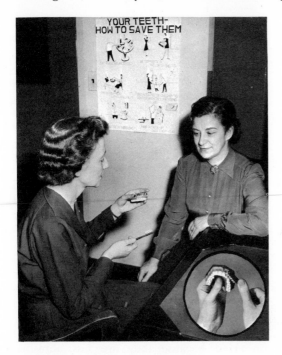

Fig. 145

The correct method of brushing the teeth is reviewed with a patient. Equipment for demonstration is useful in teaching.

wise motion should be reserved for the top grinding surfaces of the back teeth.

Some dentists recommend a slight vibrating motion over the gums with the brush for further stimulation before each downward or upward sweep of the brush, whereas others recommend massage of the gums following brushing. Massage is accomplished by gentle rubbing of the gums with a finger, using very gentle pressure toward the biting surfaces of the teeth. Gum surfaces may be massaged for a few minutes two or three times a day.

Dentifrices and mouthwashes are not really necessary. They simply make brushing the teeth more pleasant. Most dentists recommend any accepted dentifrice that is preferred by the patient and suggest that salt and sodium bicarbonate are much cheaper than commercial dentifrices and equally good. It is estimated that the American public pays approximately $80 million each year for mouthwashes and cleansing agents for their teeth, whereas sodium bicarbonate and salt flavored with peppermint would cost only a fraction of that amount. Ammoniated dentifrices and those containing chlorophyll are subject to much inquiry at present, but so far their benefits have not been proved. Dentifrices containing fluoride help to prevent caries, and their value has been officially recognized by the American Dental Association.

Mouthwashes do not significantly inhibit bacterial growth in the mouth. They should not be used by the patient in an effort to treat a mouth infection because they may be irritating to an infected mouth and, if used excessively, may be harmful to natural bacterial flora in the mouth. For the most part, however, they are harmless and are acceptable additions to mouth hygiene if desired by the patient and if he can afford them. Most dentists suggest warm water and salt to rinse the mouth if occasional bleeding of the gums occurs. Sodium perborate may be irritating to gum tissues and should not be used without specific medical or dental instruction. Dental floss should not be used regularly unless it has been recommended by the dentist and instruction as to its correct use has been given. It must be gently forced between the teeth with pressure exerted toward the side of the tooth so that it will not traumatize the gingival papillae. An instrument that ejects a stream of water to force food particles from between the teeth without traumatizing the gums is now available (Water Pik).

The essentials of good nutrition should be emphasized in the diet of all persons. The nurse may note signs of nutritional deficiency in the mouths of persons who have inadequate food intake since they often have bright, spongy gum margins that bleed easily.

Dental caries. Dental caries (decay of the teeth) is probably the most common, yet the most neglected, chronic ailment of modern man. The American Dental Association reports that tooth decay is occurring in the United States five times faster than it can be repaired.[9] Dental caries is a progressive disease of the teeth related to the consumption of refined carbohydrates such as candy. Within thirty minutes after eating, organisms in the mouth act upon the refined sugars left on the teeth and produce acids that eventually dissolve the enamel surface of the tooth. Decay, cavity formation, inflammation, infection, and loss of teeth follow. Malocclusion gradually develops as teeth are lost. Over 20% of children at the age of 2 years, over 50% at the age of 3 years, and over 75% at the age of 5 years have dental decay. By the age of 14 years, over 95% of children have experienced some dental caries.[7] The average tooth decay rate is about one tooth per person per year.[9] Methods that would control and prevent dental caries include good mouth hygiene, dental examinations every six months, proper foods, including the avoidance of refined sugars, and the use of fluorides.

The addition of *fluoride* to drinking water in the proportion of one part of fluoride to a million parts of water has been shown conclusively to increase the resistance of tooth enamel to bacterial action during the formative period of young children's teeth and to reduce dental caries between 48 and 70%.[18] The protection received is permanent and will last a lifetime. Repeated studies have proved that there are no harmful effects to persons who use fluoride in this concentration or even in double this concentration. There is even evidence to indicate that the small amount of fluoride retained and stored in the bones helps to decrease the incidence of fractures and osteoporosis in older people.[9] Mottling of the teeth may occur in parts of the country where the natural water supply contains two or more parts of fluoride per million parts of water, but harmful effects have not been demonstrated.

If the community water is not fluoridated, daily fluoride supplements may be given to children up to 12 years of age. The optimum daily dose for the child up to 1 year of age is 0.25 mg., for the child from 1 to 6 years is 0.5 mg., and for the child from 6 to 12 years is 1 mg.[7] Because the drug must be taken every day from infancy to 12 years of age, some children and their parents find the regimen difficult to follow. The prescription of fluoride supplements to pregnant women for prevention of decay in the teeth of the developing child is not recommended at this time, as the data regarding their effectiveness are contradictory. Vitamin-fluoride preparations are available, but there is no evidence that they help control dental caries. The use of these preparations is expensive, and the dosage of fluoride cannot be controlled.[11]

Although less effective and much more expensive than fluoridation of water, local application of fluoride to the teeth of children has been found helpful. Topical application of fluoride cannot prevent cavities from progressing, but it can reduce the development of new cavities by about 40%. It is recommended that children who are not protected by fluoridation of water supplies be given this preventive treatment. Some dentists recommend the local application of fluoride to the teeth in addition to the systemic ingestion of fluoride as an extra protection against the development of caries.[7,11] The treatment consists of one application of stannous fluoride or acid phosphate fluoride to cleaned, dry teeth. It is recommended that the treatment be done when the child is 3 years of age and again at the age of 7 years to protect both the deciduous and the permanent teeth. The treatment usually is repeated at 10 and 13 years of age, to protect teeth that appear after 7 years of age. Newly erupted enamel is able to absorb the fluoride ion and form a thin layer of acid-resistant fluorapatite on the enamel surface. Old enamel does not readily absorb the fluoride ion.[16]

The addition of stannous fluoride to dentifrices helps to prevent tooth decay if used regularly. Acid phosphate fluoride and monofluoride phosphate give evidence that they may equal or surpass the results obtained with stannous fluoride dentifrices.[11] Stannous fluoride recently has been added to prophylaxis pastes used by dentists and dental hygienists to clean and polish teeth. If this method proves effective in reducing caries, cleaning and polishing the teeth and the application of the fluoride may be accomplished in one treatment.[11]

The elimination or drastic curtailment of refined carbohydrate foods would reduce the prevalence of dental caries. In 1823 the average American consumed eight pounds of sugar per year, whereas now he uses over one hundred pounds per year. The consumption of lollipops, ice cream, hard candies, and soft drinks, which are so much a part of

American culture, should be curtailed or, preferably, eliminated. The custom of concluding a meal with a sweet dessert and/or candies contributes to tooth decay. The European custom of ending the meal with fresh fruit is an excellent one, since fresh fruit sugars and unrefined starches contain properties that inhibit bacterial enzyme action in the mouth. In fact, eating a raw apple before retiring is an excellent way to clean one's teeth.

Brushing the teeth or even rinsing the mouth with plain water immediately after ingestion of refined carbohydrate foods helps prevent decay. The times when most people brush their teeth are entirely wrong from the standpoint of prevention of dental caries. It is during the first half hour after eating refined carbohydrate that the most harm is done. Immediate rinsing of the mouth with plain water is more helpful than is thorough brushing of the teeth hours afterward when the bacterial damage has been done.

Periapical abscess. A periapical abscess is an abscess around the root of a tooth. It usually is an extension of an infection arising in the pulp caused by dental caries. The abscess may perforate along the gum margin, causing what is commonly known as a *gum boil,* or it may travel medially to form an abscess over the palate or spread directly to the soft tissues, causing cellulitis and a severely swollen face.

Periapical abscess can cause severe local pain and systemic reactions including malaise, nausea, and elevation of temperature. The treatment consists of drilling an opening into the pulp chamber of the tooth to establish drainage and to relieve pain. Penicillin may be given, and warm, saline mouthwashes usually are ordered several times a day. After the acute phase, the tooth may be extracted, or root canal therapy may be started if a sound, permanent tooth is involved. An *apicoectomy* (amputation of the end of the root) may be necessary.[7]

Periodontal disease. Periodontal disease is a disease of the tissues that support the teeth (the periodontium) and affects the gingivae, bone, cementum, and periodontal membrane (Fig. 146). Symptoms include infection, bleeding, recession of the gums, and loosening of the teeth. Deterioration of bone structure occurs, and teeth may eventually fall out or have to be extracted. After the age of 40 years, more people lose their teeth from this cause than from dental caries. Periodontal disease is receiving much more attention than formerly, partly because of the recognition of the whole field of dental health as a major public health problem. The United States Public Health Service is cooperating in studies, and most states now have preventive dental health programs that include attention to other dental diseases besides caries.

Many factors contribute to the development of periodontal disease, among them malocclusion, accumulation of tartar, poor nutrition, including eating too much soft food instead of solid food that requires mastication, poor mouth hygiene, and improper brushing of the teeth. *Malocclusion* may result in a poor bite with unequal pressure on teeth. It leads to deterioration of bony supportive structures. Removal of teeth without proper replacements permits the teeth to drift backward and alters the bite, again producing unequal pressure on working surfaces of the teeth. Premature loss of even temporary teeth in children should be referred to a dentist. The pressure and irritation of tartar, a hard, irritating substance that accumulates along gum margins of the teeth, destroys the tiny tendrils holding the tooth in the socket and leads to unhealthy receding gums with lessened tooth support (Fig. 146). Poor nutrition, improper brushing of the teeth, and local infection may augment the destruction of gums and supportive gum structures to such a degree that they recede. The leverage of daily use then becomes too great upon the teeth, and they loosen and finally have to be removed.

Treatment of periodontal disease includes maintenance of oral hygiene and nutrition, control of local irritations and infections by regular visits to the dentist, removal of accumulations of tartar on the teeth, replacement of lost teeth, and correction of malocclusion. Even if treatment has been delayed until there is already a good deal of damage, care by an *orthodontist* (one who specializes in straightening teeth) may be surprisingly helpful. Sometimes bridgework and other forms of splinting can be used so that further erosion of bone and supportive

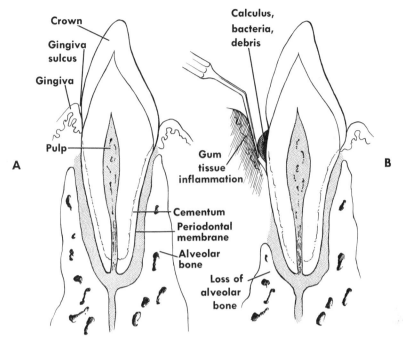

Fig. 146

A, Normal tooth with gum and root structures. **B,** The presence of foreign materials along the gum margin, which may lead to periodontal disease.

tissue can be halted even if teeth cannot be straightened and the actual bite improved.

Nutrition is so important for patients with periodontal disease that some periodontists have their patients keep weekly food-intake charts to determine what essentials of diet may be lacking. Intake should be evaluated carefully for inclusion of fresh citrus fruits and fresh vegetables, and protein consumption should be noted, since it is so important in gum healing and in gum health.

The nurse must be on the alert for opportunities to direct patients to the dentist so that periodontal disease may be treated early and the unfortunate results of neglect may be prevented. Many people do not know that malocclusion and space between teeth are of any significance beyond cosmetic effect and lessened efficiency in chewing. The patient may ask the nurse about what seems to him an expensive and possibly unnecessary yet recommended dental procedure. It has been found that people in their forties and beyond can benefit from improvement in equalizing their bite, eliminating space between teeth,

better practice in brushing teeth, care of their gums, and regular dental inspection with prophylactic care.

Artificial dentures. Artificial dentures and other dental prostheses are resisted by most people. Serious emotional reactions are manifested when the patient must give up all of his own teeth, no matter how unsatisfactory they may be. In her conversation with the patient, the nurse should stress the fact that dental prostheses need not be conspicuous, that a proper fit can be obtained in almost all instances, and that there is often cosmetic improvement. The patient should be urged to have patience in learning to use the new teeth. Many elderly people become discouraged easily and are inclined to lay artificial teeth aside and then, because they are embarrassed by their appearance without teeth, avoid people.

Artificial dentures should be cleaned at least twice daily and preferably after each meal. Salt and sodium bicarbonate, a mild tasteless soap such as Ivory, or any good dentifrice can be used. Odor should not be a problem since plastic materials have largely replaced vulcanite materials, which sometimes retained odors. A few drops of ammonium hydroxide or a drop of chlorine household bleach, which is a good deodorant, added to the water used to wash the dentures may make the teeth feel and taste fresher. When artificial teeth are removed for cleansing, the patient should massage his gums thoroughly for a few minutes. Teeth that fit snugly naturally interfere with circulation to some extent. Some dentists encourage their patients to wear their teeth both during waking and sleeping hours since facial contours may be preserved better by this means. Other dentists recommend that the dentures be removed at night to prevent irritation to underlying tissues.[19] Dentures that fit properly should not cause discomfort as soon as the general slight discomfort associated with their newness is overcome. The patient should be advised to report any persistent pressure or irritation to his dentist, since adjustment can usually be made. Any lesion in the mouth associated with the use of dental prostheses should be reported at once since it may be an early malignancy.

Very occasionally there has been so much recession and atrophy of bony structures that it is extremely difficult to fit prostheses properly. A magnetic device has been perfected that can be embedded in the palate and that, by attraction to a magnetized dental plate, helps to hold the dentures in good position.

Diseases of the mouth and closely related structures

The mouth, like the eyes and the skin, is an excellent barometer of general health, reflecting general disease and debility as well as good health. In any inspection of the mouth, the nurse should note the color of the mucous membrane and of the gum margins, the presence of broken or jagged teeth, deposits on the teeth, and any thickened, irregular areas on the tongue, the gums, or the mucous membrane of the mouth. Pernicious anemia, leukemia, and vitamin deficiencies affect the mouth. Some communicable diseases, including measles and syphilis, produce lesions on the buccal mucosa. Specific disease of the mouth most often occurs when general nutrition and mouth hygiene are poor, when people neglect their teeth, when smoking is excessive, and when broken teeth irritate the tissues.

Infections of the mouth

Stomatitis. Stomatitis is an inflammation of the mouth that may be caused by drugs such as the barbiturates, pathogenic organisms, mechanical trauma, irritants, or nutritional disorders. Symptoms may include swelling of the mucous membranes, increased salivation, pain, fetid odor of the breath, and occasionally elevation of temperature.

Catarrhal stomatitis is any mild inflammation of nonspecific origin affecting the mouth. It occurs most often in debilitated persons, and the treatment consists of improving the patient's general resistance and using mild alkaline mouthwashes. *Aphthous stomatitis* is the correct name for what are usually called canker sores. These small, painful ulcers may appear singly or in crops. They may follow biting of the cheek or lip, or they may occur spontaneously. Some persons seem to be particularly susceptible to canker sores. Although there is no specific treatment, mild alkaline mouthwashes, better oral hygiene, and more attention to improved nutrition with increased fluid intake and cessation of smoking are beneficial. Local anesthetics may reduce the pain, and topical corticosteroids may reduce the severity of the lesion.[7]

The virus causing *herpes simplex* often infects the mouths of children between the ages of 2 and 6 years. The gums are swollen and red, and they bleed easily. Vesicles, which are scattered over the tongue and oral mucosa, rupture and result in painful ulcers that interfere with eating. Treatment is supportive since the disease is self-limited to about fourteen days. If pain is severe, the physician may advise the patient to rinse his mouth with an aqueous solution of dyclonine hydrochloride (Dyclone), a topical anesthetic. He then may be able to eat in greater comfort. The use of antibiotics has not proved beneficial.

Vincent's angina. Ulceromembranous stomatitis is commonly known as Vincent's angina. During World War I it was so common that the name "trench mouth" was acquired.

It is thought to be caused by a combination of the *Bacillus fusiformis,* which resembles the spirochete of syphilis, and *Borrelia vincentii.*[1] There is some question about the communicability of this infection, since causative organisms are found in many mouths although symptoms are absent. The infection causes pain, swelling, fetid breath, and a bad taste in the mouth. Occasionally bleeding of the gums occurs and a grey membrane forms. The patient may have general lassitude and generalized pain about the jaws. If the condition is severe, antibiotics may be given. Since the anaerobic spirochete does not thrive well in the presence of high oxygen concentrations, sodium perborate mouthwashes may be ordered, or half-strength hydrogen peroxide may be applied to the gums. The patient may have to subsist on a liquid or soft diet for a few days. Strongly acid foods, highly seasoned foods, alcohol, and smoking should be avoided.

Ludwig's angina. Ludwig's angina is a rare, deep infection of the tissues of the floor of the mouth caused by the streptococcus. Symptoms include elevation of temperature, toxicity, and local edema that may quickly lead to obstruction of the throat. Once established in the soft tissues, the infection can pass rapidly between the cervical fascial sheaths and reach the mediastinum, where it can cause death. Pressure from infection and edema in the throat as the disease progresses downward can be fatal in a short time.

Treatment for Ludwig's angina requires the immediate administration of large doses of antibiotic drugs. The doctor may order hot saline solution mouthwashes hourly during waking hours and hot packs applied externally if the cervical nodes are involved. Fluids are usually given intravenously. The patient must be watched closely until acute danger is over. A rise in temperature, increased pain, and swelling usually indicate extension of infection. Increased pain on swallowing and upon movement of the neck, voice changes, and any difficulty in respiration or evidence of cyanosis must be reported to the doctor immediately. Surgical incision of the abscess often is done to relieve pressure and to prevent extension of the infection to the mediastinum. Occasionally a tracheotomy is necessary.

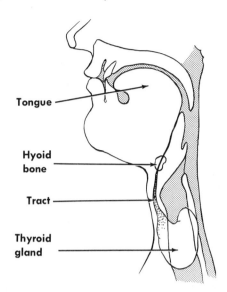

Fig. 147

Thyroglossal cyst showing fistulous tract between thyroid gland and base of tongue.

Thyroglossal cyst. Thyroglossal cyst is a somewhat rare congenital anomaly that results when certain cells at the base of the tongue do not descend completely to form the middle lobe of the thyroid gland during embryonic life (Fig. 147). The cells that are left along the way may form a cyst or a fistula that may empty near the base of the tongue or may form an external fistula anywhere along the tract. The tract is lined with mucous membrane and saliva, and organisms may enter the tract from the base of the tongue. The cyst usually appears as a painless, progressively enlarging mass in the midline of the neck just below the hyoid bone sometime between 2 and 6 years of age. It may become infected acutely or chronically. The treatment is surgical excision of the cyst and of the entire tract, including the center of the hyoid bone. The incision is made between the hyoid bone and the thyroid cartilage, and a drain usually is inserted in the wound postoperatively.

Diseases of the salivary glands

Acute infection can occur in any of the salivary glands, although the parotid gland is the one most often affected. *Parotitis* must be distinguished from *acute communicable parotitis* (epidemic mumps). Parotitis occurs in debilitated and dehydrated patients whose mouth hygiene is poor, whose mouths have been permitted to become dry, and who have not chewed solid food regularly. Elderly patients are more susceptible than younger ones. Usually the staphylococcus organism is present. The signs are pain, swelling, absence of salivation, and sometimes purulent exudate from the duct of the gland. Antibiotics often are given. Mouthwashes are used, and either warm or cold compresses applied externally may make the patient more comfortable.

Parotitis usually can be prevented postoperatively by careful attention to oral hygiene, general nutrition, and fluids. Dental prophylactic treatment preoperatively is thought to aid prevention. Having the patient chew gum at times when solid food is not permitted may prevent congestion or obstruction in the ducts of the salivary glands.

Stones may form in the ducts of the salivary glands and within the glands themselves. The submaxillary glands are most often affected. Mucous plugs or tumors may also obstruct normal salivary flow. A radiopaque substance can be injected into the duct *(sialogram),* thereby visualizing the duct and sometimes the obstruction. Patients who have an obstruction of the salivary glands should be advised to take larger amounts of fluid than usual and to pay particular attention to good oral hygiene. Sometimes probing with a fine probe or gentle massage dislodges the obstruction, but often surgical removal of the stone is necessary. If the entire gland must be removed because of a tumor, paralysis due to trauma of the facial nerve may occur. This paralysis usually disappears within about a month.

Tumors of the mouth

The lips, the oral cavity, and the tongue are prone to develop malignant lesions. The largest number of these tumors are squamous cell epitheliomas that grow rapidly and metastasize to adjacent structures more quickly than do most malignant tumors of the skin. Tumors of the mouth account for 3% of cancers in the United States and most often affect men over 50 years of age.[15] A good prognosis in treatment of malignant lesions of the

mouth depends upon early diagnosis and treatment. Every nurse has a real responsibility in interpreting the possible seriousness of any mouth lesion that fails to heal within a few weeks (two to three) and in urging immediate medical care. Pain cannot be relied upon as a signal indicating need for medical attention because many advanced malignant lesions in the mouth are painless.

Cancer of the lips usually occurs on the lower lip as a fissure or a painless, indurated ulcer with raised edges. The cause is unknown, but predisposing factors may be prolonged exposure to the sun and wind, constant irritation from the warm stem of a pipe, or chronic leukoplakia. Because metastasis to regional lymph nodes has occurred in only 10% of the patients when diagnosed, the rate of cure is high. In some instances, a lesion may spread rapidly and involve the mandible and the floor of the mouth by direct extension. Occasionally, the tumor may be a basal cell lesion that starts in the skin and spreads to the lip. Primary lesions of the lip may be treated by surgical excision or radiotherapy, depending upon the extent and size of the tumor. If extension to the jaw and mandible has occurred, excision and reconstructive surgery is necessary. A complete neck dissection usually is done if the lymph nodes are involved.

Cancer of the anterior tongue and floor of the mouth may seem to occur together because their spread to adjacent tissues is so rapid. They occur as hard plaquelike or ulcerated areas that do not heal. These cancers frequently are found on the under surfaces or lateral portions of the tongue. Irritants such as tobacco, betel leaf, jagged teeth, and poor dental hygiene may contribute to their development. Metastasis to the neck has occurred in over 60% of the patients when the diagnosis has been made. The mortality rate is high. Lesions about the base of the tongue may go unnoticed by the patient and may be far advanced when treatment is started. The prognosis is poor in the patient with this malignant lesion. Treatment depends upon the location of the lesion, its stage of development, and the judgment of the surgeon. Partial or total surgical excision of the tongue *(hemiglossectomy, glossectomy)* sometimes is done. Surgery may be followed by radiation treatment (often interstitial radiation is used, see p. 285) and/or by a radical neck dissection in which lymph nodes and adjacent tissues are removed (p. 628). Radiation treatment often is used instead of surgery, and this treatment may or may not be accompanied or followed by a neck dissection.

Leukoplakia is not a cancerous lesion, but if it is allowed to remain untreated, it so often becomes malignant that it is considered here. Leukoplakia begins as chalky, white, thickened patches on the tongue or buccal mucosa of heavy smokers. These patches are not readily removed. Conservative treatment includes good general mouth hygiene with use of mild alkaline mouthwashes, dental treatment if needed, and cessation of smoking. The lesions are watched carefully, and if they do not respond to this treatment within a few weeks, they are removed by surgical excision or by cautery. Lesions that seem thickened or papillary are removed at once since they are most likely to undergo malignant degeneration.

Preparation for therapy. The patient who is to have surgical treatment for malignancy of the mouth needs expert and sympathetic nursing care. The public is so conscious of cancer that the possibility of spread through metastasis is well known. Dealing with the entirely normal but very real sense of fear that the patient has is an essential part of nursing care.

The treatment for cancer of the mouth, whether by surgery or radiation, interferes with normal functions of the mouth. The patient and his family should be told about the changes that will occur and about the methods that will be used to help him communicate and take nourishment. For example, local excisions of the lip or tongue may affect speech to some degree, and the patient may have difficulty making himself understood. Patients having a hemiglossectomy or an intraoral mold inserted will be unable to speak. The provision of a pad of paper with a pencil, a tiny blackboard with chalk, or a "magic slate" will permit the patient to communicate with others. If a hemiglossectomy is done, taking food by mouth is impossible for a time, and the patient should know that he will be fed by other means. Because it may be difficult for patients with radon

seeds in the tongue or for those who have local excisions of the mouth to eat, parenteral fluids, fluids through a catheter or nasogastric tube, or the administration of food through a feeding cup may be necessary. The patient who is to have a hemiglossectomy should be told that suction may be used to remove saliva.

If a radical neck dissection and tracheotomy are to be done at the same time as the treatment of the primary tumor, an explanation of the patient's care after these procedures should be made (pp. 628 and 598). The patient and his family should be assured that he will be attended constantly until he is conscious and able to care for himself. The nurse should get to know the patient so that she can help judge how much he should be told about his treatment. For example, some patients who are to lose teeth and part of the jaw are relieved to know something about prosthetic devices that are available. Impressions sometimes are taken preoperatively to guide in making suitable prostheses following surgery. Other patients are so overwhelmed by the prospect of the operation itself that they are far from ready to think beyond the most immediate future.

Surgery of the mouth. The preoperative and postoperative care is similar to that discussed on p. 171. Preoperatively, oral prophylactic treatment usually is given, and antibiotics may be administered to decrease the number of bacteria present in the mouth at the time of surgery. The surgery may be done under local or general anesthesia, depending upon whether or not a radical neck dissection also is being performed. While recovering from general anesthesia, the patient may be placed in a prone position or on his side to facilitate drainage from the mouth. When he has reacted, he usually is more comfortable in Fowler's position. Bleeding and drainage from the suture line on the lip or tongue should be minimal.

Because of the vascularity of the tongue, patients who have had a wide resection of the tongue should be watched carefully for hemorrhage. If a hemiglossectomy has been performed, the patient will have difficulty in swallowing saliva or expectorating secretions, and the mouth may need to be suctioned frequently. Occasionally, a suction device such as is used by dentists is employed to carry away saliva as it accumulates. A gauze wick may be used to direct saliva into an emesis basin. The patient should be provided with mouth wipes and a bag for disposing of them. If he is unable to swallow, the nurse should attend the patient constantly until such time as he is accustomed to the situation and can help to care for himself.

The mouth may be irrigated with sterile water, a mild alkaline mouthwash, hydrogen peroxide, normal saline solution, or a solution of sodium bicarbonate, depending on the doctor's preference. Usually, sterile equipment is used even though the mouth cannot be kept sterile. A catheter may be inserted along the side of the mouth between the cheek and the teeth and solution injected with gentle pressure, or a spray may be used. Remaining fluid and mucus drains into an emesis basin or is removed with the suction apparatus. Dressings may be protected during this treatment by fitting a plastic sheet snugly over them. As soon as the patient is able to do so, he is encouraged to assist with this part of his care.

The method used to feed the patient will depend entirely upon the extent and nature of his surgery. Most patients can suction and feed themselves a few days following mouth surgery and are happier doing so. An Asepto syringe with a catheter attached may be used, and from this apparatus the patient may progress to a feeding cup with a piece of rubber tubing attached. Through practice the patient will develop confidence in caring for himself, and he is often more adept than the nurse in placing the catheter or tube in a position where fluids can be received into the mouth and swallowed without difficulty. A mirror often helps. He needs privacy when he is experimenting with the method that is best for him. He should not be hurried and should be observed very carefully to determine how much assistance he needs. As he begins to take liquids and then soft, pureed foods, he is taught to follow all meals with clear water to cleanse the mouth and foster good oral hygiene.

If the patient has had a hemiglossectomy, he may be fed through a nasogastric tube or through a soft catheter that is passed into the throat and beyond the operative site. Liquid food, 200 to 400 ml., may be given every three or four hours. The food may be a special formula or regular food that has been blended with liquids in a blender (p. 648). The patient must be watched carefully after the liquid diet is given since nausea and vomiting must be avoided. The sudden arrival in the stomach of fluid through a tube sometimes produces results different from those which occur when food and fluid are taken into the mouth and retained for a few moments during chewing. In addition, the act of swallowing causes some relaxation of the stomach. It is best to give a very small amount of fluid at first, to be certain that it is approximately body temperature, and to wait a few minutes before continuing with the procedure. Diarrhea sometimes occurs when patients must live on liquid foods. The patient should be prepared for it, and the doctor should be notified if the condition persists. Sometimes adjustments in the constituents of the liquid feedings help with this problem, and the dietitian may be called on for assistance. At other times a medication such as bismuth is added to the liquid food. If the patient goes home before feeding by these means is discontinued, he or a member of his family should be taught how to prepare the liquid diet, pass the tube, and give the feeding.

While the patient does experience some pain in the area of the incision, most of his difficulty arises from his inability to swallow and speak normally. Medications such as meperidine hydrochloride (Demerol) may be given to relieve the pain, and mouth irrigations and frequent mouth care will make him feel more comfortable. The hospital staff, other patients, and visitors should be alerted to his problem with oral communication. Conversation can be carried out so that the patient's responses can be limited to affirmative and negative gestures or to minimal written replies. The patient usually is permitted out of bed the day after surgery. There usually is no dressing applied to a mouth or lip wound.

The patient may remain in the hospital only two or three weeks, or he may be hospitalized much longer while further stages of surgery are done or while radiation treatment is given. At this time he needs constant encouragement and careful nursing care. He must be encouraged to mingle with other persons and is often happier in a room with others, provided that there are facilities for privacy when it is needed. The patient should be encouraged to take an interest in his personal appearance. Men should shave as soon as shaving is permitted by the doctor. Members of the patient's family should be encouraged to visit, and they, too, should learn how the patient may take food, how he may care for himself, what prosthetic devices are available, and how speech retraining can be accomplished if extensive resection of the tongue or palate or removal of the larynx has been necessary. (Speech training is discussed on p. 604.) Prosthetic devices cannot be fitted until healing has taken place, but pictures of persons who are wearing such devices with resultant marked improvement in their appearance are often encouraging to the patient. Prostheses are individually designed to replace portions of the palate and jaw that have been resected and to make the use of dentures possible. Plastic surgery may be done to partially replace lost tissue. Meeting and talking to other patients who have had similar operations with good results and good adjustment is very helpful to the patient.

Radiation. Tumors of the mouth may be treated by radiation in various forms. Needles or molds containing radium, radioactive cobalt, or other radioactive substances may be inserted and left in place for a prescribed time. Seeds containing emanations from radium or radioactive cobalt may be used and left in place indefinitely, or else removed. (See Fig. 61.) External radiation treatment using x-rays or other radioactive substances may be prescribed.

Whatever method of treatment is chosen should be explained fully to the patient. If needles containing radioactive elements are used, he must know that the needles are fastened to string that must not be pulled lest the dosage or direction of radiation be altered or the needle lost. He must understand that talking with the needles in place will be difficult or impossible. Radioactive needles must be checked several times each day. The nurse should know and should stress to the patient the importance of re-

porting immediately if one of the needles becomes dislodged. Auxiliary personnel and all other persons in attendance should understand the need to watch all equipment carefully for needles that have been removed or dislodged (for example, when emptying an emesis basin), lest radioactive materials be unwittingly discarded. If radiation is delivered by means of an intraoral mold, the patient must know that he will be unable to talk. He should know that any slipping or change in position of the mold will influence the dosage, so that he must report discomfort and must not attempt adjustment himself. A sling to support the chin helps to alleviate strain and discomfort in the mouth and jaw. Sometimes lying down for short periods is helpful, and occasionally sedatives may be necessary. Attention to mouth hygiene and giving food and fluids are similar to that necessary following surgery of the mouth. Suction equipment should always be ready for immediate use in the event of hemorrhage or choking. If either of these conditions should occur, the patient must be attended constantly since he may become panicky, particularly if a mold is in his mouth.

X-ray therapy usually irritates the gums and mucous membranes of the mouth and inhibits the secretions of the mucous membranes so that saliva may not be produced for months. Sloughing of the tissues may occur and cause a fetid odor in the mouth. Remaining teeth usually are extracted before x-ray therapy is begun. Dentures are not tolerated for some time thereafter because of the sensitivity of the tissues. The doctor may order the mouth irrigated once an hour with a solution of ½ tsp. of sodium chloride and ½ tsp. of sodium bicarbonate to a quart of water. Some doctors order a solution of 0.3 Gm. (5 grains) acetylsalicylic acid in 2 ounces of water as a gargle that may be swallowed. Gargling may be repeated as often as every four to six hours. Hydrogen peroxide or Dobell's solutions are ordered sometimes if there is sloughing, and Chloresium (drug preparation containing chlorophyll) may be useful for some patients. Potassium permanganate 1:10,000 occasionally is used, although its taste is objectionable to some patients. A solution of fifteen drops of common chlorine household bleach in a glass of water helps to control mouth odors and is acceptable to many patients. Inhalation of tincture of benzoin sometimes makes the mouth and throat feel pleasanter and less dry. Mineral oil may be used to relieve dryness of the lips and mouth. If infection occurs in the mouth, antibiotics may be given systemically.

Because smoke is irritating to the mucous membranes, the patient should not smoke. Hot and cold foods or fluids should be avoided because the injured mucous membranes are extremely sensitive to changes in temperature. Some patients complain of a metallic taste, which may be alleviated by sour substances such as lemon candies and citrus fruit juices. Solutions of local anesthetics such as butacaine (Butyn) may be applied to the mucous membranes, or lozenges such as dibucaine hydrochloride (Nuporals) may be prescribed if the discomfort in the mouth caused by the local irritation seriously interferes with eating. (See p. 278 for further discussion of the care of a patient having radiation therapy.)

Radical neck dissection. A radical neck dissection is used in the treatment of malignant tumors of the oropharynx and neck in an attempt to remove metastases and/or prevent the spread of cancer cells to the cervical lymph nodes. The operation usually includes wide removal of the involved tissue and lymph nodes on the affected side. The operation usually is performed in conjunction with the treatment of the primary tumor by surgery or radiation. A tracheotomy may be performed if the surgery has been so extensive that edema is likely to obstruct breathing of if a glossectomy has been performed and there is danger of aspiration during normal breathing.

The preoperative and postoperative care is similar to that discussed on pp. 171 and 193. If a tracheotomy has not been performed, an endotracheal tube will probably be in place when the patient returns from the operating room. This tube usually is removed by the surgeon or the anesthetist when the patient is able to breathe safely by himself. When the patient has recovered from the effects of anesthesia, he usually is more comfortable and breathes with less difficulty in Fowler's position. The patient should be observed closely after removal of

the endotracheal tube for signs of respiratory embarrassment caused by irritation of the tube or by edema. Internal bleeding and pressure from dressings also may obstruct the intake of air. Dyspnea, cyanosis, or changes in the temperature, pulse, respirations, or blood pressure should be reported to the doctor at once. If the superior laryngeal nerve is cut during the operation, partial anesthesia of the glottis will occur, and the patient may aspirate secretions from the mouth as well as food and fluids. Suction will need to be used frequently, and the patient must be observed carefully for difficulty in breathing.

A few hours after awakening from the anesthesia the patient is urged to sit up and cough. Coughing may be stimulated by placing the tip of the catheter used for suctioning either in the throat or, if a tracheotomy has been done, in the trachea. Coughing must often be followed immediately by suctioning of the mouth and upper throat to remove blood and secretions. If a tracheotomy has been performed, the secretions raised by coughing are suctioned through the tracheostomy tube. Two sterile catheters will be needed since different catheters must be used to remove fluid accumulations from the mouth and to suction the trachea. (See p. 598 for care of the patient who has had a tracheotomy.) The nurse can help the patient feel more secure and comfortable by placing her hands firmly in a position to support his neck as he coughs. The patient may be instructed to place his locked hands behind his neck and thus support his head and neck when he moves about. (See Fig. 170.)

Some surgeons place perforated catheters in the wound and attach them to a portable suction unit (Hemovac) to remove secretions and to draw the skin flaps down tightly. Approximately 70 to 120 ml. of serosanguineous fluid may be removed on the first postoperative day. By the third postoperative day, the amount of drainage usually has decreased to 30 ml. or less. No dressings are applied to this wound, and a plastic spray dressing such as Aeroplast may be used. Other surgeons insert one or more drains in the wound and apply massive pressure dressings to obliterate dead spaces, help prevent edema, and splint the part. The dressings are checked for signs of bleeding and for signs of constriction, which may cause edema and hamper respiration. Dressings are usually changed by the surgeon five to seven days following the operation, although the drain may be removed earlier. Some or all of the packing and some of the sutures are removed at this time, and the massive pressure dressings are replaced by a simpler dressing that permits more freedom of movement.

The patient who has had neck surgery usually receives antibiotics in addition to drugs for pain. Morphine and other narcotic drugs that depress respiration are used with caution, and an effort is made to limit their use by administering them only before painful procedures such as changes of dressings. Careful support of the neck and of the dressings when the patient sits up, a firm mattress, and gentleness in suctioning and in doing all other necessary procedures make medication for pain less necessary. Atropine sulfate is given with extreme caution because it makes secretions more tenacious and, therefore more difficult to remove.

The administration of food and fluids will depend upon the site and treatment of the original tumor. If there are no contraindications to the intake of food by mouth, it may be taken as tolerated. The patient usually is permitted to be out of bed the day after surgery has been performed.

Palliative care. Tissue necrosis and severe pain occur in advanced cancer of the mouth, either from failure in treatment or from death of tissue due to radiation. The patient is harassed by difficulty in swallowing, fear of choking, and the constant accumulation of foul-smelling secretions. The danger of severe, and even fatal, hemorrhage must always be considered. Nursing care of these patients includes the most careful and thoughtful attention to certain details; for example, secretions left in emesis basins or in suction bottles can be most upsetting to the patient. It is exceedingly difficult to induce patients with advanced carcinoma of the mouth to take sufficient nourishing fluids, and the nurse can often help by finding out specifically what fluids or foods the patient likes and believes are easiest for him to take. Relatives should be permitted to prepare and bring special dishes to the hospital if

the patient so desires. Sometimes a gastrostomy is done to permit direct introduction of food into the stomach (p. 647). Most physicians prescribe analgesic drugs freely for patients whose disease has progressed beyond medical control. The patient should be observed for signs of suicidal intent.

Since many terminally ill cancer patients are happier when cared for at home by their loved ones, an important nursing responsibility is teaching a member of the family to feed, suction, and otherwise care for the patient. Relatives may learn how to care for the patient while he is in the hospital and then are often assisted in their homes by a nurse from a community nursing agency. A carefully worded referral from the nurse in the hospital to the nurse in the community helps a great deal to make the patient's adjustment from hospital to home care an easier one.

Trauma

Fracture of the jaw. Fracture of the jaw occurs quite frequently as a result of vehicular accidents and of men's physical encounters with each other. The treatment usually is intermaxillary fixation by wiring the teeth. Preoperatively, the patient is told that he will be able to breathe normally and swallow liquids but that he will not be able to talk or to eat solid food. The jaws usually are immobilized for four to eight weeks. He should be assured, however, that he will be able to take sufficient food for health. Many times the patient with a fracture of the jaw can resume quite an active life during convalescence. Most patients are in the hospital a very short time or are treated on an ambulatory basis unless they have sustained other injuries.

The jaws are held together by wire twisted between the upper and lower rows of teeth or by tiny rubber bands attached to loops in the wiring (Fig. 148). Rubber bands are used most often since they can be removed readily and the degree of fixation can be adjusted easily.

Immediately following wiring of the teeth, the patient is watched for nausea and vomiting, which may be caused by emotional trauma, blood or other swallowed material, or anesthesia. Care must be taken to prevent

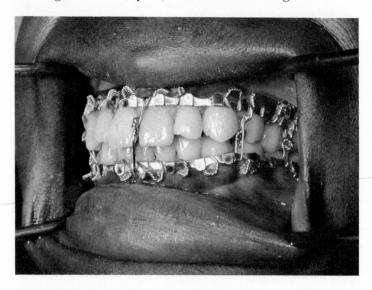

Fig. 148

One method of wiring the jaw. (Courtesy Marsh Robinson, D.D.S., M.D.)

aspiration of vomitus. Vomitus and secretions must be removed by suction since the patient cannot expectorate them through the mouth. Usually a catheter can be inserted through the nasopharynx or into the mouth through a gap created by missing teeth or in the space behind the third molar. Scissors or a wire cutter should be at the bedside so that the wires can be cut or the elastic bands released if necessary. The nurse caring for the patient must have specific orders that state, among other things, the circumstances under which wires or rubber bands should be released.

Patients who have fixation by wiring for fracture need much the same care as is needed following surgery of the mouth. They must often subsist on liquids and must learn to take a high-caloric liquid diet through a catheter, an Asepto syringe, a feeding cup, or a straw. They need instruction about mouth hygiene, and they must be instructed to report any sudden swelling, pain, or other symptoms that may occur after dismissal from the hospital. Osteomyelitis is much less common now that antibiotics are given routinely, but it can occur and is more likely to do so in the unusual cases of com-

pound fracture in which bone fragments have penetrated either the outer skin or the inside of the mouth.

Injury to soft tissue. Injuries to soft tissues within the mouth usually are caused by pressure against teeth, direct trauma from a foreign object, or protrusion of bone through the buccal mucosa following fracture of the jaw. Breaks in the skin about the mouth often accompany these injuries. Treatment consists of thorough cleansing of the wounds. Usually pHisoHex is used and is followed by irrigation with sterile normal saline solution. Skin wounds are gently debrided and sutured with an extremely fine, absorbable suture for best cosmetic results. Because of the vascularity of the scalp and face, infection is rare following traumatic injury to these areas.

Lacerations within the mouth are cleansed and sutured if their extent and location make these measures necessary. Hemorrhage must be watched for, especially if total injuries necessitate extensive dressing, which may hinder normal expectoration of blood and cause it to be swallowed. Edema may be pronounced following trauma to the mouth and may interfere with respirations. Usually the head of the bed is elevated in a semi-Fowler's position to aid in venous drainage from the area and thereby lessen edema. Tight dressings about the face must be checked carefully since they may contribute to development of edema and may cause headache.

Patients who have sustained penetrating wounds of the mouth are usually given antibiotics and tetanus serum prophylactically. The nurse should question the patient about a history of sensitivity to serum before treatment for prevention of tetanus is given. Mouth care and feeding of patients with these injuries present problems similar to those encountered following surgery or a fracture and have already been discussed in this chapter.

References and selected readings*

1 Beeson, Paul B., and McDermott, Walsh, editors: Cecil-Loeb textbook of medicine, ed. 11, Philadelphia, 1963, W. B. Saunders Co.

2 Burket, Lester W., and Castigliano, S. Gordan: Oral medicine, diagnosis and treatment, ed. 5, Philadelphia, 1965, J. B. Lippincott Co.

3 Davis, Loyal, editor: Christopher's textbook of surgery, ed. 8, Philadelphia, 1964, W. B. Saunders Co.

4 *Farr, Hollon W., and Hislop, Rhoda: Cancer of the tongue and nursing care of patients with mouth or throat cancer, Am. J. Nursing 57:1314-1319, Oct. 1957.

5 Ferber, Jack Richard: Detection of periodontal disease in the aged, J. Am. Geriatrics Soc. 2:1053-1062, Nov. 1963.

6 Frazell, Edgar L., Strong, Elliot W., and Newcombe, Barbara: Tumors of the parotid, Am. J. Nursing 66:2702-2708, Dec. 1966.

7 Gellis, Sydney S., and Kagan, Benjamin M.: Current pediatric therapy, 1966-1967, Philadelphia, 1966, W. B. Saunders Co.

8 *Hansen, Donald: The salivary glands, Am. J. Nursing 58:240-241, Feb. 1958.

9 *Hass, Robert L.: The case for fluoridation, Am. J. Nursing 66:328-331, Feb. 1966.

10 *Hayden, Mary L.: After surgery—rehabilitation for a full life, Nursing Outlook 7:21-23, Jan. 1959.

11 *Horowitz, Herschel S., and Heifetz, Stanley B.: Individual fluoridation and fluorides for the individual, Clin. Pediat. 5:103-108, Feb. 1966.

12 *Hudziak, Barbara: The nurse's role in preventive dentistry, Nursing Outlook 9:80-83, Feb. 1961.

13 *Kesel, Robert G., and Sreebny, Leo M.: Periodontal diseases, Am. J. Nursing 55:174-175, Feb. 1955.

14 *Kesel, Robert G., and Sreebny, Leo M.: Toothbrushing, Am. J. Nursing 57:186-188, Feb. 1957.

15 Masson, James K.: Radical surgical treatment of intraoral carcinoma, S. Clin. North America 43:1013-1022, Aug. 1963.

16 Nelson, Waldo E.: Textbook of pediatrics, ed. 8, Philadelphia, 1964, W. B. Saunders Co.

17 *Robinson, Marsh, and Van Volkenburg, Sue Tweedy: Intermaxillary fixation: immediate postoperative care, Am. J. Nursing 63:71-72, Jan. 1963.

18 Schlesinger, Edward R.: Dietary fluorides and caries prevention, Am. J. Public Health 55:1123-1129, Aug. 1965.

19 Schreiber, Frederick C.: Dental care for long-term patients, Am. J. Nursing 64:84-86, Feb. 1964.

20 *Stanley, Mary K., and Bader, Philip: Adult teeth can be straightened, Am. J. Nursing 62:94-97, Feb. 1962.

21 *Stark, Richard B., and Henderson, Lilian M.: Facial injuries—surgical treatment and nursing care of patients with facial injuries, Am. J. Nursing 57:450-456, April 1957.

22 *Weiss, Leonard, and Weiss, Estelle: Facial injuries and nursing care, Am. J. Nursing 65:96-100, Feb. 1965.

23 Work, Walter P.: Therapy of salivary gland tumors, Arch. Otolaryng. 83:89-91, Feb. 1966.

---

*References preceded by an asterisk are particularly well suited for student reading.

24

The patient with disease of the gastrointestinal system

Common diagnostic tests and procedures

Complaints of gastrointestinal disturbances are common and numerous. At some time in their lives, most persons experience stomach upsets and diarrhea. These disturbances may accompany other disorders such as grippe, follow dietary indiscretions, or occur with emotional upsets. Although these conditions are temporarily exhausting and uncomfortable, they are generally of short duration and may not even require medical attention. However, nausea, vomiting, or diarrhea that is severe and causes pain or is chronic and incapacitating should be reported to a doctor. Unfortunately, some diseases of the gastrointestinal system do not produce symptoms until the disease has progressed so far that medical treatment cannot cure it. As an example, cancer of the gastrointestinal tract may not produce symptoms until the condition is far advanced.

There are many laboratory tests and examinations available to help establish the presence or absence of disease in the gastrointestinal system. Some tests are done only to help establish a diagnosis when definite symptoms of disease occur, whereas others are advocated as part of a yearly physical examination for persons over 40 years of age in an attempt to detect early signs of disease such as cancer.

The common diagnostic tests and examinations used to help diagnose disease of the gastrointestinal system will be considered in this discussion. Since removal of gastric and intestinal contents may be required in the treatment of patients with many kinds of gastrointestinal disorders, these procedures also will be discussed before nursing care for specific diseases is considered.

The doctor writes an order for each test and examination. The nurse is usually responsible for working with the x-ray department and the laboratory in scheduling the tests, as well as for the instruction and physical preparation of the patient. It is the responsibility of the nurse to inform the patient about the tests he is to have. He should know what to expect, the purpose of the test, and how he may participate so that informative results can best be obtained. If some time must elapse before the results are known or if tests are to be repeated, he should be so informed. This knowledge lessens anxiety and helps the patient feel that he is participating in his treatment.

When several x-ray examinations are ordered for a patient, they should be scheduled in the following order so that the best results can be obtained with a minimum of delay: intravenous pyelogram, gallbladder series, barium enema, and gastrointestinal series. Since the tests are expensive, time-consuming, and often exhausting, it is important that the patient be properly instructed and prepared so that the examinations will not have to be repeated.

X-ray examinations

Barium enema. A series of roentgenograms taken after a barium enema has been given is used to demonstrate the presence of polyps, tumors, and other lesions of the large intestine and to reveal any abnormal anatomy or malfunction of the bowel. As the barium is instilled through a rectal tube, the roentgenologist, using a fluoroscope, observes its passage into the large intestine. The patient is asked to retain the barium while roentgenograms of the intestines are taken. He is then asked to expel

the barium, and another film is taken to see if any pockets of barium are retained.

The preparation for a barium enema includes an explanation to the patient of the x-ray procedure, of the importance of retaining the barium during the examination, and of the need for preparatory enemas. For the barium to clearly outline the lumen of the bowel, the bowel must be empty. This is best accomplished by giving enemas until the returns are clear. The nurse should find out from the doctor what he considers the maximum number of enemas. Usually no more than three are given. Repeated enemas exhaust the patient and irritate the anus and the rectal mucosa. Therefore, some doctors feel that one small enema containing a hypertonic salt solution such as disodium phosphate or monosodium phosphate is adequate. These solutions are now prepared commercially in disposable units. Food and fluids are not restricted for these x-ray examinations.

Barium that is retained in the bowel becomes hard and difficult to expel. To ensure complete evacuation of the barium from the intestinal tract after this procedure, many physicians order an oil retention enema followed by cleansing enemas. Since the patient is usually exhausted after a barium enema and the subsequent cleansing enemas, he should have rest. Petroleum jelly or, if ordered, a local analgesic ointment such as dibucaine (Nupercaine) may be applied to the anus to alleviate discomfort. If the patient is not too tired, a warm bath may also be soothing.

Gastrointestinal series. A gastrointestinal series consists of several roentgenograms of the stomach and intestinal tract and is used to detect tumors or ulcerations of the stomach and duodenum and to reveal any abnormal anatomy or malposition of these organs. As the patient swallows barium (a radiopaque substance), the roentgenologist makes a fluoroscopic examination, and then he takes roentgenograms of the stomach and the duodenum. Since the barium tastes like chalk, it is often flavored to make it more palatable. After the patient has drunk the barium, he is asked to assume various positions on the x-ray table, and the table may be tilted so that the barium will outline the stomach wall and flow by gravity into the intestinal loops as the doctor watches through the fluoroscope and takes the roentgenograms. Six hours after the initial films are taken, more roentgenograms are taken to see how much of the barium remains in the stomach. Barium will have passed through a normally functioning stomach and pylorus during this time.

In preparation for a gastrointestinal series the nurse should explain the procedure to the patient and tell him that he must not take food or fluids for six to eight hours before the examination. The presence of food in the stomach prevents the barium from outlining all of the stomach wall, and the roentgenograms will be inconclusive and misleading. If the patient eats, the x-ray examination should be postponed until the next day. The patient can be assured that the test will not cause discomfort and that he may eat as soon as the nurse is notified by the x-ray department that the series is completed. However, breakfast will probably be omitted, and lunch may be delayed. After a gastrointestinal series, a cathartic is usually ordered to speed the elimination of barium from the intestines. Retained barium may become hard and cause obstruction in the intestine or an impaction in the rectum.

Endoscopy

Esophagoscopy and gastroscopy. Esophagoscopy and gastroscopy are procedures done to visualize the esophageal and gastric mucosa. By these means, a disease process may be located and inspected, and a specimen of tissue may be obtained for microscopic study.

The conventional gastroscope is a hollow, cylindrical metal tube that permits visualization of the inner surface of the stomach mucosa except the fundus, the greater curvature, and the pylorus. The *Fiberscope,* a new type of gastroscope, has a shaft made of rubber or plastic that allows for greater flexibility and permits visualization of the greater curvature, the antrum, the pylorus, and the duodenal bulb. Glass fibers that are incorporated into the shaft of the instrument transmit light to the mucosa and the image back to the examiner. Cameras may be attached to either instrument for the purpose of taking pictures of abnormalities of the gastric

mucosa during the examination. (See Fig. 149.)

Roentgenograms of the stomach and the esophagus are taken prior to these examinations since an obstruction of the esophagus might make passing an instrument dangerous.

Although these procedures are not actually painful, patients find them extremely exhausting and uncomfortable. The nurse

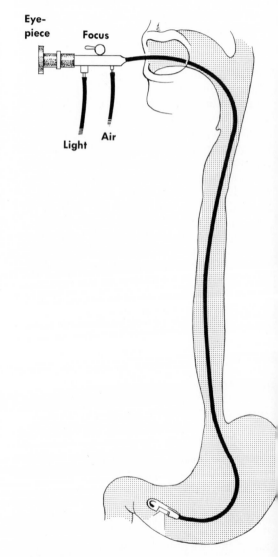

Fig. 149

By means of a Fiberscope the interior of the stomach may be visualized.

should explain the examination to the patient in simple terms, emphasizing that if he carefully follows the doctor's instructions and remains quiet during the passing of the instrument, he can help make the procedure a short and successful one. Food and fluids are withheld for six to eight hours before the examination so that the patient does not regurgitate as the tubular instrument is passed through the mouth into the esophagus and so that the lining of the stomach is visible. Occasionally an esophagoscopy or a gastroscopy must be performed as an emergency measure to remove a foreign object such as a bone or a pin. In such an emergency, the stomach cannot be emptied, but suction should be available for use to prevent aspiration of regurgitated food or fluid. Eyeglasses and dentures should be removed to prevent their being broken, and the woman patient's hair should be wrapped in a turban to keep it out of the way and to prevent its becoming soiled. The patient should void before the examination to prevent discomfort or embarrassment. Pajama bottoms should be worn to prevent inadvertent exposure during the procedure. The patient's written permission is obtained before this examination is done.

The patient is given sedatives one-half to one hour before the examination to lessen apprehension and to make him less aware of the passage of the instrument. The premedication also decreases the possibility of toxic effects from the local anesthetic. A narcotic such as meperidine hydrochloride (Demerol) and a barbiturate such as soluble phenobarbital usually are used for sedation. To decrease secretions, atropine sulfate may be given. The patient should be observed carefully for possible reactions to these drugs, and he should be protected from injury while under their influence. Before the examination begins, the doctor explains the procedure to the patient and tries to gain his full understanding and cooperation. The patient's posterior pharynx is then sprayed with cocaine or tetracaine (Pontocaine) to inactivate the gag reflex and to lessen local reaction to the instrument. In order to prevent the aspiration of medication, the patient is asked to hold his breath while the posterior pharynx is sprayed and not to swallow saliva but to

expectorate it into an emesis basin that is provided. The nurse should watch the patient for any toxic reactions to the anesthetic. An emergency tray containing barbiturates should be readily available. (See p. 185 for the toxic reactions to cocaine and Pontocaine.) When the gag reflex has disappeared (usually within five to ten minutes), the patient assumes a dorsal recumbent position on the treatment table for passage of the conventional gastroscope. For an esophageal examination his head and shoulders extend over the edge of the table, and for the passage of a gastroscope he lies on his side. The nurse supports the patient's head, and he is told again how important it is to remain perfectly still while the instrument is passed. Sudden movement at this time might cause the instrument to perforate the esophagus. Children and patients whose behavior is unpredictable should be firmly restrained if this procedure is attempted without the use of a general anesthetic. For passage of the Fiberscope the patient sits or lies on the side of the bed or table facing the doctor. If tissue is removed for pathologic examination, it should be placed immediately into a specimen bottle and correctly labeled.

When the examination is finished, the patient is instructed not to eat or drink until the gag reflex returns, lest fluid be aspirated into the lungs. The gag reflex usually returns in about four hours. In the hospital the doctor or the nurse tests for the return of the gag reflex by gently tickling the back of the throat with a cotton swab or a tongue depressor. If the patient goes home, he should check by touching his throat with a swab or his finger before he attempts to eat or drink. If there is any possibility that the esophagus may have been perforated, or if a biopsy has been taken, the doctor orders sterile water only for the first twenty-four hours, and the patient must remain in the hospital overnight.

Following an esophagoscopy or a gastroscopy, the patient may be hoarse and may complain of a sore throat. These symptoms should disappear within a few days. The patient should be so informed because he will not notice discomfort until the anesthesia wears off. Warm saline solution gargles may give some relief. Acetylsalicylic acid, 0.3 Gm. (5 grains), often is ordered to be dissolved in the mouth and then swallowed slowly. These procedures are exhausting to the patient, and provision should be made for him to rest when they are completed.

Anoscopy, proctoscopy, and sigmoidoscopy. Anoscopy, proctoscopy, and sigmoidoscopy are procedures performed to visualize the mucosa of the anus, rectum, and sigmoid. Tumors, polyps, or ulcerations may be discovered, examined, and biopsied. An anoscopy is an examination of the anus, a proctoscopy is an examination of the anus and rectum, and a sigmoidoscopy is an examination of the anus, rectum, and sigmoid. Most often, a sigmoid sigmoidoscopy is done, and this examination is routinely performed before rectal surgery and as part of the physical examination of patients who complain of chronic constipation or hemorrhoids or have any other symptoms of lower intestinal disease, such as bleeding.

The preparation for endoscopic examination of the bowel varies in different hospitals and clinics, but the patient should always receive an explanation of the procedure and of the preparation to be carried out. Usually he is instructed to eat a light evening meal prior to the examination. On the morning of the examination, soapsuds enemas may be given until the return is clear, or a small hypertonic salt solution enema may be ordered. Cathartic rectal suppositories such as bisacodyl (Dulcolax) are also used. If enemas are to be taken at home by the patient, the nurse should be certain that he knows how to carry out this procedure correctly and that he has suitable equipment. Visualization of the bowel mucosa is impossible unless all the fecal material is evacuated. Enema fluid should also be completely expelled before the examination is done since it, too, will obstruct visualization. Cathartics are seldom used in preparation for this examination because they may cause downward flow of material from the upper bowel when the test is being done. A light breakfast is usually permitted on the day of the scheduled test.

The nurse collects the necessary equipment for a sigmoidoscopy and checks the sigmoidoscope to see that it is functioning properly. Since the examination is upsetting to most patients, all possible preparations should be made before the patient is brought to the examining room to ensure a smooth-running and rapid procedure. The instrument must be checked to see that all the parts are functioning. The electric light bulb should be tested by attaching the instrument cord to the battery or to the electrical outlet. Besides the instrument, a draping sheet, gloves, lubricant, cotton swabs (12 inches in length), an emesis basin, toilet tissue, biopsy forceps, a suction machine with suction tip, and a paper bag for waste are required.

Before the examination begins, the doctor again explains the procedure to the patient. It is preferable for the patient to assume a knee-chest position, and he is draped so that only the rectum is exposed. Because it may be difficult for an elderly or a very ill patient to assume or maintain a knee-chest position, a side-lying position (Sims) occasionally may be used. (For complete description of these two positions, see p. 483.) The nurse should assist the patient in maintaining the correct position. She should encourage him to remain still, to relax as much as possible, and to take deep breaths. She should also watch him carefully, lest he become faint and fall from the table. Since the lights are turned off during the examination, it is sometimes difficult to note the patient's color. If any doubt exists about his condition, his pulse rate should be taken.

The doctor usually first examines the rectum with his gloved finger. He then inserts the lubricated instrument. After the instrument has been passed into the rectum, the solid, round-tipped inner portion (obturator) is removed. The intensity of light is then adjusted with the rheostat so that adequate light is reflected on the mucosa. If the sigmoidoscope is being used, the instrument is advanced slowly through the bowel for about 25 cm. (10 inches). The patient feels the instrument entering the rectum and sigmoid. This process may cause discomfort but should not cause real pain. Air is sometimes pumped into the bowel through the sigmoidoscope to distend the lumen of the bowel, thus permitting better visualization. The air may cause severe "gas pains." If small amounts of fluid or stool are still present

ent in the bowel, they are removed with the cotton swabs and by suctioning. A proctoscopic procedure and maintenance of a knee-chest position usually tires the patient. As soon as the instrument has been removed and the excess lubricant removed from about the anus, he should be assisted to his bed and permitted to rest. The patient who is examined in the clinic is advised to rest for half an hour and should have some food or fluid before he leaves. This is particularly important for the elderly patient.

Other diagnostic tests

Gastric analysis (with histamine). Examination of the fasting contents of the stomach is helpful in establishing a diagnosis of gastric disease. For example, an unusual amount of gastric secretions containing food ingested the night before suggest pyloric obstruction. An absence of free hydrochloric acid in the stomach contents may indicate the presence of gastric malignancy or pernicious anemia, whereas an increased amount of free hydrochloric acid suggests a peptic ulcer.

To obtain fasting stomach secretions, a nasogastric tube must be passed. The procedure must be explained to the patient, and food and fluids are withheld for six to eight hours before the test is to be done. The nurse assembles the equipment needed for the procedure and at this time gives the patient any additional information about the test that he needs.

If the patient sits up with his head hyperextended, the tube is passed more easily. This position can be maintained if the head of the bed is raised and if the pillows are arranged so that they are under the patient's shoulders, allowing his head to be supported on the mattress in hyperextension. The procedure may also be done with the patient seated in a chair. The nurse should make sure that the chair supports the patient so that he does not become unsteady if he leans backward. As the physician reviews the procedure with the patient, the nurse may draw screens about his bed and cover his gown with a protective plastic sheet or towel. He should be provided with an emesis basin and paper tissues. A nasogastric tube (Levin, No. 12, 14, or 16) is used. The tip

of the tube may be lubricated with a water-soluble lubricant, and the physician inserts it through either nostril or through the mouth. Then he gently passes it into the posterior pharynx. The patient is asked to swallow hard and repeatedly, and he may be given sips of water as the doctor quickly advances the tube into the stomach. A syringe with an adapter is then fitted onto the end of the tube, and all the stomach contents are aspirated and placed into a specimen bottle. The doctor may want to test the reaction of the aspirated secretions by using litmus paper. Blue litmus turns pink in the presence of acid. The tube is then secured to the nose and to the forehead with adhesive tape. Care should be taken that the tube does not pull or press against the nostril or cross in front of the eye. The end of the tube is closed with a clamp or with an elastic band to prevent leaking. Most patients are inclined to hold themselves very rigid while the tube is in the stomach, and they may be afraid to move. They should be encouraged to assume any position that is most comfortable.

After the fasting specimen has been collected, histamine phosphate, 0.5 mg. (1/120 grain) is given subcutaneously. This drug stimulates gastric secretions, and it causes vasodilation of the capillaries and arterioles. When histamine is given to a patient who has a peptic ulcer, there is a definite increase in the total output of gastric secretions and an increase in the amount of free hydrochloric acid in the stomach. The patient should be told that the drug may make him feel flushed and warm but that the sensation will pass quickly. Occasionally a patient may be sensitive to histamine, and go into shock because of marked dilation of the peripheral blood vessels. If shock occurs, epinephrine (Adrenalin) usually is given. After the histamine injection has been given, the stomach contents are aspirated every ten to twenty minutes until three or more specimens of gastric secretions have been obtained. These specimens are placed in correctly labeled bottles and sent to the laboratory for study.

When the test is completed, the tube is clamped and quickly withdrawn. The nurse may be asked to do this procedure. The patient should be given paper tissues because he usually has secretions in his eyes, nose, and throat. Mouth care should then be given, and if the hospitalized patient is not nauseated, breakfast may be served.

If the patient is not hospitalized, this test often is done in the doctor's office or in the clinic, and the nurse may do the entire procedure. If she is to be responsible for it, she must be very certain that she has an order to give Adrenalin at once if the patient has a reaction to histamine.

Tubeless gastric analysis. This procedure is thought to be useful as a screening technique for detection of gastric achlorhydria. The test will indicate the presence or absence of free hydrochloric acid but cannot be used to determine the *amount* of free hydrochloric acid if it is present. Quantitative determinations must be done through aspiration of stomach contents.

For a tubeless gastric analysis, a gastric stimulant such as caffeine or histamine phosphate is given to the patient. One hour later he is given 2 Gm. (30 grains) of a cation exchange resin containing 90 mg. (1½ grains) of azure A (Azuresin, Diagnex Blue) with 240 ml. of water by mouth on an empty stomach. If there is free hydrochloric acid in the stomach, upon the introduction of this resin a substance will be released in the stomach that will be absorbed from the small intestine and excreted by the kidneys within two hours. Absence of detectable amounts of dye in the urine indicates that free hydrochloric acid probably was not secreted.

Insulin tolerance test. An insulin tolerance test is another test used to evaluate the secreting action of the gastric mucosa. The test is carried out in the same way as a gastric analysis, except that instead of histamine a specified amount of regular insulin is given intravenously. The drop in blood sugar produced by the insulin stimulates the vagus nerve, and the flow of gastric secretions may be increased. A normal stomach responds only slightly to stimulation of the vagus nerve, and there will be no significant increase in the gastric secretions. In the patient with a peptic ulcer, however, there will be a marked increase in the total gastric output and in the amount of free hydrochloric acid. The insulin tolerance test may be used to deter-

mine the success of a resection of the vagus nerve in decreasing the hyperactivity of the stomach. It is, therefore, often done before and after a vagotomy. In the event that symptoms of insulin shock appear, orange or other fruit juice should be available, as well as glucose for intravenous injection.

Exfoliative cytology. Exfoliative cytology is the study of the individual cell or clumps of cells to identify or to exclude the presence of malignancy. Because malignant cells tend to exfoliate (separate from the tumor), methods of accelerating exfoliation are used by passing a Levin tube and lavaging the stomach vigorously with quantities of saline solution or by passing stomach tubes to which are attached gastric brushes or abrasive balloons to collect fragments of mucosa. Chymotrypsin may be given to digest the overlying protective coat of mucus and thereby expose the mucosa to the irrigating solution or abrasive collecting agent. All the aspirated irrigating solution, cells, and bits of tissue obtained are sent to the laboratory for study.

Peroral small bowel biopsy. Biopsy of the mucosa and of lesions of the small intestines is possible through the passage of a biopsy capsule. The capsule consists of inner and outer shells that are attached to the distal end of a Miller-Abbott tube or to special tubes constructed for this purpose. The inner shell encloses a cylindrical cavity that contains a blade. The biopsy opening is located in the distal end of the capsule. The tube with the capsule is passed as previously described, and by swallowing and peristaltic activity it reaches the biopsy site as established by fluoroscopy. At this point, the biopsy port is opened and the blade is operated by hydrostatic pressure and vacuum created by syringes attached to the double lumen openings at the other end of the tube. The specimen is guillotined off and collected in the capsule. When the tube is removed, the tissue is sent to the laboratory for study.

Stool examination. Gross, microscopic chemical, and bacterial examinations of the stool supply information that is helpful in establishing a diagnosis of gastrointestinal disease. Stools that are abnormal in color, odor, amount, consistency, and number are significant. Abnormal stools should be accurately described and a specimen saved for examination by the doctor. The doctor may order further laboratory studies to be done. Stool examinations are required for the complete evaluation of all patients with gastrointestinal complaints.

The nurse is responsible for seeing that specimens are collected. If the patient is ambulatory, she may ask him to obtain the specimen, giving him a specimen box and a spatula with which to collect the specimen. Otherwise, the specimen should be collected by the nursing personnel. The nurse should be familiar with and also inform auxiliary staff of any special techniques that are required to preserve stools for special examinations. For example, a specimen to be examined for amebae must be kept warm and taken immediately to the laboratory for examination. It can be kept warm by placing the specimen box in a pan of warm water or on a hot-water bottle. If an enema must be given to collect a stool specimen, it is important that plain tap water or normal saline solution be used, since soaps or hypertonic solutions may change the consistency of the stool and alter any abnormal contents. If the stool is to be examined for occult (hidden) blood, red meat is eliminated from the diet for twenty-four hours before the specimen is collected. The reason for this should be explained to the patient.

Gastric and intestinal decompression

Decompression of the stomach. Decompression, or removal of flatus, fluids, and other contents, from the stomach usually is accomplished by attaching a suction apparatus to a nasogastric tube. It may be used to prevent and to treat postoperative vomiting and distention caused by the lessening of peristalsis following anesthesia, by manipulation of the viscera during surgery, or by obstruction from edema at the site of operation. In pyloric obstruction it is used to relieve dilation of the stomach, and in gastric hemorrhage it may be used so that the blood loss can be accurately measured and replaced. When a nasogastric tube is to be used to keep the stomach deflated postoperatively, it usually is inserted before the patient goes to the operating room, since

it is easier to pass at that time. (Passage of the nasogastric tube is described on p. 637.)

The length of time that the tube remains in the stomach depends on the reason for its use and the doctor's opinion of the physiologic effects of intubation on electrolyte balance and the psychologic effects upon the patient. It may be left until normal peristalsis returns postoperatively (about forty-eight to seventy-two hours), it may be removed soon after surgery and reinserted only if distention or vomiting occur, or it may be removed and reinserted once or twice a day to aspirate stomach contents. When the nasogastric tube is used in the treatment of pyloric or intestinal obstruction, it usually is left in place until the obstruction is relieved. The tube used in conjunction with gastric or esophageal surgery is carefully placed by the surgeon during the operation so that it does not intrude upon the suture line. The nurse should never manipulate this tube, lest injury be caused. If there is some question about the tube's position or function, the surgeon should be consulted. If the tube is inadvertently removed or pulled out by the patient, the doctor may decide not to reinsert it because of the danger of perforating or otherwise injuring the anastomosis.

The need for continuous intubation should be explained to both the patient and his family. If the purpose of the tube is not fully understood, its use may cause apprehension and fear. Acceptance by the patient usually facilitates passage of the tube, and there is less possibility that he will pull it out. The presence of the tube in the nasopharynx soon causes local discomfort, and the patient may complain of a lump in his throat, difficulty in swallowing, a sore throat, hoarseness, earache, or irritation of the nostril. He may also expectorate and wish to blow his nose often because the irritation of the tube causes an increase in mucous secretions. Many patients report that discomfort from the tube far exceeds that from the incision. To lessen this discomfort, the tube should be secured so that there is no pressure against the nostril. Excess secretions from around the nares should be removed, and a water-soluble lubricant such as K-Y jelly should be applied to the tube and to the nostril to prevent crusting of secretions. When the tube is in the nos-

639

tril, the patient tends to breathe through his mouth, and his lips and tongue may become dry and cracked. Frequent mouth rinses and the application of petroleum jelly or cold cream to the lips help prevent dryness. Fluids usually are restricted, but the patient may be permitted to chew gum to increase salivation or to suck small pieces of ice. Warm saline solution gargles may relieve dryness and soreness of the throat, and the physician may order steam inhalations or throat lozenges. He also may spray the throat with a local anesthetic such as Pontocaine. Frequent changing of the patient's position helps to relieve pressure from the tube on any one area in the throat. The patient often is inclined to be tense and fearful. The nurse should assist him with turning and physical care, showing him how much activity is possible without displacing the tube. Sedatives, if ordered, should be given to the patient who is seriously disturbed by the tube.

Nasogastric tubes usually are attached to suction to ensure drainage, since the stomach contents must flow against gravity. The nurse should understand how the suction apparatus functions. Before the tube is attached, the nurse checks the suction apparatus to be sure that it is working properly. Various types of apparatus may be used. Regardless of the type, if, after it has been assembled and turned on, it will draw up water from a container, it can be assumed that it is working properly. The tubing from the suction apparatus is then connected by a connecting tube to the nasogastric tube, permitting observation of the fluid being removed from the stomach. A clamp or pin should be used to support the weight of the additional drainage tubing so that tension is not placed on the nasogastric tube. Sufficient tubing should be attached so that the patient can turn freely, and the pin or clamp used to secure the tubing to the bed should be placed so as not to obstruct the drainage or inhibit the patient's movement.

Mechanical failure of the suction apparatus or blockage of the drainage tubing or of the nasogastric tube itself may stop the suction, impeding drainage and causing distention, discomfort, and sometimes vomiting. The apparatus should be checked frequently to minimize this possibility. The physician may wish the tube irrigated with small amounts (30 ml.) of normal saline solution at specified intervals to keep the lumen of the tube open and free from plugs of mucus or clots of blood. After the fluid is inserted into the tube, it should be aspirated, if possible. The amount of fluid inserted and withdrawn from the tube should be recorded accurately. Fluid that is instilled but not immediately withdrawn will be removed by suction, and if the irrigating fluid is not taken into consideration, the measurement of the total gastric drainage will be inaccurate. If the fluid does not flow easily into the tube or if it does not return at irrigation, the physician should be consulted.

When continuous gastric suction is used, the gastric secretions collected in the drainage bottle should be measured every twenty-four hours, since the total amount of fluid and the electrolytes lost through drainage must be replaced by the parenteral routes. It is the responsibility of the nurse to see that the drainage is collected and measured and that there is a record of all fluid intake and output.

Decompression of the stomach may also be accomplished by attaching a gastrostomy tube that is in place in the stomach to suction. Decompression by this method is used when gastric or intestinal distention is anticipated following extensive operations such as radical resection of obstructing carcinoma of the colon and total colectomy for ulcerative colitis. Some surgeons use a gastrostomy after limited gastric resection combined with vagotomy. The tube is inserted through the abdominal incision into the stomach at the time of surgery, and suction is maintained postoperatively until the hazard of paralytic ileus is over. The patient is much more comfortable than with nasogastric suction, especially if the need for suction is prolonged, and there also is less danger of respiratory complications. Irrigation of the tube, care of the suction apparatus, and measuring and recording of the drainage are carried out as described previously.

Decompression of the intestinal tract. Decompression, or deflation, of the intestinal tract is accomplished by attaching a tube passed by way of the mouth and stomach into the intestine to the suction apparatus. This procedure is used to drain fluids and gas that accumulate above the mechanical intestinal obstruction, to deflate the intestines during paralytic ileus, and to deflate the bowel before or after intestinal surgery.

The tubes most often used for intestinal decompression are the Miller-Abbott tube and the Cantor tube. The length of these tubes permits their passage through the entire intestinal tract. There is a small balloon on the tip of each, which, when inflated with air or injected with water or mercury, acts like a bolus of food. This balloon stimulates peristalsis, which advances it along the intestinal tract. If peristalsis is absent, the weight of the mercury in the balloon will usually carry it forward.

The choice of tube depends on the physician's preference. The Miller-Abbott tube is a double tube. One tube leads to the balloon and the other to the "eyes" along its course, permitting drainage of intestinal contents and irrigation. The external end of the tube contains a metal adapter with two openings—one for drainage of secretions and the other for inflating the balloon. (See Fig. 150.) In irrigating this tube, the nurse must be careful that the correct opening is used—the one marked "suction." The other opening is for use by the doctor for inflating or deflating the balloon. It should be clamped off and labeled "do not touch."

The Cantor tube is a single tube with only one opening, which is used for drainage. Before the tube is inserted, the balloon is injected with mercury with a needle and syringe. The needle opening is so small that the globules of mercury cannot escape through it. The mercury can be pushed about so that the balloon is elongated for easy insertion.

Another intestinal tube, the Harris tube, is a single tube also, and similar to the Cantor tube except that there is a metal tip on the end of the tube, which is followed by the small bag containing the mercury. Other modifications of intestinal tubes may be used (p. 206).

Intestinal tubes are passed in the manner described under gastric analysis. The addition of the balloon on the tip of the tube makes its insertion through the nose doubly difficult for the patient. The tube can be mechanically inserted only into the stomach. Its passage along the remainder of the gastro-

Fig. 150

The tips and the ends to be attached to suction for the various types of tubes used for gastrointestinal intubation. **A,** Rubber nasogastric tube. **B,** Cantor tube. **C,** Rehfuss tube for duodenal drainage. **D,** Plastic nasogastric tube. **E,** Miller-Abbott tube.

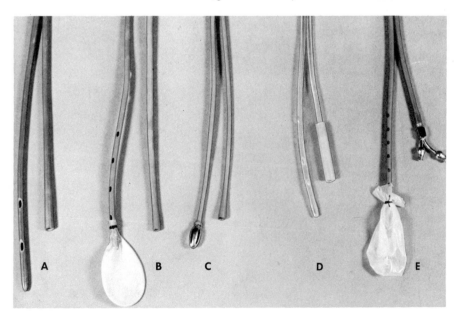

intestinal tract is dependent upon gravity and peristalsis. The weight of the mercury in the balloon helps propel the tube through the intestines. After the tube reaches the stomach, its passage through the pylorus and into the duodenum can be facilitated in many ways. Position and activity aid in its passage. After passage of the tube, the patient is usually encouraged to lie on his right side for two hours, on his back in a Fowler's position for two hours, and then on his left side for two hours. Passage of the tube through the pylorus is usually ascertained by x-ray or fluoroscopic examination. After the tube has passed the pylorus, the patient may be encouraged to walk about to increase peristalsis and to speed the advancement of the tube through the intestines with the help of gravity. During this time the doctor or the nurse advances the tube 7 to 10 cm. (3 to 4 inches) through the nose or mouth at specified intervals. The intestinal tube should not be secured to the face until it has reached the desired point in the intestines, since taping the tube will prevent it from advancing with peristalsis. Extra tubing should be coiled on the bed or, if the patient is up, pinned to his clothing.

Decompression is accomplished by attaching a suction apparatus to the tube either as the tube advances or after it has reached the obstructed portion of the bowel. Drainage should be measured every twenty-four hours, and the fluid and electrolytes lost are replaced by the parenteral routes. If the tip of the tube is far down in the intestine and if the patient is not nauseated or vomiting, he may be permitted light foods such as clear or cream soups, custards, gelatins, milk, or fruit juice, all of which can be absorbed in the upper part of the small intestine. The doctor may wish the tube irrigated at intervals with normal saline solution or tap water to check its patency. Because the fluid has a longer distance to travel than in a nasogastric tube, it is difficult to aspirate the solution used. The nurse should record the amount instilled into the tube. If no return flow can be obtained, only a small amount of solution should be used. If she is able to aspirate the fluid, this also should be recorded.

The intestinal tube is usually left in the intestine longer than the nasogastric tube remains in the stomach. It is often left in

for from four to six days after intestinal surgery, depending upon the amount of edema around the anastomosis and the return of peristalsis. In most cases of intestinal obstruction, the tube must be left in for seven to ten days, but the amount of time in which the tube remains depends upon the disease and the patient's response to treatment. Nasal and pharyngeal discomfort usually is pronounced, and the nursing measures described under gastric intubation should be employed. Signs of the return of peristalsis and of the reduction of edema at the operative site, such as the passage of gas by rectum or a spontaneous bowel movement, should be reported to the physician since they usually indicate that the tube is no longer needed.

The intestinal tube is always removed gradually, several centimeters at a time. Some resistance may be felt as it is withdrawn because of the pull against peristalsis. The patient may feel a tugging sensation and become nauseated. When the tip of the tube reaches the posterior nasopharynx, it may be brought out through the mouth so that the balloon and mercury can be removed. The tube is then pulled through the nose. Since the tube usually has a fecal odor and may cause nausea the tubing should be removed from sight at once, and the patient should be given mouth care as soon as it is removed. For several days after removal of an intestinal tube, the patient's throat may be sore and he may be hoarse. Gargles, lozenges, and steam inhalations should be continued until these symptoms subside.

Occasionally the balloon of an intestinal tube may extrude from the anus. If this occurs, the upper end of the tube is usually cut off and the tube is removed through the rectum. Removal is usually done slowly and with the help of peristaltic action.

The patient with disease of the upper gastrointestinal system

The following discussion considers the more common diseases of the upper gastrointestinal system as well as specific medical treatment and related nursing care.

Esophageal disorders

Achalasia (cardiospasm, aperistalsis)

Achalasia is an abnormal state in which there is a failure of the lower esophagus to relax with deglutition (swallowing). The cause is unknown, but the disorder is a direct result of disruption of the normal neuromuscular mechanism of the esophagus. Anxiety and tension seem to aggravate the symptoms and bring on exacerbations. It may occur at any age, but it causes most distress among adults.

In the early phases of achalasia there is no gross lesion, but as the disease persists, the portion of the esophagus above the constriction dilates, and the muscular walls become hypertrophied. The dilated area becomes atonic, and esophageal peristalsis may be absent, so that little or no food can enter the stomach. While varying degrees of the condition exist, in extreme cases the esophagus above the constriction may hold a liter or more of fluid.

The patient may first complain of substernal fullness following the hasty ingestion of bulky or cold foods. He may have to make a determined, conscious effort to pass food beyond the constricted area. As the condition progresses, vomiting occurs. The older patient may aspirate stagnant esophageal contents into the trachea or bronchi during sleep, and atelectasis or pneumonia may develop. The diagnosis is confirmed by roentgenograms taken as the patient swallows barium and by esophagoscopy.

If the constriction is not severe, the patient usually is advised to eat a bland diet, avoiding bulky foods. Meals should be eaten slowly, and drinking fluids with meals helps the food to pass through the narrowed opening. Frequent changes of position during eating may also help. The patient should sleep with his head elevated to avoid the possibility of aspiration of esophageal residue.

If the patient cannot pass food beyond the constriction, forceful dilation of the narrowed opening with the specific purpose of tearing some of the muscle fibers in the area may be done.[22] This procedure is accomplished by passing graduated mercury-tipped bougies, passing tubes with bags attached that can be inflated under pressure, or passing a mechanical (Starck) dilator. The generally accepted surgical procedure is a cardiomyotomy. The muscular layer is incised longitudinally down to, but not through, the mucosa. The incision is so done that two-thirds of its length is in the esophagus and the remaining one-third is in the stomach.[43] This permits the mucosa to expand so that food can pass more easily into the stomach.

Postoperatively, the nursing care is the same as the routine care given any patient who has had chest surgery. A rare complication is accidental perforation of the esophageal mucosa so that leakage may contaminate the mediastinum. Regurgitation occasionally occurs after the operation but can usually be controlled by the administration of antacid medications.

Esophageal diverticulum

An esophageal diverticulum is the bulging of the esophageal mucosa and submucosa through a weakened portion of the muscular layer of the esophagus. It is most often located at the pharyngoesophageal junction or in the lower end of the thoracic esophagus. As food is ingested, some of it may pass into the diverticulum. After a sufficient amount has accumulated in the pocket, it overflows into the esophagus and is regurgitated. There is always danger that some of the regurgitated material may be aspirated into the trachea and lungs. The patient may complain of pain on swallowing, of gurgling noises in the area, and of a cough due to tracheal irritation. His breath usually has a foul odor caused by decomposition of food in the diverticulum. The odor can be alleviated somewhat by frequent brushing of the teeth and the use of aromatic mouthwashes.

If the symptoms become severe, surgery is performed. The herniated sac is excised, and the resultant esophageal opening is closed. These procedures are well tolerated, and the administration of antibiotics makes postoperative infections rare. If a supraclavicular approach has been used, fluids are usually permitted as soon as nausea subsides, and a bland diet is given soon afterward. If a transthoracic approach is used, chest drainage may be used, and the patient usually is not allowed anything by mouth for several days.

Chemical burns

The deliberate or accidental swallowing of caustic materials such as lye may cause serious strictures in the esophagus as the mucosa heals. Often these strictures are so severe that no food can pass into the stomach. The patient has excruciating pain after swallowing the caustic material, and he may go into shock. Immediate neutralization of the swallowed fluid should be attempted, and treatment for pain and shock is begun at once. (For details concerning prevention and emergency treatment, see p. 249.)

Unfortunately many of the patients are small children, and they may suffer from the effects of such an accident for the remainder of their lives. Although the patient may be able to swallow fluid for a while after the accident, strictures develop as healing occurs, and sometimes no food can pass into the stomach. Careful attempts are made to dilate the stricture by passing bougies. Usually this is done under the fluoroscope so that danger of causing damage that would result in further stricture formation is lessened.[37] If the destruction of the esophageal mucosa is extensive, a *gastrostomy* (permanent opening into the stomach) may be performed. Braided silk thread is then inserted through the mouth and esophagus into the stomach and brought out through the gastrostomy opening. The two ends of the thread are tied together to form a complete loop, and the thread is used for pulling bougies or beads tied to it through the esophagus to dilate it and to prevent complete closure of the lumen. Such treatment may be necessary for months or years after the ingestion of a caustic substance. Care of the patient with a gastrostomy is discussed later in this chapter.

Tumors

Carcinoma is the most common condition causing obstruction of the esophagus and is the cause of about 2% of all cancer deaths in the United States and in the United Kingdom.[4] The tumor may develop in any portion of the esophagus, but it is most common in the middle and lower thirds.

The only possible hope for successful treatment lies in very early diagnosis and surgical treatment. The nurse should urge any patient who has difficulty in swallowing, no matter how trivial it may seem, to seek medical advice at once. This applies particularly to persons over 40 years of age since cancer of the esophagus occurs more often in middle and later life than at younger ages.

The patient who has cancer of the esophagus initially complains only of mild and intermittent dysphagia. Gradually he finds it extremely difficult to swallow solid food, and by the time he seeks medical attention he often has resorted to strained foods and liquids. He may regurgitate after eating and has gradual weight loss. Pain in the back may indicate that the growth has extended into surrounding structures. Unfortunately, even if the patient reports to a doctor when the first symptoms appear, the disease is often already well established, has metastasized, and is incurable. Diagnosis is made by roentgenograms of the esophagus taken as the patient swallows barium (Fig. 151).

Treatment for cancer of the esophagus is surgical. If the lesion has been diagnosed too late and cannot be entirely removed, surgery may be palliative to permit the patient to eat normally or to provide artificial means of getting food to the stomach. If possible, an *esophagectomy* is done. The tumor is widely excised, and the adjacent lymph nodes are dissected. The procedure is done through a transthoracic incision, and as in other surgery in which the chest cavity is entered, endotracheal anesthesia is used. The anastomosis of the free end of the esophagus after resection requires bringing the stomach up into the thoracic cavity. If the growth is located in the lower third of the esophagus, a portion of the cardiac end of the stomach may be removed because of its anatomic proximity to the lesion. This procedure also requires bringing the stomach up into the chest cavity and is called an *esophagogastrostomy*. A more recent procedure involves removal of the lesion and the adjacent esophagus and use of a section of the colon as a substitute for it. Plastic materials have also been used in attempts to find a relatively effective substitute for a portion of the esophagus.

If the patient cannot tolerate major surgery, a *gastrostomy* may be performed. This procedure is usually done under local anesthesia. An opening is made into the stomach through a small upper left abdominal incision. The anterior wall of the stomach is ex-

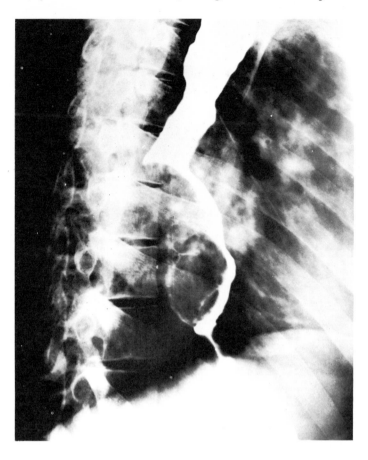

Fig. 151

This roentgenogram, taken after the patient
had swallowed barium, shows the location
of a lesion in the esophagus as
it approaches the stomach.

posed, drawn forward, and sutured to the
anterior abdominal wall about the incision,
thus preventing the stomach contents from
entering the abdominal cavity. A small incision is then made into the stomach, and a
20 or 22 Fr. catheter is inserted into it.
The opening is sutured tightly around the
catheter so that leakage of stomach contents
cannot occur. Food can then be introduced
directly into the stomach. Instead of a catheter, a special prosthesis (Barnes-Redo) may
be used (Fig. 152).

**Nursing care of the patient
having an esophagectomy or
an esophagogastrostomy**

Preoperative care. Because the nutritional
status of most patients with esophageal cancer is poor, an attempt is made preoperatively to improve nutrition and to reestablish fluid and electrolyte balance.

Fluids, electrolytes, and vitamins usually
are prescribed to be given intravenously.
An accurate record of the intake and output
should be kept since this information is important in ordering fluids to be given parenterally. If food and fluids can be taken by
mouth, they should be high in protein and in
total calories. Occasionally a temporary gastrostomy may be done to supply food preoperatively. It is closed a few weeks after
the esophageal resection if this operation
has been successful in reestablishing a communication between the esophagus and the
stomach.

645

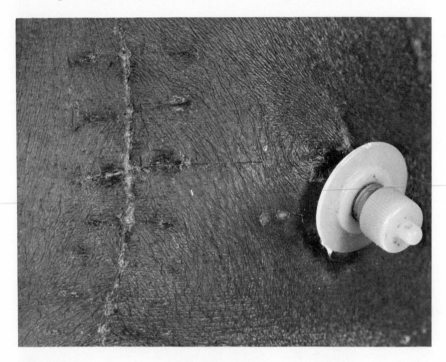

Fig. 152

The Barnes-Redo prosthesis is sutured into
the gastrostomy opening. The cap can be
unscrewed easily for tube feedings.
(Courtesy Dr. William Barnes and Dr.
Frank Redo, The New York Hospital–Cornell
Medical Center, New York, N. Y.)

The patient with esophageal cancer requires special skin care to prevent decubiti. Protection of bony prominences, frequent massage of dependent parts of the body, and frequent change of position are necessary. Because of weakness, malaise, and depression, the patient may forget to change position as often as necessary unless he is reminded to do so.

Since the breath may be foul, special mouth care should be given. The patient may raise a mixture of pus, blood, and decomposed food. He must be assured privacy when he is attempting to clear his throat and particularly when he is attempting to get food and fluids past the obstruction. The emesis basins should be changed often, and a cover should be provided. Mouthwashes, including Dobell's solution, hydrogen perox-

ide (1%), and solutions containing chlorine such as household bleaches are useful in controlling odors and in making the mouth feel fresher. Mouthwashes should be offered the patient before he attempts to take food. They should be varied from time to time unless the patient has one he prefers, because sometimes the flavor of the solution becomes identified with the unpleasant throat secretions and becomes almost as distasteful as the secretions.

Preoperative teaching should include instructions for the patient about chest drainage, coughing and turning after the operation, postoperative exercises, restriction of fluids by mouth, oxygen, frequent observation of his pulse and his blood pressure, intravenous injections, and the nasogastric tube. This teaching is described in detail in the chapters concerned with preoperative care of the general surgical patient and the patient undergoing chest surgery (pp. 174 and 577). The nasogastric tube is usually inserted immediately preoperatively if the esophagus is not completely obstructed.

Postoperative care. The immediate postoperative care for the patient who has had esophageal surgery centers about the maintenance of an airway, observation for circulatory or respiratory difficulties, protection from injury, care of the chest drainage system, and care of the nasogastric tube (as described earlier in this chapter).

Small amounts of bright red blood may drain from the nasogastric tube for a short time (six to twelve hours). The color of the drainage should then become greenish yellow. Because esophageal tissue is very friable and because the anastomosis may be under tension, the tube is usually left in until complete healing of the esophageal anastomosis has occurred. If the tube is removed, fluids by mouth are not permitted for several days. Fluids are given parenterally to meet fluid, electrolyte, and caloric needs. When fluids are permitted by mouth, a small amount of water (30 to 60 ml.) is given hourly, and the patient is observed for such signs of leakage of fluid into the mediastinum as pain, a rise in temperature, and difficulty in breathing. If no untoward symptoms occur, foods are introduced and gradually increased until the patient is receiving several small meals of bland food daily. If the stomach has been brought up into the chest cavity, the patient may complain of a feeling of fullness in the chest or difficulty in breathing after eating. Serving smaller meals more frequently may help to relieve these problems.

When the cardia of the stomach has been removed, some patients complain of nausea and vomiting. This difficulty is usually caused by irritation of the esophageal mucosa by the gastric juices. After this operation (resection of the lower esophagus and the cardia of stomach), the gastric secretions can readily flow into the esophagus when the patient lies flat. He should be advised to rest his head and shoulders on pillows when he lies down.

Resumption of activity must be gradual. Since surgery for cancer of the esophagus is extensive, the patient may require several months of convalescence. In addition, since the malignant lesion is seldom completely removed, only a small percentage of patients live more than five years after the operation, and many are chronic invalids during that time. The doctor usually informs the family of the patient's prognosis, and sometimes the patient is also told. Both the patient and his family should be told of the need for close medical supervision. Upper respiratory infections should be carefully avoided, and medical help should be sought at once if signs of even minor indisposition occur. Usually it is advised that the patient and his family be referred to the social service department while the patient is in the hospital so that a relationship may be established that may be useful to the family at a later time, when institutional care may become necessary.

Many patients with cancer of the esophagus receive terminal care at home and are cared for by a public health nurse and by members of the family under the nurse's supervision. The patient and his family should always be asked if they would like to have a nurse visit the patient in his home. Occasionally the nurse also helps the family to prepare for the patient's return home. The nurse who goes into the home can often give helpful suggestions regarding the preparation of suitable food, care of the mouth, rest, and prevention of accidents. (See p. 290 for care of the terminally ill cancer patient and p. 234 for description of home care programs.)

Some patients with cancer of the esophagus are not found to be suitable candidates for esophageal surgery. Their skin care, mouth care, and nutrition are similar to that described for the patient being prepared for esophageal surgery; sometimes a gastrostomy is done as a palliative procedure.

Nursing care of the patient who has a gastrostomy

It is usually very difficult for the patient to accept the need for gastrostomy—probably partly because of the deep psychologic significance of food and of eating. After a long period of vomiting, discomfort, and inability to eat, however, the patient may become so debilitated that both he and his family are willing for the operation to be done.

After a gastrostomy the catheter is secured to the abdominal wall by a suture or adhesive tape to prevent its slipping out. A clamp is applied to the end of the catheter to prevent leakage of gastric secretions onto the skin. A small dressing covers the incision, and there should be very little bloody drainage postoperatively.

The skin around the gastrostomy should be inspected frequently, because if there is leakage of gastric secretions around the tube, the skin will become irritated and excoriated from the action of the digestive enzymes. The skin should be kept clean with frequent use of soap and water and should be kept dry; a protective ointment such as zinc oxide and a dressing of oiled silk and gauze may be applied around the tube (Fig. 103). After about ten days to two weeks the tube may be removed and reinserted only when food is given. The patient is taught to do this procedure for himself. The tube is kept clean by washing it with soap and water after each meal. It is inserted 10 to 15 cm. (4 to 6 inches). To prevent leakage of secretions onto the skin between meals, a finger cot plugged with cotton may be inserted into the opening. The finger cot must be attached to the skin with adhesive tape to prevent its being drawn into the stomach. There is less likelihood of leakage if the patient lies flat for a short time after the meal and if the meals are not too large.

When the Barnes-Redo prosthesis is used, the problems of feeding and skin care are somewhat simpler. The prosthesis consists of a cap that unscrews, an external and internal flange, and a nylon shaft that is 4 to 6 cm. (1.6 to 2.5 inches) long. When foods are to be introduced, the cap is unscrewed and an 18 Fr. whistle-tip catheter is inserted into the shaft of the prosthesis as far as it will go. After the feeding is completed, the cap is replaced. Drainage is minimal, and skin care consists of keeping the area between the skin and the flange clean and dry. The prosthesis protrudes somewhat from the abdomen, but is not noticeable under loose clothing (Fig 152).

Soon after the operation, fluid nourishment may be given through the catheter. The initial meal, consisting of a small amount of tap water or glucose in water, is usually given by the surgeon. Fluids are given every four hours at first. If there is no leakage of fluid around the tube and if the patient appears to tolerate the clear fluids, foods blended into a mixture may be added until a full diet is eventually given through the tube. The meal should be warmed to room or body temperature before it is given, and it should be diluted if it is too thick. It

should be given with screens drawn about the patient for privacy if he does not occupy a single room. A funnel or glass syringe is used to introduce the liquid into the catheter. Before the meal is given, a small amount of water should be introduced through the tube to make sure it is patent. The fluid should flow in by gravity. Sometimes a small amount of pressure from the bulb of the Asepto syringe on the barrel of the glass syringe is necessary to pass thicker fluids through the tube. The usual amount of each meal is 200 to 500 ml. and should take ten to fifteen minutes to flow through the tube. If the patient feels "full" or nauseated, meals may be decreased in amount and their frequency increased. A small amount of water is instilled to cleanse the tube at the end of the meal.

The meals may be a special formula or regular food blended so that it will pass through the tube. The use of regular foods helps maintain the patient's nutritional state, prevents diarrhea that often accompanies the use of specially prepared tube feedings that are high in fat, and makes it easier for the patient and his family to prepare his food at home. Food that is normally cooked should be cooked until it is soft, and the juices from cooking should be included since they contain essential vitamins and minerals. Solid and liquid foods are blended into a mixture with a food blender, fork, potato masher, or egg beater and are strained. Water should be given through the tube between feedings so that approximately 2,500 to 3,500 ml. of fluids are received daily. If diarrhea occurs, camphorated tincture of opium (paregoric) may be ordered and given with the meal.

The patient should see, smell, taste, and chew small amounts of food before taking his feeding, in order to stimulate the flow of gastric secretions and give him some of the satisfaction of normal eating. It is sometimes recommended that the patient chew his food normally and then deposit it into a funnel attached to the gastrostomy tube. If he can accept this sensible although somewhat unesthetic procedure, it is unquestionably beneficial because saliva is mixed with the food. The teeth and mouth also maintain better health. Privacy must, of course, be assured the patient who takes his meals in this way.

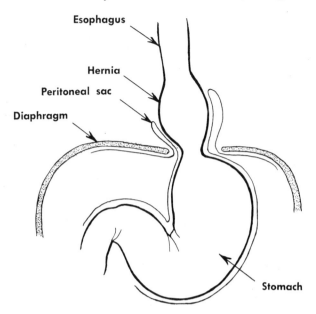

Esophagus

Hernia

Peritoneal sac

Diaphragm

Stomach

Fig. 153

Displacement of a portion of the cardia of the stomach through the normal hiatus into the thoracic cavity (sliding hiatus hernia). (From Newton, Kathleen, and Anderson, Helen C., Geriatric nursing, ed. 4, St. Louis, 1966, The C. V. Mosby Co.)

If the patient is not upset by sitting down to meals with his family when he cannot eat, he should be encouraged to do so since this socializing usually helps his digestion and is good for his morale.

The psychologic trauma of not being able to eat normally is usually severe. The patient may become depressed, and he needs a great deal of encouragement. Most patients, however, as they become proficient in feeding themselves, gradually accept this method of obtaining nourishment as inevitable and adjust remarkably well.

Both the patient and his family should learn how to care for the skin and the tube and how to prepare the liquid meals as well as how to insert the tube and instill the nourishment through it. They should be told of the need for close medical supervision, and they should be encouraged to consult the doctor, the nurse, or the dietitian when problems arise. It may be desirable for a public health nurse to visit the patient at home to supervise the initial preparation of food and giving of the feeding and to answer any other questions in regard to the patient's care.

Hiatus hernia (esophageal hernia)

There are three variations of hiatus hernia, but the *sliding hiatus hernia* is by far the most common and is now known to be one of the most common pathologic conditions of the upper gastrointestinal tract (Fig. 153).[9] In this condition, part of the stomach "slides" or follows the normal path of the esophagus through the hiatal opening into the thorax. The cause of this sliding may be trauma, congenital weakness, or a gradual weakening of the musculature due to age. Hiatus herniation can occur at any age but is more often found in persons who are middle-aged or elderly. The condition is often misdiagnosed, or diagnosis is delayed. Sometimes it is not apparent upon test by swallowing barium unless the patient is placed in a Trendelenburg position.

When a hiatus hernia develops, the function of the cardioesophageal sphincter is lost, permitting a reflux of unneutralized gastric juices into the esophagus, which in turn produces inflammation of the lower esophagus. If this condition persists over weeks and

649

months, ulceration occurs, with hemorrhage and formation of fibrous tissue. An occasional complication is incarceration of a portion of the stomach in the chest, with constriction of blood supply and possibly necrosis, causing peritonitis and mediastinitis. Another problem may be caused by regurgitation of gastric contents during sleep and subsequent aspiration into the lungs. The elderly patient may visit his doctor with signs of pneumonitis, since, because his reflexes are less acute, he aspirates fluid into the lungs more easily than the younger person.

Symptoms of hiatus hernia vary greatly. Some small hernias may cause no symptoms, whereas others cause the patient serious difficulty. Often the patient will complain of heartburn after meals and during the night. Heartburn and pain beneath the sternum may occur after meals, upon physical exertion, particularly when bending forward is entailed, or upon any sudden change of posture. Food may be regurgitated several hours after meals, and the patient may complain of the sensation of food "sticking" as he swallows (dysphagia).

Hiatus hernias are usually treated medically before surgery is recommended. The paraesophageal type, however, in which the stomach ascends beside the esophagus, which remains fixed, responds poorly to medical treatment.[7] Medical treatment of hiatus hernias includes a regular schedule of meals, with the avoidance of highly seasoned foods, coffee, and fruit juices. The patient is advised to eat small meals and to sit in an erect position during meals and for some time thereafter. The patient in the hospital for other causes should have the head of his bed elevated so that he can sit up straight for meals and should remain in this position for a half hour following his meal if his other medical problems make this possible. Antacids such as aluminum hydroxide gel may be prescribed to be taken a half hour after meals and at bedtime. If a patient is obese, weight reduction is advised.

The problem of regurgitation of food during sleep can be minimized by elevating the head of the bed on four-inch to six-inch blocks. The patient is often advised to avoid wearing tight, constricting clothing about the waist, such as a corset. He should be taught to go about usual activities with thought given to changes in posture, particularly if they involve sharp forward bending. For example, in picking up an object from the floor, he should stoop rather than bend from the waist. Kneeling rather than bending or even stooping may be better for some activities.

Hiatus hernia can be corrected surgically by a repair that may involve entering the abdominal and/or the thoracic cavity to return the stomach to the abdominal cavity and to repair the diaphragm. Many patients, however, are not sufficiently good operative risks because of their age to make surgery advisable.

Gastric disorders

Gastritis

Gastritis is an inflammation of the gastric mucosa and is the most common pathologic condition of the stomach. It may be acute or chronic.

Acute gastritis follows the ingestion of large amounts of alcohol and injudicious eating. Occasionally it may be caused by certain drugs. The gastric mucosa becomes red, congested, inflamed, and edematous, and may be covered with thin gray or green patches that may exude a white, purulent material. The main symptom of acute gastritis is severe and sometimes prolonged vomiting. (Symptoms and care of persons suffering from gastritis accompany food poisoning with organisms such as the *Staphylococcus aureus* and often accompanied by diarrhea is described on p. 251.) The treatment is to withhold everything by mouth until vomiting ceases. When food can be tolerated, tea, milk, gelatin, toast, and simple bland foods are given until a normal diet can be resumed. Drugs to relax smooth muscle, such as the atropine derivatives and propantheline bromide (Pro-Banthine), may be ordered.

Chronic gastritis is diagnosed only after tests and examinations have eliminated the possibility of other gastric diseases. The patient usually gives a history of prolonged dietary indiscretions such as eating large amounts of very hot, spicy foods or drinking alcoholic beverages excessively. Symptoms may range from chronic gastric distress to massive gastric hemorrhage. The patient is placed on a bland diet, given antacids such as aluminum hydroxide gel, and instructed to avoid foods and situations that have brought on symptoms in the past.

Peptic ulcer

A peptic ulcer is an ulceration involving the mucosa and deeper structures and is due in part to action of the acid gastric juices. It occurs in the distal esophagus, stomach, and upper duodenum and in the jejunum (following a gastroenterostomy) (Fig. 154). It is believed that probably as many as 15% of all people suffer from this condition at some time during life.[11] At the present time in the United States and Canada about 10,000 persons die from the complications of peptic ulcers each year (6,500 from gastric ulcers and 3,500 from duodenal ulcers).[11] Although a peptic ulcer can occur at any age, symptoms develop most often between 20 and 40 years of age. Gastric ulcer, however, is fairly common in old age.[11]

The cause of peptic ulcer is not known, but it is believed that there are three factors that greatly influence its development: a source of irritation, such as an increase of hydrochloric acid with a decrease of alkaline mucus secreted by the surface cells; a breakdown of the local tissue resistance and defense mechanisms; and the influences of heredity, hormones, and personality. The hormones appear to have some effect on ulcer formation since ulcers are more prevalent in men than in women. Certain so-called ulcerogenic drugs such as corticotropin and the adrenocorticosteroids, the salicylates and phenylbutazone (Butazolidin) are known to contribute to the development of peptic ulcers in some patients. The tendency for ulcers to occur runs in families. It has been demonstrated that emotional factors influence the function of the stomach and cause changes in the gastric mucosa. Persons who are under continuous pressure and who are nervous, tense, perfectionists, and unhappy may develop symptoms of peptic ulcers. It has not been proved, however, whether these symptoms truly follow or precede the development of the ulcer.

Acute ulcers usually are superficial, involving only the mucosal layer. In most cases they heal within a relatively short time, but they may bleed, perforate, or become chronic.

A chronic peptic ulcer is a deep crater with sharp edges and a "clean" base. It involves both the mucosa and the submucosa. If the ulcer penetrates the stomach wall and becomes adherent to an adjacent organ such as the pancreas, the organ may become the base of the ulcer.

Peptic ulcers are described as gastric or duodenal, depending upon their location. An ulcer (usually of the jejunum) occurring near the site of anastomosis is termed a *marginal ulcer*. Most gastric ulcers occur on the lesser curvature of the stomach. Such ulcers tend to be larger and deeper than duodenal ulcers, and they have a tendency to undergo malignant changes. Duodenal ulcers are not so well defined as gastric ulcers, but the pathology is the same. Most of them occur on the first part of the duodenum.

The patient who has a peptic ulcer usually complains of pain that is characteristic in its nature, intensity, radiation, location, and periodicity. Initial attacks of pain often occur in the spring and the fall, last for a few weeks, and then disappear. Each succeeding attack is more severe and more prolonged than the preceding one. The pain is described as gnawing, aching, or burning. It is usually located in the upper abdomen,

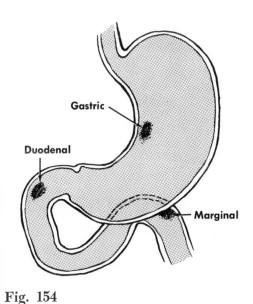

Fig. 154

The most common locations of peptic ulcers.

near the midline, and it is confined to a small area. However, it may radiate around the costal border or through to the back. Pain from a duodenal ulcer is usually located in the right epigastric area, whereas that from a gastric ulcer is usually located in the left epigastric area. Pain usually starts one or two hours after eating, when the stomach begins to empty, and it may disappear spontaneously, after the ingestion of food, or after the ingestion of an antacid medication such as aluminum hydroxide gel. If the ulcer is severe, it may cause pain at night. Although pain is felt at the site of the existing lesion, it is known that normal stomach mucosa does not have pain sensation. It is thought, therefore, that the inflamed mucosa around the ulcer must be sensitive to the gastric secretions because inflammation lowers the pain threshold.[4] Eructation is common in peptic ulcer but differs from that occurring in gallbladder disease in that it occurs more often when the stomach is empty and does not follow the ingestion of fatty foods. If edema around the lesion obstructs the pylorus, gastric retention, with dilation of the stomach, may occur, causing nausea and vomiting. This occurrence, however, is not common in peptic ulcer.

The diagnosis of peptic ulcer is made from the patient's history, a gastrointestinal series, a gastric analysis, gastroscopy, and stool examinations for occult (hidden) blood.

Treatment is directed toward relief of symptoms, healing of the ulcer, and prevention of recurrence. The majority of peptic ulcers heal under medical treatment. Surgery is used most often in the treatment of complications.

Medical treatment and nursing care. Ulcer management consists of rest and sedation, a bland diet, restriction of irritating substances such as coffee, alcohol, and tobacco, the use of antacids and anticholinergic medications, and an attempt to relieve undesirable emotional stimuli by medical counseling or psychotherapy. When the defect is covered with normal mucosa, the ulcer is considered healed. Healing may occur in a few weeks, or it may require months.

Rest. Because complete mental and physical rest is necessary for healing of a peptic ulcer, the patient may be removed from his home environment if it is believed that it

aggravates his condition. Hospitalization for a few weeks is usually recommended provided the financial burden does not increase the patient's worries too much. It may take the combined efforts of the physician, the nurse, the family, and the social worker to help the patient understand the need for complete rest and to secure his cooperation in achieving it. The patient should be on bed rest and removed from activity and disturbing noise. Usually he is permitted visitors and is allowed to participate in activities that keep him interested and occupied but that do not involve physical or mental effort (such as playing games with other patients or watching television). The nurse can gain the confidence of the patient by giving thoughtful, intelligent nursing care, by explaining procedures, and by promptly attending to his needs. Although the patient may appear outwardly calm, his emotional makeup may make him react strongly to the slightest unfavorable stimulus. Foresight on the part of the nurse will prevent the occurrence of incidents that aggravate the patient. Nursing care that provides a regular, smooth routine is best for the patient. Meals, medications, and treatments should be given at correctly spaced intervals and on time. Noise, rush, confusion, and impatience on the part of members of the staff should be avoided. The nurse should plan to spend time listening to the patient in an attempt to obtain clues to problems that should be relayed to the doctor.

When symptoms of peptic ulcer are severe and acute, large doses of sedatives such as phenobarbital and the tranquilizers may be given to help the patient rest. These drugs may make him so drowsy that close supervision will be necessary to prevent circulatory and respiratory complications. He should be turned from side to side at frequent intervals and encouraged to move his legs and arms and to take several deep breaths every one or two hours. Side rails should be placed on the bed of a heavily sedated patient to prevent falling and injury. The patient's skin should be inspected frequently for rashes that might indicate a toxic reaction to barbiturates or other drugs.

Diet. There are several approaches to dietary treatment of patients with peptic ulcers. Some physicians feel that rigid dietary restrictions result in no more rapid healing of the ulcer than does a liberal diet. Food is both an antacid and a stimulus for acid secretions, and the neutralizing action of food (especially protein) is soon overcome by an increased rate of acid secretion that irritates the ulcer and produces pain. For these reasons, physicians may prescribe a liberal, bland diet, restricting only those foods that cause the patient distress and dividing the total food intake into five or more meals if full-sized meals, three times a day, make him uncomfortable.

Other physicians prescribe a modified Sippy diet based on the fact that the acid-combining power of food proteins neutralizes the free hydrochloric acid secreted by the stomach. Theoretically, the ulcer will then heal since it is no longer constantly irritated by the gastric juices. Constant dilution of stomach contents and neutralization of acid are achieved by giving whole milk, skim milk, or half milk-half cream punctually every hour. Vitamins and minerals are usually ordered to help make up for the nutritional deficiencies of this diet. Gradually small meals of cereal, soft-cooked eggs, white toast, creamed soups, and other bland foods are added until three meals are substituted for some of the liquid nourishment. The liquid nourishment of milk or milk and cream is still taken between meals.

Patients on either regimen should avoid chemically irritating foods that stimulate the flow of gastric juices and that may cause pain. These foods include meat extracts, meat soups, gravies, certain spices, and beverages containing alcohol and caffeine, such as coffee, tea, and cola products.

When hourly feedings are an essential part of the patient's treatment, the nurse must see that they are taken as prescribed. If the patient objects to the taste of milk or tires of the sameness of his diet, small amounts of strawberry, malt, maple, or other flavoring may be added to the mixture. If the patient is acutely ill or has received much sedation, the responsibility for the hourly feedings must be assumed entirely by the nursing staff. If the patient is reliable and capable, a pitcher of milk may be left at his bedside so that he can take his own nourishment. When this is done, it is important that the nurse not forget about the patient. The patient with a

peptic ulcer needs attention as much as he needs food, and he benefits from a kindly inquiry from the nurse as to whether or not he has taken the feeding, whether there is enough milk in the pitcher, and whether or not it is sufficiently cool. Many patients find that the feedings give them relief from discomfort and therefore anticipate a quick cure with such treatment. They are very upset if meals are delayed. Since much of the patient's time is spent thinking about himself and his treatment and about the implications of his illness for his family, it is understandable that he becomes irritable when the schedule is not carefully adhered to.

It may be necessary to administer the milk and the antacids by a continuous drip tube feeding so that the gastric secretions will be continuously neutralized. This type of feeding is also better for the patient who needs to be kept very quiet since it obviates the need for disturbing him every half hour. This is particularly important during night hours. The nasogastric tube is passed in the manner described earlier in this chapter. A Kelly flask or an infusion bottle containing the milk and the antacids is connected by plastic tubing to the nasogastric tube. A screw clamp regulates the flow of solution through the tube. A prescribed amount of fluid is usually allowed to run into the stomach over a twenty-four-hour period. It should include enough water to supply the patient's daily needs. To prevent the milk from becoming sour, the nurse should keep only a small amount of mixture in the bottle at any one time. The flask should be changed frequently and should be washed and boiled before reuse. Special pump machines are now available and are described in periodic literature.[16]

Drugs. Drugs that are given to lower the acidity of the gastric secretions include calcium carbonate, magnesium carbonate, magnesium oxide, aluminum hydroxide gel (Amphojel), and magnesium trisilicate. These drugs reduce gastric acidity by physical absorption or by chemical neutralization. They are poorly absorbed from the stomach and therefore do not alter the pH of the blood or interfere with normal acid-base balance. When they are prescribed in the initial stages of treatment for an ulcer, they are given hourly. Because milk may be given hourly, a schedule is usually set up in which the milk is given every hour on the hour and the antacids every hour on the half hour. In order to maintain this schedule, it is important that the patient be well instructed so that he can assume some responsibility for this regimen under close nursing supervision.

Since sodium bicarbonate is readily absorbed from the intestine into the bloodstream, patients should be advised against taking it when gastric pain occurs. If a large quantity is taken, the acid-base balance of the blood will be upset. Also, the reaction of sodium bicarbonate and hydrochloric acid forms carbon dioxide, which may increase distress by causing distention.

Drugs used to decrease gastric motility are alkaloids of belladonna and propantheline bromide (Pro-Banthine). Tincture of belladonna has little effect upon the amount and character of gastric secretions, but it does decrease gastrointestional motility, muscle tone, and peristalsis. Some antispasmodic drugs are methscopolamine bromide (Pamine), methscopolamine nitrate (Skopolate), and Donnatal (containing atropine sulfate, hyoscyamine sulfate, phenobarbital, and hyoscyamine hydrobromide). Pro-Banthine may cause blurring of vision and urinary retention. The nurse should check for urinary output of patients receiving this drug, and untoward signs should be reported to the doctor. Other anticholinergic drugs sometimes ordered are tridihexethyl chloride (Panthilon chloride), hexocyclium methylsulfate (Tral), and isopropamide iodide (Darbid).

Patients who are on milk diets or who are receiving drugs such as Amphojel and anticholinergic drugs often become constipated. The doctor may order a mild cathartic, but no cathartic should be taken without a doctor's order since it may increase gastrointestinal motility when it is undesirable.

Preventive health teaching. To prevent exacerbations of an ulcer, the patient must learn to avoid the foods and situations that tend to reactivate the ulcer. The doctor usually evaluates the problems or pressures in the patient's home life or at work that may bring about attacks of ulcer pain. If the patient cannot be removed from his environ-

mental influence, he may be given help in accepting stressful situations. He should be encouraged to allow time for periods of rest and relaxation in his daily schedule. Occasionally the doctor may advise the patient to have psychotherapy so that he may understand his problems better and thus be more able to cope with them.

The patient should practice moderation in diet, work, and play. He should be aware that he has had an ulcer and that excesses may cause the ulcer to become reactivated.

The planning, preparation, and serving of food should be thoroughly discussed with the patient and his family, and cultural and religious preferences should be considered. Highly seasoned foods, very hot or cold food, fried foods, raw fruits and vegetables, coffee, and alcohol should be avoided. The patient should learn to eat slowly in a quiet environment, and he should try to avoid situations that cause emotional disturbance before and during meals. It is usually necessary for him to remain on a bland diet for at least a year. It is common for him to want to resume his former eating pattern as soon as pain disappears, but he should know that doing so may cause an immediate return of symptoms. The patient's work sometimes makes the selection of suitable meals difficult. If the selection of food is limited, the patient can take milk with him in a vacuum bottle to supplement the limited selection. If the patient becomes emotionally upset by situations at work or at home, he should learn to eat a bland diet and to drink milk between meals. These measures may prevent a serious exacerbation of the ulcer.

There seems to be a relationship between smoking and irritation of a peptic ulcer. Therefore, most doctors believe that the patient who has a peptic ulcer should give up smoking permanently. To do so is often very difficult for the patient, since often his life and work situations, as well as his personality makeup, are such that a change of this sort is a major one. The patient needs constant encouragement and understanding when he is endeavoring to give up smoking if the habit is well established.

For the successful treatment of an ulcer and the prevention of future exacerbations, the doctor must have the complete confidence of the patient. The nurse can often help to augment the patient's confidence in his doctor and in the prescribed treatment. She can also learn about doubts and worries of the patient and report them to the doctor so that reassurance or explanation may be given as needed. If every consideration is given to adjusting the prescribed regimen to fit the patient's physical, economic, and social pattern, he will be better able to follow the treatment. When plans are being made by the health team for the patient's discharge from the hospital, the patient and his family should be included. In this way, existing problems can be discussed realistically in relation to future care.

The patient who has had a peptic ulcer must remain under medical supervision for about a year. He may have periodic x-ray examinations of the stomach to determine the extent to which the ulcer has healed. After that time, if healing is complete, he should be advised to report to his doctor at once if symptoms reappear since peptic ulcers can recur after the patient has enjoyed several years of good health.

Complications requiring surgery. Emergency surgery is necessary when a peptic ulcer perforates and causes peritonitis or erodes a blood vessel, causing severe hemorrhage. Elective surgery may be performed if an ulcer does not respond to the medical regimen and continues to produce symptoms, if it causes pyloric obstruction, or if a chronic recurring gastric ulcer is thought to be precancerous. Whereas only 10 to 20% of duodenal ulcers require operation, 30 to 75% of gastric ulcers require surgery.[11] Immediate response of a peptic ulcer to medical treatment is about 90%, whereas the long-term response is only approximately 50 to 60%. The most common reason for operation is the tendency of the ulcer to recur.[4]

Perforation. Acute perforation of a peptic ulcer is a surgical emergency and accounts for 65 to 85% of the deaths from peptic ulcers.[4] After the perforation occurs, gastric contents pour into the peritoneal cavity, causing peritonitis. Both gastric and duodenal ulcers may perforate.

The patient who has a perforated ulcer has symptoms similar to those occurring when any abdominal organ or other part of the gastrointestinal tract perforates. The extremely irritating qualities of the gastric contents released into the abdominal cavity, however, may be quite overwhelming and lead to prostration and severe shock in a short time. There is a sudden sharp pain that spreads quickly over the abdomen. Characteristically, the patient bends over with pain and draws up his knees to prevent pull on the abdominal wall. He is reluctant to move, holds himself tense, and protests against having his abdomen touched. Upon palpation, the abdomen is found to be boardlike and very tender. The patient usually perspires profusely, and his facial expression is one of agony and apprehension. Since his breathing is rapid and shallow to prevent pull on abdominal muscles, he may be cyanotic. The patient's temperature is usually elevated but may be normal or subnormal. His pulse is usually rapid and weak. A positive diagnosis is made by making a roentgenogram of the abdomen with the patient standing. If the ulcer has perforated, air under the diaphragm is visible on the film.

Any perforation of the alimentary tract should be closed surgically as soon as possible. The longer the perforation exists, allowing the irritating (and infected) gastrointestinal secretions to pour into the abdominal cavity, the higher the mortality rate becomes.[4]

Before operation for a perforated ulcer, a nasogastric tube is passed into the stomach and attached to a continuous suction apparatus to drain the gastric secretions. Parenteral fluids are given to combat fluid and electrolyte imbalance, and antibiotics are administered. The patient is kept in a low Fowler's position so that the gastric contents that have escaped will collect in the pelvic cavity and will be more accessible surgically.

The operation used to close a perforation consists of suturing the opening and reinforcing the area with an omental graft; it is known as a *plicating* operation. The gastric contents that have escaped into the peritoneal cavity are aspirated by suction during the operation. A solution containing antibiotics may be placed in the abdominal cavity before the abdomen is closed.

Routine postoperative care is carried out as described on p. 191. As soon as the patient recovers from anesthesia, however, he is returned to a low Fowler's position. Large doses of antibiotics are given, and the nasogastric tube is left in place until peristalsis returns. Fluids are given parenterally, and antibiotics may be given as well. Drainage from the nasogastric tube is greenish yellow, and there is usually no blood present. Nursing care of patients with nasogastric tubes in use was discussed earlier in this chapter.

Postoperatively the patient should be watched carefully for signs of continuing peritonitis and for abscess formation. Elevation of temperature, respiratory distress, continued abdominal pain, and signs of paralytic ileus, such as distention and the inability to pass flatus or stool, should be reported to the doctor. The doctor may also perform periodic rectal examinations to determine the presence of pelvic masses caused by abscess formation. Such an abscess may need to be incised and drained. The nurse should explain to the patient why the rectal examinations are necessary. (A full discussion of the complications of peritonitis is given later in this chapter.)

When the nasogastric tube is removed, the patient is given small amounts (30 to 60 ml.) of clear fluid by mouth each hour. If this amount of fluid is well tolerated, he usually is given 90 ml. of milk every hour and, after two or three days, a bland diet with milk between meals. Most patients are discharged from the hospital on a medical regimen for ulcers. The nurse should review this regimen carefully with the patient who has never had this treatment and also with the patient who has been on this regimen previously.

Chronic peptic ulcers. Patients who have chronic peptic ulcers often require surgery. Even under medical treatment some ulcers persist or keep recurring. Others do not respond to medical treatment and cause the patient so much pain that he is unable to work, sleep, or eat. These intractable chronic ulcers usually occur in the middle-aged or older patient. Surgery is also indicated in gastric ulcers that do not respond to medical treatment quite rapidly, since many of them become cancerous if allowed to persist, and many times it is impossible to diagnose the condition with certainty even with the many diagnostic measures available.

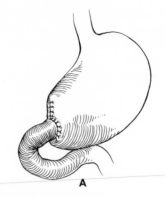

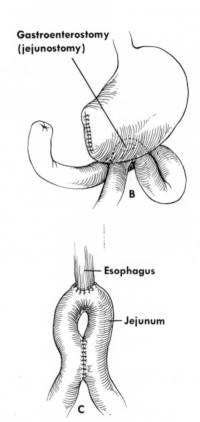

Fig. 155

Types of gastric resections and anastomoses. **A,** Gastric resection with anastomosis of the remaining segment of the stomach with the duodenum (Billroth I type). **B,** Gastric resection with closure of the duodenum and anastomosis of the remaining segment of the stomach to the jejunum (Billroth II type). **C,** Total gastrectomy with anastomosis of the esophagus to the jejunum. The duodenum has been closed.

Several different operations may be used in the treatment of chronic peptic ulcers (Fig. 155). The *Billroth II* operation, or variations thereof, (such as Polya, Hofmeister) consists of the removal of one-half to two-thirds of the stomach *(subtotal gastrectomy)*. In this type of gastric resection, the ulcer and a large amount of acid-secreting mucosa are removed. The duodenal stump is closed, and the remaining segment of the stomach is anastomosed to a loop of jejunum *(gastrojejunostomy, gastroenterostomy)*. Gastric contents now will pass directly from the stomach to the jejunum. Since the distal end of the duodenum still connects with the jejunum, bile now flows from it to the jejunum to mix with the food.

The *Billroth I* operation (or variations thereof) consists of the removal of the lower half to two-thirds of the stomach. The remaining portion of the stomach is anastomosed to the duodenum *(gastroduodenostomy)*.

An *antrectomy* consists of the removal of the entire antrum (area between the fundus and the pylorus) of the stomach and the anastomosing of the remaining stomach to the duodenum *(gastroduodenostomy)*. A *vagotomy* is performed by resecting the vagus nerve branch to the stomach 6 to 7 cm. above the junction of the esophagus and the stomach. An antrectomy with a vagotomy may be done. Theoretically, resecting the entire antrum of the stomach removes the source of the hormone, gastrin, and the gastric hormonal phase of gastric hypersecretion is eliminated. (See Fig. 156.) In addition, by eliminating the cerebral stimuli to the stomach by a vagotomy, the motility of the stomach muscle and the volume of gastric secretions are lessened.

A *gastrojejunostomy* (gastroenterostomy) or a vagotomy combined with a gastrojejunostomy may be the treatment of choice for elderly patients who cannot tolerate extensive surgery, for very young patients, whose nutritional state suffers irreparably from removal of large amounts of stomach, or for patients with penetrating ulcers of the duodenum or with a deformed duodenum where a Billroth I type of anastomosis would be technically difficult to perform. In a gastrojejunostomy (gastroenterostomy), the je-

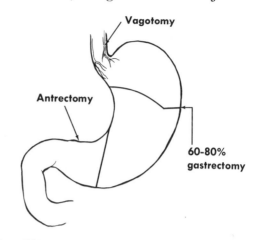

Fig. 156

Some surgical approaches used in treatment of peptic ulcer.

junum is pulled up and anastomosed with the stomach. A new opening for the food to pass from the stomach is then made between the stomach and the jejunum without removal of any portion of the stomach.

After a gastric resection procedure, the *"dumping syndrome"* sometimes occurs. Mild symptoms occur in approximately 50% of all patients and usually disappear in a few months to a year. They remain troublesome in approximately 5 to 15% of all patients who undergo gastric resection.[4] After eating, the patient complains of weakness, faintness, palpitations of the heart, and diaphoresis. A feeling of fullness, discomfort, and nausea often occurs, and diarrhea may also develop. The symptoms are thought to be due to the entrance of food directly into the jejunum without undergoing usual changes and dilution in the stomach. The food mixture, more hypertonic than the jejunal secretions, causes fluid to be drawn from the bloodstream to the jejunum. The reaction appears to be greater after the ingestion of highly concentrated and refined carbohydrate foods. Fear of symptoms makes the patient reluctant to eat, and he may lose weight. He should be advised to avoid concentrated carbohydrates such as heavily sweetened cereals and sweet desserts that are rapidly dissolved into a concentrated solution. A diet high in protein and high enough in fat to compensate for the carbohydrate restriction should be encouraged. The patient should lie down after eating, should eat frequent, small, dry meals, and should avoid drinking fluid for two or three hours after meals. The "dumping syndrome" may be a serious postoperative complication that severely hampers the patient in his work and in many other experiences of normal living. The nurse should observe all patients for early signs of this condition following a gastrectomy and report her observations to the surgeon. This may help him to treat the patient early and prevent the discomfort, malnutrition, and psychic reactions to the entire experience, which compound the difficulty of treating this condition satisfactorily.

Pyloric obstruction. Pyloric obstruction may be caused by edema of tissues around an ulcer or by scar tissue from a healed ulcer located near the pylorus. It may be only partial and cause dilation of the stomach, or it may be complete. Patients with this complication may have severe projectile vomiting that may or may not be preceded by nausea. A positive diagnosis is made by a gastrointestinal x-ray examination. If the obstruction is thought to be due to edema about the pylorus, medical treatment is given. A nasogastric tube is inserted and milk or a protein hydrolysate solution such as Aminosol is given by continuous drip to neutralize the stomach secretions and to permit the inflammation to subside. A prescribed amount of the solution is permitted to run into the stomach over an eight-hour period. The feeding is then discontinued for about fifteen to thirty minutes, and the stomach contents are aspirated to determine how much of the feeding has not passed through the pylorus. If the patient does not vomit during the eight-hour period, and if the gastric retention becomes less in each eight-hour period, it is usually assumed that the stenosis is temporary and that it will continue to respond to medical treatment. Antacids may be added to the tube feeding. Propantheline bromide (Pro-Banthine) and sedatives may be given by injection, and if the patient is vomiting or is unable to tolerate food by mouth, fluids may be given parenterally.

If the obstruction does not respond to medical treatment, surgery is necessary. The operation performed is usually the Billroth

II type or a gastroenterostomy and vagotomy, as already described.

Hemorrhage. Peptic ulcers cause bleeding in at least 25% of all persons who have the disease.[4] If the ulcer has perforated a major blood vessel, the patient may have a severe hemorrhage, vomiting large amounts of blood and passing tarry stools. Vomiting of blood usually occurs with a gastric ulcer, whereas tarry stools are more common with a bleeding duodenal ulcer. Both symptoms may be present in either conditions. The patient may also complain of feeling faint, dizzy, and thirsty. He may become dyspneic, apprehensive, and restless as the blood volume is reduced, and the blood pressure drops, the pulse rate increases, and signs of shock become apparent. The systemic signs of hemorrhage may appear before (or without) hematemesis and before passage of blood or tarry stools.

The patient with a bleeding ulcer is placed on bed rest and is usually given a sedative such as phenobarbital sodium to alleviate restlessness and apprehension. Morphine sulfate may be used since it aids rest and also helps to slow down intestinal peristalsis. The doctor usually orders that the blood pressure, pulse rate, and respirations be checked and recorded frequently (as often as every fifteen minutes when acute bleeding is suspected). Blood transfusions are often given to raise the blood volume. They are given slowly to avoid increasing the blood pressure and thereby increasing the bleeding.

If the patient is not vomiting and only a small amount of blood is being passed by rectum, he usually is given milk every hour, and antacids are prescribed. A full bland diet may be ordered because it maintains nutrition, neutralizes gastric acidity, reduces absorption of the formed clot, and slows peristalsis. If the patient is vomiting blood, however, he is given nothing by mouth. All bloody vomitus should be measured and described. The doctor may wish it saved for his inspection. A nasogastric tube may be passed and attached to a suction apparatus to collect the blood so that it can be more accurately measured and replaced by transfusion. The fluid and electrolyte balance are maintained by infusions. Sometimes there is an order to irrigate the tube with iced physiologic saline solution. If so, the irrigating fluid usually must be suctioned back, as the iced fluid causes blood to clot not only in the stomach but also within the tube. The patient who is vomiting blood will need special mouth care. A weak solution of hydrogen peroxide may be used to more easily remove blood from the tongue and the teeth and gums.

The number of tarry (or currant jellylike) stools should also be recorded, and they may be saved for laboratory examination. Since the patient may be alarmed at the sight of blood, all evidence of bleeding should be quickly removed from the bedside, and the linen should be changed as needed without disturbing the patient any more than necessary. The patient should be told that he is receiving blood transfusions to replace the blood he has lost and that rest and quiet will help stop the bleeding. The sedative or narcotic should be given regularly to allay anxiety and apprehension. If large doses of sedative and narcotic drugs are given, attention must be taken to turning the patient hourly and to encouraging him to breathe deeply to prevent the possibility of respiratory congestion.

If massive hemorrhage occurs, a gastric resection is usually done as soon as the blood volume is raised to a level at which surgery can be performed safely. The portion of the stomach containing the ulcer is removed. This usually is a Billroth II type of operation, as described for chronic peptic ulcers.

The general principles of nursing a patient after gastric surgery that are discussed later are applicable. The drainage from the nasogastric tube is usually dark red for about six to twelve hours after surgery. It should turn greenish yellow within twenty-four hours. The patient may continue to pass tarry stools for several days postoperatively, but this is usually because the blood from the hemorrhage before operation has not yet passed completely through the gastrointestinal tract.

Gastric hypothermia. Some physicians now use local cooling in the treatment of massive gastric hemorrhage. They also believe that hypothermia is effective in the treatment of some patients with peptic ulcers because the cooling suppresses gastric secretions and digestion, relieves symptoms, and permits the ulcer to heal. A double-lumen tube with a large balloon is passed through the mouth into the stomach. The coolant, a mixture of alcohol and water, is gradually instilled into the balloon until it contains approximately 600 to 850 ml. of solution and touches all of the gastric mucosa. Pumps circulate the solution at a temperature of $-17°$ to $-20°$ C. ($2°$ to $-4°$ F.). After an hour, the tube is removed. The patient is permitted to eat approximately two hours after the treatment is ended. This procedure is apparently well tolerated by patients and may be repeated at intervals if symptoms recur. The effectiveness of the treatment is still being studied, and it is not widely used at this time.[42]

Gastric irradiation. Radiation therapy to the stomach to reduce activity of the acid-producing glands may be used for selected elderly patients who cannot be operated upon and who do not respond favorably to any other form of medical treatment.

Nursing care of patients having gastric surgery

Except in emergencies, all patients who are to have gastric surgery undergo extensive diagnostic studies before surgery is done. If the patient is to have surgery for an ulcer, he is maintained on a medical regimen during the preoperative period. The nursing responsibilities related to caring for patients undergoing diagnostic procedures have already been described. Specific nursing responsibilities related to caring for patients with intestinal obstruction and with gastrointestinal hemorrhage are discussed in the appropriate sections. The general preoperative instructions and preparation are those given any patient preceding major surgery (p. 173). Special instructions for the nursing care of patients in whom a chest approach is used are discussed on p. 577.

Routine postoperative nursing care is given as described on p. 193. Because the incision is made in the upper abdomen, the patient is inclined to breathe shallowly to limit pain in the incision. The prescribed medications for pain should be given as necessary, and special attention should be given to encouraging the patient to breathe deeply and to cough productively. The patient with a high abdominal midline incision is usually more comfortable in a modified Fowler's position. Drainage from the nasogastric tube after gastric surgery usually contains some blood for the first twelve hours, but bright red blood, large amounts of blood, or excessive bloody drainage should be watched for and its occurrence reported to the surgeon at once. While the nasogastric tube is used, and until peristalsis resumes, fluids by mouth are restricted. Mouth care, therefore, is needed frequently to keep the mucous membranes of the throat and mouth moist and clean. Until the tube is removed and until the patient is able to drink enough nutritious fluids, fluids are given parenterally. The average patient is given about 3,500 ml. of fluids intravenously each day (2,500 ml. for his normal body needs plus enough to replace fluids lost through the gastric drainage and vomitus). It is important that gastric drainage and urinary output be accurately measured and recorded. Vitamins are usually prescribed until the patient is eating a full, well-balanced diet. Fluids by mouth are usually restricted for about twelve to twenty-four hours after the nasogastric tube is removed. The patient may be given 30 ml. of water every hour the first day, 60 ml. every hour the second day, and 90 ml. every hour the third day. If water is well tolerated, small amounts of bland food may be added until the patient is able to eat six small meals a day and to drink 120 ml. of fluid every hour between meals. This dietary regimen, however, usually must be adapted to the individual patient since some patients tolerate increasing amounts of food and fluids better than others. Regurgitation after meals may be caused by eating too fast, by eating too much, or by postoperative edema about the suture line that prevents the food from passing into the intestines. If regurgitation occurs, the patient should be encouraged to eat more slowly, and the size of the meals should be decreased temporarily. If the gastric retention continues, it is probably caused by edema about the suture line, and food and fluids by mouth usually are discontinued for a time. A nasogastric tube may be passed and attached to a suction apparatus, and fluids may be administered parenterally until the edema subsides.

After most gastric surgery, drainage on the dressings is minimal. If a total gastrectomy is performed, however, drains are usually inserted from the site of the anastomosis, and there may be serosanguineous drainage. The patient usually gets out of bed the day after surgery, and his activity is increased progressively thereafter.

The patient is usually discharged from the hospital two or three weeks after surgery. Before discharge, a gastrointestinal series is often done to observe the functioning of the gastroenterostomy. The patient still may be eating six small meals a day, or he may tolerate three larger meals of bland food. He should be advised to eat slowly and to decrease the size of the meals if he is uncomfortable after eating. The remaining stomach gradually is able to accept larger amounts of food and fluids. Within six months to a year, the patient is usually able to eat three regular meals. He requires about three months to convalesce before he regains his strength completely and is able to resume full activity. After discharge, he needs medical supervision and should be advised to keep appointments either in his doctor's office or in the hospital clinic. During these visits the nurse can help to determine the patient's understanding of his condition. He may need to discuss problems about his diet with the dietitian.

Cancer

Cancer of the stomach is responsible for approximately 18,000 deaths each year in the United States, or a little less than 10% of all deaths from cancer.[1] The incidence has decreased in the United States over recent years, although the cause for this is unknown. It is found more often after the age of 45 years and is more common in men than in women. There is no known cause for this disease, but it is believed that heredity is a factor in its development and that chronic gastritis and chronic gastric ulcer may be precursors of cancer of the stomach.

Cancer may develop in any part of the stomach but is found most often in the distal third. It may spread directly through the stomach wall into adjacent tissues, to the lymphatics, to the regional lymph nodes of the stomach, to the esophagus, to the spleen, and to the pancreas or through the bloodstream to the bones. Involvement of regional lymph nodes occurs early and is found in about 60 to 70% of all patients, who would seem to be curable at the time of operation.[11]

Unfortunately, the patient with cancer of the stomach usually has no symptoms until the growth spreads to adjacent organs. Symptoms may occur only after the disease has become incurable. Vague and persistent symptoms of gastric distress, flatulence, loss of appetite, nausea, gradual weight loss, and loss of strength may be the only complaints of the patient. These vague symptoms should never be ignored. If the nurse knows of anyone with them, she should encourage him to seek immediate medical advice. However, since such symptoms are not necessarily symptoms of cancer, the patient should not be unduly frightened. Pain does not appear usually until late in the disease, and the absence of this symptom is often the reason for the patient's delay in seeking medical help. If the disease progresses untreated, marked cachexia develops, and eventually a palpable mass can often be felt in the region of the stomach. Often no early gastric symptoms appear, and fatigue and persistent anemia may be the only signs. Cancer of the stomach occurs three times more frequently in persons who have pernicious anemia than in others.

A positive diagnosis of gastric carcinoma is usually made by means of a gastrointestinal series. The tumor may not be evident in its early stages, and the x-ray examinations may have to be repeated at intervals. An absence of free hydrochloric acid in stomach secretions obtained by gastric aspiration is suggestive of a gastric neoplasm. When other examinations are negative, cytologic studies may demonstrate the presence of malignant cells in the stomach. Occult blood is frequently found in the stools.

The operative treatment for cancer of the stomach is either a subtotal gastrectomy or a total gastrectomy. Whichever procedure is used, the omentum and the spleen usually are also removed because of the common occurrence of metastasis to these areas. A subtotal gastrectomy has already been described. When the cancer is spread diffusely throughout the stomach, when it extends high in the lesser curvature, or when it arises in the cardia, a *total gastrectomy* is done. The entire stomach is removed, and then continuity of the gastrointestinal tract is reestablished by anastomosis of a loop of the jejunum to the esophagus (Fig. 155). The two portions of the jejunum meeting the esophagus are then sometimes joined to form a reservoir for food.[11] A total gastrectomy is never done when signs of metastasis to other abdominal organs such as the liver are evident. A palliative resection of the stomach is usually done for patients who have cancer of the stomach with metastases.

The nursing care of a patient who has had a total gastrectomy differs in some ways from that of patients undergoing other types of gastric surgery. Since the chest cavity must be entered, the patient will have a catheter for chest drainage, and the nursing care will be that of the patient who has had chest surgery (p. 277). There is little or no drainage from the nasogastric tube because there is no longer any reservoir in which secretions may collect, and there is no stomach mucosa left to secrete. When normal peristalsis returns, the patient is given clear fluids hourly, and if after two or three days there is no evidence of leakage through the anastomosis, the diet is increased to several small meals (usually six) of bland foods a day. An elevation of temperature or dyspnea should make one suspect leakage from the anastomosis, and all oral intake should be stopped until the doctor has been consulted.

Following a total gastrectomy, the maintenance of good nutrition is difficult because the patient can no longer eat regular meals and because the food that is taken is poorly digested and therefore poorly absorbed from the intestines. Since the patient also becomes anemic, ferrous sulfate is often prescribed. Patients who have had a total gastrectomy rarely regain normal strength. Most of them are semi-invalids as long as they live. Survival rate for gastric cancer is unusual beyond five years because of early and extensive metastasis. X-ray therapy is sometimes used, but for cancer in this location it is of limited use.

Pyloric stenosis

Pyloric stenosis is one of the most common conditions requiring surgery in infancy. It occurs most often in tense infants of tense, apprehensive parents, and is seen most often in firstborn children. Pyloric stenosis causes vomiting that usually is forceful and occurs soon after the formula is taken. Vomiting is followed immediately by eagerness to take food. As the condition persists and loss of weight occurs, peristaltic waves can be seen passing across the abdomen from right to left and reversing immediately prior to vomiting. Symptoms usually appear in the second or third week of life and seldom develop after 3 or 4 months of age. The cause of this condition is hypertrophy of the sphincter muscle of the pylorus, which often may be felt as a tumor mass in the right upper quadrant of the infant's abdomen.

Pyloric stenosis is treated medically before surgery is considered. If it is treated early before hypertrophy is pronounced and malnutrition is severe, surgery may often be avoided. Medical treatment consists of giving small amounts of sedative drugs such as phenobarbital or the alkaloids of belladonna such as atropine in regular doses several times a day and usually preceding meals, and modifying the diet. Smaller amounts may be given at more frequent intervals, and cereals may be substituted for some of the milk, since solid foods are less easily vomited. The infant needs a quiet, relaxed environment. In the hospital the nurse should see that all his needs, such as for a change of diapers or for extra warmth, are met at once so that he does not become upset. Very gentle rocking prior to and immediately following meals sometimes helps. If the infant is at home, the public health nurse can often help the family to ensure a more relaxed environment for the infant. Sometimes, for example, it appears that a mother's fears about whether or not she is properly caring for her baby contribute to the infant's difficulties.

Surgical treatment for pyloric stenosis is used when the condition does not respond to medical treatment alone. It consists of incision into the sphincter muscle of the pylorus, i.e., pylorotomy (Ramstedt operation), and the response to this treatment is almost uniformly good. All the measures described in Chapter 10 relating to surgery in infancy and childhood should be considered. Usually a nasogastric tube is passed and stomach contents are aspirated just prior to surgery. Since only the muscle layers are cut and the stomach is not entered during the operation, many surgeons permit the infant to have water and sometimes formula almost as soon as he has reacted completely from the anesthesia.

The patient with disease of the lower gastrointestinal system

Many disease conditions affect the lower gastrointestinal system. Only some of the more common ones and the related nursing care will be discussed here.

Appendicitis

In the United States there are still many deaths each year from appendicitis. If symptoms had not been neglected or if the patient had not been given a cathartic, some of these deaths might have been prevented. It is important, therefore, that the nurse continue to help teach the public that symptoms of right lower quadrant or periumbilical pain accompanied by loss of appetite, elevation of temperature, and possibly nausea, vomiting, and diarrhea should be reported to a physician. Patients with these symptoms should not be treated at home by local heat, enemas, or cathartics.

Appendicitis is an inflammatory lesion of the vermiform appendix. It is more common among men, and it occurs most frequently between the ages of 10 and 30 years. It may occur at any age, however. Although there is no certain cause of the disease, occlusion of the lumen of the appendix by hardened feces (fecaliths), by foreign objects, or by kinking of the appendix may impair the circulation and lower resistance to organisms within the body such as the colon bacillus or the streptococcus. A small part of the appendix may be edematous, inflamed, or necrotic, or the entire appendix may be so involved. An abscess may develop in the appendical wall or in the surrounding tissue. The serious danger is that the appendix will rupture and cause a generalized peritonitis.

The typical symptoms of acute appendicitis are pain about the umbilicus and throughout the abdomen (which may soon become localized at a point known as *Mc-Burney's point*, exactly halfway between the umbilicus and the crest of the right ilium), nausea, anorexia, and often vomiting. Acute appendicitis is remarkable for the suddenness of its onset. The patient may have felt quite well an hour or two before the onset of severe pain. The temperature is usually moderately elevated and there is moderate leukocytosis. These symptoms are present in about 60% of all patients with acute appendicitis.[11] Other patients have less well-defined local symptoms because of the location of the appendix. It may be retrocecal, or it may lie adjacent to the ureter. If the patient has questionable symptoms, a urinalysis and an intravenous pyelogram may be made to rule out an acute pyelitis or a ureteral stone. There are many other diseases that produce symptoms similar to appendicitis, and they sometimes need to be ruled out before a positive diagnosis can be made. Some of these are acute salpingitis, regional ileitis, mesenteric lymphadenitis, and biliary colic. The older patient with acute appendicitis may experience only dull pain. Children who develop appendicitis may have only slight abdominal pain, although usually they vomit. Because the abdominal omentum is not well developed in children, if the appendix perforates, peritonitis can easily develop because the infection cannot be walled off so quickly. It is recommended, therefore, that the ill child who refuses food and who vomits be taken to a physician for diagnosis and treatment. He should *never* be given a cathartic for these complaints.

Medical treatment and nursing care

When appendicitis is suspected, the patient usually is hospitalized at once and placed on bed rest for observation and the necessary diagnostic procedures that must be done. Since an operation may be done shortly after admission, the patient is not given anything by mouth while reports of the blood count are awaited. Parenteral fluids may be given during this time. Narcotics are not given until the cause of the pain has been determined. Sometimes an ice bag to the abdomen is ordered to help relieve pain. A rectal examination is done to help establish the diagnosis, and the patient should be given an explanation as to why the procedure is necessary.

An appendectomy is usually scheduled as an emergency operation. The patient is given a general or regional anesthetic, and the appendix is removed through a small incision over McBurney's point or through a right rectus incision. The incision usually heals with no drainage. Drains are used when an abscess is discovered, when the appendix has ruptured and peritonitis has developed, and sometimes when the appendix appears edematous and ready to rupture and is surrounded by clear fluid.

Bowel function is usually normal soon after surgery. Nausea and vomiting disappear with surgical treatment, and the patient is permitted food as tolerated. Convalescence is usually short. The patient gets out of bed the day after surgery and may resume normal activity within two to four weeks.

Meckel's diverticulum

Meckel's diverticulum is a fibrous tube or cord located usually about 50 cm. (20 inches) above the ileocecal valve. It is the remnant of a duct used in fetal life and is found in about 2% of the population.[22]

The diverticulum can become inflamed, causing symptoms similar to those of appendicitis or hemorrhage from the bowel. Differential diagnosis is particularly difficult in children. The diagnosis is usually made at operation. At this time the diseased diverticulum and the involved intestine are resected.

Mesenteric vascular occlusion

Mesenteric vascular occlusion is common, occurring frequently in patients with extensive arteriosclerosis or serious heart disease. Often the patient is elderly. It also may occur in patients who are recovering from recent abdominal surgery. Thrombosis of the mesenteric vein may occur as a complication of cirrhosis of the liver, following splenectomy, or as a result of an extension of a thrombophlebitic process in the ileocolic veins. The superior mesenteric arteries usually are occluded.

The blood supply to the lower part of the

jejunum and ileum usually is interrupted by a mesenteric vascular occlusion. The walls of the intestine become thickened and edematous, then reddened, and finally black and gangrenous. The patient complains of an acute onset of sharp abdominal pain, nausea, and vomiting. He has disturbed bowel function and may pass blood from the rectum or may have no bowel action. The white blood cell count is elevated. The patient goes into shock quickly and may be in shock when first seen by a doctor even when the condition is reported at the onset of symptoms. The patient is hospitalized at once. Nothing is given by mouth, and a nasogastric tube is inserted and attached to a suction apparatus. Parenteral fluids may be started. The treatment is always immediate surgery before the dead tissue can cause peritonitis and before symptoms of obstruction become overwhelming. The gangrenous bowel and its attached mesentery are removed, and the remaining sections of the bowel are anastomosed.

The preoperative and postoperative care of patients having a bowel resection is described later in this chapter. The patient who has a resection for vascular occlusion usually is given heparin and bishydroxycoumarin (Dicumarol) to prevent further clot formation. This treatment not only requires close medical supervision but also careful nursing care, as discussed on p. 372. The patient may also be given antispasmodic drugs such as papaverine hydrochloride. He is very ill both preoperatively and postoperatively and needs constant nursing care. Close relatives usually are permitted to visit, and provision should be made for their comfort, especially during night hours. The mortality rate from mesenteric vascular occlusion is high, particularly among elderly patients.

Regional ileitis

Regional ileitis is a nonspecific inflammation of the distal loops of the small intestine. It is characterized by cobblestone-like ulcerations along the mucosa, a thickening of the intestinal wall, and the formation of scar tissue. The disease usually occurs between the ages of 20 and 30 years. Its cause is unknown. The inflammation begins at the ileocecal valve and extends upward, sometimes skipping whole areas of intestinal mucosa. The ulcers are likely to perforate and form fistulas that connect with the abdominal wall or with any hollow viscus such as the colon, sigmoid, bladder, or vagina. Scar tissue may form as the ulcers heal, preventing the normal absorbtion of food, and strictures may form and cause intestinal obstruction.

The patient with an acute regional ileitis usually has severe abdominal pain or cramps localized in the right lower quadrant, moderate fever, and mild diarrhea. The white blood cell count is elevated. Often the disease is diagnosed as acute appendicitis, but when the patient is operated upon, he is found to have a normal appendix but an inflamed ileum.

Chronic regional ileitis is characterized by a long history of diarrhea, abdominal pain, loss of weight, anemia, fistula formation, and, finally, intestinal obstruction. The diarrhea may consist of three or four semisolid stools daily containing mucus, pus, and sometimes undigested food. Bowel movements are accompanied by abdominal cramps. A mass sometimes can be felt in the area of the appendix or cecum.

The treatment for both acute and chronic ileitis is essentially medical. The patient is given a low-fat, high-protein bland diet, together with vitamins to help maintain good nutrition. Patients with regional ileitis utilize fats poorly and do not tolerate high-fat diets well. Transfusions and iron compounds may be necessary to treat anemia. Anticholinergic drugs such as propantheline bromide (Pro-Banthine) may be given. Intestinal antibiotics such as phthalylsulfathiazole (Sulfathalidine) and salicylazosulfapyridine (Azulfidine) may be given by mouth, and antibiotics may be given systemically for control of secondary infections. Steroid therapy may be used in acute stages of the disease.

If intestinal obstruction occurs or if there are fistulas, surgery is necessary. Occasionally an ileostomy is done above the involved bowel. The diseased bowel may be resected and the remaining segments anastomosed, or it may be left and a "short-circuiting" operation performed. This operation consists of dividing the ileum, closing the distal portion with sutures or removing it, and anastomosing the proximal portion to the transverse colon (*ileotransverse colostomy*). If the diseased bowel is adherent to the surrounding organs and tissues, an ileotransverse colostomy may be performed. The inflammation is treated with antibiotics.

Ulcerative colitis

Ulcerative colitis is an inflammatory disease of the colon. Although its cause is unknown, it is thought to be the result of either an infectious process or a psychogenic disturbance, although more recently an autoimmune factor has been suspected. None of the possible causes, however, has been proved. Many patients with this disease have personality disorders, and they often are perfectionistic, sensitive, frustrated, and dependent people.

Ulcerative colitis may occur at any age in either sex, but it is found most often between the ages of 20 and 30 years. The disease varies in severity, and the patient may be symptom-free between periods of acute distress. A severe attack may be brought on by an acute infection, an emotional upset, or unknown factors.

In the early stages of ulcerative colitis, only the rectum or rectosigmoid is affected, with the rectal mucosa containing many superficial bleeding points. As the disease progresses, advancing up the colon, the bowel mucosa becomes edematous and thickened. The superficial bleeding points gradually enlarge and become ulcerated. The ulcers may bleed or perforate, causing abscess formation or peritonitis. The edematous mucosa may undergo changes and form pseudopolyps, which may become cancerous. The continuous healing process, with formation of scar tissue between the frequent relapses, may cause the colon to lose its normal elasticity and its absorptive capability. It becomes thickened, normal mucosa is replaced by scar tissue, and it becomes rigid and pipelike. The diagnosis is based on the patient's history and symptoms, on results obtained from barium enemas from proctoscopic and sigmoidoscopic examinations, and on failure to find any causative organisms in the stools.

The main symptom of an acute attack of ulcerative colitis is diarrhea. The patient may pass as many as fifteen to twenty or more liquid stools a day. They contain blood, mucus, and pus. Abdominal cramps may or may not occur before the bowel movement. The patient may have loss of appetite, low-grade fever, and, occasionally, nausea and vomiting. As these symptoms persist, the patient becomes weak, dehydrated, debilitated, and cachectic. Ulcerative colitis is a serious disease with a fairly high mortality rate. The personality makeup of many patients with this disease seems to be such that they accept the disease stoically but are unable always to conform to the regimen that is prescribed; for example, it may be impossible for the patient to eat the foods that he knows are necessary.

Medical treatment for ulcerative colitis is directed toward restoring nutrition, combating infection, reducing the motility of the inflamed bowel, and treating the psychogenic factors that may be involved. Blood transfusions are given for anemia. If the patient is vomiting and is severely undernourished and dehydrated, parenteral fluids may be given. A high-protein, high-caloric, high-vitamin, and low-residue diet is usually urged to help the patient regain nutritional losses and to foster healing. Since there is no conclusive evidence that the diet affects the condition, the patient may be permitted to eat what he chooses. Sedatives such as phenobarbital are prescribed to alleviate nervous tension, and antispasmodic drugs such as belladonna preparations and propantheline bromide (Pro-Banthine) are given to slow down peristalsis. Drugs such as kaolin and bismuth preparations (bismuth subcarbonate) are used to help coat and protect the irritated intestinal mucosa and give better consistency to the stools, and opium preparations such as paregoric may be used to lessen the frequency of stools. Antibiotics may be ordered to prevent or to treat secondary infection.

ACTH and the adrenal steroids such as prednisone are now being used widely in the treatment of ulcerative colitis. They often produce dramatic results in severe cases of the disease by decreasing the toxemia and fever, diminishing diarrhea, bleeding, and rectal urgency, and promoting a sense of well-being in the patient. The explanation of these effects is not known, but patients on these drugs maintain a more active life and a more normal program. (For the nursing care of patients receiving steroid therapy, see p. 63.)

About 20% of patients with ulcerative colitis require surgery because of complications such as hemorrhage or perforation.[4] A resection of the large bowel may be done in an attempt to cure the condition when the disease is so incapacitating that it makes an invalid of the patient and when no improvement has been obtained from medical treatment over a period of time. Choice of surgery depends on the individual patient and on the physician. It is recognized that surgery does not remove the basic condition that led to development of the disease. Many patients, however, seem to recover almost completely following a large bowel resection and are able to lead normal, useful lives.

Nursing care of the patient with ulcerative colitis

The patient with ulcerative colitis may be admitted to the hospital for immediate supportive treatment during an acute exacerbation of the disease or for preparation for surgery during a remission. In either instance, if the disease is of long duration, the patient is usually thin, nervous, and apprehensive and is inclined to be preoccupied with his physical condition. These qualities, which are caused by the illness, are superimposed on the basic personality pattern of many patients with this disease—sensitivity, insecurity, and dependence are common characteristics. This makes it hard for the nurse to get to know the patient and sometimes hard for her to understand him. Yet, in the nursing care of no other patient are understanding and acceptance more necessary. The nurse should not hesitate to seek guidance from the physician in her approach to the patient. Sometimes specialized medical nursing consultation is available. All members of the nursing staff should have the same approach to the patient. Although the patient may accept treatment and nursing care, he may remain restrained and withdrawn; often he is depressed even though he appears resigned to his problems. Acceptance of his behavior, together with gentle, intelligent nursing care, will help the nurse gradually gain the patient's confidence and will increase his ability to accept certain essentials of his treatment, such as food.

All procedures and treatments should be carefully explained to the patient. Telling him, for example, that medication is available to him for controlling bowel movements sometimes seems to reduce his need. The nurse should listen carefully to the patient's own report of things that seem to stimulate peristalsis and cause frequency of bowel movements. If he has found that certain foods or combinations of foods cause diarrhea, this fact should be noted on the nursing care plan and reported to the dietitian. Other information, such as best time for bathing, whether soon after a meal (to permit a long rest period afterward) or later (when food is partially digested), should be on the plan.

The acutely ill patient may have bed rest prescribed. If he is very thin, care must be taken that bony prominences are protected. An alternating air-pressure mattress provides the best protection. If it is not available, a large piece of sponge rubber should be placed under the buttocks. Sponge rubber mattresses are also useful in the prevention of pressure sores. Areas of friction against linen should be watched for. If the patient braces himself on the bedpan by leaning on his elbows, thereby causing pressure areas, these areas should be massaged frequently with a lubricant. If the patient spends most of his time on the bedpan, it should be padded with sponge rubber. If he uses the commode, it can also be protected with a piece of sponge rubber or with a rubber ring.

A record must be kept of the number, amount, and character of the stools, and specimens of stool should be sent to the laboratory as requested. Although each bowel movement may be very small, the commode or bedpan should be emptied as often as it is used. The patient wants the bedpan accessible at all times. He may even insist on keeping it in bed with him, and usually he is permitted to do so. Air-Wick or electric deodorizers are sometimes used to dispel unpleasant odors in the room. Linen should be kept fresh, and the patient's perineum, buttocks, and anal region should be washed thoroughly several times a day.

Dibucaine (Nupercaine) or other prescribed ointment may be applied to the anus to relieve discomfort. Tub baths are beneficial to the skin and circulation and are often permitted once a day provided that the patient is carefully protected from chilling.

The patient should be kept warm, and drafts and chilling must be avoided. Extra covers should be provided so that the patient may use them as he wishes. Heat in the room and covers should provide enough warmth and protection to permit regular airing of the room to help remove odors and to supply fresh air.

Seeing that the patient eats the prescribed foods in adequate amounts and takes supplementary nourishment are essential parts of nursing care. Protein foods are very important. The ingenuity of the nurse will often be taxed in getting the patient to eat enough since sometimes a real distaste for food is a symptom of this disease. Any concession or consideration that promises to increase food intake should be made. The family may be permitted to prepare favorite foods at home and to bring them to the patient provided that the foods are bland and otherwise conform to the prescribed diet.

If infusions and transfusions are necessary, these procedures must be carefully explained to the patient since they often cause apprehension. Because the patient's blood pressure is often low and his veins poor, and because he tolerates the annoyance of these procedures poorly, care is taken to anchor the needle securely and to use an arm board so that the needle does not become dislodged.

As the nurse cares for the patient during convalescence from an acute exacerbation of ulcerative colitis, she should be alert for any suggested problems. Since the physical causes of this condition are unknown and since the condition itself cannot be cured but only alleviated by the variety of treatments available, effort is made to learn of and to control the emotional components of the disease. The doctor may ask the social worker to talk to the patient and attempt to learn of social, economic, or other problems that are bothering him. The public health nurse may make a home visit before the patient leaves the hospital to determine whether or not he can be cared for properly at home and to report any other pertinent information. The family should be guided in ways to help the patient when he is at home, such as preparing food and thus helping to maintain nutrition, and understanding and accepting the disease and the patient's behavior.

Surgical treatment and nursing care

An ileostomy usually is an operation that the patient accepts so that he may again be an active member of society without the constant annoyance of the symptoms of ulcerative colitis. An *ileostomy* is a permanent opening of the small intestine (ileum) through the abdominal wall to the outside. Fecal material no longer passes through the large bowel to the rectum but is discharged through the opening in the abdominal wall. Special bags have been developed to collect this drainage since the contents of the ileum are semiliquid. Preoperative visits and talks with patients who have made successful adjustments to ileostomies are helpful and tend to make the patient less fearful of the operation and its consequences. Persons who have had this operation sometimes gladly offer their services, and filmstrips about ileostomy care are available.

A few days before the operation, the patient is placed on a low-residue diet, and for twenty-four hours before surgery he receives only fluids. This decreases intestinal residue. Intestinal antibiotics such as Sulfathalidine or neomycin are given to lower the bacterial count of the intestine, which helps to prevent postoperative infection of the suture line. Immediately preoperatively, a nasogastric or intestinal tube is passed to keep the bowel decompressed.

An ileostomy and a *total* or *subtotal colectomy* (removal of all or part of the colon) are usually performed at the same operation. After a subtotal colectomy, the patient returns from the operating room with two openings, sometimes called buds or stomas, on the abdominal wall. The proximal opening, which is usually on the right side, is the ileostomy from which liquid stool will flow. The distal opening, usually on the left side, leads to the remnant of lower bowel that has not yet been removed. If a total colectomy was performed, the patient will have only an ileostomy since the large bowel and rectum are removed.

Ileostomy bag. A *temporary ileostomy bag* is placed over the opening to keep fecal drainage from running over the abdomen and onto the incision while the wound is healing. The first few days after surgery the amount of drainage from the stoma may be very small. However, as soon as peristalsis returns and the patient begins to eat, fecal drainage begins. Enzymes in the contents of the small intestine can digest skin. The bag prevents these enteric enzymes from draining onto the skin and

causing ulcerations that are difficult to heal and that make later use of a permanent collection appliance less successful.

If the ileostomy bud, or stoma, has been made so that it protrudes approximately 2.5 cm. (1 inch) above the surface of the abdomen, the opening of the bag should be large enough so that it does not constrict the ileostomy but small enough so that fluid cannot escape onto the skin. It takes about six weeks for postoperative edema to disappear and for the stoma to shrink to its permanent size with this type of bud. A permanent ileostomy bag may then be applied. If the ileostomy bud has been made so that it is flush or level with the skin, the opening of the bag should be cut so that only the stoma is exposed to the drainage. A permanent ileostomy bag may be applied before the patient is discharged from the hospital.

The temporary ileostomy bag usually is a disposable type (Fig. 157). It is held to the skin with skin adhesive. If the skin is intact and the bag properly applied, it will remain in place until pulled off or removed with ether or benzene. It usually needs to be changed every three or four days. Be-

Fig. 157

Various types of drainage bags are available for patients with an ileostomy or a colostomy.
A, Temporary disposable drainage bag; the opening may be enlarged to fit any orifice.
B, Permanent ileostomy bag. **C,** Permanent colostomy bag. **D,** Colostomy bag with metal frame and disposable bag.

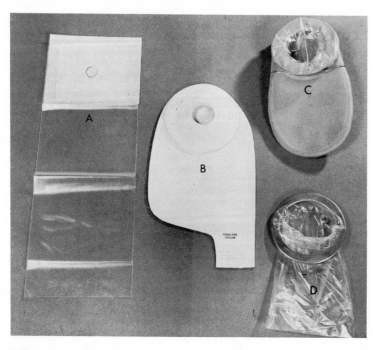

cause the skin must be clean and dry for the application of the skin adhesive and the bag, the bag should be applied before the patient eats or several hours after eating, when there is likely to be little or no drainage from the ileostomy. If a temporary bag is not available, a protective dressing of oiled silk and a gauze dressing similar to that used for urinary drainage can be applied around the ileostomy opening (Fig. 103). If the patient's skin does become irritated, ointments or powders such as karaya gum powder protect the skin from further irritation and permit healing of the erosion. Some patients use the powder as an adherent although it is not as secure as latex cement.

A permanent ileostomy bag is usually made of plastic material and lasts for one to two years. Bags are now available that can be discarded after each use. The patient should be taught how to change the bag and how to care for the skin and bag. Many patients leave the bag in place for several days. They usually wear a belt to hold it securely. It can be emptied without being removed from the body. The elastic band at the bottom of the bag is removed and the contents allowed to flow into the toilet bowl. Then, with the use of a small glass syringe or an Asepto syringe, the inside of the bag may be washed with lukewarm water and soap and rinsed. When the bag is changed, the skin under it should be washed well. Most patients keep at least two bags so that the one most recently worn can be washed and soaked in a weak solution of vinegar or chlorine household bleach (1 tsp. to 1 quart of water) and then aired thoroughly. This care will prevent odors and increase the life of the bag.

Many patients are concerned lest the bag show under their clothing. If loose, full clothing is worn, the bag is not noticeable at all. In fact, many women patients wear a girdle over the bag and are able to wear fitted clothes. As the patient gains weight and his strength returns, he may engage in any activities he wishes. Many engage in active sports, and even swimming is possible. If a woman wears a bathing suit with a full skirt and a man wears loose trunks, no one will notice the bag. Some women have become pregnant and had normal antenatal courses and normal deliveries after having an ileostomy.

Preparation for discharge and for secondary procedure. Some patients have difficulty in adjusting to the care of the ileostomy and need a great deal of encouragement and instruction. The patient should be able to care for his ileostomy before he leaves the hospital. However, if he seems reluctant to learn self-care, it may be advisable to teach a member of his family. Later, when the patient feels better physically, he usually takes over his own care. Groups of patients who have ileostomies have banded together to form "ileostomy clubs" in various parts of the country (Q.T. clubs). They hold regular meetings to discuss mutual problems.[*] The patient who is too far away to attend club meetings may want to arrange for the magazine to be sent to him. It will keep him aware of new developments in the care of ileostomies. He should be urged, however, to discuss any changes he contemplates making with his physician. Although most patients learn to accept their ileostomy and to care for it during a small part of their day, an occasional patient, unfortunately, will center most of his time and attention upon it.

Diet. There are few dietary restrictions for persons who have an ileostomy. However, the patient needs to know that some foods, such as corn, will come through the ileostomy undigested and that foods such as cabbage will cause flatus. Certain foods, such as fresh fruits, usually make the stool more liquid and profuse and therefore should be taken in small amounts or avoided. Each patient learns what foods cause him difficulty and avoids them. Any food that has caused diarrhea or flatus before the operation probably should be avoided. Before the patient leaves the hospital his food intake should be reviewed carefully with him. He should know how to plan his meals so that the essential foods are included. Much good illustrative material is available and can be secured from local health departments and voluntary agencies such as the National Dairy Council.

---

[*]A directory of ileostomy organizations can be obtained from Ileostomy Quarterly, 10 Arlington St., Boston 16, Mass.

Complications. Gastrointestinal upsets are much more serious for patients with an ileostomy than for other people. Fluid and electrolyte balance is easily upset, and the patient may develop acidosis or alkalosis (p. 96). If nausea, vomiting, and diarrhea continue, medical attention should be sought.

Medical and nursing supervision. The patient who has an ileostomy must remain under medical supervision for some time. He may be readmitted to the hospital several months later to have the remainder of the large bowel and the rectum removed. This is done as an abdominoperineal resection, and in some instances this operation alters the ability of male patients to function sexually. The operation and the nursing care of the patient undergoing an abdominoperineal resection are described later in this chapter. After the second operation the patient's general condition and appearance are usually improved. His mental outlook is also better, and he may participate in a normal social life.

Before the patient who has had an ileostomy leaves the hospital after either the first or the second operation, he should be advised to have a public health nurse visit him in his home. She can assist in his adjustment and can supervise his health needs. The patient often does better if he knows that there is someone in the community to whom he may turn for advice and help in the simple details of daily care. He may have trouble with skin irritation, in obtaining new equipment, and in deciding on use of a new paste for the skin. He may have questions related to marriage, work, or recreation. The nurse can help him decide which of his questions and problems he should take to his doctor. It must be remembered that the basic personality of the patient is not changed by the operation, although the activities that the operation may make possible often produce remarkable changes in his attitudes and reactions toward himself and toward his problems.

Amebic dysentery

Amebic dysentery is caused by the protozoan parasite *Entamoeba histolytica*, which primarily invades the large intestine and secondarily invades the liver. The active, motile form of the protozoa, the trophozoite, is not infectious and, if ingested, is easily destroyed by digestive enzymes. The inactive form, or cyst, however, is highly resistant to extremes in temperature, most chemicals, and the digestive juices. When the cyst is swallowed in food or water, it easily passes into the intestines, where the active trophozoite is released and enters the intestinal wall. Here, it feeds on the mucosal cells, causing ulceration of the intestinal mucosa. Although the disease varies in severity, the onset is usually acute, with symptoms developing within two to four days of exposure. Weakness, prostration, nausea, vomiting, and a gripping pain in the right lower quadrant of the abdomen and tenesmus usually occur. Each day the patient has numerous semi-fluid, foul-smelling stools containing mucus and pus.

Prevention

It is estimated that at least 10% of the population of the United States have amebiasis in the acute, chronic, or asymptomatic stages.[4] Although the disease exists chiefly in the tropical countries, it also prevails wherever sanitation is poor. The cyst, which is the infectious agent, can survive for long periods outside the body, and it is transmitted by direct contact from man to man, by insects, and by contaminated water, milk, and other foods. For this reason, people traveling in tropical countries should drink only boiled water and eat only cooked foods. The most infectious agent is the "carrier," who, although having a few or no symptoms of the disease, passes the cysts in his stools. If his hygienic habits are poor and if he is a food handler, he can easily transmit the cysts to the food he prepares for consumption by others.

Treatment and nursing care

If either the trophozoite or the cyst can be found in the stool, a positive diagnosis of amebiasis can be made and definitive treatment started. It is easier to find the parasite in the stool during the acute stage of the disease than later. Immediately after defecation, a warm stool should be sent to the laboratory for examination. Several stool specimens from successive bowel movements may be requested. If the laboratory is at a distance, the specimen container should be transported on a hot-water bottle or in a pan of warm water.

The patient with a mild form of amebiasis is treated on an outpatient basis; 90% of all patients usually respond to a course of amebicidal therapy.[4] The nurse should be familiar with drugs that are given for this disease and should know their effects upon the patient. If the halogenated hydroquinolines such as diiodohydroxyquin (Diodoquin) are given, the patient may have some diarrhea caused by them. Oral antimicrobials such as chlortetracycline (Aureomycin) and oxytetracycline (Terramycin) irritate the gastric mucosa and often produce gastrointestinal symptoms such as nausea, vomiting, and diarrhea. These drugs should be given after meals or with milk and crackers.

Emetine hydrochloride may be used in the treatment of the disease, especially when liver involvement is suspected. The patient receiving emetine hydrochloride is placed on strict bed rest, and pulse rate and blood pressure are watched carefully since the drug is very toxic. Some of the many signs of toxicity to this drug include nausea, vomiting, diarrhea, generalized weakness, cardiac irregularity, fall in blood pressure, neuritis, desquamation of the skin, loss of the sense of taste, and mental depression. Emetine hydrochloride usually is given only for a few days and is followed by a course of antibiotics and then Diodoquin treatment. Finally, carbarsone may be given. It may cause gastrointestinal symptoms, skin eruptions, and occasionally jaundice. The patient must remain on restricted activity for some time after having emetine hydrochloride since, although it is given only for a short time, it is slowly excreted, and cardiovascular symptoms may be late in appearing. Recently paromomycin (Humatin) has been used in the treatment of amebiasis.

Amebiasis is a disease with remissions and exacerbations, and it may persist for years. During acute exacerbations, the patient may become dehydrated, exhausted, or anemic and require hospitalization. During these times the nurse gives general care and assists with special treatments such as infusions and blood transfusions. She should review the patient's diet with him. He should eat a bland, low-residue diet, and may be advised to avoid alcohol and tobacco.

A careful record of the patient's intake and output should be kept, and he should be encouraged to take generous amounts of fluid by mouth. The number and character of the stools should be described, and the bedpan should be sterilized after each use. In handling the bedpan, precautions should be taken since some cysts are usually passed. Cleanliness should be stressed, and the patient should know why it is so important to wash his hands after bowel movements. Particular emphasis should be placed upon careful washing of hands before meals to avoid reinfection.

Salmonellosis

The salmonella infections are a group of acute infections caused by variations of the motile gram-negative salmonella bacillus. They have increased in occurrence in recent years; 15,390 cases were reported in 1963 and only 1,233 in 1950.[22] There are several hundred strains of the bacillus, and all are pathologic for man and many are pathologic for animals. The bacillus causing typhoid fever *(Salmonella typhosa)* is now considered one of the salmonella group. The incidence of typhoid fever, however, is low in this country because of effective programs of immunization. Other acute illness caused by the salmonella organisms include enteric or paratyphoid fever caused by the *Salmonella schottmuelleri,* gastroenteritis caused in most cases by the *Salmonella typhimurium,* and bacteremia often caused by *Salmonella choleraesuis.* Mortality is highest when bacteremia occurs, and complications that may develop include cholecystitis, osteomyelitis, endocarditis, meningitis, pneumonia, and pelvic or perineal abscesses.

Infection with salmonella organisms is acquired through the oral route. The source of infection may be through milk, water, ingestion of infected animal tissues, or ingestion of other foods handled by persons who have the organisms on their hands. Eggs have been found to carry the organisms on some occasions. Persons with subclinical disease and carriers can pass the infection to others who are more susceptible. Bone meal fertilizer and domestic animal and pet foods

671

have been known to harbor the organism.

Gastroenteritis usually appears within eight to forty-eight hours of ingesting the organisms in large numbers. It is more common in children than in adults. Enteric fever and bacteremia usually appear within one to ten days of exposure and last from one to three weeks. In both of these conditions the patient's temperature may be elevated markedly, and he may have nausea, vomiting, and other signs of a severe systemic infection. In bacteremia blood cultures will be positive for the organism, and in both enteric disease and in bacteremia due to salmonella organisms, the stools are usually positive one or two weeks after acute symptoms appear.

The treatment of salmonella infections depends upon the patient's symptoms. Fluids are usually forced, and a diet that is bland and largely liquid is ordered. If the patient is unable to take sufficient fluids and calories by mouth, fluids are given parenterally. If the patient has enteric fever or bacteremia, one of the tetracycline drugs or chloramphenicol will probably be given. The dosage of chloramphenicol is 50 to 60 mg. (¾ to 1 grain) per kilogram of body weight in twenty-four hours given in four to six divided doses.[4] This regimen is continued for seven to ten days. Penicillin in dosages of 40 to 100 million units is given if serious complications are thought to be developing.

Nursing care of the patient with salmonellosis depends upon the severity of the infection and the symptoms present. Excreta may need to be disinfected. Precautions should be taken in handling all body discharges. Other aspects of nursing care depend upon the symptoms and may include general nursing measures for headache, excessive diaphoresis, restlessness, and poor mouth hygiene, as well as depression and discouragement.

The nurse has a responsibility in teaching the prevention of salmonella infections. Prevention can be accomplished best by adequate washing of the hands before eating and by all who handle food, adequate refrigeration of uncooked and prepared foods, and thorough cooking of meats, eggs, and egg products. Because of the increased incidence of these infections, the use of uncooked eggs is no longer widely recommended. At the present time no immunization is being given for any of the salmonella group except *Salmonella typhosa*. It is believed that large numbers of the organisms are needed before disease occurs and that disease may occur if large numbers of organisms are ingested even if immunization were available.[4]

Trichinosis

Autopsy reports show that at least 5% of the population of the United States is affected with trichinosis. No immunization is possible and no specific treatment is available, yet the disease could be eradicated with the knowledge that we now possess.[4] The disease is caused by the larvae of a species of roundworm, *Trichinella spiralis*, which become encysted in the striated muscles of man and hogs and other animals, particularly those (such as rodents) that consume infected pork in garbage. Trichinosis is transmitted through inadequately cooked food. Pork is the most common source of infection. When infected food is eaten, live encysted larvae develop within the intestine of the host, mate, and produce eggs that hatch in the uterus of the female worm. The larvae are discharged in huge numbers (approximately 1,500 per worm) into the lymphatics and lacteals of the host's small intestine at the rate of about two an hour for about six weeks. They pass to the muscles of the host, where they become encysted by the reaction of the host's body and may remain for ten years or longer.

Signs and symptoms of trichinosis are varied. Although the reason is unknown, edema appears as puffiness about the eyes, particularly involving the upper lids. If a very large number of larvae have been ingested, nausea, vomiting, and diarrhea due to intestinal irritation usually occur about four days after the infected food has been eaten. On about the seventh day, when the larvae migrate throughout the body to the muscles, there are usually muscle stiffness, weakness, and remittent fever. The extent of these symptoms depends upon the number of larvae present and the resistance of the host. There may be pain in the back, the muscles of the eyeballs, the muscles of chewing, and elsewhere in the body. Muscles of the diaphragm are often affected, causing pain on breathing. An increase in the eosinophil count is a characteristic finding in trichinosis and persists for several weeks after the onset of acute symptoms. Trichinosis can cause death, which usually occurs from pneumonia or cachexia from four to six weeks following the onset of symptoms.

The incidence and prevalence of trichinosis are higher in the United States than in any other country in the world. It occurs much more often in hogs that have been fed garbage than in those fed on grain. Using only garbage that has been cooked has reduced the incidence somewhat.[4] Only about 70% of the pork in this country is processed in plants that are under close supervision, and it is known that at least 10% of the sausage sold in large city markets is infected.[4] The larvae do not form cysts in pork. Therefore they are not visible to the naked eye and cannot be seen by food inspectors.

Basic scientific facts necessary for the complete prevention of the disease in human beings have been known for years. Trichinae can be killed by cooking and by freezing at a temperature of $-18°$ C. ($0°$ F.) for twenty-four hours. They are not killed by smoking, pickling, or other methods of processing. Sausage and other infected pork products carelessly prepared in eating places are a common source of infection in man. Other meats ground in the same machine without thorough cleaning or cut on the same meat block may also cause infection. The nurse has an important responsibility to teach the need for thorough cooking of all pork products consumed at home regardless of how sanitary the local meat market may appear to be. A safe rule to follow is never, under any circumstances, eat pork products in a restaurant—only at home, where adequate cooking can be assured—and never eat other ground meat without thoroughly cooking it.

Diverticulosis and diverticulitis

A diverticulum of the large bowel is an outpouching caused by weakness of the muscular layers of the bowel wall. The presence of many diverticula in the sigmoid and the descending colon is called *diverticulosis.* If diverticula become inflamed, the term *di-* *verticulitis* is used. The cause of diverticula is unknown. At least 10% of the total population has this condition, which is much more common in middle-aged and elderly persons than in the young. In itself, a diverticulum is a benign condition usually causing no symptoms. It may, however, become impacted with feces and become irritated, inflamed, and infected. Diverticulitis may sometimes be prevented by care in selection of food and avoidance of constipation. A fairly bland, low-residue diet is usually recommended, and mineral oil may be prescribed.

The patient with diverticulitis complains of general discomfort or pain in the left lower quadrant. There may be local tenderness, leukocytosis, and fever. Hemorrhage occurs in about 10 to 20% of all patients and may be chronic and mild or severe. The patient is usually treated conservatively with a low-roughage diet, daily doses of mineral oil or a demulcent such as metamucil, antispasmodics, and sedation. More recently, smooth but bulky foods have been prescribed with good results. Antibiotics are given when there are signs of infection.

A possible complication of diverticulitis is perforation, with resultant abscess formation or generalized peritonitis. The inflammatory process may also cause bowel obstruction. The patient may require surgery for treatment of these conditions, and occasionally surgery is also done to remove a portion of the seriously involved bowel. A colostomy is sometimes necessary.

Cancer of the colon

Malignant tumors of the large bowel and rectum are expected to cause 43,000 deaths in 1966.[1] They are thought to be increasing in frequency because of the increase in the life-span. More people are now living to the age when cancer is common, and consequently more diagnoses of cancer are being made than was true years ago. Although the cause of cancer of the colon is unknown, isolated polyps are known to undergo malignant changes. *Familial polyposis,* therefore, may predispose to the development of cancer of the lower bowel. Because, in the early stages, symptoms of cancer of the colon are vague and may be absent, it is now recommended that the yearly physical examination of persons over 50 years of age include examination for the presence of this disease. Since carcinoma of the lower bowel is more common in men than in women, it has also been recommended that all men over 40 years of age have this examination. In some cancer-detection clinics, proctoscopic examinations are made routinely on all men past 35 years of age.

Anyone in whom constipation, diarrhea, or alternating constipation and diarrhea develops should seek medical attention at once. Changes in the shape of the stool, the passing of blood by rectum, and any change in bowel habits also should be reported. Weakness and fatigue are sometimes the first signs of cancer of the colon since constant loss of blood in the stool may go unnoticed, and a severe anemia may develop.

Early discovery of the growth and its immediate removal offer a fairly good chance for cure. Cancer of the colon usually grows slowly and remains localized for a relatively long time. Eventually, it spreads either directly into the peritoneum or into abdominal organs or indirectly through the lymphatics into the surrounding lymph nodes and through the blood vessels to the liver and other structures.

Symptoms of cancer of the colon vary with the location of the growth. Carcinoma of the colon on the right side (ascending colon) usually is a large cauliflower-like growth. It causes severe anemia, nausea, vomiting, and alternating constipation and diarrhea. A mass is usually palpable on the right side of the abdomen. There are no symptoms of obstruction as a rule, because the fecal contents in this portion of the colon are still liquid and able to flow past the growth.

Carcinoma of the colon on the left side (descending colon) often produces symptoms of partial obstruction. Although tumors in this area are usually smaller than those found in the colon on the right side, they proliferate fibrous tissue which, as it contracts, causes narrowing of the lumen of the bowel. Because the stool in the bowel on the left side is formed, it has difficulty passing by the tumor and through the stenosed area. The patient becomes progressively constipated, the stool may be small or flattened, "pencil-shaped," or "ribbon-shaped." Blood, mucus, and pus may be passed with the bowel movement. The abdomen may become distended, and rumbling of flatus and fluid may be heard. Fifty percent of the cancers of the lower bowel occur in the sigmoid part of the colon.[11]

Diagnosis of cancer of the colon is made by physical examination, sigmoidoscopy, and barium enema examination. The treatment is always surgical, and the tumor, surrounding colon, and lymph nodes are resected. If possible, the remaining portions of the bowel are anastomosed. If cancer of the ascending colon is found, the colon on the right side is entirely removed (*right colectomy*), and the ileum is anastomosed to the transverse colon (*ileotransverse colostomy*). Growths of the descending colon or upper sigmoid are removed by a *left colectomy*, and the remaining sigmoid is anastomosed to the transverse colon. If the cancerous growth is such that it is not resectable, or if the growth has caused an obstruction with accompanying inflammation, an opening may be made into the cecum (*cecostomy*) or into the transverse colon (*transverse colostomy*) as a palliative measure to permit the escape of fecal contents. When the edema and the inflammation around the tumor subside, the growth is resected, the bowel sections are anastomosed, and the cecostomy or colostomy usually is closed. The preoperative and postoperative nursing care of patients who have resection of the bowel, a cecostomy, or a colostomy is discussed later in this chapter.

Occasionally carcinoma of the colon causes a complete obstruction, and the acute symptoms of obstruction may be the first indication that anything is wrong. Occasionally the tumor perforates into the peritoneal cavity and peritonitis occurs before any other signs of illness have been noticed by the patient.

The patient with a hernia

A hernia is a protrusion of an organ or structure from its normal cavity through a congenital or acquired defect. Depending of its location, the hernia may contain peritoneal fat, a loop of bowel, a section of bladder, or a portion of the stomach. If the protruding structure of organ can be

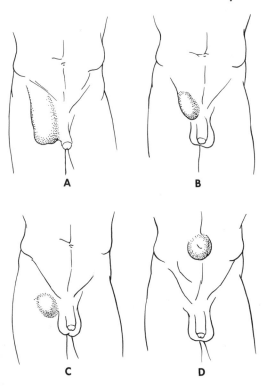

Fig. 158

Types of hernias: **A,** large indirect inguinal hernia; **B,** direct inguinal hernia; **C,** femoral hernia; **D,** umbilical hernia.

returned by manipulation to its own cavity, it is called a *reducible* hernia. If it cannot, it is called an *irreducible* or an *incarcerated* hernia. The size of the defect through which the structure or organ passes (the neck of the hernia) determines largely whether or not the hernia can be reduced. When the blood supply to the structure within the hernia becomes occluded, the hernia is said to be *strangulated.*

The patient with a hernia complains of a lump in the groin, around the umbilicus, or protruding from an old surgical incision (Fig. 158). The swelling may have always been present, or it may have suddenly appeared after coughing, straining, lifting, or other vigorous exertion. Age, sex, and obesity are contributory causes in the development of a hernia.

A hernia may cause no symptoms except swelling that disappears when the patient lies down and reappears when he stands up or coughs. If pain is present, it may be due to local irritation of the parietal peritoneum or to traction on the omentum. An incarcerated hernia may become strangulated, causing severe pain and symptoms of intestinal obstruction such as nausea, vomiting, and distention. These complications require emergency surgery, and a portion of bowel may have to be resected if it has become gangrenous from impairment of its circulation.

Unless there are contraindications due to age or physical condition, most hernias can be treated successfully by an operation. When the patient is in good physical condition and when the hernia is causing little or no discomfort, elective surgery may be done. Surgery obviates the serious complications of untreated hernias such as strangulation and incarceration. Patients who have unusual abdominal protrusions or enlargements, therefore, should be advised to seek medical advice. If a hernia is found during a pre-employment physical examination, employment may be deferred until the hernia is repaired. This is particularly likely when the work involves physical labor. Since the hernias that appear after employment begins are compensable, the time and money involved in their treatment are of economic concern to the employer. Unfortunately, the patient too often seeks medical attention only if the protrusion becomes troublesome, if he fears it is malignant, or if he must have it repaired before he can be accepted for employment.

An *indirect inguinal hernia* is one in which a loop of intestine passes through the abdominal inguinal ring and follows the course of the spermatic cord into the inguinal canal. The descent of the hernia may end in the inguinal canal, or it may proceed into the scrotum (and occasionally into the labia). It is caused by the intestines being forced by increased intra-abdominal pressure into a congenital defect resulting from failure of the processus vaginalis to close after the descent of the testes in the male and after fixation of the ovaries in the female. Indirect hernias comprise 60% of all hernias[11] and are much more common in men than in women. This higher incidence in men may be explained in part by their participation in more vigorous exercise and by the size of the testes, which must pass through the inguinal ring during fetal life.

A *direct inguinal hernia* is one that passes through the posterior inguinal wall. It is caused by increased intra-abdominal pressure against a congenitally weak posterior inguinal wall. These hernias are more common in men. They are the most difficult to repair and are likely to recur after operation.

A *femoral hernia* is one in which a loop of intestine passes through the femoral ring and down the femoral canal. It appears as a round bulge below the inguinal ligament and is thought to be due to a congenital weakness in the femoral ring. Increased intra-abdominal pressure due to pregnancy or obesity probably causes the herniation through weakened muscle. Femoral hernias are more common in women than in men. This is thought to be because of the inclination of the female pelvis.

An *umbilical hernia* is one in which a loop of intestine passes through the umbilical ring. It is caused either by the failure of the umbilicus to close at birth or by a congenital defect in the umbilical scar, which opens in adult life under conditions causing increased intra-abdominal pressure, such as pregnancy, intestinal obstruction, or a chronic cough. Infantile umbilical hernias occur frequently in Negro babies. Umbilical hernias that occur in adults are seen most often in elderly, obese women.

An *incisional hernia* is one that occurs through an old surgical incision. It is caused by the failure of the resected and approximated muscles and fascial tissues to heal properly because of wound infections, drains, or poor physical condition. As a result of increased intra-abdominal pressure a portion of the intestine or other organs and tissues may protrude through the weakened scar.

Treatment

The patient can very often reduce the hernia (return it to its normal position) by lying down with his feet elevated or by lying in a tub of warm water and pushing the mass gently back toward the abdominal cavity. If his physical condition does not per-

mit an operation, the doctor sometimes advocates the use of a *truss* to keep the hernia reduced. However, this device is not a cure, and its use is somewhat rare. A truss is a pad made of firm material that is placed over the opening through which the hernia protrudes and is held in place with a belt. The truss should be applied before the patient gets out of bed and after the hernia has been reduced. If the hernia cannot be reduced, the truss should not be applied and the patient should seek medical treatment. The truss should be applied next to the body, since underclothing worn under it causes it to slide and decreases its effectiveness. Irritation of the skin under the truss can be overcome by daily bathing and the use of talcum powder. Unless the patient has a chronic cough, the truss should be removed when he is in bed.

The only cure for a hernia is surgical treatment. The herniating tissues are returned to the abdominal cavity, and the defect in the fascia or muscle is closed with sutures (*herniorrhaphy*). To prevent recurrence of the hernia and to facilitate closure of the defect, a *hernioplasty* may be done using fascia, filagree wire, tantalum mesh, stainless steel mesh, or a variety of newer plastic materials to strengthen the muscle wall.

Nursing care

The preoperative preparation for a hernia repair includes examination to detect any diseases of the respiratory system that postoperatively might cause increased intra-abdominal pressure. A chronic cough due to excessive smoking or other causes or excessive sneezing due to an allergy might cause weakening of the repair before the incision has completely healed. The operation is postponed until the patient recovers from any respiratory disorder that is discovered. The nurse should report to the surgeon any signs of incipient upper respiratory infection since such an infection may occur after he has examined the patient.

In addition to good general postoperative care, the nurse, in caring for the patient who has had an operation for a hernia, should prevent tension on the newly repaired tissues. Postoperatively the nurse should be alert for signs of respiratory infection. If a cough occurs, medications are usually prescribed to depress the cough reflex. They should be given as ordered to prevent paroxysms of coughing and subsequent strain on the repair. The patient should be instructed to hold his hand firmly over the operative area when coughing or sneezing.

Since urinary retention may occur after a herniorrhaphy, appropriate nursing measures should be taken to prevent the bladder from becoming overdistended. Catheterization is sometimes necessary. The patient is usually permitted to get out of bed to void on the operative day, and after the first day he has full ambulatory privileges.

The patient who has elective surgery for a hernia usually is permitted a full diet as soon as it is tolerated. If a spinal anesthetic is used and the abdominal cavity is not entered, there is usually no loss of peristalsis, and the patient is able to eat normally at once. If a general anesthetic is used, the fluid and food are restricted until peristalsis returns. When an umbilical or a large incisional hernia has been repaired, a nasogastric tube attached to suction may be used to prevent postoperative vomiting and distention with subsequent strain on the suture line. Fluids are given parenterally, and food and fluids are restricted by mouth. Abdominal distention following a hernia repair should be reported to the doctor at once. He may pass a nasogastric tube, or he may order a rectal tube inserted. Mild cathartics may be prescribed since straining during defecation increases intra-abdominal pressure and should be avoided.

Because of postoperative inflammation, edema, and hemorrhage, swelling of the scrotum often occurs after repair of an indirect inguinal hernia. This complication is extremely painful, and any movement of the patient causes discomfort. It is difficult to turn, to get into or out of bed, and to walk. Ice bags help to relieve pain. The scrotum is usually supported with a suspensory or is elevated on a rolled towel. Narcotics may sometimes be necessary for pain, and antibiotics may be given to prevent the development of epididymitis. When a patient has this condition, the nurse must check his voiding carefully. He may delay voiding because moving about increases pain and discomfort.

Wound infection occurs occasionally. It interferes with healing, and if it is not recognized early and treated adequately, the repair may weaken. Infections are treated with antibiotics systemically and with dressings or packs locally (p. 71).

The patient who has had elective surgery for a hernia is usually hospitalized for only seven days, but he is restricted from strenuous activity for at least three weeks. He should be advised to consult the doctor about when he may return to work. If his work entails lifting, he should be certain that the doctor knows this, and he should be instructed in good body mechanics.

Peritonitis

Peritonitis is an inflammatory involvement of the peritoneum caused by trauma or by rupture of an organ containing bacteria, which are then introduced into the abdominal cavity. Some of the organisms often found are *Escherichia coli*, streptococci (both aerobic and anaerobic) staphylococci, pneumococci, and gonococci. Peritonitis also can be caused by chemical response to irritating substances such as might occur following rupture of the fallopian tube in an ectopic pregnancy, perforation of a gastric ulcer, or traumatic rupture of the spleen or liver. Inflammation due to chemical causes, however, is so closely followed by invasion of blood-borne bacteria that it is only a few hours before organisms may be isolated from most fluids that accumulate in peritonitis.

Local reactions of the peritoneum include redness, inflammation, edema, and the production of serous fluid that becomes purulent as the condition progresses and as bacteria become more numerous. Peristalsis is halted by the severe peritoneal infection, and all the symptoms of acute intestinal obstruction may occur. They include nausea, vomiting, pain in the abdomen, electrolyte imbalance, severe distention, rigidity of the abdominal wall, and failure to pass anything by rectum. The patient's white blood cell count is usually high. Peritonitis also causes serious systemic symptoms, including high temperature, tachycardia, weakness, diaphoresis, pallor, and all other signs of severe systemic reaction and of shock. Peritonitis is a very serious disease that had an extremely high mortality rate before antimicrobial and bacteriostatic drugs and other modern treatment became available.

Medical treatment and nursing care

Treatment usually consists of emergency measures to combat infection, to restore intestinal motility, and to supply lost electrolytes and fluids. Massive doses of antibiotic drugs are given parenterally. Intestinal or gastric intubation is usually ordered at once, the tubes are attached to suction, and a rectal tube is inserted. Fluids and electrolytes are given intravenously, and the patient may be prepared for surgery. He is not given anything by mouth, and narcotics and sedatives are given for severe pain and apprehension as soon as the diagnosis is confirmed and there is no danger of masking symptoms.

Nursing care of the patient having gastric and intestinal intubation was discussed earlier in this chapter. The patient who has acute peritonitis needs constant nursing care since he is extremely apprehensive. Pain and discomfort may also be so severe that he cannot be expected to use good judgment in leaving the nasogastric tube in place and in keeping his arm still on a board when an infusion is being given. The patient should be given mouth care, and protection is needed to prevent drying and cracking of the lips since dehydration is usually marked.

Usually the patient is placed in a semi-Fowler's position so that gravity may help localize pus in the lower abdomen or the pelvis. Also, in this position the patient can take deeper breaths with less pain, which helps to prevent respiratory complications. Heat may occasionally be applied to the abdomen, but some doctors feel that heat is not advisable.

Natural barriers are used in the body's attempt to control the inflammation. Adhesions quickly form in an attempt to wall off the infection, and the omentum helps to enclose areas of inflammation. These processes may result in involvement of only part of the abdominal cavity and may finally narrow the infected area to a small, enclosed one (abscess). As healing occurs, fibrous adhesions may shrink and disappear entirely so that no trace of infection can be found upon exploration of the abdomen at a much later date, or else they may persist as constrictions that may permanently bind the involved structures together. Sometimes they cause an intestinal obstruction by occluding the lumen of the bowel. If abscesses form, they are usually in the lower abdomen. They may, however, be walled off elsewhere. For example, abscess formation following a ruptured appendix may develop under the diaphragm (Fig. 17), and may even perforate that structure and cause an empyema.

Surgery is usually done as soon as the patient's condition permits if the peritonitis is due to a perforated structure that is releasing irritating or infected material into the abdominal cavity. However, if the patient is in shock, it may be several hours before shock can be relieved and before surgery can be safely performed. The operation usually consists of closure of the abnormal opening into the abdominal cavity and removal of the fluid that has accumulated. (See discussion of perforated peptic ulcer for further details of nursing care, p. 655.) If peritonitis is due to the rupture of a fallopian tube, as in an ectopic pregnancy, the tube must be removed (p. 502).

Intestinal obstruction

Intestinal obstruction develops when intestinal contents cannot pass through the lumen of the bowel. It may be due to mechanical causes, neurogenic causes (paralytic ileus), or vascular abnormalities (Fig. 159). *Mechanical obstruction* is most often caused by strangulated hernias and adhesions, although cancer of the large bowel accounts for 70% of the cases of mechanical obstruction in the colon.[11] Other mechanical causes are *volvulus* (a twisting of the bowel) and *intussusception* (telescoping of a segment of the bowel within itself, most common in emaciated infants and small children). Volvulus occurs most often in elderly persons, and the sigmoid loop of the large bowel is usually affected. Bands, strictures, and adhesions that cause obstruction of the bowel lumen may be congenital but usually result from previous abdominal operations or from peritonitis.

In *neurogenic obstruction* there is interference with the innervation of the bowel, which causes peristalsis to cease or to be markedly retarded. Paralytic ileus may be

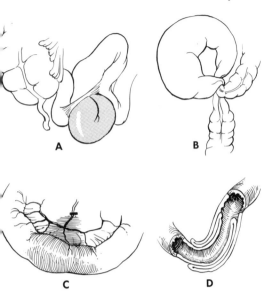

Fig. 159

Some causes of intestinal obstruction: **A,** constriction by adhesions; **B,** volvulus; **C,** mesenteric thrombosis; **D,** intussusception.

becomes obstructed, there is an increase in peristalsis above the occlusion in an attempt to move intestinal contents past the obstruction. As the peristaltic waves become more forceful, they cause sharp intermittent or cramping abdominal pain. The increased peristaltic activity also injures the intestinal wall, causing edema around the obstructed area, and the intestine proximal to the obstruction becomes distended. Normally most of the fluid in the intestinal tract is absorbed through the intestinal wall, helping to maintain fluid and electrolyte balance. When the intestine is obstructed, however, the normal absorptive power of the intestinal mucosa is lacking because of irritation from hyperactivity and/or impairment of circulation. Most of the gas consists of swallowed air that contains about 79% nitrogen and is slowly absorbed from the intestinal tract. The combined presence of fluid and this gas in the bowel causes increased tension and may occlude the blood supply, causing gangrene to develop. The bowel distal to the obstruction remains empty and constricted so that there is no passage of gas or stool by rectum.

Vomiting that occurs with intestinal obstruction may be frequent, abrupt in onset, copious, often spontaneous, and foul in odor (often fecal). Such vomiting is caused by reverse peristalsis, as the intestinal contents are regurgitated into the stomach, from which they are ejected. In general, the higher the obstruction, the earlier and more severe is the vomiting. If the obstruction is in the large bowel, vomiting may not occur as the ileocecal valve permits fluid to enter the colon but prevents its passage back, into the ileum.

Intestinal obstruction is an extremely serious condition which, if not treated promptly, can cause death within a few hours. Failure of the normal absorptive powers of the intestinal wall to continue and the loss of fluid through vomiting cause severe fluid and electrolyte imbalance. Bacteria and toxins escaping through the affected bowel may cause toxemia and peritonitis. The patient develops all the signs of shock and requires immediate treatment.

a complication of peritonitis, acute medical illness such as pneumonia, or changes in circulatory supply to the bowel. Other causes of paralytic ileus include handling of the bowel during surgery, spinal cord lesions, electrolyte imbalance, or toxic conditions such as uremia.

Obstruction due to vascular disease is relatively rare and usually occurs in persons who have evidence of other vascular disease. Occlusion usually occurs in the superior mesenteric vessels, cutting off the blood supply to a large segment of the bowel. When the affected portion of the bowel is unable to perform its muscular function, peristalsis ceases, and the bowel quite rapidly becomes distended with fluid, gas, and food residue, and finally becomes gangrenous.

The symptoms of intestinal obstruction vary according to the degree and site of obstruction. In general, sudden acute mechanical occlusions located high in the intestinal tract produce more intense and earlier symptoms than those occurring lower in the system.[4] When the lumen of the bowel first

Medical treatment and nursing care

The treatment for intestinal obstruction is intestinal intubation, the administration

679

of fluids and electrolytes by infusion, and the relief of mechanical and vascular obstruction by surgery. Paralytic ileus is not treated surgically unless gangrene of a portion of the bowel has occurred. The operative procedure varies with the cause and the location of the obstruction and the general condition of the patient. If constricting bands or adhesions are found, they are cut, and it may be necessary to resect the occluded bowel and to anastomose the remaining segments. It may be necessary to do a temporary cecostomy or colostomy and, later, when the patient is in better physical condition, a resection and anastomosis of the bowel may be performed.

Nursing care includes caring for the intestinal tube, maintaining intestinal decompression, and keeping an accurate record of all intake and output. Intravenous fluids are ordered to maintain fluid and electrolyte balance. Good supportive care must be given. Pain and vomiting often leave the patient physically and emotionally exhausted. He may need assistance in simple activities such as turning in bed, and he needs encouragement and assurance that the intubation and other treatment usually result in lessening of symptoms within a short time. Skin and mouth care are essential. Any vomitus should be immediately removed from the bedside since its foul odor may increase nausea. Ventilation should have the nurse's careful attention. Since intestinal distention may cause respiratory distress, the patient usually is more comfortable in a Fowler's position. He should be encouraged to breathe through the nose and not to swallow air because it increases the distention and discomfort. A hot-water bottle or an electric heating pad may be ordered, and a rectal tube may be used to provide relief from lower abdominal distention. Enemas or colonic irrigations may be ordered, and the nurse must carefully observe the results of these treatments. She should be alert for signs that peristalsis has returned, and she should report the passage of flatus and any abnormal substances such as blood or mucus. Urinary retention due to pressure on the bladder may occur, and the patient should be observed for this and the amount at each voiding recorded. A total twenty-four-hour urinary output below 500 ml. should be reported to the physician.

Nursing care of the patient having surgery of the lower gastrointestinal tract (resection and anastomosis of the bowel)

Preoperative care. Preoperative preparation of the patient who is to have surgery of the bowel varies in some aspects from that of preparation for other abdominal surgery. During the preoperative period the patient is usually given a low-residue diet so that the bowel will have little or no stool when surgery is done. Vitamins and supplementary meals of food high in protein are usually given. Twenty-four hours before operation, the diet is usually changed to liquids and sometimes even to clear liquids. The reason for the diet changes should be explained to the patient so that he does not eat food other than that served to him.

Antibiotics specific for organisms found in the bowel are given beginning three to five days before surgery in an attempt to decrease the bacterial count of bowel contents, which helps to decrease the incidence of postoperative wound infection. Oral antibiotics used to "sterilize" the bowel are succinylsulfathiazole (Sulfasuxidine), phthalylsulfathiazole (Sulfathalidine), neomycin, streptomycin, and chlortetracycline (Aureomycin). These drugs are poorly absorbed from the gastrointestinal tract and thus their concentration in the bloodstream is low. A cathartic such as magnesium sulfate may be given before they are administered, and then the drugs are given in large doses every four hours until the operation is done. The patient may also receive a daily cathartic or enemas followed by instillation of phthalylsulfathiazole into the bowel.

A nasogastric or intestinal tube is inserted before the operation. Since the passage of a tube into the intestines may take as long as twenty-four hours, intestinal intubation is usually started the day before operation. As the tube passes through the small intestine, the bowel becomes "threaded" on it and thus is compactly held together and shortened while the operation is performed. Before and after surgery, the intestinal tube is usually attached to a suction apparatus for the aspiration of intestinal contents. This prevents the accumulation of gas and intestinal fluid around the suture line. If a nasogastric tube is used, it is inserted the morning the operation is scheduled.

Postoperative care. Until peristalsis returns and the anastomosis is partially healed, the nasogastric or intestinal tube is used, and special attention must be given to keeping the tube draining and to maintenance of fluid and electrolyte balance. The doctor carefully checks the amount of solutions needed and reviews the daily output from voiding and from aspiration through the tube. The nurse must be very certain that recording of these fluids are accurate and that all fluids given as infusions or by other means the previous day are also carefully included in the patient's record. The patient should have mouth care frequently, and an antibiotic solution may be ordered for this care, since colon bacteria may reach the mouth perhaps via a "wick action," especially when an intestinal tube is used.

Since the patient may have some difficulty in voiding after bowel surgery, nursing measures should be instituted to prevent urine retention. A Foley catheter may be used (p. 443). Pain in the incision may be severe and may interfere with full respiratory excursion. The patient should be given narcotics as necessary for pain and must then be encouraged to cough and to breathe deeply. He must also be encouraged to change his position every hour or two and often needs encouragement and assistance in doing so during the first day or two postoperatively.

A rectal tube occasionally is sutured in the anus to be certain that it will be in place to facilitate the passage of flatus. This tube is attached to a drainage bottle. The nurse must be sure that drainage is possible by having an extra opening in the bottle for an air vent if a cork is used and that there is enough tubing to allow the patient to move about freely in bed without traction on the tube. Discomfort from suturing of this tube can be severe and may require the use of analgesic drugs. Often the tubing is anchored firmly to the thigh with wide bands of adhesive tape. Drugs to stimulate expulsion of flatus such as dexpanthenol (Ilopan) or neostigmine (Prostigmin) may be given. Since ambulation is of great assistance in starting peristalsis, the patient may be assisted out of bed a day or two after surgery, even while the rectal tube and the

nasogastric or intestinal tube are still in use. The passage of gas or stool by rectum should be reported to the surgeon at once, since it usually indicates the return of peristalsis and means that the patient may begin to take something by mouth and that the intestinal tube can be removed.

Until the intestinal tube is removed, the patient is not given anything by mouth, and total food and fluid needs are met by the parenteral route. After the tube is removed, the patient gradually is given additional foods until he has a full diet, although occasionally bland foods may be given for some time after surgery. It is not unusual for patients who have had a resection of the bowel to have some diarrhea after peristalsis returns. It is only temporary and soon disappears. When the stool becomes normal, the patient is advised to avoid becoming constipated because a hard stool and straining to expel it could possibly injure the anastomosis, depending upon its location. If he has a tendency to develop constipation postoperatively, he should try drinking fruit juice and water before breakfast or taking a glass of prune juice daily. He should not take laxatives without medical approval. The doctor may recommend mineral oil or some other mild bulk cathartic such as psyllium (Metamucil).

Nursing care of the patient having a cecostomy

Although the treatment of choice for growths in the ascending colon is a resection and anastomosis or a transverse colostomy, a temporary cecostomy is occasionally performed to relieve obstruction if the patient cannot tolerate major surgery. With the use of local anesthesia to control pain, an opening is made into the cecum through a small incision in the right lower quadrant of the abdomen, and a catheter is inserted into the bowel. The catheter is sutured to the skin and provides an outlet for feces, which is still fluid in the ascending colon. Tubing is attached to the catheter, which is attached to a bottle that is capped to control odors but that is provided with an air vent so that drainage can occur. The tubing should be long enough so that the patient can move about freely. In order to keep the tube open, it is usually irrigated every four hours with physiologic solution of sodium chloride. The fluid is allowed to run in by gravity and flows out by inverting the syringe or funnel or by aspiration.

The dressings around the tube should be changed as frequently as necessary, and the skin should be kept clean and dry. After the tube is removed, skin care and changes of dressing should be continued until all drainage ceases (Fig. 103). Occasionally an ileostomy bag is used to keep drainage off the skin (Fig. 157). Water-soluble chlorophyll derivative (Chloresium) may be applied for its soothing, antipruritic, and deodorizing effects.

Nursing care of the patient having a colostomy

A colostomy is an operation in which an artificial opening is made into the colon. It is done to permit escape of feces when there is an obstruction of the large bowel or a known lesion, such as cancer, that will eventually cause an obstruction. It also may be done to permit healing of the bowel distal to it after an infection, perforation, or traumatic injury since it diverts the fecal stream from the affected area. It may be done as a palliative measure in the treatment of an obstruction caused by an inoperable growth of the colon, or, if the rectum must be removed to treat cancer it may be done to provide a permanent means of bowel evacuation.

When the doctor first tells the patient of the probable need for a colostomy, the patient's immediate response is likely to be one of shock and disbelief. Whether the colostomy is to be temporary or permanent, he finds it very difficult to accept. Knowledge that it is a lifesaving measure, confidence in the surgeon, and sometimes explanation and acceptance of the proposed operation by members of his family may convince him to consent to the operation. It is not unusual for the patient to be sad, withdrawn, and depressed. So great is the emotional reaction that some women patients cry throughout most of their hospital stay. Occasionally a patient commits suicide in the hospital or abruptly signs himself out of the hospital when he knows that a colostomy is necessary. The nurse should anticipate and prepare for possible events and should help auxiliary nursing personnel to understand the emotional turmoil the patient is experiencing. The patient's reaction to a proposed colostomy will be based on the way he sees it affecting his life, his physical stature, his place in his family, his economic welfare and that of his loved ones, his social life, and many other situations that have meaning for him. His response will depend on his social and cultural background and on his emotional makeup, as well as on a number of other circumstances.

The nurse should be prepared to supplement any information given to the patient by the doctor, and she should try to determine how much information to give him preoperatively on care of the colostomy. Some patients definitely benefit from discussing the care, reading materials, seeing equipment, and talking to persons who are living normal lives following a colostomy. Others find this approach upsetting. The patient should, however, have at least superficial knowledge of the changes a colostomy may cause in his daily living pattern.

Some hospitals have prepared printed materials for patients who have had a colostomy. Booklets on colostomy care also may be packaged with colostomy bags and equipment sold commercially. If printed material is used, it should be carefully discussed with the patient before it is left with him. After he has perused it, the nurse should plan to spend additional time answering any questions he may have. One of the advantages of this type of material is that the patient has a reference available after his discharge from the hospital. It adds to his security in caring for himself.

Members of the patient's family should be encouraged to visit him often since it is essential that the patient who has had a colostomy feel loved and accepted despite his misfortune. During the preoperative period, effort should also be made to augment the patient's confidence in the members of the medical and nursing staff, since the patient who has complete confidence in the persons who will treat and care for him is more likely to accept his situation postoperatively and be more willing to start to learn self-care. The patient watches every facial expression or gesture of the nurses and is extremely sensitive to evidence of distaste. If other persons accept the colostomy as not unusual, it helps the patient to feel that it is not a calamity that has happened to him alone.

Occasionally a patient may reject the colostomy completely postoperatively and will make no attempt to learn to care for it. With help however, most patients will learn to care for themselves. Beginning in the immediate postoperative period, the nurse should take every opportunity to have the patient look at the colostomy and to assist her in small ways as she gives him care. In this way, fear and distaste for the task can usually be gradually overcome. Every effort should be made to keep the patient as clean and dry as possible. He may become emotionally upset and depressed at the sight of fecal drainage and particularly when the drainage is liquid and soils the bed and his gown in addition to dressings. Soiled dressings and linen should be disposed of neatly and quickly. They make the patient depressed, interfere with his activity and his desire to eat, and delay his acceptance of the colostomy. Soiling of the bedclothes and the patient's clothing should be prevented if at all possible, but the patient should understand that, until defecation through the colostomy has been regulated, occasional soiling of bedclothes may occur. He should be reassured that it is not of major importance and that he should not let fear of continuous drainage keep him from moving about freely in bed. This is very seldom a problem in colostomy care. If it is, however, a disposable colostomy bag should be tried.

Although it is useless and even detrimental to urge the patient to participate in his own care before he is able to accept self-care, the nurse should quietly, calmly, but persistently encourage increasing participation. Usually, a major psychologic hurdle for the patient is seeing the colostomy for the first time and observing while it is cared for. The nurse should observe the patient's physical and emotional status and determine how much participation she should expect from him. It is sometimes necessary to work with a member of the family and to teach him to care for the patient. If this is not possible or if there are no relatives, plans may need to be made for care in a nursing home or for a public health nurse to visit the home to give part of the regular care.

Transverse colostomy

A transverse colostomy eliminates function of all the bowel distal to it and is performed to relieve an obstruction, to divert the fecal stream and thus permit healing of a portion of the bowel, or as a palliative measure to prevent obstruction in inoperable lesions of the lower bowel. Two types of procedures may be done. The transverse colon may be divided and the ends brought out at the margins of the skin incision. This type is called a *double-barreled colostomy*. The proximal opening, or stoma, in the right margin of the incision is the outlet for the stool, and the distal left opening (stoma) leads to the now nonfunctioning lower bowel. This type of colostomy may begin to drain feces as soon as peristalsis returns after surgery.

In another method, a loop of the transverse colon is brought out into the abdominal wall, and the skin and underlying tissues are sutured *(loop colostomy)* (Fig. 160). A glass rod, the ends of which are connected to a piece of rubber tubing, usually is placed between the loop of the bowel and the skin to prevent the bowel from slipping back into the abdominal cavity. The rod is left in place until the wound is well healed and the loop of bowel has become adherent to the abdominal wall. This takes about ten days. The bowel usually is not opened to permit the escape of intestinal contents for three to five days after the operation, which allows the skin incision to heal and prevents contamination of the abdominal cavity. A nasogastric tube is used until the loop of bowel is opened, and the passage of gas and stool indicate the return of peristalsis. The bowel is usually opened by an incision made with a scalpel. The lumen is exposed but is not divided completely. It may also be opened with an electric cautery to minimize bleeding. The colostomy is usually opened in the treatment room since it does not cause pain and no anesthetic is necessary. Since the bowel has no sensory nerve endings, the patient may be assured that he will have no pain. If cauterization is done, however, the odor of burning flesh may disturb the patient

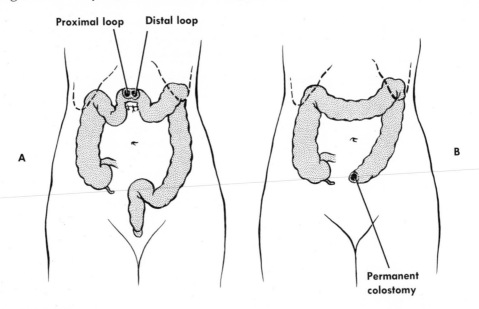

Proximal loop   Distal loop

A

B

Permanent
colostomy

Fig. 160

A, Transverse colostomy that may or may not be permanent. **B,** Permanent colostomy following an abdominoperineal resection.

and may cause nausea. The opened bowel now has a proximal opening leading to the functioning gastrointestinal tract from which stool and flatus will flow and a distal opening leading to the colon and rectum similar to the double-barreled colostomy. Since it may be difficult to establish which is the proximal (usually on the right) and which is the distal opening, the nurse who assists the doctor in opening the bowel or with the first irrigation should obtain this information and make a drawing on the nursing care plan, indicating the proximal and distal openings. However, if such information has not been recorded, inspection will reveal the opening from which fecal material is coming; this is the proximal opening.

Care of a transverse colostomy. Because semiliquid drainage from the opening may be fairly constant, the skin should be washed with soap and water, and the dressings should be changed as often as necessary to prevent skin irritation. A piece of plastic film or other waterproof material, cut large enough to envelop the dressings and with an opening in the center cut to fit snugly around the colostomy bud yet not compress

it, may be used to prevent fecal contents from getting onto the skin and staining the patient's gown or bed linen. This dressing is similar to that used for patients who have had ureteral surgery (p. 459 and Fig. 103). Montgomery straps may be used to hold the dressing in place and obviate the need for frequent removal and application of adhesive tape. Petroleum jelly gauze or a protective ointment is sometimes placed around the opening to keep the skin from becoming irritated. However, the ointment must be removed at frequent intervals to ascertain that the skin under the protective coating remains in good condition. The use of ointments may make the appearance of the colostomy more objectionable to the patient.

The patient's bedside unit should be equipped with supplies needed for changing the dressings. It is best to keep the equipment on a tray that is easily available to both the patient and the nurse. The tray should be stocked with paper bags or newspapers for disposal of waste, gauze for dressings, cotton for cleansing the skin, abdominal pads for extra protection over the dressings, petroleum jelly gauze or protective ointments and tongue blades for their application, tincture of benzoin, and extra Montgomery straps.

As soon as the patient is physically able, he should be encouraged to assist in changing the dressings. Since this procedure is not a sterile one, washed, used gauze or unsterile pieces of gauze may be used. The gauze should be rolled and placed about the opening in doughnut fashion, thus preventing drainage from easily seeping out the bottom and sides of the dressing. If the gauze is opened and fluffed, it will be more absorbent than a flat piece.

A colostomy irrigation may be done regularly through the proximal opening. However, elimination through the opening rarely can be completely regulated so that there is no drainage between irrigations. The irrigation procedure is described in the discussion on care of the patient who has had a permanent colostomy. A colostomy bag usually is necessary for the patient who has a transverse colostomy. Without it, he may have difficulty in engaging in daily activities. Often it is when the bag is to be worn that the patient first takes an interest in his own care. The bag tends to give him a feeling of security. If disposable bags are not used, the colostomy bag must be cleansed daily and immediately following its removal. It should be washed throughly with soap and water, dried, powdered to prevent the two surfaces from sticking together, and allowed to air for at least twelve hours. If this procedure does not remove odors, the patient may be advised to soak the bag for a half hour in a weak solution of chlorine household bleach or vinegar.

Materials needed for the colostomy should be obtained early so that they will be available for use before the patient leaves the hospital. He should not be discharged from the hospital until he or a member of his family is competent in caring for the colostomy or until other arrangements for his care have been made. This is extremely important since it may color the patient's ultimate adjustment to his situation. It is advisable to ask a public health nurse to visit the patient in his home (if he agrees) to evaluate the adjustment he has really made and to give him and his family additional help if necessary. The public health nurse should report her findings to the doctor or the nurse in the hospital or clinic. Most patients welcome the suggestion that a nurse may be available to visit them at home. The patient should remain under medical care and should feel that there is a nurse in the doctor's office, the hospital clinic, or the public health agency to whom he can turn for help in overcoming problems related to normal living following the colostomy.

Closure of a transverse colostomy. If the colostomy was done to relieve obstruction or to divert the fecal stream to permit healing of a portion of the bowel, the patient will be readmitted to the hospital at a later date for a further examination and for possible resection of the diseased portion of the bowel. The opening may subsequently be closed.

In preparation for a resection of the bowel and closure of the colostomy, the doctor may order irrigations of the distal loop. Fluid, usually normal saline solution, is instilled into the distal loop through a catheter attached to a funnel or Asepto syringe. For this irrigation the patient should sit on the bed pan or on the toilet since, unless there is complete obstruction, the solution may be expelled through the rectum. Mucus and shreds of necrotic tissue may be passed. The returns should be inspected before they are discarded. A nonabsorbable sulfonamide derivative, such as Sulfathalidine, dissolved in a small amount of water may be slowly instilled into the distal loop and rectum after the irrigation. The patient should be asked to retain this solution as long as possible since the antibiotic lowers the bacterial count of the bowel contents and lessens the risks of postoperative infection.

Permanent colostomy

A permanent colostomy is usually performed in conjunction with an abdominal perineal resection for cancer of the rectum. After the sigmoid colon is resected, the proximal end is brought out through the abdominal wall and sutured to it to become the permanent opening for the elimination of feces. Although there is no sphincter control, bowel movements from a sigmoid colostomy can be regulated or controlled by regular habits of eating and by giving an enema at a specific time each day. The stool in the sigmoid is formed and is of normal consistency.

At the time of the operation, the proximal end of the resected sigmoid may be brought out through the incision and sutured to the skin so that the opening, called a stoma or bud, is flush or level with the abdominal wall. The patient returns from the operating room with a dressing over the colostomy. There is usually no drainage from the opening until peristalsis returns, approximately twenty-four to forty-eight hours after the operation. In other instances, the proximal end of the resected sigmoid is brought through the incision and sutured so that approximately 2.5 to 3.75 cm. (1 to 1½ inches) of the colon protrudes above the level of the skin. This type of stoma shrinks after several weeks to become a small, pink bud of mucosa on the abdominal wall. The patient with this type of stoma usually returns from the operating room with the opening clamped off. The clamp is usually removed at the end of three days.

As soon as peristalsis returns, as evidenced by the passage of gas or stool, the nasogastric tube is removed. The patient may then progress from a liquid to a regular diet as tolerated. The dressing should be changed as frequently as necessary, and the skin should be kept clean and dry, as described in the discussion of care of a transverse colostomy. The incision may be protected with collodion or a water-soluble tape.

Colostomy irrigation. About the fifth to the seventh postoperative day the doctor usually does the first irrigation through the artificial opening. If the returns are satisfactory and the opening is unobstructed, the nurse then assumes responsibility for subsequent irrigations. It is a nursing function to teach the patient how to establish regularity of evacuation through the colostomy and how to irrigate it.

Equipment needed for the irrigations should be assembled on a tray, and the patient should be encouraged to keep it in a convenient place when he returns home. While commercial irrigation sets are used by most patients, it is possible to improvise equipment, for example, a soft plastic container from the grocery store may be used as an irrigating cup. Various types of commercial irrigation sets are available, but the

principles of all are the same. The cup that fits over the opening has a small hole in the center through which to insert the catheter. It is usually plastic so that returns can be easily seen, and it is held snugly in place against the abdominal wall with elasticized straps. Outlet tubing attached to the cup allows drainage of the fecal material into the toilet or into a bucket if the patient does the irrigation in bed. The irrigator prevents uncontrolled drainage of the fluid and feces. The nurse should know that special cups are available for the patient who has an unusually large or high opening, although in modern practice the opening is made to be flush with the skin so that no protrusion should exist. Representatives of the various manufacturers are glad to give advice and assistance in such matters. In addition to the irrigator, the patient needs a 2-quart enema can or bag, tubing 2 feet long, a glass connecting tip, a 16 or 18 Fr. catheter (usually a whistle-tip catheter is used), a tubing clamp, a pitcher for extra water, toilet tissue, petroleum jelly to lubricate the catheter, a paper bag or newspaper, dressings, and an irrigating pole or a hook on which to hang the bag. The patient may install a hook in his bathroom at home or he may use a clotheshorse. The hook should be so placed that there are no more than eighteen to twenty-four inches between the irrigating fluid and the colostomy opening. A small table or shelf on which to place equipment within easy reach should also be provided.

As soon as the patient is ambulatory, the irrigation should be done on a commode or on the toilet. Bathrooms that have poor ventilation and that do not afford privacy should be avoided since the procedure is a long one, taking at least one hour and often longer at first, and the patient is extremely self-conscious. At first it may be necessary to pad the toilet seat with sponge rubber and to provide some support for the patient's back. Several bath blankets in a pillowcase can be used. When the equipment has been assembled, water obtained for the irrigation, privacy assured, and the patient comfortably settled on the toilet, the dressing is removed, and the area around the colostomy is cleansed with reclaimed gauze or with disposable tissues that can be discarded in the toilet. Warm tap water, about 40.5° C. (105° F.), is used, although recently, cool water has been used because it is believed to stimulate peristalsis and thereby lessen the time necessary for the procedure.[38] After the air has been expelled from the tubing, the lubricated catheter is inserted through the opening in the cup and through the colostomy opening into the bowel. The cup is fastened snugly against the skin, and the outlet tubing is allowed to hang between the patient's legs into the toilet bowl. When the catheter is inserted 10 to 20 cm. (4 to 6 inches), the clamp on the tubing is released and the solution is allowed to flow into the bowel. After about one-third or one-half of the solution has run into the bowel, the inlet tubing should be clamped until the fluid and fecal contents drain out. If, during the insertion of the fluid, the patient has abdominal cramps, the inflow should be clamped for several minutes. Excessive cramping usually means that the irrigating can is too high and the fluid is running in too rapidly. This should be avoided in order to lessen discomfort and because markedly increased peristalsis may hamper passage of material through the intestine. The procedure is continued until a normal amount of fecal material is expelled. For some patients, this may require only 500 ml. of fluid, whereas others may need more fluid.

The patient usually benefits psychologically from sitting on the toilet during the irrigation. Discarding tissues into the toilet and draining the bag directly makes him feel that his situation is not so far from normal as he had feared. If possible, the same nurse should assist the patient with this procedure for several successive days (Fig. 161). This saves the patient embarrassment and enables the nurse to give appropriate encouragement, reassurance, and assistance without the patient's having to repeat his particular difficulties and problems.

When the irrigation is completed, the patient should be encouraged to massage the abdomen, to bend forward and from side to side, and to stand up once or twice before the cup is removed. Considerable variation in the time necessary for an irrigation exists among patients. Since it may take twenty minutes or longer for the bowel to completely empty, some patients read during

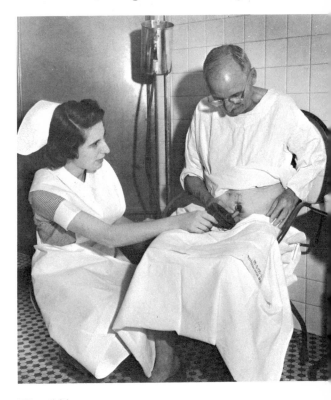

Fig. 161

The nurse assists the patient in learning to irrigate his colostomy. (From Newton, Kathleen, and Anderson, Helen C.: Geriatric nursing, ed. 4, St. Louis, 1966, The C. V. Mosby Co.)

that time. Most patients leave the cup on and clamp off the bottom of its outlet while they take a shower, do household chores, or shave since there may be a small amount of drainage after they start to move about. If elimination has been regulated, only a small dressing such as a piece of cleansing tissue needs to be worn over the colostomy. This dressing prevents the clothing from being stained with the small amount of mucus that may drain from the opening. When elimination is well regulated, it is preferable that the patient not wear a colostomy bag, thus obviating any possibility of odors. Some patients, however, worry lest they have drainage and can become regulated only when a bag is worn. Since emotional upsets and worry hinder regulation, it is not always advisable to insist that the patient with a permanent colostomy go without a bag.

As the nurse helps the patient with the irrigations, she should explain what she is doing. Gradually the patient should take over one step of the procedure after another until, before discharge from the hospital, he is assembling his own equipment, doing the irrigation, and cleaning the equipment. The nurse should continue to do some part of the procedure occasionally so that the patient will feel that she is interested in his welfare.

Regularity of evacuation through the colostomy depends upon setting up and maintaining a regular routine in its care. Before irrigations are started in the hospital, the nurse and the patient should try to determine the time of day it will be most convenient for him to do the irrigations when he returns home. He should remember that the procedure will probably prevent use of the bathroom by others for some time, and he must plan for his family's needs as well as his own. If possible, the irrigations should be done in the hospital at the time that will be best to do them at home, so that a pattern of regularity will not have to be reestablished when the patient goes home. Since the amount of solution needed to completely empty the bowel and to prevent any leakage until the next irrigation varies among individuals, it must be tested for each patient. After the irrigation, the nurse should note any incontinence. If incontinence has occurred, the amount of fluid should be increased. Some patients need to irrigate the colostomy every day, whereas others may need to do so only every two or three days. The latter is likely to be true if the patient normally has not had a bowel movement every day. An occasional patient may not have to irrigate at all. He may find that at the regular time for evacuation the colostomy empties spontaneously.

A permanent colostomy may need to be dilated because of narrowing of the opening due to shrinkage during and after healing. The procedure is usually initiated by the surgeon after the intestines become adherent to the abdominal wall, usually within ten days postoperatively. If the surgeon wishes the patient to dilate the opening routinely or periodically, the nurse should instruct the patient to insert his forefinger (or little finger if his hands are especially large), covered with a lubricated finger cot, gently into the opening. The finger should remain in the opening for a few minutes and be carefully rotated. It is usually more convenient to do this dilation just before the irrigation is started.

The patient may eat the food that he enjoys and that he was accustomed to before his operation. However, he should avoid foods that have caused diarrhea in the past. Most patients who have had a colostomy avoid gas-forming foods such as beans and cabbage, since the flatus is not retained by the artificial opening, which has no real sphincter.

When the skin incision is healed and the patient is physically able, he may bathe, swim, work, and engage in any physical or social activities he chooses. The convalescent period usually lasts from two to four months. However, the care of the colostomy should be mastered and regularity should be established within two to four weeks. The patient should be encouraged to have a public health nurse visit him in his home since he often finds that some unanticipated adjustments need to be made after he is home.

The family is not always able to accept the patient who has a colostomy. There may be strong feelings of disgust or revulsion at the colostomy and its function, fear of cancer, or less well defined rejection of body mutilation. If difficulties of this kind seem apparent for any patient, the nurse should discuss them with the doctor. Sometimes the social worker can help to work out a solution for the patient in the hospital, and often a public health nurse can help in the transition from hospital to home.

Perineal colostomy. Sometimes the loop of sigmoid can be brought out onto the perineum so that the colostomy opening is located in more nearly the normal position of the anus. The care of this type of colostomy is the same as for any permanent one except that it is more difficult to care for immediately after surgery. The problems are similar to those of patients with uncontrolled incontinence (p. 157). Once the patient learns to care for his colostomy, he may find the perineal opening more acceptable and its care not too awkward.

The patient with disease of the rectum and anal canal

Patients having surgery involving the rectum and anal canal may present special nursing problems. After these operations, the tissues around the anus may be very sensitive to pain. Careful attention to this area is needed to provide maximum comfort for the patient while healing takes place.

Cancer of the rectum

Cancer of the rectum and lower sigmoid is quite common. It occurs most frequently in men between 50 and 60 years of age. Cancer of the rectum metastasizes slowly, since the tumor extends by direct spread through the rectal wall to surrounding tissues before metastasis through the lymphatic and venous systems occurs.

The most common symptoms of cancer of the rectum and sigmoid are the passage of small amounts of bright red blood in the stool and alteration in bowel habits. Either constipation or diarrhea may occur, or these two conditions may alternate. Early diagnosis and treatment are possible only if the patient reports early symptoms to a doctor. The importance of reporting these seemingly unimportant but most significant symptoms cannot be overemphasized to the public, since pain does not occur until the disease is far advanced. Cancer of the rectum can be accurately diagnosed by pathologic examination of a biopsy of the lesion taken during a proctoscopic examination.

Abdominoperineal resection of the bowel

Malignant growths in the rectum are removed by an operation known as an abdominoperineal resection of the bowel. The operation is performed through two incisions: a low midline incision of the abdomen and a wide circular incision about the anus. Through the abdominal incision, the sigmoid colon is divided and the lower portion is freed from its attachments and temporarily left beneath the peritoneum of the pelvic floor. The proximal end of the sigmoid is then brought out through a small stab wound on the abdominal wall and becomes the permanent colostomy. Through the perineal incision the anus and rectum are freed from the perineal muscles, and the anus, the rectum containing the growth, and the distal portion of sigmoid are removed. The perineal wound may be closed around Penrose drains, or it may be left wide open and packed with gauze and a rubber dam to cause it to heal slowly from the inside outward.

Preoperative care. Preoperative nursing care of the patient who is to have an abdominoperineal resection of the bowel is similar to that given the patient having other intestinal surgery. Such care is described earlier in this chapter. Some surgeons pass ureteral catheters preoperatively so that the ureters are not inadvertently tied off during surgery. A Foley catheter is inserted into the bladder and is attached to a straight drainage system to keep the bladder empty during surgery and thus prevent operative injury.

Postoperative care. Postoperatively the patient has a permanent sigmoid colostomy. The care of this colostomy is discussed earlier in this chapter. Because a large amount of tissue is removed at this operation, the patient is frequently in shock immediately postoperatively. Blood pressure, pulse rate, and respiration should be noted frequently, and urinary output may be checked hourly. An hourly urinary output below 30 ml. per hour may indicate impending renal failure, which may necessitate fluids and other means to elevate the blood pressure and thus the pressure of blood flow through the kidneys. Rectal dressings should be watched carefully for signs of excessive bleeding. The usual drainage is serosanguineous and profuse. The mattress, therefore, should be adequately protected, and pads that can be changed without unduly disturbing the patient should be used. The dressing may need to be reinforced during the first few hours postoperatively. After the doctor has changed the first dressing (usually twenty-four hours postoperatively), the nurse may be requested to change the dressings as necessary. Since the dressing requires frequent changing, a T binder gives the best support without causing skin irritation.

Bed rest may be prescribed for several

days because of the effect of the extensive surgery upon the patient. The surgeon may also wish to avoid having the patient get up too soon so that the pelvic floor can heal partially and the danger of a perineal hernia can be avoided.

Since the patient usually has severe pain while lying on his back, and since he finds it very difficult to turn, he usually prefers to lie on one side and remain there. He must, however, be encouraged to change his position frequently, to breathe deeply, and to cough productively. During the first few days the nurse should assist him in turning as necessary and should help him to do exercises in bed. For example, he must be encouraged to straighten out his knees, to dorsiflex the feet, and to tense the muscles of the legs. In her efforts to make the patient comfortable, the nurse must see that positions, such as flexion of the knees, that may predispose to development of postoperative thrombophlebitis, are avoided. Pillows should be used to add to the patient's comfort, but the nurse *must* assist him to change position at regular and frequent intervals. Some patients are comfortable in a flat position lying on a rubber air ring. Others find that this position causes a pull on the incision. The patient is most comfortable on a firm bed with pieces of sponge rubber placed to relieve pressure on weight-bearing areas and to support the perineal dressing when he is lying on his back.

The patient usually needs a narcotic for pain at regular intervals for the first two or three days postoperatively. If he is in the older age group, however, the narcotic should be given judiciously so that respirations and physical activity are not decreased too much. Smaller doses may be sufficient for older patients. If the nurse finds that the dose appears to depress the patient too much, she should discuss this problem with the surgeon.

The Foley catheter usually is left in the bladder postoperatively to prevent the bladder from becoming distended and from pressing against the repaired pelvic floor until it heals. Its use also eliminates the need for women patients to use the bedpan to void (a very painful procedure after this operation) and prevents contamination of the wound and dressings with urine. The catheter, however, fairly frequently causes irritation and infection of the bladder. After it is removed, the patient may be unable to void or may void inadequately. It may then have to be reinserted for several more days, or the patient may be catheterized at specified intervals as necessary until he is able to void normally. It is not unusual, following this operation, for the male patient to require a prostatectomy for benign prostatic hypertrophy. Antibiotics and large amounts of fluid are given when a catheter is used. Special care should be taken that the catheter drains constantly so that residual urine does not remain in the bladder. (See p. 442 for discussion of care of patients needing catheters.)

If the perineal wound has been packed, the packing is removed gradually. When this process is completed, the wound is irrigated once or twice a day to remove secretions and tissue debris from the wound, to prevent abscesses from forming in the dead space that may be left, and to help ensure healing of the wound from the inside outward. The nurse should ascertain from the doctor how deep the catheter can be inserted and in what direction to insert it. Precise directions as to how to do the irrigation should be recorded on the nursing care plan.

Normal saline solution or diluted hydrogen peroxide is frequently used as the irrigating solution. When the patient is permitted out of bed, sitz baths may be substituted for the irrigations, and as drainage from the wound decreases, a perineal pad may be substituted for the dressing. A rubber ring should be used when the patient takes a sitz bath so that water can flow freely around the incision. The response in healing is often quite remarkable when this is done. Since the patient is usually ready to leave the hospital before the perineal wound has completely closed arrangements must be made for him to continue to take sitz baths at home. If he does not have a bathtub available, a large basin may be used. A public health nurse should always be called upon to assist the patient and his family in procedures of this kind to avoid accidents and to give the patient the assurance of professional help as he cares for himself.

Because a longer time on bed rest may be

necessary than following many operations, the patient is usually weaker than most patients when ambulation is attempted. He should be very carefully assisted and closely observed until he is strong enough to get about alone with safety. If a plastic-covered pillow, a piece of sponge rubber, or a rubber air ring is placed on the chair, the patient is usually more comfortable and is able to sit up for a longer time.

Convalescence after an abdominoperineal operation is prolonged, and may require months. During this time the patient should remain under close medical supervision. A well-prepared and detailed interagency referral from the nurse in the hospital to the nurse in the public health agency helps a great deal in assuring continuity of care for the patient. By this means the nurse in the home may contact one of the nurses who gave the patient care in the hospital or the doctor to discuss problems she encounters as she gives guidance and assistance to the patient and to his family. This helps to prevent minor differences in procedures or in other instructions which may be upsetting to the patient.

Disease conditions of and about the anus

Although most conditions of the anus usually do not endanger the life of the patient, they are often a source of chronic discomfort and concern. They may cause a great deal of pain because the anus is well supplied with nerves. These diseases may prevent the patient from walking or sitting comfortably, may increase or initiate constipation, and may even cause so much local discomfort that the patient is unable to work. Even after treatment, local discomfort may continue for some time, and although the treatment is minor, the patient may have difficulty in readily resuming normal activity. The nurse should be aware of the problems that patients with disease of the anal area encounter, and she should try to anticipate nursing care that will prevent and relieve discomfort.

Hemorrhoids

Hemorrhoids are one of the most common afflictions of man, and they cause an enor-

mous amount of pain and discomfort. Congestion occurs in the veins of the hemorrhoidal plexus and leads to varicosities within the lower rectum and the anus. The cause for the development of this condition is not definitely known, but many factors seem to be involved. Heredity, occupations requiring long periods of standing or sitting, the erect posture assumed by man, structural absence of valves in the hemorrhoidal veins, increase of intra-abdominal pressure caused by constipation, straining at defecation, and pregnancy all are factors predisposing to development of hemorrhoids.

Internal hemorrhoids appear above the internal sphincter and are not apparent to the patient unless they become so large that they protrude through the anus, where they may become constricted and painful. Internal hemorrhoids often bleed on defecation, and although the amount of blood lost may be small, continuous oozing over a long period of time may cause anemia. *External hemorrhoids* are those which appear outside the anal sphincter. They bleed relatively rarely and seldom cause pain unless a hemorrhoidal vein ruptures and a so-called thrombosis occurs. If this occurs, the hemorrhoid becomes inflamed and exquisitely painful.

Many patients have both internal and external hemorrhoids. Constipation often predisposes to the development of hemorrhoids and usually becomes worse after they occur because the patient tries to restrain bowel movements that produce pain or bleeding. Other people resort to laxatives without competent medical supervision. Although hemorrhoids rarely undergo malignant degeneration, constipation and bleeding may be symptoms of cancer of the rectum. Since cancer of the rectum is fairly common all patients with these symptoms should have medical attention. The nurse is often in a position to advise persons who have what they assume to be painless bleeding hemorrhoids of long duration to visit their doctor.

Medical treatment and nursing care. The treatment of hemorrhoids consists of local treatment, sclerosing by injection, and surgery. The local application of ice, warm magnesium sulfate compresses, and analgesic ointments such as dibucaine (Nupercaine) give temporary relief from pain and reduce the edema around external hemorrhoids or prolapsed internal ones. Sitz baths are also extremely helpful in relieving pain. The doctor may prescribe mineral oil to lubricate the anal canal and to soften the stool. Thrombosed external hemorrhoids usually respond to this treatment with lessening of pain and absorption of the confined blood. Finally, only a painless skin tag remains, and it is not removed surgically unless it causes strictures or its presence interferes with cleanliness enough to aggravate the patient seriously. If a thrombosed external hemorrhoid does not respond to medical treatment, it may be incised to release the encased blood. This procedure usually is done in a doctor's office and results in immediate relief of pain.

Injection is used in the treatment of moderate-sized internal hemorrhoids that cause bleeding or are protruding. A sclerosing solution such as 5% phenol in oil is injected carefully *under* the mucosa, where it causes scarring and reversal of symptoms. It is never injected directly into the hemorrhoids since this results in the formation of an ulcer and does not correct the basic condition.

Surgical excision is the treatment most often used for almost all external hemorrhoids that are causing difficulty and for the internal ones that are large or that recur after injection has been done. Preoperatively the patient may be given a laxative, and he is encouraged to eat a full, normal diet until a few hours before the anesthetic is given. Mineral oil is often given to soften the stool and facilitate its passage through the rectum postoperatively, and a bulk laxative such as metamucil may be given to increase the bulk of the stool.

To prevent pressure on the anal area following a hemorrhoidectomy, the patient may be placed on his abdomen, although many patients prefer to lie on the back, with a support such as a rubber air ring under the buttocks. Since the patient may have severe pain postoperatively, ice packs, warm wet compresses, analgesic ointments, and narcotics may be given. Since the operation is usually considered minor and dressings may not be used, the tendency may be to minimize this operative procedure. In reality it can cause the patient more discomfort than some more serious operations. The patient may be permitted out of bed the evening of

surgery or the day after, and sitz baths usually are ordered to be taken twice a day. They often give relief from pain and discomfort. They should be supervised by nursing personnel until the patient can manage safely alone.

The patient often has difficulty voiding after a hemorrhoidectomy. This difficulty can usually be overcome by getting the patient out of bed to urinate. Sitz baths are also very helpful in stimulating voiding.

If the patient is not nauseated, a full diet is permitted immediately after surgery. Mild laxatives such as mineral oil are continued as preoperatively, and the patient is encouraged to have a bowel movement as soon as the inclination occurs. Passing a stool of normal consistency as soon as possible after surgery prevents the formation of strictures and preserves the normal lumen of the anus. The incidence of wound infection is slight after rectal surgery due to local tissue resistance to the bacteria normally present in the rectum. It is most likely to occur if bowel action has been delayed and healing tissues have become adherent. If the patient complains of much pain about the area and is fearful of having a bowel movement, the doctor often orders medication such as dextropropoxyphene hydrochloride (Darvon), in dosages of 65 mg. (1 grain) or Darvon Compound (1 capsule), to be taken a short time before a bowel movement is attempted. The patient needs careful nursing attention when he attempts the first bowel movement since it may cause dizziness and even fainting.

If a spontaneous bowel movement does not occur within two or three days postoperatively, laxatives are increased and an oil-retention enema followed by a cleansing enema may be given through a small rectal tube. The patient is advised to take a sitz bath after each bowel movement to keep the operative area clean and to relieve local irritation. This practice should be continued until he returns to the doctor (usually within one or two weeks).

Following a hemorrhoidectomy, the patient is advised to avoid constipation by eating a diet containing adequate fruit and roughage, exercising moderately, drinking plenty of fluids, and establishing a regular time for daily bowel movements. The doctor may prescribe mineral oil or another mild laxative to be taken daily or every other day for a time.

Anal fissure

An anal fissure is a slitlike ulcer resembling a crack in the lining of the anal canal at or below the anorectal line. Usually it is the result of trauma caused by passage of hard-formed stool. The ulcer does not heal readily. Defecation initiates spasm of the anal sphincter, and the patient has severe pain that lasts for some time. Slight bleeding may occur, and constipation is usually caused by the patient's restraining his bowel movements to avoid pain.

Anal examination causes muscle spasm of the sphincter. Since spasm results in pain, the fissure must be examined under anesthesia. Treatment usually consists of digital dilation of the sphincter under anesthesia, or the anal ulcer may be surgically excised.

Local pain and spasm sometimes can be relieved by warm compresses, sitz baths, and use of analgesic ointments. Mineral oil is usually ordered to lubricate the canal and to soften the stool. Postoperatively the care is similar to that given the patient who has had a hemorrhoidectomy.

Anal abscess

An anal abscess is located in tissues around the anus. It is caused by infection from the anal canal and may follow an anal fissure. If the abscess involves the anal, para-anal, or perineal tissues, there is throbbing local pain caused by pressure on the somatic sensory nerves in the perineum and local signs of inflammation. The patient finds it difficult to sit or lie on the area. In fact, any position is uncomfortable since he suffers from reflected pain.

If the abscess is located deep in the ischiorectal tissues, however, the patient is aware only of vague discomfort until the disease spreads into an area where there are nerve fibers. The patient with an *ischiorectal abscess* is usually very ill. He has fever, chills, and malaise. The abscess must be incised and drained.

Postoperative care. Postoperatively the patient usually prefers to lie on his side or abdomen. Since most patients have some

difficulty voiding, nursing measures should be initiated to prevent bladder distention. To void, the female patient needs to lie on her abdomen. This position prevents pain and contamination of the wound. A small child's bedpan or an emesis basin is more comfortable for the patient to use in this position.

There is usually a large amount of seropurulent drainage from the wound, and the physician may order that the dressings be changed as necessary. The wound is usually packed with gauze, and the nurse may be asked to wet the pack with warm normal saline solution or to repack the wound with warm normal saline dressings at specified intervals. The packs should be inserted into the bottom of the wound since it is important that it heal from the inside outward. The skin around the wound should be protected with petroleum jelly to prevent irritation from drainage. The wet dressing should be covered with oiled silk or plastic material to prevent wick contamination and to prevent wetting the bed. The dressing can be held in place by Montgomery straps or a T binder.

As healing progresses, sitz baths are usually ordered. If the wound is located near the anus, the patient is advised to cleanse the area carefully after defecation and to take a sitz bath after each defecation. Until healing is complete and all drainage disappears, a small dressing should be worn over the wound. Mineral oil may be given to prevent or to treat constipation. Antibiotics usually are given.

The patient is often discharged from the hospital before the wound has completely healed. He should continue to take sitz baths at home. If any difficulties are encountered he should report them to the doctor.

Anal fistula

An anal fistula is an inflammatory sinus or tract with a primary opening in an anal crypt and with a secondary opening on the anal, para-anal, or perineal skin or in the rectal mucous membrane. It results from the rupture or drainage of an anal abscess. The patient has a periodic drainage that stains his clothing. An anal fistula is usually a chronic condition, and unfortunately many patients attempt to treat themselves with patent remedies before they seek competent medical care.

The treatment of an anal fistula is a *fistulectomy* or a *fistulotomy*. A fistulectomy consists of an excision of the entire fistulous tract. The overhanging edges, if any, are trimmed away to leave an open, saucer-shaped wound. This procedure is usually performed when the fistula is quite straight and somewhat superficial. When a fistulotomy is performed, the entire tract is laid open, and the overlying skin margins are excised to leave a wide, saucer-shaped wound. The membranous lining of the remaining half of the fistulous tract quickly acquires a covering of granulation tissue. This procedure is usually used when a deep fistulous tract exists.

Postoperatively, patients with both procedures usually have warm, wet dressings applied. They generally are permitted to get up to void. Mineral oil may be given by mouth daily until the first bowel movement occurs, and sitz baths are prescribed to keep the area clean and to relieve discomfort. The patient who has had an operation for a fistula is more comfortable sitting on a protected pillow or a piece of very thick sponge rubber rather than on a rubber ring.

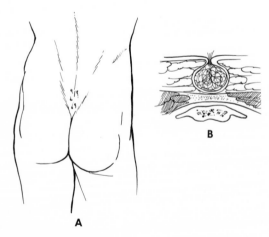

Fig. 162

Pilonidal sinus showing, **A,** opening in skin over sacrococcygeal area; **B,** cross section through cyst and pilonidal opening.

Pilonidal disease

Pilonidal cysts occur in the sacrococcygeal area and are thought to be congenital in origin. The cyst is lined with epithelium and hair. Pilonidal means "nest of hair." The cavity of the cyst communicates with the overlying skin by means of one or more short channels, each opening onto the skin in the midline. (See Fig. 162.) The lining of the channel or sinus is the same as the cyst, and tufts of hair are often seen protruding from the opening on the skin. These cysts or sinuses cause no symptoms unless they become infected. The patient then complains of pain and swelling at the base of the spine. An abscess forms, and it may rupture spontaneously or may require surgical incision and drainage. If the infection becomes chronic and the sinuses continue to drain, surgery becomes necessary.

Several types of operations may be done. The cyst may be excised and the wound closed. The patient remains in bed for several days after this procedure. To prevent contaminating the wound, the woman patient should void while lying on her abdomen. It is best if she practices this procedure before the operation. The patient should be observed for complications of bed rest such as urinary retention and should be encouraged to cough, breathe deeply, and move his arms and legs often. Ambulation is gradual. The patient should not take large steps, and he should not sit for long periods since these activities cause tension on the incision. A low-residue diet is usually given, and foods, such as orange juice or prune juice, that may stimulate peristalsis are avoided for the first few days. Defecation usually is delayed several days if possible, and a small oil retention enema is sometimes ordered before the first defecation takes place. When the patient does have his first bowel movement, the surgeon usually wishes to be notified so that the dressing can be changed. Antibiotics are usually given prophylactically, and narcotics may be needed for pain.

The cyst may be excised and the wound left open to heal by secondary intention. The wound is packed, and the patient remains in bed until the packing is removed twenty-four to forty-eight hours later. The patient is then permitted out of bed, and the wound is dressed daily. Sitz baths may be prescribed to be taken three or four times daily and after each bowel movement.

If an exteriorization operation or marsupialization is performed, the cyst cavity and all the channels are opened. The overhanging margins of skin are excised down to the base of the wound, providing a flat, saucer-shaped wound, the floor of which is formed by the deep half of the lining of the cyst or channel. The area to be covered by granulation tissues is thus decreased, and healing will occur in less than six weeks. The wound is packed, and the patient usually remains in bed until the packing is removed twenty-four hours later. Wet dressings are then applied, and sitz baths may be prescribed.

References and selected readings*

1 American Cancer Society, Inc., 1966 cancer facts and figures, New York, 1965, American Cancer Society, Inc.

2 *Amshel, Albert Livingston: Hemorrhoidal problems—medical and surgical treatment; Sheridan, Brigid Ann: After hemorrhoidectomy—postoperative nursing care, Am. J. Nursing 63:87-91, Dec. 1963.

3 Barton, Kenneth M., and Kirsner, Joseph B.: Gastric ulcer—individualization in diagnosis and therapy, M. Clin. North America 64:103-115, Jan. 1964.

4 Beeson, Paul B., and McDermott, Walsh, editors: Cecil-Loeb textbook of medicine, ed. 11, Philadelphia, 1963, W. B. Saunders Co.

5 *Behrend, Albert: Changing trends in appendicitis, Am. J. Nursing 63:88-89, Oct. 1963.

6 Bergersen, Betty S., and Krug, Elsie E.: Pharmacology in nursing, ed. 10, St. Louis, 1966, The C. V. Mosby Co.

7 Boros, Edwin: Hiatus hernia, Am. J. Gastroenterol. 37:438-441, April 1962.

8 Cole, Warren H., and Zollinger, Robert M.: Textbook of surgery, ed. 8, New York, 1963, Appleton-Century-Crofts.

9 Dagradi, Angelo E., and Stempien, Stephen J.: Symptomatic esophageal hiatus sliding hernia, Am. J. Digest. Dis. 7:613-633, July 1962.

10 Davidsohn, Israel, and Wells, Benjamin B.: Todd-Sanford clinical diagnosis by laboratory methods, ed. 13, Philadelphia, 1963, W. B. Saunders Co.

11 Davis, Loyal, editor: Christopher's textbook of surgery, ed. 8, Philadelphia, 1964, W. B. Saunders Co.

12 Dericks, Virginia C.: Rehabilitation of patients with ileostomy, Am. J. Nursing 61:48-51, May 1961.

13 Drummond, Eleanor E., and Anderson, Mary L.: Gastrointestinal suction, Am. J. Nursing 63:109-113, Dec. 1963.

14 *Eisenberg, Samuel W., Napoli, Rita P., and Radding,

Beatrice: Proctosigmoidoscopy, Am. J. Nursing 65:113-115, Jan. 1965.

15 *Frenay, Sister Mary Agnes Clare: A dynamic approach to the ileal conduit patient, Am. J. Nursing 64:80-84, Jan. 1964.

16 Friedrich, Helen N.: Oral feeding by food pump, Am. J. Nursing 62:62-64, Feb. 1962.

17 Fuerst, Elinor V., and Wolff, LuVerne: Fundamentals of nursing, ed. 3, Philadelphia, 1964, J. B. Lippincott Co.

18 Gabriel, William B.: The principles and practice of rectal surgery, ed. 5, Springfield, 1963, Charles C Thomas, Publishers.

19 Goldstein, Franz: Newer approaches to the management of peptic ulcer, M. Clin. North America 49:1253-1270, Sept. 1965.

20 Gordon, John E., editor: Control of communicable disease in man, ed. 10, New York, 1965, American Public Health Association.

21 Hardy, James D.: Diaphragmatic hernias, Am. J. Surg. 103:342-351, March 1962.

22 Harrison, T. R., and others, editors: Principles of internal medicine, ed. 4, New York, 1966, Mc-Graw-Hill Book Co.

23 Holmes, George W., and Dobrushin, Dorothy Jean: Diaphragmatic hernia and diaphragmatic hernia nursing care, Am. J. Nursing 56:183-186, Feb. 1956.

24 Jay, Arthur N.: Colitis, Am. J. Nursing 59:1133-1135, Aug. 1959.

25 *Jay, Arthur N.: Is it indigestion? Am. J. Nursing 58:1552-1554, Nov. 1958.

26 Jones, H. Leonard, and Nielsen, Orville F.: Colitis: management based on pathologic mechanisms, M. Clin. North America 49:1271-1294, Sept. 1965.

27 *Kaplan, Murrell H., Bernheim, Edmundo J., and Flynn, Besse McCoy: Esophageal varices, Am. J. Nursing 64:104-108, June 1964.

28 Katona, Elizabeth A.: Learning colostomy control, Am. J. Nursing 67:534-541, March 1967.

29 *Klug, Thomas J., Magruder, Lucinda, and others: Gastric resection—and nursing care, Am. J. Nursing 61:73-77, Dec. 1961.

30 *Kurihara, Marie: The patient with an intestinal prosthesis, Am. J. Nursing 60:852-853, June 1960.

31 Littman, Armand, and Dunphy, James V.: Management of the complications of duodenal ulcer, M. Clin. North America 48:93-102, Jan. 1964.

32 McHardy, Gordon, editor: Current gastroenterology, New York, 1962, Harper & Row, Publishers.

33 *McKittrick, John B., and Shotkin, Jane M.: Ulcerative colitis, Am. J. Nursing 62:60-64, Aug. 1962.

34 *Rynbergen, Henderika J.: In gastrointestinal disease—fewer diet restrictions, Am. J. Nursing 63:86-89, Jan. 1963.

35 *Steigmann, Frederick: Are laxatives necessary? Am. J. Nursing 62:90-93, Oct. 1962.

36 Steigmann, Frederick, and Shlaes, William H.: The treatment of amebiasis, M. Clin. North America 48:159-175, Jan. 1964.

37 Terracol, J., and Sweet, Richard H.: Diseases of the esophagus, Philadelphia, 1958, W. B. Saunders Co.

---

*References preceded by an asterisk are particularly well suited for student reading.

38 Turell, Robert, and others: Symposium on new perspectives in colorectoanal surgery, S. Clin. North America 45:1067-1329, Oct. 1965.

39 U. S. Bureau of the Census: Statistical abstracts of the United States, 1965, ed. 86, Washington, D. C., 1965, U. S. Government Printing Office.

40 U. S. Department of Health, Education, and Welfare, Public Health Service: Proceedings, National Conference on Salmonellosis, March, 1964, Washington, D. C., 1965, U. S. Government Printing Office.

41 *Usher, Francis C., and Matthews, Joan: Surgery: treatment of choice for hernia, Am. J. Nursing 64:85-87, Sept. 1964.

42 Wangensteen, Owen H., and others: Can physiological gastrectomy be activated by gastric freezing? Ann. Surg. 156:579-591, Oct. 1962.

43 Warren, Richard: Surgery, Philadelphia, 1963, W. B. Saunders Co.

44 *Werrin, Milton, and Kronick, David: Salmonella control in hospitals, Am. J. Nursing 66:528-531, March 1966.

45 White, Dorothy Ruth: I have an ileostomy, Am. J. Nursing 61:51-52, May 1961.

46 *Woldman, Edward E.: Peptic ulcer: current medical treatment, Am. J. Nursing 59:222-223, Feb. 1959.

47 Wolfman, Earl F., Jr., Flotte, C. Thomas, and Hallburg, Jeanne C.: Carcinoma of the colon and rectum and the patient with surgery of the colon, Am. J. Nursing 61:60-66, March 1961.

48 *Woodward, E. R., and Eisenberg, M. M.: Gastric physiology, with special reference to gastric and duodenal ulcers, S. Clin. North America 45:327-343, April 1965.

49 *Zimmermann, W. J., and Brandly, Paul J.: The current status of trichiniasis in U. S. swine, Public Health Rep. 80:1061-1066, Dec. 1965.

50 Zuidema, George D., and Klein, Marilyn Kitching: A new esophagus, Am. J. Nursing 61:69-72, Sept. 1961.

25

The patient with disease of the liver and adjacent structures

Study questions

1 Review the main functions of the liver.
2 Review the anatomy of the biliary system. What are the important constituents of bile? What is its function in digestion?
3 What are the practices in your hospital regarding use and sterilization of needles and syringes? Are sterile syringes used to draw blood? How are needles sterilized?
4 List some drugs you have learned about that are toxic to the liver.
5 Review procedure and the nursing care given when a paracentesis is done.

The liver and the biliary system are affected by a variety of diseases. In this chapter nursing related to diagnostic tests and to general problems commonly seen in patients with hepatic and biliary diseases will be discussed before specific nursing care in some of the more common diseases is considered.

Since the public is becoming better informed about diseases such as viral hepatitis, fear is usually present when disease of the liver is suspected. Many people have friends or acquaintances who have died of a hepatic disease or who have been handicapped for long periods of time because of it. However, certain diseases of the liver need not necessarily occur, and the nurse can help in their prevention. For example, the spread of viral hepatitis can be controlled substantially if the public is taught to use good hygienic practices and proper sterilization techniques. Certain degenerative diseases of the liver can be prevented if people are informed about the proper use of substances, such as carbon tetrachloride, that are harmful to hepatic cells. Serious damage to hepatic tissue may be prevented by referring persons with signs of disease of the liver, such as dark urine, light stools, and jaundice, to the doctor promptly.

Diagnostic examinations and tests

Several tests are used to determine whether or not disease of the liver is present and to distinguish the various causes of symptoms if some derangement of the liver or of the biliary system is evident. They include tests of hepatic function, procedures that demonstrate the amount and distribution of bile pigment, and roentgenograms that may show biliary malfunction. The patient should be told the purpose of each test, what preparation is necessary, and what to expect during the test or examination.

Liver function tests

Liver function tests are used to determine the presence and the extent of hepatic damage and to check the progress of disease of the liver. They are of great importance in determining whether or not signs and symptoms are due to disease of the hepatic cells themselves (hepatocellular) or to pathology outside the hepatic cells (extracellular). Since the liver has many functions that are closely interrelated, single tests of liver function usually give information about the efficiency of several of the organ's activities. This is particularly true when metabolic functions are considered.

Most liver function tests involve taking samples of the patient's blood, and many require that he fast preceding the test, causing inconvenience and discomfort for the patient. If the nurse makes sure that the tests are scheduled as ordered, laboratory slips are filled in correctly, blood samples are correctly labeled, urine specimens collected on time, and food withheld as necessary, she can help prevent the need for repetition of the tests. Since the rules of laboratories vary as to whether or not fasting should precede the taking of blood for some tests, the nurse should learn the practice in her hospital. If in doubt, it is usually best to have the patient fast, although the importance of regular meals for persons with disease of the liver must be kept in mind.

Tests based on bilirubin metabolism. Tests may reveal the functional capacity of the liver in breaking down, reusing, and excreting bile pigment by measuring the amount of bilirubin present in the blood, stools, and urine. Bilirubin, the pigmented end product

of hemoglobin breakdown, is formed in the liver. Normally, it is excreted with bile into the duodenum and is broken down by bacteria in the lower intestines into urobilinogen. Most of the urobilinogen is excreted in the feces, becoming urobilin, which gives the characteristic brown color to stools. The remainder returns to the liver, where it is reconverted to bilirubin, or it is eliminated in the urine. Only minute amounts of bilirubin are found in the blood and urine of well persons. When the hepatic and biliary ducts become blocked for any reason, however, bilirubin is no longer excreted into the bowel. It then is absorbed into the blood (*jaundice*) and excreted by the kidneys (*bilirubinuria*). Under these circumstances, urobilinogen in the blood and urine is decreased or absent.

The *quantitative van den Bergh* test for *serum bilirubin* is one that measures the total serum bilirubin in the blood. The total serum bilirubin content indicates the intensity and progress of jaundice; determination of the amount by the direct or by the indirect method gives some indication as to the cause of the jaundice. For example, the bile pigment in the serum of patients with hemolytic jaundice is determined by the indirect test (indirect-reacting bilirubin), whereas in obstructive jaundice, there is bile in the blood serum, and values can be obtained without extraction with alcohol (direct method, or direct-reacting bilirubin). Normal values for total serum bilirubin range from 0 to 1 mg. per 100 ml. Fasting is not necessary for this test.

The *icterus index* occasionally is used to determine the amount of bile pigment in blood serum. The normal reading is 4 to 6 units, but it may reach 15 units before jaundice is evident. Fasting usually is required for this test. Carrots eaten the day before the test will interfere with results because they color the blood serum.

Changes in the color of urine or stools may be early specific signs of hepatic or biliary disease. If the nurse observes a change in the color of either the urine or the stool, she should examine both and report her findings to the doctor.

Urine containing abnormal amounts of bilirubin has a characteristic mahogany color, and if the specimen is shaken, a yellow foam appears (the *foam test*). Urobilinogen in a fresh urine specimen is colorless but turns to brown urobilin on standing. The normal amount of *urinary urobilinogen* ranges from 0 to 4 mg. a day. This amount is increased in nonobstructive liver disease and will cause the urine to be darker than usual. If the flow of bile into the intestines is obstructed, urobilinogen is not formed and it disappears from the urine. All urine voided in twenty-four hours may be needed to determine the amount of bilirubin or urobilin being excreted in the urine.

The normal range for *fecal urobilinogen* is from 40 to 280 mg. daily. In hemolytic jaundice, as much as 4,000 mg. may be excreted per day.[5] A decrease in or absence of urobilinogen in the stool (acholia) would suggest an obstruction to the flow of bile that prevents it from reaching the intestines. The stool gradually becomes lighter and may be clay-colored or almost white.

Tests based on protein metabolism. Some of the most important functions of the liver are concerned with protein metabolism, including the deamination of amino acids and the maintenance of normal levels of albumin, globulin, and fibrinogen in the blood. Determination of the *ratio of serum proteins* (A/G ratio) is a measure of hepatic function. An alteration in the normal ratio may indicate degenerative disease of the liver. The serum albumin tends to drop below 4 grams per 100 ml. of blood, whereas the serum globulin tends to rise above 2.4 grams per 100 ml. of blood in patients with disease of the liver. No fasting is necessary for this test.

The *cephalin-cholesterol flocculation test* is performed to distinguish jaundice due to disease of the liver from obstructive jaundice. and to screen for early detection of subclinical disease of the liver. A colloidal suspension of a cephalin-cholesterol mixture shows distinct flocculation and sedimentation when serum from the blood of a patient with liver damage is used. The latter is caused by failure of the diseased liver to make certain changes in the protein constituents of the plasma. A reading of 1+ at the end of twenty-four hours or 2+ at forty-eight hours is considered a positive test.

The *thymol turbidity* test depends upon the presence in the serum of increased amounts of gamma globulin, beta globulin, and serum lipids. The test is particularly valuable in acute hepatitis in determining the degree of hepatic damage and in following the course of the disease through the late convalescent stages.

Since prothrombin (and fibrinogen), necessary for blood clotting, is manufactured by the liver, the *prothrombin level* may be determined when disease of the liver is suspected. Normal plasma clots in twenty seconds or less. A prothrombin-complex activity below 80% is considered abnormal; when below 40%, it may be associated with bleeding.[5] The prothrombin level is often lowered in cirrhosis of the liver and in metastatic carcinoma of the liver. Failure of a low prothrombin level in a patient with jaundice to respond to bile salts given by mouth and to parenteral administration of synthetic vitamin K indicates that the jaundice may be due to liver damage and not to biliary obstruction. Fasting is not necessary for this test.

Since most of the ammonia resulting from protein catabolism is converted into urea in the normal liver, a high concentration of *ammonia* in the blood is a good indicator of potential or existing hepatic coma. The normal levels range from 40 to 70 mg. of ammonia nitrogen per 100 ml.

Tests based on carbohydrate metabolism. There is a decreased ability to use both glucose and galactose when hepatic cells are damaged. If performed within the first two weeks of jaundice, the *galactose tolerance* test is one of the most specific tests for differentiating hepatocellular jaundice and extracellular jaundice. The galactose tolerance test is done as follows: The patient is given nothing by mouth on the morning of the test. The first morning specimen of urine is discarded, and the patient drinks 40 mg. of galactose dissolved in 500 ml. of water and flavored with lemon juice. After ingestion of this solution, urine specimens are collected hourly for five hours, numbered, and sent to the laboratory. The urine is examined for the total amount of sugar excreted. An excretion exceeding 3 Gm. of sugar is considered indicative of disease of the liver. This test may also be performed by giving the galactose intravenously; 1 ml. of 50% solution of galactose per kilogram of body weight is given after a sample of blood has been drawn. Another blood sample is taken seventy-five minutes after injection of the galactose. A test on normal blood should reveal under 5 mg. of sugar per 100 ml. of blood in this blood sample. Patients with hepatic disease have higher levels. The glucose tolerance test is described in relation to care of the patient with diabetes (p. 745).

Tests based on serum lipid metabolism. The liver is the main source of *serum cholesterol* and *serum phospholipids* and influences the concentration of other blood lipids.

A *quantitative determination of serum cholesterol* helps to determine hepatic function. It is known that patients with hepatic disease have a decrease in cholesterol esters in relation to total cholesterol. The normal blood serum cholesterol is between 140 and 220 mg.%, approximately 70% of which is the cholesterol ester. In suspected or known hepatic disease, a figure of 40% or lower in cholesterol esters or a steady decrease in cholesterol esters are indicative of progressive disease of the liver with poor prognosis, whereas an increase in the cholesterol esters indicates improvement in the condition. Fasting usually is required for this test.

The concentration of *serum phospholipids* tends to be low in severe hepatocellular disease and increased in diseases associated with obstruction to the flow of bile. An elevation of serum phospholipids reflects corresponding elevation in cholesterol. The normal range of serum phospholipids, expressed as lecithin, is 110 to 250 mg. per 100 ml.

Tests based on detoxification. The detoxifying capacity of the liver may be tested by means of the *hippuric acid test*. Hippuric acid results from the synthesis of benzoic acid and glycine by the liver and is normally excreted at a regular rate in the urine. The test is done as follows: The patient is given a light breakfast of toast and coffee. One hour later, 6 Gm. of sodium benzoate, dissolved in 30 ml. of water and flavored with oil of peppermint, cherry syrup, or lemon juice is given by mouth. This may be followed by 100 ml. of water. The patient is then asked to void immediately, and this specimen is discarded. Then he fasts and voids each hour for four hours. The specimens are labeled, numbered, and sent to the laboratory. Normal excretion should total 3 Gm. of hippuric acid in the four specimens.

In the intravenous hippuric acid test, 1.77 Gm. of sodium benzoate is administered after the patient has voided and taken a glass of water. One urine specimen is collected an hour later and should contain more than 0.7 Gm. of hippuric acid. Abnormal findings may show poor hepatic function such as occurs in hepatitis, cirrhosis, and malignant disease of the liver. In conditions in which jaundice is the result of obstruction in the biliary passages and in which the liver has not yet been damaged, the test is normal.

Tests based on dye excretion. Since one of the functions of the liver is excretion, tests that measure the rate with which a dye such as *Bromsulphalein* (BSP) is removed from the bloodstream are useful. Fasting is necessary for this test. The patient is weighed, and the dosage of the dye is calculated on the basis of 5 mg. per kilogram of body weight. The dye is injected slowly into the vein, and a blood sample is taken in forty-five minutes from the opposite arm. Blood values are raised above 4% in diseases of the liver. The nurse participates in the scheduling of tests and should know that phenolsulfonphthalein tests for kidney function should not be scheduled for at least twenty-four hours after dye for a liver function test has been given. Rose bengal or indocyanine green also may be used as a dye for a test of liver function.

Tests based on serum enzyme determinations. Necrosis of liver cells, such as occurs in hepatitis, brings about an increase in serum enzymes. Two enzymes frequently studied are the *serum glutamic oxaloacetic transaminase* (SGOT) and the *serum glutamic pyruvic transaminase* (SGPT). While SGPT is specifically elevated in diseases of the liver, SGOT is raised in myocardial infarction, pulmonary embolism, and other diseases, as well as in hepatic diseases (pp. 311 and 573).

Serum cholinesterase is believed to be synthesized in the liver and involved in protein metabolism. Its activity is depressed in cirrhosis particularly.

The *alkaline phosphatase test* is significant in that the level is only slightly elevated in diseases of the liver such as hepatitis and cirrhosis but is markedly elevated in biliary obstruction. Depending upon the method used, normal levels range from 0.5 to 4.0

Bodansky units or 3 to 13 King-Armstrong units.[21] Fasting is usually requested for this test.

Tests based on hemagglutination. A substance or substances found in the blood of a large number of patients in the acute phase of viral hepatitis will agglutinate the erythrocytes of a day-old chick or those of a Macaca rhesus monkey. The mechanism of the agglutination reaction is not completely understood. There is evidence that a specific antibody reaction may be involved.[5] There is no hemagglutination reaction in the blood of patients with obstructive or hemolytic jaundice.

X-ray examination

X-ray examinations are used to diagnose diseases of the liver, the portal system, the gallbladder, and the biliary ducts, and to determine the ability of the gallbladder to concentrate bile and to expel it through the common bile duct into the duodenum.

Cholecystography. A normal liver will remove radiopaque drugs such as iodoalphionic acid (Priodax), iopanoic acid (Telepaque), and iodipamide methylglucamine (Cholografin methylglucamine) from the bloodstream and store and concentrate them in the gallbladder. Because the roentgen rays cannot penetrate the dye, the dye-filled gallbladder shows up as a dense shadow upon x-ray examination (*cholecystogram, gallbladder series*). A satisfactory gallbladder shadow would indicate a functioning gallbladder. A total absence of opaque material in the gallbladder would suggest a nonfunctioning gallbladder. After ingestion of a fatty meal, a functioning gallbladder should contract and expel the radiopaque dye along with the bile through the common bile duct into the duodenum. X-ray examination at this point would outline the bile ducts. Stones, which are not radiopaque, show up as dark patches on the film. Visualization of the gallbladder depends upon absorption of the dye through the intestinal tract, isolation of it by the liver, and a free passageway from the liver to the gallbladder. Therefore, if the results show a nonfunctioning gallbladder, sometimes the test is repeated to be sure that failure to visualize the gallbladder by x-ray examination was not due to insufficient dye.

On the evening before cholecystography is scheduled, the purpose of and preparation for the test should be explained to the patient. The importance of following instructions regarding food restriction the morning of the test as well as the need for the high-fat meal, which may cause nausea, should be discussed.

The average adult dose of both Priodax and Telepaque is 3 Gm. (45 grains) given orally following a low-fat evening meal, after which no food is given. These drugs may cause nausea, vomiting, and diarrhea in some people. The nurse should check dosages accurately and watch carefully for toxic signs, which should be reported to the doctor. If vomiting occurs soon after ingestion of the drug, the doctor may ask that the tablets be repeated when nausea subsides, or he may delay the test for several days. If the patient cannot tolerate the drug by mouth, a radiopaque substance such as Cholografin may be given intravenously by the doctor in the x-ray department. The radiopaque dyes are organic iodine compounds and may cause allergic reactions when given intravenously. Symptoms may include dyspnea, chills, diaphoresis, faintness, and tachycardia and are identical to symptoms that can occur when radiopaque substances containing iodine are injected intravenously for other tests such as pyelography or arteriography. (See p. 426 for a discussion of precaution and care.)

On the morning of the examination the patient may have only black coffee, tea, or water. One or more enemas may be given to help remove gas from the intestinal tract so that it will not interfere with a clear roentgenogram. The patient goes to the x-ray department, where two roentgenograms are taken during the morning. He is then given a high-fat noon meal, after which another roentgenogram is taken. Ingestion of fat should stimulate flow of bile and emptying of the gallbladder. The dye is finally excreted in the urine, and some patients report slight temporary pain on urination following the test.

Cholangiography. Cholangiography is the x-ray examination of the bile ducts to demonstrate the presence of stones, strictures, or tumors. The radiopaque substance may be administered intravenously or injected directly into the common bile duct with a needle or catheter at the time of surgery. Following operations on the common bile duct, the radiopaque drug may be instilled through a drainage tube, such as the T tube, to determine the patency of the duct before the tube is removed. The dye also may be injected through the skin and abdominal wall into a bile duct in the main substance of the liver *(percutaneous transhepatic cholangiography)*.

Portography. If radiopaque dye is injected into the portal vein or one of its tributaries, part or all of the portal venous system may be visualized by x-ray examination *(portal portography)*. The injection of the radiopaque solution through the skin into the spleen is the most commonly employed method *(percutaneous splenic portography)*.

Radioisotope scanning. The liver may be outlined by radioisotope scanning techniques. After radioactive isotopes such as colloidal gold (Au^{198}), molybdenum (Mo^{99}), or rose bengal tagged with radioactive iodine (I^{131}), all of which selectively localize in the liver, are administered, the patient assumes a supine position and a scintillation detector is passed over the abdomen in the area of the liver. The radiation coming from the isotopes immediately beneath the probe is detected, amplified, and recorded by photoscanning. This technique helps differentiate nonfunctioning areas from normally active liver tissue and helps identify hepatic tumors, cysts, and abscesses. It is not as helpful in diagnosing cirrhosis of the liver. As reactions to the drugs usually do not occur, the procedure is considered safe and does not cause the patient any discomfort. Only small amounts of the radioactive material are given, and precautions are not necessary. Radioisotope scanning techniques are used to detect diseases in other tissues of the body, such as the kidney (p. 424).

Duodenal drainage

In this test, also known as the biliary drainage test, bile obtained from the duodenum is examined for occult blood, pancreatic enzymes, tumor cells, leukocytes, cholesterol crystals, and pigment granules. It may be done when the patient is ambulatory or while he is hospitalized. The patient should be prepared for a somewhat lengthy procedure, but he should know that once the tube has been passed he will have little or no discomfort. The preparation is similar to that for a gastric analysis (p. 637). The patient is not permitted anything by mouth except small sips of water for twelve hours. A slender tube weighted at its tip with metal, and marked with a series of rings to indicate the distance it travels to the cardia, pylorus, and duodenum, respectively, is passed through the patient's mouth (Fig. 150). Other modified gastroduodenal tubes are available and may be used for this purpose. After the tube is in the stomach, the patient is placed on his right side with his hips elevated about 6 inches so that gastric motility will be aided by gravity to carry the tube into the duodenum. The doctor may have to manipulate the tube into place with the aid of the fluoroscope. It may take from one to five hours for the tube to reach the duodenum. When the tube finally reaches the duodenum, several specimens are taken. The first specimen is usually light in color and consists of bile coming from the common duct. After this specimen is obtained approximately 50 ml. of magnesium sulfate (25% solution) are introduced through the tube to stimulate the flow of bile, and a second specimen is collected in ten to fifteen minutes. This specimen is usually darker and more viscid, containing bile from the gallbladder that has flowed in response to the cholagogue action of magnesium sulfate. A third specimen, containing bile coming from the hepatic duct and freshly secreted by the liver, is sometimes collected.

Olive oil may be instilled through the tube to stimulate the gallbladder to contract and expel bile into the duodenum, or cholecystokinin, a synthetic preparation of the substance normally found in the intestinal mucosa, may be administered intravenously. An intravenous injection of synthetic secretin may be given. It should cause an increase in the flow of bile and pancreatic secretions.

Biopsy of the liver

A biopsy of the liver may be taken in an attempt to establish a diagnosis. In this procedure a specially designed needle is inserted through the chest or abdominal wall into the liver and a small piece of tissue is removed for study. This procedure is contraindicated if the patient is jaundiced or has an infection of the right lower lobe of the lung, ascites, or a blood dyscrasia. To avoid hemorrhage, vitamin K may be given parenterally for several days before the biopsy is taken. The doctor should explain the procedure to the patient; for example, the patient should know that he must hold his breath and remain absolutely still when the needle is introduced. Movement of the chest may cause the needle to slip and to tear the liver covering. Most hospitals require that the patient give written permission for the procedure to be done. Food and fluids may be withheld for several hours preceding the test, and a sedative usually is given about one-half hour before the biopsy is to be taken.

The procedure usually is performed with the patient lying on his back, but sometimes it is done with the patient sitting on a treatment table or in bed with his feet over the side and firmly supported on a chair or a stool. If so, one nurse should give the patient encouragement, observe him closely, and support him if dizziness occurs, while a second nurse assists the doctor. Usually the doctor and the nurses wear masks during this procedure. The method is as follows: With the patient lying on his back, the skin over the area selected (usually the eighth or ninth intercostal space) is cleansed and anesthetized with procaine hydrochloride. A nick is made in the skin with a sharp scalpel blade. Then the patient is instructed to take several deep breaths and to hold his breath while the needle is introduced through the intercostal or subcostal tissues into the liver. The special needle assembly is rotated to separate a fragment of tissue, and then is withdrawn. The specimen is placed into an appropriate container, which is then labeled and sent to the pathology laboratory. A simple dressing is placed over the wound, and the patient usually remains on bed rest for twenty-four hours.

The dangers of this procedure, which is done relatively "blind," are accidental penetration of a small blood vessel, causing hemorrhage, and accidental penetration of a biliary vessel, causing a chemical peritonitis from leakage of bile into the abdominal cavity. Occasionally a laparotomy must be done to treat complications of liver biopsy. The nurse should check the equipment

used and the specimen very carefully for any signs of discoloration from bile and should report her findings to the doctor. The patient's pulse rate and blood pressure should be taken every half hour for the first few hours and then hourly for at least twenty-four hours. The doctor may order pressure applied to the biopsy site to help stop any bleeding. This procedure may be accomplished by having the patient lie on his right side with a small pillow or folded bath blanket placed under the costal margin for several hours after the biopsy.

General nursing care of patients with hepatic and biliary diseases

Jaundice, difficulty with nutrition because of poor appetite, nausea and poor tolerance of food, and secondary infections are problems confronting many patients with hepatic and biliary disease, regardless of its cause. Therefore, these problems and the medical and nursing care essential to alleviating them will be discussed before the nursing care for patients with specific disease is considered.

Jaundice

Jaundice is a symptom complex caused by a disturbance of the physiology of bile pigment and is present in many diseases of the hepatic and biliary system. There is an excess of bile pigment in the blood, which eventually is distributed to the skin, mucous membranes, and other body fluids and body tissues, giving them a yellow discoloration. Jaundice, caused by faulty hepatic function due to disease of the hepatic cells, is described as *hepatocellular*. When it results from intrahepatic or extrahepatic obstruction that interferes with the flow of bile, it is described as *obstructive*. *Hemolytic* jaundice presumably is caused by destruction of great numbers of blood cells, which results in the production of excessive amounts of bilirubin.

Pruritus. The presence of bile pigment in the skin causes pruritus (itching) in about 20 to 25% of the patients who have jaundice. Bathing or sponging the skin with tepid water, followed by the application of calamine lotion with 1% phenol, often helps relieve itching. Starch and sodium bicarbonate in the water may give relief, but they are drying to the skin, and their use should be followed by a gentle massage with a cream lotion. The antihistaminic drugs are sometimes used to control pruritus. Tranquilizing drugs such as chlordiazepoxide (Librium) have been effective in helping to decrease the patient's reaction to pruritus. Recently it has been found that relief from itching followed the administration of a resin, cholestyramine, which binds bile salts in the intestines and increases their excretion in feces.

Only soft, old linen should be used for the patient who has pruritus. Profuse diaphoresis sometimes accompanies jaundice, and bile-stained perspiration may color the bed linen. The linen should be changed at once for psychologic reasons as well as for physical comfort. The patient's fingernails should be cut short and his hands kept clean, since itching may be so severe that the patient may excoriate the skin by scratching and may cause skin lesions, which heal very slowly when jaundice is pronounced.

Emotional factors. The patient with marked jaundice is usually sensitive about his appearance. If he is ambulatory, dark glasses can be worn to conceal the yellow color of the sclerae. The hospital room should be kept softly lighted. White or yellowish light bulbs make jaundice much less obvious than does fluorescent lighting. If possible, mirrors should be inconspicuously removed. The patient who is particularly concerned with his appearance may rest better in a room by himself and may wish to have visitors restricted.

Hemorrhage. Because the jaundiced patient has a low blood prothrombin level, the coagulation time of his blood is prolonged and he bleeds easily. Therefore, he is a poor risk for surgery and may bleed profusely from minor medical procedures such as a venipuncture or an intramuscular injection. Normal production of prothrombin is dependent upon four things: (1) ingestion of foods that can undergo synthesis in the intestine, (2) presence of bile in the intestine, thus enabling the intestine to produce vitamin K from food constituents, (3) absorption through the intestinal wall of the vitamin K produced, and (4) use of the vitamin K by the liver in the formation of prothrombin.

Since vitamin K depends upon the presence of bile salts for its manufacture and absorption in the intestine, bile salts are often given by mouth to patients who are jaundiced. Vitamin K may be given both orally and parenterally in the hope that it will enable the liver to form more prothrombin. If vitamin K, which is not water soluble, is given by mouth, bile salts must be given as well. However, menadione sodium bisulfite (Hykinone), a water-soluble preparation of vitamin K, usually is ordered. The usual dose is 0.5 to 2 mg. (1/120 to 1/30 grain) daily, given parenterally. If the jaundice is due to obstruction in the biliary tract and not to hepatic disease, it can be treated satisfactorily. If the liver is severely diseased and unable to make use of the vitamin K provided, the prothrombin level will remain low despite the administration of bile salts and vitamin K. Fresh blood then may have to be given to provide the prothrombin essential for clotting.[3]

Since the jaundiced patient may bleed more than usual from such minor procedures as drawing blood from a vein, plans should be made for samples of blood to be taken at the same time for several tests. If an infusion is ordered, it should be started at the time blood is obtained. When giving intramuscular and hypodermic injections, the nurse should select the smallest needle that she can use safely and should be particularly careful that the needle is sharp and that, following an injection, firm pressure is exerted for longer than is normally necessary. The patient's urine and stools should be checked for either old or fresh blood, and if bleeding is suspected, specimens should be saved. Steady oozing of blood from hemorrhoids is not unusual in severe jaundice. Incisions heal more slowly when jaundice is present, and the nurse should inspect dressings frequently for bleeding. The patient's activity may be restricted until the wound has healed completely.

Nutrition. Seeing that the patient with hepatic or biliary disease eats enough of the necessary foods is one of the most important nursing responsibilities. The patient usually has difficulties with food. Disturbance of hepatic function and interference with normal flow of bile into the intestine upset the entire digestive system, causing indigestion, poor appetite, flatulence, and constipation. The patient may not tolerate fatty foods well. He may have learned over a period of months or years, or may need to be taught, to avoid high-fat foods, which tend to produce gas in the stomach and intestinal tract. Food often provokes nausea and vomiting, and the patient may be apprehensive about eating.

In recent years a great deal of attention has been given to diet and its relation to chronic degenerative disease of the liver. It is suspected that the liver's ability to excrete toxins and carry on its many other functions is seriously hampered by inadequate intake of protein and of vitamin B. If liver damage has occurred, the organ's ability to store glycogen and vitamins A, B complex, C, and D may also be lessened, and the patient may be in much greater need of regular intake of complete foods than before his illness.

A diet high in calories, protein, and vitamins, fairly high in carbohydrate (unless weight reduction is desired), with moderate amounts of fat is often ordered for patients with diseases of the liver. Many doctors believe that the patient who has hepatic damage should have 100 to 300 grams of protein per day, but it is exceedingly difficult to have the patient eat this amount. Lean beef (broiled steak if it can be afforded), broiled chicken, and fish are some of the best high-protein foods. Egg white, gelatin, and cottage cheese provide large amounts of protein and can be prepared in a variety of ways. Yeast is particularly high in protein and in vitamin B. Dried skimmed milk is very useful for fortifying drinks taken between meals and can be added to muffins, sauces, and many other foods.

The nurse should learn what the patient likes to eat, what particular foods cause him most distress, and what foods he tolerates well. She should learn what meal schedule for the day seems to suit him best. For example, does he tolerate and enjoy frequent small meals? Does he like snacks between meals? Does he like the heaviest meal at noon or at the end of the day? She should convey this information to the dietitian so that meals for the hospitalized patient may be similar to those eaten at home.

Often the patient eats best when comment about his appetite is kept to a minimum. Mouthwashes before meals help to relieve the unpleasant sensation and taste in the mouth that interfere with appetite and that are so common in patients with hepatic disease. Meals should be attractively served, with hot foods hot and cold foods cold. Diversion during meals helps to improve appetite. Some patients find that drinking effervescent fluids instead of water during the meal helps to relieve nausea and the feeling of flatulence after meals. The patient should rest for a half hour immediately after concluding a meal. Almost any exceptions in dietary regulations should be made to get what the patient needs and will eat. If the patient is hospitalized, members of his family may be permitted to bring foods that he likes and will eat, provided that these foods conform to the diet prescribed and that this practice is approved by the doctor. The dietitian should be informed if this is done. Alcohol, however, to stimulate appetite or for any other purpose is usually not ordered for patients with hepatic disease since it may be taxing to an injured liver.

Protection from infections and drugs

The patient with severe hepatic or biliary disease is a ready candidate for *infection*. His resistance is so low that infections are easily acquired and shed with difficulty. Also, infections produce toxins that must be dealt with by the liver. The patient should be protected from exposure to infection of any kind. If he is seriously ill, he should be in a single room, and no one who has a cold should be admitted, including medical and nursing staff as well as visitors.

A large number of *drugs* such as morphine sulfate and chlorpromazine are toxic to the injured liver. Furthermore, drugs such as the barbiturates may not be disposed of at the usual rate if hepatic function is impaired. Therefore, physical symptoms such as restlessness should be alleviated by nursing care so that medications can be avoided. The usual nursing measures such as a back rub, attention to ventilation, and a warm drink should be tried before resorting to sedatives for sleep, and an ice cap should be tried before codeine or other drugs are given for a headache. Even if the patient has little or no jaundice, the liver should be protected from possible additional injury by drugs.

Diseases of the liver and pancreas

Viral hepatitis

Viral hepatitis is by far the most important infection attacking the liver. Although the disease is not new, it assumed serious proportions during World War II. Since that time it has become a major public health problem in the United States as well as in many other countries and has been studied intensively.

Incidence. Viral hepatitis is a reportable disease in most states. While there is a downward trend in its incidence since 1960-1961, 37,740 cases were reported in the United States in 1964.[25] The data are not separated as to infectious or homologous serum strains, but it generally is believed that the largest number of cases are due to the infectious type. Although viral hepatitis is not a major cause of death, in 1964 it ranked second only to influenza as a cause of death from acute viral infection.[25] Homologous serum hepatitis has a somewhat higher mortality rate than infectious hepatitis, but it is thought that its higher rate may be due to the fact that many patients who are given plasma or blood transfusions are already quite ill. It is also believed that lowered host resistance, rather than a higher virulence of the virus, may be the cause of death.

It is estimated that at least 10% of all patients suffer some residual hepatic damage for as long as a year after an attack of viral hepatitis and that at least 2% have hepatic damage persisting much longer. The disease has not been under study long enough to determine whether or not cirrhosis or other severe degeneration of the liver occurs many years after the acute onset of the disease. However, Denmark, which had a large epidemic of viral hepatitis in the 1940's, has had an increase in deaths from chronic disease of the liver in the past fifteen years.

One attack of viral hepatitis confers immunity for that strain of virus infection but does not protect against attack by the other virus. However, the disease can become chronic, with acute exacerbations occurring months after the first acute symptoms have subsided. Hepatic damage following attack by one virus naturally lessens the body's defenses if attack by the second virus should occur.

Viral hepatitis seems to be most prevalent in low-income areas where there is crowding and limited sanitation. Susceptibility to the disease is highest between 6 and 25 years of age, but there is a trend toward an increased incidence in adults, particularly in the older age groups.[5] Recent studies show that pregnant women are highly susceptible to viral hepatitis during the second and third trimesters of pregnancy and that the mortality rate is extremely high in the last trimester.

Viral hepatitis is prevalent in orphanages, schools, and housing projects, where the high concentration of children produces an optimum setting for contact spread. In many ways the epidemiologic pattern of this disease resembles that of poliomyelitis. It appears to be a seasonal disease. The incidence is highest in the fall and early winter. Major outbreaks seem to occur about every seven years, although this pattern is not the same for all parts of the country. Larger epidemics seem to follow a few scattered, small epidemics among children.

Causative agents—conduct and mode of transmission. Viral hepatitis is believed to be caused by filtrable viruses. Since these viruses are not transmissible from man to experimental animals, study of the disease is difficult. The viruses of hepatitis appear to be extremely resistant to usual methods of destruction of pathogenic agents, such as drying, freezing, and exposure to various infecting agents. There is no proof that boiling for less than thirty minutes is effective in its destruction. Autoclaving is the best way to destroy the virus.

Viral hepatitis is caused by two distinct but similar viruses that produce almost identical symptoms but that vary in their incubation period and mode of transmission. These viruses are known as the "A" or IH virus (short-incubation virus), which causes infectious hepatitis, and the "B" or SH virus (long-incubating virus), which causes homologous serum hepatitis. The incubation period for the IH virus is ten to forty days, for the SH virus, probably two to six months.

The source of the virus causing *infectious hepatitis* is human blood and human feces. The infection is spread by the oral intake of food, milk, or water contaminated with the virus or by the parenteral introduction of the hepatitis virus through blood, blood products, or the equipment used for venipuncture or other procedures that require penetrating the skin. Biting insects, urine, and nasopharyngeal secretions also may be sources of the virus, but this possibility is still unproved. The virus is excreted in the feces long before clinical symptoms appear, and they may remain for long periods of time in the feces of persons who have had the disease and in carriers. It is not known whether carriers are natural carriers or whether they have had the disease in a less severe and unrecognized form. It is known that mild, subclinical disease that is not severe enough to cause jaundice can occur.

The only source of the virus that causes *homologous serum hepatitis* is the blood of persons who have the infection or who are carriers of the virus. The virus is transmitted parenterally through blood, serum, or plasma or through equipment used for venipuncture or pricking the skin. The increased use of blood transfusions in recent years has led to a higher incidence of homologous serum hepatitis, although the chance of acquiring it by this means is much less than when pooled plasma is given. In the use of pooled plasma the chances are increased proportionately by the number of donors whose plasma is used. Any immunizing or therapeutic agent made from human plasma can be a means of transmitting the disease to persons who receive the product by injection. There is no acquired immunity to homologous serum hepatitis, and anyone who is exposed may develop the disease despite age. Homologous serum hepatitis can be transmitted from infected patients to medical, nursing, and other hospital personnel by accidentally pricking the skin with needles contaminated by a patient's blood.

Prevention. It is in the area of prevention that the nurse can make her greatest contribution to the control of viral hepatitis. Since there is no specific treatment for the disease and no adequate immunization, it is only by making use of what is known about the viruses that control can be accomplished.

Methods of destroying the viruses of hepatitis are limited. Therefore, particular emphasis should be placed on *thorough washing of hands* with soap and running water after possible exposure. The patient should be taught how to wash his hands thoroughly, and should know why this is necessary, particularly after having a bowel movement. Thorough washing of all equipment that might be contaminated lessens the danger to persons who must handle it and may help protect the next patient for whom the equipment is used. Since infectious hepatitis can be transmitted by infected stool and contaminated foods and water, food handlers should be encouraged to pay careful attention to hand-washing regulations.

At the present time dry heat and steam heat under pressure (autoclaving) are the only safe ways to sterilize needles and other equipment used to penetrate the skin. The adequate boiling time is still undetermined, and for this reason many hospitals are converting to autoclave sterilization and the use of sterile, disposable syringes and needles almost entirely. Although the nurse cannot set the policy in such matters for the hospital or the public health agency where she is employed, by careful planning she can often see that almost all equipment is autoclaved and that boiling is resorted to only in emergencies. When boiling is the only way to sterilize needles and other equipment, the nurse should see that everything placed in the sterilizer is *covered completely and boiled for at least a half hour.*[10] (See fundamentals of nursing texts for the proper method of sterilizing equipment by boiling.)

Both infectious hepatitis and homologous serum hepatitis can be transmitted from one patient to another when several doses of a drug are put into one syringe and only the needle is changed between patients. Drug addicts who use communal syringes and needles are likely to be exposed to hepatitis. The use of communal syringes and/or needles is a dangerous practice under any circumstances and should never be used. Regardless of the extra expense involved and the extra time and work entailed in preparation of materials for each injection, separate needles and syringes that have been autoclaved or disposable syringes and needles should be used. School immunization programs and practices in large outpatient clinics such as allergy clinics have been affected by recent recommendations in this regard. The nurse often must help explain the need for the extra cost to administrative personnel.

If the nurse is in a postion in which she is responsible for obtaining blood specimens for laboratory tests, she should insist that only autoclaved lancets or needles be used to prick the skin and that only autoclaved or sterile, disposable needles and syringes be used in taking blood. All syringes that are to be reused should be autoclaved since a vacuum may be created when the blood is being taken that can draw contaminants such as viruses from the syringe into the patient's vein. Soaking equipment in alcohol or any of the commonly used antiseptics is useless. In fact, no chemical sterilization is safe against the virus of homologous serum hepatitis.[10]

Since there are carriers of the IH and SH viruses, all needles and other equipment that have penetrated the skin of any patient should be handled with the greatest care. Homologous serum hepatitis occurs quite frequently among hospital personnel. This is not surprising considering how often the nurse, the laboratory worker, or other member of the nursing staff may unwittingly prick himself with needles that have been used for a wide variety of parenteral treatments. The safest way to handle any needle that is to be sterilized and reused is to rinse it carefully in plain water after use and to place it in a rack that can be immersed in a solvent or soap solution. This practice is now in use in some institutions and agencies where all needles are cared for by a central sterile supply department or by a special staff. Also, special washers that provide efficient cleansing of both needles and syringes with a minimum of handling are now available. Needles from infusion sets should be removed immediately from the tubing when an infusion is discontinued so that persons cleaning the equipment at a later time will not accidentally prick themselves. Disposable syringes and needles should be collected in a closed container for disposal lest garbage handlers accidentally become injured by them and contract the disease. This practice also obviates the problem, which has been reported in some areas,

of children and even adults finding and using them for undirected purposes.

It is recommended that patients with infectious hepatitis be isolated for seven days,[1] although there is no record that the disease has been directly transmitted to persons caring for a patient in the hospital. If the patient is isolated, he should be told why isolation is necessary and how long it will last. Regardless of whether or not the patient is isolated, the greatest caution should be taken in handling his stool and in performing treatments that involve contamination of the hands. Bedpans should be isolated and should be autoclaved following the patient's discharge from the hospital. Rubber gloves are often advised when enemas are given. In most localities feces need not be treated if proper sewage disposal is available. If there is any doubt, the local health department should be consulted.

To prevent spread of IH viruses by carriers, it is suggested that individual toilet paper packages, rather than rolls, be used in any public bathroom and that toilets be cleaned with 1% aqueous iodine. The use of disposable seat covers and foot pedals for flushing the toilet would help to reduce the chances of spread of the infection.

All patients should have individual thermometers, and the thermometer used for a patient with infectious hepatitis should be discarded upon his discharge from the hospital. Since there is no really safe and satisfactory method of sterilizing a thermometer, discarding it is the only way to be certain that the disease will not spread by it. The cost of the thermometer is relatively small. For the protection of the nursing personnel, the patient's temperature should be taken by mouth whenever possible. When small children must have the temperature taken rectally, the greatest care should be given to washing hands thoroughly. Poor technique in carrying out temperature-taking procedures has been suspected as a cause of widespread infection from the IH virus in foundling homes and similar sheltered care facilities for children.

The virus of infectious hepatitis has never been found in urine; therefore, no special protection is needed in the handling of urinary excretions. However, because the virus usually is transmitted by the oral route from contaminated hands and food, special care should be taken in handling nose and mouth secretions. The patient should be instructed to use tissues, which are placed in a paper bag and burned. Disposable dishes are best to use. Food waste should be burned and dishes boiled for thirty minutes or (ideally) autoclaved. If feasible, utensils may be washed in the patient's room and autoclaved upon his discharge. Rooms should be cleaned well and aired when the patient leaves the hospital. No isolation is necessary for homologous serum hepatitis since it is transmitted only by contamination from the patient's blood and blood plasma. If any doubt exists as to which of the virus diseases a patient has, it is safest to isolate him for seven days and to take the precautions necessary in the care of patients with infectious hepatitis.

Anyone who has been exposed to viral hepatitis should be urged to report this fact to the doctor. This is especially important for a woman in the second or third trimester of pregnancy. Although the role of transplacentally transmitted viral hepatitis in causing injury to the liver in newborn infants has not been determined, the disease is believed to increase the likelihood of abortion, stillbirth, and congenital abnormalities.[5] Gamma globulin offers some protection against infectious hepatitis, but it does not protect against the SH virus of homologous serum hepatitis. However, since often it cannot be determined which of the two diseases is involved, gamma globulin usually is given in the hope that exposure was to the IH virus of infectious hepatitis. Although gamma globulin and serum albumin are obtained from the blood, they do not transmit the virus of homologous serum hepatitis. Therefore, their administration cannot expose the patient to this disease.

Recently a simple test for bilirubinuria, the *Ictotest*, has been developed. Since bilirubin is present in the urine of the person who has viral hepatitis before clinical signs appear, it has been suggested that this test be done on anyone exposed to infectious hepatitis, all schoolchildren, hospital patients and employees, blood donors, employees in public institutions and industrial plants, and food handlers as part of a disease detection program. Early recognition of the disease would make control of its spread easier. The test is done by placing five drops of urine on the Ictotest reagent tablet.

Symptoms and pathology. The clinical symptoms of viral hepatitis vary. Patients may be asymptomatic and show minimal laboratory evidence of hepatic disturbance. Some patients may have many symptoms of the disease but no jaundice. A few may have fulminating necrosis of the liver and die. In most instances, however, viral hepatitis is a mild disease, and complete recovery is the rule.[5] Symptoms and pathology in infectious hepatitis and homologous serum jaundice are almost identical, except that acute symptoms may be more severe in infectious hepatitis. Symptoms usually appear from four to seven days before jaundice is apparent and may consist of headache, anorexia, nausea and vomiting, chills, elevation of temperature, aches and pains, malaise, and tenderness over the liver. Often the patient who smokes has a sudden distaste for tobacco. Examination of blood cells reveals a leukopenia. The temperature usually returns to normal when jaundice appears, but the anorexia and nausea persist. Children usually have a milder, nonicteric form of infectious hepatitis with symptoms predominantly those of an intestinal or respiratory illness.

Viral hepatitis causes diffuse degeneration and necrosis of liver cells. Inflammatory reaction and regeneration also occur, and all processes may be going on simultaneously. Because the pathologic process is usually distributed evenly throughout the liver, biopsy has been particularly useful in studying and diagnosing the disease. In most instances of nonfatal viral hepatitis, regeneration begins almost with the onset of the disease. The damaged cells and their contents eventually are removed by phagocytosis and enzymatic reaction, and the liver returns to normal.[5] The outcome of viral hepatitis may be affected by such factors as the virulence of the virus, the amount of hepatic damage sustained during the patient's life before exposure to the virus, his natural barriers to damage and disease of the liver, and the supportive care he receives when symptoms appear. The disease may take several courses, and different terms describe each of them.

Fulminating viral hepatitis designates a sudden and severe degeneration and atrophy of the liver. This condition may follow acute poisoning, but it most often is associated with an overwhelming infection with the hepatitis virus that progresses rapidly to cause death. The liver may shrink in size to as little as 600 grams, in contrast to a weight of 1,500 grams in a normal adult.

Subacute fatal viral hepatitis causes acute massive necrosis, which, even though it is not evenly distributed throughout the organ, finally destroys enough of the liver to cause death. This form of the disease may vary in duration from several weeks to several months, with apparent short remissions followed by exacerbations. In its late stages subacute fatal viral hepatitis is almost impossible to distinguish from cirrhosis of the liver in clinical manifestations and in liver function tests. However, history of exposure to viral hepatitis and symptoms of acute infection aid in diagnosis.

Chronic forms of the disease are still not well understood. Signs of chronicity may persist in biopsied hepatic tissue when liver function tests show no abnormality and when no clinical signs are evident. However, the opposite may be true. Acute exacerbations of chronic viral hepatitis can progress to acute fatal hepatic necrosis.

Cholestatic hepatitis is a condition in which stasis occurs in the bile canaliculi, while bile ducts within and outside the liver remain normal. It is thought to be due to viral hepatitis, although the same or very similar pathologic changes occur in the liver after ingestion of some drugs, such as chlorprozamine (Thorazine). Cholestatic hepatitis is presumed to be caused by increased permeability of the cholangioles (ductules that carry the bile to the intrahepatic ducts), causing bile to be regurgitated into the blood. Obstruction of the cholangioles follows since not all constituents of the bile are absorbed. Cholestatic hepatitis is more likely to occur in older patients. Jaundice is present and the stools are acholic. Itching may be a major complaint.

Medical treatment and nursing care. There is no specific medical treatment for viral hepatitis. Physical activity is restricted during the acute phase, and the patient is kept in bed. General care, including attention to good oral hygiene, skin care, and elimination, is necessary. Special attention should be paid to protecting the patient from infection. The nurse who cares for the patient in his own home should observe carefully for changes in the color of urine and stool and for jaundice and should report her findings at once to the physician.

During the acute stage of the disease, fluids are encouraged by mouth if nausea is not a problem. The desirable fluid intake usually is considered to be at least 3,000 ml. per day. If the patient's temperature is high and nausea and vomiting are severe, infusions containing glucose are given, and occasionally solutions containing other electrolytes and protein hydrolysates are ordered. Fluid intake and output are recorded. Occasionally a record of daily weight is requested to determine whether there is water retention in acute stages of the disease. When chronic disease has developed, the patient is weighed daily if ascites or edema is suspected.

When the appetite has returned to normal, a diet high in calories, proteins, and moderate carbohydrates usually is ordered. Fats may or may not be limited, and vitamins may be given. If necessary, all the nursing measures described on p. 705 should be used to encourage the patient to eat.

During the first few days after the onset of symptoms, the patient feels ill, and keeping him contented in bed is not difficult. However, restlessness becomes a nursing problem if the patient must remain in bed several weeks. When the patient begins to feel well, he becomes anxious to resume normal living and is irritated by the circumstances requiring enforced inactivity. His irritation may be expressed, for example, by tiring of the hospital menu, regardless of the quality of the food. The family should realize that in the home he may also be critical of food for the same reason. Wheeling the patient in his bed to the recreation area, where he may view television or converse with others, often helps him pass the day without boredom. Occupational therapy activities that can be brought to the bedside are useful in keeping the patient relatively content during the tiresome convalescent period.

There is a trend toward earlier ambulation of patients with viral hepatitis. When acute symptoms subside and the jaundice begins to recede, the patient may be permitted to walk about in his room with periods of rest after each meal. Activities are increased gradually, and if there are no adverse effects, the patient may be permitted to convalesce at home under close medical supervision. Recurrence of anorexia, enlargement or tenderness of the liver, or lack of progress as shown by studies of hepatic function indicate a need to return to bed rest. Some patients are cared for at home from the onset of symptoms to complete recovery. With the assistance of a public health nurse, many families are able to care for the patient safely and adequately.

Abscess of the liver

The most common cause of an abscess of the liver is infection with *Entamoeba histolytica,* the causative organism in amebic dysentery. Signs of hepatic involvement may appear several months after an attack of amebic dysentery. An abscess of the liver also may be caused by a variety of pyogenic organisms, such as *Escherichia coli* or *Staphylococcus aureus,* which are carried by the bloodstream or travel from the biliary ducts. Occasionally an infection in abdominal organs or other structures such as the appendix may lead to an abscess in the liver.

Nausea, vomiting, and jaundice are frequent symptoms of abscesses of the liver. Chills and sweats are common and are followed by temperature elevation, malaise, and dull, constant pain in the area of the liver. Most pyogenic abscesses can be prevented by prompt treatment of intra-abdominal infections with surgery and antibiotics. The treatment of a single abscess consists of drainage of the abscess and administration of antibiotics. Emetine hydrochloride and chloroquine are used in the treatment of the amebic hepatic abscess, followed by aspiration or drainage as indicated. (See p. 670 for discussion of treatment of amebiasis.)

Carcinoma of the liver

Primary carcinoma of the liver is exceedingly rare. Secondary carcinoma, however, is very common and occurs in about one-third of all patients in whom carcinoma has not been controlled by surgery before metastasis occurs. Metastasis to the liver should always be suspected when a patient with a history of carcinoma develops anorexia, weakness, loss of weight, secondary anemia, pain in the right upper quadrant and general ill health. Jaundice and ascites are signs that the process is quite far advanced. The patient may live only a short time after their onset.

Until recently there was no treatment for carcinoma of the liver beyond symptomatic medical and nursing care. Now, provided that the growth is limited to a single lobe and there is no evidence of metastases elsewhere, a *hepatic lobectomy* may be done to remove metastatic as well as primary carcinoma. The remarkable regenerative capacity of the liver permits resection of 70 to 80% of the organ.[5] Preoperatively, the patient is given massive doses of vitamin K, blood volume is ascertained and necessary blood given, and preparation of the bowel is done as for intestinal surgery. Postoperative care may include the care of a patient who has had chest and abdominal surgery plus the general care needed by any patient with dysfunction of the liver. A nasogastric tube usually is inserted and attached to suction. Nothing is given by mouth for several days. Cortisone may be given to enhance liver regeneration. The patient is acutely ill following this surgery and must be attended constantly, with the most careful attention given to changes in vital signs. Hemorrhage is the complication most feared, and myocardial infarction seems to occur readily.

Following surgery of the liver, the patient may be out of bed by the third postoperative day, but he must be attended constantly, and his pulse, blood pressure, and respiratory rate must be checked before, during, and after any exertion, since complications such as hemorrhage may occur.

If the growth has spread throughout the liver, irradiated yttrium or radioactive gold (Au^{198}) may be injected into the metastatic tumor masses through the abdominal wall (percutaneous route). Continuous infusions of antitumor agents such as methotrexate or 5-fluorouracil (5-FUO) into the liver through a catheter inserted into the hepatic artery also may cause regression of the tumor and alleviate symptoms. (For further details and for care of the terminally ill cancer patient, see p. 290.)

Trauma to the liver

Trauma to the liver is fairly commonly associated with automobile accidents or other injuries. There may be rupture of the liver with severe internal hemorrhage and death. Attempts are sometimes made to operate and suture the ruptured organ or to apply local pressure to stop the bleeding.

Trauma to the liver can cause severe contusion, with subsequent degeneration of injured hepatic cells. Prognosis depends upon the amount of tissue damaged and other factors, and the final outcome for the patient may not be known for many years after the injury has been sustained.

Degeneration of the liver

Degeneration of the liver can follow injury, infection, and damage by toxic agents such as incompatible blood. It can be caused by obstruction of biliary passages with subsequent pressure and damage to hepatic cells. It can also be due to the ingestion of substances toxic to the liver, to faulty nutrition, and possibly to other factors not yet understood.

Prevention. The nurse can help in the prevention of degenerative liver disease by teaching the danger of injudicious use of materials that are known to be injurious to the liver and by emphasizing the need for a diet that is protective to the liver.

Since cleaning agents, solvents, and related substances sometimes contain products that are harmful to the liver, the public should read instructions on labels and should follow them implicitly. Dry-cleaning fluids may contain carbon tetrachloride, which can cause injury if warnings to avoid inhalation of the fumes and to keep windows open are not heeded. If people must use these agents inside their home, a good practice is to open the windows wide, clean the materials as quickly as possible, and then vacate the room, the apartment, or the house for several hours, leaving the windows open.

The "do-it-yourself" movement has increased the danger of hepatic damage from poisons. Many solvents that are used to remove paint and plastic material and to stain and finish woodwork contain injurious substances and should be used outdoors and not even in the basement, since dangerous fumes may spread throughout the house. Cleaning agents and finishes for cars should be applied with the garage door open or outdoors. Nurses in industry have a responsibility to teach the importance of observing regulations to avoid industrial hazards. Nitrobenzene, tetrachlorethane, carbon disulfide, and dinitrotoluol are examples of injurious compounds used in industry.

Some drugs that are known to cause mild damage to the liver must be used therapeutically. However, the nurse should warn the public regarding the use of preparations that are available without prescription that may be injurious. Many drugs reach the market before dangers of their extensive use have been conclusively ruled out; for example, chlorpromazine, which was being widely used to control "nerves," is known to cause stasis in the canaliculi of the liver, which may lead to serious hepatic damage. A safe rule to follow is to avoid taking any medication except that specifically prescribed by a physician for a specific ailment.

For many years alcohol has been incriminated as the cause of cirrhosis. While this may be true in certain susceptible persons, the most probable cause of cirrhosis is an inadequate protein intake resulting from the haphazard fashion in which the alcoholic eats. This inadequate diet results in degenerative changes in the liver and subsequent blockage of the portal blood vessels, causing cirrhosis. Since many people have poor eating habits, teaching the principles of proper nutrition and checking on eating habits is an important nursing function for prevention of hepatic damage.

Toxic hepatitis

Toxic hepatitis results from the effects of noninfectious agents such as arsenic and other poisons of infinite variety. Signs and symptoms are not clear-cut, and the disease may resemble viral disease and also degenerative liver disease.

The treatment for toxic hepatitis is to remove or stop the cause if it is known. Rest in bed and general supportive care are presently all that can be done beyond the general measures used for patients with any hepatic disease. Some patients who have severe toxic hepatitis recover with apparently little, if any, residual hepatic damage. Others have severe permanent damage and may develop all the signs and symptoms of cirrhosis of the liver. The patient who recovers from an attack of toxic hepatitis should be instructed to avoid additional injury for the rest of his life.

Cirrhosis of the liver

Cirrhosis of the liver usually refers to portal cirrhosis and also is called *Laennec's cirrhosis.* There is no question that cirrhosis of the liver and alcoholism often appear together. The National Institute of Statistics reports that France, a country that has been plagued with the problem of alcoholism during recent years, had 14,176 deaths from cirrhosis in a population of 43 million, or 32.5 fatalities per 100,000 population, in 1956. Of all alcoholics who died in France during that year, 80% had a diagnosis of cirrhosis of the liver.[19] However, the relationship between alcoholism and cirrhosis is not absolute. There are many persons who drink heavily but who do not develop cirrhosis, and almost half of those who develop cirrhosis have never consumed alcohol. It is believed that malnutrition is a primary cause of cirrhosis, although other factors, such as previous damage from toxins or from infections such as viral hepatitis and schistosomiasis, may contribute. Cirrhosis sometimes follows rigid dieting by women who are intent upon retaining a slim figure but who do not choose proper foods. For many patients, there is no known cause.

Incidence. Although cirrhosis is considered a disease of late middle life, it may occur in younger persons. It is not common in children in the United States but occurs relatively frequently in children in the Orient and Near East. In 1964, cirrhosis of the liver was the tenth leading cause of death in the United States.[25]

Pathology. The symptoms of cirrhosis are caused by the progressive destruction of hepatic cells. The resultant regeneration and proliferation of interstitial tissue with fibrosis causes obstruction of the portal vein, which the body attempts to circumvent by establishing collateral circulation. *Ascites,* or fluid in the abdomen, usually follows obstruction of the portal vein and occasionally is one of the first signs of cirrhosis, although it usually does not occur until the disease is quite far advanced and jaundice has become marked.

Once the disease is established, it usually advances slowly to cause death. Many patients, however, can be helped to live for years if they follow instructions to protect their liver from further damage. The liver has remarkable powers of regeneration. Sometimes sufficient collateral circulation can be established and sufficient repair of hepatic tissue can be accomplished so that symptoms subside for long periods of time. At other times the patient appears to be doing fairly well when the liver suddenly gives up its battle and the patient dies in coma within a few days.

Signs and symptoms. The patient with cirrhosis may have a long history of failing health, with vague complaints of gastrointestinal distress, fatigue, and low resistance to mild infections. There may be weight loss, depression, headache, and slight elevation of temperature. As the disease advances, typical signs of severe anemia, including malaise and memory loss, may occur. Venules on the head and upper body become markedly distended, and spider angiomas (tiny, bright red, pulsating arterioles that disappear on pressure) frequently appear. Veins may be prominent in the lower extremities as the patient loses weight. The skin becomes thin and dry, and edema appears in the lower trunk and lower extremities. Sometimes jaundice, first apparent in the sclerae of the eyes, is the first sign that something is wrong. Increased pressure may develop in the portal system. This pressure, in turn, increases the pressure in the esophageal veins, and varicosities may develop in them. Occasionally, gastric hemorrhage following rupture of a varicosed esophageal vein and drainage of blood into the stomach are the first indications that the patient has advanced cirrhosis of the liver.

Medical treatment and nursing care. There is no specific treatment for cirrhosis of the liver. Rest, moderate exercise, avoidance of exposure to infections, and protection from toxic agents of any kind are emphasized in treatment, and alcohol usually is forbidden. As the disease progresses, more and more effort must be made to compensate for the failure of the several functions of the liver. Vitamins may be given to compensate for the organ's lost ability to store vitamins A, B complex, D, and K. Bile salts are usually given if the patient is jaundiced because absorption of fat-soluble vitamin A and synthesis of vitamin K are poor due to insufficient bile salts in the intestine. Transfusions may be given to combat marked anemia. Diet is the most important part of treatment and is the most difficult with which to cope. The patient needs constant encouragement to eat enough protein and carbohydrate.

To achieve a remission of threatened hepatic failure in cirrhosis may take a long time. There may be setbacks and periods where there is no improvement. The patient and his family often become discouraged and require encouraging support from the doctor and nurse. Upon discharge from the hospital, visits from the public health nurse

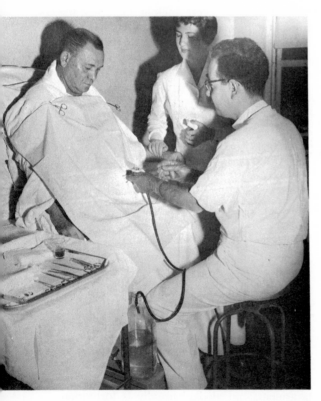

Fig. 163

Careful observation is necessary during a paracentesis. Note the pillows supporting the back and arms of the patient.
The patient's feet are resting on a stool.

may be requested to give whatever care, supervision, and support that seem necessary. The patient must be taught to avoid substances potentially toxic to the liver, such as alcohol and chlorpromazine (Thorazine).

Complications. *Ascites,* or the accumulation of fluid in the abdominal cavity, is a fairly common complication of advanced hepatic disease. This condition may cause discomfort and difficulty in breathing and may require treatment by paracentesis. (For details of this procedure and the nursing care involved, see texts on fundamentals of nursing.) A paracentesis is not without danger to the patient with advanced hepatic disease (Fig. 163). Besides the usual complications that might occur, such as perforation of the bladder, there is danger of hemorrhage from the wound because of the low prothrombin level. In far-advanced cases, fluid may form so fast that it exerts pressure on the wound, preventing its healing, and fluid may drain continuously. This drainage is uncomfortable for the patient and predisposes to infection in the wound. If paracenteses must be done at intervals, it is necessary to supply additional protein. One liter of ascitic fluid contains almost as much protein as 200 ml. of whole blood.[2]

Restriction of sodium aids greatly in limiting the formation of ascitic fluid in disease of the liver. The patient with cirrhosis usually is on a low-sodium diet. The lack of salt in the food makes it less palatable, and the patient may not consume enough protein and total calories. The nurse should report the patient's food intake to the doctor and dietitian, as adjustments may need to be made in the salt restriction. Salt substitutes such as potassium gluconate may be permitted.

Many physicians try to control edema and fluid accumulation in the abdomen by giving diuretics. Removal of fluid through the kidneys has the advantage of usually not removing essential body protein, which is contained in fluid removed from the abdominal cavity. Since a single diuretic usually is not successful, a combination is used. The mercurials, such as meralluride (Mercuhydrin), and the thiazides, such as chlorothiazide (Diuril), inhibit the reabsorption of sodium in the proximal renal tubules. If there is no response to these drugs, spironolactone A,

(Aldactone A) may be added to prevent the absorption of sodium in the distant tubules. Occasionally, one of the glucocorticoids, such as prednisone, may be added. Complications do occur from the administration of these drugs but can be prevented in some instances. For example, the loss of potassium due to the administration of the thiazides can be compensated for by increasing the intake of potassium in foods. Aldactone A may increase the amount of potassium in the blood, and it may be necessary to decrease the potassium intake. The nurse should list the food and fluids that are high in potassium for the patient and his family so that they can make the necessary adjustments in his diet. (See p. 123.[15,20])

Esophagogastric varices are varicosities occurring in the cardiac end of both the stomach and the esophagus and are caused by pressure within the portal venous system with subsequent backing up of venous blood. Esophagogastric varices occur in approximately 30% of all patients with cirrhosis of the liver.[8] The varices may rupture, with flow of blood into the stomach. Severe hematemesis and resultant shock follow, requiring emergency treatment.

Medical treatment. Before shock can be treated adequately, the bleeding must be stopped. Since raising the blood pressure increases the bleeding, drugs and transfusions are used, but only along with mechanical efforts to stop the bleeding. This is done by passing a nasogastric double-balloon tube (Blakemore-Sengstaken tube) within an hour of onset of hemorrhage, if possible (Fig. 164). The tube is passed through the nose into the stomach with the balloon deflated. The tip of the tube has several openings through which stomach contents can be aspirated. When the tube is in the stomach, the distal balloon is inflated with 100 to 150 ml. of air, and the tube is pulled back so

Fig. 164

The esophageal balloon (Blakemore-Sengstaken tube). **A,** Lumen leading to the esophageal balloon. **B,** Lumen leading to the gastric balloon. **C,** Lumen for gastric suction. (See text.)

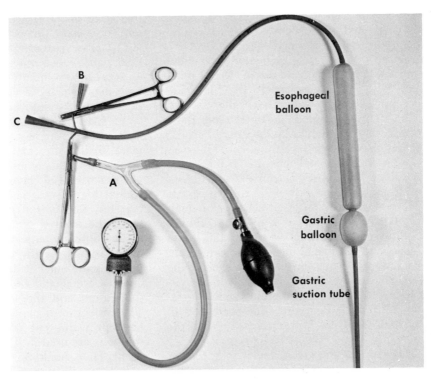

that the balloon is held tightly against the cardia of the stomach. The esophageal balloon is then inflated until the pressure in the balloon, as indicated by the mercury manometer, is raised above the patient's portal venous pressure. A pressure of 20 to 25 mm. Hg or more is usually used. If the bleeding is from esophageal varices, blood will no longer be aspirated from the stomach. If there is blood, the gastric balloon is inflated with 300 to 400 ml. of air, and a 2-pound weight is suspended from the end of the gastric tube for traction and to maintain pressure. Usually this will stop gastric varices from bleeding. Instead of air, a solution of iced alcohol and water may be used to inflate the balloons. The solution is circulated continuously through them and provides hypothermic vasoconstriction as well as pressure. The esophageal balloon can be left inflated up to ninety-six hours without tissue damage or severe discomfort for the patient. The fully inflated gastric balloon with traction exerted on it, however, compresses the stomach wall between the balloon and the diaphragm, causing ulceration of the gastric mucosa, and is severely uncomfortable for the patient. It should be removed within twenty-four hours if at all possible, even though emergency gastric surgery to ligate the varicosed vessels and control bleeding may have to be performed.

A second tube should be in the patient unit ready for immediate use in case of damage to the one being used (the tubes are not reused). The tubes have the date of manufacture stamped on them, and those over a year old should be discarded because of deterioration of the rubber.

As soon as the balloons are in place and bleeding has been controlled, transfusions of fresh blood are given to combat shock. Fresh blood usually is used because the damaged liver may not be able to metabolize citrate from the sodium citrate used in stored blood, and citric acid intoxication can result. Patients who have cirrhosis also excrete the sodium poorly. Refrigerated blood is virtually devoid of prothrombin, which is essential for clotting, and the patient with cirrhosis needs fresh prothrombin to halt the bleeding.

Oxygen may be given, and if so, a tent or catheter is used most often. A saline cathartic such as magnesium sulfate may be given through the nasogastric tube to hasten the expulsion of blood that has passed from the stomach to the intestine, and enemas may also be given. This is in an effort to lessen bacterial action on the blood in the intestinal tract. This action produces ammonia, which passes to the bloodstream and in turn puts a burden on the liver, which must detoxify it to form urea. An antibiotic that destroys intestinal bacteria, such as neomycin, also may be given to lessen their activity in the decomposition of protein in the intestine.

Before removal of the tube, the balloons are deflated gradually, and the tube is then gently withdrawn by the doctor. The patient then should be observed closely for any indications of renewed bleeding.

Nursing care. The patient with bleeding esophagogastric varices is acutely ill and extremely apprehensive. He must be attended constantly, given reassurance, and kept absolutely quiet. All procedures and his part in them should be quietly and calmly explained to him and carried out with the minimum of activity. The family generally is very frightened and should be given as much information as necessary to relieve their concern. Some member of the family should be permitted to see the patient or to stay with him for a short time.

The nurse is responsible for checking the vital signs, which may be observed as often as every fifteen minutes until there are signs that hemorrhage is controlled. The blood pressure cuff should be left on the arm deflated, and care should be taken to inflate it only a few degrees above the anticipated level. In this way many patients may sleep through the taking of blood pressure. The nurse must also check the manometer attached to the esophagogastric tube. If the pressure rises or falls below the prescribed level, the amount of air or solution in the balloon must be adjusted. Often this adjustment is made by the doctor, but it may be made by the nurse if there are orders to that effect. Care should be taken to see that the transfusion and the infusions are running. The patient in shock may feel cold and must be kept warm but not perspiring. If iced solutions are used in the balloons, chills may occur. They should be reported to the doctor.

Because the inflated esophageal balloon

occludes the esophagus, the patient cannot take anything by mouth or even swallow his saliva. He should be provided with cleansing tissues and an emesis basin. The patient needs frequent mouth care, and all blood in his mouth should be removed. If he is very weak or if he is not permitted to move at all, gentle suctioning of the mouth and throat may be needed to prevent aspiration of saliva. The nostrils should be kept clean, lubricated, and protected so that tissues do not sustain injury because of pressure from the tube. A commercial disk that fits against the nares and through which the tube is inserted gives good protection. Cotton may be used and should surround the tube as it leaves the nostril. A tiny piece of sponge rubber may also help prevent pressure. Care must be taken not to disturb the tube, and the nurse should consult with the doctor as to how much movement the patient is permitted. Passive moving of extremities usually is allowed.

Surgical treatment and nursing care. Since bleeding from esophageal varices usually is caused by portal hypertension due to obstruction of blood flow somewhere in the portal venous system, curative treatment is aimed at locating the site of obstruction by x-ray examination and then reducing the flow of blood through that portion of the portal system. Depending on the location of the obstruction, various operative procedures may be employed. If the splenic vein is blocked, a *splenectomy* may be done. If the block is intrahepatic, a *portacaval anastomosis* (portacaval shunt) may be done. The portal vein is anastomosed to the inferior vena cava so that the blood from the portal system bypasses the liver (Fig. 165). When the portal vein is blocked, the spleen may be removed and the splenic vein anastomosed to the left renal vein. This procedure is called a *splenorenal shunt* and relieves pressure on the portal vein since approximately 30% of the blood in the portal vein comes from the splenic vein.[8] If there is no portal hypertension, the varicosed vessels may be ligated through a thoracotomy incision.

Careful preoperative preparation is necessary since it must be remembered that the patient with liver damage severe enough to cause bleeding varices is not a good operative risk. If he also has marked ascites, the operation is not attempted. The patient is usually apprehensive about the recommended operation, yet in selected cases it is known that the operative risk is much less than the risk from recurring hemorrhage. Vitamin K, antibiotics, and transfusions are usually given preoperatively.

Following surgery the patient needs close observation and often constant nursing attention. Narcotics should be given for severe pain, but sedative drugs usually are avoided because of the disease of the liver. The patient must be encouraged to breathe deeply and to cough hourly. Fluid intake and output must be recorded accurately, and lessening of output must be reported since renal function sometimes decreases for a time following this operation. Hemorrhage may occur since prothrombin levels may be lowered.

Some surgeons do not pass a nasogastric tube because of danger of injury to the varices. Others pass a soft rubber tube and attach it to suction postoperatively since it is believed that postoperative distention may predispose to thrombosis of the portal vein. In either instance the patient is fed intravenously and given nothing by mouth until signs of active peristalsis are apparent. The patient is observed closely for pain, distention, fever, and nausea, which may be signs of thrombosis at the site of anastomosis. *Regional heparinization* may be employed to prevent thrombus formation at operation. A fine polyethylene catheter is inserted into the right gastroepiploic vein, brought out through the wound, and attached to a continuous drip of heparin and saline solution. The surgeon determines the rate of flow. The catheter may be left for five to seven days, and during this time the nurse must see that it is not obstructed or subjected to tension in any way. During heparinization, the patient remains in bed or sits by the bedside. Particular attention should be paid, therefore to exercising the lower extremities in an attempt to prevent thrombi from developing.

Some surgeons prefer to keep the patient flat in bed for several days until the anastomosis is healed. Others have their patients get out of bed on the day after the operation. Leg and arm exercises are begun on the day after surgery. The lower extrem-

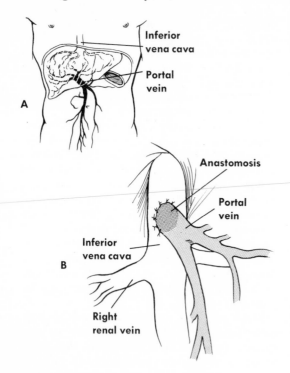

Fig. 165

Portacaval shunt. **A,** the normal relationship of the portal vein to the inferior vena cava. **B,** the anastomosis of the portal vein to the inferior vena cava.

ities must be observed carefully for signs of edema, which may follow the sudden increase of blood flow into the inferior vena cava. Elevation of the lower extremities may be ordered, and the length of time the patient spends standing and walking should be medically prescribed.

After a shunting procedure, none of the venous blood passes through the liver, and protein end products are not completely detoxified. For this reason, the patient is occasionally placed on a low-protein diet. Neomycin or chlortetracycline (Aureomycin), or both of which destroy the bacteria in the intestine, may be given so that fewer bacteria remain to break down protein.

Hepatic coma

Hepatic coma, or liver coma, is a serious condition caused by failure of the liver to perform certain of its metabolic functions. It may occur as a complication of bleeding esophogeal varices or of operative procedures such as portacaval shunt, or it may occur in far-advanced hepatic disease of any cause. Often it comes on suddenly, and the prognosis is then poorer than if the onset were gradual. Signs and symptoms include changes in personality and behavior, lethargy, confusion, twitching, and a characteristic flapping tremor of the extremities, dizziness, stupor, and coma. A peculiar sweetish odor can frequently be detected on the breath (fetor hepaticus). The patient's temperature may rise markedly. Symptoms may follow a sudden increase in jaundice or in ascites.

Most patients in hepatic coma have been found to have increased ammonia in the blood. The ammonia is formed in the intestine in the breakdown of protein by bacteria and normally would be converted by a functioning liver to urea. Treatment includes eliminating protein from the diet completely for several days, giving carbohydrates by mouth or nasogastric feedings, and administering antibiotics, such as neomycin, that destroy bacteria in the intestine and subsequently reduce the amount of ammonia formed. Cathartics such as magnesium sulfate are given in most cases. Some physicians prefer to rely upon cathartics and upon the use of cation exchange resins to help remove toxic substances from the bowel rather than to give the antibiotics. These antibiotics destroy bacteria, which are active in the manufacture of vitamin K, and the absence of bacteria causes diarrhea and other symptoms.[27] (See p. 432 for care when exchange resins are used.) Sodium glutamate and L-arginine are sometimes given intravenously in a solution of glucose in an attempt to stimulate the formation of urea and reduce the amount of ammonia in the blood, but these two substances have not been proved to be of definite benefit.[2] Large doses of adrenal steroids are sometimes effective in reversing the process if hepatic cell destruction has not been overwhelming.

The supportive nursing care required by any patient with hepatic disease as well as by any unconscious patient should be given. If the patient survives, long-term care as discussed for the patient with cirrhosis of the liver should be planned. The patient who has had definite or threatened hepatic coma may be kept indefinitely on a diet low in protein.

Pancreatitis

Pancreatitis is an inflammation of the pancreas. There may be edema of the tissues, suppuration and abscess formation, necrosis, or hemorrhage, depending upon the cause and the severity of the disease. The chief cause is the obstruction of the pancreatic duct by stones, tumors, or inflammatory strictures that prevent the free flow of pancreatic secretions into the duodenum. Regurgitation of bile through the pancreatic duct and activation of proteolytic enzymes in the pancreatic juice also cause pancreatitis. It may be caused by infection carried by the bloodstream or traveling from the biliary system or the duodenum. Many of the patients with acute pancreatitis have associated disease of the biliary tract or are chronic alcoholics.[8]

The most common type of *acute pancreatitis* is known as the edematous type and often is associated with chronic biliary tract disease. The patient has constant pain radiating to the back which may be so severe that he is unable to lie on his side. The pain may be so excruciating that it causes shock. Nausea and vomiting, elevation of temperature, and elevation of white blood cell count often are present, and jaundice may occur. Elevated serum and urine amylase levels often help the doctor to distinguish acute pancreatitis from other acute conditions of the abdomen or from coronary artery disease.

Meperidine hydrochloride (Demerol) combined with nitroglycerin or papaverine may be given for pain and to relieve spasms of the sphincter of Oddi. Occasionally, the intravenous administration of procaine hydrochloride or a splanchnic nerve block may be necessary to relieve the pain. Nothing is permitted by mouth because of nausea and because it would stimulate pancreatic secretions and aggravate symptoms. Propantheline bromide (Pro-Banthine bromide) or atropine sulfate may be given parenterally to depress vagal stimulation of pancreatic secretions. Antibiotics may be administered to control infections. A nasogastric tube usually is inserted and attached to suction. Intravenous

fluids and appropriate electrolytes are administered. If shock is present, it may be treated with transfusions of blood, plasma, or dextran.

An exploratory laparotomy may be performed in acute pancreatitis when a diagnosis cannot be established and the possibility of general peritonitis, perforation of an organ, or a bowel obstruction cannot be excluded. If cholecystitis or cholelithiasis are present, an operation may be performed when the patient can tolerate surgery. An operation also is sometimes done in an attempt to divert or increase bile flow at the sphincter of Oddi (entrance to the duodenum) and thereby reduce regurgitation of bile into the pancreatic duct.

A much less common but more severe form of acute pancreatitis is known as acute hemorrhagic pancreatitis. This fulminating process may cause severe necrosis of pancreatic tissues with destruction by its own enzymes and hemorrhage into the gland with release of blood exudate into the abdominal cavity. The patient goes quickly into shock, which must be treated immediately. An operation may be done to drain blood or other fluid from the abdominal cavity. Despite intensive medical treatment and the best of nursing care, the mortality rate is high.

Pancreatitis can become *chronic* with calcification and fibrous replacement of normal duct tissue. Nausea, persistent pain, loss of weight, and occasionally jaundice occur. The danger of addiction to narcotics becomes a problem with patients who have chronic pancreatitis, particularly alcoholics. If there is extensive damage to the islet cells, diabetes mellitus may complicate the disease.

Tumors of the pancreas

Tumors of the pancreas are usually malignant and occur most often in the head of the pancreas, causing jaundice and obstruction. Men are affected much more often than women. Usually the patient is past middle life, and obvious signs such as severe pain and jaundice may have been preceded by vague anorexia, nausea, and weight loss over a period of months. Surgery is usually done in an attempt to remove the tumor from the head of the pancreas.

If the tumor is operable, a pancreaticoduodenal resection (Whipple procedure), which includes removal of the head of the pancreas, the lower end of the common bile duct, the duodenum, and the distal stomach, may be done. The common bile duct and the remaining portion of the pancreas and stomach are then anastomosed to the jejunum. If the tumor is not resectable, a palliative operation, such as a cholecystojejunostomy, a choledochojejunostomy, or a palliative gastrojejunostomy, may be done to help restore temporarily a normal flow of bile and some pancreatic enzyme to the intestinal tract. The type of procedure performed depends on the involvement found at operation. Palliation of the symptoms also may be achieved by the administration of chemotherapeutic agents such as 5-fluorouracil.[8]

In addition to routine postoperative care following abdominal surgery, the patient who has had pancreatic surgery must be watched for signs of peritonitis, gastrointestinal obstruction, and jaundice until sufficient time for healing has elapsed and until it is determined that all the anastomoses are secure and patent. Stools should be observed, and frothy, light-colored stools containing conspicuously undigested fat should be reported. If most of the pancreas was removed, the patient may have to take pancreatic enzymes in tablet form by mouth to aid the digestion of fat. The patient should be watched for signs and symptoms of diabetes mellitus following this procedure, although it rarely occurs unless the entire pancreas has been removed. If hypoinsulinism occurs, treatment with insulin will be necessary for the remainder of the patient's life (p. 746). The average duration of life after the Whipple procedure is about a year.

Occasionally a patient may have an islet cell tumor of the pancreas. It is a benign lesion in the tail of the pancreas and results in overproduction of insulin, causing symptoms of hypoglycemia (p. 753). Surgical removal of the tumor relieves symptoms.

Disease of the biliary system

There are no specific means to prevent disease of the biliary system. However, since disease of this system occurs much more often in obese persons, it is reasonable to suppose that control of obesity may con-

tribute to its prevention. Women are more often affected than men, and the description, "fair, fat, and forty," is a fairly accurate one. Married women who spend most of their time at home may add more calories than they realize by "eating up leftovers." In all health education, the nurse should stress the importance of avoiding excess weight. Patients with biliary tract disease are usually advised to keep fat intake to a fairly low level for the remainder of their lives, although no rigid dietary regulations are needed. Patients who tend to form stones in the ducts are usually advised to be particularly careful of their fat intake and to take generous amounts of fluids. The nurse should emphasize the doctor's instructions in this regard.

Cholecystitis

Inflammation of the gallbladder is called cholecystitis. This condition may be acute or chronic and usually is associated with gallstones or other obstructions of bile passage.

A large variety of organisms may contribute to acute disease of the gallbladder. Colon bacilli, staphylococci, streptococci, salmonellae, typhoid bacilli, and many other organisms have been found. Infection may reach the gallbladder through the bloodstream, the lymph system, or the bile ducts. Inflammation may be confined to the mucous membrane lining, or the entire wall of the gallbladder may be involved. Sometimes damage to the wall of the gallbladder results from distention caused by obstruction of bile flow and from contractions of the smooth muscle as it attempts to dislodge a stone occluding the lumen of one of the bile ducts. Cholecystitis is more common in women than in men, the ratio being 2.5:1. Sedentary obese persons are affected most often, and the incidence is highest in the fifth and sixth decades of life. The incidence of cholecystitis and the mortality rate are high in the elderly.[22]

Acute cholecystitis may be abrupt in onset, although the patient often has a history of intolerance to fatty foods and some general indigestion. Nausea and vomiting usually occur, and there is severe pain in the right upper quadrant of the abdomen. The patient's pulse rate and respiratory rate are increased, and temperature and white blood count are elevated. The chronic form of the disease is usually preceded by several acute attacks of moderate severity, and the patient gives a history of having learned to avoid fried foods and certain other food, such as nuts, that are high in fat.

The treatment for cholecystitis is surgical. The decision as to when to operate depends largely on the age and condition of the patient and the way he responds to treatment. Although some surgeons favor conservative treatment until the acute infection has subsided, others believe that the danger of rupture and subsequent peritonitis is so great that immediate surgery to drain the gallbladder is advisable (*cholecystostomy*). Both recommended removing the gallbladder (*cholecystectomy*) when the acute condition has subsided. Infection may spread to the hepatic duct and liver, causing inflammation of the ducts, with subsequent strictures that may cause obstruction of bile flow and that are exceedingly difficult to correct surgically.

Medical treatment includes the administration of antibiotics and infusions of glucose and appropriate electrolytes. Food is withheld until acute symptoms subside. If vomiting persists, a nasogastric tube is passed and attached to suction. Meperidine hydrochloride (Demerol) may be given for pain, although it is thought by some authorities to increase spasm of the biliary sphincter. The inhalation of amyl nitrite may diminish intestinal and biliary spasms.

When food is tolerated, a reducing diet and careful avoidance of too much fat usually are recommended by the doctor. Patients who have had acute attacks are more strongly motivated to follow dietary instructions, and the nurse may be of real help to them in planning attractive dishes that are low in fat and total calories.

Cholelithiasis

Cholelithiasis means the presence of stones in the biliary tract. The stones are composed largely of cholesterin crystals, although some contain calcium. Cholelithiasis may occur in either sex at any age, but it is more common in middle-aged women. The incidence increases gradually thereafter, and one out of every three persons who reach the age of 75

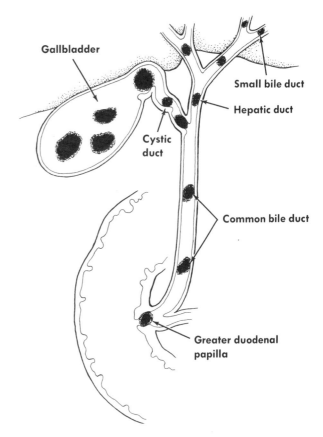

Fig. 166

Common sites of gallstones.

years will have gallstones.[8] It is not known why stones form in the gallbladder and in the hepatic duct. They may be present for years and cause no inflammation. Sometimes they appear to be preceded or followed by chronic cholecystitis. Chronic cholelithiasis is aggravated by pregnancy, perhaps because of the increased pressure in the abdomen.

Gallstones vary in size and number. The small stones are more likely to cause attacks of acute biliary colic, since they pass more easily into the ducts. Stones may lodge anywhere along the biliary tract, where they may cause an obstruction which, if unrelieved, leads to jaundice, or they may cause pressure and subsequent necrosis and infection of the walls of the biliary ducts (Fig. 166). Occasionally a stone, because of its location, blocks the entrance of pancreatic fluid and bile into the duodenum at the ampulla of Vater. This condition is difficult to differentiate from obstruction due to malignancy.

There may be no signs of cholelithiasis until a stone becomes lodged in a biliary duct, although the patient often gives a history of indigestion after consuming rich, fatty foods, occasional discomfort in the right upper quadrant of the abdomen, and more trouble than the normal person with gaseous eructations after eating. Gaseous eructations in cholelithiasis characteristically occur almost immediately following meals, in contrast to those associated with gastric ulcer, which occur when the stomach is empty (usually several hours after a meal).

Gallstone colic, or *biliary colic,* can cause what is probably the most severe pain that can be experienced. The pain may come on suddenly and is probably caused by spasm of the ducts as they attempt to dislodge the stone. There is severe pain in the right upper quadrant of the abdomen, and it radiates through to the back under the scapula and to the right shoulder. Pain may be so severe that the patient writhes in agony despite large doses of analgesic drugs. Morphine sulfate and Demerol are avoided if possible because they are thought to increase spasm of the biliary sphincters and increase pressure, which can cause further trauma to the walls of the biliary passages. Nitroglycerin or inhalations of amyl nitrite are sometimes helpful, and papaverine hydrochloride, atropine, and calcium gluconate often are given to help produce relaxation of the biliary ducts. The patient usually has nausea and vomiting, profuse diaphoresis, tachycardia, and occasionally complete prostration. A nasogastric tube attached to a suction apparatus often helps to relieve distention in the upper gastrointestinal tract and thereby lessens the pain. Occasionally, following an acute attack of biliary colic, the stools are saved to determine whether or not a stone has passed into the intestines. The stools may be sent to the laboratory, or they may be strained for examination on the patient unit.

The treatment for cholelithiasis is surgical removal of the gallbladder and exploration of the common bile duct as soon as the acute attack subsides and the patient can withstand an operation safely.

Carcinoma

Carcinoma can occur anywhere in the biliary system, and unfortunately at present there is no way of diagnosing early carcinoma in the abdominal viscera. Jaundice may be the first sign and indicates that the lesion has developed sufficiently to obstruct bile passage at some point. The treatment for carcinoma of the biliary system is surgical, and an operation is performed as soon as the patient's condition warrants it in the hope that complete surgical removal of the lesion is possible. Patients often benefit from surgery even when cure of the carcinoma is impossible, since various operations that help to restore the flow of bile into the gastrointestinal tract produce remarkable relief of symptoms, and the patient may feel relatively well for a time.

Biliary atresia

Biliary atresia is a condition in which there is a congenital absence or obliteration of the biliary bile ducts. There is no known cause. Jaundice appears about two to three weeks after birth and progresses until the infant is a greenish bronze color. Tears and saliva may be pigmented, the urine is dark, and the stools are white or clay-colored. The child may not be alert and may move slowly, but he usually has a good appetite. The treatment consists of an operation to establish a pathway for bile into the intestines. As surgery is possible for only a small percentage of these children, the prognosis is poor.

SURGICAL TREATMENT AND NURSING CARE
Terminology

The terminology used to indicate specific biliary tract surgery sounds somewhat complicated but actually is self-explanatory. *Cholecystectomy* is the removal of the gallbladder, whereas *cholecystostomy* refers to the creation of a new opening into the gallbladder for decompression and drainage. *Choledochotomy* is a surgical incision into the common bile duct, usually for removal of a stone (*choledocholithotomy*). When carcinoma has been found or when strictures in the ducts make other methods of treatment unsatisfactory, *choledochoduodenostomy* and *choledochojejunostomy,* which refer to anastomoses between the bile duct and the duodenum and between the bile duct and the jejunum, respectively, also may be done. *Cholecystogastrostomy* is the surgical formation of an anastomosis between the gallbladder and the stomach.

Preoperative care

A general medical examination done prior to biliary surgery includes a roentgenogram of the chest, x-ray study of the gallbladder, and examination of the urine and stools. Usually an electrocardiogram is ordered to detect heart damage. Various tests of hepatic function may be made if disease of the liver is suspected, and if the patient is jaundiced, tests are done to determine the cause. The prothrombin level usually is checked preoperatively.

If there is jaundice, the prothrombin level usually is low, and vitamin K preparations such as phytonadione (vitamin K_1, Mephyton) may be given preoperatively. Occasionally when the prothrombin level is quite low, yet surgery is imperative, transfusions of whole blood may be given immediately preoperatively to provide prothrombin, which is essential for blood clotting. If the patient is taking food by mouth poorly, infusions containing glucose and protein hydrolysates may be given in an effort to protect the liver from potential damage and to ensure wound healing. Signs of upper respiratory disease should be reported at once since upper respiratory infections can lead to serious complications following surgery of the biliary tract. A nasogastric tube may be inserted before the patient goes to the operating room.

Postoperative care

The patient is usually placed in a low Fowler's position upon his recovery from anesthesia. Because the wound is fairly high in the abdomen, breathing is painful, and the patient may hold his breath and take shallow breaths in order to splint the incision and lessen pain. Analgesic medications for pain should be given fairly liberally during the first few days, and the patient should then be urged to cough and to breathe deeply at regular intervals. He must also be helped and encouraged to change his position and to move about in bed frequently. If

a nasogastric tube is in use, it is attached to suction equipment. Because essential electrolytes, as well as gas, are removed by this procedure, it is discontinued as soon as possible—usually within twenty-four hours. Infusions of 5% glucose in distilled water usually are administered. Sometimes solution containing electrolytes and protein hydrolysates are ordered. When the nasogastric tube is removed, the patient is given clear fluids by mouth. Sweet, effervescent drinks usually are tolerated best at first. Within a few days the patient usually is able to eat a soft low-fat diet. Appetite will probably remain poor if bile is not flowing into the duodenum.

The nurse should check the dressings as often as every fifteen minutes for the first few hours postoperatively because, although hemorrhage from the wound is rare, it can occur. Internal hemorrhage also occasionally follows surgery of the gallbladder and bile ducts, particularly when the inflamed gallbladder was adherent to the liver and was removed with difficulty. Lowering of blood pressure, increase in pulse rate, and other signs of hemorrhage should be reported to the surgeon at once.

The nurse should know exactly what surgical procedure has been done so that she may care for drains and check dressings intelligently. If the gallbladder is removed, the cystic duct is ligated and a drain usually is inserted near its stump and brought out through a stab wound. This tube drains bile and small amounts of blood and other serous fluid or exudates onto the dressings. It usually is removed within five to six days when drainage has largely subsided.

If a cholecystostomy has been performed, a self-retaining catheter is inserted through an opening in the gallbladder and is attached to straight drainage. Bile will drain out through this tube until it is removed, usually between six weeks and six months.

If exploration of the common duct has been done, a T tube, with the short ends placed into the common duct, will probably be used (Fig. 168). The long end of this soft rubber tube is brought through the wound and sutured to the skin. The section of the T tube emerging from the stab wound may be placed over a roll of gauze anchored to the skin with adhesive tape to prevent it

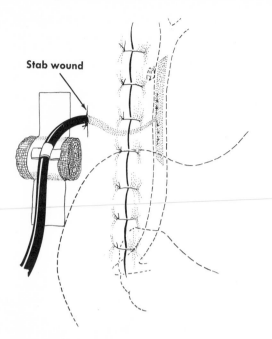

Fig. 167

The section of the T tube emerging
from the stab wound may be placed over
a roll of gauze anchored to the skin
with adhesive tape to prevent its
lumen from being occluded by pressure.

and blood-stained fluid during the first few hours, but drainage of more than a small amount of blood should be reported to the doctor. After this, the amount should be measured and recorded each day. At first, the entire output of bile (normally 500 to 1,000 ml. daily) may flow through the tube, but within ten days most of the bile should be flowing into the duodenum.

Usually the T tube is removed in ten days to two weeks. Before this is done, a *burette test*, similar to that described prior to removing a nephrostomy tube (p. 455), is done to determine the patency of the biliary system (Fig. 168). If the common bile duct is patent, the pressure readings will fluctuate

from occluding (Fig. 167). The T tube is inserted to preserve patency of the common duct and to ensure drainage of bile out of the body until edema in the common duct has subsided enough for bile to drain into the duodenum normally. If the T tube was clamped while the patient was being transported from the recovery room, it must be released *immediately* upon arrival in his room. The nurse should check the operative sheet carefully and make inquiries if directions are not clear. The tube usually is connected to closed gravity drainage similar to that used to drain the urinary bladder. Sufficient tubing should be attached so that the patient can move without restriction. The purpose of the tube should be explained to the patient, and he should be told why it must not be kinked, clamped, or pulled. The drainage should be checked for color and amount at least every two hours on the operative day. The tube may drain some blood

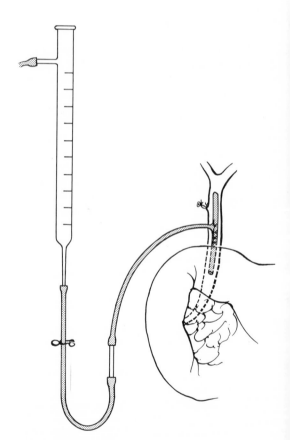

Fig. 168

A T tube placed in the common bile duct
and attached to a manometer for a burette
test. The common bile duct has been
brought from its normal position
for better visualization of the T tube.

very little from the initial reading, unless the patient is moving, coughing, talking, or laughing just prior to the reading. If the common bile duct is still obstructed, the level of bile will rise in the burette beyond the set point, usually 15 cm. above the level of the common bile duct. If this happens, the doctor should be notified. A cholangiogram usually is made following the burette test to confirm the patency of the duct (p. 701). Following the removal of the T tube, the patient may have chills and fever, but they usually subside within twenty-four hours. They are caused by edema and a local reaction to the bile. Occasionally flow of bile into the abdominal cavity causes peritonitis, and therefore, any abdominal pain should be reported at once.

Postoperatively the bile should either drain out through the drainage tubes or flow into the intestine. If it does not do so, it can be assumed that the flow of bile is obstructed and that bile is being forced back into the liver and into the bloodstream. The nurse should observe the patient closely for jaundice, particularly in the sclerae. Urine should be examined grossly for the brown color that is indicative of bile pigment. A specimen should be saved for the doctor's inspection when bile pigment is observed in the urine. The nurse may observe the patient's progress by noting the stools: a light color is usual if all the bile is flowing out through the drainage tubes (unless bile salts are being given by mouth), but the normal brown color should gradually reappear as drainage diminishes and finally disappears.

The patient should be told about any drainage tubes that have been used. He should know if much bile is expected on the dressings so that he will not become alarmed by soiling of dressings, his gown, or bedclothes. Outer dressings usually need to be changed frequently when there is excessive drainage, since the drainage is irritating to the skin and wet dressings interfere with the patient's comfort and rest. Soap and water will remove bile from the skin. Montgomery straps make the changing of dressings much easier.

The patient usually is permitted out of bed the day after the operation. If a T tube or a cholecystostomy tube is present, it may be attached to a small drainage bottle to permit greater freedom of movement. It may be placed in a pocket of the patient's bathrobe or attached to his robe below the level of the common duct. The patient may need help and encouragement because dressings are uncomfortable and he fears "spilling" the drainage when he moves about. He may still be receiving infusions, and transporting the infusion bottle is necessary (p. 200). He often benefits from a regular schedule of getting up and sitting in a chair or walking with assistance.

Special diets are seldom prescribed by the doctor following biliary surgery, but the patient is advised to avoid excessive fats in his meals. The nurse should help to teach the patient the essentials of good nutrition, with emphasis on foods that are low in fat.

Occasionally, if excessive drainage through the T tube or cholecystostomy tube continues for a long time, the bile collected in the drainage bottle is administered to the patient through a nasogastric tube to improve digestion. If this is done, the funnel or Asepto syringe should be covered, and the bile should be in a receptacle so that the patient does not see it. Sometimes the bile may be diluted with grape or other juices to disguise its appearance. The patient generally is not told that he is receiving bile.

Usually from ten days to two weeks of hospitalization are required following biliary surgery when no complications occur. The length of convalescence depends on the individual patient, but usually at least a month is needed before normal activities can be resumed safely. The nurse should emphasize to the patient the importance of keeping medical appointments as requested.

References and selected readings*

1 American Public Health Association: Control of communicable disease in man, ed. 10, New York, 1965, The American Public Health Association.

2 Beeson, Paul B., and McDermott, Walsh, editors: Cecil-Loeb textbook of medicine, ed. 11, Philadelphia, 1963, W. B. Saunders Co.

3 Bergersen, Betty S., and Krug, Elsie E.: Pharmacology in nursing, ed. 10, St. Louis, 1966, The C. V. Mosby Co.

4 *Bielski, Mary T., and Molander, David W.: Laennec's cirrhosis, Am. J. Nursing 65:82-86, Aug. 1965.

---

*References preceded by an asterisk are particularly well suited for student reading.

5 Bockus, Henry L.: Gastroenterology, vol. III, ed. 2, Philadelphia, 1965, W. B. Saunders Co.

6 *Cunningham, Lyda Martin: The patient with ruptured esophageal varices, Am. J. Nursing 62:69-71, Dec. 1962.

7 Davidsohn, Israel, and Wells, Benjamin B.: Todd-Sanford clinical diagnosis by laboratory methods, ed. 13, Philadelphia, 1963, W. B. Saunders Co.

8 Davis, Loyal, editor: Christopher's textbook of surgery, ed. 8, Philadelphia, 1964, W. B. Saunders Co.

9 *Eisenmenger, William J., Uhl, Marilyn, and Lydon, Joan: Viral hepatitis, Am. J. Nursing 61:56-59, Nov. 1961.

10 Fuerst, Elinor V., and Wolff, Luverne: Fundamentals of Nursing, ed. 3, Philadelphia, 1964, J. B. Lippincott Co.

11 Gelb, Donald, West, Michael, and Zimmerman, H. J.: Serum enzymes in disease. IX. Analysis of factors responsible for elevated values in infectious mononucleosis, Am. J. Med. 33:249-261, Aug. 1962.

12 *Glenn, Frank: Surgical treatment of biliary tract disease, Am. J. Nursing 64:88-92, May 1964.

13 Harrison, T. R., and others, editors: Principles of internal medicine, ed. 5, New York, 1966, McGraw-Hill Book Co.

14 *Henderson, Lillian M.: Nursing care in acute cholecystitis, Am. J. Nursing 64:93-96, 1964.

15 Jones, Philip N., and Cappa, Richard B.: The management of hepatic coma, M. Clin. North America 48:37-51, Jan. 1964.

16 Krause, Marie V.: Food, nutrition, and diet therapy, ed. 4, Philadelphia, 1966, W. B. Saunders Co.

17 Linton, Robert: The treatment of esophageal varices, S. Clin. North America 46:485-498, June 1966.

18 McCollum, Robert W.: Epidemiologic patterns of viral hepatitis, Am. J. Med. 32:657-664, May 1962.

19 *Molander, David W., Brasfield, Richard D., and Virgadamo, Barbara T.: Liver surgery and care of the patient with liver surgery, Am. J. Nursing 61:72-76, July 1961.

20 Nelson, Waldo E.: Textbook of pediatrics, ed. 8, Philadelphia, 1964, W. B. Saunders Co.

21 New York Times, Aug. 4, 1957.

22 *Schaffner, Fenton, and others: Symposium: liver disease, J.A.M.A. 191:466-486, Feb. 8, 1965.

23 Schiff, Leon, editor: Diseases of the liver, ed. 2, Philadelphia, 1963, J. B. Lippincott Co.

24 Stahl, William M.: Major abdominal surgery in the aged patient, J. Am. Geriatrics Soc. 11:770-780, Aug. 1963.

25 *Stokes, Joseph, Jr.: The control of viral hepatitis, Am. J. Med. 32:729-733, May 1962.

26 U. S. Department of Health, Education, and Welfare: Monthly vital statistics report, annual summary, vol. 13, no. 13, July 2, 1964.

27 U. S. Department of Health, Education, and Welfare: Morbidity and mortality, weekly report, Annual supplement, vol. 13, no. 54, released Sept. 30, 1965.

28 Warren, Kenneth W., McDonald, William M., and Veidenheimer, Malcom C.: Trends in pancreatic surgery, S. Clin. North America 44:743-760, June 1964.

29 Warren, Richard, and others: Surgery, Philadelphia, 1963, W. B. Saunders Co.

Study
questions

1 Where is each of the endocrine glands located? Review the hormones secreted by each.
2 In what way does giving a large amount of a hormone to a patient who already is producing a normal amount affect his own production of the hormone? Why does this reaction take place?
3 What is the difference between secretion and excretion?
4 What vitamin is essential for the body to use calcium efficiently? Why is it necessary?
5 List the signs and symptoms of respiratory obstructions that might be caused by pressure on the trachea.
6 How would you explain to a patient who has a high basal metabolic rate that he needs increased amounts of foods? Name some foods that are high in carbohydrates.
7 Review the procedure for giving a medication by hypodermic injection, and outline a plan for teaching this procedure to a patient.
8 What is the price of a bottle of protamine zinc insulin? Of NPH insulin? If the patient is to take a daily dose of 30 units, how long would one bottle of insulin last? What would be the monthly cost?
9 Review the physiologic action of the sympathetic nerves.
10 Where is the hypothalamus located?
11 Review the physiology of stress in Chapter 4.
12 In what ways would the nursing needs of a patient having a hypophysectomy as treatment for cancer of the breast be likely to vary from those of a patient having a hypophysectomy to control the vascular complications of diabetes mellitus?

The endocrine glands are special glands, or groups of cells, located in various parts of the body. Knowledge as to exactly how they function is still incomplete, but more is being learned about them each year. They are known to secrete and release highly specific chemical compounds (hormones) into the bloodstream. These substances are synthesized in the endocrine glands under genetic control, and they are continually lost from the body either by excretion or by metabolic inactivation. None are secreted at a uniform rate; some seem to have a rhythmic pattern (daily or periodic), while others seem to be secreted in response to the blood level of a specific substance such as sugar, sodium, water, or another hormone.

The hormones, in conjunction with the nervous system, communicate information about conditions in the internal and external environment to all parts of the body and help the body maintain a homeostatic state. It still is unclear exactly how hormone production is stimulated or how the hormones act in the cells. They probably do not initiate any physiologic processes, but by a complex yet unified action they seem to augment and regulate many vital functions, such as energy production, metabolism of foodstuffs, water and electrolyte balance, growth and development, and reproductive processes. They also integrate the responses of the body to stress.

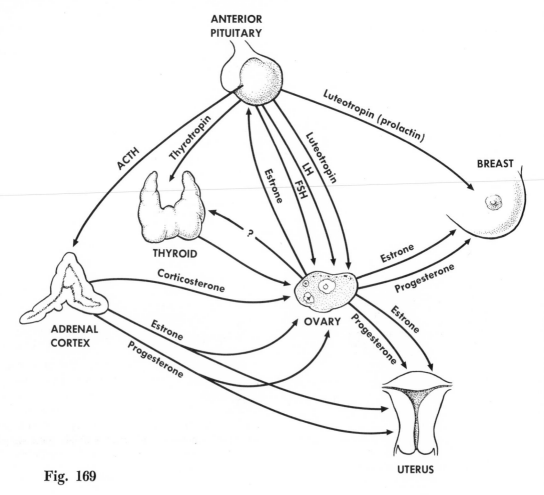

ANTERIOR PITUITARY

Luteotropin (prolactin)

ACTH

Thyrotropin

Luteotropin

LH

FSH

Estrone

BREAST

THYROID

?

Estrone

Corticosterone

Progesterone

ADRENAL CORTEX

Estrone

Progesterone

OVARY

Progesterone

Estrone

UTERUS

Fig. 169

Site of origin of some of the important hormones and the organs they affect.

Authorities now believe that the production of most hormones is directly or indirectly under the control of the nervous system.

The anterior pituitary gland, often called the "master gland" because it seems to be the regulator of the whole hormone environment, secretes two types of hormones—one type that affects specific tissues directly, and another (the tropic hormones) that regulates the output of hormones from other glands (Fig. 169). One of the tropic hormones, adrenocorticotropic hormone (ACTH), stimulates the secretion of glucocorticoids by the adrenal cortex. (Aldosterone also is secreted by the adrenal cortex, but it does not seem to require pituitary stimulation since its production continues when the pituitary gland is excised.) Thyroid-stimulating hormone (TSH), secreted by the anterior pituitary gland, causes the secretion of thyroid hormones. The gonadotropic hormones stimulate secretion of testicular and ovarian hormones. The growth-stimulating hormone (GH) produced by the anterior pituitary gland seems to interact with other hormones such as thyroxin and insulin, produced by the islands of Langerhans in the pancreas, to regulate the body's growth and development. The posterior pituitary gland secretes antidiuretic hormone (ADH), pituitrin, which stimulates smooth muscles of the blood vessels and intestine to contract, and oxytocin, which stimulates uterine contraction. The adrenomedullary hormones seem to control the emergency system for quickly mobilizing the body defense system, including the activation of other hormones. Further information as to the action of each hormone and what stimulates its secretion is included with the discussion of diseases of the endocrine gland producing it.

The actions of the endocrine glands are interrelated (Fig. 169). Many hormones seem either to oppose or to supplement one another. For example, insulin lowers the blood sugar, while the glucocorticoids elevate it. The tropic hormones stimulate production of certain other hormones, but these other hormones, in turn, inhibit production of the tropic hormones. The growth and thyroid hormones must work together for normal growth and development. The two thyroid hormones have similar actions, varying only in degree, and both the glucocorticoids and aldosterone can regulate sodium balance. Probably no vital function occurs without the interrelated action of at least several hormones.

In health, the amount of each hormone in the blood is kept within definite limits. Disturbance in the functioning of an endocrine gland may be caused by malfunction in the regulatory mechanism or by failure of the body processes to respond to regulation. Because the endocrine system is so closely interrelated and because the production of each hormone is dependent not only upon other hormones but upon nervous stimulation, genetic controls, enzymatic action, and available energy and nutrients, it is obvious that endocrine dysfunction can arise from diverse causes. Dysfunction of one gland is likely to affect the function of one or more of the others. The structure and thus the function of an endocrine gland may be changed by abnormal embryonic development of the endocrine tissue, deprivation of blood supply to the gland, infection of the gland, tumor (benign or malignant) growths in it, overstimulation of it, or overgrowth of its tissues (hypertrophy and hyperplasia). In *hyperplasia*, the size of the gland increases because it is continuously overstimulated, and there is a proliferation of active secreting cells. In *hypertrophy*, there is an increase in the size of the gland, caused by the increase in functional demands upon it. Hypertrophy may or may not be accompanied by hyperplasia. *Hypoplasia* is a decrease in the amount of functioning tissue, and consequently, there is a decrease in the amount of hormone produced. It may be caused by anything that inhibits tissue growth. It is believed that both the production of hormones and the effect of hormones upon body cells can be affected by age, race, sex, season, climate, and disease.

Disease of an endocrine gland usually causes a decrease or an increase in the secretion of its hormones, and the symptoms are those of increased or decreased regulation of the processes normally controlled by it. Owing to the diverse physiologic functions under hormonal control, symptoms of endocrine dysfunction may be reflected in many parts of the body, and because many of the functions controlled are vital ones, endocrine disorders may be extremely serious.

The specific treatment of endocrine diseases consists basically of decreasing the output of hormones from hyperactive glands and supplying or compensating for deficient hormones. Occasionally, in hypofunction, treatment may be designed to lessen the need for the hormone or to stimulate its production. Overproduction of a specific hormone often can be controlled by resecting part of the gland secreting the hormone or, if a tumor is stimulating the gland, by removing the tumor. However, sometimes the entire endocrine gland must be removed surgically or destroyed. Occasionally the pituitary gland may be removed or destroyed if it stimulates the secretions of the overactive gland. Sometimes radiation of either the specific endocrine gland or the pituitary gland destroys enough tissue to bring the symptoms under control. If endocrine glands are completely removed or destroyed, essential hormones must be supplied regularly for the remainder of the patient's life. Regular replacement also is necessary to control disease when there is hypofunction of the endocrine gland.

Only a few of the more common diseases of the endocrine system will be discussed in this chapter. Those occurring less often should be reviewed in appropriate specialized texts. Since replacement of hormones is common to most endocrine diseases, replacement therapy will be discussed before some specific diseases are mentioned.

Hormonal replacement therapy

Long-term replacement. The patient who requires hormonal substitution for the remainder of his life often presents a serious rehabilitative problem. His prognosis may depend largely on his acceptance of the situation and his understanding of his limitations and his treatment. Although hormonal replacement treatment may seem to restrict the patient's life seriously, the person who has been helped to accept his limitations and live within them is able to have a relatively normal life and is far less restricted than he was with the uncontrolled disease. It is important for the patient to have the support of the members of his family and for them to understand and be willing to assume responsibility for his treatment should he be unable to do so himself.

The patient must know that his treatment cannot be discontinued for a single day without specific direction from the doctor and that it does not usually provide for the excessive hormonal demands produced by unusually stressful physical or emotional situations. Because of this he should strive to recognize and to avoid stress-producing situations such as tensions on the job, family quarrels, and sudden bouts of unaccustomed exercise. Fasting, extremes of temperature, and fatigue should be avoided also. If any infection, no matter how minor, or any illness occurs, the person should seek medical advice. Pregnancy produces stresses and therefore, the physician should be consulted about family planning; additional hormones may be needed during the period of gestation and delivery. Because sudden, unexpected, stressful situations such as accidents or incapacitating illness may occur, the patient receiving hormones regularly always should carry an identification card on which is noted his name and the name of his doctor, with address and telephone numbers and the prescribed hormone being taken, with the dosage to be used in event of an emergency.

Even in the absence of stressful situations, the normal person has changing needs for hormones. In replacement therapy, how-

ever, a specified amount of hormone must be given. Therefore, it is not unusual for the patient to develop symptoms of hypofunction or hyperfunction of the gland for which the hormone is being given. Both the patient and his family should be able to recognize symptoms of dysfunction of the gland and know what to do about them. If there is a means of compensating for too much or too little of the hormone, such as taking sugar for insulin shock, the method should be taught. If this is not possible and the symptoms are acute, the patient must be taken at once to his doctor or the emergency department of a hospital. Many times, if medical advice is sought at the first evidence of even minor symptoms of dysfunction, the dosage of the hormone can be adjusted and further trouble avoided.

Patients receiving hormone replacement always should have at least a two-month supply of the special drugs and equipment they need, lest an emergency prevent them from obtaining supplies. As new supplies are bought, they should be kept in reserve and the old ones used. Continuous hormonal therapy is expensive. If the patient finds it difficult to pay for the drugs he needs, help should be sought from the social service department in the hospital or from an appropriate social agency in the community.

Temporary replacement. The patient requiring only temporary replacement of hormones may be at home while he is taking them, and if so, he must be taught the importance of taking the prescribed dosage regularly. Usually the dosage is reduced gradually and finally discontinued. While therapy is being tapered off, the patient should be observed for symptoms of hypofunction of the gland that produces the hormones that have been given. The patient and his family should know the signs and symptoms of hormonal deficiency and should understand the need to seek immediate medical attention if these symptoms occur. They also should know that symptoms of hypofunction of the gland may occur even after the therapy has been discontinued. Regular medical follow-up should be continued until the doctor determines that it is no longer needed. Glands that have been partially destroyed by radiation or partially removed by surgery eventually increase in size so that their function is normal. The patient usually is advised to lead a less stressful life than usual until normal function has returned.

The patient with disease of the thyroid gland

An oversimplified description of the function of the thyroid gland is that it is the regulator of the rate of metabolic processes in the body. Thyroid hormones are essential for normal physical and mental growth and development of a child. It is thought that when there is need for an increased rate of cellular oxidation, nerve fibers carry the message to the hypothalamus, which, in turn, stimulates the anterior pituitary gland to secrete thyroid-stimulating hormone. The thyroid gland then secretes thyroxin and triiodothyronine. These hormones have a similar action but differ greatly in their rate of action. Thyroxin takes eight to ten days to produce its full effect, but it lasts about three weeks. Triiodothyronine's action is much more rapid (one to three days) but lasts only about a week.[41] Iodine is essential for the production of thyroid hormones, and the thyroid gland alone contains approximately 80% of all the iodine in the body. Several enzymes also are essential for the thyroid to synthesize its hormones.

Diseases of the thyroid gland include functional hyperplasia and hypoplasia, hypertrophy, neoplasms, infections (thyroiditis), and anomalies. Symptoms of disease consist primarily of changes brought about by derangement of the thyroid gland's function as a regulator of metabolism.

Tests used in diagnosing diseases of the thyroid gland will be described before some of the more common diseases and their related nursing care are discussed.

Diagnostic tests

The *basal metabolism test* determines the amount of oxygen used by a person at rest during a given period of time. It is a crude indicator of thyroid function. Results of the test are compared with the mean values obtained from testing a group of normal people of the same age, sex, and size (body surface). The results are expressed in percentage of deviation from the mean values. Thus, if the patient needs 10% more oxygen

than the control group, he has a basal metabolic rate (BMR) of plus 10%. Normal basal metabolic rate ranges from minus 15% to plus 15%.[41] Although this test is still used, newer and more accurate diagnostic measures are now available.

The patient does not have to be hospitalized for a basal metabolism test. If he is, he should be given time to become adjusted to the hospital routine before the test is scheduled, since the mere fact that he is in a hospital may increase metabolism. The patient must have eight to ten hours of sleep before the examination, but no sedation should be taken. If the patient is hospitalized, special precautions need to be taken to ensure his having a quiet room and to prevent him from being disturbed prior to going for the test. Whether he is at home or in the hospital, the patient should omit most of the personal care he usually carries out in the morning and he should avoid hurry. If he is at home, he should be urged to dress slowly and to have someone drive him to where the test is to be done. No food or fluid should be taken after the evening meal.

During the test the patient lies on a bed, his nostrils are closed with a clamp, and he is asked to breathe through his mouth from a tube that supplies oxygen. A drumlike apparatus beside the bed will measure the amount of oxygen he uses.

Accuracy of results depends on how carefully the patient is prepared and follows instructions during the test. Therefore, the nurse should give him a detailed explanation of what to expect during the test and explicit instructions as to preparation for it.

Achilles tendon reflex recording is a simple method of estimating thyroid function. Electrodes attached to a recording drum are applied to the patient's ankle. The physician taps the ankle tendon, and the response time for the reflex is recorded on the drum. A slow ankle jerk correlates with an underactive thyroid, and a rapid one correlates with an overactive thyroid.

The *protein-bound iodine test* determines the thyroid function by measuring iodine that can be precipitated with plasma proteins in the blood. The normal range is from 3.5 to 8 μg per 100 ml. of serum.[41] The blood for this test can be taken without regard to food intake, emotional state, or activity, but the patient should receive no medications containing iodine during the week before the test lest the readings be abnormally high. Cough syrups containing iodine, as well as specific iodine preparations, should be avoided. Tests in which iodine preparations are used, such as x-ray series of the gallbladder or intravenous pyelograms, also interfere with accurate results. Estrogens cause readings to be abnormally high and therefore should be discontinued prior to the test. Mercury causes readings to be abnormally low. Mercurial diuretics should be omitted for twenty-four to forty-eight hours before the test.

A *blood cholesterol test* may be used in diagnosing thyroid diseases, but there is variation in opinion on its reliability. When the test is ordered, food should be withheld until the blood sample has been obtained. The normal cholesterol reading is from 150 to 250 mg. per 100 ml. of blood.[41] In hyperfunction of the thyroid, the blood serum cholesterol level usually tends to be subnormal, whereas in hypofunction it usually is increased.

There are several tests of thyroid function using radioactive iodine. For a *radioactive T-3 red cell uptake*, a sample of the patient's blood is taken, and I^{131}-labeled thyroid hormone (thyroid hormone tagged or identified with radioactive iodine) is added to it in the laboratory. The amount of binding of the hormone by the red cells is measured. With normal thyroid function, 11 to 19% of the radioactive-labeled thyroid hormone is taken up by the red blood cells; less is taken up in hypofunction, and more in hyperfunction.[41] Estrogen and anticoagulants cause false estimates and must be discontinued prior to the administration of the test. This test is now used widely since it has the advantages that the patient need not be given radioactive material and that a sample of blood is obtained easily.

The *radioactive iodine uptake test* determines the ability of the thyroid gland to accumulate iodine that is ingested. A tracer dose of radioactive iodine (I^{131}), which is colorless and tasteless, is given by mouth, either diluted in distilled water or contained in a capsule. The drug is absorbed from the gastrointestinal tract and accumulated in the

thyroid gland, and the excess is excreted by the kidneys. Approximately two, six, or twenty-four hours following the administration of I^{131}, a shielded Geiger counter or a scintillation detector is placed over the neck in the region of the thyroid gland, and the amount of accumulated radioactive iodine is calculated. The normal thyroid usually will accumulate 15 to 50% of the drug within twenty-four hours. If the patient has thyrotoxicosis, 55 to 60% may be shown. Most patients with thyrotoxicosis excrete from 5 to 40% of the drug within twenty-four hours.[41] Determination of how much radioactive iodine is excreted usually is desired. Therefore, all urine voided during the test period may be collected. This test is not done if the patient has poor renal function, since the results are unreliable.

Since food delays the absorption of the iodine preparation, the patient should fast or have only fruit juice and toast before taking it. Preceding the test no antithyroid compound should be given for at least three days and no medications containing iodine or foods with particularly high iodine contents, such as seafood, should be given for a week preceding the test. Thyroid extract should be omitted at least three weeks prior to the test, and no test using dyes containing iodine should have been done for several weeks prior to it. Apprehension at the thought of taking a radioactive substance usually is allayed by explanations, but the nurse should report to the doctor any fears the patient expresses so that further reassurance can be given if necessary. No isolation for radioactivity is necessary.

The *thyroid "scan"* test is used to determine if there are elevated concentrations of iodine in a particular node or portion of the thyroid gland or in adjacent tissue. The procedure is similar to that for a radioactive iodine uptake test except that the scintillation detector moves back and forth across the neck, recording on a drum a picture of the distribution of radioactivity.

When hyperthyroidism is suspected but other tests for it are inconclusive, a *thyroid uptake suppression test* may be ordered. A radioactive iodine uptake test is done first to establish a base line. A fast-acting thyroid hormone is given for eight days, and then the uptake is retested. Failure of the hormone to suppress the uptake indicates hyperthyroidism, since normally the excess thyroid hormone in the blood should depress the secretion of thyroid-stimulating hormone from the anterior pituitary gland.

When hypothyroidism is suspected but other tests for it are inconclusive, *thyroid-stimulating hormone* (TSH) is given by injection after a base line radioactive iodine uptake has been obtained. After the injection the uptake is repeated. A person with a normal thyroid will have a marked increase in iodine uptake, whereas a person with hypofunction of the thyroid gland will have no increase in iodine uptake. If the hypothyroidism is due to failure of the anterior pituitary gland to secrete thyroid-stimulating hormone, the uptake will be normal.

Simple goiter

Any enlargement of the thyroid gland is spoken of as a goiter. A goiter may be caused by various disorders, such as congenital metabolic defects that prevent synthesis of thyroid hormones or chronic thyroiditis. Simple goiter, or hyperplasia due to inadequate iodine, with subsequent overwork of the thyroid gland to produce adequate amounts of thyroid hormones, is one of the most common forms. It frequently is seen in girls, appearing at puberty, when the metabolic rate is highest and the body's need for thyroid hormones is greatest. It may diminish or disappear spontaneously after the age of 25 years. In temperate climates, the greatest incidence of simple goiter occurs in late winter and in spring, and it may be an endemic or a sporadic disorder. The incidence of simple goiter in the United States is greatest in the Great Lakes Basin, Minnesota, the Dakotas, the Pacific Northwest, and the Upper Mississippi Valley, because of the limited amount of iodine in the water and food supply of these regions. Iodine normally is found in seafood, and small amounts of iodine are found in green leafy vegetables that have been grown where iodine is present in the water and soil. Using iodized table salt is an easy and inexpensive way of assuring sufficient iodine intake, since the average adult can obtain more than twice his daily iodine requirement from the amount of salt he normally uses.

A simple goiter may grow unnoticed, or the patient may ignore it unless it becomes nodular or symptomatic. Toxicity or difficulty in breathing, resulting from pressure of the goiter on the trachea, may occur, and occasionally malignancy develops. In the early stages of simple goiter, one drop of saturated solution of potassium iodide a week usually provides enough extra iodine for the thyroid gland to use to produce thyroid hormones, and the hyperplasia will decrease gradually. If the goiter is moderately large, it may be necessary for the patient to take thyroid extract as well as iodine to decrease its size. When the goiter is causing symptoms of pressure, it may have to be removed surgically. Very large goiters also may be removed surgically for cosmetic improvement.

The nurse can help to prevent simple goiter by teaching the importance of eating foods that contain iodine. When reviewing any person's diet, she should ask about the quantity of leafy vegetables and seafoods he eats and the kind of table salt he uses. Encouraging use of iodized salt is important in parts of the country where there is a known deficiency of iodine in the natural water. The nurse should notice the contour of the neck whenever giving care to any patient. If there seems to be enlargement, the patient should be questioned as to his awareness of it and asked whether he has consulted a physician about it. If not, he should be encouraged to do so.

Cancer of the thyroid gland

Although cancer of the thyroid gland is less prevalent than other forms of cancer, about 1,000 people in the United States die of it each year. It usually is first diagnosed by palpation of a hard nodule on physical examination, but it sometimes is first recognized because it produces symptoms of hyperthyroidism. The treatment is total thyroidectomy. Radioactive iodine in large doses may be given in conjunction with surgery, but it is not usually effective when used without surgery. Regular administration of thyroid hormone is started following the operation, and it must be continued throughout the patient's life.

The nurse should urge people to have yearly physical examinations since this may help to detect cancer of the thyroid gland in its early stages. The nursing care of the patient is the same as that for any patient having an operation on the thyroid gland (p. 737). (The care given to the patient who is being treated with radioactive iodine is described on p. 735.)

Hyperthyroidism

The disease characterized by hyperactivity of the thyroid gland commonly is known as hyperthyroidism, but it may be called *thyrotoxicosis, toxic goiter, Graves's disease,* or *Basedow's disease.* In this condition the gland usually enlarges, and it always secretes excessive quantities of thyroid hormones, speeding up all metabolic processes. More oxygen is used, more fuel is burned, and heat output rises markedly. The patient becomes nervous and jittery, tense, overly alert, and irritable. His reactions to situations may be exaggerated, and he may weep or laugh out of proportion to what is expected normally. There is a fine tremor of the hands, and the patient may drop articles easily and may appear awkward or clumsy in his movements. He usually complains of weakness and fatigue, and he often loses weight, although he may eat enormous amounts of food. There is heat intolerance and increase in perspiration. The palms of the hands typically are warm and moist. Palpitations and breathlessness sometimes occur. Gastrointestinal motility is increased, and diarrhea may occur. Today the patient usually seeks treatment fairly early, and his only obvious signs may be nervousness and slight weight loss. Hyperthyroidism is a serious disease which, if not checked, can lead to death from heart failure.

Exophthalmos, or protrusion of the eyeballs, is a characteristic although not uniformly present sign of hyperthyroidism. This condition may become so severe that the eyes cannot be closed. In this event the eyes should be protected to prevent irritation and possible corneal ulceration. Until a more permanent measure, such as a plastic operation on the lid, can be done, the patient should wear protective glasses in the daytime and sleep with an eye covering (p. 165). Control of the thyroid hyperactivity stops the progress of exophthalmos, but it never regresses.

Hyperthyroidism is more common in women than in men, the ratio being 4:1. It can occur at any age, but it is most likely to occur at puberty, following pregnancy, or at the menopause. Emotional trauma, such as loss of a parent, divorce, or financial crisis sometimes precedes thyroid hyperplasia, but it is not clear whether emotional trauma precipitates the hyperplasia or whether the presence of hyperplasia may cause the severe emotional responses to crises. Toxic thyroid disease often occurs in persons who have other endocrine disturbance such as diabetes mellitus.

Every nurse should be alert to early signs and symptoms of hyperthyroidism. The public health nurse, particularly, may encounter people with beginning signs and symptoms. Physical signs may be obvious, but the patient's expressed complaints about his or her changes in behavior and management of usual activities may give many additional clues. Since the disease gradually becomes more serious, and treatment is more effective and less difficult in the initial stages, people suspected of having hyperthyroidism should be urged to seek medical attention early. If treatment is started early, hospitalization may not be necessary.

Treatment for the patient with hyperthyroidism is directed toward reducing the output of thyroid hormones as well as the need for them. Since the advent of antithyroid drugs, this is accomplished more easily than previously. These drugs interfere with the conversion of iodide to iodine (necessary for the synthesis of thyroid hormones) by the thyroid gland and therefore decrease the production of thyroid hormones. The drugs may produce regression of the hyperthyroid state in some patients. If not, they usually temporarily reduce the production of hormones to normal so that surgical or radiation therapy can be carried out safely. Until the symptoms are controlled, measures to keep the patient emotionally and physically quiet and thus reduce his metabolic needs are necessary. The patient often is given a diet high in calories to provide adequate fuel for the increased energy requirements and to prevent further weight loss, as well as to replace weight already lost.

Drugs. Propylthiouracil and *methimazole* (Tapazole) are the most commonly used *antithyroid drugs.* The action of these drugs is slow, and it usually takes two weeks to a month before improvement is noticeable. The patient usually is started on a relatively large dose of an antithyroid drug, and then the dosage is gradually reduced to a maintenance dose. When antithyroid drugs are used as the primary therapy, they usually are continued for six to eighteen months.[41] It is important to give the drugs at regularly spaced intervals since their effect wears off in about eight hours. Patients should know this. The patient should be instructed to look for toxic signs of the drug, such as fever, sore throat, and skin eruptions. He should call his doctor if they appear. If toxic reaction occurs, blood counts may show leukopenia. Continued use of antithyroid drugs may not be tolerated by some patients.

Large doses of antithyroid drugs taken during the third trimester of pregnancy may cause the baby to be born with a goiter, but it usually disappears spontaneously. Breast feeding by the mother who is taking these drugs is contraindicated because it produces hypothyroidism in the infant.

In addition to the antithyroid drugs, preparations of *iodine,* such as Lugol's solution (strong iodine solution), are still widely used in the treatment of hyperthyroidism. They reduce glandular vascularity and help to prevent postoperative hemorrhage when a partial thyroidectomy is necessary. They also are used when the metabolic rate must be reduced rapidly, because their action is more rapid than that of the antithyroid drugs, although less sustained. When Lugol's solution is ordered, it is more palatable given in milk or fruit juice. It should be taken through a straw because it may stain the teeth. A brassy taste in the mouth and sore teeth and gums are signs of toxicity, but this complication rarely occurs.

Occasionally, as when the patient is unable to tolerate antithyroid drugs, *thyroid hormone* may be given to reduce the hypersecretion of the thyroid glands and prepare the patient for surgery. The rationale for this treatment is that if a high blood level of the hormone is maintained, thyroid-stimulating hormone will not be released from the anterior pituitary gland. Sometimes when antithyroid drugs are being taken preparatory to surgery, thyroid hormone may be used instead of iodide preparations to reduce the vascularity of the thyroid gland. There are four preparations of thyroid hormone currently used. Desiccated thyroid, thyroglobulin (Proloid), and levothyroxine sodium (Synthroid sodium) are slow-acting preparations, producing their full effect in about ten days and gradually declining in effect on discontinuance. Sodium liothyronine (Cytomel) has a rapid onset and a brief duration of effect. It must be given at least twice daily.

When antithyroid drugs are not tolerated or do not produce permanent remission of hyperthyroidism, *Radioactive iodine* is now widely used for treatment unless the patient is pregnant or under 25 years of age.[41] It is suspected that radioactivity may injure the germ plasma, and the tendency of radioactive substances to stimulate carcinogenic activity has not been excluded. I^{131} is the preparation most often used. Usually a single dose of the drug is given, and the dosage is calculated on the basis of 0.16 millicurie per gram of estimated thyroid weight. As in the iodide uptake test, the drug is given by mouth (a radioactive "cocktail"). If a large dose of radioactive iodine is given, the patient usually is hospitalized and isolated for radioactivity for eight days (the half-life of radioactive iodine [I^{131}]). Following administration of large doses of radioactive iodine, the patient must be watched for thyroid storm (p. 737). Patients requiring only small amounts of the drug may go directly home, and no precautions are advised. It takes about three weeks for the symptoms of hyperthyroidism to subside and over two months for thyroid function to become normal. Occasionally remission is not achieved with one dose, and the treatment is repeated after an interval of several months. Hypothyroidism also may result if too much glandular tissue has been destroyed, and the patient will then need to take thyroid hormones either temporarily or permanently. The patient must be urged to keep appointments with his doctor or with the hospital clinic, since it is important that he be followed medically for months to be certain that a normal rate of function remains.

Patients who receive radioactive iodine for hyperthyroidism need to have the treatment explained to them with special care, and they usually need repeated reassurance that the radioactive properties are quickly dissipated. Since they often are more highly emotional than other patients, they sometimes think they are experiencing reactions to the drug long after this is possible.

General care. Since the advent of the antithyroid drugs and the trend toward early treatment, most patients with hyperthyroidism can be cared for at home. Although patients allowed to stay at home usually are not particularly overactive, they are likely to be very nervous and irritable. It is important for the patient's family and friends to understand that extreme sensitivity and excessive irritability are part of the disease. Otherwise, they may become upset with the patient and aggravate the situation. Plans for maintaining a quiet environment should be made with the patient and his family. The patient who must be hospitalized usually is *very* restless, overactive, and jittery, and his behavior must be explained to the nonprofessional nursing staff as well as to his family and friends. Special adjustments in routine nursing measures may be needed to help the patient rest.

The physical and emotional environment of the patient with hyperthyroidism should be kept as quiet and restful as possible. Whenever possible the patient should have his own room, and it should be kept cool. Patients with this disease often tolerate heat poorly. Often the patient will want no top bedding, and he may want the windows wide open even in cold weather. His wishes should be granted because the patient with hyperthyroidism is generating enough heat to keep from being chilled. If the patient is extremely restless, the base of the bed may need to be made with two full-sized sheets so that it can be tucked in securely at both the head and foot. This measure usually obviates the need for frequent straightening of the bed, which may be embarrassing and upsetting to the patient. The linen may need to be changed frequently because the patient with hyperthyroidism often perspires profusely. Lightweight pajamas are preferable to nightgowns because covers can then be left off or thrown off as necessary.

If the patient is very nervous, he may drop articles or may not be able to handle objects securely. This usually upsets him, and may become a source of real frus-

tration. Therefore, it may be necessary to do small things for the patient that he may seem physically able to do for himself. For example, he may need water or other beverages poured for him, and some patients may even need help in buttoning their clothes and tying shoelaces. This help should be given as inconspicuously as possible.

Rest. The greatest nursing problem in care of patients with severe hyperthyroidism is providing enough rest. The actitivites around the patient should be quiet ones, but some limited and guided activity may help the patient more than enforced absolute quiet and rest. Quiet activity, such as nonintricate handicrafts or reading, keeps the patient occupied and actually may provide rest. The unoccupied patient who is allowed out of bed may use a great deal of energy in wandering about. If he is hospitalized, he may have upsetting contacts with other patients, who may misunderstand him, and he may disturb others. Modifying routines also may be necessary. For example, if the patient on bed rest becomes very upset by having to use the bedpan, he may expend less energy in walking to the bathroom, and orders permitting him to use the bathroom may be needed. Visitors should be restricted if they seem to make the patient more overactive, and the patient should be protected from surprise visits or disturbing news. Persons around the patient, either personnel or family, should try to remain calm, and discussion of controversial subjects should be avoided. When the patient has real difficulty resting, a sedative such as phenobarbital may be ordered to be given regularly. Consistently assigning a staff member who has established good rapport with the patient to care for him also may help to lessen his anxiety and permit him to rest.

Diet. Since appetite usually is increased in hyperthyroidism, the nurse should see that the patient is getting sufficient food. If weight loss has occurred, extra protein may be needed to help rebuild lost tissues, and extra carbohydrate is needed to meet the increased fuel requirements brought on by the disease. Stimulating drinks such as tea and coffee should not be given unless withholding them upsets the patient. Decaffeinated preparations may be substituted for patients who are accustomed to a hot liquid with meals.

The patient should know that persons around him understand his increased need for food, so that self-consciousness does not keep him from eating as much as he really needs. Occasionally the patient's appetite is not good, and yet he needs extra food. Finding out what he likes to eat and trying to obtain it often helps. The patient should be given repeated helpings of foods he likes, and he should be given food between meals.

Treatment of thyroid storm. A rare but life-threatening disorder known as thyroid crisis, or thyroid storm, may occur in patients with uncontrolled hyperthyroidism in response to the stress of surgery, infection, or physical or emotional trauma. Increased amounts of thyroid hormones are released into the bloodstream and metabolism is markedly increased. The patient's temperature may rise to 41° C. (106° F.) as the body becomes unable to release the heat formed with increased metabolism. The pulse may be very rapid, and there is marked apprehension, restlessness, irritability, and prostration. The patient may become delirious and finally comatose, with death resulting from heart failure. Treatment may include oxygen by tent; hypothermia, alcohol sponges, or ice bags to lower temperature; antithyroid drugs; intravenous fluids as necessary; narcotics; sedative drugs; and cardiac drugs such as digitalis preparations or quinidine, as indicated by the heart action. Cortisone and prednisone may be given to decrease the body's own output of adrenocortical hormones, since it appears that cortical hormone action may play some part in thyroid crisis.

Operative treatment of diseases of the thyroid

Part or all of the thyroid gland may be removed surgically, depending upon the purpose for which the operation is done. In the case of a malignancy, the gland may be removed completely *(total thyroidectomy)*, and the patient must then take thyroid hormones regularly for the remainder of his life. When antithyroid drugs do not correct the hyperthyroidism and treatment with radioactive iodine is contraindicated, hyperthyroidism may be treated surgically by removing approximately five-sixths of the gland *(subtotal thyroidectomy)*. In most cases this operation permanently alleviates symptoms, while the remaining thyroid tissue provides enough hormones for normal function.

Postoperatively, the patient who has had either a total or a subtotal thyroidectomy should be protected from strain on the suture line, helped to raise secretions from the lungs, and observed closely for complications such as hemorrhage, obstruction of breathing, and calcium deficiency, each of which requires immediate medical treatment. He also should be helped to swallow by using measures to relieve the sore throat that usually lasts for several days.

Care related to the incision. As soon as the patient has reacted from anesthesia, he usually is placed on his back in a low Fowler's or semi-Fowler's position, with the head, neck, and shoulders supported so that the neck is neither flexed or hyperextended. This position prevents strain on the suture line and avoids the sensation that "the neck is falling off." The patient should be cautioned not to flex or hyperextend his neck, and the nurse should support it while he turns, sits up, or lies down. Support can be given by placing a hand on either side of the neck. As soon as the patient is able (usually by the second postoperative day), he is taught to support his own neck by placing both hands at the back of his head (Fig. 170) when he changes position. After the sutures or clips and the tissue drain have been removed from the incision (usually two to four days postoperatively), and when the doctor feels that sufficient healing has occurred, the patient should begin gradually to practice full-range neck motion (Fig. 2) to prevent permanent limitation of head movements. At this time the doctor also usually wants the patient to begin daily lubrication of the incision with cold cream to soften the tissues.

General care. As soon as postoperative nausea subsides, the patient should take high-carbohydrate fluids by mouth and a soft diet if tolerated. Since the throat usually is sore for several days following surgery, the patient may have some difficulty taking nourishment. Analgesic throat lozenges or a narcotic may be ordered. These medications should be given as necessary to relieve

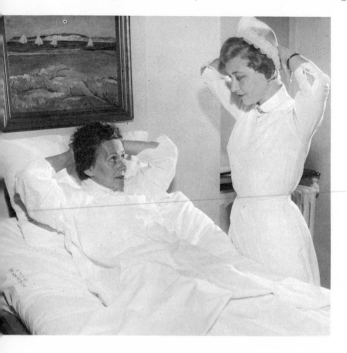

Fig. 170

The nurse is teaching the patient who has had a thyroidectomy how to support the weight of her head as she attempts to sit up in bed.

the discomfort, which may be severe and prevent the patient from raising secretions, but the time of administration should be planned so that a dose can be given about a half hour before meals to make swallowing easier. Benzoin or plain steam inhalations may be used in the room to soothe the mucous membranes of the throat and trachea and thus relieve discomfort.

Postoperative complications. The complications following thyroid operations are extremely serious, and if they are not recognized and treated at once, they can result in death. Complications that the nurse should be alert for are recurrent laryngeal nerve injury, hemorrhage, tetany, and respiratory obstruction. Since the thyroid gland partially surrounds the larynx and trachea, there is danger of respiratory obstruction from a variety of causes, and a tracheotomy set should be kept readily available.

Hemorrhage. The patient's pulse rate,

respirations, and blood pressure usually are checked every fifteen minutes for several hours postoperatively and then, if they continue within normal limits, at longer intervals. The dressings should be watched for signs of hemorrhage. Since blood may drain back under the patient's neck and shoulders, the nurse should slip her hand gently under the neck and shoulders each time she observes the patient to be certain that any bleeding will be detected early. A choking sensation, difficulty in coughing and swallowing, or tightening of the dressing usually means there is bleeding into the surrounding tissues, causing pressure on the trachea and epiglottis. If these symptoms occur, the dressing should be loosened at once and the doctor notified. If loosening the dressing does not relieve the respiratory difficulty and a doctor will not be immediately available, the surgeon may instruct the nurse to remove the clips or sutures from the wound to relieve pressure on the trachea. The procedure to follow should be ascertained from the doctor whenever the nurse is caring for a patient having a thyroidectomy. When the doctor arrives, an emergency tracheotomy may be necessary, and the patient often must be taken to the operating room for retying of the blood vessels and resuturing of the wound.

Respiratory obstruction. The patient and his family should know that he will be a little hoarse and have some difficulty swallowing after the operation due to irritation caused by the endotracheal tube through which the anesthesia was given. This condition is temporary and will subside after local irritation and edema disappear. Although slight hoarseness is normal, the nurse should observe the patient for any increase in it and for any respiratory difficulty accompanying it, since these conditions may be caused by injury to the recurrent laryngeal nerves, hemorrhage, or excessive edema about the vocal cords and larynx. The most common condition to suspect when the patient has difficulty in speaking or breathing is edema, but if the recurrent laryngeal nerves have been injured during an operation on the thyroid gland, the patient may have vocal cord spasm. If the nerve to one vocal cord only is injured, hoarseness may develop. If the nerves on both sides are injured, the vocal cords will become tight and close off the larynx, causing the patient to show signs of respiratory obstruction. As he attempts to pull air in through tightened vocal cords, a crowing sound is made and the tissues around the neck are retracted (appear sucked in). To recognize early symptoms of recurrent laryngeal nerve injury, the nurse should ask the patient to speak as soon as he has reacted from anesthesia and at intervals of from thirty to sixty minutes. The patient with any hoarseness should be observed closely for any other symptoms, such as crowing respirations or retraction of the tissues of the neck, and they should be reported to the doctor at once. A tracheotomy usually is necessary. The injured nerve heals within a few weeks. Respiratory problems disappear and the patient's speaking voice becomes normal. The singing voice, however, often is permanently affected by a recurrent laryngeal nerve injury. A very rare complication of surgery on the thyroid gland is severance of the nerves supplying the vocal cords, which results in permanent loss of speech.

Tetany. A rare but serious complication following thyroid surgery is the accidental removal of one or more of the parathyroid glands. This may cause symptoms of calcium deficiency (tetany), which is fully described on p. 100. This complication may appear from one to seven days postoperatively. If not treated in time, it can cause contraction of the glottis, respiratory obstruction, and death. Calcium gluconate is given intravenously as immediate treatment. Daily oral doses of calcium chloride are then started. If not all of the glands are removed, the remaining ones hypertrophy, so that the hyperthyroidism is only temporary. If all are removed, the patient must have medical treatment for hypoparathyroidism for the rest of his life.

Special needs of the patient with hyperthyroidism. The patient with hyperthyroidism usually undergoes a fairly lengthy program of medical treatment before surgery is scheduled. This treatment may be given at home or in the hospital. The acutely toxic patient usually has a short period of hospitalization and then returns home for a time. The medical regimen of antithyroid drugs, hormones or iodine preparations, rest, and diet,

and the nursing needs of the patient on this regimen are described under the discussion of hyperthyroidism. The patient usually is considered ready for surgery when thyroid function has returned to normal (euthyroid) and the patient has a consistent weight gain and a marked diminution of signs of thyrotoxicosis, such as tachycardia. An electrocardiogram is made before surgery in order to detect evidence of heart damage. Patients with heart damage are preferably treated with radioactive iodine.

Postoperatively, the patient with hyperthyroidism may be placed in an oxygen tent for the first twenty-four hours. The tent is used not only to supply extra oxygen but also for its cooling effect in hot weather. The intravenous fluids given postoperatively may contain Lugol's solution to keep the metabolic rate lowered. A narcotic such as morphine sulfate or meperidine hydrochloride (Demerol) may be given at regular intervals to ensure rest and therefore slow metabolism. However, it must be given judiciously; respirations should not go below 12 per minute. The patient should be observed for signs of thyroid storm, which occasionally occurs following surgery in patients who have severe thyrotoxicosis and who may have undergone too short a period of preoperative medical treatment.

Hypothyroidism

The patient with hypothyroidism has signs and symptoms almost directly opposite to those of the patient with a hyperactive thyroid gland. There is a general slowing up of the body's activities. This condition may occur at any age and is caused by reduction in the secretion of thyroid hormones due to physiologic atrophy, overtreatment for hyperthyroid states, or total removal of the gland for a neoplasm.

Congenital absence or atrophy of the gland in infancy leads to the condition known as *cretinism,* in which both physical and mental growth is stunted. Early recognition and treatment prevents retarded physical growth, but it does not seem to prevent mental retardation.

The adult with hypothyroidism may notice that he is more sensitive to the cold than in the past, that he perspires little, and that his skin and hair are dry. If the condition has come on slowly, the hair may have become thin. He may have become forgetful and slow to grasp new situations, and he may have noticed that he is slowing up at work, falling asleep in the evening, and perhaps having an increase in minor accidents. Very often family members misjudge the person and feel that he has grown lazy, or a new acquaintance may consider him slow mentally. Speech is slowed, and the patient may have to plan sentences before speaking. All changes may occur so gradually that family members scarcely notice them. Since the gastrointestinal tract becomes sluggish, as do all other body functions, constipation with fecal impactions can ocur. Even though appetite may be decreased, the patient tends to gain weight. Some added weight may be due to accumulation of water, but increased weight is due also to the lowered metabolic rate. Menstrual disorders such as anovulation, amenorrhea, functional menorrhagia, and infertility are common in women, and the normal sexual drive is reduced in men.

Most adults have *myxedema* as a complication of hypothyroidism. This general or localized nonpitting edema is caused by accumulations in the tissues of mucopolysaccharides, which are chemical substances that hold water. Periorbital edema and puffy hands and feet are rather common. The tongue often is edematous and may protrude slightly. Edema of the vocal cords may cause the patient to be hoarse. The tissues of the heart also frequently become edematous, and this condition may cause cardiac symptoms.

Treatment of hypothyroidism is the administration of the deficient thyroid hormone. (See p. 734 for the preparations used.) It is important that dosages be increased gradually because a sudden increase in metabolic rate can cause death from heart failure. The daily maintenance dose of thyroid hormones required varies widely. The correct dose for each patient is determined by a remission in the symptoms of hypofunction. The nurse should carefully note and report all changes that may indicate either excessive or inadequate dosage. Adults with hypothyroidism respond quickly to the administration of thyroid hormones. Changes in appearance and physical symptoms occur within two or three days. If hypothyroidism is caused by malfunction of the thyroid gland itself and if treatment is started early, men-

tal and physical characteristics may be restored even though treatment must be continued throughout the patient's life. When derangement of the adrenocortical and pituitary hormones is also involved, treatment is more complicated and sometimes less successful.

General nursing care for the patient with hypothyroidism is determined by his symptoms. The family should be helped to understand the patient's behavior and to meet his needs. They must give the patient time to carry out any activity since he is almost always slow but not necessarily incapable. Provision should be made for extra warmth, and if the patient complains of drafts, his bed should be moved to avoid them. A minimum of soap should be used for bathing, and creams and lotions should be used to keep the skin in reasonably good condition. If constipation is a problem, the diet should consist largely of foods that are high in roughage. The doctor usually orders a diet fairly high in protein and low in total calories. If myxedema is a problem, fluids may be restricted.

Since the early symptoms of hypothyroidism in both children and adults are rather vague, people may not recognize them, or if they do, they may not consider them significant enough to require medical attention. Regular physical examinations by the same doctor should be urged, since he may be able to recognize symptoms of hypothyroidism earlier than would otherwise be possible.

The patient with disease of the parathyroid glands

The parathyroid glands are four or more tiny glands located in close proximity to the thyroid gland. The secretion, parathyroid hormone, regulates the level of calcium and phosphate ions in the body fluids by increasing the rate of release of calcium from the bones, enhancing its absorption from the intestine, and increasing the renal excretion of phosphorus and the renal absorption of calcium. Its secretion is thought to be stimulated by a fall in the level of blood calcium.

As with other endocrine glands, the parathyroid glands may become hyperactive or hypoactive. Benign neoplasms are the most frequent cause of hyperfunction, but malignant tumors and hyperplasia may occur. Inadvertent removal of all or some of the parathyroid glands during surgery on the thyroid gland or during other surgery in the region and ideopathic atrophy are the commonest causes of hypofunction. Any upset in the function of the parathyroid glands causes symptoms of electrolyte imbalance. (See the discussions of hypocalcemia and hypercalcemia, p. 100.)

Hypoparathyroidism

When there is insufficient hormone production or hypofunction of the parathyroid glands, blood calcium decreases and neuromuscular symptoms appear. (These symptoms are described on p. 100.) They appear because a certain level of calcium in the body fluids is essential for the normal transmission of nerve impulses. As the level decreases, the irritability of all the muscles increases, and tetany may develop. Spasm of the laryngeal muscles may cause hoarseness of the voice. Manifestations of prolonged hypocalcemia are prematurely gray hair with alopecia (loss of hair), enamel defects of the teeth, and the development of cataracts in the lenses of the eyes.

The patient with hypoparathyroidism is usually given calcium salts or dihydrotachysterol (Hytakerol) by mouth daily until the serum calcium level stabilizes, and then once a week for the remainder of his life. A diet high in calcium and vitamin D must also be taken. Vitamin D appears to be the principle regulator of the level of calcium ions in the body fluids and consequently is essential. Because of the danger that hypercalcemia will develop, serum calcium level tests or the Sulkowitch test for calcium in the urine must be done at intervals.

Immediate treatment of tetany is the intravenous administration of calcium gluconate. Maintenance doses of calcium carbonate and calcium lactate may then be given by mouth, and vitamin D may be given to ensure efficient use of the calcium by the body. Nursing care of patients with tetany includes careful observation of beginning symptoms of neuromuscular disorders so that prompt treatment can be given and severe reactions such as convulsions can be prevented. If the patient does have a convulsive seizure, he should be protected against physical injury, and his tongue should be prevented from slipping backward in his throat, preventing passage of air. (See care of the patient with convulsions, p. 871.)

Hyperparathyroidism

In hyperparathyroidism, too much parathyroid hormone is released into the bloodstream, causing the serum calcium to be higher than normal and the serum phosphorus level to be lower than normal. There is increased urinary excretion of both calcium and phosphorus, and renal calculi frequently develop. Other symptoms are anorexia, nausea, vomiting, and constipation, all of which may be due to electrolyte imbalance. If the calcium intake is not increased, calcium is removed from the bones and *osteoporosis* (a demineralization of the bones) results. Osteoporosis causes the bones to become fragile and to fracture easily. Pathologic fractures (fractures resulting from weight-bearing or pressure, and not from trauma) often occur.

Treatment for hyperparathyroidism is the surgical removal of part or all of the glands. If the parathyroidism is caused by an adenoma, this tumor is excised. If there is generalized hyperplasia, a subtotal parathyroidectomy is performed. All of the parathyroid tissue may be removed if the patient has a malignancy of the gland, and he then must be treated for hypoparathyroidism for the remainder of his life.

Following surgery the patient must be watched carefully for signs of hypoparathyroidism, especially tetany. Dihydrotachysterol or calcium salts are usually given in decreasing doses for several weeks following surgery, and a high-calcium diet supplemented with vitamin D is continued for many months.

Until treatment is well under way, the patient needs to take generous amounts of fluid so that the calcium is less likely to precipitate out in the urine, causing renal calculi. Until the bones have become recalcified, special care needs to be taken to prevent injury, as described later in this chapter.

Diabetes mellitus

Diabetes mellitus is a chronic metabolic disease involving a disorder of carbohydrate metabolism and subsequent derangement of protein and fat metabolism. Disturbance in production, action, or metabolic rate of insulin, a hormone secreted by the islands of Langerhans in the pancreas, is involved in the disease.

Cause

Normally, insulin facilitates the conversion of glucose to fat in adipose tissues, speeds the conversion of glucose to glycogen in the liver and the muscles, and speeds the oxidation of glucose in the cells. It is uncertain how insulin actually acts to accomplish these activities, but the most generally accepted theory is that it facilitates the transport of glucose across cell membranes. The secretion of insulin is stimulated by a rise in the glucose level in the blood and inhibited by a fall in it.

In diabetes mellitus there always is insufficient insulin available for use in carbohydrate metabolism. It is now known that this insufficiency may be caused by at least three factors: a failure in production of insulin, blockage of its use, or its destruction by the body. The beta cells in the islands of Langerhans may fail to produce enough insulin. The need for insulin may be greater than the available supply, usually because metabolism is increased excessively for some reason. The use of insulin by the cells may be prohibited by some antagonistic factor such as the growth hormone from the anterior pituitary gland or adrenocortical glucocorticoids. It may be bound to gamma globulin fractions in the serum (anti-insulin activity) so that it is not available for use. Insulin also may be destroyed by the liver or other tissues. It is felt that anti-insulin activity (a sensitization to the protein in insulin) may be a factor in the adult type of diabetes, and that years of hyperfunction of the insulin-producing cells in the pancreas also may be a cause. Children are thought to have a primary derangement in the insulin-producing cells, or in some other hormonal or enzymatic activity necessary for regulating the secretion or the utilization of insulin.

The predisposition to develop diabetes is known to be hereditary and transmitted as a mendelian recessive characteristic. If both parents have diabetes, all their children, if they live long enough, will eventually develop the disease. If a person with diabetes marries one with no inherited tendency to the disease, none of the children will have diabetes although they will carry the recessive trait and in turn pass it on to their own children.

From 70 to 90% of adults with diabetes mellitus have a history of obesity; this is not true in children. According to one theory, obesity presents an increased demand for insulin, the special cells within the pancreas that secrete insulin become exhausted, and diabetes develops. Diabetes mellitis is more common in women than in men, and it is thought that this may be due to the higher incidence of obesity among women. It is also more common among married than among single women. This may be linked to the frequent occurrence of obesity in women who have borne children or to hormonal influences related to pregnancy.

Signs and symptoms

The most common and characteristic symptoms of diabetes mellitus are increased appetite (polyphagia), increased thirst (polydipsia), and increased urine (polyuria). The signs and symptoms are directly related to faulty oxidation of carbohydrate and the chain of events that follows. Normally, glucose is oxidized by the body to form carbon dioxide and water, with production of energy to meet body needs. Any excess is changed to glycogen in the liver and is stored in the liver and in the muscles, or it is converted to fat and stored. However, insulin is needed for the formation of glycogen. In diabetes, glucose remains in the bloodstream and cannot be converted to glycogen because the insulin is not present or is unusable. The amount of sugar in the blood increases (hyperglycemia) and some of it is eliminated in the urine (glycosuria), after being diluted by the kidneys to cause the polyuria. Pruritus vulvae, caused by the irritating effect of the urine with its high sugar content, may occur.

Since the patient with untreated diabetes mellitus is unable to utilize carbohydrates satisfactorily, large amounts of fat, including body fat, are oxidized to produce energy. Fats on oxidation form ketone bodies (fatty acids), which in normal amounts are neutralized with bases such as bicarbonate in the blood plasma to maintain the normal acid-base balance of the body. When excessive amounts of fat are burned, the bases in the blood plasma may become exhausted. Acidosis (ketosis) develops (p. 101) and acetone bodies are then excreted in the urine. Despite having a large appetite, the patient often loses weight. Weakness and fatigue are common, and normal resistance to infection is lowered.

The onset of symptoms in the young person often is rapid, but in the older, obese patient, the onset usually is insidious. Complications often cause the elderly patient to seek medical care. Diabetes in children frequently is diagnosed when severe acidosis develops during the course of an acute infectious illness.

Incidence

Diabetes mellitus is found most frequently in persons over 40 years of age who are obese and who have a family history of diabetes, although the disease is fairly common in children and in young adults. The incidence increases steadily until the seventh decade of life. Elderly persons usually have a much less severe form of the disease than younger ones, although complications may be severe. An estimated 2 million persons in the United States have diagnosed diabetes, and it has been estimated that there are approximately 1.5 million persons with undiagnosed disease.[12] The incidence is higher among Jewish than among non-Jewish people.

In general, the increased incidence of diabetes can be attributed to the longer lifespan with more people in the older age group, to the lower mortality rate among young people with diabetes mellitus since the discovery of insulin, to the increase in the number of persons with diabetes who now marry and have children, to the public's increased awareness of the disease, and to the availability of detection facilities. In 1964, diabetes was the seventh cause of death in the United States.[12]

Significance as a public health problem

The fact that diabetes mellitus probably occurs in 1 out of 55 persons presents a sizable public health problem of particular economic and social significance. The estab-lishment of community diabetes programs is being urged by the United States Public Health Service. These programs should be directed toward (1) detection of diabetes and follow-up of suspected cases to confirm the diagnosis and to give treatment, (2) prevention or correction of obesity, (3) keeping patients with diabetes under medical supervision and their condition under control, (4) promotion of understanding of diabetes mellitus through education of professional groups, the patient, his family, and the community as a whole, and (5) mobilization of community resources such as medical, nursing, social, and nutrition groups to aid persons who have diabetes.

The American Diabetes Association, Inc., which is composed of physicians, furthers patient education, professional education, diabetes detection, public education, and research. It publishes a professional journal* that helps to keep physicians informed and a bimonthly magazine† for persons with diabetes. Each year there is a National Diabetes Week. This week is sponsored by the Association to stimulate early case finding in persons who do not know that they have diabetes and to educate the public about the disease. The Association has fifty local groups that work in their own areas. They sponsor camps for diabetic children and cooperate on nationwide projects. The National Institute of Arthritis and Metabolic Diseases at Bethesda, Maryland, as part of the program of the United States Public Health Service, contributes greatly to research in diabetes.

Local health departments have established multiphasic screening programs to detect diabetes. A test of the blood for sugar level or a test of the urine for sugar is used to detect diabetes, but the blood tests are considered best. Urine testing may give inaccurate results.[19] Case finding programs can be carried out in health department clinics, hospital outpatient clinics, doctors' offices, industry, or in the community (at health fairs or by mobile testing units). Selected groups or whole communities can avail themselves of these services. Follow-up of any positive findings is essential for a successful program. Public health nurses can

---

*Diabetes.

†American Diabetes Association Forecast.

help by making home visits if diabetes is definitely established, if retesting needs to be done, if individuals have indicated that they have no physician or are under no medical supervision, or if persons being tested request home visits by a nurse at the time of the first testing. Through her visits, misunderstandings about retesting can be clarified, and family reactions to the possibility of diabetes can be determined.

Prevention

Since the cause of diabetes mellitus is unknown, specific measures for primary prevention are limited. However, much can be done by every nurse if she is aware of the hereditary nature of the disease and its probable association with obesity. If diabetes is part of a family history, the nurse can explain to relatives of the patient the significance of periodic testing for detecting the disease early and can encourage all members of the family to maintain normal weight. Women who have had large babies also should be urged to avoid gaining weight and to have periodic tests for diabetes. Statistics show that 17% of mothers with babies weighing over 9 pounds develop diabetes later in life, and 80 to 90% of those with babies weighing over 13 pounds do.[34]

Studies of women with diabetes have shown that there is a high fetal and neonatal death rate, a high proportion of large babies with a high mortality rate, and a great tendency toward other abnormalities in pregnancy.[43] Thus, early prenatal care should be emphasized. It has been suggested that studies be done on women who have glycosuria during pregnancy to determine if the administration of insulin or oral antidiabetic drugs during this time might help to produce a more successful outcome of pregnancy and delay or prevent development of diabetes in them.[43]

It has also been discovered that women who have repeated spontaneous abortions, although giving no signs of carbohydrate intolerance by a regular glucose tolerance test, often show evidence of a decreased insulin reserve when cortisone is given prior to the glucose tolerance test. A significantly large number of relatives of persons with diabetes also respond in this manner. Therefore, it is suspected that these people may need close

medical supervision during stress situations such as pregnancy, extensive surgery, or serious illness to determine a need for insulin or oral antidiabetic drugs.[9] The nurse should look at the medical history of patients and watch those with family histories of diabetes mellitus closely for symptoms of the disease.

There is much the nurse can do to prevent complications in the person with known diabetes. These measures will be discussed as part of nursing care.

Diagnostic tests

Urine tests. Urine testing is familiar to most of the public. Testing of urine for sugar is part of a complete urinalysis, and the urine of patients with known or suspected diabetes mellitus is tested frequently for sugar and acetone by one of the following methods. Patients with known diabetes mellitus may be asked to do the tests themselves at regular intervals as an indication of adequate control of the blood sugar level.

The *Benedict test,* a copper reduction method, is a standard way to test urine for sugar; 5 ml., or approximately 1 tsp., of Benedict's solution is placed in a test tube, and eight drops of urine are added. The urine and Benedict's solution are mixed and then either placed over a direct flame or in a water bath and allowed to boil for five minutes. A color chart then is used to compare the color of the specimen with a standard, and it is graded as follows: if the solution remains blue, there is no sugar; green is considered 1 plus; yellow, 2 plus; orange, 3 plus; and red, 4 plus.

Clinitest is another copper reduction method of testing the urine for sugar. It comes in a compact kit and is convenient for use because it is small and easy to carry and store. The kit contains a test tube, a medicine dropper, caustic tablets, a small pinch forceps, and a color chart. Ten drops of water and five of urine are placed in the test tube, and a tablet is added. The tablet generates heat, and the color of the solution is graded just as in the Benedict test.

Dreypak is also a copper reduction method used to detect sugar in the urine. A urine-impregnated strip of filter paper is dipped into boiling Benedict's solution. Color changes are the same as for the Benedict test.

Galatest is a bismuth reduction method for detecting sugar in the urine. The testing substance comes in powder form. A drop of urine is placed on the powder, and the color changes are shades of gray to black. Since shades of gray are difficult to distinguish, this test is not widely used.

Tes-Tape and *Clinistix* are both enzymatic tests for sugar. In the Tes-Tape test, a strip of paper impregnated with the testing ingredients, which convert the glucose in the urine into gluconic acid, is dipped into the urine specimen. Clinistix is similar to a book match and is also dipped into the urine. Positive colors for sugar in both tests are green or blue.

Although single specimens of urine may show the presence of sugar, the physician may wish to find out what time of day the most sugar is excreted and prescribe insulin accordingly. To determine this, *fractional* or *group urines* may be collected. All the urine voided from before breakfast to just before lunch is collected, and a sample is tested for sugar. This is the first specimen; the second is collected from before lunch to just before dinner; the third, from dinner to before bedtime; and the fourth, from bedtime until the next morning.

Twenty-four-hour urine collections also may be obtained to determine the quantity of sugar excreted in a day. In this collection the first specimen of the morning is discarded. All urine excreted for the next twenty-four hours is collected in a gallon bottle and sent to the laboratory. It is important that the patient knows he must add the first urine voided the next morning to the specimen.

There are several *tests for acetone* in the urine. In one method (*Gerhardt's test for acid bodies*) 10% ferric chloride is added drop by drop to 5 ml. of urine in a test tube until sediment no longer forms. A wine-red color indicates presence of ketones (acetone). If the patient has been taking aspirin or salicylate drugs, the specimen should be divided, one part boiled, and then compared with the other part. If the color in the boiled specimen has disappeared, acetone is present; color due to drugs does not disappear when the urine is heated.

In the *Lange method,* or *sodium nitroprusside test,* five drops of Lange's solution (glacial acetic acid and sodium nitroprusside) are added to 5 ml. of urine in a test tube. From ten to fifteen drops of ammonia are added slowly along the side of the tube to cover the surface of the solution. If a purplish ring forms between the solutions, the test is positive for acetone.

Testol or *Acetest* tablets may be used to test for acetone. Urine is dropped on the tablet. If acetone is present, a purple color appears and can be compared with a color chart for intensity.

Ketostix is a paper strip that is dipped into the urine specimen and one minute later compared with a color chart to detect the presence of acetone.

Blood sugar tests. Blood sugar levels are determined when diabetes mellitus is suspected or to check on the effectiveness of the treatment for diabetes. The normal fasting blood sugar ranges from 80 to 120 mg. per 100 ml. of blood. The blood specimen for sugar usually is taken when the patient is in a fasting state, but occasionally the specimen is taken an hour or two after a heavy meal (a postprandial specimen).

Glucose tolerance test. This test is done to detect abnormalities of carbohydrate metabolism such as may be present in hypoglycemia, diabetes mellitus, and adrenocortical disease. No food is allowed after midnight the night before the test. Samples of blood and urine to test for sugar are obtained at the beginning of the test, and the patient is then asked to drink a mixture containing glucose, water, and lemon juice. The amount of glucose administered is proportional to body weight. Samples of blood and urine are taken at intervals of one-half hour, one hour, and two hours following the ingestion of the glucose mixture. Within one-half hour of ingestion of the glucose, the blood sugar normally rises to above 150 mg. per 100 ml. of blood, and within two hours it will drop to a normal fasting level. There will be no sugar in the urine. Usually when the blood sugar level exceeds 140 mg. per 100 ml. of blood, sugar will appear in the urine.

In patients with hypofunction of the adrenal cortex, the initial rise in the blood sugar is less than normal, and it returns rapidly to normal levels. The blood sugar of a person with diabetes mellitus or hyperfunction of the adrenal cortex goes up rapidly and will remain high for a longer time than normal. The patient who has hypoglycemia may have a drop in his blood sugar much below normal levels and must be watched during the test for signs of hypoglycemic reaction (similar to insulin shock).

Cortisone-glucose tolerance test. This test is more sensitive than a glucose tolerance test and is used when the results of the glucose tolerance test are inconclusive. It is frequently used to detect prediabetic states in women who are pregnant and in relatives of persons with known diabetes. It is performed by a method similar to the glucose tolerance test except that cortisone, which is known to cause an abnormal rise in the blood sugar level of people who are predisposed to diabetes, is administered at the start of testing. It is considered positive when the blood sugar is 140 mg. or more per 100 ml. of blood at the end of two hours.

Medical treatment and nursing care

Control. Although diabetes cannot be cured, it can be controlled to a large extent by regulating the diet and giving insulin or oral antidiabetic drugs. There are two schools of thought on the control of diabetes. One medical group believes that the patient's urine must be kept sugar free and the blood sugar at a normal level. The other theory is that the disease can be controlled in the presence of an above-normal blood sugar and of sugar in the urine provided enough insulin is taken and enough food is eaten to meet metabolic needs. This is demonstrated by disappearance of signs and symptoms such as loss of weight and fatigue. There is evidence that complications such as retinal damage occur more often in persons who are not under medical supervision and treatment than in those whose disease is diagnosed and who remain under medical care.[1]

Emotional factors. The emotional response to a diagnosis of diabetes is often severe and is not easily dealt with. Part of this may result from fear of disability and eventual death. Since diabetes is so widespread, many people know of relatives and friends who have had the disease and who have eventually had amputations or have become blind. Perhaps an even greater cause of emotional reaction is that diabetes affects the patient's life pattern in regard to food.

Food and eating have meaning beyond the actual meeting of nutritional needs, and changes in eating habits are extremely hard for patients to accept. Adolescents, perhaps more than any other age group, find restriction in eating almost intolerable and need much understanding in their early adjustment to the disease.

Getting started on a suitable plan of care for diabetes will often make a great difference in how the patient continues with care. It can help him and his family avoid undue stress and concern that may make it difficult to control the diabetes. Since most patients with diabetes are now treated in a doctor's office or a hospital clinic, the public health nurse may need to help them with the initial adjustments. Patients who are particularly difficult to control (*brittle diabetics*), those with complications such as infection, and those who are unusually apprehensive often are hospitalized for a period of time. The hospital nurse should work closely with these patients to try to help them adjust to their disease. On discharge from the hospital, they, too, often need to be visited by the public health nurse.

The patient's response to the persons who work with him, at the time the diagnosis is made and shortly thereafter, is tremendously important in determining his attitude toward his disease and, in turn, his ability to accept the treatment and restrictions that are necessary. Most medical authorities believe that the patient must know the potential seriousness of untreated diabetes. On the other hand, they believe that the more simply and easily the necessary changes can be made, the better for all concerned. If the patient with diabetes mellitus continues with the prescribed dietary regimen, takes the medication ordered, follows other instructions, and has periodic medical checkups, his life can be very much like that of anyone else. Only occasionally do adjustments in the patient's work need to be made, although it is preferable that patients with diabetes work regular hours. If they must rotate shifts, plans should be made to avoid the 12 midnight to 8 A.M. rotation, because the temporary change in the eating pattern tends to upset control of diabetes. The patient who takes insulin regularly, is difficult to regulate, and consequently may have hypoglycemic reactions (insulin shock) should not work where there is danger of injury to himself or others. He therefore may occasionally need vocational rehabilitation.

General nursing care. Whether care and teaching are done in the hospital, in the clinic, or in the patient's home, it is important that the nurse get to know the patient. The patient should be given an opportunity to express what he thinks having diabetes will mean to him, and the nurse should attempt to learn what the patient knows about the disease. In the clinic, provision should be made for every newly diagnosed patient to have a conference with the nurse, preferably in a private conference room. Plans should always be made with him for future teaching conferences.

Since diabetes is a chronic disease and patients often must take daily medication and must adhere to a diet, both children and adults are taught early to take care of these particular needs for themselves unless this is not possible for some reason. Children as young as 6 or 7 years of age can begin to learn to take care of their particular needs.

The nurse works out a plan for the patient for self-administration of medication, self-testing of urine (if it is necessary), preparation and measurement of food, regular exercise, and recognition of unusual symptoms. She also has the responsibility to review with him the general rules of good hygiene and of healthful living. The patient is taught special care of the feet since circulatory difficulties of the lower extremities often occur, especially in elderly patients. The family members should always be included in the teaching plan even though they may not take an active part in the procedures involved. This helps them to understand what is necessary and to encourage the patient to carry out instructions and enables them to take over if necessary.

The teaching plan should be arranged so that the patient is not rushed and has enough time for sufficient practice in self-care. If a

Fig. 171

The public health nurse discusses some information regarding the treatment of diabetes with both the patient and her mother.

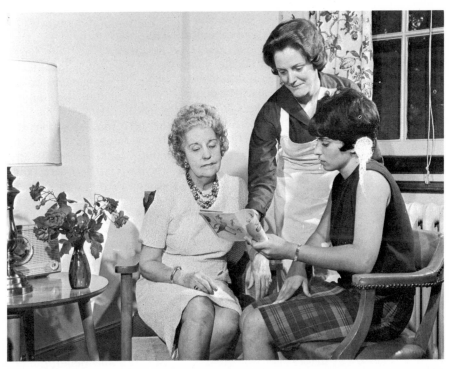

member of the patient's family is to learn to give the care, arrangements may need to be made for this person to come to the hospital or the clinic at other than regular hours. Work or home responsibilities may make attendance at the usual times impossible. A public health nurse may need to be asked to give this instruction in the home (Fig. 171).

Group teaching, combined with individual conferences, is desirable whenever possible and when the patient's physician agrees to this plan. Patients as well as family members often gain reassurance and consolation from contact with others who have similar problems. Emphasis in teaching, in groups or individually, however, should be on the fact that the patient is essentially a *normal* person and quite capable of living a completely *normal* life if he follows a few simple rules of health and adheres closely at all times to the prescription for insulin or other medication and to the diet given to him by his physician. Filmstrips such as *Taking Care of Diabetes*° or *Just One in a Crowd*† are useful for group sessions. They should be followed by a question period. Booklets are available to supplement teaching, and patients often find them helpful. *Facts About Diabetes*‡ and *A Pocket Reference for the Diabetic*§ are especially useful, but nonessential aspects for individual patients should be deleted. A bimonthly publication, *ADA Forecast*,‖ is helpful for some patients. For young people, *Keith and Ellen Win a New Look at Life*¶ depicts in comic-strip fashion two people's acceptance of diabetes and the regimen compatible with normal living.

As she works with each patient, the nurse should give him encouragement and note

---

°Produced by the American Diabetes Association, Inc., 1 East 45th St., New York, N. Y., 1951.
†Produced by the United States Public Health Service, 1965, and available from Public Health Service Audiovisual Facility, Communicable Disease Center, Atlanta, Ga.
‡Published by the American Diabetes Association, Inc., 1 East 45th St., New York, N. Y., 1956.
§Published by Eli Lilly & Co., Indianapolis, Ind., 1954.
‖Published by the American Diabetes Association, Inc., 1 East 45th St., New York, N. Y., 1956.
¶Vic Herman Studio Productions, New York, N. Y., vol. 1, Eli Lilly & Co., Indianapolis, Ind., 1954.

how he appears to be accepting his disease. The necessity of having to take injections and perhaps to limit his diet for the rest of life is more than some patients can face. The patient may feel that he is different and must live a life different from that of other people. He may tend to dissociate himself from friends because he can no longer engage in many activities without fear of having insulin shock. He may be self-conscious about eating with others because he must avoid certain foods. Each patient will need individual understanding and help to live as normal a life as possible. Satisfactory arrangements can usually be made in his social life. Help in learning diet substitution will aid him in overcoming unnecessary embarrassment when eating meals away from home. He also often can be assisted in planning a schedule for injections that will keep his diabetes under control yet allow him as much freedom as possible. Throughout this adjustment period the patient needs emotional support and interest from his family and from medical personnel who are familiar with his particular needs.

If the nurse is assigned to care for a patient with diabetes in the hospital, she should know whether the diagnosis is recent or whether the patient has had diabetes for some time. Patients who have diabetes often enter the hospital for treatment of another condition. If so, the nurse should find out early the usual diabetic regimen of the patient. If his general condition permits, she usually should help him continue self-care, such as giving his own insulin and making his own food selection. If he is not allowed to continue his routine, he may have difficulty readjusting to it upon discharge from the hospital. Self-care, however, is not always desirable. Some patients need to be dependent when a new illness occurs and want others to assume complete responsibility for their care. The nurse should help to determine whether it is best for him to be allowed to be dependent in this aspect or whether he should be urged to continue self-care, while providing for his dependency needs in other ways. Some patients may be seriously ill and actually physically unable to continue self-care.

Diet. Depending upon the physician's experience and belief, the patient is placed on a weighed or measured diet or on an un-weighed, unmeasured diet with elimination of concentrated sweets. The patient on a *weighed diet* actually weighs out specific amounts of food on a small scale. Food can be weighed for a day at a time. However, if the patient eats away from home, practice in estimating usual weighed amounts will be necessary. Specific amounts of carbohydrates, protein, and fat are prescribed. A usual diet consists of 150 to 200 grams of carbohydrate, 75 to 100 grams of protein, and fat in an amount that will make up the needed number of calories. A *measured diet* is one in which the amounts are calculated according to household measurements or usual-sized portions. It is important to use reasonable-sized portions to avoid confusion and to simplify preparation for the patient and his family. If the patient has a *self-chosen, unmeasured diet*, he should eat a well-balanced selection of food in moderate quantity and should avoid overindulgence in sweets. On this regimen the young patient usually must take insulin every day. He should eat regularly and at the accustomed time without skipping or delaying meals.

The nurse can do much to help the patient with diabetes to understand food values and to follow his prescribed diet. In each instance the patient's age, activity, medical condition, and general nutritional state should be considered when planning his meals. His social and economic background, as well as his eating habits and emotional needs, should be considered. For example, a patient who requires or normally has eaten a low-caloric diet should not have a 2,500-calorie diet planned unless for some reason this is prescribed by the doctor. The patient who is used to the foods of a specific culture should have his diet planned around them. Working people may find that they need to increase their caloric intake on return to work since they use more of their food for energy, causing the blood sugar level to drop and leaving an excess of insulin, which may cause signs of insulin shock. Extra food is also often necessary after unexpected exercise or emotional stress.

It must be emphasized repeatedly to all patients who have diabetes that insulin or oral antidiabetic medications, if ordered, *must* be taken, the usual amount of daily exercise *must* be taken, and meals *must* be eaten. Regulation of the blood sugar level depends on maintaining a balance of these three factors. A decrease or an increase in physical activity seems to change the need for glucose and thus the need for insulin or antidiabetic drugs. Normally, the body would adjust its secretion of insulin to the changes, but regulation of the insulin level is not possible when standardized doses must be given.

Many patients assume that medications for diabetes and food can be safely omitted if they have a cold or other minor ailment and do not feel like eating. This is not so. Full-liquid or clear-liquid diets can be prepared to provide the essential food for a short time, and the patient and his family should know how to prepare them. Any patient taking medication for diabetes who cannot eat or who is physically incapacitated should consult his physician at once.

In any situation in which a clinical dietitian is available, she may initiate or participate in the diet teaching program. However, the nurse often must give the diet instructions. If the dietitian does the teaching, the nurse should work closely with her to assure adequate follow-up supervision. A good time for teaching the patient is during his meal. Current periodic articles contain many useful suggestions for teaching the patient about his diet.[7,11]

In planning the patient's diet, the six food-exchange lists prepared jointly by the American Diabetes Association, The American Dietetic Association, and the Public Health Service are useful and should be available to the nurse. These lists have been published in a booklet* and are available for patients. They are set up according to calories and show how each food listed is equal in nutritional value to any other food on the list and they give suggested menus. The exchange lists allow for substitution of one food for another, depending upon the patient's likes or dislikes or the general menus for the day. Exchanges are set up in seven categories: foods not needing measurement, vegetables, fruits, cereals, meats, fats, and

---

*Meal planning and exchange lists, 620 North Michigan Ave., Chicago, Ill., The American Dietetic Association, Inc.

milk. The patient may take as much as de-sired of foods not needing measurement such as coffee, tea, bouillon, sour pickles, aspara-gus, cabbage, celery, cucumber, greens, lettuce, and tomatoes. He must be cau-tioned not to use sugar, cream, or dressings on these foods, however, without planning for these "extras" in the total intake. A new substitute for sugar is now available. It is a combination of glycine and saccharin and is reported to be less bitter than saccharin. It comes in granulated form. Each packet (2 tsp.) does contain 0.5 mg. of sodium, so that use of the product may be contraindicated if a low-sodium diet is necessary.

If the nurse can help with menu plan-ning on a weekly basis, she can demon-strate how the patient can have variety and foods that he likes even though restric-tions are necessary. Most patients find it helpful to see food portions, especially such "unmeasurable" things as a small potato, an ounce of meat, or a slice of cheese. When possible, foods are measured using standard household measures such as an 8-ounce mea-suring cup, a teaspoon, or a tablespoon. All measurements are level, and cooked foods are measured after cooking. The patient with diabetes usually does not need to buy special foods but can select his diet from the same foods purchased by the rest of the family. Canned fruits that are packed in water rather than in syrup should be suggested since sugar can be added by others as necessary. Vegetables can be prepared with those for the rest of the family except that the patient's portion should be removed before such things as extra butter, milk, flour, or cheese are added. Meats should be baked, broiled, or boiled. Any fat used must be accounted for in the measurements for the meal. A spe-cial cookbook[4] with recipes that can be used for diabetics as well as for other members of the family is now available. It may help pa-tients make meals more varied and appetiz-ing. Special diabetic foods are expensive, and the patient should be reminded that they usually are not calorie-free and need to be reckoned in the daily dietary allowance.

Medications used to control diabetes. Either oral (antidiabetic drugs) or parenteral (insulin) medications may be used to treat diabetes mellitus. Use of oral drugs is par-ticularly helpful for elderly patients who have failing vision and shaky hands, making the administration of insulin difficult. These drugs are a boon, too, for the patient whose emotional reactions make the taking of in-jections almost impossible. Diabetes, how-ever, cannot be controlled in all patients with oral medication. When oral medications fail to control the condition, insulin must be used. The oral drugs are most likely to be effective in treating elderly patients who have a mild form of the disease. They are rarely successful in treating diabetes in the young or in middle-aged or older persons whose blood sugar fluctuates widely. They are useless in treating diabetic acidosis.

If patients are taking oral antidiabetic medication instead of insulin, they often feel that they do not need to be as careful about taking the prescribed dosage of the drug, following the prescribed diet, maintaining the usual amount of exercise, testing their urine for sugar, or taking general health pre-cautions. This is particularly true of the elderly patient. However, the dangers are the same. Patients on both types of medication may develop hypoglycemic reactions, keto-acidosis, and all the other complications of diabetes. In fact, the patient on oral medi-cations needs to be especially cautious if he develops an infection or is subjected to great stress. Oral medication usually becomes in-effectual then, and he will need to take in-sulin at least temporarily to control his blood sugar level. Many doctors want patients with diabetes to learn to give themselves insulin even if they are taking oral antidiabetic drugs. The nurse may need to supervise the care of the patient taking oral medication even more closely than that of the one on insulin.

Insulin. Insulin, which is obtained from the pancreas of sheep, hogs, or cattle, is used in the treatment of 50 to 70% of the patients with diabetes in the United States. There are now six types of insulin in general use, and each is effective in the lowering blood sugar level by aiding in the metabolism of carbo-hydrates. Insulins are either rapid acting or slow acting. Rapid-acting insulins include regular insulin and crystalline insulin. Food must be taken within at least an hour of the injection of rapid-acting insulin to prevent insulin shock. *Regular insulin* is a clear liquid that begins to act approximately forty-five minutes to an hour after injection, reaches the peak from the third to the fifth hours, and loses effectiveness in six hours. *Crystalline insulin* looks the same as regular insulin but is a more refined product. It remains effective one hour longer than regular insulin and is less likely to cause local reaction at the site of injection.

Four types of insulin contain material to slow their action. *Globin zinc insulin* is a clear but slightly amber solution that becomes effective in two hours, reaches its peak action at eight hours, and is effective for twenty-four hours. *Protamine zinc insulin,* a milky-appearing solution, begins to act from four to six hours after injection, reaches the height of activity between eighteen and twenty hours, and is effective for twenty-four hours. *Neutral protamine Hagedorn insulin* (NPH) is another type of protamine zinc insulin. It reaches maximum action from six to ten hours after injection and lasts from twenty-four to thirty hours. NPH insulin is often used when an intermediate action is desired. Most patients receiving NPH insulin need an afternoon snack to prevent a hypoglycemic reaction. *Lente insulin* is a new kind of insulin made without the use of protamine, to which some patients become sensitized. It is a milky-appearing solution, and its "time action" is the same as that of NPH insulin. Similar precautions must be taken to prevent hypoglycemic reaction.

Protamine zinc insulin, NPH insulin, and Lente insulin all separate into layers if allowed to stand. To obtain an accurate dose of the active ingredient, the solution should be mixed by gently rotating the bottle between the palms of the hands. It should not be shaken or allowed to become frothy.

Each individual patient has his own particular insulin need, and suitable amounts as well as types are carefully selected by the doctor. Patients receiving only rapid-acting insulin need more than one injection a day to enable them to use the carbohydrates eaten. Many patients are given the slower-acting insulins since they eliminate the need for several doses during the day. Other patients may need a combination of regular insulin and a protamine insulin.

It is important that the nurse understand the type and the rate of action of each kind of insulin prescribed, It is imperative that she know that the the patient must take food soon after the administration of rapid-acting insulin. A supplementary meal at bedtime is usually necessary for the patient taking slow-acting insulin.

TEACHING THE PATIENT TO ADMINISTER INSULIN. Typical trays for the injection of insulin can be set up for use in demonstrations and for patients to use in practice. The materials are gathered in a cardboard box or on a tray. The nurse can discuss boxes or trays that the patient might have at home or suggest suitable purchases. She can suggest that when the equipment is not in use, it be covered. She should remind the patient that the set should be stored on a shelf or in a closet out of the reach of children. The timesaving value of having all necessary equipment in one place and accessible is obvious.

Equipment needed for the *injection of insulin* includes an insulin syringe, several No. 25 hypodermic needles, a small jar for cotton or a box roll of cotton, a bottle of alcohol, and a small saucepan of sufficient depth to boil the syringe and needle. Disposable syringes and needles may be used. Many public health nursing agencies include a strainer that can be set into the saucepan, making it easier for the patient to drain and handle the equipment without breakage or contamination.

The patient first can learn to prepare the needle and syringe for injection and can practice injecting water into an orange. Then, on a gradual daily plan, he can proceed to inject himself, using the thighs as sites. The use of sterile, disposable syringes and needles facilitates the administration of the medication and teaching of the patient. If the patient cannot afford to use disposable equipment, he should be taught proper techniques of sterilizing and caring for the needle and syringe. (See fundamentals of nursing texts for this procedure.)

Since repeated injections are necessary, *the site of injection must be rotated* to assure proper absorption of medication. Irritation from repeated injections at the same site can cause induration of the tissue, so that the insulin is absorbed too slowly or not at all. Injections should never be given in any one spot oftener than every two weeks, and a safe rule to follow is not to use the same site oftener than once every thirty days. A diagram of the thighs with the possible sites numbered can be made as a guide. The site of injection is then rotated according to the plan.

It may be necessary for a patient to take two types of insulin. If so, the nurse may teach him to *mix the two insulins* in the same syringe so that they may be given in one injection. A simple way of mixing insulin in the same syringe is first to insert a hypodermic needle in each of the bottles to be used. This equalizes the pressure within the bottle and will prevent the plunger of the syringe from being drawn in when the needle is inserted in the bottle, or, if the plunger of the syringe is loose, it will prevent pressure within the bottle from blowing the plunger out and perhaps causing breakage. It also eliminates the necessity of having to inject air into the syringe equivalent to the amount of insulin to be removed. There is danger of accidentally mixing one type of insulin with the other in the bottle if the pressure is not equalized before beginning. Regular insulin and one of the zinc insulins is the usual mixture. After placing the needles in the bottles, the syringe should be attached to the needle in the regular insulin

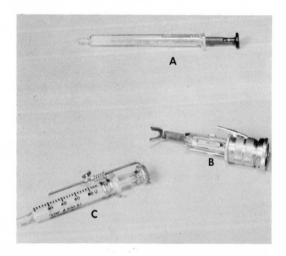

Fig. 172

Special syringes are available for the diabetic patient who has visual difficulty. **A,** Regular insulin syringe. **B,** Automatic injector. **C,** Tru-Set syringe.

bottle without any air in the syringe. The correct amount of regular insulin is withdrawn, and the needle and syringe are withdrawn. Then the needle is taken from the zinc insulin bottle. The needle attached to the syringe containing regular insulin is inserted into the zinc insulin bottle, and the correct amount of insulin is withdrawn. The syringe should be rotated gently to obtain a well-distributed solution. The injection is then given in the usual manner.

At times *modification in methods of administration of insulin* may be necessary because of particular problems; for example, the patient may be elderly, may have unsteady hands, or may have failing vision. In these instances, measurement of insulin, as well as proper injection technique, will require close attention, and adaptation of equipment may be necessary (Fig. 172). The usual 40 to 80 unit insulin syringe may be too slender to grasp, and numbers may be too small for the patient to read easily. The True-Set syringe has a capacity of 1 ml. and an adjustable metal marker that can be placed in the correct-amount position. This prevents the plunger from drawing farther back. The patient draws up insulin until the plunger of the syringe will not go any farther. Even with very limited vision he can tell by feeling that he has the correct amount. Patients who have failing vision also may use a small magnifying adapter (C-Better Magnifier) that can be clipped to a syringe. The numbers on the syringe are magnified, and the patient can see that he has the correct amount of insulin in the syringe. These special syringes and other aids usually are available from surgical supply houses. Some very practical suggestions as well as information as to sources of equipment are available in the publication *Aids for the Blind.*

Patients with poor vision have the danger of drawing air instead of insulin into the syringe. They must be cautioned to invert the bottle completely and to insert the needle only a short distance. Often they are advised to use only about two-thirds of the bottle of insulin and to have on hand another full bottle. Some patients have a public health nurse

---

*Prepared by the American Foundation for the Blind, Inc., 15 West Sixteenth St., New York, N. Y.

or a friend withdraw the last doses in a bottle of insulin for them or go to a clinic for the last few injections.

Some patients are reluctant to put the needle through their own skin. This is difficult even for the calm, matter-of-fact person and may be impossible for the tense, nervous person. An automatic injector, however, can be used (Fig. 172) and is a great help to some patients. It can be attached to a regular 2 ml. syringe. When the medication is drawn up into the syringe, the automatic spring is set, and the patient can wipe the site of injection with alcohol, pinch the skin, and press the spring release. The needle automatically and quickly enters the skin, and the injection can then be given slowly.

Many elderly patients have a tremor of the hands that makes handling the equipment and giving themselves insulin quite difficult. Usually the patient has less tremor at certain times of the day, and plans usually can be made with the physician so that the patient can take his insulin at the time of day that is best for him. A member of the patient's family may have to give the insulin. A family member should always know how to do this in case impending coma or other illness makes it impossible for the patient to give the insulin to himself.

Oral antidiabetes medications. Several oral medications are now available for use in controlling the blood sugar levels in diabetes mellitus. They are not hormones such as insulin, but they stimulate release of insulin from the pancreas, retard the release of glucose from the liver, or aid in the uptake of glucose by cells. Sometimes combinations of oral drugs are used.

Tolbutamide, commonly referred to by the trade name *Orinase,* is a sulfonamide derivative that appears to be helpful in the treatment of some elderly patients who have a mild form of diabetes. Its exact action is unknown, but it appears to increase the ability of the pancreas to secrete insulin. The usual dose is 1 to 2 Gm. (15 to 30 grains) taken daily after an initial dose of 3 Gm. daily for two to eight days.[3] Toxic reactions to tolbutamide may occur, and include skin reactions, depression, and urticaria.

Chlorpropamide (Diabinese) is also a sulfonamide derivative, and its use is similar to that of tolbutamide. Patients needing more than 500 mg. (7½ grains), however, cannot use this drug since it is slowly excreted and produces hypoglycemic reactions. Jaundice occasionally occurs when this drug is used. Another sulfonamide derivative is *acetohexamide (Dymelor).*

Phenformin (DBI, DBI-TD) is a new antidiabetes drug useful for middle-aged and elderly patients who respond to tolbutamide. Its mode of action is not fully understood, but it does not stimulate the pancreas to secrete insulin. It is also used as a supplement for insulin in younger patients, serving to reduce the insulin requirement. If more than 200 mg. (3 grains) of this drug are taken daily, nausea, vomiting, and diarrhea may occur.

Hypoglycemic reaction (insulin shock). All persons with diabetes and their immediate family should know the signs and symptoms and the treatment of hypoglycemia (too much insulin for the available glucose in the blood). Even if the patient follows his usual schedule of medication for diabetes and the prescribed diet, he may have slight reactions at times. Severe reactions, however, are usually caused by too large a dose of insulin or oral antidiabetic drug, or too little food. If the patient does not eat all of his food or if he skips between-meal and bedtime supplements of food that have been prescribed, he may have a reaction. Some patients alter the dose of medication to cover excesses in eating, which may cause them to have a reaction. Vomiting, diarrhea, added exercise, or emotional stress may also be the cause of insulin shock. Every person who has diabetes should carry a card giving his address, the name and address of his doctor, the fact that he has diabetes, and his daily insulin or oral hypoglycemic (antidiabetes) drug dosage.

If for any reason the patient feels shaky, is slightly nervous, perspires, is irritable, or feels dizzy, he should take or be given additional food. These difficulties are the beginning signs of too much insulin. He may also feel weak or hungry, may have headache, palpitation, tremor, blurring of vision, or numbness of the lips or tongue. Many persons with diabetes carry lump sugar or hard candies to be eaten in such emergencies. If the patient is at home, he should drink a glass of orange juice or other fruit juice, which should be available at all times. Sometimes the reaction comes on suddenly, and the patient may not sense early signs. In such an instance a family member may have to give the orange juice or some other sweet fluid. If impending hypoglycemia is not treated immediately, the patient becomes stuporous and unconscious. Occasionally the tremor is very severe, and convulsions may occur. When this happens and when the patient is unconscious, glucose may be given intravenously. Glucagon, a hormone produced by the noninsulin-secreting alpha cells of the pancreas, is now available. It can be given parenterally and is very effective in the emergency treatment of hypoglycemia.

Teaching the patient to test urine for sugar. The urine-testing equipment used will depend upon the doctor's orders and the patient's wishes and finances. He may use a compact set such as Clinitest, or Benedict's solution, which is cheaper. If the latter is used, he needs a clean, empty can in which to place the tube for boiling, two or three test tubes, a teaspoon, a medicine dropper, and a bottle of Benedict's solution. A piece of wire can be bent to fasten over the sides of the pan and looped in the center to hold the tube in an upright position. The patient must be cautioned to avoid vigorous boiling, which may cause the fluid to sputter and burn him. The open end of the test tube must be directed *away* from the patient. A clock can be used for timing. Each patient who must test his urine should be provided with a color chart. Charts are available from pharmaceutical firms or are enclosed in the kits for testing urine. A helpful color guide can be made easily by any resourceful nurse. She uses a piece of cardboard or paper and crayons and refers to a good laboratory textbook for accuracy of color.

What the patient *does* if his test is abnormal depends entirely upon the particular patient and the instructions from his doctor. They should be in writing. The doctor may, for example, instruct the patient to do nothing except repeat the test again during the same day and keep a careful record of urine reactions, increase or decrease his insulin or oral drug dosage, increase or decrease his food intake, or get in touch with him at once. Some doctors may want certain patients to show a trace or even a plus one sugar in

their urine once daily as evidence that the blood sugar is not going too low, whereas for other patients this would not be considered good control. The age of the patient and the stability of his disease affect the doctor's decision in advising a course of action. The nurse must emphasize to the patient that he must follow the doctor's instructions *exactly*. Some patients, particularly young adults, take it upon themselves to alter dosage of insulin or oral antidiabetes drug and diet for themselves and get into serious trouble by so doing.

Skin care. Since patients with diabetes are more susceptible to infection and since healing is generally slow, attention should be given to skin care. Oral hygiene and care of the nails, as well as overall cleanliness, should be stressed (Fig. 173). The legs and feet of the patient with diabetes are particularly vulnerable to infection. Bumps or bruises on the lower extremities should be avoided. If they do occur, they should be observed carefully, and if they do not heal readily, medical attention should be sought. Maintenance of good circulation is extremely important for all adults who have diabetes. (For complete discussion of measures to improve and maintain circulation and to give good general care to the feet, see p. 366.)

If the patient has pruritus vulvae, cleanliness should be stressed. The area should be sponged after each voiding, then thoroughly dried by blotting with a soft towel. Cornstarch can be used as a powder. Sitz baths may be ordered to be taken two or three times a day. Calamine lotion is sometimes helpful, and medicated ointment may be prescribed. When the diabetes is under treatment and the excretion of sugar and abnormal amounts of urine are decreased, the pruritus usually subsides.

Diabetic coma

Diabetic coma is a complication of undiagnosed or neglected diabetes and is the result of prolonged and increasing acidosis. The series of events leading to the development of acidosis are difficult to describe, and many questions regarding the metabolic processes involved have not yet been answered. As has been stated previously, the defect in carbohydrate metabolism is followed by derangement in protein and fat metabolism. For example, nitrogen is excreted in the urine of the poorly controlled diabetic patient, presumably because of the altered ability to store protein normally in the absence of insulin. There then follows an abnormally rapid breakdown of fats into acetoacetic acid and beta-hydroxybutyric acid. These acids cannot be used by the body at the rate in which they are produced. Their accumulation in the bloodstream leads to ketoacidosis and all the signs and symptoms of acidosis appear. These include a fruity odor of the breath, deep respirations, flushed, dry skin, softness of the eyeballs, and eventual loss of consciousness (p. 101).

Before the discovery of insulin, diabetic coma often caused death. *Immediate* care and treatment is still necessary, but with this care the outcome is usually good. The patient or his family should contact their physician at once if any signs or symptoms of acidosis occur. Carrying a card which states that he has diabetes helps to ensure prompt treatment in the event that coma develops while the patient is away from home. Such a card also helps prevent this condition from being mistaken for head injury, cerebrovascular accident, or drunkenness.

The patient in diabetic coma usually is given emergency treatment in the hospital emergency room or clinic, although he may be admitted to a ward. He is given fluids, glucose, and insulin intravenously. The amount of glucose and insulin is prescribed carefully by the doctor, and changes are based on the blood sugar and urinalysis findings. The patient should be kept warm. Epinephrine may be given to raise the blood pressure. Hourly urine specimens may be obtained by catheterization and examined for sugar and acetone. As soon as the patient can take fluids by mouth, he is given salty broth to help maintain electrolyte balance, then orange juice or other sweet fluids. Insulin then is given subcutaneously.

Continued care

The nurse in the hospital or in the home should always pass information along to other medical personnel as to what care has been given, what teaching has been accomplished, and probable future needs of the patient. This information enables the nurse

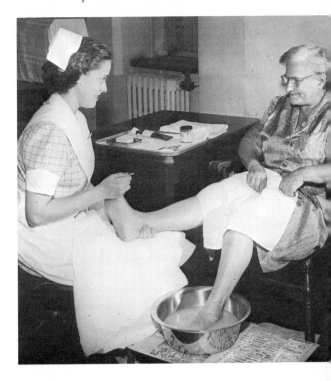

Fig. 173

During visits to the clinic, the elderly patient with diabetes may learn to care for herself. Here the nurse is teaching the patient the proper care of her feet.

and patient to continue his care without delays and repetition. Sometimes the patient may not be capable of learning the care he needs to give himself. If the patient lives alone and has no relative or neighbor who can be taught to give daily injections of insulin and to check on other aspects of care, it may be necessary for a nurse to visit the home to carry out these procedures.

In teaching the patient with diabetes, the nurse should stress the need for him to have enough medication, equipment, and foodstuffs so that he can withstand any unexpected situation. He should also know that the stress of such a situation may easily change his need for medication since more glucose will be used, leaving a surplus of insulin in the blood. Therefore, it will be imperative for him to test his urine for sugar frequently so that he may regulate his medication according to his doctor's instructions or seek medical assistance for regulating the dosage.

Complications of diabetes mellitus

Most medical authorities believe that persons with diabetes who are under treatment and who are reasonably well controlled may develop complications later than those less well controlled. Atherosclerosis, often affecting the coronary arteries, and arterial changes involving particularly the lower extremities, pyelonephritis, retinopathy, neuropathy, and intercapillary glomerulosclerosis (Kimmelstiel-Wilson syndrome) are the common complications.

The alert nurse can help prevent the occurrence of complications in the lower limbs by teaching the patient to protect and make the best use of his limited vascular resources. Ulcerations heal very slowly in these patients, and amputation may be necessary if gangrene occurs. All patients with peripheral circulatory damage also have lessened nerve acuity. They need to be cautioned about possible traumatic injury from lack of sensitivity and taught how to protect the lower extremities from injury (p. 367).

Kimmelstiel-Wilson syndrome, a nephrotic syndrome with albuminuria, edema, and hypercholesterolemia, has an unfavorable prognosis. Treatment is the same as for nephrosis from other causes. Pyelonephritis is treated with antibiotics.

Patients with retinopathy may have serious handicaps because failing vision makes it difficult, if not impossible, for them to inject insulin, test urine, prepare their own food, and give themselves general care. Helping them to accommodate to visual changes presents a great challenge to the nurse. (See discussion of diabetic retinopathy on p. 841.)

Patients with diabetes mellitus are particularly susceptible to tuberculosis infection. They are treated for both diseases with as few modifications in treatment of each disease as possible.

Hypoglycemia

Hypoglycemia is a relatively common disorder characterized by low blood sugar level. The blood sugar falls more rapidly than normal after eating and may drop to abnormally low levels several hours after a meal or after exercise. The patient usually has a sudden onset of faintness, hunger, weakness, and tremor. Headache and feeling of anxiety sometimes occur. In more severe cases, pallor, diaphoresis, rapid pulse, and even twitching, convulsions, and coma can occur. The symptoms may be intermittent, being relieved by food, or they may last for hours or for days.

Hypoglycemia is often functional with no known cause demonstrable. It may also be due to a pancreatic adenoma, causing extra insulin to be released, by liver disease, causing inability to store glycogen, or by pituitary or adrenal dysfunction. If possible, the primary cause is treated.

A high-protein, low-carbohydrate diet often relieves symptoms. Carbohydrates are used quickly, but protein in excess of the normal body needs is converted gradually to glycogen. This helps to maintain the blood sugar at a more nearly normal and more stable level from meal to meal. The patient should eat meals that are spaced regularly and should carry lump sugar or candy with him at all times for immediate use if faintness occurs.

Diseases of the adrenal glands

Each kidney is capped by an adrenal gland consisting of two parts, the medulla and the cortex. When stimulated by the sympathetic nervous system, the *adrenal medulla* secretes two hormones, epinephrine and norepinephrine. (Their physiologic action is described on p. 80.) Both are apparently secreted continuously in small amounts, but their output is markedly increased by any stressful situation. When they are secreted in large amounts into the bloodstream, they rapidly stimulate the physiologic functions needed for responding to emergency situations in both the internal and the external environment. However, they are not essential to life because the sympathetic nervous system produces similar though slower and less extensive responses.

The *adrenal cortex* is essential to life. Without its hormones, the corticosteroids, the body's metabolic processes seem to respond inadequately to even minimal physical and emotional stresses, such as changes in temperature, exercise, or excitement. Severe stresses, such as those caused by serious infections or extreme anxiety, may result in shock and death. Although in recent years many steroid compounds have been isolated from the adrenal cortex, only a few appear to affect metabolism significantly. Hydrocortisone, cortisone, corticosterone, and aldosterone seem to be produced in the largest amounts. Small amounts of the sex hormones, especially androgens, also are secreted. The physiologic actions of the corticosteroids are complex and affect a wide variety of vital functions. In fact, it is felt that they may influence the function of all body cells. The corticosteroids are classified according to their major physiologic action as *glucocorticoids* (hydrocortisone and cortisone), *mineralocorticoids* (aldosterone), and *adrenosterones* (sex hormones secreted by the adrenal cortex). All the corticosteroids to some degree cause sodium (and therefore water since it is always held by sodium) to be retained in the body and potassium and chloride to be excreted by the kidneys. However, this seems to be the primary function of the mineralocorticoids.

The glucocorticoids seems to affect numerous metabolic processes, although their exact actions are not known. They apparently enhance protein catabolism and inhibit protein synthesis, and they appear to be insulin antagonists and to increase the synthesis of glucose by the liver. These actions all tend to raise the blood sugar level. They also seem in some way to influence the defense mechanisms of the body. High concentrations of glucocorticoids in the blood suppress inflammation, inhibit the formation of scar tissue, and may prevent allergic responses. Because of this action, they are useful in treating inflammation (p. 63). In man, glucocorticoids seems to be essential in the body's adjustment to stress, and they appear in some way to influence emotional responses. For example, patients with adrenal insufficiency typically are depressed and anxious Patients receiving large doses of cortisone over a long period of time may become euphoric (unrealistically optimistic and cheerful). Glucocorticoids also apparently play a role in the regulation of melanin metabolism, which determines the pigmenta-tion of the skin and mucous membranes. When there is a deficiency of glucocorticoids, such as in Addison's disease, the skin takes on a bronze coloring.

The action of the adrenosterones apparently is identical to that of the sex hormones that are secreted by the sex glands. Therefore, in treating conditions such as cancer of the breast, in which inhibition of secretion of all sex hormones is considered essential for controlling metastasis, bilateral adrenalectomy may be done.

The secretion of the glucocorticoids and the adrenosterones seems to be stimulated by adrenocorticotropic hormone produced by the anterior pituitary gland, and a high blood level of glucocorticoids suppresses the secretion of adrenocorticotropic hormone. Secretion of aldosterone does not seem to be dependent on hormones from the anterior pituitary gland, but rather is regulated by the concentration of sodium and potassium in the body fluids. When the sodium level in the body fluids is low, the secretion of aldosterone is increased, causing the body to retain salt and also water. A high sodium level inhibits its secretion and allows the kidneys to excrete sodium and water and to retain potassium.

Diseases of the adrenal cortex

Diseases of the adrenal cortex usually are related to *hyperfunction* or *hypofunction* of the cortical portion of the adrenal glands. The malfunction may be from a variety of causes both within and without the gland.

Since the adrenal cortex affects so many physiologic functions, tests that are diagnostic for many disorders may be done. Chemical analyses of the blood usually are ordered to ascertain the stability of electrolyte balance. A glucose tolerance test may be done to determine the ability of the patient to use carbohydrates. Tests of renal tubular function may be done to determine the ability of the kidneys to concentrate and dilute urine and thus maintain water balance. X-ray films of the kidney area may be taken to delineate any adrenal tumor. The doctor usually orders urine collected so that he may study the *urinary excretion of 17-ketosteroids* (androgenic components) *and 17-hydroxycorticoids* (glucocorticoids and related fractions). A twenty-four-hour urine specimen must be obtained for this test. If the original test showed the excretion to be less than normal, adrenocorticotrophic hormone (ACTH) is given and a second collection made. Excretion of more of the substances than normal is diagnostic of hyperfunction of the adrenal cortex. Excretion of less than the normal amount may be diagnostic of adrenocortical insufficiency, but a return to normal excretion after the administration of ACTH indicates a malfunction of the anterior pituitary gland rather than the adrenal cortex. The eosinophil count also may be determined before and after the administration of ACTH *(Thorn test)*. No change in the eosinophil count after the administration of ACTH is diagnostic of adrenocortical insufficiency. In a normal or a hyperplastic gland, ACTH will cause an outpouring of corticosteroids with a resultant decrease in the eosinophil count within four hours. ACTH for these tests usually is given intravenously in a sterile normal saline solution.

Only two of the most common, yet rare, diseases of the adrenal glands will be discussed here. Other related diseases are fully discussed in specialized texts.[16,44]

Addison's disease. In Addison's disease, there is insufficient secretion of adrenocortical hormones *(hypofunction)*, resulting in widespread metabolic malfunction including failure of the body to maintain a normal sodium and potassium balance, loss of body fluids, and inability to withstand stress. It usually is caused by tuberculous or other infectious invasion of the cortex, but occasionally, tumors and idiopathic processes cause atrophy of the cortex.[3] The primary disease occurs in only one person in 100,000 population.[3] However, adrenal insufficiency may be caused by surgical excision of the adrenal glands (total adrenalectomy).

Usually Addison's disease is slow in onset and becomes chronic. Early symptoms and signs may be so nonspecific that the patient either fails to notice them or feels that they are not severe enough to warrant medical attention. They include lassitude, ease of fatigue, weight loss, amnesia, nausea, diarrhea, gastrointestinal discomfort, tension, irritability, and depression. Brown pigmentation of the skin, particularly over the knuckles and other joints, is often the first sign observed. The skin may appear tan or bronzed at first

and then become muddy brown and unwashed in appearance. Occasionally an acute addisonian crisis may be the first sign of adrenal insufficiency. It may accompany or follow other acute illness that increases the body's need for cortisone.

Addison's disease usually can be effectively treated by giving cortisone and fluorohydrocortisone. The patient usually must take cortisone (or hydrocortisone) in doses of 25 to 37.5 mg. (⅜ to ⅝ grain) daily; 25 mg. of the drug are given by mouth at 8 A.M., and 12.5 mg. are given at 3 P.M. Taking the second dose after 4 P.M. may lead to excitability and sleeplessness. Usually less difficulty is encountered if the patient takes the larger dose in the morning. Because cortisone and hydrocortisone often cause gastric irritation, the morning dose should be taken with breakfast and the afternoon dose with a snack or a glass of milk. (See p. 63 for further important information the nurse should have before giving cortisone to any patient.)

Since cortisone and hydrocortisone control food metabolism but do not control salt depletion and water balance in Addison's disease, the patient must have additional treatment to avoid hypotension and dehydration. Taking extra salt each day sometimes suffices, but usually deoxycorticosterone or fluorohydrocortisone (synthetic aldosterones) must be taken to regulate retention of sodium and excretion of potassium. Daily doses of 9-α-fluorohydrocortisone, 0.1 to 0.2 mg. (1/600 to 1/300 grain), are now most widely used because they can be given by mouth. Deoxycorticosterone acetate in oil is available for intramuscular injection. It may be given daily, or a long-acting form may be used. Deoxycorticosterone pellets also can be inserted under the skin for slow absorption over months.

The patient on the usual therapeutic dose of cortisone for Addison's disease rarely has symptoms of overdose of the hormone, such as "moonface," hypertension, or hirsutism. Signs of overtreatment with deoxycorticosterone and 9-α-fluorohydrocortisone, however, occur more easily and include the signs of potassium depletion (p. 99).

The patient with Addison's disease should be taught about his disease, about the hormones he must take, and how he can safely live with his disease (Fig. 174). If he adheres to his medical prescription and does not indulge in physical, mental, or emotional stress of any kind, he can, as a rule, live a perfectly normal life. If he becomes ill with an acute infection or suffers serious stress of any kind, he needs more of the hormone, just as the person who suffers from diabetes mellitus needs more insulin.[3] Therefore, he must be urged to guard against all stresses and any acute infection and should report even minor indispositions to his physician. In acute illness, the dosage of cortisone may be increased to as much as 75 to 150 mg. (1¼ to 2½ grains).[3] The patient with Addison's disease should carry a card stating his disease, the name and address of his physician, and what should be done in the event of sudden injury and unconsciousness.

Addisonian crisis. Addisonian, or adrenal, crisis is really a severe exacerbation of Addison's disease. It is a very serious condition in which there is severe hypotension, shock, coma, and vasomotor collapse, and it quickly leads to death. It may occur in any person with an insufficient amount of adrenocortical hormones, regardless of the cause, and may be precipitated by strenuous activity, infection or other stressful situations, or by failure to take prescribed steroids. It often is a complication of surgery or other treatment of the pituitary or adrenal glands. The signs of impending crisis are those of the disease in exaggerated form.

When addisonian crisis occurs, a large dose of hydrocortisone is given immediately by the intravenous route. Continuous infusions of normal saline solution and glucose are started to provide for the maintenance of fluid balance and the administration of drugs. Cortisone is given intramuscularly also. The patient must do *absolutely nothing* for himself. If he is conscious, the nurse should caution him not to attempt to turn or otherwise help himself. He should be attended constantly. An hourly temperature recording may be requested since hyperthermia is common. Blood pressure recording may be requested every fifteen minutes, and if hypotension is extreme, the nurse should anticipate that levarterenol bitartrate (Levophed) may be prescribed. The patient may be placed in shock position. The patient often complains of severe headache; an ice

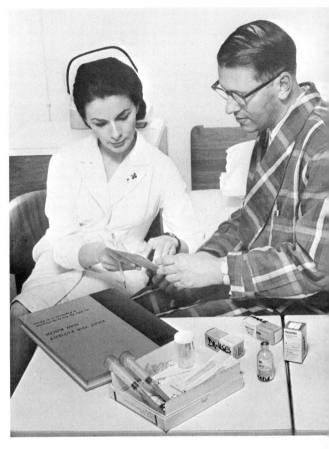

Fig. 174

The patient with Addison's disease should be taught about his disease, about the hormones he must take, and how he can live safely with his disease. (Reprinted, with permission, from Shea, Kathleen M., and others: Am. J. Nursing **65**:80-85, Dec. 1965.)

bag may be used to relieve it. The patient has an extremely low resistance to infection, and medical isolation usually is used to protect the patient from exposure to infection. He always must be protected from anyone, including members of his family and from hospital personnel, who has a cold or other infection. Sometimes antibiotics are given prophylactically.

Cushing's syndrome. Cushing's syndrome is a rare disease that occurs more often in women than in men. It sometimes follows pregnancy. There is excessive secretion (*hy-*

perfunction) of the 11,17-oxygenated corti-
coids, (hydrocortisone and cortisone) by the
adrenal cortex.[3] This oversecretion results in
disruption of normal metabolic processes.
Excessive amounts of water and salt may be
retained in the body; the potassium level in
the body fluids is reduced and other electrolyte balances, such as the calcium-phos-
phorus balance, are upset; protein catabolism
is increased; the blood sugar level rises and
insulin production decreases; the eosinophil
count decreases, predisposing the patient to
hemorrhage; and there are changes in the
secondary sex characteristics. The most common cause of this disease is hyperplasia of
the adrenal cortex, although a tumor may be
found. It may also be caused by a tumor in
the anterior pituitary gland, which causes
excessive stimulation of the adrenal cortex.
The condition is then called *Cushing's
disease.*

Signs and symptoms of Cushing's syndrome include muscle wasting with resultant
weakness, susceptibility to hemorrhage, peculiar fat distribution with deposition of fat
in the face (moon face), neck, and trunk.
Osteoporosis is also common, and fracture of
vertebrae may occur. The patient usually has
hypertension and is irritable and changeable
in mood. Diabetes mellitus may develop.
Women patients show signs of masculin-
ization, and the menses often cease. Adolescent or preadolescent boys may have precocious sexual development. Resistance to
infection is often lowered and may lead to
death.

Treatment of Cushing's syndrome depends
on whether it is caused by primary adrenocortical hyperfunction or by a tumor of the
pituitary gland. If a tumor of the adrenal
cortex is the cause, the tumor may be surgically resected. When there is hyperplasia of
the adrenal cortex, one of the adrenal glands
may be surgically removed; sometimes part
of the other gland also must be resected.
Pituitary tumors usually are irradiated, but
they also may be removed surgically. All these
procedures lessen the glandular activity.

The patient with Cushing's syndrome
needs skilled nursing care and the utmost
consideration. The patient usually is seriously ill and debilitated. Helping him to
maintain adequate nutrition, some level of
emotional balance, and an acceptance of his

situation will challenge the best efforts of
all members of the nursing staff. The nurse
should notice and record on the nursing care
plan those situations which seem to upset
the patient, and all staff members should be
reminded to avoid them if possible.

Diseases of the adrenal medulla

Pheochromocytoma is a tumor (usually
benign) of the adrenal medulla. It causes
hypertension but is curable by surgery. The
symptoms are those of hypertensive heart
disease, and the care during the preoperative period is similar to that for the patient
with hypertensive heart disease (p. 337).

In making the diagnosis, a *Regitine* test
is frequently done. In this test, after recording the blood pressure, the physician administers an antipressor agent such as phento-
lamine (Regitine), benzodioxane, or dibenamine intravenously. Blood pressure readings
are taken at prescribed intervals until the
pressure returns to its pretest level. A hypotensive effect, lasting ten to fifteen minutes,
is diagnostic of pheochromocytoma of the
adrenal medulla, but a negative response
does not necessarily rule out such a lesion.
The patient should be in bed during this
test since the decrease in blood pressure may
cause him to faint. Pressor drugs such as
Levophed should be available for immediate use if necessary.

Surgery of the adrenal glands

Both adrenal glands may be removed surgically *(total adrenalectomy)*. In this procedure all the adrenal cortical and medullary
tissue is removed. Usually the glands are removed at separate operations. A total adrenalectomy is done most often for patients
with cancer of the breast with metastasis, but
occasionally it is used for patients with cancer of the prostate with metastasis. Only
one adrenal gland or a part of one may be
removed *(subtotal adrenalectomy)*, or a tumor and the tissue immediately surrounding
it may be resected from either the cortex
(adrenocortical tumor resection) or the medulla *(adrenal medullary tumor resection)*.

*General care needed by patients having
adrenal surgery.* When any surgery on the
adrenal glands is planned, treatment with
steroids usually is discontinued for several
weeks preoperatively to prevent the danger

of infection after surgery (p. 64). This also allows postoperative control of blood levels of steroids to be more accurately regulated. If antihypertensive drugs have been used, they, too, are discontinued since the surgery may cause a rather severe drop in the blood pressure. Phenobarbital may be given for sedation during this time.

The operative incision for any type of adrenal surgery is made in the flank close to the diaphragm. Therefore, special care should be taken postoperatively to have the patient turned frequently and to encourage him to breathe deeply and to cough. Usually a narcotic is ordered and it should be given about a half hour before coughing is attempted; the incision should be supported. Dyspnea or sudden chest pain should be reported at once because a spontaneous pneumothorax may occur. A nasogastric tube is often passed and attached to suction to relieve the abdominal distention that may accompany this surgery.

Usually the patient remains in bed for two or three days postoperatively and is kept flat during this time. When he is permitted out of bed, elastic bandages may be applied to the lower extremities because of the instability of the vascular system. The patient's blood pressure must be taken every fifteen minutes when ambulation is first attempted. If the blood pressure drops, he should be assisted back to bed, and orders for further attempts at ambulation must be obtained from the doctor.

Special care needed by patients having adrenocortical surgery. The immediate postoperative care for patients having any type of adrenocortical surgery is quite similar. Adrenocortical function is very labile when part of the adrenocortical tissue is removed and, of course, it is labile when all the tissue is removed since maintenance of the hormonal level then must be controlled completely by replacement therapy. The patient's special needs center around maintaining appropriate amounts of adrenocortical hormones in the blood. The patient undergoing a total adrenolectomy also requires the care needed by a patient with surgery of the adrenal medulla, which is described below.

Immediately after surgery, replacement of corticosteroids is started. Cortisone is given continuously by intravenous drip, and dosage is adjusted at intervals according to the clinical findings. Since hormonal replacement is delicately regulated on the basis of continuous observations of electrolyte balance, metabolic functions, and blood pressure determinations, the patient, following any adrenal surgery, needs to be given constant nursing attention until hormonal stability is regained or a maintenance regimen established. Drugs to raise the blood pressure may be given. The rate of infusions containing vasopressor drugs such as Levophed is regulated in accordance with frequent blood pressure readings (usually every fifteen minutes). The nurse is responsible for taking accurate blood pressure readings and adjusting the rate of flow according to the doctor's orders. When there is no order to decrease or increase the flow, the doctor must be notified at once about any significant changes in blood pressure. The nurse should also observe the patient carefully for signs of *hypoglycemia* (p. 756). This condition is likely to occur if the patient had diabetes mellitus as a symptom, but it can occur in any patient. Intravenous solutions containing glucose are usually ordered. If the patient is able to eat, the nurse should check to see that he has eaten the food served. If not, the doctor should be notified since the diet is prescribed to meet the patient's particular needs and the doctor may wish to give nourishment intravenously. Hypoglycemic reactions are most likely to occur in the early morning, and they may follow any unusual physical activity or any emotional upset. The nurse also should be alert for symptoms of *addisonian crisis*, which requires immediate treatment. *Markedly increased* urinary output may indicate the need for Pitressin to control excessive diuresis.

If the patient had hyperfunction of the gland, his preoperative symptoms will continue for several weeks following surgery. The nursing care started in the preoperative period, therefore, must be continued.

Most patients will require adrenocortical hormones at least temporarily even after being discharged from the hospital. Those who have had a total adrenalectomy must take adrenocortical hormones regularly for the remainder of their lives. All patients usually must take cortisone, and many must take fluorohydrocortisone. Testosterone may be given to the patient who has had surgery for Cushing's syndrome, especially if she continues to have muscle weakness and lethargy. Testosterone is never given to the patient whose surgery has been done for cancer of the breast or prostate because the purpose of the surgery was to remove this hormone.

Special care needed by patients having adrenal medullary surgery. Marked hypotension often follows removal of a medullary tumor. It is well to remember that these patients have usually had hypertension, and, therefore, a blood pressure reading within normal limits may represent hypotension for them. Changes in the blood pressure are more significant when several readings are considered. Infusions containing vasopressor drugs such as Levophed always are given until the blood pressure stabilizes, and very accurate and frequent regulation of the infusion, similar to that described under adrenocortical surgery, is required. Cerebrovascular accidents and circulatory collapse may complicate the postoperative course. The nurse caring for these patients should review the care of the patient with hypertension, heart failure, cerebrovascular accident, and shock.

Diseases of the pituitary gland

The pituitary gland, located deep in the cranial cavity at the bifurcation of the optic chiasm, is made up of two parts, the anterior pituitary lobe and the posterior pituitary lobe. The functions of some of the better known hormones secreted by this very important gland are described in a simplified way early in this chapter. Actually the action of each hormone is complex and incompletely understood, and it is felt that not all the hormones probably have even been isolated. New information about the pituitary gland is being learned each year, and each new fact seems to reemphasize the complexity of this gland. What initiates the secretion of pituitary hormones is not clearly understood. It is known that the tropic hormones are secreted in response to lowering of the blood level of the hormones whose secretions are stimulated by them. It also is known that the antidiuretic hormone is secreted in response to a decrease in the blood volume. How this information reaches the anterior pituitary lobe, however, is still not known, but it is generally believed that the hypothalamus of the brain may be involved.[2]

Because of the influence of the anterior pituitary hormones on other endocrine glands, dysfunction of the anterior pituitary gland may cause symptoms of malfunction in the glands whose secretions are dependent upon its tropic hormones. By irradiating or surgically removing the pituitary gland, the secretion of hormones from other glands can be reduced. Sometimes this is done rather than performing a total adrenalectomy, as in treatment for metastatic cancer of the breast or prostate gland.[20] Recently, the pituitary gland has been irradiated or surgically removed in an attempt to decrease the need for insulin in selected patients with diabetes. This seems to reduce the severity of renal and retinal vascular complications.[20,42] Because of its location near the optic chiasm, tumors of the pituitary gland may press on the optic nerves and cause visual changes.

Hypofunction—anterior lobe

Hypofunction of the anterior lobe of the pituitary gland may result from compression of the gland by a tumor within the gland itself or tumors associated with contiguous structures. Metastatic carcinoma or inflammatory disease such as meningitis also can damage it, or it may be congenitally malfunctioning.

If a tumor is present, the patient may have visual disturbance caused by pressure on the optic nerve, severe headache due to increased intracranial pressure, and symptoms associated with disturbance of the gland itself. These symptoms may vary according to which hormone insufficiency is manifested. One result of hypofunction is the effect upon body growth. In the adolescent, sexual growth and development may be arrested. If the thyroid-stimulating hormone is decreased, symptoms of hypothyroidism may occur. If ACTH secretions is impaired, the patient may have symptoms of Addison's disease. A combination of many endocrine deficiency diseases may be present. *Dwarfism* results from congenital deficiency of the growth hormone.

Treatment of anterior pituitary gland disorders depends upon their cause. Pituitary xtract has been used successfully in some patients with dwarfism, but at present this hormone is extremely hard to obtain and very costly. Tumors causing pressure on the gland are removed surgically if possible. Some tumors of the gland itself, such as chromophobe adenoma, are amenable to radiation therapy. Sometimes a hypophysectomy (removal of the entire gland) must be done.

Hyperfunction—anterior lobe

Congenital hypersecretion of the growth hormone from the anterior pituitary gland causes excessive growth *(gigantism)*. Hyperfunction of the anterior lobe of the pituitary gland in the adult results in *acromegaly* and usually is caused by a tumor in the eosinophil cells. The main symptoms or signs of both acromegaly and gigantism are those of excessive body growth. In gigantism, symptoms become apparent soon after birth, and since the child is in the growth period, the bones enlarge both in length and in width. In acromegaly, bones enlarge transversely. The features become coarse and heavy, with the lower jaw becoming particularly large. Frontal sinuses are pronounced. Hands and feet become conspicuously wider, necessitating larger-sized gloves and shoes. Lips are heavier, and the tongue is enlarged. Striking changes in the patient's appearance may be noticed in comparing his appearance with pictures of him taken before the onset of symptoms. Patients may be asked to bring pictures of themselves to the hospital to help in diagnosis.

During diagnosis and treatment, the patient and his family need understanding care. Changes in appearance often produce emotional reactions. Since physical changes are irreversible even if the disease is arrested, they may be doubly difficult to accept.

Sometimes it is possible to ameliorate the disease with external radiation to the hypophyseal gland (pituitary). Recently, it has become possible to irradiate the hypophyseal gland internally by implanting yttrium-90, a radioactive substance, through the nose and sphenoid sinuses and into the gland.[20] The location of the pituitary gland makes surgical removal of a tumor very difficult. Consequently, if the condition is treated by surgery, a hypophysectomy is usually done.

Hypofunction—posterior lobe

Diabetes insipidus is a disease caused by failure of the posterior lobe of the pituitary gland to secrete antidiuretic hormone. Primary diabetes insipidus is a rare disease, but its symptoms are seen fairly frequently since they may occur when a tumor develops in the gland and because they follow surgical removal or irradiation of the hypophyseal gland, which are procedures that are now being performed.

The antidiuretic hormone increases reabsorption of water from the renal tubules, and in its absence a very large amount of urine is excreted; as many as 15 liters may be excreted daily. This causes fluid and electrolyte imbalance. Patients with diabetes insipidus also have insatiable thirst (polydipsia), anorexia, weight loss, and weakness.

Specific treatment for diabetes insipidus usually consists of giving extracts of the posterior pituitary lobe. Vasopressin tannate (Pitressin tannate) in oil, 5 units, given intramuscularly, will give relief for up to forty-eight hours and is usually used for immediate treatment. This hormone also is available as a powder which the patient sniffs to deposit it on the nasal mucosa, where it is absorbed. It should not be inhaled. The patient is taught to use this powder whenever he notices polyuria or polydipsia.

Hypophysectomy

A hypophysectomy is the complete removal of the hypophyseal gland. Production of both the anterior and the posterior pituitary hormones ceases as soon as the surgery is done. To minimize the danger of serious complications resulting from sudden removal of the hormones that stimulate the secretion of cortisone and thyroxin, these hormones are usually given preoperatively. A craniotomy must be done to remove the gland.[13]

Following a hypophysectomy the patient must be attended constantly for several days. In addition to giving care needed by any patient having a craniotomy (p. 892), the most alert attention must be paid to detect early signs of thyroid crisis, addisonian crisis, or sudden electrolyte imbalance, all of which require immediate treatment. Cortisone and Pitressin are given throughout the postoperative period and, of course, must be continued throughout the patient's life. Thyroid extract usually is not restarted until several weeks after surgery, since the action of thyroxin continues for about three weeks. The operation causes gonadal function to cease and thus causes sterility. Testosterone is ordered frequently for the impotence that occurs in men. Since women rarely have severe menopausal symptoms as a result of this surgery, they usually are not given sex hormones. If the hypophysectomy has been done to treat metastatic cancer of the breast or prostate gland, sex hormones are never given.

Any patient who is hospitalized for this type of surgery has been given explicit information as to its results by the doctor. The nurse should listen attentively to the patient as he or she expresses feeling about it both preoperatively and postoperatively. Any misunderstandings or misgivings should be reported to the doctor. Most patients appear to accept their limitations surprisingly well, especially if the symptoms of metastasis or of other disease are ameliorated. They always should be observed closely for the need of emotional support, however, and appropriate help for them should be obtained. The patient and his family must, of course, be taught the precautions he must observe in taking the hormones.

Internal radiation of the hypophysis

The care of the patient who has yttrium-90 implanted is completely described in a recent journal article.[20] The care is not very different from that following a hypophysectomy, except that the symptoms of hormonal deficiencies develop slowly, and therefore the patient must be carefully observed so that replacement of hormones can be started or increased as necessary. The precautions used for any radiation therapy also must be observed. The patient has not had cranial surgery, but meningeal infection may be a complication. The patient also needs attention similar to that given a patient who has intranasal surgery of the sinuses. The patient having this treatment usually is hospitalized for a much shorter time than is the one having a hypophysectomy. Therefore, special care must be taken to ensure that he is adequately instructed in self-care either in the hospital or by a nurse visiting him at home.

External radiation of the hypophysis

Both anterior and posterior pituitary function may be temporarily or permanently impaired by external radiation of the pituitary gland. Therefore, replacement of cortisone and Pitressin may be essential. However, these hormones are given only if symptoms develop. The nurse should very carefully note and report changes in the vital signs, the patient's general appearance, weight, emotional state, and mental alertness. The urinary output should be measured carefully and recorded every two hours for several days, and an output of 300 ml. or more in any two-hour period should be reported to the physician at once. Pitressin must be started before serious fluid and electrolyte imbalance develop. Prolonged replacement therapy with various hormones may be necessary after external radiation of the pituitary gland, especially if most of the glandular tissue has been destroyed.

Osteoporosis

Osteoporosis is an exceedingly common yet poorly understood disease in which there is a defect in the bone matrix formation, with resultant decrease in bone substance and in the ability of the bones to withstand normal stresses. A variety of hormonal derangements are known to cause osteoporosis, including hyperthyroidism, acromegaly, diabetes, hyperparathyroidism, and Cushing's syndrome, as already mentioned in this chapter. By far the larger number of patients with osteoporosis, however, have the condition either associated with disuse of the bones or occurring after the climacteric in the absence of other obvious endocrine dysfunction. It is known that lack of the anabolic steroids permits a negative nitrogen balance to occur and that osteoporosis is a disease primarily of protein metabolism and not of use of calcium. Although unproved, it is believed that hormones (notably estrogen) in some way affect bone metabolism and that their lack permits the resorption of bone at an increased rate.

Osteoporosis is much more common in women than in men and occurs frequently in women in their sixties. It is so common that it has almost been considered "physiologic" when it occurs in women after the menopause, and little attention has been paid to it.[3] So frequent is the condition in elderly women that it has been listed as the most commonly seen abnormality of the vertebral column upon roentgenographic examination and exceeds even arthritis in incidence. It is now believed likely that almost all elderly women have some osteoporosis, since approximately 40% demineralization of the bones occurs before roentgenograms show pronounced disease.

Osteoporosis (other than that caused by bone disuse) develops most often in the vertebrae and in the pelvis. By far the most common symptom is low back pain. Many times, however, the patient has no knowledge that anything is wrong until a fracture occurs, or until severe symptoms follow collapse of a vertebra. Pain occurs when bone changes have altered alignment so much that pressure occurs or strain is placed on nerves and supportive structures. Sometimes compression of the vertebral bodies occurs, and this may decrease the height of the trunk and increase the curve of the thoracic spine. A feeling of lack of stability, noted most when walking on uneven surfaces, and difficulty in maintaining balance may also be described by the patient. The nurse should advise any elderly person with any of these signs and symptoms to visit his doctor so that treatment, if needed, can be started before a fracture occurs or other serious limitations develop.

Treatment of osteoporosis usually consists of measures to prevent further damage if possible. Daily exercise is felt to be imperative, and many doctors insist that the patient do some walking each day. If severe pain occurs from further collapse or from injury, it usually is treated with the judicious use of muscle relaxants and analgesics, and with rest on a firm bed. Even if a fracture is sustained, it may be treated by applying a cast and having the patient mobilized. Estrogen and androgen therapy has been effective for many patients and is widely used at this time. Even when administration of estrogens seems to produce no marked regeneration of bone as seen by roentgenogram, their use often lessens pain and enables the patient to be more active. Usually an estrogen preparation such as Premarin is given for one week out of four. A diet high in protein, calcium, and vitamin D may be ordered, although some physicians believe that the

person taking a normal, adequate diet receives enough of these essentials, provided he is helped to use them by the administration of hormones.

Most physicians prescribe a firm corset or brace. Whether it is worn continuously or only during periods of special activity depends upon the individual patient and the doctor. Usually the corset or brace enables the patient to be more active than would otherwise be safe or comfortable for him. A firm bed for sleeping hours and rest periods is always prescribed, and a careful balance between rest and activity to avoid overfatigue is usually advised.

The patient with osteoporosis must guard against accidents. Walking on uneven surfaces and when lighting is poor should be avoided, and often the use of a cane is recommended. The patient should be taught the correct method of stooping to pick up an object from the floor and to avoid direct bending, which places pressure upon lumbar vertebral bodies. The patient should not lift any heavy object and should distribute any small weight he carries between his two arms to lessen strain on one side of the body. Since his future well-being depends upon his being up and about, the patient with osteoporosis should be taught to give special attention to care of his feet and selection of his shoes. Any difficulties should be discussed with his doctor.

The nurse who cares for any aged patient should bear in mind that the patient may have undiagnosed osteoporosis. Since the condition can be made worse by confinement in bed, all elderly patients who have been in bed for some time, regardless of the cause, should be treated with the greatest care when mobilization is permitted.

References and selected readings*

1 Adler, Francis Heed: Textbook of ophthalmology, ed. 7, Philadelphia, 1962, W. B. Saunders Co.

2 Bard, Philip, editor: Medical physiology, ed. 11, St. Louis, 1961, The C. V. Mosby Co.

3 Beeson, Paul B., and McDermott, Walsh, editors: Cecil-Loeb textbook of medicine, ed. 11, Philadelphia, 1963, W. B. Saunders Co.

4 Behrman, Deaconess Maude: Cookbook for diabetics, New York, 1959, American Diabetes Association.

*References preceded by an asterisk are particularly well suited for student reading.

5 Bergersen, Betty S., and Krug, Elsie E.: Pharmacology in nursing, ed. 10, St. Louis, 1966, The C. V. Mosby Co.

6 Bowen, Rhoda G.: The effects of organized instruction given by registered professional nurses for patients with the diagnosis of diabetes mellitus, The Nurse and Groups of Patients or Clients, no. 10, New York, 1962, American Nurses' Association.

7 *Caso, Elizabeth K.: Diabetic meal planning—a good guide is not enough, Am. J. Nursing 62:76-78, Nov. 1962.

8 *Coates, Florence Cuozzo, and Fabrykant, Maximilian: An insulin injection technique for preventing skin reactions, Am. J. Nursing 65:127-128, Feb. 1965.

9 Conn, Jerome W., and Fajans, Stefan S.: The prediabetic state, Am. J. Med. 31:839-850, Dec. 1961.

10 Conner, J. F., and Miller, B. H.: Clinical experience with oral hypoglycemic agents in an institutionalized group of elderly diabetics, J. Am. Geriatrics Soc. 10:467-472, June 1962.

11 *Coultas, Rita Nied: Patients use props to plan diabetic menus, Am. J. Nursing 63:104, Aug. 1963.

12 Diabetes statistics, Am. J. Nursing 64:103, Nov. 1964.

13 Fager, Charles A.: Surgical ablation of the pituitary gland, S. Clin. North America 65:697-703, June 1965.

14 Gaspard, Nancy J.: Summer camp for diabetic children, Am. J. Nursing 63:108-109, June 1963.

15 Greenblatt, Robert B., and others: Addison's disease and nursing care of the patient with Addison's disease, Am. J. Nursing 60:1249-1255, Sept. 1960.

16 Grollman, Arthur: Clinical endocrinology and its physiologic basis, Philadelphia, 1964, J. B. Lippincott Co.

17 Hamolsky, Milton W.: Hypothyroidism—its manifestations and treatment, M. Clin. North America 46:1213-1227, Sept. 1962.

18 Hatch, F. E., and others: Diabetic glomerulosclerosis, Am. J. Med. 31:216-230, Aug. 1961.

19 Haunz, E. A.: The role of urine testing in diabetes detection, Am. J. Nursing 64:102-103, Nov. 1964.

20 *Hawken, Patty: Hypophysectomy with yttrium-90, Am. J. Nursing 65:122-125, Oct. 1965.

21 *Jackson, Helen: Helping a blind diabetic patient become self-dependent, Am. J. Nursing 62:107, Nov. 1962.

22 Jay, Arthur N.: Hypoglycemia, Am. J. Nursing 62:77, Jan. 1962.

23 Krosnick, Arthur: Diabetic neuropathy, Am. J. Nursing 64:106-108, July 1964.

24 *Krysan, Germaine S.: How do we teach four million diabetics? Am. J. Nursing 65:105-107, Nov. 1965.

25 *Lanes, Phyllis: Primary aldosteronism, Am. J. Nursing 61:46-47, Aug. 1961.

26 Locke, Raymond K.: Foot care for diabetics, Am. J. Nursing 63:107-110, Nov. 1963.

27 *Lonergan, Robert C.: Osteoporosis of the spine, Am. J. Nursing 61:79-81, Jan. 1961.

28 *Long, Phyllis J.: The diabetic child at home, Nursing Outlook 12:55-56, Dec. 1964.

29 *MacNeil, Ann: Urine testing when the diagnosis is diabetes, Am. J. Nursing 61:67-69, Nov. 1961.

30 *Mannix, Henry, Jr., and Glenn, Frank: Hypertension in Cushing's syndrome, J.A.M.A. 180:225-229, April 21, 1962.

31 Marlow, Dorothy R.: Textbook of pediatric nursing, ed. 2, Philadelphia, 1965, W. B. Saunders Co.

32 *Martin, Marguerite M.: Diabetes mellitus: current concepts, Am. J. Nursing 66:510-514, March 1966.

33 Martin, Marguerite M.: Insulin reaction, Am. J. Nursing 67:328-331, Feb. 1967.

34 Martin, Marguerite M.: New trends in diabetes detection, Am. J. Nursing 63:101-103, Aug. 1963.

35 *Martin, Marguerite M.: The unconscious diabetic patient, Am. J. Nursing 61:92-94, Nov. 1961.

36 Moore, Mary Lou: Diabetes in children, Am. J. Nursing 67:104-107, Jan. 1967.

37 Nelson, Waldo E., editor: Textbook of pediatrics, ed. 8, Philadelphia, 1964, W. B. Saunders Co.

38 *Nordyke, Robert Allan: The overactive and the underactive thyroid, Am. J. Nursing 63:66-71, May 1963.

39 *Pearson, Olaf H., and Lubic, Ruth Watson: Adrenalectomy and hypophysectomy and nursing care, Am. J. Nursing 62:80-86, April 1962.

40 Pearson, Olaf H., and others: Hypophysectomy for the treatment of diabetic retinopathy, J.A.M.A. 188:116-122, April 13, 1964.

41 Pfizer Laboratories' Spectrum and Basic Systems, Inc.: Current concepts of thyroid disease (a programmed study for physicians), New York, 1965, Chas. Pfizer & Co., Inc.

42 Ray, B. S.: Neurosurgeons' new interest in pituitary, J. Neurosurg. 17:1-21, Jan. 1960.

43 Rouse, George P., Jr.: Pregnancy and diabetes, Am. J. Nursing 58:100-101, Jan. 1958.

44 Sawyer, Janet R.: Nursing care of patients with urologic diseases, St. Louis, 1963, The C. V. Mosby Co.

45 *Shea, Kathleen M., and others: Teaching a patient to live with adrenal insufficiency, Am. J. Nursing 65:80-85, Dec. 1965.

46 Soffer, Louis J., and others: Cushing's syndrome, Am. J. Med. 30:129-146, Jan. 1961.

47 Vital Statistics of the United States, Washington, D. C., 1962, U. S. Government Printing Office.

48 White, Priscilla, editor: Diabetes, M. Clin. North America 49:857-1161, July 1965.

49 Yount, Ernest: Metabolic diseases. In Johnson, Wingate M., editor: The older patient, New York, 1960, Paul B. Hoeber, Inc.

27

The patient
with
skin disease

Study questions

1 Review the anatomy and physiology of the skin. What are its main functions?
2 What have you learned in fundamentals of nursing about skin care for the elderly patient, the malnourished patient, the dehydrated patient, the emaciated patient, and the obese patient?
3 Review techniques for bandaging various parts of the body.
4 What drugs may fairly often cause skin eruptions?
5 Review the various forms in which external medications can be applied. What are some good features and some limitations of each?

People vary in their resistance to skin disease. Some are born with tough skins that can resist irritation and infection quite well, whereas others have delicate skins that have little resistance to trauma, irritation, and infection. Usually, the person with blond coloring has a more delicate skin than the person with a dark complexion.

General condition of the skin, color, and texture provide an excellent barometer of the state of a person's general health. Many conditions existing within and outside the body affect the skin. Nutritional and vitamin deficiencies predispose to skin disease and slow the rate of healing. Hormonal influences are believed to have a part in the progress of some skin diseases. A very nervous person may develop skin lesions. For example, nervousness may lead to itching and to subsequent scratching; infection may then be introduced. Occupational exposure to irritating substances and the removal of natural skin secretions also predispose to skin diseases. For example, a person who handles fabrics or who washes dishes steadily may develop chapped hands and susceptibility to infection unless natural skin oils are replaced by creams and lotions. He may also develop a sensitivity to substances such as dyes and soaps.

The skin is affected by age. The skin of a baby is very delicate, thin, and vascular.

It may become irritated easily. In the elderly person, the skin undergoes atrophy of underlying tissues and hardening of superficial arterioles that nourished the skin during youth. Sebaceous glands are less active, and the skin is thin, dry, and easily traumatized. Infections occur easily and often heal slowly.

General skin care and prevention of disease

The nurse can contribute to the prevention of skin disease by teaching good care of the normal skin and by encouraging people to seek medical attention for abnormal skin conditions. This can be done as she encounters people at work, in their homes, in school, in the hospital, and elsewhere in the community.

Cleansing

The old saying that cleanliness is next to godliness is probably not entirely true. People from cultures who do not have high standards of cleanliness do not necessarily have more skin disease than others. The outer layer of skin cells and the perspiration are acid in reaction, and their presence inhibits the life and growth of bacteria. Strong soaps that are alkaline in reaction may neutralize this protective acid condition of the skin. They may also remove the oily secretion of the sebaceous glands, which lubricate the outer skin layers and contribute to their health. However, mechanical removal of dead skin and excess oil appears justified because they can coat bacteria and prevent the antibacterial action of perspiration. Also, since these substances have an unpleasant odor after undergoing bacterial decomposition, bathing is necessary for esthetic reasons.

The skin should be washed often enough to remove skin excretions and prevent odors but not often enough to cause drying and irritation. Detergent cleansers that are neutral in reaction probably are better than soaps for cleansing the skin. Both soaps and detergents may cause skin reaction in some people, however. There is a great deal of individual variation in the bathing necessary to ensure cleanliness without causing skin irritation. The person who has an oily skin and who perspires freely may need to bathe twice daily in warm weather and wash his face several times, whereas the person who has a dry skin may have to use creams and lotions to protect the skin even when he bathes but once a day.

Skin secretions are decreased during cold weather so that most people need to use protective creams and lotions to prevent skin irritation at this time. There are many bath oils on the market today. They leave a residue film of oil over the entire body and may relieve itching from dryness. However, many dermatologists discourage their use because the oily film may prevent normal excretion from the pores. Hard, thickened skin areas should be rubbed daily with a substance such as cold cream, lanolin, or vanishing cream that contains a small amount of salicylic acid and helps to soften dry, thickened skin. Elderly people need to take special precautions in the care of their skin (p. 43).

Observation of abnormalities

Care of the normal skin should include regular observation of pigmented skin areas, moles, or other apparently minor skin lesions. Any change in size, color, or general appearance should be reported to a physician at once. Pigmentation (lentigo) occurs on the face, neck, and backs of hands and arms of elderly people (Fig. 175). These freckles, which are a source of annoyance to many elderly women, are harmless. They can be removed by abrasion, but so-called "freckle creams" are useless.

Dangers of self-treatment

People should be urged to seek competent medical help when skin conditions develop. Although skin diseases rarely cause death, they do account for much human discomfort and for serious interruption of work and other activities. Many persons are inclined to rely upon the advice of friends or of the local druggist or upon medications they may have on hand. Each individual's skin reacts differently to treatment, and the skin that is already irritated or diseased may respond violently to inexpert treatment. Since the skin changes, medications prescribed even for a similar skin ailment in the same patient some time previously may not produce a favorable response. Also, drugs may deterior-

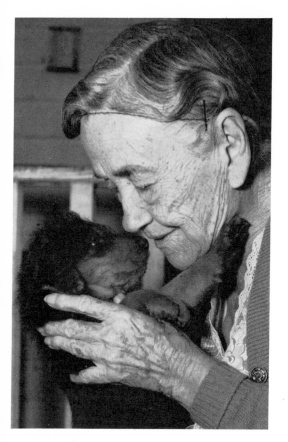

Fig. 175

Elderly patients have skin changes. Note discolored spots on skin and the tiny raised area on this woman's eyelid. (VanDerMeid from Monkmeyer Press Photo Service.)

ate, and for this reason old medications are not safe. The patient may be spared much discomfort and expense if he turns to a specialist when symptoms first develop and before a mild skin condition becomes really troublesome. He should be advised to present himself to the doctor without changing dressings or otherwise "cleaning up" the lesion.

General nursing care of patients with skin conditions

Certain general principles of nursing care apply to most skin conditions and will be discussed before a few of the more common diseases are mentioned. Most nursing care is directed toward making the patient as comfortable as possible, controlling pain and itching, and encouraging healing of the lesions.

Relief of pruritus

Pruritus, or itching, was defined centuries ago as a disagreeable sensation that stimulates the urge to scratch. Actually, very little is known about the physiologic mechanism by which pruritus is caused. It is believed to be closely associated with the nerve mechanism that causes pain. The sensation arises in the nerve endings in the skin. It is unknown in lesions in which skin layers have been destroyed. Pruritus is known to be aggravated by dilation of capillaries, tissue anoxia such as occurs in venous stasis, and presence of abnormal constituents such as bile pigment in the skin. Some skin diseases, such as tumors and tuberculous and syphilitic lesions, are not accompanied by pruritus.

Pruritus can be exhausting and demoralizing to the patient. It is useless, however, to tell him not to scratch, for he may be unable to comply with this advice. Admonishing the patient may only increase his frustration and may make the pruritus worse. It is safe to assume that the normal person who has pruritus will stop scratching when the condition has been sufficiently controlled. Antihistaminic drugs often are prescribed for treatment of pruritus, and the adrenocorticosteroids are used widely. External medications with antipruritic action and colloidal baths also may be ordered and are discussed later in this chapter.

Trauma from scratching can be partially prevented by cutting the fingernails short and by urging the patient to try such measures as pressing the itching lesion with the finger or with the back of the fingernail instead of using the ends of the nails. Hands should be kept scrupulously clean so that danger of introducing infectious organisms is reduced. Infants and young children may need protective mittens or elbow restraints.

Diversions may take the person's mind off the urge to scratch. Sedatives may be given since they help to make the person less irritable. Irritability increases the urge to scratch and decreases willpower. By counting to one hundred before scratching, some patients are able to control the urge until the strongest impulse is dissipated.

Cool, light clothing or bedclothes may help to allay itching. It is well known that wool is particularly likely to cause itching even in persons who have no skin disease but who have somewhat dry skins. Any clothing that constricts, rubs, or retains body moisture and heat in local areas should be avoided.

Soft, old sheets should be used on the bed, and sometimes *"neutral"* linen is necessary. It is prepared by rinsing the linen in a mild acid solution, which counteracts the excess alkaline of ordinary laundry soap. A tablespoon of vinegar to a quart of water may be used in the home.

Pruritus usually increases when the body temperature goes up. Therefore, the patient with pruritus should be kept quiet. Activities of all kinds, both physical and mental, increase metabolism and increase body heat. Activities causing perspiration should be avoided also, because perspiration moistens the skin and increases pruritus, particularly under dressings and on parts of the body where skin surfaces touch each other. Excessive drying of the skin caused by high room temperature and low humidity can also increase pruritus. It occurs easily in the elderly patient who already has a dry skin. Usually a room temperature of 20° to 21° C. (68° to 70° F.) and a humidity of 30 to 40% are best for the patient with pruritus.

Gentleness in handling

Gentleness in treatment and handling of all skin lesions is important. Skin lesions should be patted, never rubbed, and irritation of the area surrounding the lesion should be avoided, because it stimulates circulation and leads to increased warmth and pruritus. Touching, rubbing, scratching, removing dressings, and inspecting the lesion are activities that interfere with healing and yet are a temptation to the patient both in the hospital and at home.

Skin lesions may be overtreated easily. The conscientious, ambitious nurse and the patient and his family should know that too much cleansing and treating can do more harm than good. The nurse must be certain that she understands exactly how much treatment the physician wishes. Usually, the more acute the skin disease, the gentler the treatment should be.

Warmth in special situations

The patient who has a generalized flush, or erythema, and the one who has an extensive exfoliative dermatitis may be losing body heat at an abnormally increased rate and may need a room temperature of 32.2° C. (90° F.) or more to maintain normal body temperature. Care must be taken to avoid chilling, particularly after baths and when compresses are used or when parts of the body are exposed. It is surprising how much body heat can be lost when cool, moist compresses are applied to even a relatively small portion of the total body surface. For example, the patient who has cool compresses on a hand and arm or who has an uncovered weeping skin condition of one limb may suffer from generalized chilling if adequate covers are not provided for the rest of his body, and if the room is not kept sufficiently warm.

Rest

All dermatologic patients need sleep and rest, yet skin conditions often interfere with these requirements. Skin ailments and accompanying pruritus tend to become worse at night when surroundings are quiet and there are fewer distractions. The patient needs the benefit of nursing measures to induce sleep, such as a warm drink, a back massage, elimination of light and noise, and attention to ventilation. Every effort should be made to help him get enough sleep without the aid of drugs, since they may cause further pruritus or may even cause increased restlessness, which is harmful. A sedative such as chloral hydrate, which seldom causes skin reaction, or a tranquilizing drug sometimes is given.

If the patient awakens, he should be urged to call the nurse, or to turn on the light and read or otherwise occupy himself while resisting the temptation to scratch the skin lesions. It may be necessary for the patient to have a private room in the hospital, but he should be taken to the sun porch or recreation room during part of the day so that he will have contact with others. This not only helps to keep him happier, but it may divert his attention from the itching. If he sleeps during the day, however, he should not be disturbed.

Emotional support

Because many skin lesions are unsightly and slow in healing, the patient often becomes discouraged and upset. He may fear that he is not accepted, not wanted, and not liked by others, particularly if there are unsightly lesions on exposed parts of the body. This response may be due in part to the idea that unsightly complexions often are linked with unwholesome living and communicable disease. Such a response also may be due to the fact that no one likes to be conspicuous. Members of the patient's family may need interpretation of the patient's reactions.

The nursing staff should try to make the patient feel that he is socially acceptable to persons about him. Care must be taken not to show any distaste or rejection no matter how difficult care of the skin lesions may be. When the lesion, despite its appearance, is not communicable, the use of equipment such as gowns and rubber gloves is bad for the patient's morale and should never be employed.

The nurse must know each patient and plan individual care accordingly. For example, one patient may be happier if he is permitted to change his own compresses and otherwise care for himself, whereas another patient, because he needs the attention and reassurance of having things done for him, may feel discriminated against if self-care is suggested. However, in almost all instances the nurse should give some care to the skin lesion, even though the patient may attend to his other needs. It affords her an opportunity to observe the lesion carefully, and it helps the patient to feel accepted.

Occupational and diversional therapy is helpful in the care of most dermatologic patients. Any activity that keeps the patient busy and thus distracts his attention from the skin ailment or its feared consequences is justified. A program including occupational therapy during the day will often help the patient sleep during the night. Occupational therapy should be carefully prescribed, however, because in some instances the patient may be sensitive to materials used in the activities.

Bathing and cleansing

The patient with skin disease should not be bathed until he has been examined by a physician. Clothing, dressings, and the lesions themselves with crusts or exudates should be left undisturbed unless a definite order has been given for their care.

After the initial inspection by the physician, oil may be ordered for cleansing the skin. Mineral or cottonseed oil may be used. It should be warmed slightly and applied with a soft pledget, with care taken not to rub or irritate the lesions or the surrounding skin. Gauze should not be used because of the danger of trauma. Hard crusts or thickened exudates often are soaked with physiologic solution of sodium chloride, peroxide, pHisoHex in water, or a mild solution of tincture of green soap in warm water. Whether or not a sterile technique is used depends upon the lesions, but in any event clean techniques should be used. Care should be taken to avoid reinfection from soiled outer dressings or other sources.

Regular bathing is seldom permitted for dermatologic patients. Tepid sponge baths without the use of soap are often ordered, and the genital area usually can be cleansed as often as necessary. The water may be softened with a handful of bran or oatmeal or a tablespoon of uncooked laundry starch to a basin of water. Borax and sodium bicarbonate are sometimes used to soften water and allay itching, but they are drying and therefore are seldom ordered if the patient is elderly or has a dry skin.

Many patients simply do not feel clean and are greatly distressed when not permitted a shower or tub bath for several days. Although perfumed cleansing preparations also are usually prohibited, some of the detergents, pharmaceutically approved rose ointment, and cold cream may be permitted by the dermatologist. The use of these products may make the patient feel more comfortable and acceptable to himself and to others.

Colloidal baths are often ordered. Some colloid substances make the enamel surface of the tub slippery. Therefore, a rubber mat should be placed in the tub before the patient steps into it. Usually the patient should stay in the bath only for twenty to thirty minutes. Occasionally when itching is particularly severe, he may remain for over an hour. In this event, small amounts of hot water should be added to the bath at intervals to prevent its becoming too cool. The patient must be watched closely for signs of fatigue and should not be left unattended.

After the bath, the skin should be patted dry with a soft towel. Skin medication should be conveniently placed so that it may be applied immediately, since pruritus may otherwise recur with intensity. Following a bath, the patient should remain in bed for at least a half hour to avoid chilling.

An *oatmeal, soybean,* or *bran bath* may be prepared as follows: (1) add 2 cups of cereal to 2 quarts of boiling water and stir while boiling for five minutes; (2) fill tub to three-fourths of capacity with tepid water, 35° C. (95° F.); (3) pour the cooked cereal into a mesh or gauze bag and stir the bag about in the bath of a few minutes. The bag may also be used as a mop to gently pat the skin and remove crusts and debris.

A boiled-starch bath is prepared by pouring 2 quarts of boiling water over a cup of cornstarch or laundry starch moistened with cold water and stirring as it thickens. This solution may be added directly to the bath without straining through a mesh bag. Cold uncooked starch also may be used in the same quantity.

Several simple packaged preparations such as *Aveeno* (oatmeal-bran extract) are now available, although their cost is relatively high. *Sodium bicarbonate,* ¼ to ½ cup, may be added to any colloidal bath if ordered by the doctor for its drying action on the skin. *Camomile tea* (approximately two handfuls steeped in 2 liters [2 quarts] of water) added to a sitz bath is often prescribed in the treatment of severe pruritus ani.

If the skin lesion is infected, such as might occur in severe neglected eczema, following burns, or in advanced pemphigus; *medicated baths* may be ordered. Potassium permanganate 1:40,000 and a hexachlorophene preparation such as pHisoHex often are used.

Compresses and dressings

Dressings often are referred to in dermatologic practice as open, closed, or fixed dressings. *Open dressings* are ones for which no outer covering is used. *Closed dressings* have an outer covering such as bandages. *Fixed dressings* may have a covering of collodion starch paste, gelatin paste, or other material.

Compresses may be either sterile or unsterile, depending upon the skin condition, but regardless, every effort must be made to prevent new infection of skin lesions by thoroughly washing the hands before any procedure is begun. Hot compresses are used to increase circulation and to hasten healing. If it is safe to do so, the basin of solution may be kept hot by placing it on an electric plate at the patient's bedside. Cold compresses are used to reduce inflammation and to lessen itching. A solution of 3% aluminum acetate (Burow's solution) or 5% magnesium sulfate is often used for cold compresses in the treatment of conditions such as poison ivy dermatitis. Ice may be added to the bowl of solution for unsterile compresses. If it is used, the solution must be changed frequently since it will become diluted. In applying sterile cold compresses the basin containing the solution can be placed in a bowl of crushed ice. For either hot or cold sterile compresses, two pairs of forceps with which to wring them are needed. Sterile compresses are usually discarded after each use.

Equipment for compresses may be placed at the patient's bedside so that he may help with the treatment if he is able and wishes to do so. If sterile compresses are used, the patient needs special instruction before participating in his care.

Wet dressings are used to soften crusts, to promote and remove drainage, to combat infection, to allay itching, and to provide constant protection to healing tissue. A few of the many solutions used for wet dressings are potassium permanganate 1:10,000, hydrogen peroxide and mineral oil in equal parts, acetic acid or vinegar, and physiologic solution of sodium chloride. Sometimes the entire dressing must be changed each time it is moistened because remoistening the original dressing would increase the concentration of the drug used more than is advisable.

If the wet dressing can be safely remoistened without being changed, an Asepto syringe may be used. Care should be taken to avoid contaminating the dressing, how-

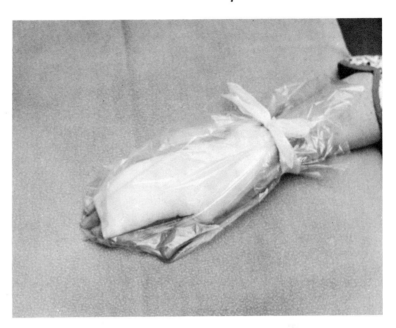

Fig. 176

A plastic bag can be used to cover wet dressings and protect the patient's clothes and bed.

ever. Care also must be taken to moisten all parts of the inner dressing and yet to prevent fluid from running through outer dressings to other parts of the patient's body or onto the bed. The frequency with which complete change of dressings is necessary depends upon the type of lesion and the amount of drainage. Any skin maceration (softening and withering) should be reported to the doctor. Wet dressings may be alternated with either powder dressings or exposure to the air with or without a heat lamp.

Pieces of worn-out linen are best for wet dressings, since they do not stick or hold heat. If linen is not available, gauze is the best substitute. Cotton becomes soggy and uncomfortable and tends to hold heat and cause itching. Several thicknesses of material should be used, and the compress may be covered with waxed paper or oiled silk. Rubberized or plastic materials tend to hold in heat and increase itching but are sometimes used (Fig. 176), depending upon the nature of the lesion being treated. An outer wrapping sometimes is used. Old Ace bandages that have lost their elasticity make satisfactory outer wrappings.

Either dry or moist dressings may be covered with *boiled starch dressings.* These rather bulky dressings are made of gauze dipped in thick boiled starch and then wrapped about the part and allowed to dry. They provide a firm protection for the healing lesion. Such an outer dressing may be ordered when the physician suspects that the skin lesion may be self-inflicted or that the patient has an active part in preventing its normal healing. This circumstance is most likely to occur in patients with industrially associated skin lesions, in young children, or in patients with strong attention-seeking motives. The adult patient who is suspected of disturbing a lesion purposefully needs close observation to prevent him from doing it. He should be given special consideration since his need for attention is greater than that of the usual patient.

Paste dressings such as an Unna paste boot may be used in the treatment of stubborn eczematous lesions, stasis dermatitis, and ulcerations of the legs. (This dressing is described on p. 387.)

A large variety of *dressing materials* are needed in caring for dermatologic patients. The effectiveness of medications and dressings may depend largely upon the imagination and resourcefulness of the nurse. The nurse in a dermatologic unit often becomes a collector. She collects old linen, table napkins, muslin, binders, stockings, gloves, and the like, which may be cut up to prepare suitable dressings for every conceivable location on the body. The cheaper and older the dressings, the better for everyone concerned since they may become lost in the laundry or so soiled or stained that it seems best to destroy them. A white stocking makes an excellent head dressing when shortened and tied with attached chin straps. Old white cotton gloves or mittens are often better than dressings for lesions on the hands, and stockings with the foot cut off make excellent circular dressings for arms or legs. The stockinette used in the plaster

room may be useful for arm and leg dressings. Suits of long underwear, long stretch stockings, and pajamas may be used when large portions of the body must be treated. Pieces of worn-out sheet may be cut into 4- or 6-tailed bandages, which are useful in securing dressings under the jaw, on the chin, or on the scalp (Fig. 177). Old pillowcases can be used to make a mask to cover the face. The knitted finger dressings used in treating minor surgical wounds are useful in securing dressings on fingers and toes.

External medications and their application

External medications are used in dermatology for many purposes and in many different forms. The list of drugs available is endless. The nurse should know the purpose for which a local application is ordered, the drug (or drugs) contained in the preparation, and any toxic signs that may occur from its use. For detailed descriptions, the student is referred to texts on pharmacology and to specialized medical texts on skin diseases and their treatment.[2,17]

Fig. 177

Ointment may be spread on a piece of discarded sheet that is to be used as a mask to cover the face. Note that the ointment is applied to the dressing rather than to the patient's skin. In actual practice, the table would be protected from soiling.

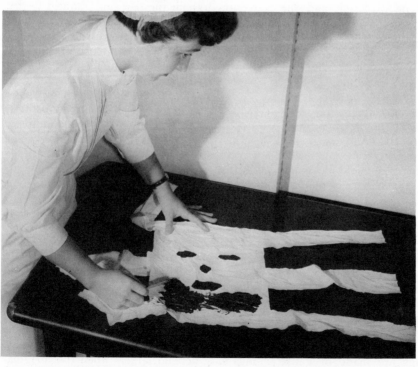

Action of external medications. External medications have many actions, and frequently the single preparation ordered has several actions. Preparations used to treat skin disease may be *antiseptic*. Ammoniated mercury ointment, 5%, is one example, and bacitracin and many other antibiotic drugs are used. Penicillin and sulfa preparations are generally not used locally because local use may lead to a sensitivity that would prevent their future value to the patient if severe illness should require their use systemically. Preparations may be *cooling* and thus lessen inflammation and discomfort—cold cream is an example of a cooling preparation—or they may be *astringent*, constricting local blood vessels and thus lessening inflammation, congestion, pruritus, and general discomfort. Burow's solution (aluminum acetate) is widely used for its cooling and astringent effects. Preparations such as calamine lotion or Lassar's paste (zinc oxide ointment) may be *soothing*, thus lessening pruritus or pain and thereby fostering healing. Other preparations such as coal tar ointments may be *stimulating* and even mildly *irritating* and thus may foster healing. Some drugs, such as salicylic acid in Whitfield's ointment, are *keratolytic* in their action and soften outer skin so that it may be removed, thus permitting other drugs to be effective. Some drugs, such as coal tar and dibucaine (Nupercaine), are *antipruritic* in their action.

Hydrocortisone and its related preparations are now widely accepted as useful drugs in dermatologic treatment and have proved of great value in the medical management of stubborn pruritus. Triamcinolone acetonide (Aristocort ointment) has proved especially effective. There is some danger of systemic absorption when fluorohydrocortisone preparations are used topically, but usually not enough of the drug is used to produce a systemic reaction. Occasionally these preparations may be injected directly *into* the skin lesion.

Forms of external medications. External medications are incorporated into various media so that suitable selection for the particular skin ailment can be made. *Powders* are widely used for their cooling and drying effect and as vehicles for antibacterial or disinfectant drugs. Thymol iodide (Aristol) and sulfanilamide powder are examples.

When large areas must be covered, *lotions* or powders suspended in liquids are often used for their cooling, refreshing, and antipruritic effects. One such preparation, calamine lotion, is widely used in the treatment of eczema, hives, and insect bites. It may be used with phenol, 1%, which has an anesthetic effect and allays itching. Care must be taken in using preparations containing phenol, however, since it may burn people with sensitive skins. Infants, old people, and persons with open skin lesions tolerate it poorly. *Liniments* are prepared with a medication and an oily substance emulsified in water. They facilitate the application of medication to large areas when dressings are not desired. Liniments are widely used by the general public for discomfort following vigorous exercise, for massage, and for their counterirritant effect. *Ointments* usually are made with medications added to a base of petrolatum, lanolin, white wax, tallow, or cold cream. Ointments may be protective or antiseptic or have a variety of other uses. They may contain a keratolytic agent (salicylic acid) to soften the outer skin layers and enable other drugs to be effective. Some, such as tar ointments, are antipruritic. *Pastes* have 50% or more of powder in the ointment base. *Cold cream,* in which water is emulsified into the ointment base, gives a cooling reaction when in contact with the skin.

Application of external medications. The nurse should know exactly how much medication is necessary for therapeutic effects so that waste is avoided and so that excessive amounts may not be left on the skin to cause caking, stickiness, and discomfort. Before new medication is applied, any old medication that is on the skin often must be removed. This should be done once or twice daily unless otherwise specified by the doctor. Cleanliness and gentleness are important in removing it.

Lotions and *liniments* must be shaken well, and those that do not appear to mix thoroughly with shaking should not be used. Lotions should be applied with clean hands or with gauze. Gauze, not cotton, should be used because cotton holds the powder solute. A paintbrush also may be used. A firm, gentle pressure should be exerted with it so that "tickling" is avoided (Fig. 178).

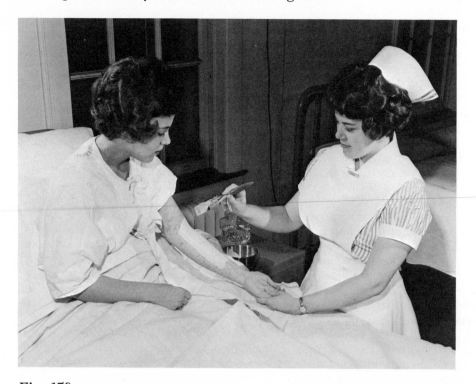

Fig. 178

Lotions may be applied to the skin with a paintbrush.

Fig. 179

When pruritus is severe, ointments can be applied to the dressing, which is then placed directly on the skin.

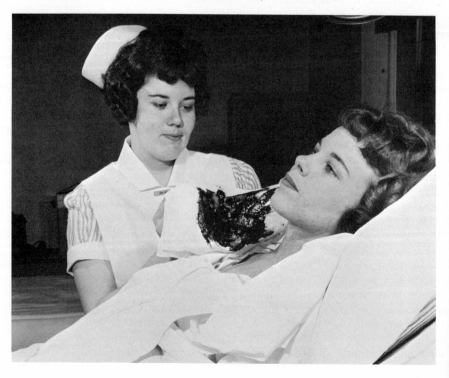

Powders should be used sparingly, as their excessive use on moist surfaces leads to caking and hardening, which may cause trauma upon removal. Care should be taken not to spread powder in the air, since sensitivity to inhaled powders is common.

Ointments should be carefully applied in small amounts, using a tongue depressor or clean fingers. They should be removed at prescribed intervals with the solvent ordered. Trauma may be avoided in applying ointment by spreading the ointment or paste on a linen, muslin, or gauze dressing and then applying the dressing to the lesion (Fig. 179). Care should be taken to estimate correctly the size of dressing needed. Many healing ointments, such as scarlet red, and some liniments contain dyes that stain linen. Therefore, the oldest bed linen available should be selected for patients receiving this treatment.

Drugs and other preparations used for skin ailments often are costly. The nurse should know the cost of the preparation used, and if the patient is caring for himself at home, she should direct him to use only enough for therapeutic benefit. In the hospital it is well to have individual jars of ointment for each patient to prevent contamination between patients and to avoid waste of medication kept in large jars. Sometimes it is best to use clean fingers to apply costly ointments. When external medications are used on infants and young children, special care must be taken to ensure that they are not ingested. Sometimes a bulky external dressing can be used and will prevent the child from getting to the medication. At other times, elbow restraints or even wrist or ankle restraints must be used.

Teaching the patient

Many patients with skin diseases are not hospitalized. In the home and in the clinic the nurse must be specific in her instruction to the patient and/or the family member who will be responsible for his care. It is often best to write out instructions specifically. A common mistake that patients make when at home is to believe that if some is good, more is better. While a skin ailment may respond to an ointment rubbed on very gently and lightly, trauma from vigorous rubbing may counteract all benefit and may

even make the condition worse. The patient, in his eagerness to cure the condition, may not realize how vigorous his own administrations are. The nurse can help the patient to improvise equipment that he needs. She may need to teach him how to apply ointment and how to sterilize linen for dressings by scorching it with an iron and then folding it inward until ready for use. The inside is then applied next to the lesion. Heating the dressing in the oven at 500° F. for twenty minutes also sterilizes it. It should be folded before sterilization.

Diseases of the skin

Some of the many causes of skin disease are fungal and parasitic infections, response to bacterial organisms and viruses, reactions to ingestion of toxic substances, sensitivity to substances taken internally or encountered externally, and new growths. Some skin diseases are of unknown cause. Others are part of a systemic disease that may or may not be communicable. Only a brief description of a few of the more common skin diseases can be given here, and grouping must be somewhat arbitrary in a book of this kind.

Dermatology is a complex subject with a vocabulary all its own. *Dermatoses* is the term used to designate conditions of the skin that are largely noninflammatory, whereas *dermatitis* is the term used to designate inflammation of the skin whether due to infection, irritation, or any other cause. Considerable time and effort must be spent in learning terminology if the specialty of dermatology is to have meaning for nurses. The following are some of the more common skin lesions.

macule a circumscribed, discolored area, usually small, and not causing skin elevation
papule a circumscribed area that is elevated, although usually not over 0.5 cm. in diameter
vesicle a papule that is filled with clear fluid held beneath superficial skin layers
pustule a circumscribed area containing pus and not usually over 0.5 cm. in diameter
bulla a large elevation of outer skin layers containing either serous or purulent fluid
nodule a large elevation of the skin usually involving the deeper skin layers and subcutaneous tissue
excoriation a break or abrasion in the skin surface
crust a dry exudate over a lesion

scar a fibrous tissue covering of a lesion after healing and repair

ulcer the erosion of skin substance

scale the outer layer of epithelium as it loosens from the skin surface

lichenification a leathery thickening of the outer skin layers

Pruritus is a symptom, not a disease, and the best treatment is to remove its cause. Causes may include systemic disease, such as liver disease with jaundice or diabetes mellitus in which sugar is not fully metabolized. Pruritus of the vulva, for example, may herald the onset of diabetes since sugar in the urine causes irritation and itching. Emotional stress is a real factor in the cause and control of pruritus, and even persons who have an average amount of emotional reserve will develop localized areas that itch excessively during periods of emotional strain. Pruritus is present in a very large proportion of all dermatoses and in almost all cases of dermatitis.

Insect pests

Several kinds of pediculi attack human beings: *Pediculus humanus* (capitis, or *head louse,* and corporis, or *body louse*) and *Phthirus pubis (pubic louse).* Other lice from animals may bite human beings, but they have a short life unless the animal host is nearby. Head and pubic lice attach themselves to the skin and live on the victim's blood. Their eggs are laid along the shafts of the hair, along with a substance that encircles the hair shaft to secure them. The substance is dissolved fairly readily by an alkaline solution or by an acid solution such as vinegar.

The person infested with lice has itching of the area involved. This is caused by the lice biting him to obtain blood. On inspection the skin in the area may appear reddened and bites may be seen. The lice and eggs (nits) also may be seen. *Pediculus humanus* var. *capitis* is grayish in appearance, 0.15 cm. ($\frac{1}{16}$ inch) long, and often can be found on the nape of the neck, where it is most likely to lay its eggs. Pubic lice are about the same size, brownish, and crab-shaped. They may occasionally be found in the axilla and on the eyebrows, as well as in the pubic region. Body lice, about 0.3 cm. ($\frac{1}{8}$ inch) in length and dark in color, attach themselves to the underwear of the host,

usually along the seams. The nits are yellowish and are laid in clumps along the seams of clothing. They are easily removed after they have been killed.

Pediculi are most often found among individuals who have poor personal hygiene habits. They may, however, be easily acquired in city living. Many children get head lice from their classmates or in crowded buses. Pubic lice may be acquired from toilet seats. Pediculi produce much more consternation on the part of the patient or his family than is warranted. They are easily killed. One or more applications of 1% benzene hexachloride in vanishing cream, when massaged thoroughly into the skin, usually destroys head and pubic lice. Preparations containing DDT also are available. A powder containing 10% DDT dusted on bedclothes and on inner surfaces of underwear is usually sufficient to destroy all body lice and nits. Underwear and bedclothes should be changed and boiled or autoclaved. Outer clothing that cannot be autoclaved or washed should be dry-cleaned. Pressing the inner surface or lining with a hot iron sometimes suffices for clothing that cannot be washed or cleaned. Sometimes shaking clothing in a pillowcase or laundry bag containing DDT powder is adequate.

Bedbugs are dark brown, oval-shaped insects, about 0.45 cm. ($\frac{3}{16}$ inch) in length, which have an unpleasant odor. They usually hide in bed frames and mattresses in poor housing units. However, they may also be acquired on crowded city buses.

Bedbugs usually bite at night. The victim awakens with itching bites, and he may notice tiny spots of blood on the bedding. The presence of bedbugs often can be detected if the bedcovers are thrown back at night in a lighted room. They may also be found along the seams of mattresses and in cracks in the bed frame.

Bedbugs are destroyed by the same drugs that are effective in destroying pediculi. Mattresses should be autoclaved. If this is not possible, spraying with DDT solution or benzene hexachloride and extended airing in sunlight are usually sufficient. Bed frames and baseboards should be thoroughly cleaned and sprayed with DDT.

Scabies caused by the itch mite *Sarcoptes scabiei,* usually is found in persons who live in unhygienic surroundings and who bathe infrequently. The female burrows under the skin, leaving a dark trail behind her and causing the skin to itch. It is by the trail that a diagnosis is often made. The mite prefers the delicate skin areas such as the inner surfaces of the forearm and thighs, under the breasts, and between the fingers. Scabies responds readily to benzyl benzoate and DDT preparations. One application of benzene hexachloride ointment, 1%, thoroughly applied from head to foot usually is effective also. The patient may be sensitive to the medications used or may have irritation and infection from damage done by the insect pests. Usually mild antiseptic ointments or lotions such as calamine lotion are prescribed for the irritation. Antibiotics may be given systemically if the lesions become infected.

An important problem in treating patients with insect infestations is reinfestation. In large, crowded families where there may be inadequate facilities for segregation of clothing, every member of the family may be affected and must be treated.

Fungal infections

Fungal infections can be either deep or superficial. The deep fungal infections, *actinomycosis* and *blastomycosis,* are extremely serious conditions and often lead to death. Fortunately they are quite rare. They usually involve other body tissues besides the skin. Invasion of the lungs and gastrointestinal tract is common. Tissues gradually thicken and then break down and suppurate. Potassium iodide, arsphenamine, and x-ray therapy are used to treat deep fungal infections, and some encouraging results have been obtained with corticosteroids.

Barber's itch (tinea barbae) is an extremely unpleasant superficial fungal infection causing lymph gland enlargement and swollen, boggy skin tissue with softening of the hairs of the beard. It is treated with copper undecylenate or ammoniated mercury preparations. X-ray therapy is used to remove the hairs. Barber's itch is entirely preventable by rigorous attention to cleanliness in barber shops.

Tinea of the scalp (tinea capitis), often incorrectly referred to as *ringworm,* is a disease seen most often in children. The condition often starts as a small, reddish papule, although it may begin as a localized area of apparent dandruff with thinning of the hair. Sometimes scaling and pustule formation with matting of the hair and crusting are the first signs. As the roots of the hair become involved, the hairs drop out, leaving bald patches. Since tinea capitis is a disease of children, it is advisable to keep small boys away from barber shops as long as possible, because it is in these establishments that the disease is often spread. The condition is highly infectious among schoolchildren, so that children with tinea capitis are often kept away from school.

It is important to diagnose the condition and begin treatment at once. An important aid to diagnosis and determination of the extent of involvement is the Wood's light, obtained by a special filter from an ultra violet lamp. The infected hairs fluoresce, or appear luminous, under the light. The doctor or technician usually works under the light and removes all infected hairs. These hairs are loose and may be removed easily. X-ray therapy may also be used to help remove infected hairs. The area is then treated with a variety of drugs. Often a preparation of copper undecylenate is used with success. An antifungal drug, griseofulvin, has been found to be effective in treating tinea capitis when comparatively large amounts are taken orally.[13] Clothing should be boiled or destroyed and the scalp protected with a stocking cap during treatment. If the treatment has been adequate, hair will eventually return in the affected area.

Epidermophytosis (athlete's foot; dermatophytosis) is a superficial fungal infection that is widely spread through the use of showers, swimming pools, and common bath mats and by direct contact with persons who have the infection. It thrives in moist skin areas. Often the first lesion appears as a crack between the fourth and fifth digits of the foot. The disease may spread to the entire foot and cause peeling, cracking, and itching of the skin. The groin, hands, and other parts of the body may become involved. Extensive involvement occurs easily in elderly patients, possibly because of poor circulation in the feet and legs. This condition can incapacitate a person.

The keynote to management of epidermophytosis is prevention. It has been said that the fungus cannot thrive on a dry skin. Therefore, after the daily bath the feet should be carefully dried, including between each toe, and then ordinary talcum powder should be dusted between the toes. Medicated powders such as those containing zinc undecylenate (Desenex) are considered even more effective. Persons who exercise vigorously, who stand for long periods at work, and whose feet perspire excessively should have two pair of shoes, which they wear on alternate days, leaving one pair to air and dry between uses. During hot weather, shoes with straw or nylon mesh insets, which permit ventilation to the feet, are desirable. It is inadvisable ever to walk in public showers with bare feet. Even the foot bath placed before the public shower at swimming pools is not sufficient protection. Paper slippers or one's own shoes should be used. The habit of sharing bath towels even among the closest of friends also should be discouraged. Athlete's foot is common among adolescents, and they should be given instruction in its prevention.

Many agents have been used in the treatment of epidermophytosis. At the present time propionate-propionic acid and undecylenate-undecylenic acid ointments are widely used. They are applied generously at night and removed in the morning. Powder is used during the day. Application of ointment may be preceded by soaks in potassium permanganate 1:10,000, which is an old and effective method of treatment. Cotton socks or stockings, which absorb perspiration better than rayon or nylon, should be worn during treatment and should be changed and washed daily. Every effort should be made to keep the feet dry. If it can be arranged, direct exposure to the sun is effective treatment. Underclothing of the person with epidermophytosis involving the body should be boiled. Shoes should be destroyed or treated with formaldehyde fumes. Drying and sunning of shoes is not sufficient to kill the fungus. Bath mats and bedclothes should be boiled, and tubs and showers should be scrubbed with 0.1% bichloride of mercury or 0.2% creosol.

Diseases caused by and associated with bacterial infection

Furuncles (boils) are purulent lesions of the skin involving sebaceous glands and hair follicles. They often occur in crops *(furunculosis)* and are caused by the staphylococcus

organism in most instances. *Carbuncles* are also caused by the staphylococcus organism and differ from furuncles in that they are much larger and involve not only the skin but also the subcutaneous tissues. Furuncles are likely to occur on the face, neck, forearms, groins, and legs, whereas carbuncles are usually limited to the nape of the neck and the back. They occur most often in poorly nourished, fatigued, or otherwise susceptible persons whose hygiene may be poor, in debilitated elderly people, and in persons who have inadequately treated diabetes mellitus.

A furuncle usually begins as a small pustule at the base of a hair follicle, while a carbuncle develops at the base of several hair follicles. Local swelling and redness soon occur, and there is severe local pain, which can be helped by moving the involved part as little as possible. Within three to five days the lesion becomes elevated, or "points up," the surrounding skin becomes shiny, and the center or "core" turns yellow. A carbuncle has several cores. The boil will usually rupture spontaneously but it may be surgically incised and drained. As drainage occurs, the pain is immediately relieved. The drainage soon changes from a yellow, purulent material to a serosanguineous discharge. All drainage usually subsides within a few hours to a few days, and the redness and swelling gradually subside. As the boil drains, care must be taken to keep the infected drainage off the surrounding skin, because organisms may be harbored in hair follicles and furunculosis may recur.

Hot, wet dressings are used to help bring the boil "to a head," but the patient should be warned to discontinue them as soon as drainage starts. They tend to macerate the skin, making it easily infected. The patient also should be cautioned to keep his hands away from the draining area to prevent spread of the infection.

If the patient is hospitalized, he usually is isolated strictly until the drainage subsides lest the organism be carried to others. The nurse should be sure to wash her hands thoroughly after caring for the patient, and she should avoid getting the drainage on her own skin. If she does, she should wash it thoroughly. The patient who is at home must be taught to be scrupulously careful about accidentally passing organisms to others in his family or to persons at work. It is not uncommon for entire families to have some type of staphylococcal infection after one member has had a boil.

Furuncles and carbuncles tend to recur in susceptible individuals, and the staphylococci causing them often are resistant to local treatment and to antibiotics. Sunshine, autogenous vaccine, and pHisoHex to cleanse the skin are used, although their benefits are uncertain. The patient with furuncles must avoid additional infection by washing his hands thoroughly before treating the lesions and by keeping drainage from other skin surfaces. He must be cautioned never to manipulate a lesion about the nose and mouth lest infection be carried to the cranial venous sinus and cause a sinus thrombosis or a brain abscess.

Acne vulgaris is one of the most troublesome and most common skin conditions of adolescence. It is a condition about which the nurse must be informed, since she is often called upon in the home, the school, and the community to advise in the total management of young persons with this difficulty. Lack of cleanliness is often blamed for the development of the condition by the patient or his family. In reality, cleanliness plays no part in the initial development of the condition.

Acne vulgaris is definitely known to have a relationship to hormonal activity. It usually makes its appearance at puberty, and in girls its activity can be clearly related to gonadal activity during different parts of the menstrual cycle. Hormonal activity produces hyperkeratosis of follicular orifices, which leads to blocking of the secretions (sebum) and the formation of discolored fatty plugs or blackheads (comedones). After the blackhead forms, there is hypertrophy of the sebaceous glands, and secondary infection occurs. A microorganism called the acne bacillus may contribute to this, and it is known that staphylococci are present in large numbers in the pustules that form. Sometimes cysts and nodules then form, and unsightly scars result despite the best treatment.

Unfortunately there is no specific treatment for acne vulgaris, although a wide variety of treatments are tried with varying success in individual patients. The face should be washed from three to five times a day with a mild soap, but the vigorous scrubbing so often undertaken by the patient in his effort to cure the condition often only makes it worse. A blackhead may be safely removed by applying hot compresses for fifteen minutes to a half hour and then removing it with an instrument with a hole in a rounded metal tip that is especially made for this purpose. Pustules should never be squeezed or broken by the patient. He should be taught to avoid touching his face with his hands, since this may cause more infection by grinding dirt and organisms into open pores. It is often difficult for the patient to carry out this instruction, since he may try to hide his face with his hands and may develop the habit of resting his chin in his hands.

Hormones are sometimes given but may cause undesirable systemic effects. The antibiotics are widely used and often produce marked improvement in the secondary infection, but their use must be continued over too long a period to be a satisfactory treatment. Staphylococcal toxoid also is sometimes used. Often a quartz lamp is ordered for use in the home, and direct exposure to sunshine is thought to be helpful in destroying infection on the skin and improving its general resistance to organisms.

A variety of diets and other hygienic measures are usually advocated with varying success. Most authorities are in agreement that a diet low in carbohydrates, condiments, and fat is advisable and that certain foods, particularly chocolate and nuts, should be avoided. Rest apears to foster improvement in the condition. Regular elimination is stressed, although there is no evidence that autointoxication from faulty elimination has anything to do with the condition.

Probably most important is emotional support to the patient in the acute stages of the condition and assistance in his adjustment to any scarring that may occur. Unfortunately this condition appears at a time in life when the patient is adjusting to become an adult, and disfiguring blemishes sometime precipitate serious emotional reactions. The greatest understanding on the part of all members of the family is necessary. The pancake makeup used by many adolescent girls in an attempt to hide the affliction often makes it worse. Among adolescent boys there is sometimes the mistaken belief that masturbation leads to acne. Some people believe that acne is aggravated by sexual abstinence and that it will be cured by marriage. This is not so, although acne is largely a self-limiting disease that tends to disappear at the marriageable age. Persons who have residual scars should know that a procedure known as *dermal abrasion,* or *planing,* often helps tremendously in removing scars (p. 220).

Acne rosacea is a skin condition that usually affects people over 25 years of age. The actual cause is unknown. It begins with redness over the cheeks and nose, which is followed by papules, pustules, and enlargement of superficial blood vessels. Many persons who have acne rosacea are of unstable emotional makeup. Achlorhydria has been found in many patients with this condition, and some favorable response has been obtained by giving hydrochloric acid. The treatment for acne rosacea is nonspecific and often not very satisfactory. Some patients respond to ultraviolet light treatment, and preparations containing naphthol and sulfur produce striking results in some. The condition is often accompanied by some pruritus, and the patient must be cautioned against touching the face since this may cause infection and aggravate the condition.

Impetigo contagiosa is a superficial skin disease produced by a form of streptococci often in association with staphylococci. It is largely a disease of children and may be endemic in nurseries unless special precautions are taken. The disease begins as a vesicle usually in the area of the mouth or nostrils, but it can be anywhere on the body. It becomes pustular and dries to form a honey-colored crust, which comes off as the lesion heals. Scarring does not result unless superimposed infection or trauma occurs. Greatest care must be taken to isolate the patient and to prevent reinfection with fingers and clothing. There is no common agreement as to treatment, but penicillin is now usually ordered either locally as ointment or systemically, or both locally and systemically. Other antibiotics may also be given. Ammoniated mercury ointment and gentian violet are old, reliable methods of treatment.

Erysipelas is caused by the hemolytic streptococcus. It is an acute febrile disease in which there is localized inflammation and swelling of the skin and subcutaneous tissues, usually of the face. A bright, sharp line separates the diseased skin from the normal skin. Elderly people with poor resistance are most often affected. Erysipelas was a serious disease before the advant of antibiotic and sulfonamide drugs, but it responds quickly to these drugs.

Viral diseases

Verrucae (warts) are caused by a filtrable virus that may be transmitted from one person to another. Warts should be removed to prevent crops of them from developing. Electrodesiccation (drying by electric current) is one of the better methods of treatment. It is safer than the use of acids, such as nitric acid, which may injure normal tissue. Warts sometimes disappear spontaneously, and this unexplained characteristic leads to the many tales of their being charmed by a variety of means. Warts may grow inward on the soles of the feet and cause severe pain and incapacity. These are known as *plantar warts* and are treated by x-ray therapy or are removed surgically.

Herpes simplex, or the common *cold sore,* is caused by a virus thought to be related to the virus of encephalitis. A cluster of vesicles appear on a reddened, swollen base, usually under the nose or on the lips. The lesion is painful and frequently cracks open. However, a crust gradually forms and the lesion heals in about ten days. It is probable that canker sores in the mouth and herpetic lesions about the genitals are of the same origin.

The treatment of herpes simplex is not specific nor too satisfactory. Some patients have excellent results from the application of copper sulfate to canker sores in the mouth. Hot compresses sometimes relieve the discomfort from lesions on the lips and on the genitals. Lip lesions sometimes respond to application of spirits of camphor. Small tubes of lip ice containing camphor can be used. Tincture of benzoin also helps to dry the lesions. Sometimes smallpox vaccination is tried when the lesions recur frequently and are very troublesome to the patient.

Herpes zoster, or *shingles,* is thought to

be due to a virus related in some way to that causing chickenpox. Clusters of small blisters usually form along the waistline. They follow the course of the peripheral sensory nerves and often are unilateral. Since they follow nerve pathways, the lesions never cross the midline of the body. Nerves on both sides, however, can be involved. Itching and severe pain usually precede the development of the blisters by several days and continue throughout the course of the disease. Herpes zoster can be a serious condition in any adult and may even lead to death from exhaustion in elderly debilitated individuals. It is one of the most drawn-out and exasperating conditions found in elderly patients and leads to discouragement and demoralization. One attack of this aggravating condition, however, usually confers immunity.

Treatment of herpes zoster consists of keeping the blisters dry and using local applications to allay itching. Calamine lotion with phenol is often prescribed. Alcohol injection of the offending nerves may be tried in an attempt to allay pain and itching, and general systemic medications, including sedatives and analgesics, are often necessary. Even after the blisters have crusted and disappeared, there may be severe pain and itching in the surrounding tissue. In extreme cases, death and sloughing of involved tissue occur.

Dermatitis due to sensitivity to internal and external toxic agents

Dermatitis is inflammation of the skin that usually goes through the stages of redness or erythema, vesicle or blister formation with oozing, and crusting, scaling, and thickening of the skin. *Eczema* is actually the name for a symptom complex designating skin reaction to an irritating factor of endogenous origin and not acquired from the external environment. In the strictest sense of the word, eczema most accurately describes the skin lesions of sensitive persons who often also have asthma or hay fever. Infantile eczema, for example, often occurs soon after birth and may be outgrown only to be replaced by asthma or hay fever. The tendency to develop these conditions is inherited. (For a discussion of allergic reactions, see p. 74.)

Contact dermatitis identifies the acute skin inflammations and reactions caused by contact with irritating factors in the environment. Skin conditions caused by industrial products fall into this group. Primary irritants such as acids affect persons who must have their hands and arms in solutions during the larger part of their working hours. Sensitivity to chemical products such as nylon and plastics plagues many workers in the dye and solvent industries. People whose work demands constant wetting of the skin often develop dermatitis. Use of detergents, petroleum products, tars, and resins may cause either direct irritation or sensitivity that may lead to contact dermatitis. Biologic products cause contact dermatitis in some persons. Nurses and doctors have been known to become so sensitive to penicillin and streptomycin that they must wear rubber gloves when handling the drugs. Some people have had to abandon working where the drugs are used. In the home, there are many materials that may lead to the development of contact dermatitis. Nail enamel and various cosmetics and related products such as deodorants and depilatories are examples. Some women develop contact dermatitis from contact with metal such as nickel, which may be used in the clips of earrings or in other jewelry. A common form of contact dermatitis is caused by contact with the oil of certain plants. *Poison ivy, poison oak,* and *sumac* are the most common offenders. This condition is known as *dermatitis venenata.*

The symptoms of contact dermatitis vary from redness, with itching and burning to blister formation and severe edema followed by secondary infection. Its treatment consists of finding and removing the cause. In the home a large number of household cleaning agents, plastic products, and related materials must be considered. Occasionally the person who develops a sensitivity to materials encountered in his daily work must change his mode of employment permanently.

Dermatitis venenata is largely preventable. Everyone should be taught to recognize the shiny leaves of the poisonous plants that are commonly found in his part of the country. Sensitivity to poisonous resins varies with individuals. Almost all people, however, are sensitive to some extent, and everyone should wear clothing that protects his skin if he is knowingly in contact with poisonous plants. Some persons are so sensitive that minute particles of the irritating oil carried in smoke or borne in the air after someone has crushed the plant are sufficient to cause a severe skin reaction. Pets may carry the irritating resin to their masters. The resin can remain on clothing for several days.

If there has been known contact with the oleoresin of a poisonous plant such as poison ivy, the skin should be washed thoroughly with alkaline laundry soap and then sponged with alcohol. Preferably this should be done within ten minutes of exposure. To relieve the symptoms, cool compresses dipped in Burow's solution (aluminum acetate) in a 1:20 dilution are often applied for ten to twenty minutes every few hours, and a lotion such as calamine may be alternated with the compresses. The greatest care must be taken not to involve new areas by contact with the exudate from active lesions. Although the condition usually does not last over a week, it may persist in some sensitive individuals for weeks and even months. Corticosteroids may be given. They seem to hasten the drying of lesions and limit the progress of the condition. Self-treatment in cases of extensive exposure to poisonous plants is dangerous since secondary infections may occur. The public should be taught this fact.

Neurodermatitis (atopic eczema) is an inflammation of the skin of neural origin. There usually is no lesion of the skin but only redness. Pruritis often is severe. Thickening and hardening (lichenification) of the skin occurs. Tar ointments are often used in an attempt to allay itching. Changes in the emotional life of the patient and in his general environment often are of most help in correcting this troublesome and stubborn condition.

Dermatitis medicamentosa is the name used to designate reactions of the skin to drugs taken internally. Bromides are frequent offenders, and in recent years a large number of patients have suffered severe, prolonged drug reactions as a result of treatment with penicillin and other antibiotics. Iodides, barbiturates, and sulfonamide drugs frequently cause skin eruptions. The skin lesions vary in dermatitis medicamentosa. In some instances they are highly colored and sharply defined, whereas in others they may resemble urticaria, with large, flat wheals almost covering the entire body.

The treatment for drug sensitivity consists of finding and discontinuing the offending medication. Pruritis must be relieved and infection prevented. It is important to reassure the patient since he may become panicky when a generalized eruption is superimposed on the illness for which the drug was given. The skin lesions sometimes disappear as suddenly as they appeared.

Exfoliative dermatitis is usually caused by drugs containing heavy metals such as mercury, bismuth, or arsenic. The condition is seen less often since the antibiotics and the bacteriostatic drugs have largely replaced drugs containing the heavy metals. Signs include redness, edema, and massive desquamation (shedding of epidermal cells). The patient may lose the entire outer layer of skin from the soles of his feet and the palms of his hands. Colloidal baths are often used to allay the itching. Lotions may be used to reduce itching and to make the erythema and desquamation less conspicuous. Patients with exfoliative dermatitis should be reassured that the loss of skin is not harmful and will not cause scarring.

Urticaria, or hives, is a disease of the skin characterized by *wheals*, which may vary in size and appearance. The condition can be acute or chronic. When the lesions are very large and are accompanied by large areas of edema that do not pit upon pressure and that occur most often about the eyes, mouth, hands, and genitalia, the term *angioneurotic edema* is used. Urticaria is generally conceded to be caused by the body's reaction to some foreign substance to which it is sensitive. In some instances the cause is easily determined. Many people, for example, develop hives immediately after the ingestion of certain foods such as eggs, strawberries, and shellfish and after receiving drugs such as penicillin. In other cases the cause of hives is obscure. Urticaria may disappear spontaneously after a few minutes or may persist for hours or days. Usually there are severe itching, redness, and local heat. Calamine lotion is used for local relief of the pruritis, and the antihistaminic drugs are often given. Epinephrine (Adrenalin) and corticosteroids also may be used.

The only real danger from this condition is the possible occurrence of giant hives in a vital area, such as on the mucous membrane of the larynx or glottis. Patients who have repeated attacks of hives that do not respond to an antihistaminic drug are advised to take (and are taught to give themselves) an injection of Adrenalin when the hives appear or at the first sign of respiratory difficulty.

Other toxic skin reactions

Erythema multiforme is a skin condition in which round, reddened, slightly raised, and painful lesions appear along the shins and sometimes on the arms and thighs. It may be accompanied by headache, elevation of temperature, and joint pains. It may be of unknown cause or may be a general systemic response to disease elsewhere in the body. The treatment is primarily detection and treatment of the original pathology. Local treatment includes baths, soaks, and dressings. Fluids are forced, and the patient is encouraged to take a high-caloric diet. Lesions may appear in the mouth. If so, special care is needed, including frequent mouth irrigations with hot salt solution or alkaline solutions such as Dobell's solution.

Communicable diseases such as measles, chickenpox, smallpox, scarlet fever, and typhoid fever produce skin reactions. Nodes and hemorrhagic spots in the skin also accompany severe acute rheumatic fever.

Dermatoses of unknown cause

Psoriasis is a very common benign skin disease of unknown origin. It causes a dry, scaly eruption on any part of the body but occurs most often on the elbows, back, shins, scalp, and chest. For some unknown reason psoriasis is often found in persons suffering from atrophic arthritis. The lesions have a shiny, metallic (fish scale) appearance.

A variety of medications is used in local treatment of psoriasis, but tar ointment is perhaps the most satisfactory in the majority of cases. Fluorinated hydrocortisone creams, applied under closed dressings, are now used widely. In severe cases triamcinolone acetone, a corticosteroid, may be given systemically or injected into the lesions. (See p. 63 for side effects and precautions.) A short course of therapy with an antimetabolite such as methotrexate may be tried. This drug is contraindicated in pregnancy and for anyone with a history of a peptic ulcer. No precautions need to be taken in bathing. In fact, bathing is beneficial in removing the scales.

Lesions may fade with treatment, only to recur eventually in the same area or elsewhere. The patient should know that the condition is not contagious, that it is benign, and that while it probably will not get worse, it probably will never be cured. If the patient does not know these things, he may lose confidence in his physician and may seek a quick cure. Because psoriasis is so common (it comprises about 5% of all skin disease) and so stubborn in response to treatment, manufacturers of patent remedies find a lucrative field for their products among persons who have the disease. Anyone who reads the daily papers regularly has seen numerous promises of cure. The patient should be warned lest he takes these advertisements seriously and waste his money.

Pemphigus is a skin condition characterized by enormous pustules called bullae, which appear all over the body and on the mucous membranes. The lesions break and are followed by crusts that heal and leave scars. The cause of pemphigus is unknown. The condition may appear to clear up, and there may be remissions, but lesions eventually appear in such large numbers that a large part of the skin surface is raw and oozing and becomes infected. It is finally fatal. Cortisone and ACTH (adrenocorticotropic hormone) cause marked improvement in symptoms and may produce remissions lasting for months or even years.

Nursing care of a patient with pemphigus is very difficult. Bradford frames or Stryker frames may be used in an effort to move the patient as painlessly as possible and prevent weight-bearing on raw surfaces. Dakin's solution compresses may be applied to oozing lesions to help control odors and infection. Special mouth care, including frequent gargles with normal saline solution or alkaline mouthwashes, may be necessary if the lesions appear in the mouth. In an attempt to prevent secondary infection, reverse isolation may be used (p. 61).

Emotional support and encouragement of both the patient and his family are extremely important. The patient may fear that he is so repulsive that no one will take care of him. He needs constant reassurance that the nursing staff is interested in him and will care for him. The family and friends should be prepared for the patient's appearance before they visit him if they have not seen him recently. The family should be encouraged to visit often and to behave as normally as they possibly can. Fortunately pemphigus is a relatively rare disease, for it taxes the resources of the patient's family and medical personnel to the utmost.

Degenerative skin diseases

Corns are thickened skin lesions with a center core that thickens inwardly and causes acute pain upon pressure. They are often caused by the pressure of ill-fitting shoes and occur on the toes. A corn is best treated by correction of shoes and by placing a small felt pad with a hole in the center over it to relieve pressure. Popular corn remedies seldom produce a cure, since their active ingredient is usually salicylic acid, which only dissolves the outer layer of skin. As soon as the medicated pad is removed, a new layer of skin forms unless pressure is relieved.

Soft corns occur between the toes where the skin is moist. They are extremely painful and difficult to treat. Sometimes x-ray treatment is required to effect a cure.

Calluses, or thickening of circumscribed areas of the horny layer of the skin, often appear on the plantar surface of the foot when the metatarsal arch has fallen and there is constant pressure against the sole of the shoe. They are often successfully treated by relief of the pressure and by regular massage with softening lotions and creams. They must be distinguished from plantar warts.

Stasis dermatitis is a common skin condition of the lower extremities in older persons. It is usually preceded by varicosities and poor circulation. With the reduction in venous return from the legs, substances normally carried away by the circulation remain in the tissues and irritate them. The skin is often reddened and edematous. Pruritus may be quite severe. Breaks in the skin are often caused by scratching, and infection then is introduced by the hands, clothing, and other sources.

The most important treatment for stasis dermatitis is prevention by careful attention to the treatment of peripheral vascular conditions and preventing the constriction of the circulation to the extremities (p. 370). Unna paste boots (Fig. 82) are often ordered for this condition.

Seborrheic keratoses occur most often in persons past middle age. The lesions resemble large, darkened, greasy warts and are often found around the trunk, on the back, and under the breasts. They seldom become malignant but should be observed at intervals for any change. They often can be removed easily with dichloracetic acid or carbon dioxide snow.

Angiomas are tufts of blood vessels that may occur spontaneously either as tiny bright red lesions or as purplish vascular lesions. The lesions should be watched closely, for although they do not usually become malignant, thay may suddenly develop extensive vascular channels that may be difficult or impossible to remove surgically.

Malignant and premalignant lesions

Malignancies of the skin are more accessible to treatment than are those in any other part of the body. Education of the patient in reporting suspicious lesions and prompt action by nurses and doctors when such lesions are reported should make malignancies of the skin a largely controllable disease. By far the best treatment is early and complete surgical removal of the lesion.

Leukoplakia occurs as raised, even shiny areas of various sizes on the mucous membrane of the mouth and also of the genitals in women. About 25% of the lesions become cancerous if not removed. Surgical removal is the treatment of choice. However, if the lesions are too extensive to be removed by surgery, radiotherapy or electrodesiccation may be used. In the early stages leukoplakia of oral mucosa may be controlled by careful mouth hygiene. The patient who smokes should stop smoking. Smoking is definitely known to aggravate the condition. Any loose or jagged teeth are removed, periodontal treatment is given if necessary, and frequent mouth irrigations with an alkaline solution are advised.

Senile keratoses usually begin as scaly raised lesions in exposed parts of the body. The lesion is firm to pressure, and there is usually an elevated surface or border that bleeds easily. Senile keratoses require prompt surgical treatment because they may undergo malignant degeneration and become basal cell carcinomas.

Basal cell carcinomas involve the lower or basal layer of skin cells. They grow and metastasize slowly but may progress extensively over a period of years while unnoticed. A typical form known as a *rodent ulcer* often develops from senile keratoses. The lesions frequently ulcerate, crust over, and heal, leaving a small scar, and then recur at the same site.

Pigmented moles are often precancerous. These skin lesions may be present at birth or may appear at any time of life. The darker the lesion, the more dangerous it seems to be. The blue or greenish black type (melanotic nevus) is the most dangerous of all. Yellow and brownish moles are less likely to become malignant. Blue or black moles should be removed even if they are not raised above the normal skin surface. Most physicians agree that any mole that shows signs of growth or that is in a part of the body where it is traumatized by clothing should be removed at once. The *malignant melanoma*, deriving its name from the melanin, or pigment, in the basal layer in the skin, is the most dangerous of all cancerous skin lesions. The mortality is extremely high, and often wide metastasis has occurred before the lesion is noticed.

Squamous cell carcinomas originate in the outer prickly or squamous layer of skin cells. Usually the lesion begins as a warty growth with a hard, horny outer layer that breaks down to form an ulcer. The lesions often occur in areas of irritation such as on the bridge of the nose in persons who wear glasses or on the lower lip in those who smoke pipes. If they are not diagnosed and treated early, squamous cell carcinomas metastasize rapidly.

Sarcoma and *fibrosarcoma* are lesions that may develop quite suddenly from seemingly innocuous nodules somewhere in the skin. Unfortunately metastasis often occurs before the original node shows much change. For this reason any nodule in the skin should be reported to a physician at once.

Mycosis fungoides is one of the most dreaded of all skin diseases. It begins as an itching, thickened lesion in the skin and progresses to a tumor stage, which finally breaks down and destroys the skin. A large, soft, mushy vegetative lesion develops that destroys all the normal adjacent structures. Lesions may break out in several parts of the body. While the patient lives, all resemblance to his normal self is lost, and the disease is invariably fatal. X-ray therapy is sometimes used to allay itching in the early stages, and nitrogen mustard is sometimes given intravenously. Cortisone delays the process somewhat but does not affect the final outcome. In the late stages, the nursing care for mycosis fungoides is similar to that required for pemphigus.

References and selected readings*

1 Beeson, Paul B., and McDermott, Walsh, editors: Cecil-Loeb textbook of medicine, ed. 11, Philadelphia, 1963, W. B. Saunders Co.

2 Bergersen, Betty S., and Krug, Elsie E.: Pharmacology in nursing, ed. 10, St. Louis, 1966, The C. V. Mosby Co.

3 *Bozian, Marguerite Wilkinson: Nursing care of patients having dermatologic conditions, Am. J. Nursing 52:873-875, July 1952.

4 *Cahn, Milton: The skin from infancy to old age, Am. J. Nursing 60:993-996, July 1960.

5 *Carney, Robert G.: The aging skin, Am. J. Nursing 63:110-112, June 1963.

6 *Cormia, Frank E.: Acne vulgaris, Am. J. Nursing 57:198-201, Feb. 1957.

7 *Edwards, Elizabeth: Mycosis fungoides, Am. J. Nursing 61:61-63, Feb. 1961.

8 *Goldman, Leon: Prevention and treatment of eczema, Am. J. Nursing 64:114-116, March 1964.

9 *Iverson, Preston C., and Staneruck, Isabella D.: Dermal abrasion, surgical care and nursing care after dermal abrasion, Am. J. Nursing 57:860-864, July 1957.

10 *Jeghers, Harold: Herpes zoster, Am. J. Nursing 54:1217-1219, Oct. 1954.

11 Marlow, Dorothy R.: Textbook of pediatric nursing, ed. 2, Philadelphia, 1965, W. B. Saunders Co.

12 Nelson, W. E., editor: Textbook of pediatrics, ed. 8, Philadelphia, 1964, W. B. Saunders Co.

13 Osment, Lamar S.: Tinea capitis, Am. J. Nursing 60:1264-1266, Sept. 1960.

14 Piper, William N.: Poison ivy, poison oak and poison sumac, Am. J. Nursing 54:814-816, July 1954.

15 *Samitz, M. H.: The industrial dermatoses, Am. J. Nursing 65:79-82, Jan. 1965.

16 Sauer, Gordon G.: Manual of skin diseases, Philadelphia, 1959, J. B. Lippincott Co.

17 Sulzberger, Marion B., and others: Dermatology, diagnosis and treatment, ed. 2, Chicago, 1961, The Year Book Publishers, Inc.

18 *Torrey, Frances: Care of the normal skin, Am. J. Nursing 53:460-463, April 1953.

19 *Wechsler, Harry L.: Psoriasis, Am. J. Nursing 65:85-87, April 1965.

*References preceded by an asterisk are particularly well suited for student reading.

28

The patient
with burns

**Study
questions**

1 What are some of the precautionary measures you have already learned that must be observed when applying heat to the skin?
2 From your knowledge of anatomy and physiology, list the harmful effects of loss of a large area of skin.
3 From your notes in fundamentals of nursing review the principles and techniques of surgical asepsis.
4 Name some ways of helping a patient increase fluid intake. What kinds of food are high in protein? What are some ways in which high-protein foods may be given to the critically ill patient?

Burns are wounds caused by excessive exposure of the body to heat, radiation, x-rays, electricity, and certain chemicals such as strong acids. Heat in various forms, such as flame, air, water, and steam, is the most common cause of burns. This chapter is devoted mainly to the nursing care of patients who have been burned by heat.

Burns are classified as first, second, and third degree, depending upon their depth. First- and second-degree burns are classified as *partial thickness*, whereas third-degree burns are *full thickness*. A *first-degree burn* is one in which the outer layer of skin is injured and reddened without blister formation; mild sunburn is a good example. A *second-degree burn* is one in which a blister, or bleb, forms beneath the upper layer of skin and in which deeper layers are not destroyed; thus regeneration of epithelium can occur. First-degree and second-degree burns are likely to be painful because nerve endings have been injured and exposed. A *third-degree burn* is one in which all layers of skin are destroyed, thus making regeneration impossible. Nerves, muscles, and bone also may be injured or destroyed in third-degree burns. If the nerves are destroyed, the wound is painless. Because epithelization is impossible, areas that have sustained third-degree burns eventually must be covered either by skin growing from normal skin around the edges of the burned area, by scar tissue, or by skin grafts.

Approximately 7,700 persons died of burns in the United States in 1964.[1] Many of these deaths could have been prevented. Nurses can help prevent accidental burns from occurring by participating in general health education and by promoting legislation that would control some of man's thoughtless practices and make his working and living environments safer. Public health nurses are in an unusually advantageous position to recognize unsafe practices in the home and to help families develop safe habits of living.

Accidental burns in and about the home are common and primarily are caused by ignorance, carelessness, and the curiosity of children. Approximately one-half of those burned in the home are under 20 years of age—infants and young children being the most common victims.[20] Young children should be supervised in their play and should never be left at home alone. Children should be taught at an early age about the hazards of fire. Parents must carefully check play areas for all fire hazards, such as live extension wires, matches, and unprotected floor heaters, and should remove them. Serious burns to children often result from pot handles that project beyond the stove top. A large number of children have been burned to death or maimed for life by fireworks. Legislation in many states now prohibits the sale of fireworks, but violations of the law and accidents still occur.

Kerosene or lighter fluid used to light stoves indoors and charcoal broilers or wood fires outdoors cause many burns by igniting clothing. Explosions resulting from defective gas stoves and heaters also lead to many deaths each year. Smoking in bed and falling asleep in an upholstered chair with a lighted cigarette are two of the most easily preventable, yet most common causes, of fatal burns in the home. Increase in the use of electrical equipment, in the use of plastic materials, some of which may be inflammable, and smoking among both patients and personnel has made the danger of fires in hospitals very real.

Each year brings increased demand for careful inspection and regulation of places in which the ill and infirm are housed. Aged persons frequently are housed in old and poorly equipped structures and many of them have been burned to death. Attention is being focused on places where large numbers of people congregate. Laws now require that doors in public buildings be hinged to swing outward, that draperies and decorations be fireproof, and that stairways with special fire doors be used in new apartment buildings and hotels. These laws have been passed as a result of serious fires in which many persons have lost their lives. Rigid enforcement of laws requiring that industrial products be labeled when known to be flammable and that new products be tested carefully for their flammable qualities before being placed on the market is further evidence of government effort to protect the public from accident by fire.

Sunburn should be cautioned against, as even a relatively mild first-degree burn of a large part of the body can cause change of fluid distribution and kidney damage. Camp nurses should keep this in mind in their educational programs for children and camp counselors. (For further discussions of sunburn, see p. 253.)

Emergency care

The nurse may be called upon to assist with injuries at the scene of a fire. If flame is involved and the victim's clothing is on fire, his first panic reaction is to run, which only fans the flame. Rolling the burning person in a blanket on the ground to exclude oxygen, thereby putting out the fire, is one of the best procedures. The person whose clothing is aflame should never stand since this increases the danger of breathing flames, heat, and smoke into the lungs.

As soon as the burning clothing is extinguished, immediate arrangements should be made to transport the patient to a hospital or doctor's office. A layman or nurse should never attempt to estimate the degree or severity of burns, but should assume that all burns are more severe than they may appear to be. All patients with burns, regardless of their superficial appearance, should be seen by a doctor. The hospital or physician should be notified, in order that preparations can be made for the arrival of the patient, since a well-prepared and well-equipped team of personnel is needed to care for the severely burned patient.

While awaiting transportation to a medical facility, the patient should be kept quiet and lying down. Loss of natural body heat may be prevented in part by covering the victim with blankets, coats, or whatever is available. External heat should not be applied since this may cause dilation of blood vessels and further loss of body heat. If clothing adheres to the burned surface, it should not be removed. Exposed burned surfaces should be covered with sterile dressings or with the cleanest material available. *Oils, salves, and ointments should not be used on burns* since these materials hamper treatment. Cold water or ice packs help to ease the pain and reduce the edema in minor burns. Pain in extensive burns is best controlled by gentle and minimal handling and by the application of dressings to exclude air from the burned skin surfaces. Occasionally, deep, third-degree burns are almost painless, since nerve endings have been destroyed, and for the first few minutes the patient may appear not too badly affected. Usually, however, some part of the body has sustained first-degree and second-degree burns that cause pain.

If the distance to reach medical aid is long, and the burn is not too extensive, warm fluids (preferably containing salt) may be given by mouth, provided the patient can tolerate them. If the patient is nauseated or vomits, nothing should be given by mouth.

Burns occurring about the eyes should be lavaged with copious amounts of cold, clean water, and if the burn was caused by acids, the procedure should be repeated in from ten to fifteen minutes. A few drops of any mild oil such as mineral oil, castor oil, or olive oil should then be put into the eyes, and a doctor should be consulted at once.

Physiologic changes occurring in severe burns

The lives of many badly burned patients are now being saved, since, in recent years, much has been learned about the physiologic changes occurring in patients with severe burns. When tissues are burned, vasodilation, increased capillary permeability to proteins, and changes in the permeability of tissue cells in and around the burn area occur. As a result, abnormally large amounts of extracellular fluid, sodium chloride, and protein pass into the burned area to cause blister formation and local edema or escape through the open wound. Visible fluid loss makes up only a small part of the fluid lost from the circulating blood and other essential fluid compartments (Table 4). Most of the fluid loss occurs deep in the wound, where the fluid extravasates into the deeper tissues. Burns of areas such as highly vascular muscle tissue or the face are believed to cause greater fluid losses than comparable burns of other parts of the body. Fully one-half of the extracellular fluid of the body can shift from its normal distribution to the site of a severe burn. The extracellular fluid constitutes about 20% of the body weight. Three-fourths of it surrounds the cells and one-fourth is found in blood plasma. (See Table 4.) For a person weighing 67.2 kg. (150 pounds) this means that from 10 to 15 pounds, or from 5,000 to 7,500 ml., of fluids may be removed from the interstitial spaces and bloodstream. The result is a tremendous drop in blood pressure, shock, inadequate blood flow through the kidneys, which in turn leads to further shock and anuria, and death within a short time if treatment is not given promptly or is inadequate.

In addition to dehydration, hypoproteinemia, sodium depletion, and shock, other changes take place. Hyperkalemia (excessive amounts of potassium in the blood plasma) occurs as a result of injury to the epithelial and red blood cells and from a diminished urinary output. Anemia develops as red blood cells trapped in the burned area are destroyed and the injured cells continue to hemolyze. Renal damage and hematuria may occur as a result of reduced blood volume and the passage of the end products of hemolyzed cells through the glomeruli. Blood concentration develops because of loss of fluid from the bloodstream and hematocrit levels are elevated. Burns increase the production and loss of heat, and water vapor is lost through the open wound; these, in turn, cause increased metabolism and weight loss. Electrolyte imbalance may develop, particularly in children, following the administration of sodium chloride solutions. There often is evidence of adrenocortical hyperfunction for a few days after a burn.

Medical treatment and nursing care

The severely burned patient presents one of the most taxing assignments that doctors and nurses can encounter; full-time efforts of both doctors and nurses are needed. The following discussion of care in the early stages refers primarily to treatment and nursing care of the severely burned patient. When 20% or more of the body surface of an adult or 12% of a child is destroyed, the burn is considered severe. Modifications are made for the patient with less damage and also for other individual factors such as age. For example, when burned severely, the very young child or the elderly person responds poorly to treatment.

Immediate treatment

When the patient arrives at the hospital, his clothes are removed carefully and his condition and injuries evaluated by the doctor. A tracheotomy may be performed if he has difficulty in breathing, has extensive burns of the face and neck, or has inhaled hot gases such as steam, smoke, or flames. Oral fluids usually are withheld, and a Foley type catheter is inserted. Morphine sulfate or meperidine hydrochloride may be given intravenously for pain. Subcutaneous injections often are absorbed poorly in severely burned patients because they usually have alterations in fluid distribution and low blood pressure. Large doses of sedatives and analgesics are avoided because of the danger of respiratory depression and because they may mask other symptoms. The patient should be weighed. This measurement will be used to determine fluid therapy and to evaluate his progress. Blood samples are taken to determine protein, electrolyte, and red blood cell levels.

In evaluating the severity of the burn, the doctor considers such factors as the extent of the body surface areas burned. For adults, the "rule of nine's" is used (Fig. 180). These calculations are modified for infants and children under 10 years of age because of their relatively larger heads and smaller extremities. (See pediatric textbooks for these figures.[19]) The depth of the burn (first, second, or third degree) also is considered. The age of the patient is important in estimating

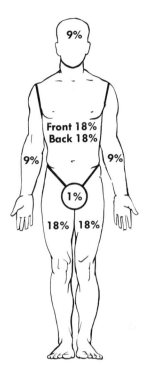

Fig. 180

The "rule of nine's" is used to estimate the amount of skin surface burned.

the severity of the burn. Infants tolerate burning poorly and the mortality in this group is high, even with small burns. In burns involving up to 30% of the body surface in older children and in adults under the age of 50, the mortality rate is quite low. As the age of the patient increases beyond 50, the mortality rises even in burns of less than 30%.[2] The anatomic location of burns is important. Burns on the hands, feet, face, neck, and most joint surfaces may produce the most serious loss of function and the most conspicuous disfigurement. Preexisting diseases of the heart and kidneys and associated injuries, such as fractures, also influence treatment.

Fluid therapy

Replacement of fluids and electrolytes is an essential part of the treatment and is instituted as soon as the extent of the burn and the patient's condition have been determined. Ideally, fluid therapy should be started within an hour following a severe burn. A cutdown in a vein usually is done and a polyethylene catheter inserted.

Three types of fluid are considered in calculating the needs of the patient: (1) colloids, including whole blood, plasma, and plasma expanders such as dextran, (2) electrolytes, such as physiologic solution of sodium chloride, Ringer's solution, Hartmann's solution, and Tyrode's solution, and (3) nonelectrolyte fluids, such as distilled water with 5% glucose.[5] Medical authorities do not agree as to the proportion of colloid and electrolyte fluids needed. Several formulas are described in medical literature to guide physicians in determining the type and amount of fluids to be administered, based upon the patient's weight and age and the percentage of the body burned.[5,16] The present trend is to administer balanced salt solutions (such as Ringer's), water, and plasma and to use whole blood only if a large number of red cells are destroyed or if anemia develops.

Fluid needs for the first twenty-four hours are calculated from the time of the burn. Usually the patient receives one-half of the total amount in the first eight hours, one-fourth in the second eight hours, and one-fourth in the third eight hours. One-half of the total amount given on the first day is given in the second twenty-four hours. If vomiting occurs or if a nasogastric tube is inserted and attached to suction, additional fluids containing electrolytes may be given intravenously. Hydrocortisone may be given intravenously to patients who do not respond to fluid therapy.

The amount of fluids required after the first forty-eight hours usually is determined by the sodium concentration in the plasma. Normal figures for this are 132 to 138 mEq./L., and an increase over these figures indicates water depletion and a need for additional water. The amount of water required to keep a severely burned patient well hydrated may range from 4,000 to 6,000 ml. per day.[5] Solutions containing sodium usually are discontinued when the normal flow of urine is established, the danger of shock is passed, and the patient is able to eat.

The patient often complains of severe thirst, but this usually is relieved by the fluids given parenterally. The nurse should give fluids by mouth only in the amounts ordered and should record them accurately. Unlimited oral intake and failure to measure it may result in too much fluid in the circulating blood and in water intoxication.

Renal function

The rate of urinary output is probably the most reliable measure of determining the adequacy of fluid therapy during the first forty-eight hours. Hourly checking and measuring of urinary output is one of the most important responsibilities of the nurse. Usually a retention catheter (Foley catheter) is inserted and drained into a calibrated bottle. The amount of urine in the bottle is measured and recorded every hour. The care of the patient with an indwelling catheter is discussed on p. 444. The color of the urine should be observed, and the doctor should be notified if hematuria occurs. A urine flow of 30 to 50 ml. per hour is adequate for an adult.[5] The urine flow should be at least 15 ml. per hour for infants and 25 ml. per hour for older children.[12] If the urinary output rises above or falls below these figures, the doctor should be notified immediately. Fluid therapy will need to be adjusted accordingly. Lack of urinary output may indicate insufficient fluids or acute renal failure. The administration of too much fluid may cause pulmonary edema.

After the first forty-eight hours the urinary output is no longer a reliable guide to fluid needs, since water deprivation may occur even when the urinary output for adults is 1,000 ml. or more per day. Severely burned patients require a large fluid intake to compensate for the loss of fluid into the tissues and from the wound. Fluid needs then are determined by measuring the sodium concentration of the plasma. Fluids administered during the first forty-eight hours to patients with small, uncomplicated burns are excreted rapidly. Excretion of fluids by patients with extensive, deep burns may be delayed for several weeks as the fluids move to other portions of the body and are excreted slowly through the kidneys and wound exudate.[5]

Observation

The severely burned patient needs constant nursing observation and attendance. The nurse must check the general condition of the patient and report any changes promptly. Persistent vomiting should be noted and the amount recorded, since this loss must be considered in estimating the total amount of fluid needed. If a sphygmomanometer can be applied, blood pressure should be taken as often as every fifteen minutes. Rate and volume of the pulse should be carefully noted. Skin color and level of consciousness are often important in determining whether or not progress is favorable. Restlessness is always significant, and mania is indicative of a poor prognosis. Signs of water intoxication should be watched for and include tremor, twitching, nausea, diarrhea, salivation, and disorientation. The patient who has been burned by hot air or steam must be closely watched for signs of respiratory complications. Difficulty in breathing, coughing and expectoration of blood, and cyanosis are signs that the trachea and the lungs may have been burned. These signs must be reported immediately. Depending upon the severity of the symptoms, emergency treatment may include oxygen, suctioning, and postural drainage. Tracheotomy may be necessary if severe edema of the throat develops.

Prevention of infection

Every effort is made to prevent introduction of infection to the burned area. Local and systemic infections (septicemia) are the most common complications of burns and are a major cause of death, particularly in burns covering more than 25% of the body.[15] The primary source of bacteria appears to be the burn wound. The organisms that usually infect burn wounds are *Staphylococcus aureus*, *Pseudomonas aeruginosa (pyocyanea)*, and the coliform bacilli. Antibiotics may be given prophylactically, or they may be withheld until an infection does occur. Cultures of the nose, throat, wound, and skin of the patient may be taken upon admission and at intervals to determine the bacteria present and their sensitivity to antibiotics.

All who attend the patient should wear masks to prevent the introduction of their organisms into the wound. Personnel with upper respiratory infections should not be permitted to attend the patient. Good aseptic surgical techniques should be used in the emergency room. Sterile gloves should be used when doing dressings. Sometimes the patient is transferred to the operating room, where sterile surgical techniques can be carried out. The extent of local cleansing depends upon the severity of the burn and the judgment of the doctor. Sometimes soap and detergents such as pHisoHex are used, and a rather extensive debridement may be carried out at the initial cleansing. The wounds then are treated by methods that will be described later in this chapter. If the exposure method is used, strict isolation technique is observed when caring for the patient. Some hospitals use a specially built isolation system (bubble) in order to protect the patient from the hospital environment.[13] (See p. 62.) If silver nitrate dressings are used, the patient is not isolated and clean technique is used.

Tetanus toxoid and/or antitoxin is usually given to the patient who has received extensive burns. The patient may receive both a booster dose of toxoid (0.5 ml.) and 3,000 units of antitoxin if he has not been immunized or has had no booster dose in the previous four years.[5]

Local treatment

At the present time, there is no completely satisfactory method of treating the burned area. New methods are being tried and are reported in medical literature but, while favored by a few, have not replaced the occlusive dressings or exposure method. A brief description of the latest method advocated for the treatment of the burned site (silver nitrate dressings) is included in this discussion.

Occlusive dressings. The occlusive dressing method of treating burns came into wide use during World War II. Today the occlusive or absorptive dressings are used primarily for hand burns. They help maintain the hand in a position of function and allow for elevation, support, and compression of dead spaces. Occlusive dressings also may be used in the treatment of burns of the lower limbs to facilitate nursing care. The use of this type of dressing permits the patient to move about more freely and to be out of bed sooner. Mobilization improves circulation, speeds healing, helps to prevent deformity, and contributes to the patient's morale. The moist, dark, protected area under occlusive dressings is, however, conducive to bacterial growth, especially in hot, humid weather. Local antibiotic treatment is believed to be of dubious value for this.[5] Treatment of burns with occlusive dressings is very time consuming, and the materials are expensive. It has been pointed out that, in the event of major disaster such as atomic attack, it would be impossible to procure sufficient dressings despite stockpiling of equipment for initial dressings.

In applying an occlusive dressing a single layer of lightly impregnated petrolatum, xeroform, or dry, fine mesh gauze is applied first. A very absorptive, bulky layer of fluffed or washed gauze is placed next to the first layer and is followed by several large abdominal pads. The dressing then is covered with a cotton elastic bandage, stockinette, or a conforming bandage.[5]

When assisting with the application of occlusive dressings, the nurse should help to see that the affected part is placed in such a position that a deformity, such as foot drop, will not occur. If dressings are changed frequently, position should be altered somewhat from time to time. If the nurse is responsible for the dressings, she must be sure that no two skin surfaces are left in contact to prevent their healing together. Petroleum jelly gauze can be placed between toes and fingers, between the ears and scalp, and between genital folds.

After the occlusive dressing is applied, the nurse watches for signs of impaired circulation such as numbness, pain, and tingling. Signs of infection, such as odor on the dressings and increased pulse rate and temperature, are reported to the doctor. Since elevation of the extremity hastens the absorption of fluid, the patient is advised not to stand for more than a very short time if lower limbs are involved and to elevate a bandaged arm when sitting or lying down.

Dressings are changed every four to ten days. This treatment is continued up to the time when skin grafting is done, which may sometimes be as early as one week after the initial burn. When large areas are involved, the patient may be taken to the operating room and a general anesthetic given while a change of dressings is carried out. The need for anesthesia in many instances is a disadvantage of this method of treatment.

Exposure method of treatment. The exposure method of treatment was accidentally discovered to be effective in 1888 when, during a serious steamboat fire on the Mississippi, those in attendance ran out of bandages and later observed that the neglected persons fared better than those who received more intensive local treatment.[9] Today, the exposure method is used most often in the treatment of burns involving the face, neck, perineum, and broad areas of the trunk. The burned area is cleansed and exposed to the air. (See Fig. 181.) The exudate of a partial-thickness burn dries in forty-eight to seventy-two hours and forms a hard crust that protects the wound. Epithelization occurs beneath this crust and may be complete in fourteen to twenty-one days.[5] The dead skin of a full-thickness burn is dehydrated and converted to an *eschar* (black, leathery, dead-tissue covering) in forty-eight to seventy-two hours. The eschar acts as a protective covering until it is removed and a skin graft is applied. A dry environment hastens the formation of a protective crust. All efforts must be made to prevent injury to the crusts or eschar since cracks permit the entrance of bacteria. The crusts or eschar must be removed if infection occurs.

To decrease the possibility of infection, the patient with exposed burn wounds should be placed in a unit or room where only "clean" surgical cases are cared for. He usually is placed on sterile linen. A cradle may be used since no clothing or top bedclothes are allowed directly over a burned area. In summer months, screen doors and window screens should be used to keep out flies, which may introduce direct infection or lay eggs in the open wounds. Sterile cornstarch can be sprinkled on the bed to help prevent sticking caused by drainage from cracks in the crust as the patient moves about. Infants may need to have their hands restrained to prevent them from picking off crusts. Until the wounds are healed, children's toys need to be sterilized to prevent them from causing infection.

The nurse caring for the patient should wear a sterile gown and mask. In most hospitals it is fairly simple to make up a "burn pack" to be autoclaved. This pack can include sheets for the canopy and bed, loin cloth and halter, bath blankets, pillow-

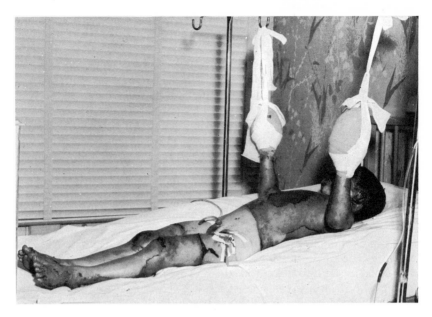

Fig. 181

The open method of treating burns is now widely used. (From Baker, T. J., and Peterson, J. E.: Plast. & Reconstruct. Surg. 24:209-213, Aug. 1959.)

cases, towels, washcloths, and bedpan covers, as well as gowns and masks for those in attendance.

During the first twenty-four to forty-eight hours, patients having exposure treatment complain of pain and chilling, but they usually are more comfortable after the crusts have formed. Pain may be relieved by administering morphine sulfate, meperidine hydrochloride (Demerol), barbiturates, or propoxyphene hydrochloride (Darvon) as ordered. Discomfort can be decreased if drafts are avoided and the temperature of the room is kept at 24.4° C. (76° F.). Patients lose more heat from burned surfaces than from the normal skin surfaces, since there is no vascular bed to contract and retain heat in the body, but too warm an environment must be avoided because it promotes the growth of bacteria. The humidity of the room also should be controlled. A humidity of 40 to 50% usually is considered satisfactory. Portable electric humidifiers and dehumidifiers can be used to achieve and maintain this level. A high humidity may cause the crust to soften and separate prematurely, whereas a humidity that is too low may cause crusts to crack more easily when the patient moves. This causes pain and may permit infection to be introduced. Many patients prefer to turn themselves, and, if dress-ings are used to cover small areas, they may wish to help remove the dressings. They should be permitted to help themselves since this is often less painful and more acceptable to them.

If the burn is extensive, the patient may be placed on a burn bed, which is prepared by draping a Balkan frame with sheets to make a tent. A thermometer should be hung within the canopy, and a small section of the canopy should be left open to prevent humidity from rising and softening the crust; the temperature in the tent should be maintained at about 24.4° C. (76° F.). Electric lights may be strung up inside the tent to maintain the temperature, using small bulbs. The bulbs should be enclosed in wire frames for safety and should be placed out of the reach of children. If the lights are used and there are no burns about the face, sometimes patients rest and sleep better when wearing sunglasses. Others find that cloth eyeshades are helpful in keeping the light from their eyes. The burned patient can be kept from embarrassing exposure and can be kept warm in the tent while wearing only a halter and loin cloth. Maximum freedom is provided for him to get on or off the bedpan, move about, and perform exercises for the prevention of contracture and the improvement of circulation.

Silver nitrate treatment. The use of thick gauze dressings saturated with a silver nitrate solution (0.5%) is being used by some physicians in the treatment of the burn wound.[16,21] These dressings are said to decrease mortality, lessen pain, eliminate odor, and have a bacteriostatic effect. The dressings are kept wet so that the solution remains in continuous contact with the wound surfaces. The thick dressings are used to retain moisture and heat and to reduce evaporation. The dressings are removed every 12 or twenty-four hours and the patient is placed in a bath of salt solution with the temperature carefully maintained at the same level as the body. When skin grafts are done, silver nitrate dressings are placed over the graft and donor sites on the first postoperative day. Because the silver nitrate solution is hypotonic, electrolytes are lost into the wound. Therefore, throughout treatment, frequent determinations of blood sodium levels are necessary, and sodium lost may need to be replaced.

Isolation technique is not required when the burn is treated with silver nitrate dressings, but clean dressings and sterile gloves and instruments usually are used. Because everything that comes in contact with the silver nitrate solution is stained black, the nurse must wear a gown and gloves when applying the solution, to protect her skin, nails, and clothing. Although linen can be specially treated to remove stains, great care must be taken to prevent splashing the solution on the furniture, walls, and floors.[15]

Dressings and soaks. Local applications may be ordered to stimulate healing of burned areas. While sterile petrolatum or a local anesthetic cream may be applied to first-degree burns, ointments, particularly those containing antibiotics, are not being used as often as formerly in the treatment of severe burns. Mafenide hydrochloride (Sulfamylon), mafenide acetate (Sulfamylon acetate), and gentamicin (Garamycin) cream are being used by some physicians in the

local treatment of burn wounds.[14,16] If ointments such as nitrofurazone (Furacin), cod-liver oil, scarlet red, and balsam of Peru are used, old or discarded linen should be used for bandages, since most of these agents will stain.

Saline dressings may be used to treat small infected areas, and it is important to keep them moist, because drying causes the dressing and the exudate to shrink. This shrinkage produces pain and may cause hemorrhage from newly developed superficial blood vessels.

Tub baths at 37.7° C. (100° F.) may be used to soak off extensive dressings over infected areas. Although the water in the tub cannot be kept sterile, many patients benefit a great deal from its cleansing effects and from the fact that dressings are removed so much more easily and less painfully. Salt may be added as ordered to the water and occasionally antiseptics such as potassium permanganate 1:40,000 or a hexachlorophene preparation such as pHisoHex is used. The patient must receive careful personal care before being placed in the tub so that fecal contamination is minimal. Those in attendance should wear gowns and gloves until the wounds are healed. The patient should never be left unattended during this procedure because fainting and injury may occur.

Skin grafts. Skin grafts are applied to cover the burn wound and speed healing, to prevent contractures from occurring, and to shorten convalescence. Successful grafting reduces the patient's vulnerability to infection and prevents the loss of body heat and water vapor from the open wound or eschar. Most skin grafts are done between the fifth and twenty-first day after the initial injury, depending upon the depth and extent of the burn. Small areas of third-degree burns, such as those that occur on the dorsum of the hand, may be excised and skin grafted during the first twenty-four to forty-eight hours to hasten healing and to help restore function more quickly. The wound is prepared for the graft as described on p. 214.

Split-thickness grafts usually are used. These grafts include the upper layer of the skin and part of the under layer, but are not taken so deep as to prevent regeneration of the skin at the site from which they were taken (donor site). They grow as normal

dies or sloughs within one to three months. (See p. 212.)

The donor site, which presents an oozing, painful surface, may be covered with sterile gauze and a pressure dressing or it may be covered with a fine mesh gauze and left exposed to the air. The drainage from the wound dries and serves as a protective covering. The wound usually heals within two weeks. Many patients complain of quite severe pain in the donor site, and the nurse should not hesitate to give medications that are ordered for pain. The pain should subside within a day or two. Sometimes an odor develops from dead tissue at either the donor site or the recipient site, which is distressing to the patient, and should be reported to the doctor. If infection has developed, antibiotics may be administered and the wound treated with wet dressings.

Nutrition

To meet the increased metabolic needs, to maintain the patient's nutritional state, and to repair and replace tissue destroyed or injured by the burn, the protein, fluid, and vitamin and mineral intake must be increased as well as the total caloric intake. A diet containing from 125 to 150 grams of protein and from 3,000 to 5,000 calories is necessary to meet the needs of severely burned adults.[10,16] The caloric requirement for children usually is estimated as follows: for children up to 1 year, 100 calories per kilogram of body weight; for children from 1 to 3 years of age, 90 calories per kilogram of body weight; and for children between 4 and 12 years of age, 70 calories per kilogram of body weight.[19] Supplemental vitamins, particularly ascorbic acid to aid in wound healing and vitamin B complex to meet the increased metabolic needs, also are required, as well as iron preparations, such as ferrous gluconate. Depending upon the extent of the burned area and serum electrolyte levels, sodium chloride, potassium, and calcium preparations also may be administered intravenously or orally.

The patient who is burned may have nausea and vomiting to such an extent that nutrition must be provided entirely by the intravenous route. Paralytic ileus also may occur, and peristaltic action may be absent for a few days. Food and fluids are withheld

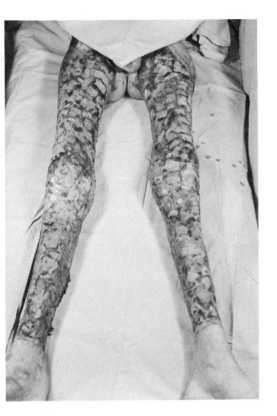

Fig. 182

Postage stamp grafts have been cut from split-thickness graft and have been used to partially cover large burned areas on lower limbs. (From Artz, C. P., and Reiss, E.: The treatment of burns, Philadelphia, 1957, W. B. Saunders Co.)

skin on the burned areas (recipient sites). These grafts are removed with a dermatome from almost any unburned part of the body. They may be removed in strips or small squares (postage stamps) (Fig. 182). Grafts may be laid on the burn wounds and held in place with dressings or sutured into place. Pressure dressings may be applied to secure the graft, provide even compression, and act as a splint. If the loss of skin is so great that life is threatened, the skin of other persons is taken to cover burned surfaces. However, this is a temporary measure since, with the exception of identical twins, the skin of another person is incompatible and

until peristalsis returns. A solution containing 3 to 4 Gm. (½ tsp.) of table salt and 1.5 to 2 Gm. (1½ tsp.) of sodium bicarbonate in 1,000 ml. (1 quart) of water (Haldanes' solution) flavored with lemon juice and chilled can often be retained when other fluids would be vomited. It supplies electrolytes as well as fluid. Effervescent beverages are also an acceptable means of supplying some necessary electrolytes as well as sugar. Sodium citrate (packaged in envelopes) to be added to water has been stockpiled for use in treating severely burned patients in the event of a major disaster. Salty solutions, such as meat broths, often are given to help replace sodium chloride that is lost into the tissues and in wound exudate, but broths or fruit juices that contain potassium are withheld for forty-eight hours or until the serum potassium levels go down.

The diet is advanced as quickly as possible to a regular one but, because of the patient's poor appetite, the utmost imagination and ingenuity on the part of the dietition and the nurse are needed to persuade him to eat what he needs. Sometimes relatives are helpful in suggesting favorite foods, and the patient's knowledge that special preparations are being made in the hospital may motivate him to take more food. If the patient is able to feed himself, it may help to improve his appetite. It is important that painful and disagreeable changes of dressings and other treatments be timed so that they do not immediately precede meals.

The high-protein powdered milk preparations are valuable in masking the amount of protein taken and often seem to leave the patient with less of a feeling of oversatiation than may result from large servings of meats such as chops, which are often high in fat. They are also valuable because the very ill patient can take fluids more easily than he can chew and swallow solid foods.

Bulk foods and fruit juices must be stressed in the diet of the severely burned patient, because they aid in elimination. Fecal impaction is a common problem for burn patients. Bulk-forming laxatives, such as preparations of the psyllium seed (Metamucil), may be given, or a fecal softener, such as dioctyl sodium sulfosuccinate (Colace), may be ordered.

Prevention of contractures

Contractures are among the most serious long-term complications of burns. Many patients must undergo painful reconstructive surgery as a part of rehabilitation, which would not have been necessary if those in attendance had been alert to the prevention of contractures. A large responsibility for the prevention of contractures rests with the nurse, who is with the patient more than anyone else and she should note whether or not the patient's position has been changed regularly during the day and night. Early skin grafting prevents many contractures by mobilizing the patient sometimes months earlier than would otherwise be possible.

Burned patients often have severe pain as healing progresses. They are anemic, debilitated, and very often in a state of depression. The nurse's temptation may be to leave them in what appears to them the most comfortable position, promising herself that change will be made tomorrow. The nurse must never let her sympathy for the patient lead her to overlook her concern for his ultimate good. She must make gentle, but determined, efforts to have the patient maintain range-of-joint motion and thus prevent scars from healing in positions that will result in deformity. The problem is even worse in children, since normal skin and normal tissues grow while scar tissue shrinks. Thus, what begins as a minor deformity in childhood may become a major one with increased growth.

For a definite interval of time each day, patients with burns should lie prone and also flat on their backs with no pillow or elevation of the head of the bed. This can be accomplished more easily if the patient is placed on a Stryker frame, a Foster bed, or a CircOlectric bed. Prolonged rest in a semi-Fowler's position or with the pillow pushing the head forward must be avoided. Many patients like this position because it enables them to see about the room better. The resourceful nurse can often turn the bed so that the patient can look about without having to assume positions that may lead to the formation of contractures. It is often advisable to change the bedside table from one side of the bed to the other at intervals. Mirrors help these patients keep in better touch with their environment, provided that view-

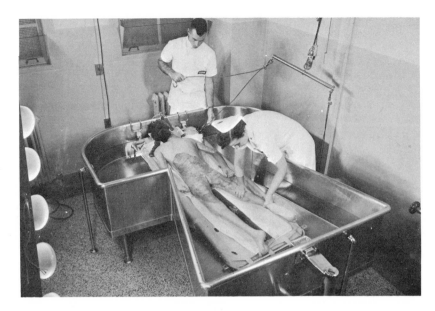

Fig. 183

If the burn has healed sufficiently, the patient may be placed in a Hubbard tank, where exercises are done more easily under water. (From Artz, C. P., and Reiss, E.: The treatment of burns, Philadelphia, 1957, W. B. Saunders Co.)

Fig. 184

Stryker frames are used in the care of some severely burned patients since they facilitate turning and caring for the patient. (From Artz, C. P., and Reiss, E.: The treatment of burns, Philadelphia, 1957, W. B. Saunders Co.)

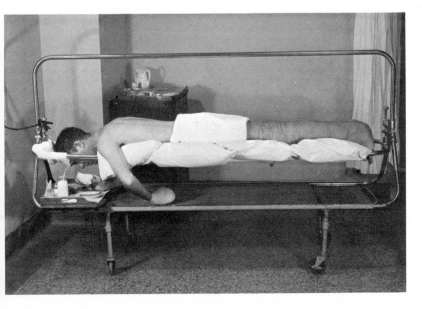

ing disfiguring burns on the face can be avoided.

If burns have been sustained about the neck, chin, and face, the patient should lie in a position of hyperextension of the neck for a period of time each day. A pillow may be placed under his shoulders and the bed lowered to a level position. Facial exercises are encouraged to prevent scars from tightening as they form. Chewing gum and blowing balloons provide exercise for this purpose.

Burns on the hands can easily result in contractures unless the part is kept in a position of hyperextension at least part of each day. If the patient has only one hand burned, he can be taught to exercise it, using his other, unaffected hand. Tight scarring in the axilla may be prevented by bandaging the arm loosely to the head of the bed in a position of external rotation for a period of time each day. Splints and shell casts may be used to prevent contractures of knees and plantar flexion deformity of the foot. These deformities can result from poor position during sleeping hours.

Exercises for prevention and correction of contractures are often supervised by a physical therapist. When the burned areas have healed sufficiently, exercises may be done more easily in an occupational therapy or physical therapy department where the patient also may benefit from a change in environment. In the department of physical medicine exercises often are done in water. A Hubbard tank may be used for this (Fig. 183). The occupational therapist may help the patient to improve his range of motion in a satisfying and efficient fashion by teaching him crafts suitable for his particular needs, such as typing, weaving, or a host of other activities. The nurse must know what the patient is being taught by the physical therapist and the occupational therapist so that progress can be continued when he returns to his room.

The patient who is not hospitalized and the one who returns home early due to skin grafting needs instruction in how to prevent contractures from developing. If public health nursing services are available, a physical therapist may be called upon to assist the patient at home. If this service is not available, the nurse in the hospital or the public health nurse may have to take responsibility for teaching the patient how he may prevent contractures from developing.

Special beds to facilitate care

Stryker frames, Foster beds, and CircOlectric beds are used in the care of some severely burned patients, since they facilitate the use of the bedpan and urinal, permit change of position with a minimum of handling, and permit larger skin surfaces to remain free from body pressure than is possible when the patient lies in bed. These special beds are particularly useful when both back and front of the trunk, thighs, and legs have been burned. They allow turning of the patient with a minimum of handling and thus help to decrease pain. (See Fig. 184.) A regular schedule for turning the patient must be set up to prevent thrombophlebitis, emboli, contractures, and decubiti. (For details of use of these beds, see textbooks on orthopedic nursing.)

Emotional aspects of care

The emotional impact of severe burns is enormous. During the first few days the patient is too ill to fully comprehend what has happened, but then comes the long healing period and the realization of endless implications. The patient's reaction is determined by his own personality make-up, by his degree of total adjustment to life, and by the extent and location of the burns. Burns on the face make adjustment particularly difficult. All kinds of fears arise to harrass the patient. Will my husband (or wife) still care for me? Can I ever let my children see me? To the adolescent, the thought of being different or conspicuous may be unbearable. Fears about not being taken back on the job often haunt the wage earner who is badly burned. If possible, the patient should not see facial burns until a good deal of healing has taken place or until skin grafting has been done. One way to reassure a patient is to show him pictures of patients with burns in the early stage and several years after treatment. The recovery is almost unbelievable in some instances. He should be told that the redness that accompanies both burns and newly healed skin will often fade a great deal within a few months.

Patients who are severely burned usually

are exhausted and often demoralized by the pain, treatment, and frequent dressing changes. Anticipation of painful procedures may upset and frighten the patient. The pain can be minimized in many instances by giving medication before the dressings and treatments are scheduled, explaining the necessity of the procedure to the patient and gaining his cooperation, using careful technique, and permitting the patient to participate in the treatment whenever possible. Depending upon the age of the patient and the extent of the burn, television, games, puzzles, weaving, and painting may distract him from the pain and also provide occupational therapy.

The patient should have an opportunity to talk about his problems and his fears. He may discuss these with the nurse when he cannot express them to relatives, and she must take time to listen. Almost every burned patient needs the help of the social case worker for himself and for his family. The nurse should recognize this need and initiate the referral. Visiting hours can be used to gather information from relatives that would aid in understanding the patient and his particular needs.

Long-term problems and rehabilitation

Complete recovery and rehabilitation of the severely burned patient may be a long and costly process. Many industries have compensation insurance to cover part of the cost, and the patient should be encouraged to discuss his financial problem with his doctor and with the social case worker if one is available. If the patient is under 21 years of age, he will be eligible for care financed in part by the Children's Bureau through its aid to states for their programs for crippled children. This care will cover surgical procedures and care, special rehabilitative services, and social service.

Patients who have been burned should have medical checkups at regular intervals indefinitely and should be advised to report any unusual change in the burn scar to their doctor at once. There is a fairly high frequency of malignant degeneration of scar tissue following burns. This is particularly true when the burn is caused by electricity or by x-rays.

References and selected readings*

1 Accident Facts, Chicago, 1965, National Safety Council.

2 American College of Surgeons, Committee on Trauma: Early care of acute soft tissue injuries, ed. 3, Philadelphia, 1965, W. B. Saunders Co.

3 Artz, Curtis P., editor: Research in burns, Washington, D. C., Philadelphia, 1962, American Institute of Biological Sciences and F. A. Davis Co.

4 *Artz, Curtis P., editor: The burn patient, Nursing Forum 4:87-92, 1965, No. 3.

5 Artz, Curtis P., and Reiss, Eric: The treatment of burns, Philadelphia, 1957, W. B. Saunders Co.

6 *Baker, Thomas J., Rhodes, Verna A., and Shannon, Anna M.: Open technique in the management of burns and nursing care of the burn patient, Am. J. Nursing 59:1262-1268, Sept. 1959.

7 *Bennett, Herman J.: Burns—first aid and emergency care, Am. J. Nursing 62:96-100, Oct. 1962.

8 Brantl, Virginia M., and others: The care of patients with burns, Nursing Outlook 6:383-387, July 1958.

9 Cockshott, W. P.: The history of the treatment of burns, Surg., Gynec. & Obst. 102:116-124, Jan. 1956.

10 Cooper, Lenna F., and others: Nutrition in health and disease, ed. 14, Philadelphia, 1963, J. B. Lippincott Co.

11 Davis, Loyal, editor: Christopher's textbook of surgery, ed. 8, Philadelphia, 1964, W. B. Saunders Co.

12 *Farmer, A. W.: Management of burns in children, Pediatrics 25:886-895, May 1960.

13 Haynes, B. W., Jr., and Hench, Miles E.: Hospital isolation system for preventing cross-contamination by staphylococcal and Pseudomonas organisms in burn wounds, Ann. Surg. 162:641-649, Oct. 1965.

14 Larson, Duane, and Gaston, Rita: Current trends in the care of burned patients, Am. J. Nursing 67:319-327, Feb. 1967.

15 *Maxwell, Patty, and others: Routines on the burn ward, Am. J. Nursing 66:522-525, March 1966.

16 Moyer, Carl A., and others: Surgery, principles and practice, ed. 3, Philadelphia, 1965, J. B. Lippincott Co.

17 Nelson, Waldo E.: Textbook of pediatrics, ed. 8, Philadelphia, 1964, W. B. Saunders Co.

18 Rubin, Maxine: Balm for burned children, Am. J. Nursing 66:296-302, Feb. 1966.

19 Silver, Henry K., Kempe, C. Henry, and Bruyn, Henry B.: Handbook of pediatrics, ed. 6, Los Altos, Calif., 1965, Lange Medical Publications.

20 Stark, Richard B.: Plastic surgery and burns, Surg. Gynec. & Obst. 120:285-287, Feb. 1965.

21 *Wood, MacDonald, Kenney, Helen A., and Price, William R.: Silver nitrate treatment of burns, Am. J. Nursing 66:518-521, March 1966.

*References preceded by an asterisk are particularly well suited for student reading.

29

The patient
with disease
of the breast

**Study
questions**

1 Review the anatomy of the breast and adjacent structures.
2 What are some of the psychologic reactions to be expected when a patient faces disfiguring surgery?
3 Review the normal range of motion of the shoulder joint. What daily activities involve the full use of this joint?
4 Describe how you would teach a person to apply a sling.
5 Review the physiologic processes controlled by the hormones secreted by the ovaries, testicles, adrenal glands, and the anterior and posterior lobes of the pituitary gland. What are the effects of insufficiency of any of these hormones?

The most common diseases of the breast are dysplasia (fibrocystic disease), carcinoma, and fibroadenoma. These conditions occur almost entirely in women, and are known to surgeons as the "big three" of breast disease. Carcinoma is by far the most important, and the nursing care for this disease will be discussed in some detail before the other two.

Carcinoma of the breast

The nurse plays a vital role in regard to carcinoma of the breast. Her responsibilities include educating women so that breast cancer may be discovered and treated early; caring for the patient who has had a cancerous breast removed, and assisting with physical and emotional rehabilitation; helping the patient and her family in the home or in the hospital when the lesion is inoperable or when metastasis has occurred.

Incidence, cause, and prognosis

Carcinoma of the breast is the most common malignancy in women; of 26,162 deaths from this cause reported in 1964, 20,663 occurred between the ages of 35 and 75. It is estimated that one out of eighteen women in the United States is destined to develop carcinoma of the breast, with the probability increasing steadily with age.[7] The American Cancer Society estimates that, in 1966, 63,000 new cases will have been discovered, and approximately 27,000 women will have died from breast cancer.[3] Unfortunately, the present five-year survival rate for all patients with cancer of the breast, whether treated or untreated, is approximately 50%. This low survival rate is due in part to the frequent failure to detect the lesion before regional involvement occurs and failure to seek medical treatment as soon as a lesion is discovered. Studies show that approximately 82% of women treated when the lesion appears localized have a five-year life expectancy, compared with 47% of those with obvious regional involvement at the time of treatment.[3] However, survival at the end of five years cannot be considered synonymous with cure. Many women treated before regional involvement is apparent die of the disease after five years, and the ten-year survival rate for these patients is only approximately 40 to 45%.[7]

Although carcinoma of the breast occurs quite often in young women, it often immediately precedes or follows the menopause, and also develops in those past the climacteric. Most tumors of the breast in women past the menopause are malignant. Benign fibroadenomas occur largely in younger women, and dysplasia (fibrocystic disease), in those between 30 years of age and the menopause.

Causes of carcinoma of the breast are not known. However, studies have disclosed that it is found more often in women in the higher economic levels, in those who have a family history of breast cancer, and in those who have a late menopause. Although it had been thought that hormonal secretions had some relationship to the development of breast cancer, recent studies now show that perhaps the estrogenic hormones and progesterone are prophylactic rather than causative factors. Individuals differ as to rate of growth and the probability of metastases, and this "genetic determination" can be an extremely important factor in controlling the outcome for the patient.[7] It is believed that injury does not lead to breast cancer, although a lump in the breast is often discovered after a minor injury has been sustained, perhaps because the one injured feels her breast at the time of injury and may note a mass that was already present. There is little evidence that dysplasia (fibrocystic disease) predisposes to the development of carcinoma, although the presence of this condition may make it much more difficult to diagnose an early carcinoma.[7]

Prognosis in carcinoma of the breast depends to a great extent upon early diagnosis and complete surgical removal of all tissues containing malignant cells before metastasis occurs. It is estimated that approximately 40% of all patients who seek medical attention for cancer of the breast are incurable at the time of the initial examination.[7] Since the disease develops in a relatively accessible part of the body, it is unfortunate that early diagnosis is not made more often so that more lives might be saved. At the present time, the only hope for cure lies in complete, early removal of the entire breast and its surrounding tissues.

Making an early diagnosis

Carcinoma may develop anywhere in the breast or on the nipple, although the upper outer quadrant is the most commonly affected area. The early lesion may be discovered by careful examination of the entire breast. Attempts are being made, by means of roentgenograms *(mammograms)*, to detect lesions before they become palpable. It has been reported that skilled roentgenologists can detect areas of increased density due to tumors with a fair degree of accuracy. The practicability of this procedure for use in early diagnosis has not been demonstrated at this writing. An additional, potential screening device is *thermography,* which photographically portrays the temperature of the skin over the area in the breast where a malignant lesion is located. An infrared scanner is used to detect the abnormal variations in the natural infrared heat emissions coming from the breast.

Self-examination of the breasts. For years, surgeons have been urging women to learn to examine their own breasts for lesions, since it is not practical to see a physician for these frequent, routine examinations. Authorities[2] feel that a self-examination should be made at least once a month, although women over 30 years of age with a familial history of breast cancer should have a medical examination at least twice a year. All women should have a complete examination that includes palpation of the breasts at least once a year.

The nurse working in industry, in the clinic, in the doctor's office, or in the community nursing agency has the responsibility of teaching women how to examine their breasts and of explaining why it is necessary. A movie prepared by the American Cancer Society, describing one method of self-examination is available for loan from local chapters of the Society. In most large cities the local committee of the American Cancer Society will arrange for showing the film to an audience of fifty or more. In smaller communities the film may sometimes be obtained through the local health department.

Self-examination of the breasts should be done regularly each month. The best time is at the conclusion of, or a few days following, the menstrual period. Some women have engorgement of the breast premenstrually, and the breasts may have a lumpy consistency at that time. This condition usually disappears a few days after the onset of menstruation, although occasionally lumpiness and tenderness may extend throughout the menstrual cycle. Because of this possible change, it is important that the breasts be examined at the same time each month in relation to the menstrual cycle. Women who have passed the menopause should check their calendars and examine their breasts on the same day each month. (See Fig. 185.)

Self-examination of the breasts as outlined by the American Cancer Society,* should include the following steps:

Step 1. Sit straight before a mirror, arms relaxed at sides. Study the contour of the breasts. Has there been a change since the last examination?

Step 2. Next, raise the arms high above the head and observe whether there is any deviation from normal in size or shape of the breasts or abnormal puckering or dimpling of the skin.

Step 3. Lie down, place folded towel under shoulder, and raise arm above head on the side being examined. With flat of the fingers, feel gently the inner half of the breast.

---

*Leaflets on self-examination of the breasts are available free of charge from local chapters of the American Cancer Society, Inc., for distribution to all women.

Step 4. Then, bring the arm down to side and feel gently the outer half of the breast, giving special attention to the upper outer section. Examine the other breast in the same way.

Some women need help in learning to examine themselves; they may, for example, feel a rib when examining the lower half of the breast and become alarmed. However, most women learn quite readily. If a lump of any kind is discovered, it should not be rubbed or touched excessively. It should be left alone, and the advice of a physician should be sought at once.

Signs and symptoms. The only early sign of carcinoma of the breast is a small palpable mass. Pain is seldom a symptom of early cancer. Dimpling of the skin (orange rind appearance) over a hard lump, puckering of the skin, changes in the color of the skin over the lesion, alteration of contour of the breast, raising of the nipple, serous or bloody discharge from the nipple, and unusual scaling or inversion of the nipple are signs that the lesion is well established and has invaded surrounding tissues. In the advanced phases of neglected cases there may be ulceration of the skin, with subsequent infection in necrotic tissue. Spread to the axillary lymph nodes occurs early. Because of the distribution of the lymph vessels and because there are no lymph nodes between the two breasts to delay spread of malignant cells, these carcinomatous cells may spread rapidly through the lymph vessels with metastasis occurring in the opposite breast and in the mediastinum. Sometimes discovery of enlarged lymph nodes or pain in the ribs or vertebrae is the first indication to the patient that anything is wrong, particularly when the lesion is deep in the breast tissue and routine palpation of the breast has not been carried out.

Paget's disease is a condition in which there is a shiny-appearing scaling of the nipple. This progresses to bleeding and ulceration of the nipple and areolar structures. This lesion is precancerous in its early stages, but, if untreated, it always becomes malignant. The treatment is total mastectomy as soon as a diagnosis is established.

Fear of diagnosis. The woman who finds a lump in her breast should not become panicky and decide that she has cancer. She

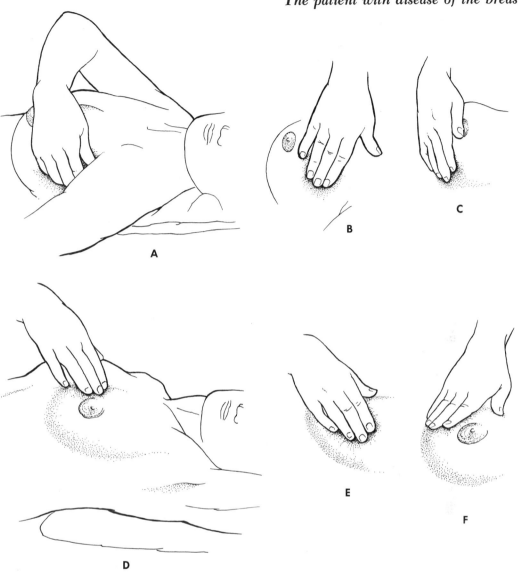

Fig. 185

Every woman should examine her breasts each month.
The drawing illustrates one method.

should know that there are other causes for a mass in the breast besides cancer. The lump may be caused by a benign tumor or by a cyst; only the doctor can determine this. All women should know that a malignant tumor in the breast does not, as a rule, cause pain. Tenderness in a mass in the breast usually suggests dysplasia (fibrocystic disease).

Women should be taught that the prognosis for cancer of the breast is likely to be much better *if the cancer is discovered early, and treatment instituted immediately.* Although 95% of all breast cancers are discovered by self-examination, many are not reported for several months. Fear of mutilation or of death are the two main reasons why some women delay seeking medical advice and treatment and hesitate to risk confirmation of their fears when a tumor is discovered. National statistics on deaths from cancer of the breast are widely publicized, and, as a result, many women fear the disease and have a negative attitude, causing delay in seeking medical help. Also, some women may have had a relative or a friend who has died from the disease, which causes the fear to be even more acute. Unfortunately, the average woman may tell only her closest friends when a breast has been successfully removed for cancer. As a result, deaths from the disease are much better known than cures by surgery with no recurrence. Some women wish to avoid the expense or embarrassment of an examination, or rationalize that their trouble would appear trivial to the busy doctor. Sometimes they seek the advice of nurses. It then becomes the responsibility of the nurse to stress the urgency of getting medical advice at once. A safe rule to follow is to suspect that any lump in the breast may be cancerous until proved otherwise.

Medical treatment and nursing care

Although doctors can develop remarkable skill in distinguishing benign from malignant tumors by inspection and palpation, the only way to determine this conclusively is by microscopic examination of a section of the tumor obtained by biopsy. Sometimes, as when axillary lymph nodes can be felt, the diagnosis of malignancy can be made with relative certainty before operation, and an axillary node may be excised for microscopic study. Most surgeons believe that, if there is the slightest possibility of cancer, it is safer to remove the entire mass rather than risk permitting a malignant tumor to remain. Pieces of a tumor are seldom removed surgically because there is danger of releasing malignant cells into the blood and lymphatic systems at the time of the operation.

Emotional preparation. The surgeon usually discusses the entire situation with the patient and sometimes with her family. This may be done in the doctor's office prior to admittance to a hospital or in the hospital a day of two before surgery is scheduled. The physician explains the operation, why it is necessary, and what he hopes can be accomplished. The nurse should report to the physician if she feels the patient does not fully understand his explanation, and thus alleviate needless anxiety. The patient who comes to the hospital for removal of a breast tumor is always worried and upset, although she may try to hide her fear. She needs the greatest understanding from all who care for her preoperatively. Visits from her husband and other close members of her family should be permitted at any time. The nurse must observe the patient closely and be guided by what she learns. If a mastectomy is almost a certainty, some women benefit from a short visit by a patient who has had a mastectomy and has made a satisfactory adjustment. Some patients are helped by a concise discussion of breast prostheses, whereas others are much too upset at this time by the thought of the loss of a breast or the threat to life to even talk with others or consider the use of an artificial breast.

In our culture the breasts have become a primary source of women's identification with femininity. Since much emphasis is placed on the female breast as a symbol of attractiveness, the thought of loss of a breast becomes almost intolerable to many women. This is particularly true of those who depend largely on physical attractiveness to hold the esteem of others and to secure gratification of their emotional needs. Psychologists have pointed out that there is a symbolic connection between the breasts and motherhood which is severely threatened when a breast must be removed.[19] All women, including single women and those past the menopause, are seriously threatened emotionally by the loss of a part of the body that is so closely associated with sexual attractiveness and motherliness. Carcinoma of the breast often occurs at the menopause or soon after when some women may feel that they have lost much of their sexual attractiveness, or when normal women take stock of their relative degree of satisfaction with their own femininity. Although the surgical removal of a cancerous breasts may save a woman's life, it may endanger her own appraisal of her femininity. The single woman or the married woman who has had no children may feel even greater privation than the married woman with children, who can be assured that her breasts have served their essential function. Surgeons often discuss the implications of the loss of a breast with the patient's husband since his attitude and behavior can help in the patient's acceptance of the decision regarding surgery and in her future rehabilitation.

Preoperative care. The preparation for surgery is similar to that discussed in Chapter 10. If a diagnosis of a malignancy is almost a certainty, x-ray examinations may be ordered to rule out the possibility of metastases to other areas of the body. Preparing the patient for certain procedures that will take place before and after surgery is of the utmost importance in allaying her fears, as well as setting the stage for successful rehabilitation. Should a radical mastectomy be indicated, the patient can be prepared for what she will experience *postoperatively*. She should be told that a pressure dressing may be applied to the incision and that a catheter attached to suction may be used. She should also be told whether or not she will be able to move her arm, or if it will need to be elevated. She should know that she will probably be able to get out of bed the day after the operation. She should know that, if the breast is removed, there will be a tendency for her shoulder to droop on the opposite side because of the inequality of weight and that it can be prevented by close attention to posture. Poor posture may give more evidence that a breast has been removed than will a slight inequality in the breast contours. While padding and prosthetic devices are used to take the place of the breast and restore normal contours to the upper body, stooped, awkward posture cannot be hidden. Exercises that will strengthen muscles and help to improve posture should be discussed with the patient before surgery. Telling the patient about the exercises helps to give her the feeling that there is something in the situation that she can control and contribute to and thus aids in a positive attitude toward rehabilitation.

The operation. At the time of surgery, the tumor is removed and a frozen section of the tissue is examined under the microscope. If the tumor is malignant, the first incision is closed. Drapes, instruments, and gloves are changed to help prevent possible spread of cancer cells and the more extensive operation is then performed.

If there are no gross signs of extension of the carcinoma, the entire breast, the pectoral muscles, the axillary lymph nodes, and all fat, fascia, and adjacent tissues are removed in one piece. This is a *radical mastectomy*. The judgment of the surgeon regarding the amount of overlying skin that can safely be left to cover the defect determines whether or not a skin graft is to be done. Preoperatively, the surgeon may order the skin of the anterior surface of a thigh shaved and prepared surgically in case need for a graft should arise. If the lesion is located in the medial quadrant of the breast, particularly the upper medial quadrant, an *extended radical mastectomy* may be performed to include removal of the parasternal lymph nodes. Lesions in the medial quadrants tend to metastasize to the internal mammary chain of lymph nodes. The nodes may be exposed by splitting the sternum or by dividing the costal cartilages of the second through the fifth ribs. Results of the five-year survival rate following this procedure are promising but inconclusive at this time.[16] A *simple mastectomy* (removal of breast tissue without lymph node dissection) sometimes is performed if cancer is believed to be limited to the breast or as a palliative measure to remove an ulcerated carcinoma of the breast in disease that is known to be advanced.

Following removal of the breast and adjacent tissue, some surgeons make a stab wound near the axilla and insert a catheter, which is attached to gentle suction. Its purpose is to remove serous fluid that may collect under the skin, delaying its attachment and predisposing to infection. There usually is very little drainage from the incision where the catheter is inserted, and a dressing is not always necessary.[7] Pressure dressings rather than a catheter may be used to help prevent the accumulation of fluid under the skin. These dressings may be made of gauze, marine sponge, rubber sponge, or cotton reinforced with mechanic's waste. They may be held in place with adhesive tape, Ace bandages, or binders.

Postoperative care. The operative site should be inspected to determine the type of dressing applied and the presence of drains, if any. The catheter should be attached to gentle suction as ordered. Sometimes a small portable suction unit (Hemovac) is attached to the catheter in the operating room so that constant suction is maintained while the patient is being transported to her room. This unit should be emptied of the collected fluid, in accordance with specific directions of the manufacturer, because the pressure becomes equal to that in the wound if not properly emptied and this prevents further drainage. If the wound is draining properly, fluid will not collect under the skin. The nurse should inspect the wound for swelling if it is not covered with a dressing. Since a dressing may become tight as fluid collects, any swelling should be reported to the doctor. The catheter usually is removed within three to five days, depending upon the amount of drainage.

The wound or the dressing should be checked every fifteen minutes for the first few hours to detect hemorrhage or excessive serous oozing. The bedclothes under the patient must be examined for blood that may flow from the axillary region backward. Any evidence of bleeding should be reported to the surgeon.

Pressure dressings should be checked to be certain that they do not hamper circulation. Signs of circulatory obstruction such as swelling and numbness of the lower arm or inability to move the fingers must be reported at once. The nurse, however, should never loosen dressings without specific instruction from the surgeon.

If a graft has been taken from the thigh, this area may be covered with a firm pressure dressing or fine mesh gauze may be used and the wound exposed to the air. The patient may complain of severe discomfort in this donor site as soon as she responds from anesthesia.

Dressings over the breast area and the donor site usually are not changed for several days after the operation. The skin sutures closing the breast and axillary incision are often removed on the sixth to the eighth postoperative day.

The patient must be encouraged to take deep breaths and to cough deeply at frequent intervals since this helps to prevent congestion in the lungs. The patient may complain of a feeling of constriction over the chest that is painful, causing her to take short, shallow breaths. Supporting the area next to the wound while the patient breathes

deeply or coughs may lessen the pain (Fig. 133). If the pain is severe, narcotic drugs should not be withheld for the first few days following a radical mastectomy, provided deep breathing and coughing are done routinely every few hours. Because the patient may be drowsy from sedation, it is best to remain with her to see that she takes deep breaths at specific intervals.

When the patient recovers from the effects of anesthesia, she usually is more comfortable lying on her back with her head elevated. If the arm on the operated side is not elevated, incorporated in the dressing, or supported by a sling, a pillow placed under the lower arm and elbow will help prevent muscle strain and reduce discomfort. Pillows can also be used to support the arm when the position is changed to minimize her general discomfort. A firm mattress will help to splint the chest wall and lessen pain when the patient moves. The patient may be more comfortable sitting up straight while getting back care since turning toward the affected side may be exceedingly painful. A pull rope attached to the foot of the bed will help the patient to raise herself to a sitting position.

The patient should be encouraged to take fluids by mouth as soon as she has completely reacted from anesthesia. Her time of voiding postoperatively should be noted.

The patient usually is told by the doctor that the breast was removed when she has recovered from the effects of anesthesia. It usually is her first question and she will try to determine the fact by feeling the dressing. Reactions such as crying, withdrawal, or anger are to be expected and should be accepted, and the nurse should respond with tact and understanding. Most patients are helped by a kindly, yet matter-of-fact, attitude toward loss of the breast and by the assumption that there need be no change in outward appearance or mode of living. Mention of ways by which clothing can be adjusted to preserve normal contours often helps. The patient may be told that bathing suits and low-cut dresses can be worn without the incision's being seen if there is evidence that this information will be of comfort.

Ambulation. The patient usually is allowed out of bed the day after a mastectomy. She needs help when she gets up to use the

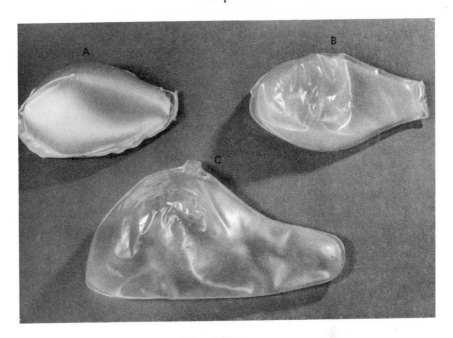

Fig. 189

Several types of breast prostheses are available. **A**, Foam rubber prosthesis. **B**, Prosthesis containing fluid. **C**, Prosthesis containing air.

remember to wash her hands thoroughly before doing this, and she must be careful not to cut the skin. Creams help to keep the skin in a healthy condition. Gloves should be worn during activities in which there is danger of trauma or gross contamination of the hand. Hangnails or any other infections of the hand or arm should be cared for by the doctor.

Treatment when metastasis occurs

In advanced carcinoma of the breast the treatment is palliative—that is, it affords relief but does not effect a cure. Although some of the procedures may seem radical, they produce temporary regression of the tumor, lessen pain, and permit the patient to remain more active. There are several types of treatment. Radiotherapy is often used in conjunction with surgery; it may also be used instead of surgery when the tumor is large, ulcerated, and inoperable. It tends to decrease bleeding, stimulate healing, and may diminish the size of the tumor.

Other treatments are used only when the lesion and symptoms are no longer amenable to surgery or radiation therapy. They are often used in specific sequence and only after recurrence of distressing symptoms of metastasis. The choice of procedure depends upon the patient and whether or not she has experienced the menopause. Because carcinoma of the breast is largely affected by estrogenic hormones, a bilateral oophorectomy may be performed to remove the major source of estrogens and thus suppress the growth of the tumor in women who are not past the menopause. This procedure is usually followed by giving a hormone such as testosterone. Bilateral oophorectomy may also be done as a prophylactic measure when the patient is considered to have a good prognosis following a radical mastectomy.

If the patient is more than five years past the menopause, bilateral oophorectomy is seldom done, but estrogens or androgens may be given. At this age, these hormones seem to produce a regression of the tumor in some patients.[7] The reason they do so is not known, although hormonal therapy does prevent physiologic secretion of estrogen from the adrenal gland. Hormonal treatment may be followed later by either an adrenalectomy or a hypophysectomy. Both of these pro-

813

cedures curtail further the output of the woman's own estrogenic hormones. It is important to remember that not all patients respond to these forms of treatment, but if the patient gets relief from hormonal treatment, there is reason to believe she will get further relief from the further curtailment of her own hormone production by means of surgery. The treatment is determined on the basis of the type of lesion, the side effects of the treatment, and the response of the individual patient to previous treatment.

Chemotherapy is usually used as a last resort when procedures to curtail endocrine function have failed to slow the progress of the disease. (For details of the drugs given and the nursing care involved, see p. 288.)

Radiotherapy. Radiotherapy may be given if there is suspected or known metastasis. Treatment can be started as soon as the day after surgery and may be continued on an ambulatory basis after the patient leaves the hospital. (For details of care of patients receiving radiation treatment, see p. 281.) Radiotherapy is also used to treat painful metastatic bone lesions, which occur in the spine, ribs, hips, and pelvis of about 30% of all patients who develop metastasis from carcinoma of the breast, and to treat lesions in the brain, which occur in about 10% of all cases of metastasis. If pleural or peritoneal effusions occur, radioactive isotopes such as radioactive gold (Au^{198}) or radioactive phosphorus (P^{32}) may be instilled into the chest or abdominal cavities to attempt to control the formation of fluid. (See p. 287 for discussion of this treatment.)

Hormone therapy. Estrogenic, androgenic, and corticoid hormones are used to treat advanced carcinoma of the breast. They seem to be particularly effective in controlling the pain and also the progress when there has been metastasis to the bones. For example, bone cells may be regenerated in decalcified areas in the spine, and pathologic fractures may heal as a result of hormone treatment. It is estimated that, with hormone treatment, patients with metastases who are responsive to the effects of the hormones have relief of symptoms for one year or more. Testosterone propionate is the androgen most often used and may be given in doses of 50 mg. (¾ grain) intramuscularly twice a week for an indefinite period. Much larger doses may

also be given. Treatment with testosterone will cause secondary changes which are distressing to the patient. These include deepening of the voice, coarsening of the skin, and appearance of hair on the face and the rest of the body. The patient usually gains weight. She should be warned that these changes may occur, and she may need to pay greater attention to details of personal grooming than formerly was necessary.

Diethylstilbestrol (stilbestrol) is the estrogen commonly used. It may be given in oral doses of 15 mg. (¼ grain) daily. If estrogenic therapy continues for a long period, the patient may develop uterine bleeding (p. 496). The corticosteroids may produce regression of the tumor in some patients. However, the use of these hormones may cause undesirable side effects. (See p. 63.)

Surgical procedures. Since estrogens are believed to enhance the growth of malignant cells in women who are not past the menopause, several operative procedures are now used to remove the estrogen supply from the body in an attempt to prolong the life of the patient. These include *bilateral oophorectomy* (p. 510) and *bilateral adrenalectomy,* done when the effect of the oophorectomy has subsided. After an adrenalectomy, the patient needs special nursing care. (See p. 761 for a discussion of this care.) Removal of the pituitary gland, or *hypophysectomy,* suppresses the function of both the ovaries and the adrenal glands. (See p. 763 for a discussion of this procedure and the special nursing needs of the patient undergoing it.)

Psychologic considerations. The patient who has metastasis needs encouragement and help to continue to carry on her normal work either in the home or elsewhere for as long as possible. Some patients who have had to wear a brace because of metastasis to the spine have returned to their jobs for a year or more. Nothing contributes more to the patient's morale than continuing to work and participate in life around her. Appetite improves, and probably the resultant general improvement in health delays complete invalidism for some time. Patients may even continue to work or to carry on normal social activities when they have severe pain that requires regular narcotic or other analgesic treatment.

814

Nonmalignant disease of the breast

Dysplasia and fibroadenoma

Dysplasia (fibrocystic disease). Dysplasia is characterized by thickened nodular areas in the breast which usually become painful during or prior to menstruation. The process is almost always bilateral. A variety of changes take place in the breast tissue, which in some cases includes the formation of cysts. The condition is thought to be caused by hormonal imbalance. There is failure of normal involution following the reaction of the breasts to the cyclic activity of the female sex hormones. The nodules or cysts may be singular or multiple. They may increase in size or remain the same. Usually they are fairly soft and tender on palpation and are freely movable, sliding under the examining fingers. The woman who discovers such a mass (or masses) in her breast should seek the advice of her doctor, who will decide whether or not the lesion should be measured and checked at frequent intervals or whether the administration of hormones or surgery should be considered. There is little, if any, evidence that dysplasia predisposes to the development of malignancy, but the presence of nodules in the breast makes the early detection of malignant lesions much more difficult.

Fibroadenoma. Fibroadenomas are usually firm, round, freely movable, nontender, and encapsulated. They occur most often in women under 25 years of age and are caused by an overgrowth of fibrous connective tissue. The woman who discovers such a mass should not delay in seeking medical consultation. Usually the tumor will be removed under local anesthesia and will be examined microscopically to be sure it is not malignant. Although the hospital stay for excision of an adenoma is short and the patient returns to the doctor's office or clinic for the sutures to be removed, she needs thoughtful nursing care since she usually is extremely fearful of cancer.

Infections

Infection of the nipple. Infection usually follows cracks in the nipple during lactation. This condition is less common than previously since women are taught to "toughen" the nipple during pregnancy so that cracking is less likely to occur.

Infection of the breast. An infection can occur in the breast by direct spread from cracked or infected nipples and following congestion or "caking" during lactation when a portion of the breast becomes engorged from blockage of gland ducts. Manual expression of excess milk and hormone treatment for women who are not going to nurse their infants have reduced the incidence of infections of the breast. The microorganisms causing the infection may be transmitted to the mother's breast from the nasopharynx of the newborn infant who has been exposed to infected infants and hospital personnel or from the hands of the patient or those of hospital personnel. Staphylococcal infections are the most common. Infections in the breast can also occur with no specific cause and perhaps follow infections elsewhere in the body. These infections can occur at times other than during pregnancy or lactation.

Infections of the breast cause pain, redness, swelling, and elevation of temperature. The treatment is usually conservative. Antibiotics are usually given systemically. Sometimes local heat is used, and at other times ice packs may be prescribed. If the condition does not subside with conservative treatment and becomes localized to form an abscess, surgical drainage is necessary. To help prevent infections of the breast from occurring, there is a continued need for strict aseptic technique in nurseries for newborn infants and the prevention of all infected persons (carriers) from contact with patients.

Gynecomastia. Gynecomastia is a hyperplasia of the stroma and ducts in the mammary glands in the male that occurs during puberty and after the age of 40. It is thought to be due to an abnormally large estrogen secretion. It also frequently is seen following estrogen therapy for carcinoma of the prostate. Gynecomastia is a nonmalignant lesion, but doctors may suggest a biopsy of the breast since men occasionally develop carcinoma of the breast.

References and selected readings*

1 *Alexander, Sarah E.: Nursing care of a patient after breast surgery, Am. J. Nursing 57:1571-1572, Dec. 1957.

2 *American Cancer Society, Inc.: A cancer source book

*References preceded by an asterisk are particularly well suited for student reading.

for nurses, New York, 1963, The American Cancer Society, Inc.

3 American Cancer Society, Inc.: 1966 cancer facts and figures, New York, 1965, The American Cancer Society, Inc.

4 Britton, Richard C., and Nelson, Paul A.: Causes and treatment of postmastectomy lymphedema of the arm, J.A.M.A. 180:95-102, April 14, 1962.

5 Connell, James F., and others: Thermography in the detection of breast cancer, Cancer 19:83-85, Jan. 1966.

6 Crile, George, Jr.: Treatment of breast cancer by local excision, Am. J. Surg. 109:400-403, April 1965.

7 Davis, Loyal, editor: Christopher's textbook of surgery, ed. 8, Philadelphia, 1964, W. B. Saunders Co.

8 Egan, Robert L.: Mammography, Am. J. Nursing 66:108-111, Jan. 1966.

9 Galante, Maurice, Fournier, Dudley J., and Wood, Davis A.: Adrenalectomy for metastatic breast carcinoma, J.A.M.A. 163:1011-1016, March 23, 1957.

10 *Gold, Mitchell A.: Causes of patients' delay in diseases of the breast, Cancer 17:564-577, May 1964.

11 Haagensen, C. D.: Diseases of the breast, Philadelphia, 1956, W. B. Saunders Co.

12 *Higginbotham, Sarah: Arm exercises after mastectomy, Am. J. Nursing 57:1573-1574, Dec. 1957.

13 *Kennedy, B. J.: Hormone therapy for advanced breast cancer, Cancer 18:1551-1557, Dec. 1965.

14 Kennedy, B. J., and French, Lyle: Hypophysectomy in advanced breast cancer, Am. J. Surg. 110:411-415, Sept. 1965.

15 *Lewison, Edward F.: The treatment of advanced breast cancer, Am. J. Nursing 62:107-110, Oct. 1962.

16 Moyer, Carl, and others: Surgery, principles and practices, ed. 3, Philadelphia, 1965, J. B. Lippincott Co.

17 *Quint, Jeanne C.: The impact of mastectomy, Am. J. Nursing 63:88-92, Nov. 1963.

18 Randall, Henry Thomas: Oophorectomy and adrenalectomy in patients with inoperable or recurrent cancer of the breast, Am. J. Surg. 99:553-561, April 1960.

19 *Renneker, Richard, and Cutler, Max: Psychological problems of adjustment to cancer of the breast, J.A.M.A. 148:833-838, March 8, 1952.

20 *Smith, Genevieve Waples: When a breast must be removed, Am. J. Nursing 50:335-339, June 1950.

21 U. S. Department of Health, Education, and Welfare, National Center for Health Statistics: Monthly vital statistics, Advance Report, Final Mortality Statistics, 1964, vol. 14, no. 10, Supplement, Jan. 14, 1966, Washington, D. C.

22 Williams, Marjorie J.: Gynecomastia, Am. J. Med. 34:103-112, Jan. 1963.

23 Wilson, Robert A.: The roles of estrogen and progesterone in breast and genital cancer, J.A.M.A. 182:327-331, Oct. 27, 1962.

30

The patient
with
disease of the eye

Study questions

1 Review the anatomy of the eye.
2 Locate and explain the functions of the three coats of the eyeball. Review the location of the vitreous humor. How does it differ from the aqueous humor? What is the function of the lens?
3 Is there an organization in your community that is concerned primarily with aid to blind persons? If so, how it is financed?
4 From what you have learned in hygiene classes or elsewhere in school, list some measures that everyone should take to preserve eye health.
5 Review the technique for application of sterile eye compresses.

Vision is one of man's most priceless possessions. It is essential to most employment and is necessary in countless experiences that make life enjoyable and meaningful. Yet in the United States an estimated 90 million persons have some ocular malfunction. More than 3.5 million Americans have a chronic, noncorrectable visual defect. Of these persons, 1 million are functionally blind and cannot read, even with glasses. Thirty thousand more become totally blind each year. The incidence of blindness has increased 350% since the 1940's and is still increasing. Care of the blind already costs the nation about $1 billion annually.[14]

Public education in the prevention of eye disease and help in ensuring early medical care when disease symptoms appear are responsibilities of every nurse. Therefore, this chapter deals with health education, as well as general nursing, in eye disease. At the conclusion of the discussion on general nursing, specific nursing procedures for a few of the more common eye conditions are discussed.

Health education in care of the eyes and in prevention of disease

Nurses should be able to explain the complex structure of the eye, to teach people to care for their eyesight, and to direct them to the proper specialist. A nurse also should recognize signs suggestive of eye disease and teach them to others.

Care of the eyes

Normal healthy eyes do not need special local treatment. The secretions of the conjunctiva are protective and should not be removed by frequent bathing with unprescribed solutions. Boric acid solution and numerous trade preparations recommended to cleanse the eyes are usually unnecessary. Although these preparations are generally harmless, some proprietary solutions contain substances that may cause allergic reactions in sensitive persons.

Many people believe that eyestrain causes permanent eye damage. Eyestrain actually refers to strain of the ciliary muscles when there is difficulty in accommodation. It causes a sense of fatigue but does not produce serious damage to the eyes. However, a good light should be used when reading and doing work that requires careful visual focus, and extremely fine work should not be done for long periods of time without giving the eye muscles periodic rest. Looking at distant objects for a few minutes helps to rest the eyes after close work. The eyes should be protected by goggles or special dark glasses from prolonged exposure to very bright light, such as sunlight over snow. They also need special protection from sudden flashes of light and heat that occur in some industrial occupations. Nurses often are asked the effect of television on the eyes. A moderate amount of television viewing should not damage normal eyes provided that the television screen is at eye level, the room is not so dark as to exaggerate the contrast between the room and the screen, the vision of the screen is in focus, and viewing the screen is done directly and not from an angle. An eye examination is needed if headache or eye discomfort occur with moderate viewing of television under these conditions.

In the school and in the home, as well as in health agencies, the close relationship between diet and good eye health should be taught. One extensive ten-year study gave the amazing information that fully two-thirds of a large group of boys and girls had eye difficulties related to dietary deficiencies.[34] Older persons and teen-agers are perhaps the worst offenders in this respect. Teen-age boys and girls may eat poorly because of poor habits established in early childhood and because of adolescent notions and group preferences; an example is the diet consisting mainly of soft drinks, frankfurters, potato chips, and ice cream. Elderly people may not have the energy or the incentive to prepare and eat proper meals. Persons of all ages should be taught the essentials of good nutrition and should be encouraged and assisted to change their diet pattern (Chapter 5).

Care should be taken not to irritate the eyes or introduce bacteria into the eyes by rubbing them. Children sometimes develop the habit of rubbing their eyes, and this habit may persist into adulthood. Rubbing the eyes is a natural response of many persons under nervous strain. It may, however, be due to eczematous scaling, infection of the lids, or, occasionally, to louse attachment on the lashes. Prevention of accidental injury to the eyes should be stressed in child and parent education. Slingshots, BB guns and even the seemingly harmless rubber bands and paper wads can be dangerous. The nurse can help physical education teachers and others to be alert to hazards to the eyes in gymnasiums and on playgrounds.

First-aid measures necessary in the event of eye injury should be known by everyone; these measures may be taught in schools and in industry. The sight of many persons could be saved each year if everyone understood the need for immediate copious flushing of the eye with water when an acid or other irritating substance has been accidentally introduced. Much damage is done by the layman's well-intentioned efforts to remove foreign bodies from the eye and by not obeying the important rule of always washing the hands before attempting to examine the eye or to remove a foreign body. Everyone should know that a person who has a foreign object lodged on the cornea must be referred to a physician; the layman should never attempt to remove it. The eye should be closed to prevent further irritation, the lids held shut and loosely covered with a dressing or patch anchored with a piece of cellophane or adhesive tape, and the patient should be taken to a doctor at once.

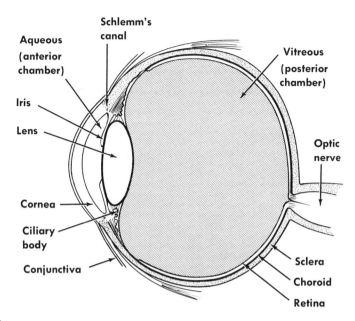

Fig. 190

Anatomy of the normal eye.

The eye is extremely complicated (Fig. 190) and seldom is absolutely perfect even when its function appears within normal limits. The eyes should be examined by an ophthalmologist at regular intervals throughout life. Many authorities believe the child should have his eyes examined before starting school, at age 10 approximately, and in early adolescence. The young adult should consult an ophthalmologist at least every five years. After the age of 40 years the lens becomes firmer and less resilient. The individual begins to hold written material at a distance for better vision, and close vision may become blurred. Medical specialists recommend an eye examination every two years after the age of 40.

Eye specialists now realize that examination of the eyes without examination of the rest of the body is unwise. The eyes cannot be considered alone since they are often profoundly affected by conditions within the rest of the body. In fact, nearly all diseases of man cause some eye change that is diagnostically important. The nurse who is teaching eye health must be aware of total health. When apparently minor disease or abnormality of the eyes occurs, she must be particularly alert for other signs of illness. Many serious medical conditions, such as diabetes, renal disease, and generalized arteriosclerosis, may be diagnosed through early recognition of eye symptoms and examination of the eyes by a medical specialist.

There is widespread confusion and misunderstanding on the part of the public as to the proper specialist to consult about visual problems. People who demand the best care when other medical and surgical problems arise may fail to seek help from an ophthalmologist when they have eye difficulties. Many persons do not understand the difference between the *orthoptist,* who directs eye exercises, the *optician,* who grinds and fits lenses, the *optometrist,* who adjusts lenses to changes in accommodation of the eye, and the *ophthalmologist* or *oculist,* who has had intensive medical training and experience in the diagnosis and treatment of eye diseases. In their search for help, a surprisingly large number of people respond to radio advertising and may even purchase glasses from store counters or use glasses originally prescribed for friends or relatives. These people need to understand that eye conditions cannot always be remedied simply by the purchase of a pair of glasses or a change of lenses.

Recognition and care of eye diseases

A nurse should recognize signs of eye disease, and without making the persons unduly apprehensive, she should guide them in seeking appropriate treatment. Nurse-teachers and schoolteachers should be alert to changes in the eyes and vision of children during the school year. If changes occur, the child should be referred to an ophthalmologist as soon as possible. If an individual complains of itching or burning of the eyelids after reading, or of the sensation of needing to "wash out his eyes," he should consult an ophthalmologist. Frowning, squinting, rubbing the eyes, covering one eye or tilting the head, blinking excessively, headache, fatigue, and irritability upon doing close work with the eyes also are signs that medical care may be needed. Constant dull pain in the eyes, blurring of vision, spots before the eyes, rings around lights, and noticeable changes in visual acuity are signs that eye function is affected and should be investigated. Frequent changes of lenses and history of repeated visits to optometrists for lens changes indicate the need for complete medical examination.

Another detriment to good eye care is the natural human tendency to put things off, to reject any obvious fact that is unpleasant or disturbing, and to assume that an eye condition will "clear up" within a few days. Although the average person thinks of loss of vision as a major catastrophe, he is careless in giving early attention to eye difficulties which, if neglected, may become serious. The danger of procrastination must be stressed since some eye diseases progress rapidly, and irreparable damage may occur quickly. Neither the patient nor the nurse can know, for example, whether an irritation of the eyes is a simple conjunctivitis or an incipient acute glaucoma. The patient must never be permitted to postpone treatment and thus risk further infection or progress of disease.

One of the most tragic areas of neglect is that of *strabismus* in young children. Parents are naturally reluctant to face the fact that

something about their child may not be quite normal. They are likely to believe and hope that the child will outgrow the conditions, and they often believe that no accurate medical examination can be done until the child is able to read. An infant should have acquired binocular vision at about 6 to 9 months of age. He should have some ability to fix upon an object at 4 months and definite ability to grasp a single object visually at the age of 1 year.[1] If he does not, the mother should be advised to mention it to her doctor. Strabismus can be treated with glasses, exercises, or surgery, or a combination of these. Self-treatment of the eyes is dangerous, and much valuable time for treatment can be lost thereby. Nevertheless, people frequently treat eye ailments with proprietary remedies or with eye drops and other medications which the patient or others have used at some time in the past. Many persons fail to realize that there are many disorders that can affect the eyes and that many different drugs are used, each of which has a specific purpose. For example, two drugs may have completely opposite effects. Since liquids may evaporate and drugs may deteriorate, use of preparations that the patient or his friends may have on hand can contribute to actual damage.

Glasses and special lenses

Eyeglasses are prescribed to improve vision and to relieve discomfort resulting from use of the eyes. Acceptance of glasses seems to be influenced by personality and the improvement of vision demonstrated by their use. The preschool child may reject glasses but almost always accepts them upon entering school. There is some stigma attached to wearing glasses, and the child does have to become accustomed to being different. The vogue for attractive frames makes the wearing of glasses more acceptable to teen-age boys and girls. All persons should be encouraged to wear their glasses as prescribed and to have periodic examinations of their eyes by an ophthalmologist. Instructions for persons who wear glasses should include how to keep their glasses clean, how to protect them from being scratched or broken, and how to care for them when they are removed.

Sunglasses should be carefully ground and

should be large enough to exclude bright light around their edges and dark enough to exclude about 30% of the light. Their excessive use is questioned by some specialists since it is believed that their use may lessen the sensitivity of the eye in response to light. Glass tinted in colors such as rose or green is of no particular value. The person who wears glasses regularly should have dark ones made from his prescription. Eyestrain can occur if correctly prescribed glasses are not worn by persons who need them even though they wear dark glasses when in bright sunlight.

Light *plastic lenses* are useful for some persons who must wear thick lenses that are heavy when made of glass. Plastic lenses are useful for individuals engaged in vigorous activities since they do not break and splinter, and they do not fog easily in cold weather; they are often prescribed for active children. Plastic lenses must be carefully cleansed with soap and water. Abrasive materials such as those contained in cleansing papers should not be used since they may scratch the plastic material. *Shatter-resistant safety lenses* are advocated for all persons who wear glasses constantly. It is felt that they are needed particularly by children and by persons whose occupation has a high potential for eye injuries, such as laboratory work.

Contact lenses are thin shells of transparent, ground, plastic material designed to be worn over the cornea (microlenses) or the cornea and sclera (scleral type) to replace eyeglasses. They are inserted after being cleaned thoroughly and immersed in a wetting agent such as methylcellulose. The lenses usually are worn for prescribed periods of time, removed, and then reinserted. Conjunctival secretions provide the lubrication needed for the lenses to be worn in comfort, and the lenses are held in place by capillary attraction and by the upper lid. Although some people wear the lenses continuously, others can never physiologically or psychologically tolerate the constant presence of a foreign object in the eye. Contact lenses sometimes are prescribed for persons who have a cone-shaped deformity of the cornea (keratoconus), which may prevent satisfactory fitting with conventional glasses. Elderly patients who have lenses removed because of cataracts benefit from wearing contact lenses but may have difficulty adapting to their use. Contact lenses may be used by persons who engage in sports because they do not fog or break easily, or they may be worn for cosmetic reasons. They are expensive, costing about $125. Care must be taken when the lenses are worn that substances such as dirt or dust do not concentrate behind the lens to irritate the cornea. Therefore, they are prohibited in some industrial occupations. Occasionally, acute, painful corneal abrasions or erosions occur. Although improvements are made each year, many ophthalmologists still believe that contact lenses should not be prescribed generally. Persons interested in wearing contact lenses should be encouraged to consult an ophthalmologist and to accept his recommendations regarding their use. Contact lenses usually are not prescribed for children under 15 years of age unless indications of possible benefit are quite strong.[24]

General ophthalmologic nursing

Examination of the eyes

Refraction is one of the most common eye examinations. This procedure reveals the degree to which the various light-transmitting portions of the eye bring light rays into correct focus on the retina. Refractive errors account for the largest number of impairments to good vision. The refractive error is tested by means of trial lenses and the Snellen chart. Suitable glasses are then prescribed.

Some specific terminology must be understood before refractive studies can be meaningful. *Emmetropia* refers to a normal eye, whereas *ametropia* indicates that a refractive error is present. *Accommodation* is the ability to adjust vision from near to far objects. This is normally accomplished by the ciliary muscles, which, by means of contraction or relaxation, can cause the lens to flatten or thicken as need arises. *Myopia*, or nearsightedness, is caused by an abnormally long anteroposterior dimension of the eyeball, which causes light rays to focus in front of the retina. *Hyperopia*, or farsightedness, is caused when the anteroposterior dimension is too short, causing light rays to focus behind the retina. *Astigmatism* is a condition caused by asymmetry, or irregular curvature, of the cornea, so that rays in the horizontal and perpendicular planes do not focus at the same point. In *presbyopia,* which occurs in persons past 40 years of age, the lens becomes more firm and responds less to the need for accommodation in viewing near and far objects. Blurring of near objects results, and those who require different lenses for distant and for close vision must obtain bifocal lenses.

Before refraction is performed, the nurse may be asked to instill a cycloplegic drug into the eyes to dilate the pupil and temporarily paralyze the ciliary muscles. Cyclopentolate (Cyclogyl) usually is used since it is effective in a half hour, and the effect wears off completely by the end of six hours. Homatropine occasionally is used for adults and atropine for children, but both of these drugs require longer to take effect, and their effects persist longer. Atropine must be instilled at intervals for three days prior to examination and persists in its action for about ten days. Persons over 40 years of age are usually given eye examinations without the use of cycloplegic drugs, because the power of accommodation has become sufficiently weak to permit satisfactory examination without their use. Small, active children may be given a sedative before their eyes are examined.

The nurse who works in a clinic, in an ophthalmologist's office, or in schools must know how to do *vision screening tests* and how to teach other to do them. Distance vision is usually determined by use of a Snellen chart (Fig. 191). Examination is done with the patient standing 20 feet from the chart. The chart consists of rows of letters, numbers, or other characters arranged with the large ones at the top and the small ones at the bottom. The uppermost letter on the chart is scaled so that it can be read at 200 feet, and the successive rows are scaled so that they can be read by the normal eye at 100, 70, 50, 40, 30, 20, 15, and 10 feet, respectively. Visual acuity is expressed as a fraction, and a reading of 20/20 is considered normal. The upper figure refers to the distance of the patient from the chart, and the lower figure indicates the distance at which the smallest letters can be read by the person being tested. For example, the person

who is able to read, at 20 feet, only the line that should be readable at 70 feet has 20/70 vision in that eye.

The distance from the chart to where the patient stands must be carefully measured. The person doing the testing usually stands beside the chart and points to the line to be read so that no mistake occurs. Each eye is tested separately, and its performance is carefully recorded. When testing vision, it is best to have the person being examined hold a piece of cardboard over his unused eye rather than have him attempt to read the line with first one and the the other eye closed. The Snellen chart examination is only a basic screening test. Additional detailed procedures must be done to test for nearsightedness, color blindness, and many other abnormalities.

The instrument used most often by the ophthalmologist is the *ophthalmoscope.* It magnifies the view of the back of the eye so that the optic nerve, retina, blood vessels, and nerves can be seen through the dilated pupil. The examination usually is made with the patient seated. The examination is not painful, but the head must be held still. The ophthalmoscope presumably would be damaged by boiling or autoclaving, but it may be wiped clean with alcohol or benzalkonium chloride. If the instrument is contaminated with known infectious organisms, it may be exposed to the sun or air for twenty-four hours after having been cleaned with a solution such as benzalkonium chloride.

An instrument known as a *tonometer* has been devised for measuring ocular tension and is helpful in detecting early glaucoma. Some ophthalmologists suggest that tonometric readings be taken by the medical internist or the family doctor as part of a regular, annual physical examination. The most common indentation tonometer in clinical use is that of Schiötz. The procedure is performed with the patient lying down and looking upward at some fixed point. The eye may be anesthetized with one or two drops of tetracaine (Pontocaine), 0.5 to 1% or proparacaine (Ophthaine), 0.5% after which the tonometer is placed on the cornea. (See Fig. 192.) The weight of the tonometer is supported by the cornea, and the amount of indentation that the plunger of the instrument makes in the cornea is measured on the at-

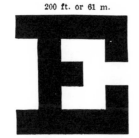

200 ft. or 61 m.

100 ft. or 30.5 m.

70 ft. or 21.75 m.

50 ft. or 15.24 m.

40 ft. or 12.19 m.

30 ft. or 9.14 m.

20 ft. or 6.10 m.

15 ft. or 4.57 m.

10 ft. or 3.05 m.

A

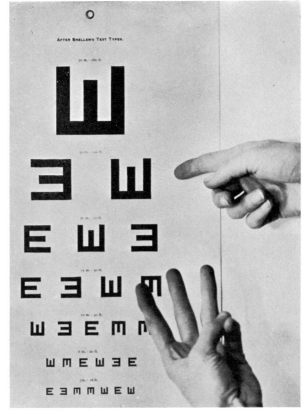

B

Fig. 191

A, Snellen's chart, used in testing vision. B, Modified Snellen's chart
for testing vision of small children and persons who are not
familiar with the English alphabet. (From Parkinson, Roy H.: Eye, ear,
nose, and throat manual for nurses, ed. 8, St. Louis, 1959, The C. V. Mosby Co.)

tached scale. This reading is used to determine the pressure within the eye. Readings over 30 mm. Hg (Schiötz) suggest glaucoma, but tests usually are repeated because temporary increases sometimes may be caused by such things as emotional stress.

Although the tonometer cannot be boiled or autoclaved, it is cleansed with soap and water and wiped clean with a solution such as benzalkonium chloride. If alcohol is used for cleansing, it must be removed thoroughly because it is irritating to the cornea.

Areas of opacity within the eye may be detected by means of a fine beam of light projected through the eye from a *slit* lamp. The limitation of visual field is determined

823

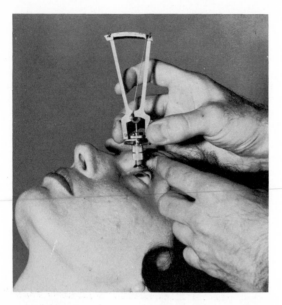

Fig. 192

Measurement of intraocular pressure with a tonometer. (From Havener, William H., Saunders, William H., and Bergersen, Betty S.: Nursing care in eye, ear, nose, and throat disorders, St. Louis, 1964, The C. V. Mosby Co.).

by *perimetry*. The patient is seated in a darkened room at a specific distance from a dark-colored chart on which a dot of light is flashed at consecutive points. Pins are placed on the chart to indicate each dot of light seen by the patient. The placement of the pins describes his field of vision. The tracing can be transferred to the patient's chart for reference. Neither of these two eye examinations requires specific nursing assistance.

Local treatments

Accuracy in the administration of medications and treatments is essential. Irreparable damage can follow instillation of unprescribed or deteriorated preparations into the eyes. All medication bottles must be checked frequently for smearing or obliteration of labels. Solutions that have changed in color, are cloudy, or contain sediment should not be used. The nurse must know the usual dosage and strength of medications she uses. The following is a safe rule: Question any dosage that is over 1% in strength

824

unless one is completely familiar with the drug, with the patient, and with ophthalmologic nursing. The nurse who is assigned to care for patients with eye disease should immediately familiarize herself with the drugs most commonly used, the therapeutic dosages of these drugs, and their toxic signs. In the home the patient should be protected from the use of incorrect drugs from the family medicine cabinet. Medications for the eyes should be placed carefully in a separate part of the cabinet, and dangerous drugs should be removed if the patient is to select and administer his own medications.

Drugs. A large variety of drugs are used for treatment of eye diseases, and most of them are applied locally as drops, irrigations, or ointments. *Mydriatics* are drugs that dilate the pupil. Phenylephrine (Neo-Synephrine), 10%, and hydroxyamphetamine (Paredrine), 1%, are often used. *Cycloplegics* are drugs that not only dilate the pupil but also block accommodation (focusing of the eye) by paralyzing the ciliary muscle. Common cycloplegics are cyclopentolate (Cyclogyl), 1%, bistropamide (Mydriacyl), 1%, homatropine, 2%, and atropine sulfate, 1%. These drugs are used to keep the pupil dilated as part of the treatment for diseases of the cornea and for inflammatory diseases of the iris and ciliary body, after certain operations, and for eye examinations. *Miotics* are drugs that constrict the pupil. They include pilocarpine, 0.5 to 2%, physostigmine (also known as eserine salicylate), 0.25%, carbachol (Carcholin), 0.75% and isoflurophate (Floropryl), 0.25%. Their widest use is in the treatment of glaucoma. Local topical anesthetics such as tetracaine (Pontocaine), 0.25 to 1%, and proparacaine (Ophthaine), 0.5%, are used frequently for treatments and operations on the eye. Procaine hydrochloride (Novocain), 1 or 2%, and lidocaine hydrochloride (Xylocaine), 1 or 2% are the common injectable anesthetics used. Epinephrine (Adrenalin) 1:50,000 may be used in combination with local anesthetics to prolong the duration of anesthetics by constricting blood vessels so that the drug remains longer in the injected area and its absorption is delayed. Hyaluronidase (Wydase), which makes cell membranes more permeable, often is mixed with local anesthetic solutions to increase the diffusion of the anesthetic through the tissues. Physiologic solutions of sodium chloride or mild silver protein (Argyrol) are used as cleansing agents. Ophthalmologists may employ uncommonly used antibiotics such as bacitracin, polymyxin B, and neomycin for ocular instillation because bacteria are less likely to be resistant to them. Penicillin causes ocular allergy in about 5% of adult patients.[23] A lubricant such a methylcellulose, 0.5% may be used for dryness of the cornea and conjunctiva that is caused by deficiency in production of tears or faulty lid closure due to unconsciousness or nerve involvement. *Antiseptic* drugs include silver nitrate solution, 1% and boric solution, 2%, administered as drops, and yellow oxide of mercury, 1 to 2%. Cortisone and hydrocortisone as drops and in ointment, 0.5 to 2.5%, are used postoperatively as well as for a variety of conditions involving the eyelids, the conjunctiva, and the cornea to contol inflammatory and allergic reactions. Steroids also may be given systemically for the treatment of acute or subacute infections such as those of the iris and choroid. *Astringents* such as zinc sulfate preparations are often useful in chronic conjunctivitis, and the dye fluorescein is employed to stain and thereby outline penetrating injuries of the cornea.

Techniques. Nursing techniques for doing irrigations, applying compresses, and instilling eye drops are fully described in texts on fundamentals of nursing, and therefore techniques will not be discussed in detail here. Gentleness is extremely important in performing all treatments. The natural sensitivity of the eye and the reluctance of the normal person to have anything done to his eyes are increased by pain, discomfort, and fear. Nature's powers of repair may be retarded by trauma resulting from pressure on the irritated or inflamed tissues. Hands must be thoroughly scrubbed before doing any eye treatment, and all materials placed in the eyes should be sterile. If the patient is being treated for an active infection, individual medicine bottles, droppers, tubes of ointment, and other equipment should be used. This precaution is also necessary when an infected eye is being treated with an antibacterial drug such as bacitracin and the same medication is ordered prophylactically for the other eye. Many eye medications to be instilled as drops now come in bottles with droppers attached to the stopper. These medications can be used safely to dilate the eyes for examination and to treat noninfectious conditions such as glaucoma since the dropper does not touch the patient when proper technique is used. A good light is necessary when giving treatments, but care must be taken to protect the patient's eyes from direct light.

Eye pads are worn to absorb secretions and blood, to limit movement of the eyes after certain operations or injuries, to protect the eye from light, to eliminate double vision, or to conceal a deformity of the eye. The use of an eye pad is contraindicated in the presence of an eye infection because it enhances bacterial growth. An eye pad is secured with two pieces of tape placed diagonally, one on each side of the pad. Cellophane tape and the newer plastic tapes usually are used because they are easy to remove and do not cause allergic irritations. If an eye closes poorly, a drop of a lubricant such as methylcellulose may be ordered to be placed in the eye before it is covered with a dry pad to prevent scratching the cornea. After an operation on the anterior portion of the eye, a metal eye shield may be worn over the dressing to protect the eye from injury until it heals.

Compresses. Hot compresses are used in the treatment of surface infections of the cornea, conjunctiva, or eyelid and after many types of eye surgery to help cleanse the eye, relieve pain, and promote healing. Compresses may be sterile or unsterile, depending upon the eye condition, and should be large enough to cover the entire orbit. If both eyes are involved and the condition is infectious, separate trays must be prepared and the hands carefully washed between treatment of each eye. The temperature of the solution used for compresses should not be over 49° C. (120° F.), and the treatment usually lasts for ten to twenty minutes and is repeated hourly or several times a day. Great care must be taken not to exert pressure on the eyeball when applying compresses. If there is evidence of irritation of the skin about the eyes from the hot water, a small amount of sterile petrolatum can be used, but it should not be allowed to enter the eyes. Compresses may be heated in a basin placed on an electric plate at the patient's bedside, or they may be heated in a strainer placed in steam and then applied with sterile forceps.

Another method of preparing heat applications for the eyes is by means of a *Hydrocolator*, which is an electric water heater with a thermostatic control. It is equipped with special pads to fit the eye that are encased in folds of toweling material for protection from contamination. This convenient piece of equipment can be placed beside the patient's bed.[40] Moist heat also may be applied to the eye by using a clean washcloth soaked in hot water and squeezed free of excess moisture. When the cloth cools, the process is repeated.

Cold compresses often are ordered to help control bleeding immediately following eye injury, to prevent or control edema in allergic conditions, and to attempt to prevent spread

of infection in the early stages of such conditions as conjunctivitis. A small basin of sterile solution may be placed in a bowl of chipped ice at the bedside. Sterile forceps are used to wring out and apply the compress. If the compress does not need to be sterile, a washcloth or compresses may be placed on pieces of ice in a basin at the patient's bedside. A rubber glove packed with finely chipped ice may be adjusted to the eye and necessitates fewer changes of compresses. A piece of plastic material loosely filled and secured with a rubber band is effective also.

Irrigations. Eye irrigations are done to remove secretions, to cleanse the eye preoperatively, and to supply warmth. Pillows should be protected with waterproof material, and irrigations should always be done with the patient lying comfortably toward one side so that fluid cannot flow into the other eye. A rubber bulb syringe is usually used unless a very large amount of fluid is needed (Fig. 193). If only a small amount of fluid is needed, sterile cotton balls may be used. Physiologic solution of sodium chloride is most often used because it is less likely to

Fig. 193

When irrigating the eye, the fluid is directed along the conjunctiva and over the eyeball from the inner to the outer canthus.

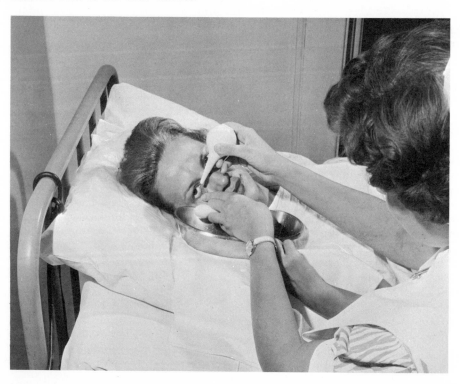

cause pain. This solution is isotonic, and it does not remove from the eye secretions the electrolytes necessary for normal action of the eyes. Irrigating fluid is directed along the conjunctiva and over the eyeball from the inner to the outer canthus. Care is taken to avoid directing a forceful stream onto the eyeball and to avoid touching any eye structures with the irrigating equipment. If there is drainage from the eye, the nurse may wrap a piece of gauze about her index finger to raise the lid and ensure thorough cleansing.

Instillation of medications. Eye drops should be sterile. Each patient should have his own bottle of medication. However, if stock solutions are used, only enough fluid should be drawn out for use at one time. If the bottle is small, it may be warmed slightly by holding it in the hands for a few moments. Eyedroppers must be sterile. Blunt-edged eyedroppers are available and should be used for children. The dropper is held downward so that medication does not flow into the rubber bulb since foreign material from the bulb can contaminate the solution. When instilling drops, the patient is asked to tilt his head back and look toward the ceiling. The lower lid should be pulled gently outward, and the dropper should approach the patient's eye from the side and not directly (Fig. 194). Drops are placed on the lower conjunctiva. Care must be taken not to touch the eyelids, the conjunctiva, or the eyeball with the dropper. The eyelids should then be closed. The patient should be reminded not to squeeze the eye shut, as this action causes the medication to escape. Absorbent tissue or cotton held against the cheek will prevent the drops from running down the patient's cheek.

To instill ointment, the nurse asks the patient to tilt his head back and to look toward the ceiling. The lower lid is gently pulled down and the ointment is expressed directly onto the exposed conjunctiva from a small, individual tube. Care is taken not to touch the tissues with the tube. A small, sterile glass spatula may also be used to apply ointment to the eye.

The patient's environment

Most patients with eye conditions are more comfortable in a darkened room, provided it is not dreary and depressing. Screens or cur-

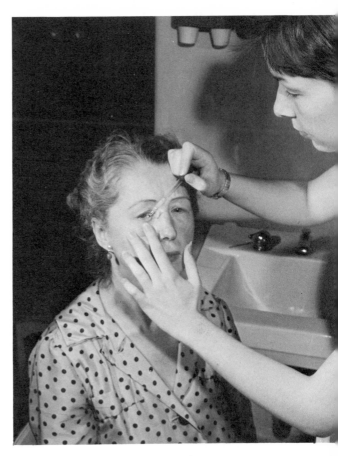

Fig. 194

When instilling eye drops, the lower lid should be gently turned outward, and the dropper should be held so as not to be directed at or into the eye.

tains should be arranged so that bright light does not enter the room. Bright artificial lighting should be shaded. The patient in the hospital is usually happiest in a room with other patients, especially if both eyes are covered or if he is unable to see. The sound of voices and normal activity around him tends to relieve the feeling of isolation that the blinded person experiences. He benefits from having others around him who may, for example, share newspaper headlines with him. Radios also help the patient to keep up with everyday events.

Accidents present a real hazard when eye disease occurs, especially if an eye is covered or there is loss of vision. If the onset of visual loss is slow, the patient and his family may have sufficient time to eliminate common household hazards such as stairs without banisters. The partially blinded person who receives care on an ambulatory basis is taught to have someone accompany him to the doctor's office or clinic because he may need additional help for a short time after certain treatments. In the hospital, special measures to prevent accidents are necessary. Side rails are usually needed on beds, and low beds are safer, particularly for older patients who may forget that they are in a hospital bed. Particular effort should be made to have the space around the patient's bed and chair uncluttered; for example, gooseneck lamps and electric plates used for compresses must have short cords that do not fall to the floor. If the patient has serious visual difficulty, hot plates for compresses are not kept at the bedside because the patient may burn himself. Furniture should be firmly anchored with casters locked. Rails along hallways and in bathrooms are also helpful.

Emotional factors in loss of sight

Emotional reactions to temporary or threatened loss of sight are often severe. Even if the individual has been careless with his eyes, he is much disturbed at the thought of losing his vision. Fear of the diagnosis may lead the patient to reject danger signs and delay medical attention. Worries over finances and family support and fear of being conspicuous among others may be added to concern over losing vision. The patient may not act rationally, he may be impatient and demanding, or he may be withdrawn and depressed. While he adjusts to his loss, patience, acceptance, and understanding are necessary from all persons who come in contact with him.

Sudden or jerky movements must be avoided in caring for any patient with eye disease since the natural reaction, blinking, may be painful or impossible. Jerky movements and haste tend to make the patient "on edge" and hamper release of tension and rest. Treatments should be done on time, because delay in treatments is of vital significance to the patient even when adherence to a rigid schedule may be irrelevant from a therapeutic point of view.

The person who has loss of vision depends upon sound and tactile sensation to maintain his feeling of security and kinship with those around him. He must be spoken to frequently in a quiet and reassuring voice. This is particularly important when he is in a strange hospital environment and awaiting diagnostic procedures and perhaps surgery. It is upsetting for the patient who cannot see to be touched without first being addressed; such an occurrence can be irritating and humiliating as well as actually dangerous. The nurse must teach all persons who attend the patient the importance of making their nearness known to the patient before touching him. They should introduce themselves and explain why they are there. On leaving the room, they should inform the patient so that he is spared the embarrassment of talking to someone who is not there. A small bell often is given to a patient with visual loss instead of a call signal. It gives the patient who can hear the assurance that his request has been made. The patient who is also deaf presents a real problem. If one cannot direct conversation into his ear and have it heard, there is no alternative but to touch him gently to make one's presence known, and if he is to remain in contact with his environment, frequent physical contact must be made with him. Elderly persons who use hearing aids are urged to bring them to the hospital.

Life for the patient who has both eyes covered should be made as normal as possible. If he is used to smoking, he should be permitted to smoke, although someone must be in attendance to prevent a fire. Visitors should be allowed, though sometimes they need assistance in learning how to conduct themselves when they are with the patient who cannot see. They should be as natural as possible; for example, they should not make a conspicuous attempt to avoid such common phrases in speech as "see what I mean." Common sense makes it obvious that gifts should appeal to other senses than vision; scented colognes and soaps or a small bouquet of highly scented favorite flowers should be brought, for instance, instead of a large display bouquet of flowers.

Restraints are sometimes necessary to prevent the patient from disturbing his dressings during sleep. They can be psychologically traumatizing unless carefully explained to the patient. The patient should be told that the restraints are used only to cause him to awaken and recall where he is and what has happened so that he will not touch his dressings. The use of side rails should be explained in the same fashion. They are primarily to assist the patient in carefully shifting his position and to remind him not to get out of bed. They are not used to keep him in bed forcibly.

Preoperative care

Routines for preoperative treatment and care vary with the part of the country, the institution, and the eye surgeon. If a complete medical examination has not been given before hospitalization, the patient usually spends a few days in the hospital preoperatively. The patient's general condition and his reaction to the anticipated surgery should be observed closely and reported. He should meet the staff in the unit and get to know other patients, particularly if he is to have both eyes covered following surgery. The patient should know whether his eyes are to be covered postoperatively, and he should be given an opportunity to become familiar with his immediate environment. He should be prepared for the routines necessary for his care following his return from the operating room. The patient often benefits from meeting and talking to another patient who has successfully recovered from a surgical treatment such as he is to receive. The child should practice having his eyes covered so that he will not be too frightened or restless postoperatively. If possible, the child's mother should be permitted to stay with him before the operation.

The preparation of the patient on the evening before surgery is similar to that described on p. 178. If the patient has his eyes covered, the side rails must be up and his call light should be available. The older patient becomes disoriented with his eyes covered, and he should be visited frequently. The child may become frightened and may need to be comforted if his mother is not with him.

The preparation of the eye on the day of surgery consists of the instillation of a combination of drugs, such as atropine sulfate, 1%, Cyclogyl, 1%, and Neo-Synephrine, 10%, into the eye at various intervals to dilate the pupil. Topical anesthesia is begun with the instillation of such drugs as (Pontocaine), 0.5%, Butacaine sulfate (Butyn), 2%, or phenacaine hydrochloride (Holocaine), 1%. Argyrol, 10%, may be instilled also to stain mucous shreds and surface debris so that they can be easily identified and removed during surgery. The medications must be given at the prescribed times so that the eye is prepared at the time of surgery. After the anesthetizing drops are instilled, the patient is asked to close his eye, and a pad is applied to protect the insensitive eye from injury due to rubbing, dryness, or dirt and dust. If only one eye is to be operated upon, a mark may be placed on the forehead over that eye so that it can be identified easily in the operating room.

If a local anesthetic is to be used, chloral hydrate, pentobarbital sodium (Nembutal), or meperidine hydrochloride (Demerol) may be given preoperatively, and the patient with false teeth may continue to wear them so that facial contours will be maintained. Atropine sulfate may be included if a general anesthetic is to be administered. When possible, general anesthesia is avoided because the patient may be restless upon reacting and disturb the eye dressing, and the strain of vomiting may increase the tension on the suture line. Children, however, require general anesthesia and must be supervised closely until they have reacted fully. If the operation is to be done while the patient remains in his bed, he is placed head to foot in bed to facilitate the work of the surgeon.

The eyelashes usually are cut by the surgeon, who uses a straight, sharp scissors with fairly short blades that have been lubricated with petrolatum jelly to help prevent the cut lashes from entering the eye. After the skin preparation has been completed and the eye has been irrigated, if local anesthesia is being used, additional anesthetic drugs such as Xylocaine may be injected into the operative area at this time. If general anesthesia is given, either intravenous or inhalation agents may be used.

Postoperative care

It is impossible to outline specific routines for postoperative care following eye surgery since they vary so much in different locations and change so rapidly as new techniques are developed. However, a few general principles of postoperative care will be included here.

Immediately after the operation, the patient should keep his head still, and he should try to avoid coughing, vomiting, sneezing, or moving suddenly. He should lie with the unoperated side down to prevent pressure on the operated eye and to prevent possible contamination of the dressing with vomitus. A pillow placed along his back will help keep the patient on his side. During the first four to twenty-four hours, the head of the bed usually is elevated gradually, and the patient may turn from his back to the unoperated side, but he may not lie on his stomach or on the operated side.

Postoperative confusion is a problem, particularly in elderly persons and in persons who have had both eyes covered. If confusion does occur, the surgeon may decide that the danger of activity due to confusion is worse than activity resulting from having one eye uncovered. For this reason, many surgeons no longer cover the unoperated eye.

Side rails are placed on the bed immediately postoperatively and are kept on while both eyes are covered, if the patient cannot see, or as long as necessary for his protection. The bedside table should be placed on the side of the unoperated eye so that the patient can see it without excessive movement of his head.

Care should be taken that the dressing is not loosened or removed. If the patient is not reliable, he should be attended constantly. Restraints may occasionally need to be applied if the patient does not understand or cannot cooperate and if it is not possible to have him attended constantly. Restraints should be very light in weight and loosely attached to the wrists; usually a 2-inch gauze bandage is used, but a boxing-glove type of hand restraint may be applied. Elbow restraints usually are satisfactory for infants, but if not, the clove-hitch bandage may be used. If the dressings are removed, they should be replaced and the doctor should be notified. It is usual for some bleeding and serous drainage to occur, but it should be minimal. The lid is edematous, but

this condition subsides within three or four days. A sensation of pressure within the eye is abnormal and suggests hemorrhage, and sharp pain is suggestive of infection or hemorrhage. These complaints should be reported at once to the surgeon.

Postoperative ambulation depends upon the type of operation, whether or not it was performed for the first or second time, the general condition of the patient, and the surgeon's preference. The patient may be up on the first postoperative day, or he may be in bed five or six days after surgery. Whatever the regime, supervision and assistance should be given by the nurse to be sure that the patient is able to walk without sustaining injury. Because he cannot see out of the covered eye, he must try to avoid bumping into things and jarring the operative site. To avoid falls, he should not sit down until he has located both arms of the chair with his hands. He usually is advised not to bend or stoop or to lift objects for several weeks after the operation in order to prevent increasing intraocular pressure, which might nullify the surgery. Slippers or shoes that he can slip into without tying or buckling are preferable during this time. Patients who have both eyes covered should be led to their destination. (See Fig. 195.) They should be informed of obstacles in their path, alerted when to turn before the turn appears, and told when to move to *their* right or left.

If the patient must remain in bed, he will require the postoperative care discussed on p. 194 to keep him comfortable and to prevent postoperative complications from developing. During this period of inactivity, visits from other patients, family, and friends and listening to the radio or television may help to distract the patient and pass the time. Volunteers may be available to read to patients and to answer their mail. The child will benefit from having his mother with him, listening to stories, and playing with passive games and toys that are familiar to him. Mineral oil or milk of magnesia often are given postoperatively to lessen difficulty in having bowel movements since straining increases intraocular pressure and should be avoided. Discomfort in the eye usually is relieved by acetylsalicylic acid (aspirin), 0.6 Gm., Demerol, 50 to 75 mg., or dextropropoxyphene hydrochloride (Darvon), 32 mg.

A soft diet may be ordered for a few days postoperatively, although some doctors feel that a diet which permits moderate chewing will decrease distention and discomfort. If both eyes are covered, the patient must be fed. Otherwise, whether or not he needs assistance depends on the amount of vision he has and his general condition. When feeding the patient who cannot see, the nurse should remember that it is important to identify the kind of food he is to receive. She must not allow feeding a patient to become a routine procedure, and she must not appear hurried. If the patient is to have visual limitation for some time, he must be helped to learn to feed himself. Very exact descriptions of the kind and location of food and equipment and guiding the patient's hands so that he may feel the outline and placement of dishes helps. It is important that, if possible, the bed patient have the bed raised so that he may sit in a somewhat normal position for eating. Having him go through the motions a few times with an empty utensil helps to give him a correct feeling for distance. The patient should have privacy until he learns to handle food in a fairly normal way.

The nurse must help the patient and his family develop patience. The operation may not cure the patient's eye condition. The eye condition may never be cured but only improved, and the patient should be informed of this possibility. It also may take weeks and even months for him to become accustomed to the type of glasses he must wear. This demands understanding by both the patient and his family.

After surgery the patient should follow his doctor's instructions carefully and keep appointments as specified. Many patients must return to the doctor's office or the clinic periodically for a long time, some indefinitely. The nurse caring for the patient in the hospital has a responsibility to teach him this when he is most receptive to teaching. The nurse working in the community can be invaluable in arranging for clinic care and in helping the patient and his family to avoid discouragement, to administer medications as prescribed, and to report to the doctor regularly.

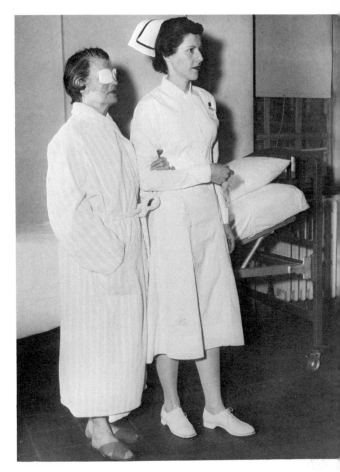

Fig. 195

Ambulation of a patient who cannot see. Note that the patient holds onto the nurse's arm and is thus led to her destination without being held.

Disease conditions and related nursing care

Trauma

Trauma may damage the eyelids and adjacent structures, the outer surface of the eyeball, and the deep structures of the eye. (For details of first aid in event of eye injury, see p. 255.) Lacerations of the eyelids should be treated by an eye specialist, because there is danger of scar formation as healing occurs. Any injury to the eyeball should be referred immediately to the specialist.

Patients with *ecchymosis* of the eyelids and surrounding tissues (black eye) should be examined to rule out coexisting skull fractures. Cold compresses will help to control the bleeding, and subsequent hot compresses will speed up the reabsorption of blood from the tissues. The disfigurement will last about two weeks and can be covered with cosmetics. *Lacerations* of the eyelid may need to be sutured after the bleeding is controlled and any foreign material is removed. Antitetanus serum usually is given to all patients who sustain eye wounds. *Corneal injuries* are serious since resistance to infection is low in the cornea and scars that form can impair vision. *Injuries to the ciliary body and sclera and injuries involving the orbit* are critical because adjacent tissues usually are also injured and there may be escape of contents of the eyeball and possible infection of the interior of the eye. If these injuries result in wounds that are small and clean, treatment consists of bed rest, antibiotics given systemically and topically, suturing the wound, instilling atropine to put the iris and the ciliary body at rest, and a firm dressing. If the injury is extensive and if sight is lost, enucleation (removal of the eyeball) is performed at once.

The most dreaded sequela to eye injury is *sympathetic ophthalmitis*. This complication is a serious inflammation of the uveal tract (ciliary body, iris, and choroid) in the sound eye that follows a penetrating injury to the other eye. The cause of this condition is unknown, but it may be due to an allergic reaction to the uveal pigment that is set free in the bloodstream at the time of the injury. Children are especially susceptible, but it may occur at any age. The uninjured eye becomes inflamed, there is photophobia and lacrimation, dimness of vision, and pain in the eye. Sympathetic ophthalmitis may appear three to eight weeks after the eye injury or months or years later, but it never appears if the injured eye is removed within a week of the injury. The decision as to whether or not the involved eye should be removed rests with the surgeon and often depends on the amount of damage to the uveal tract. Before the use of cortisone, sympathetic ophthalmitis usually resulted in total or almost complete loss of vision of both eyes. When cortisone has been given immediately following the injury or at the first sign of involvement of the good eye, it has saved the vision of many patients. Because of increased medical skill in treating perforating wounds and the administration of cortisone at the earliest suggestion of inflammation, sympathetic ophthalmitis has become a rare disease in recent years.

Tumors

Tumors involving the eyelids and structures about the eye as well as the eyeball itself are not unusual. Often they are malignant, thus endangering both vision and life. Tumors within the eyeball are often silent except for a bloodshot appearance of the eye. Yet, as in all malignant tumors, the prognosis depends upon early diagnosis and prompt treatment. Retinoblastomas occur in infants and children under 5 years of age. There is a hereditary influence, and a number of children in one family may be affected. These malignant growths arise from the posterior part of the retina, grow rapidly, and spread backward along the optic nerve and invade the brain. Malignant melanomas occur in the choroid of adults. They grow slowly, but due to the vascularity of the choroid, they metastasize early to the liver and lungs. Medical treatment of tumors of the eye may include enucleation, radiation treatment, use of chemotherapeutic agents, and plastic surgery.

The emotional response to a tumor of the eye is perhaps even greater than to malignancies elsewhere. The surgeon may advise immediate enucleation of the eye in the hope of saving life. If both eyes are involved, the most involved eye may be removed and the lesion in the other eye treated more conservatively in the hope of arresting its growth and possibly saving vision. (See p. 842 for a discussion of enucleation.) Both the patient and his family need to be encouraged to talk about their feelings and concerns and helped to readjust their lives in the face of this serious situation.

Infections and inflammation

Infections and inflammation can occur in any of the eye structures and may be caused by organisms, mechanical irritation, or sensitivity to some substance.

Styes. Styes (hordeola) are relatively mild

but extremely common infections of the small lubricating glands of the lid margins of children and young adults. Staphylococci are often the infecting organisms. Patients should be taught not to squeeze styes because the infection may spread and cause cellulitis of the lids. If warm, moist compresses are used, styes usually open and drain without surgery. These infections often come in a series (recur at intervals), affecting persons who use their eyes a great deal and those who need glasses but do not use them. Poor nutrition and lowered resistance to infection may also be contributing causes.

Chalazion. A chalazion is a cyst caused by an obstruction in the ducts of the sebaceous glands (meibomian glands) located in the connective tissue in the free edges of the eyelids. The cysts present a hard, shiny, lumpy appearance as viewed from the inner side of the lid, and they may cause pressure on the cornea. Small chalazions need not be removed and may disappear after the application of an antibacterial ointment followed by massage and hot compresses. If they are large or become infected, they usually require a surgical incision and curettage. Chalazions usually are removed in the doctor's office or the clinic under local anesthesia. An antibacterial ointment such as neomycin sulfate may be applied to the conjunctiva, and a pad worn for a day or two.

Conjunctivitis and blepharitis. Conjunctivitis, or inflammation of the conjunctiva, and blepharitis, or inflammation of the eyelids, are common infections and have a variety of causes. They may result from mechanical trauma such as that caused by sunburn, or infection with organisms such as staphylococci, streptococci, gonococci, or viruses may be the cause. Inflammation is often due to allergic reactions within the body or to outside irritants such as poison ivy. Pinkeye (conjunctivitis caused by the Koch-Weeks bacillus) is common in schoolchildren and is highly infectious. Conjunctivitis is always accompanied by hyperemia, which varies in degree and distribution and increased secretions.[15] The secretions may be watery, due largely to an increased secretion of tears, or mucoid, mucopurulent, or purulent, depending upon the cause.

Treatment for conjunctivitis depends upon the cause. Specific antibacterial drugs may be used systemically and locally. Compresses, irrigations, eye drops, and ointments often are prescribed. The patient must be cautioned not to touch his eyes since the inflamed tissues are susceptible to new infection, and trauma delays healing. If only one eye is involved, he must be cautioned to leave his good eye strictly alone. The good eye may be covered for its protection. Patients with blepharitis or conjunctivitis rest better in a darkened room than in a well-lighted one. They should be observed carefully for progress of the eye condition. Infections of the conjunctiva can be stubborn and may even lead to involvement of the cornea, with serious consequences to vision, and blepharitis can extend to the conjunctiva.

Corneal ulcer. A corneal ulcer indicates either an abrasion or an infected lesion on the surface of the cornea. The cornea has many pain-transmitting fibers, and damage to its epithelium is easily recognized because of the pain that follows. The ulcer may be caused by trauma or by infections of the conjunctiva that have spread to the cornea. Persons with a low resistance to infection may develop ulcers from little apparent cause (for example, the individual who has diabetes). The extent of the ulcer can be outlined by using sterile fluorescein, a green, harmless dye. The ulcer may be self-limiting, it may spread across the cornea, or it may penetrate into its deeper layers.

Nonpenetrating ulcers such as those caused by fingernail scratches heal readily unless infected. Antibiotic drops may be instilled to prevent infection, and a protective dressing may be worn for a few days. Ulcers that penetrate to the deep layers of the cornea may be cleansed with an antiseptic solution, cauterized, treated with antibiotics locally and systemically, and covered with a firm dressing. Atropine sulfate may be instilled to keep the pupil dilated and to put the ciliary body and iris at rest, thus reducing pain. Hot compresses may be applied to help clear the infection, and cortisone may be administered to control the inflammation. Depending upon their location, infected ulcers may destroy corneal tissue, causing partial or total blindness.

Keratitis. Inflammation of the cornea is called keratitis. It causes severe pain in the eye, photophobia, tearing, and blepharo-

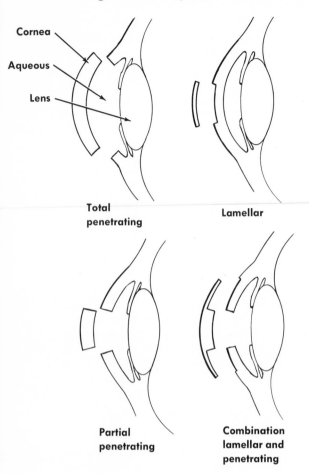

Total
penetrating

Lamellar

Partial
penetrating

Combination
lamellar and
penetrating

Fig. 196

The types of corneal grafts now being
used. Note that in the lamellar graft
the defect does not penetrate the
entire thickness of the cornea.

spasm (spasm of the eyelids). Uncontrolled
keratitis can result in loss of vision due to
impairment of corneal transparency or destruction of the eye by corneal perforation.
Keratitis may be acute or chronic and superficial or deep (interstitial). It may be associated with a corneal ulcer or be caused by
disease such as tuberculosis and syphilis.
Allergic reactions, vitamin A deficiency, or
viral diseases such as mumps, measles, and
herpes zoster may contribute to its development in children. If possible, the systemic
cause is found and treated. Cortisone may be

used to control the inflammation, and antibiotics may be given to treat the infection.
Atropine sulfate will keep the iris and ciliary
body at rest, and hot compresses will help
promote healing. Idoxuridine (IDU) applied locally has recently been found to be
effective in helping to clear keratitis caused
by herpes zoster. The eyes usually are covered to limit eye movements, and the patient
generally in placed on bed rest.

Corneal grafts (keratoplasty). Loss of vision caused by an opaque or destroyed cornea may be restored by replacing the damaged layers with a corresponding corneal
graft obtained from the eye of a fetus or
new cadaver or from an eye freshly removed
by operation because of a tumor or other
causes. For the best results, the corneal transplant must be removed within six hours of
death and should be used within forty-eight
hours. Transplants preserved for longer periods may be used for lamellar grafts. The
present practice is to keep a waiting list of
persons who need grafts, since eye banks
are not able to keep up with the demand.
Eye Bank for Sight Restoration, Inc.,* is a
nonprofit organization that collects and distributes donated eyes throughout the country. Donors or their relatives usually make
arrangements for donating the eyes before
death.

Corneal transplantation cannot be done if
there is any infection, and it is usually performed under local anesthesia. The kind of
corneal graft used depends upon the depth
and size of the damaged part that must be
replaced (Fig. 196). Corneal transplants, or
grafts, may involve the entire thickness of
the cornea (total penetrating), only part of
the depth of the cornea (lamellar), or a
combination of these, in which a small
part of the graft involves the entire thickness of the cornea (partial penetrating).
Obviously the penetrating graft is the more
difficult to accomplish and requires the more
definitive care postoperatively. For the penetrating graft the eye surgeon seldom uses a
donor eye that is over forty-eight hours old.

Because a large amount of tissue is removed and replaced, the patient who has
had a penetrating graft transplant usually
remains in bed with both eyes bandaged for

---

*210 East 64th St., New York, N. Y. 10021.

834

forty-eight hours so as not to disturb the graft. The patient who has had a mixed or partial penetrating graft usually has both eyes bandaged and is kept very quiet for at least twenty-four hours, whereas the patient who has had a lemellar graft only may not have the unaffected eye covered at all and may be out of bed and able to feed himself on the day of the operation. Corneal grafts heal very slowly because of the lack of blood vessels in the cornea and require at least three weeks to heal firmly. The patient is advised to avoid sudden, quick movement, jarring, bending, or lifting during this period in order to avoid disturbing the healing process.

There are several complications of corneal transplant operations; blood vessels may grow into the new cornea (compensatory neovascularization) so that clarity may be lost, or the new cornea may become cloudy for no apparent reason. The operation can usually be repeated, although performing a second operation depends on the condition of the patient's eye.

Iritis. Iritis (inflammation of the iris) rarely occurs alone and usually is associated with inflammation of the ciliary body. Then the term *iridocyclitis* is used. If the choroid also is involved, the infection is called *uveitis*. These infections produce pain in the eyeball radiating to the forehead and temple, photophobia (sensitivity to light), lacrimation, and interference with vision. There is edema of the upper lid, the iris is swollen owing to congestion and exudation of cells and fibrin, and the pupil is contracted and irregular as a result of the formation of adhesions. Iritis and iridocyclitis may be associated with a systemic disease such as syphilis or tuberculosis, or it may result from trauma, but usually there is no known cause. The instillation of 1% atropine sulfate or 0.2% scopolamine into the eye puts the iris and ciliary body at rest, relieves pain and photophobia, and diminishes congestion. By keeping the pupil dilated, these cycloplegic drugs prevent adhesions from forming between the anterior capsule of the lens and the iris and tend to cause those already formed to regress. Moist, hot compresses may be applied several times each day to help diminish pain and inflammation. The eyes usually are covered, and in the convalescent period,

dark glasses are ordered to be worn. The patient is on bed rest during the acute stages. Acetylsalicylic acid (aspirin) may be helpful for relieving pain, but sometimes morphine sulfate may be necessary. Cortisone preparations are of great value in controlling the inflammation in many patients, but the inflammation in other patients resists almost all forms of treatment. If a systemic cause cannot be found and treated, the injection of a foreign protein, such as the typhoid H antigen, into the body to stimulate its defense mechanism may be used. Complications of these infections of the uvea include the formation of adhesions, secondary glaucoma, and the loss of vision.

Strabismus

Strabismus, or squint, is characterized by the inability of the eyes to move simultaneously in the same direction, resulting in a crossing of the eyes. The patient will fix one eye (look straight ahead) while the other deviates. The crossing may be slight or very noticeable. If the eye is turned inward toward the nose, it is called convergent strabismus (esotropia). If the eye is turned outward, it is called divergent strabismus (exotropia). Strabismus may be paralytic or nonparalytic. Paralytic strabismus is caused by loss of function of the ocular muscle resulting from damage to the muscle or the cranial nerves (III, IV, or VI) by tumor, infection, or brain or eye injuries. Its main symptom in addition to the strabismus is double vision (diplopia). Normally, when both eyes look at the same object, the image of the object is focused by the brain into a single picture. If muscle paralysis causes the eyes to cross, the brain sees two separate pictures. The treatment is directed toward removing the cause of the paralysis, if possible, and straightening the eye.

Nonparalytic strabismus affects 1% of the population and is caused by an inherited abnormality of the fusion center within the brain.[23] When the infant with normal eyes is born, his eyes do not focus together. At the age of 6 to 8 weeks, his eyes begin to work harmoniously, and by the age of 9 to 12 months he should have developed fusion (the ability to see a separate image with each eye and fuse them into one image). The desire for binocular singular vision keeps the eye straight. Occasionally an infant is born without this ability of fusion, and it can never be acquired. In most cases of strabismus, however, fusion is present but underdeveloped. The child's eyes are crossed, and he may look straight with either the right eye or the left eye but not with both simultaneously. If he fixes (looks straight ahead) with one eye and then the other, he has *alternating strabismus*. If he prefers to use one eye to the exclusion of the other and always uses the preferred eye, he has *monocular strabismus*. *Suppression* is the ability of the brain to disregard conflicting visual images from the deviating eye. If the child never uses the crossed eye, impaired vision may result. This type of defective vision is called *suppression amblyopia*. If it is not treated by the time the child is 6 years of age, it usually will not respond to any therapy. It is the most common cause of partial blindness in children.

Early medical attention is important in strabismus both to save vision and to prevent the emotional trauma that is always associated with crossed eyes. Treatment should begin by the end of the first year of life or sooner. During early childhood, occlusion is used to improve vision. The good eye is covered with a patch, bandage, or attachment to the glasses, and the child is forced to use the weaker eye. *Orthoptics* is a technique of exercises used to train the child to use the two eyes together. It usually cannot be started until the child is about 4 years of age.

Strabismus in children who are farsighted and who accommodate excessively may be corrected by constantly wearing glasses. Glasses with harness frames can be safely worn by children 5 to 6 months of age. As the child becomes more independent, it is sometimes very difficult to get him to wear glasses consistently. When the glasses are removed, the eyes tend to cross. Long-acting miotics such as isoflurophate (DFP) instilled daily cause constriction of the ciliary muscle and help correct farsightedness. Sometimes the use of glasses and the use of drugs are combined.

Surgery is resorted to if none of the above methods correct the crossed eyes. After the age of 6 years, surgery achieves only cosmetic improvement and does not correct the already impaired vision. Surgery consists of shortening or lengthening the muscle attachments to straighten the eye. The child may wear a dressing over the eye for a few days and is permitted to move about freely and to be out of bed. Surgery usually is followed by the prescription of corrective glasses and eye exercises, depending upon the individual patient. The operation can be and may need to be repeated, and the child's family should understand this fact. Parents should be encouraged to continue with medical treatment for as long as recommended, sometimes indefinitely. They may believe that the condition is completely cured and may neglect medical attention until a conspicuous squint again appears. By this time, damage to vision may have occurred, and the condition may be exceedingly difficult to correct. The public health nurse and the school nurse should be particularly alert to notice children who show signs of strabismus and to direct them to medical care.

Glaucoma

Glaucoma is a disease that is increasing with the proportionate increase in older people in our population. It is seldom seen in persons under 35 years of age, but it is the greatest enemy to vision in older people. It is the second leading identified cause of blindness, and it has been estimated that there are about 1 million persons in the United States with glaucoma that has not been diagnosed. Treatment of glaucoma often is more difficult than treatment of cataracts, which also occur in older people.

There are several types of glaucoma, but they all have one characteristic physical sign: increased intraocular pressure that may be caused by an obstruction to the circulation of aqueous humor at the pupil or to its drainage through the angle of the anterior chamber. Increased intraocular pressure leads to destruction of the retina and blindness unless diagnosis is made early and treatment is effective and continued.

Primary glaucoma is of unknown origin. A predisposition to the disease may be inherited. Primary glaucoma occurs most often in persons who have a family history of glaucoma and who have a somewhat unstable emotional makeup. Secondary glaucoma may follow another disease, such as uveitis or a tumor.

Glaucoma may be acute or chronic, the latter being much more common. *Acute glaucoma* may cause general symptoms of nausea and vomiting in addition to eye pain and dilation of the pupil, as the iris remains dilated. Increased vascularity of the cornea may cause the patient to conclude that he has "pinkeye." There is edema of the ciliary body and the cornea and an increase of tension within the eyeball. Marked increase in tension for twenty-four to thirty-six hours may lead to complete and permanent blindness, and hence the necessity for immediate treatment. Treatment usually consists of miotics such as Pilocarpine to constrict the pupil and permit the outflow of aqueous humor, narcotics for pain, and complete rest. If symptoms do not subside within a few hours, an emergency operation such as an iridectomy may be performed to reduce the pressure by providing an outlet for the aqueous humor.

Chronic glaucoma may come on slowly, and, at first, symptoms may be absent. Chronic glaucoma gives one characteristic sign that is important: before central vision becomes affected, the peripheral visual fields are impaired so that objects to the side are ignored. Limitation of vision may not be so apparent as in other eye diseases, and much damage can occur before medical aid is sought. The patient may bump into other persons in the street or fail to see passing vehicles, yet not realize that the fault lies in his own vision. A diminished field of vision may cause the driver of an automobile to have an accident. The community nurse who recognizes this difficulty may be most helpful in early case finding and in promptly referring patients to an opthalmologist.

Chronic glaucoma usually begins in one eye, although if it is left untreated, both eyes often become affected. Symptoms are most apparent in the morning, when a persistent dull eye pain may develop. Frequent changes of glasses, difficulty in adjusting to darkness, failure to detect changes in color accurately, and slight blurring of vision are fairly early signs to glaucoma. Then follows a steamy appearance to the cornea and further blurring of vision. Tearing, misty vision, blurred appearance to the iris, which becomes fixed and dilated, headache,

pain behind the eyeball, nausea, and vomiting can then occur. Halos, resembling street lamps seen through a steamy windshield, may be seen about lights. Symptoms may be increased in some persons by watching movies or television. Early symptoms have been confused with sinus trouble, and treatment has been delayed for this reason.

There is no known cure for glaucoma; all treatment is directed toward reducing intraocular tension and keeping it at a safe level. Miotics such as pilocarpine are used to constrict the pupil and to draw the smooth muscle of the iris away from the canal of Schlemm to permit aqueous humor to drain out at this point. Acetazolamide (Diamox), a drug that tends to reduce the formation of aqueous humor, is used successfully in some types of chronic glaucoma. Surgical procedures for glaucoma are used to produce a permanent filtration pathway for aqueous fluid. A *cyclodialysis* is performed to form a channel between the anterior chamber and the suprachoroidal space. In an *iridectomy,* a portion of the iris is excised to make an opening between the anterior and posterior chambers to permit drainage. If the iris is blocking the angle of the anterior chamber, an iridectomy may be performed to relieve the obstruction. An *anterior sclerotomy* is the removal of a piece of the sclera to permit fluid to escape from the anterior chamber. An *iridencleisis* is a procedure in which a piece of iris is brought into the scleral incision to prevent it from closing, thus providing a permanent fistula for the drainage of fluid. Following surgery the patient usually is allowed out of bed at once, although one or both eyes may be bandaged for several days. Postoperative nursing care of patients having eye surgery has already been discussed.

The patient with glaucoma needs assistance in learning to accept his disease. Despite explanation from his physician, he frequently hopes that the operation will cure his condition, that no further treatment will be necessary, and perhaps that the sight he has lost will be restored. He should realize that the vision lost cannot be restored but that further loss can usually be prevented and his life can be quite normal if he continues under medical care. He should avoid anything that will increase his blood pressure and, in turn, intraocular tension. For example, he should avoid emotional situations such as arguments and quarrels, tight-fitting clothing such as constricting collars, constipation with straining at defecation, and heavy lifting. Watching movies and television, driving a vehicle, and work involving close watching of moving objects often must be limited.

The person with glaucoma should be under medical care for the rest of his life, receiving either drug or surgical therapy, or both. Following the operation he should return regularly to the doctor since one operation does not necessarily mean that drainage will be continued. Any obstruction or closing of the artificial pathway will result in reappearance of symptoms and further visual damage. The patient and his family should know specifically what to do if essential eye drops are accidentally spilled; for example, they should know what local drugstore is open at night and during holidays. The patient often is advised to have an extra bottle of medication in his home and to carry one with him if he works away from his home. It is advisable also for the patient to carry a card or other identifying information to identify himself as having glaucoma in case an accident occurs.

Cataract

A cataract is a clouding, or opacity, of the lens that leads to blurring of vision and eventual loss of sight. The opacity is due to chemical changes in the protein of the lens caused by slow, degenerative changes of age, injury, poison, or intraocular infection. Cataracts can occur at any time of life and may be associated with iritis, uveitis, and other conditions such as diabetes. They may follow the ingestion of injurious substances such as dinitrophenol, which was taken for weight reduction a few decades ago. Cataracts may be congenital, occurring most often in infants whose mothers had German measles during the first trimester of pregnancy.

Cataracts occur so often in the aged that the term senile cataract is used. At 80 years of age, about 85% of all people have some clouding of the lens. Senile cataracts are listed as the most common cause of blindness in older persons, yet the response of the condition to surgery often is excellent. Patients who are in their nineties can often be operated upon with good results.

Operative treatment is the only satisfactory treatment for cataracts. Decision as to when to remove the cataract depends largely on the individual patient and the use he makes of his eyes. If any signs of inflammation are present, surgery is not attempted. It is the nurse's responsibility to refer the patient with a cataract to an ophthalmologist and to encourage him to accept treatment as recommended.

Cataracts usually are removed under local anesthesia. Removal has been simplified in many cases by the use of the enzyme alpha-chymotrypsin, which weakens the zonular fibers that hold the lens in position. Cataracts may be removed within their capsule (*intracapsular technique*), or an opening may be made in the capsule and the lens lifted out without disturbing the membrane (*extracapsular technique*). The lens and its capsule may be frozen with a probe cooled to a temperature of $-35°$ C. ($-31°$ F.) or lower and then lifted from its position in the eye (*cryoextraction*). All these procedures usually are preceded by an iridectomy, which is performed to create an opening for the flow of aqueous humor, which may become blocked postoperatively as the vitreous humor moves forward. Usually only one eye is operated upon at a time lest some complication arise or some unexpected behavior of the patient, such as rubbing his operative eye, interfere with healing. If the patient has cataracts in both eyes, both may be removed during one hospitalization. This plan for treatment must be explained to the patient and his family or else he may feel that time is being spent in the hospital unnecessarily.

Following any cataract operation, a dressing is applied to the eye and covered with a metal shield to protect it from injury. The unoperated eye also may be covered, but usually it is left free. The patient normally is allowed out of bed the day following surgery. Dressings are changed by the surgeon in one to three days, and at the end of a week or ten days, all dressings are removed and temporary glasses may be used.

Congenital cataracts respond favorably to a simple operation known as a *discission* procedure. A very small opening is made in the capsule surrounding the lens, and a small, sharp needle knife is passed in pendulum-like manner through the lens. This procedure also is referred to as a "needling" operation. The operation permits aqueous fluid to pass into the cloudy lens, causing the cloudiness to disappear. Congenital cataracts are usually operated upon when the child is about 4 years of age or older. A general anesthetic is used, no immobilization in bed is necessary, and the child may be permitted to go home within a day or two of the operation. The results from discission of congenital cataracts in children are remarkably good.

The elderly patient sometimes finds it hard to adjust to removal of a cataract. The little remaining ability to accommodate the eye is lost when the lens is removed, and the patient must wear glasses at all times. Bifocal lenses often are ordered, and the patient must have perseverance in becoming accustomed to their use. He may be surprised to learn that he needs glasses before he can use his operated eye, that the color of objects seen with the eye from which the lens has been removed is slightly changed, that if he has the lens removed from one eye only, he will use one of his eyes at a time but not both together, and that he must wait at least three months before he can have permanent glasses prescribed. He needs to know that it will take time to learn to judge distance, climb stairs, and do other simple things.

Detachment of the retina

Retinal detachment is a separation or elevation of the retina away from the choroid. This detachment may be caused by fluid that has seeped from the vitreous cavity through tears or holes in the retina, from fluid that has extravasated from the retina or the choroid, or from fibrous bands in the vitreous that pull the retina away from its normal position. The retina is that layer of the eye which perceives light and coordinates and transmits impulses from its seeing nerve cells to the optic nerve. When it separates from the vascular choroid, loss of vision occurs at that point. As the detachment extends and becomes complete, blindness results. Myopia and myopic degeneration, trauma, and cataracts are the most frequent causes of retinal detachment in children and adults. It may also result from hemorrhage, tumor, or exudates that occur in front of or behind the retina. Detachment of the retina may follow sudden severe emotional shock or physical exertion, especially in persons who are debilitated.

The detachment may occur suddenly or develop slowly. The symptoms include floating spots or opacities before the eyes, flashes of light, and progressive constriction of vision in one area. The floating spots are blood and retinal cells that are freed at the time of the tear and cast shadows upon the retina as they seem to drift about the eye. The area of visual loss depends entirely on the location of the detachment. When the detachment is extensive and occurs quickly, the patient may have the sensation that a curtain has been drawn before his eyes.

Immediate care for the detachment of the retina includes keeping the patient quiet in bed and his eyes covered to prevent further detachment. Extended conservative treatment for detachment of the retina has not been successful, and early surgery is now the approved method of treatment. Cyclogyl or Neo-Synephrine is used to keep the pupils widely dilated so that tears in the retina may be identified during the operation. The surgery may be done under either local or general anesthesia. The surgical procedure includes draining the fluid from the subretinal space, so that the retina returns to its normal position, and closing the opening in the retina. To drain the fluid from the subretinal space, the sclera and choroid are perforated at the time of the operation. The retinal breaks are closed by various methods that produce an inflammatory reaction (*chorioretinitis*) in the area of the tear so that the adhesions will form between the edges of the break and the underlying choroid to obliterate the opening. When the tears are small or of recent origin, diathermy may be applied through the sclera with needlepoint electrodes to produce the inflammatory process. An intense beam of visible light directed to the area by means of an elaborate ophthalmoscope may be used to close retinal tears when the retina is not elevated (*photocoagulation*). The *laser* beam is used by some as a source of intense radiant heat to produce the chorioretinitis. Subfreezing temperatures ($-20°$ to $-50°$ C. [$-4°$ to $-58°$ F.]) may be applied to the surface of the sclera in the area of the hole to produce the inflammatory reaction (*retinal cryopexy*).

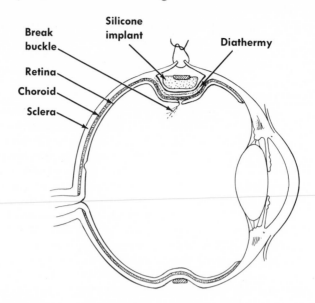

Fig. 197

One method of doing a scleral buckling operation.

Liquid nitrogen or carbon dioxide snow flowing through a tube attached to a delicate instrument are used to produce these low temperatures.

For recurrent or extensive detachments previously considered unoperable, *scleral buckling* procedures are used. The subretinal fluid is released, the break or tear is closed by one of the methods described above, and then the area overlying the treated tear is indented or "buckled" inward toward the vitreous cavity. (See Fig. 197.) To create the buckle, a fold is taken in the treated sclera and choroid and sutured into place, or a segment of the sclera is resected and shortened. This procedure may be combined with the implantation of a foreign material, such as various-shaped pieces of silicone, to cause further indentation of the choroid. By these procedures, the choroid is pushed into contact with the retinal tear during healing and vitreous adhesions that have exerted traction, or pull, on the retinal break are relaxed as the size of the scleral shell is decreased.

The patient's postoperative position will depend on the extent and location of his retinal detachment. Because postoperative routines vary a great deal, the nurse must be certain that orders for bed position and for ambulation have been written by the surgeon and that she understands exactly how much activity he wishes the patient to have. (See general discussion of the postoperative care of a patient having eye surgery.) Dressings are usually changed daily, but it is about a week before the eye can be fully examined and determination made as to whether or not the operation has been successful. It may be possible to reoperate upon eyes when surgery has not been successful, although a second operation usually is delayed for at least one or two weeks. Hemorrhage is the worst complication of an operation for detachment of the retina. It may result from electrocautery destruction of blood vessels or from trauma at the time of operation. When dressings are removed, the patient is usually required to wear pinhole glasses, which permit some vision but tend to limit eye movement. The length of time that they are necessary varies.

After operation for detachment of the retina, the patient is urged to avoid heavy lifting and straining of any kind for several months. Therefore, he may have to be away from work for a long time, or he may even have to alter his mode of earning a living entirely.

Eye disease resulting from nutritional deficiency

There seems to be a direct relationship between good nutrition and eye health. A lack of vitamin A in the diet can cause changes in the conjunctiva and corneal epithelium. Tears are reduced, and eyes and lid margins become reddened and inflamed. Sensitivity to light is often present, and some loss of visual acuity is noticed at night.

Pathologic changes can occur in the retina as a result of nutritional deficiency, particularly of vitamin B. This condition is found in persons who ingest large amounts of alcohol and who pay little attention to their diets. The disease has been thought to be caused by alcohol, and the name *tobacco-alcoholic amblyopia* is used. Patients who suffer from optic atrophy as a result of nutritional deficiency often will respond to a diet high in vitamin B, even though they may continue to take alcohol. Occasionally, when damage to the nerve tissue of the retina has been severe and prolonged, a diet high in vitamin B and all other essentials can accomplish only partial recovery. A lack of vitamin C may cause hemorrhage in the subconjunctiva, retina, and other structures of the eye.

Eye manifestations of systemic diseases

Diseases and infections that affect other parts of the body also affect the eye. Only a few of the more common conditions will be discussed briefly here. A persistent systemic *hypertension* will eventually produce such changes in the retina as hemorrhage, edema, and exudates, which, if uncontrolled, may result in the loss of sight. If the cause of the elevated blood pressure is eclampsia of pregnancy and is of short duration, the *retinopathy* (any disorder of the retina) usually subsides when the pregnancy is terminated. Retinopathy due to hypertension resulting from renal arteriolar sclerosis or diffuse glomerulonephritis is usually progressive and irreversible. The severity of the hypertension causes narrowing of the retinal arteries, and the blood flow through the retina and choroid is diminished, resulting in degenerative changes in the retina and loss of vision.

Senile degeneration of the macula is a rather common cause of diminished vision in elderly patients. The condition probably results from impaired nutrition of the retina due to changes in the blood vessels caused by senile arteriosclerosis or atherosclerosis. The patient usually loses central vision and cannot read, sew, or do other activities requiring close and intent vision. He has enough peripheral vision to function independently but requires supervision to prevent accidents.

Visual loss may follow vascular accidents to vessels anywhere in the eye or in the main blood vessels outside the eye. A cerebral vascular accident may cause hemianopia (blindness for one-half of the field of vision in one or both eyes) or total blindness, depending upon its location. Thrombosis of the central vein or arteriosclerotic involvement of the central artery of the eye may cause blindness. Generalized arteriosclerosis involving the vessels of both eyes may cause partial or complete loss of vision in both eyes.

Diabetes may affect any of the structures of the eye. Senile cataracts occur earlier in persons who have diabetes and progress more rapidly than in most elderly people. *Diabetic retinopathy* produces characteristic changes in the retina (punctuate hemorrhages, capillary microaneurysms, and a soapy or waxy exudate) that cause severe visual damage and eventually result in blindness. The incidence of diabetic retinopathy seems to depend upon the duration of the diabetes and upon its control. Persons whose blood sugar level has been kept in strict control appear less prone to develop diabetic retinopathy than those who have been less restricted. There is apparently no effective treatment to prevent the development of this condition except, possibly, adherence to a strict insulin and diet regimen.

Night blindness (nyctalopia) is a condition in which good vision is present in the daytime or with a good light but deficient at night or with a poor light. It may be a symptom of secondary optic nerve atrophy such as *retinitis pigmentosa*, which may be congenital or may develop in early childhood. Retinitis pigmentosa is a progressive disease in which the pigment epithelium degenerates and its cells migrate and deposit on the retina, causing loss of peripheral vision and then of central vision. There is no treatment for this condition, which leads to poor vision but does not cause blindness. Night blindness may also be caused by defective regeneration of the visual purple contained in the outer rods and in the pigment epithelium due to poor ocular nutrition resulting from starvation, anemia, scurvy, vitamin A deficiency, or exposure to a bright light. This condition responds favorably to the administration of a nutritious diet and vitamin A and iron preparations.

Retrolental fibroplasia

Retrolental fibroplasia is a disease of premature infants in which a dense, opaque, fibrous membrane forms in the anterior vitreous behind the lens, causing blindness. The cause of the disease is now thought to be due to too much oxygen administered to premature infants in the hospital. Since the amount and concentration of oxygen given to premature infants has been curtailed, new cases of retrolental fibroplasia are rare.

Removal of the eye

An eye, with or without its supportive structures, may be removed for four reasons: (1) in an attempt to save life when a malignant tumor has developed, (2) to save sight in the other eye when sympathetic ophthalmia is feared or threatens, (3) to control pain in an eye blinded by disease such as chronic glaucoma or chronic infection, or (4) for cosmetic reasons following blindness from trauma or disease *Enucleation* is removal of the eyeball, and *evisceration* is the removal of the contents of the eyeball, leaving only the sclera. Occasionally, the entire eye with the surrounding structures must be removed *(exenteration)* because of a disease such as cancer. If feasible, the eyeball alone is removed, leaving the surrounding layers of fascia (Tenon's capsule) and the muscle attachments. A gold, plastic, or tantalum ball or a piece of body fat is inserted into the eye socket, the cut ends of the muscle attachments are overlapped and sutured around it, and then Tenon's capsule and the conjunctiva are closed. This procedure provides a stump that supplies both support and motion for an artificial eye and therefore gives the patient whose eye has been removed a more normal appearance. The metal or plastic ball is left in place permanently.

Hemorrhage, thrombosis of blood vessels, and infection are possible complications following enucleation, exenteration, or evisceration of an eye. Pressure dressings may be used for one or two days to help control possible hemorrhage. Headache or pain in the operated side of the head should be reported at once since meningitis occasionally occurs as a complication following thrombosis of adjacent veins. The patient is usually allowed out of bed the day following surgery.

An *artificial eye* can be used as soon as healing is complete and edema has disappeared—usually six to eight weeks after operation, although many patients begin to wear an artificial eye after only three weeks. Artificial eyes are made of glass or plastic materials. Glass eyes last longer if not broken, but they are heavier. Plastic ones are more expensive and must usually be replaced every year or two because they become roughened around the edges and may be irritating to the conjunctiva. There are two kinds of artificial eyes: the shell-shaped and the hollow artificial eye. The choice for the individual patient depends on what operation has been done. Artificial eyes may be bought in shades that closely match the normal eye or they may be specially made. Stock eyes of plastic cost approximately $50, and glass ones cost $15; the prices for custom-made eyes are about $110 for the plastic and $35 for the glass. Artificial eyes that almost exactly match the natural eye can be made, but the pupil must, of course, remain fixed.

Even young children can be taught to care for their own artificial eye. Usually the eye is removed before retiring and kept either in a clean, dry place after cleansing or in a glass of normal saline solution. The eye should be cleansed immediately after its removal, and care should be taken not to scratch its surface. The eye is removed by gently pressing upward on the lower lid, being certain that the cupped hand is held against the cheek so that the eye does not fall to the floor and break or become lost. It is inserted by gently everting the lower lid,

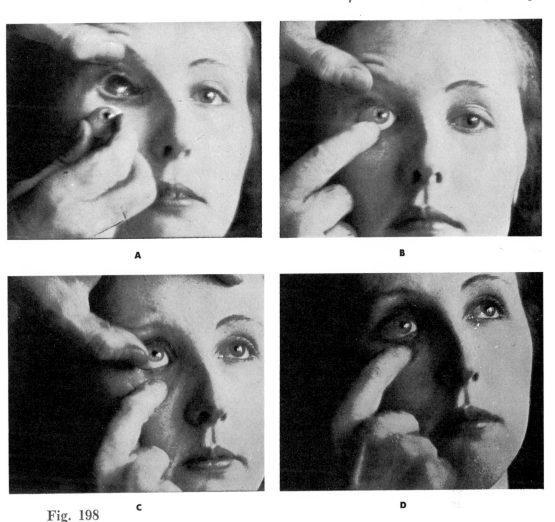

Fig. 198

Steps in inserting an artificial eye. (From Parkinson, Roy H.: Eye, ear, nose, and throat manual for nurses, ed. 8, St. Louis, 1959, The C. V. Mosby Co.)

being certain that the narrower end of the eye is place next to the inner angle of the orifice. Then, by grasping the upper lashes and gently raising the upper lid, the eye is easily slipped into place. (See Fig. 198.) Most people who wear prosthetic eyes keep an extra one in case the eye in use should be lost or broken.

More important than care of the artificial eye is care of the remaining eye. The person who has only one eye is advised to wear protective nonbreakable glasses. He is also instructed to avoid excessive strain on his eye. The patient should be prepared

for the adjustment necessary in learning to carry on normal activities with only one eye and of the accident hazards entailed. Driving a car, for example, is dangerous for the person who suddenly must use only one eye since depth perception is altered. With patience, however, almost all normal activities are possible—surgeons who have had an eye removed have even been able to learn to operate successfully.

Blindness

Despite the best efforts of all concerned, some patients will become blind. The National Society for the Prevention of Blindness estimates that there were 411,000 legally blind persons in the United States in 1964. It is likely that the number will increase in the future since glaucoma, cataracts, and degenerative diseases associated with arteriosclerosis occur in older people, and this part of our population is increasing faster than the population as a whole. According to the National Health Survey, 68% of the blind population is 65 years of age or over.

The decision as to whether or not the patient should be told of approaching blindness or of certain blindness must rest with the doctor. Usually it is considered best for the doctor to be completely honest and frank with the patient, provided he is certain that blindness will occur or is irreversible. It then becomes the responsibility of the nurse, working with other members of the health team and with the patient, to help him adjust to blindness.

When the patient has been told that he will become blind, it is to be expected that he will be depressed for a while. This is a normal reaction and is described by psychiatrists as a period of mourning for his dead eyes which the patient must undergo before he can begin to think and plan for his new life.[12] Some patients believe that becoming blind is a symbol of punishment and often need to cope with feelings of inadequacy, guilt, resentment, and loneliness.[23] Family members are extremely important throughout this period, as the patient needs to be sure that they love and accept him in spite of his disability.

The nurse can help the patient during his period of adjustment to partial or complete blindness. She can merely listen to him talk of what blindness means to him, she can report any exaggerated reactions that might indicate thoughts of self-destruction, she can direct the patient's thinking gradually along positive constructive lines, and she can help to make available to him the resources that he will need.

The child who has never known sight adjusts well and is happy provided that he is treated as a normal child and is neither overprotected nor rejected. It is chiefly the parents who have to adjust to and accept the child's handicap and be willing to use the resources available in the community to de-

velop his independence and enable him to face problems of living. Both the parent and the child may need special consultation and training in order to achieve this end.

Rehabilitation. The blind person's major handicaps are loss of mobility (moving about safely indoors and outdoors) and loss of sight. These can be overcome for the most part by training and the substitution of some of the other senses for the lack of sight. Two-thirds of the persons who are blind lose their visions after the age of 20 years, and must learn a completely new way of life. It is estimated that between 20 and 30% of those who become blind are employable. If the patient has a little time before becoming blind, he may use it to good advantage by beginning certain rehabilitative activities (for example, learning Braille).

Important contributions that the nurse can make to rehabilitation are to begin to teach the patient as soon as he becomes blind and to encourage him to carry out the activities of daily living. She can also help members of his family see the importance of letting the patient experience the satisfaction of his own independence. It is imperative that the patient be given an opportunity to preserve self-respect and esteem by caring for his personal needs. He should be urged to feed, clothe, bathe, and otherwise care for himself. The family needs expert counseling and guidance since the natural tendency is to overprotect the patient and thus render him completely helpless. The nurse can suggest ways in which the home may be arranged to prevent accidents and to permit the blinded person to get about without embarrassment. Many blinded people can learn to be completely independent and may go about in busy city traffic with only a seeing eye dog to help them* or may even go alone.

The patient will have many questions and many needs. He may, for example, want to go to the occupational therapy department of the hospital to learn to type, or he may want to know how he may arrange to learn braille and what cost is involved. The patient may be impatient to know his chances of learning a new occupation. The nurse's actual participation in giving direct help will depend on whether she works in a hos-

---

*Seeing Eye, Inc., Trenton, N. J. 08600.

pital that has a social service department and other good rehabilitation resources or whether she works in a rural public health nursing agency where she may have to seek specific answers for the patient rather than refer his questions to others. The nurse who works with patients with eye disease and blindness should familiarize herself with the local resources in her own community. Religious groups such as Catholic Charities, the Salvation Army, and others often have programs in local areas. Almost every state has a voluntary organization devoted to this need, and the nurse can learn about it by writing to the state health department. Some state health departments also have their own special programs. If the patient qualifies, help may also be available through the Veterans Administration.

National voluntary organizations. Two national voluntary organizations concerned with blindness and the prevention of blindness are the American Foundation for the Blind* and the National Society for the Prevention of Blindness.† Both organizations have literature that is available to nurses and patients upon request. The American Foundation for the Blind distributes a booklet entitled *Tools and Aids for the Blind,* which contains a list of aids for the blind and the partially blind; for example, magnifying glasses that can be carried in the pocket and used to see street signs are available, and a variety of special syringes and aids for giving injections are described for the partially blinded person who has to give himself insulin or other parenteral medication. The primary functions of the National Society for the Prevention of Blindness include research, education, and preventive services. Pamphlets and films are available for both lay and professional use. The quarterly publication of this voluntary organization, *The Sight-Saving Review,* is available to nurses and covers many aspects of sight conservation and eye health. Recordings of textbooks and educational materials are available free of charge for blind persons for educational, vocational, and professional use from Recordings for the Blind, Inc.‡

These recordings also may be obtained from many local and state libraries.

Legal blindness. A person is considered legally blind when his vision in the better eye is reduced to 20/200 or less even with the use of corrective lenses. This means that he is able to see at 20 feet what the normal person can see at 200 feet. Legal blindness entitles a person to certain federal assistance. A 1952 amendment to the Social Security Act made provision for assistance to the blind, and now all fifty states and all territories have approved plans for such aid. Assistance through this program is based on need. The Internal Revenue Act of 1948 permits blinded persons an extra deduction ($600) in reporting income. In 1943 the federal government established a counseling and placement service for the blind in the Vocational Rehabilitation Administration. It shares cost of rehabilitation with the states. The Veterans Administration provides a substantial pension for the single veteran who has enucleation of both eyes even when he has no other physical defects.

Schools. Progress has been made in improving school opportunities for the blind. It is believed now that the blind child, like any other handicapped child, does best when accepted and is in as normal an environment as possible. Blind children of school age are being educated in regular public or parochial schools, where special provisions for their individual needs are being met, or they attend special residential schools. Schools emphasize the use of auditory instruction and the development of reading skills through touch perception by the Braille system. The child needs to encounter as much of his environment as is practical in order to develop concepts that other children acquire by sight. Many states have legislated funds to provide higher education for the blind and to provide readers for them, and many blind students go on to college and compete successfully with their sighted peers.

References and selected readings*

1 Adler, Francis Heed: Textbook of ophthalmology, ed. 7, Philadelphia, 1962, W. B. Saunders Co.

2 Allen, James H.: Mays' manual of the diseases of the

---

*15 West 16th St., New York, N. Y. 10011.
†163 East 40th St., New York, N. Y. 10016.
‡121 East 58th St., New York, N. Y. 10022.

---

*References preceded by an asterisk are particularly well suited for student reading.

eye, ed. 23, Baltimore, 1963, The Williams & Wilkins Co.

3 Armstrong, Inez, and Browder, Jane J.: The nursing of children, Philadelphia, 1964, F. A. Davis Co.

4 Bellows, John G.: The application of cryogenic techniques in ophthalmology, Am. J. Ophth. 57:29-31, Jan. 1964.

5 Bledsoe, C. Warren, and Williams, Russell C.: The vision needed to nurse the blind, Am. J. Nursing 66:2432-2435, Nov. 1966.

6 *Blodi, Frederick C.: Glaucoma, Am. J. Nursing 63:78-83, March 1963.

7 *Blodi, Frederick C., and Honn, Ruth C.: Tumors of the eye—medical and nursing care, Am. J. Nursing 56:1152-1156, Sept. 1956.

8 *Brockhurst, Robert J., and O'Donnell, Catherine T.: Detachment of the retina, Am. J. Nursing 64:96-100, April 1964.

9 Brueggen, Stella L.: Eye health in industry, Am. J. Nursing 61:83-88, Sept. 1961.

10 *Burian, Hermann M.: Strabismus, Am. J. Nursing 60:653-656, May 1960.

11 Campbell, Charles J., and others: Clinical studies in laser photocoagulation, Arch. Ophth. 74:57-65, July 1965.

12 Cholden, L.: Some psychiatric problems in rehabilitation of the blind, Bull. Menninger Clin. 18:107-112, May 1954.

13 *Committee of A.M.A.: Guiding principles and procedures for nurses in care of eye injuries, J.A.M.A. 174:536-539, Oct. 1, 1960.

14 Duane, Thomas David: Ophthalmic Research USA: A Report to the Trustees of Research to Prevent Blindness, Inc. (1965), 598 Madison Ave., N. Y. 10022.

15 Duke-Elder, Sir Stewart: Parson's diseases of the eye, ed. 14, New York, 1964, The Macmillan Co.

16 Esposito, Albert: Contact lenses, Am. J. Nursing 57:462-463, April 1957.

17 Fullington, Sandra Musick: The child with bandaged eyes, Am. J. Nursing 61:98-99, May 1961.

18 *Gamble, Richard C.: The medical eye examination, Am. J. Nursing 57:1590-1592, Dec. 1957.

19 Gellis, Sydney S., and Kazan, Benjamin M.: Current pediatric therapy 1966-1967, Philadelphia, 1966, W. B. Saunders Co.

20 *Gibbons, Helen, and Cunningham, Florence: Finding and helping the partially seeing child, Nursing Outlook 7:524-526, Sept. 1959.

21 Girard, Louis J.: Cryotherapy in ophthalmology, Sight-Saving Rev. 35:87-90, Summer 1965.

22 *Gordon, Dan M.: The inflamed eye, Am. J. Nursing 64:113-117, Nov. 1964.

23 *Havener, William H., Saunders, William H., and Bergersen, Betty S.: Nursing care in eye, ear, nose, and throat disorders, St. Louis, 1964, The C. V. Mosby Co.

24 Holt, L. Beverly: Pediatric ophthalmology, Philadelphia, 1964, Lea & Febiger.

25 *Jones, Ira S., and Bosanko, Lydia: The cataract extraction operation and nursing care of the patient with a cataract extraction, Am. J. Nursing 60:1433-1437, Oct. 1960.

26 Knobloch, William H., and Abis, Paul A.: Retinal detachment surgery with preserved human sclera, Am. J. Ophth. 60:191-204, Aug. 1965.

27 Kornzweig, Abraham L.: The eye in old age, Am. J. Ophth. 60:835-842, Nov. 1965.

28 Kuhn, Hedwig S.: Questions and answers—contact lenses, J.A.M.A. 178:1055, Dec. 9, 1961.

29 *Leopold, Irving H.: Anti-inflammatory agents in ophthalmology, Am. J. Nursing 63:84-87, March 1963.

30 *Lincoff, Harvey A., and others: Modifications to the Custodis procedure for retinal detachment, Arch. Ophth. 73:160-163, Feb. 1965.

31 *Meyer, William J.: Rural glaucoma screening, Am. J. Pub. Health 52:75-79, Jan. 1962.

32 Newell, Frank W.: Current status of diabetic retinopathy, Sight-Saving Rev. 35:80-86, Summer 1965.

33 Newell, Frank W.: Ophthalmology, St. Louis, 1965, The C. V. Mosby Co.

34 News item, Field of Vision 9:2, March 15, 1954.

35 Nordstrom, Wyvonne: Adjusting to cataract glasses, Am. J. Nursing 66:1578-1579, July 1966.

36 Oerther, Barbara: The blind patient need not be helpless, Am. J. Nursing 66:2436-2439, Nov. 1966.

37 *Ruedemann, Albert D.: Headaches caused by eye defects, Am. J. Nursing 52:1093-1094, Sept. 1952.

38 Scheie, Harved G.: The management of glaucoma and cataracts in children, Sight-Saving Rev. 34:75-82, Summer 1964.

39 Schwartz, Paula: Alerting parents to eye problems of the young child, Sight-Saving Rev. 34:157-159, Fall 1964.

40 *Shepard, Mary Estelle: Nursing care of patients with eye, ear, nose and throat disorders, New York, 1958, The Macmillan Co.

41 *Stocker, Frederick W., and Bell, Ruth: Corneal transplantation and nursing the patient with a corneal transplant, Am. J. Nursing 62:65-70, May 1962.

42 Troutman, Richard C., and others, editors: Plastic and reconstructive surgery of the eye and adnexa, Washington, D. C., 1962, Butterworth, Inc.

43 *Weaver, Helen E.: Glaucoma: a problem for the public health nurse, Pub. Health Nursing 41:92-95, Feb. 1949.

44 *Weiss, M. Olga: Psychological aspects of nursing care for eye patients, Am. J. Nursing 50:218-220, April 1950.

31

The patient
with neurologic
disease

Study questions

1 Review the anatomy of the nervous system.

2 What vital centers are located in the brain? What bodily functions would be affected by pressures on these centers?

3 Outline a plan for moving and changing the position of a completely dependent patient. What nursing measures can be used to maintain normal body alignment and function?

4 Describe the procedure for giving tube feedings.

5 If a patient is unable to speak, what methods of communication could you devise?

6 From among patients on your unit or among members of your family or acquaintances, select a person who has a chronic neurologic disease. How has his disease affected family life? How has the community been affected?

The specialties of neurology and neurosurgery are complicated and demand special knowledge, skill, and experience. Before the nurse can give good nursing care to a patient with neurologic disease, she needs to have knowledge of the nervous system, of any pathology present, of the surgical procedure if one is performed, and the general nursing needs of neurologic patients. It is suggested that the student nurse review the anatomy, pathology, treatment, and nursing care needed for each neurologic patient encountered in her daily practice on any service.

Many neurologic patients have serious emotional and even psychiatric disturbances that may be related in part to their neurologic disease. Psychiatry, however, is concerned largely with functional disorders, whereas neurology is concerned largely with disorders that have a demonstrable organic, or physical, cause. There may be neurologic involvement in such general diseases as pernicious anemia, diabetes, and severe infections, but many diseases are caused by pathology that is primarily in the nervous system. Only a few of the frequently seen neurologic diseases and their nursing care will be considered in this chapter. General nursing care that is common to many neurologic diseases will be discussed before a few of the more common diseases and neuro-surgical procedures are described.

General nursing care

Loss of function and control. Neurologic disease may occur suddenly, as in cerebro-vascular hemorrhage or traumatic spinal cord injury, or may be slow in onset, as in multiple sclerosis or Parkinson's disease. The loss of some motor or sensory function is common in most neurologic diseases. There-fore, it may be difficult for the patient to carry out daily activities that require co-ordinated movement. The ability to move about at will and control one's actions is precious to every human being. Regardless of the speed of its occurrence, the loss of the ability to function independently or to predict one's movements is psychologically traumatizing. Irritability, defensiveness, fear, and other signs of threat to emotional se-curity are likely to appear and should be met with calmness, patience, and kindness by all who work with the patient.

If the patient has a nonprogressive limi-tation of function due to neurologic damage, he needs reassurance that his condition will not become worse. Unfortunately, however, cure is not possible in many neurologic dis-eases. The nurse needs to know what the doctor has told both the patient and his family about the prognosis. If assurance of arrest or of improvement of the disease can-not be given, the patient must be helped to live a relatively full life as long as possible, and it is the nurse who often gives much of this help.

The nurse can protect the patient from close observation and comment by persons who have no part in his care, particularly when he is in a general hospital or in his own home. The peculiarities of gait or man-nerisms and the loss of control so common in neurologic disease seem to interest people who should have no concern with them. The unfortunate quality of morbid curiosity in human nature must be faced. The patient should be told how common his particular condition is and that he is not alone with his affliction. The nurse can help him by making him feel that she is interested in him as a person and not primarily in his physical ail-ment. She may find that he turns to her as

someone with whom he can discuss his re-actions to his disease when he cannot dis-cuss them with his family. Listening atten-tively to the patient's problems is an essential part of neurologic nursing. Knowing when problems are too involved and beyond the nurse's sphere of knowledge is equally es-sential. A medical social worker can often be of great help to the patient in helping him to think through his feelings about his disease.

It is useless to argue with the patient or to try to talk him out of his fears. Giving a word of encouragement on small achieve-ments, changing the conversation to other topics, and introducing some diversional activity sometimes help. Emotional tension seems to be released by working with one's hands. Making something useful in the oc-cupational therapy department of a hos-pital or in his own home may be very satis-fying to the patient. The patient may receive more satisfaction from weaving a belt or making a wallet than from spending an equivalent amount of time watching tele-vision or in a similar passive, time-passing activity. He should not, however, be urged into activities that do not interest him. For example, the patient at home may receive more satisfaction from washing dishes and peeling vegetables than from making some decorative object.

The desire of the patient and his family to shop for a cure is understandable when the diagnosis of a chronic and incurable neurologic disease has been made. The nurse should help to prevent the loss of time and of financial and emotional resources which this practice usually entails. She should try to build up the confidence of the patient and his family in the doctor and in the clinic or hospital where he is receiving care. She will have to have patience and understanding in answering questions about advertised remedies, news items that may be mislead-ing, and reports from neighbors and friends. At times she may need to refer questions to the doctor. Many patients with incurable neurologic disease live out their years in the hope that a cure will be found during their lifetime. They need to feel sure that the persons responsible for their care are alert for new discoveries that may be helpful to them.

Provision for self-care. Physical facilities

should be arranged so that the patient can do as much as possible for himself to maintain his self-esteem and to give him some satisfaction. Handrails along hallways, firm locks on bed casters and bedside tables, low beds, and handrails along the sides of the tub and toilet help the patient to handle himself even though his movements are uncertain. It is important to most people to be able to feed themselves. Appetite is better and disposition improves when this is possible. Even a patient with poor coordination may be able to feed himself if food is cut into bite-sized pieces. A special spoon with a large handle may be helpful. If he is clumsy and untidy while eating, he will usually want to be protected from the scrutiny of others. The nurse should be calm about failures in attempts to master an activity or else she should ignore them. Emotional outbursts as a result of frustration should be treated in a matter-of-fact fashion. The nurse needs to know what the patient can do and should keep him aware of her faith in his ability to do these things for himself. Statements such as "You're not trying" or "You couldn't be tired yet" only add to the patient's discouragement and should be avoided. Good judgment is needed in deciding what the patient may safely do without assistance. If any doubt exists, the nurse should consult the doctor. She should know what activities are dangerous for the patient. Great frustration may result from attempting activities that are beyond his abilities because they accentuate his limitations. Activities that are steppingstones to greater accomplishments will result in satisfaction for the patient and will motivate him to further self-help.

It is fortunate that many neurologic diseases progress slowly so that the patient has time to adjust to necessary changes. As difficulty in walking progresses, the patient may benefit from special shoes. They may need to be built up in a variety of ways to provide a stable base of support. They should have low rubber heels, fit well, and give good support for the arches. As disease progresses, many patients must use a cane; this is a painful step for the patient in his acceptance of the disease, even though built-up shoes and a cane may be less conspicuous than the patient's gait would be without these aids. The nurse can help by

suggesting the activities that are safe and possible with the use of a cane. Eventually, many patients must resort to a wheelchair. The light wheelchairs now available make it possible for the quite helpless patient to get about safely in his home and to be taken in a car for trips away from home. Collapsible wheelchairs should be used only for special occasions because most of them do not give enough support to foster good sitting posture.

The nurse should help the patient to plan the necessary adjustments needed in the home so that he can continue to be at least partially self-sufficient. Furniture can be arranged to allow the patient to get about more easily in his wheelchair, cupboards and shelves can be lowered, and special equipment such as lamps and the telephone can be placed on lower tables.

If the patient has difficulty using his fingers and hands for fine movements, the use of shoes with elasticized insteps or of elastic laces instead of the usual ones and the use of metal grippers on clothing instead of buttons may help him to remain self-sufficient. When the patient is hospitalized, the activities he can perform should be noted on the nursing care plan or other equivalent record forms. If he is at home, the family should know what he can and cannot do so that he is not overprotected.

Aphasia. Aphasia is a disorder of language caused by damage to the speech-controlling area of the brain. Cerebral hemorrhage and cerebral thrombosis are the most common causes of such damage, but tumors, multiple sclerosis, and trauma may also lead to aphasia. Aphasia caused by cerebral edema following trauma is usually temporary. Occasionally a patient cannot speak following a cerebrovascular accident because the vocal cords are affected, not because of cerebral damage. This condition is not true aphasia.

A variety of abnormalities in speech can occur. The patient may be unable to comprehend the spoken or written word (sensory aphasia), or he may comprehend yet be unable to use the symbols of speech (motor aphasia). He may have both disorders at the same time. He may be able to write but not to speak; he may be able to speak but may use the wrong words or have a selective loss of words; he may be able to read but be unable to speak or to write. It is unusual for a patient to be unable to understand the spoken word or to know what he wishes to express. Sensory aphasia is much more difficult to deal with than motor involvement. Explanations are difficult, and it is hard to reassure the patient, who may become completely confused and undirected in his efforts to speak.

Each patient reacts to language difficulty in a different way, depending on his pattern of adjustment to life's problems. Most patients with aphasia become tense and anxious. They may be irritable and emotionally upset because they are unable to evoke the words they need, and they become discouraged easily in their efforts to speak. Some may quickly refuse to attempt to communicate. Others feel ashamed and withdraw from people, including even their family and close friends. Yet desire to communicate and persistence in efforts to do so are the essential ingredients in speech rehabilitation.

Nursing care is directed toward decreasing tension and should be started as soon as aphasia occurs in order to help the patient make a more satisfactory adjustment to his limitation and in order to make later rehabilitative efforts less difficult. The nurse should anticipate the patient's needs so that he will not have to make repeated attempts to ask for things. She should try to help him understand that he may relearn speech and should teach him ways in which he may communicate with others at this time. She must also help his family and friends and the auxiliary nursing staff to learn how to communicate with the patient and thus spare him humiliating experiences. She can help other patients to understand and help the patient by talking with him, avoiding any show of amusement or embarrassment, and making him feel that he is one of the group. Calmness and avoidance of hurry and impatience on the part of the nurse are essential to the patient's acceptance of his difficult program of practicing the use of relearned words and patterns of speech.

The patient's environment should be quiet. Persons who care for him should guard against speaking loudly; the patient with aphasia is seldom deaf. Although he cannot respond, he should be talked to and have procedures explained in the manner used with any patient. Recreational activities should be quiet. Music is often relaxing, and the patient may enjoy listening to the radio. If a patient is able to read and comprehend the written captions on television, watching television may be particularly gratifying. Some patients may be made irritable by radio music they do not enjoy or television programs they do not like or cannot follow. Watching the patient's facial expression may give the nurse a useful clue to the satisfaction derived from these activities.

Tests must be done to determine what language abilities have been lost. In some hospitals a trained therapist may be available to make an initial evaluation and to guide members of the nursing staff in making appropriate nursing care plans concerning the patient's speech problems. Sometimes, however, this assistance is not available, and the nurse must do simple tests that have been ordered by the doctor or, more often, devise her own tests. They may be conducted as follows. Spread several familiar objects, such as keys, a pencil, a book of matches, a penny, and scissors, before the patient: (1) ask him to name each object; (2) as you name each object, ask him to point to it; (3) ask him to write the name of each object as you point to it; (4) ask him to write the name of each object as you say the word; (5) show him a card containing the printed name of each object and ask him to read the word orally and point to the object. It may be too fatiguing for the patient to do all the tests at one time, so that some must be delayed. The patient's responses indicate the best way to communicate with him. If he can only read, one should give him cards with the words and phrases needed in asking for the most common daily necessities. Words needed by most ill persons include yes, no, bedpan, urinal, hot, cold, headache, pain, doctor, nurse, turn, sit up, lie down, bed, pillow, sheet, gown, water, thirst, hunger, comfortable, chair, light, telephone, and wife or husband. If the patient is unable to recognize the written word, he may be able to recognize pictures of objects. If he can write or draw a picture of his needs, he should be given a writing pad and pencil with which to do so.

As the nurse cares for the patient, she should name common objects and encourage the patient to handle them, to speak their names, and to write or copy their names. The patient should be helped to relearn the names of members of his family and friends. The family can supply these words and others that are particularly important for the patient. Speech retraining should be done for short periods of time because it is exceedingly trying, and fatigue tends to increase difficulty in speaking (dysphasia). The slogan of the National Hospital for Speech Disorders is "slow and easy." Praising the patient for each small improvement and encouraging him to take his mistakes good-naturedly help to make this difficult problem more bearable. The patient's progress in language retraining will depend on his level of intelligence, his age (older patients have more difficulty), the severity of the damage, and whether or not the brain lesion is a progressive one. Complete language rehabilitation may require months of painstaking work on the part of skilled therapists.*

Personality changes and prevention of accidents. Personality changes are common in neurologic disease, and occasionally their slow development is the first and only sign of a serious neurologic disorder. These changes should be watched for carefully and reported accurately. Physical changes caused by neurologic disease may affect the personality; reporting these changes may help the doctor in his diagnosis and treatment of the patient. Frustrations resulting from restrictions and attempts to get about, anxiety from increasing helplessness, and the fear of helplessness may also cause personality changes.

Changes in judgment and in intellect may become serious. The patient may make poor investments or other unwise decisions in business or family matters. Multiple sclerosis, Parkinson's disease, cerebrovascular arterio-sclerosis, and brain tumors are examples of neurologic disorders that may seriously alter judgment. Handling such a situation is extremely difficult because strong emotional reaction may follow curtailment of the patient's freedom in managing his own affairs. The problem is usually dealt with by the doctor and the family with the assistance of the medical social worker. The nurse should not tell the patient that she knows of measures taken to prevent the consequences of errors in his judgment.

Judgment defects may lead to behavior that is dangerous both to the patient and to others. It is believed that many automobile accidents are caused by persons with neurologic disease; for example, patients with multiple sclerosis may have blind spots (scotomas), and those with convulsive disorders may lose consciousness for only a few seconds—long enough for an accident to occur. Unfortunately, these two diseases appear in young people, who feel very keenly the restriction of such activities as driving an automobile. The need to avoid certain other dangerous activities must be stressed; for example, swimming is dangerous for the patient who has convulsive seizures. Emphasis must be positive, however, and must be upon the many things that the patient can do. Members of the patient's family should be helped to plan so that the necessary restrictions are not obvious; for example, hiking and camping may be substituted for swimming or horseback riding if the patient has convulsive seizures.

The neurologic patient must be protected from accidents in his daily living. Measures to prevent accidents must be carefully introduced because the patient may resent his limitations so much that he is inclined to reject precautions for his safety. Personality changes and judgment defects again may interfere with the patient's acceptance of measures that would help to ensure his personal safety. Elderly persons with arteriosclerotic brain damage are often great trials to their families; for example, they may decide to paint the outside of the house, when standing on a ladder is obviously dangerous.

The bathroom is a common location of accidents. To prevent falls in the bathtub, handrails should be installed beside the tub and the tub should be made slip-proof by

---

*Some institutions that specialize in working with patients who have aphasia are The National Hospital for Speech Disorders, New York, N. Y.; The Institute for the Crippled and Disabled, New York, N. Y.; The Institute of Logopedics, Wichita, Kan.; and the Vanderbilt University Hospital Clinic, Nashville, Tenn.

applying a rough paint to the floor of the tub or by using roughened plastic strips that also prevent slipping. They are available at most variety stores. It is often helpful to place a rubber or plastic mat in the tub, and many patients at home invest in the type of hand-rail that clamps to the side of the tub. A low box or a small commercially made seat can be placed in the tub to help the patient get out safely since rising from the seat is less difficult than from the tub bottom. One way to prevent accidents in bathtubs is to seat the patient while the tub is empty and dry and to empty it before he gets out. When limitations are severe, it may not be advisable for the patient to take a tub bath without assistance or to take a tub bath at all. Sitting on a stool or preferably in a small metal wheelchair in the shower and using a spray attached to the faucet is safer and is usually satisfactory for the patient.

Bathroom doors should not lock from the inside, since there is danger that the patient may lock himself in and, in the event of accident, prolong the time needed to reach him. This precaution is particularly important if the patient is elderly or if his sensory perception is impaired. Patients have received severe and even fatal burns from stepping into a tub of water that was too hot or from fainting or suffering a stroke or heart attack as hot water was running into the tub.

Accidents in and about the home may be prevented by special attention to causes of accidents by the nurse and the patient's family. Scatter rugs should never be used, and any upturned, curled rug edges should be nailed down. Wall-to-wall carpeting is best. Floors should not be highly waxed. Toys, lamp cords, or other accident hazards on floors should be removed. The patient should wear firm slippers or shoes. Bathrobes should have buttons instead of long cords or sashes. Good lighting is essential. Night-lights at the bedside, in hallways, and in bathrooms are desirable.

Railings and firm casements on steps and ramps often enable the patient to get about independently for a longer period. It is advisable to caution the family to lock basement doors and even front and back doors when persons who have neurologic disease with judgment defects are living in the house. They may open the wrong door and fall down basement steps or go into the street at odd hours and come to harm.

Contractures. Since muscle action is controlled by the nervous system, patients with neurologic disease are likely to develop contractures and deformities. Many changes come on so gradually that they are barely noticed by the patient until they are relatively fixed. In the home, as well as in the hospital, much can be done to prevent the progress of deformities. Warm baths often relax tightened muscles enough so that joints can be put through a range of motion. In this way, limitation of joint motion may be prevented or delayed. Since muscle and joint stiffness come from prolonged sitting or lying in one position, the patient should be advised to change his position frequently.

Failure to keep the body in good alignment, both while up and while in bed, may lead to deformity. If the patient is rational and able to help himself, the nurse can teach him to help prevent deformity and preserve his best possible function. A firm mattress and chairs that provide good support are essential. Pillows may be used to support paralyzed parts, and changes of position, both in and out of bed, help to prevent deformities from developing.

Standing for even a few minutes each day will prevent the development of contractures at the hips caused by prolonged sitting. In many communities walkers that permit the patient to stand supported may be rented or borrowed from such agencies as the local Red Cross, the public health nursing agency, the local rescue squad offices, or other volunteer groups. Many times the patient can stand safely between two sturdy kitchen chairs, providing he and his family are taught how he may manage himself in this position.

Body parts that are paralyzed must be put through the normal range of motion daily so that range will not be limited if and when the ability to move is restored. The nurse can determine the patient's range of motion as normal or limited by comparison with her own range of movement. She must allow for individual variations and for changes due to age and to any joint disease the patient may have. Since range of motion for some joints cannot be achieved with the patient in the supine (back-lying) position, it is necessary that he lie prone at least once each day. The nurse should know any special exercises prescribed for the patient so that she can assist with them at intervals during the day if this is desirable. They should be written or typed. Stick drawings help the patient to understand such details as the angle and arc of motion. (For complete range of joint motion, see Figs. 2 to 4.)

Pressure areas and skin care. When the nerve supply to a body part is affected by disease, nutrition of that part is impaired because the arterial and venous blood flow, which is dependent upon normal muscle action, is often decreased as a result of disturbance of nerve impulses. It is well to consider how often the normal person changes his position during both waking and sleeping hours. Some change is made in distribution of weight on weight-bearing parts of the body every few minutes. When the patient is paralyzed or unable to move, the pressure of body weight further curtails adequate circulation. The skin breaks down easily, and pressure sores may be difficult or impossible to cure. Therefore, the patient with a neurologic disorder who is confined to bed or chair must be reminded to change his position frequently if he is able to do so. If he cannot move himself, he must have assistance. If he is unconscious, he will sense no need to move or be moved. An important nursing responsibility is to change the patient's position at regular intervals or to remind others to do so. Light massage of the dependent areas should be given each time the patient is turned. If the patient is completely paralyzed, aged, or particularly devitalized, regular turning and massage may not be adequate to prevent decubiti, and an alternating air-pressure mattress, sponge rubber, or sheepskin under the bony prominences should be used. Attention should be given to a well-balanced diet since it helps to maintain healthy tissues.

Turning patients who are helpless or unconscious involves physical labor. The nurse and the auxiliary workers who help her need to apply the principles of good body mechanics, which will make the difference between ending the day with a feeling of normal tiredness and satisfaction and ending it with the feeling of discouragement and undue fatigue. (For principles of good body mechanics, see texts on fundamentals of nursing.)

It is necessary to keep the skin clean and dry. Incontinence is sometimes a problem in care of the patient with neurologic disease. (See Chapter 8.)

Nursing care of the patient in a respirator. Respirators may sometimes be used for patients with chronic lung disease such as emphysema, for patients with severe endocrine disorders involving the thyroid or parathyroid glands, and in other medical emergencies. Because they are used most often for patients with neurologic disease such as myasthenia gravis, toxic encephalitis, and fracture of the skull, the nursing care needed is included here. Respirators are mechanical devices used to substitute for normal respiratory action by creating a negative pressure outside the chest wall. This pressure causes air to enter the respiratory passages. A mechanical device is a poor substitute for normal respiration and therefore is usually used as a last resort. For example, the rate of inhalation and rate of exhalation are the same when a respirator is used, whereas in normal respiration the time for inhalation is less than that for exhalation.

Since respirators are used in emergencies, it is essential that they be checked often and kept in working order at all times. If they are kept on a ward or unit of the hospital, a regular day each week should be designated for their routine inspection. There are two main kinds of respirators and several manufacturers of each. The tank respirator encases the entire body except the head and imposes handicaps on persons who attempt to give nursing care. The chest respirator encloses the entire chest. Chest respirators permit the patient much greater freedom and simplify nursing care. They cannot, however, be used for long periods of time since they may not provide adequate aeration of the lungs. Several variations of equipment are available to aid breathing. Some of these respirators employ the use of a mask over the face and do not encase the body, and some can be attached to a tracheostomy (pp. 192 and 561).

Respirators can be dangerous in inexperienced hands. Too much negative pressure can cause inspiration to be too deep and thus traumatize the alevoli of the lungs. The respirator must be tested before the patient is placed in it. This is done in the tank respirator by closing all arm ports and other openings and turning the pressure gauge until approximately the desired pressure is reached. The head opening can be closed by holding a pillow firmly against it. Pressure must again be carefully regulated when the patient is in the machine.

If the patient is conscious, it is imperative that the procedure of placing him into the respirator and the purpose of this treatment be explained to him. Usually he is told that the respirator has been ordered so that he can relax and breathe more easily and thus get necessary rest and sleep. Often the patient is so exhausted from having to remain awake and consciously use his accessory muscles of respiration in an effort to breathe that he welcomes use of the respirator. Occasionally he becomes panicky and "fights" the machine so that adjustment is extremely difficult. A nurse must always remain with the patient and help him to breathe with the machine until he becomes accustomed to it.

Before the patient is placed in a respirator, provision must be made for his relative comfort and for care that will be necessary. The mattress should be covered with small sheets in sections that can be easily removed through the arm holes, and the following supplies should be in the respirator: a piece of plastice material to protect the sheet under the buttocks, bath towels, bath blankets, foot supports, and a thermometer. Soft material such as an old diaper or chamois skin should be used to protect the patient's throat and neck from the rubber collar.

The patient in a respirator must never, under any circumstances, be left alone. Patients have been known to die because an electric cord was inadvertently disconnected or because some other mechanical failure occurred. Auxiliary nursing personnel, relatives, and volunteers are often asked to stay with the patient when a nurse is unable to do so.

An important concept to remember in care of the patient in a respirator is that he needs exactly the same care as if he were not in this awkward enclosure. He needs to be turned, to have skin care, to have joints flexed and extended, to void, and to defecate regularly. He needs to take fluids and food in normal amounts. Teamwork is essential, and planning should be done so that several essential activities can be carried on at once. For example, when turning the patient to relieve pressure on the sacrum, one can also sponge the back, flex the knees, and massage the ankles, provided that equipment for these procedures has been placed in the respirator before the patient has been turned. If the patient can be out of the respirator or can breathe on his own for a short time, this time is used by several nurses and attendants to give essential care (Fig. 199).

The greatest care must be taken in helping patients to swallow when in the respirator. It is extremely difficult for anyone to swallow comfortably when lying on his back or in mild hyperextension, much less when breathing cannot be controlled. Swallowing must be done on exhalation. The patient should first try small amounts of liquid or semisolid foods; foods that tend to cause choking—for example, mashed potatoes—must be avoided. A suction machine should always be on hand when a patient first attempts to swallow when in a respirator. If the patient vomits, he must be removed from the respirator at once to prevent aspiration into the lungs.

Although some patients are overly anxious to be out of the machine, others become overly dependent upon it. Effort is made to stop the machine for a few seconds or minutes at intervals. Oxygen may be given during this time, and a nurse stands at the patient's head, encouraging him to breath normally and timing his efforts while others give physical care. At first the patient is left on the carriage of the machine so that he knows that its use is immediately available. He may then be moved to a bed, where a chest respirator may be used, or to a *rocking bed*, which tilts at a specified rate and thus assists in breathing. As the head of the bed goes down, the viscera fall against the diaphragm and assist in exhalation, while, as the head goes up, the diaphragm falls toward the abdominal viscera and assists in inhalation.

The patient's family. Few illnesses tax the entire physical and emotional resources of the patient's family as do the chronic neuro-

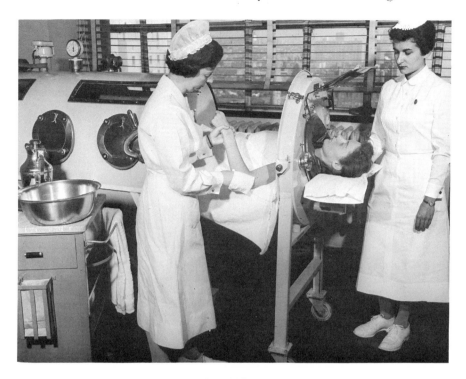

Fig. 199

A patient being weaned from a respirator needs encouragement. Short periods out of the respirator are also used to give essential care.

logic diseases. It is imperative that the family participate in long-term plans for the patient. Members of the family may have severe emotional reactions and difficulties in adjustment that may require the assistance of specially trained persons, such as a psychiatrist. A medical social worker or spiritual adviser can be invaluable in listening to close members of the family and in helping them to think through their own futures so that they may determine a constructive plan of action for caring for a loved one who has a serious neurologic disease. Both the patient and his family need time. Sometimes the enormity of the significance of the diagnosis cannot be grasped for weeks or even months by either the patient or his family. Toxic polyneuritis in a young husband and father and multiple sclerosis in a young mother are examples of problems of such magnitude that long-term plans cannot be made quickly.

The family may need help in accepting the concept of self-help and independence for the patient. Upon learning the diagnosis, their first reaction may be to do too much for the patient and thus to hasten his complete dependence upon them. Later,

when the reality of the burden becomes clearer, they may tire of the restrictions imposed upon them and become impatient or needlessly exhausted. Care of the patient may fall too much on one relative who most readily assumes the burden. Sometimes this family member eagerly takes on the greatest responsibility yet resents it. She may complain that others do not contribute, yet avoids their assistance when it is offered. By reacting in this way she may be meeting some particular emotional needs of her own. Family crises may sometimes be prevented by careful initial family planning in which each member assumes some specific part of the total responsibility. In the hospital the medical social worker may be the key person who brings about joint planning by the family. In the patient's home the public health nurse may provide this help.

The relative who is to give nursing care to a chronically ill or terminally ill person should be taught how to give it with a minimum of strain to herself and a minimum of discomfort to the patient. Sometimes the relative may enroll in a home-nursing course given by the local chapter of the American National Red Cross and thus be prepared for the time when the patient will need more physical help. In the hospital, at the bedside of the patient, or in the clinic she may learn specific techniques and procedures that will be needed. She should know that public health nurses from local agencies are available to give assistance and instruction in the home. If the patient has been in the hospital, it is well for the public health nurse to visit his home to review the plan of care with responsible relatives and to consult, if necessary, with the doctor or with nurses in the hospital. Members of the family should be prepared for anticipated changes but should not be given cause for worry about situations that may not arise.

If the patient with neurologic disease has marked personality changes, aphasia, or convulsions, the family may even be afraid of him. Because they are unaware that he may fully understand, they may make tactless remarks in his presence. When the patient is admitted to the hospital, it is often desirable to have him escorted directly to his room and then to take the family aside to ascertain their insight into the situation. This interview gives the nurse valuable information for beginning a nursing care plan, and it gives her an opportunity to help interpret the patient's actions and responses so that his family may not inadvertently upset him.

The neurologic examination

The patient with neurologic disease dreads examinations and tests more than many other patients. He may fear that certain procedures, such as a spinal puncture, will cause further disability, and he may be reluctant to have his limitations proved or exposed. He may sense a serious prognosis yet dread its confirmation. It is essential that all tests and procedures be thoroughly explained to the patient before they are begun. Even the neurologic examination itself is trying and

exhausting. Usually the patient wears little clothing, and he may be examined by more than one person. It is upsetting to him to be examined for alteration in gait, equilibrium, hand grip, and other similar abilities even when the examination is done gently and with kindliness.

The neurologic examination includes a complete history, with detail not solicited in a general physical examination. The patient should be prepared for a long and tedious procedure that is sometimes done in stages, depending on the condition of the patient and the urgency of completing the study.

Equipment needed. In addition to the necessary materials for a routine examination, the neurologic examination tray should contain the following: a straight pin that is usually stuck through a tongue blade and a safety pin to be used for testing the sensation of pain, a wisp of cotton and a fine, soft brush to test the sensation of touch, tuning forks to test vibratory sense and hearing, a dynamometer to measure hand grip, substances with distinctive odors such as peppermint, vanilla, coffee, and tobacco to test the sense of smell, test tubes for hot and cold water to test heat and cold sensations, and sugar, salt, vinegar, and quinine or cascara to test the sense of taste. A diagram of the anterior and posterior surfaces of the body on which to indicate areas of abnormal tactile sensations is needed. This diagram helps the doctor determine the nerves involved and may indicate the location of the primary lesion.

Vocabulary and definitions. Certain neurologic signs are of interest to the nurse. Also, she must learn a special vocabulary if the study of the patient's symptoms and the results of the examination are to be meaningful to her.

A positive *Kernig's sign* indicates irritation of the meninges. The sign is positive when there is pain upon extension of the lower leg while the thigh is maintained in a flexed position upon the abdomen. This sign is elicited with the patient in a back-lying or sitting position.

A positive *Brudzinski's sign* also indicates meningeal irritation. The sign is considered positive when attempts to flex the head on the chest result in involuntary flexion of the ankle, knee, or hip. This test is done with the patient lying on his back or sitting on the side of the bed.

A positive *Babinski's sign* (or reflex) indicates lesions in the pyramidal tract. The sign is positive if the great toe extends upward when the sole of the foot is stroked. Usually a broken tongue blade is used to stroke the foot.

A positive *Romberg's sign* indicates locomotor ataxia or degeneration of the posterior column of the spinal cord. The sign is positive if there is inability to maintain body balance when standing with the feet close together and the eyes closed.

An *area of anesthesia* is one in which sensation is absent. *Hyperesthesia* means that sensation is intensified, and *paralgesia* indicates a painful sensation. *Parasthesia* is an abnormal sensation such as burning, pricking, or itching.

Hemiplegia is paralysis of one-half of the body (linear division), *paraplegia* refers to paralysis of the lower half of the body, and *quadriplegia* means that all four extremities and the trunk are paralyzed.

The terms used to describe spasms and convulsive movements are as follows: *tonic movements* are fixed contractions of the muscles that usually draw joints into a position of flexion, and *clonic movements* are alternating contractions and relaxation of muscles. *Spastic* refers to a state of muscular rigidity or tenseness, while *flaccid* or flail-like means that the involved part is completely relaxed and limp. These terms usually describe the more common kinds of paralysis or partial paralysis. A *spasm* is an involuntary, sudden movement or convulsive muscular contraction that the patient cannot control. A *tic* is a spasmodic muscular contraction usually of the face, neck or shoulder muscles that may be involuntary or the result of habit. *Ataxia* means lack of coordination in attempting to perform a planned, purposeful motion.

Tests of special nerves and groups of nerves. The first cranial, or olfactory, nerve is tested by blindfolding the patient, covering each nostril in turn, and having him smell and identify certain odors such as coffee.

The second, or optic, nerve is tested grossly by having the patient count the number of fingers one holds up and more minutely by having the patient identify letters on a Snellen's chart (see p. 821 for details of examination of the eyes). Visual field examinations test not only the ability to see directly ahead but also over a broad normal field. The test, performed on each eye separately, may be done crudely by standing behind the patient and moving the fingers toward the eyes from various points above, below, and at either side of the field of vision; the patient indicates when he sees them. If the test is done in a dark room, the results may be specifically plotted on a diagram with the use of a flashlight and a special chart known as a perimetry chart. This examination identifies patients who may have lesions that press on one side of the optic nerve, cutting off half the vision of each eye.

Examination of the eyes with an *ophthalmoscope* reveals the condition of the blood vessels in the retina. Congestion of the optic nerve head (choked disc) can be seen by an ophthalmoscopic examination and is particularly indicative of increased intracranial pressure.

The third, fourth, and sixth cranial nerves are examined by noting the size and reaction of the pupils and the movements of the eye. Double vision (diplopia), squint (strabismus), and involuntary rhythmic movements of the eyeballs (nystagmus) may indicate involvement of these nerves.

The fifth cranial, or trigeminal, nerve is tested by noting sensation caused by pricking or lightly brushing the face. The patient is asked to make chewing and biting movements and to open his mouth against resistance. If the fifth nerve is involved, severe pain radiates to the midline of the face and neck in the involved side.

The seventh, or facial, nerve is tested for its motor components by having the patient raise his eyebrows, close his eyes and resist attempts to open them, show his teeth, smile, frown, and whistle. The sense of taste on the anterior two-thirds of the tongue is tested by applying liquid testing solutions along the outer part of each side of the tongue and having the patient identify the taste as sugar, salt, acid, or bitter.

The eighth, or acoustic, nerve is tested by having the patient listen to whispering, the tick of a watch, and a tuning fork at prescribed distances. Special hearing tests with an audiometer give more accurate information about the acoustic nerve. (See p. 585.)

The ninth and tenth cranial nerves are tested by noting the movements of the tongue, by noting the gag reflex, and by having the patient speak and cough. If there is involvement of the vagus nerve, the voice is weak and hoarse, and coughing is not effective.

The eleventh, or spinal accessory, nerve is tested by checking the sternocleidomastoid and trapezius muscles for atrophy or weakness, by having the patient rotate his head, and by having him shrug his shoulders against resistance.

The twelfth, or hypoglossal, nerve is tested by having the patient stick out his tongue. Lateral deviation indicates paralysis of the nerve on the side to which the tongue turns.

Motor and sensory function of the trunk muscles are checked in detail. For example, asking the patient to close his eyes and place his index finger on his nose tests both his coordination and his sense of touch and of position. Reflexes throughout the body are tested. The patellar reflex (knee jerk) and Achilles tendon reflex (foot flexion) tests are familiar to all nurses. Sense of position may be tested by having the patient close his eyes and tell the examiner where his hand or foot has been placed. Sense of touch may be tested by having the patient feel and identify materials of various textures. The autonomic nervous system is examined by noting the general appearance of the skin, whether its temperature and color are normal, and whether perspiration is either excessive or less than normal.

Special examinations

Special examinations of the nervous system include study of the cerebrospinal fluid, x-ray study of the spinal cord and brain, and measurement of electrical activity of the brain.

Examination of cerebrospinal fluid. The cerebrospinal fluid normally is a water-clear fluid that is formed in the lateral ventricles of the brain. It passes through the third ventricle, the aqueduct of Sylvius, the fourth ventricle, and finally into the cisterna magna at the base of the brain. From this location between the arachnoid and the dura mater, the fluid bathes the entire brain surface and passes down to surround the spinal cord. The main purpose of the spinal fluid appears to be to provide mechanical protection for the brain and spinal cord. The exact manner of its production and absorption is not entirely clear nor is the rate of its production clearly determined. It is thought that approximately 150 to 200 ml. of spinal fluid circulate within the system.

Spinal fluid normally is under slight positive pressure; 80 to 180 mm. of water is considered normal. It is measured on a manometer when a spinal puncture is done. When a brain tumor or other space-occupying lesion is within the cranium, the spinal fluid pressure usually is greatly increased. For this reason a lumbar puncture is not done lest the quick reduction in pressure produced by removal of spinal fluid cause the brain structures to herniate into the foramen magnum, which would put pressure upon vital centers in the medulla and might cause sudden death. The experienced neurologist often writes "no spinal tap" on the patient's chart to be certain that no other medical staff member attempts this procedure.

Normally, each milliliter of spinal fluid contains 0 to 5 lymphocytes. An increase in the number of cells may indicate an infection. Tuberculosis and viral infections may cause an increase in lymphocytes, while pyogenic infections may cause increase in polymorphonuclear leukocytes, which may be in large enough numbers to make the fluid cloudy. Bacterial infections such as tuberculous meningitis often lower the blood sugar level from the normal level of 40 to 60 mg. per 100 ml. (approximately one-half the normal level). They may also reduce the chloride level from the normal 720 to 750 mg. per 100 ml. In the presence of degenerative diseases and when a brain tumor is present, the spinal fluid protein is usually increased from the normal level of 30 to 50 mg. per 100 ml. Study of the spinal fluid may occasionally reveal the actual organism causing disease. The serologic test for syphilis may be positive in spinal fluid even when the blood serology is negative.

Blood in the spinal fluid indicates hemorrhage somewhere in the system. It may be caused by a fracture of the base of the skull that has torn blood vessels, or it may be due to the rupture of a blood vessel, which may occur, for example, with a congenital aneurysm. Occasionally, the first specimen of spinal fluid contains blood from slight bleeding at the point of the puncture. For this reason the specimens of fluid are numbered, and the first one is not used to determine the cell count.

The strictest aseptic technique is mandatory in all procedures in which the cerebrospinal fluid system is entered. The nurse is responsible for seeing that all equipment is sterile and that safe technique is used throughout the procedure. She explains the procedure to the patient and sees that a permit for treatment is signed if hospital policy requires it. If the patient is uncertain about any details of the procedure, the nurse should not hesitate to ask the physician to give him further explanation. The nurse tells the patient what to expect during the procedure and how he may help to make it as uncomplicated as possible.

Details of the *spinal puncture procedure* and a list of the equipment needed are given in texts on fundamentals of nursing. The doctor may explain to the patient that the needle will be inserted below the level of the spinal cord so that there is little danger of injury (Fig. 200). He should be helped to lie with both his knees and his head acutely flexed, and he should have constant nursing attention during the procedure. Even when a local anesthetic is used (usually 1% procaine), the patient should be prepared to feel slight pain and pressure as the dura is entered. The patient should be reminded not to move suddenly. He may be told that he may experience a sharp shooting pain down one leg. This pain is caused by the needle's coming close to a nerve and is similar to hitting one's "funnybone"; however, the nerve actually is floating in fluid and is safe from injury.

The nurse prepares the equipment, assists the doctor, watches the patient during and immediately following the procedure for signs of reaction such as pulse changes,

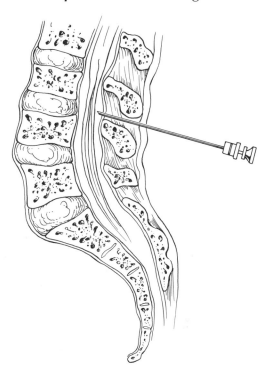

Fig. 200

The position and angle of the needle when a lumbar puncture is done. Note that the needle is in the fourth lumbar interspace below the level of the spinal cord.

arranges for suitable labeling and disposition of specimens, and replaces equipment. If she holds the manometer during the procedure, she must hold it above the point where the doctor's hands need to come in contact with it since her hands are not sterile (Fig. 201). The nurse may be asked to compress the jugular vein first on one side, then on the other side, and finally on both sides at the same time, and she may be asked to help the doctor to recall the spinal pressure under each of these circumstances. The pressure should be exerted with the fingers flat against the patient's neck, avoiding his trachea. This test, known as the *Queckenstedt test*, is simple but may alarm the patient if he has not been informed that pressure may be exerted on his neck for a few seconds.

Headache is fairly common following a lumbar puncture. Although its exact cause

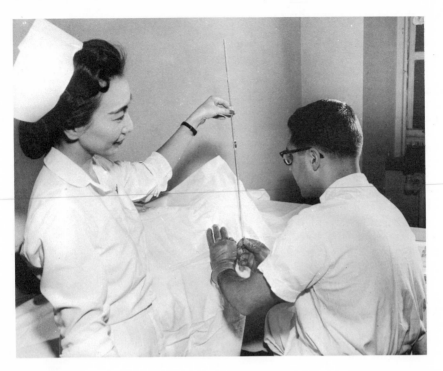

Fig. 201

The nurse assisting the doctor with a lumbar puncture may support the manometer and record essential readings.

is unknown, it is thought to be due to loss of spinal fluid through the dura. The sharpness and size of the needle used, the skill of the doctor, and the emotional state of the patient are probably the determining factors in whether or not a headache will develop. If one does develop, it is treated with bed rest, an ice cap to the head, and acetylsalicylic acid. Most headaches from this cause disappear within twenty-four hours.

Lumbar punctures are often performed on patients who are ambulatory and who go home immediately after the procedure is completed. It has been found that they suffer no more from headaches than do those who are treated more conservatively with bed rest and no elevation of the head.

In a *cisternal puncture*, the cerebrospinal fluid system is tapped by inserting a short-beveled needle immediately below the occipital bone into the cisterna magna (Fig. 202). This procedure may be more frightening to the patient than a lumbar puncture since the approach is closer to the brain. The patient should have a detailed explanation by the doctor before any head preparation is done or before he is placed in the required position. A permit for operation is usually required. The back of the patient's neck may be shaved, and he is placed on his side at the edge of the bed or on a treatment table, with his head bent forward and held firmly by the nurse or another assistant. The patient is observed immediately following the procedure for dyspnea, apnea, and cyanosis, but these complications seldom occur. A cisternal puncture is often done on children. In some outpatient departments it is commonly done because it is considered less likely to be followed by headache than is a lumbar puncture.

Pneumoencephalography. Pneumoencephalography (air encephalography or encephalography) combines a spinal or a cisternal puncture with an x-ray examination. Air or oxygen is injected (25 to 30 ml.) and rises to the ventricles, where its presence can be noted upon x-ray examination. Abnormal shape, size, or position of the ventricles or failure of the ventricles to fill with

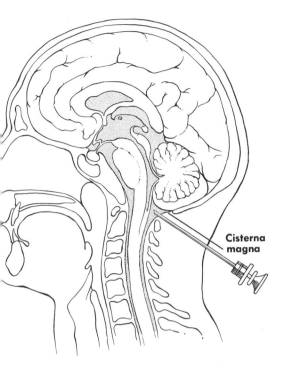

Cisterna magna

Fig. 202

The position of the needle when a cisternal puncture is done. Note the needle length and the short bevel.

the gas is diagnostically significant. (See Fig. 203.) The procedure usually is done under local anesthesia, but a general inhalation, rectal, or intravenous anesthetic may be used for nervous or unstable patients. Headache is usually severe during and following encephalography. Nausea and vomiting are not uncommon. A nurse must be in constant attendance to observe the patient while a second person assists the doctor.

The patient who is to have a pneumoencephalogram may be prepared as for surgery with no food or fluids by mouth for six hours and sedation the evening before and a half hour before the treatment is started. A permit must be signed and dentures removed (p. 179).

The procedure may be started in the patient's room or in the treatment room. The patient is then taken to the x-ray department, where the pictures are taken. The equipment needed is the same as that for a spinal puncture with the addi-

tion of a three-way stopcock, a 20 ml. syringe with which to withdraw spinal fluid and inject air, a calibrated glass to measure any fluid that is removed, and an ampule of caffeine sodium benzoate and an ampule of epinephrine (Adrenalin) for use in case of respiratory distress. Emergency oxygen equipment is also often requested.

The pressure of the spinal fluid is taken as soon as the needle is inserted into the lumbar spine. As the procedure is carried out, the patient is watched carefully for headache, nausea, and vomiting, and his pulse rate, respiratory rate, blood pressure, and color are noted and recorded. The head of the bed or table is gradually raised, and some physicians like to have the patient's head gently rotated after the air has been injected in the belief that this gives better filling of the lateral ventricles.

Upon return from the x-ray department the patient is placed in bed with the head flat. Usually he is more comfortable without a pillow. If a general anesthetic has been given, he is kept on his side and constantly attended until awake. Blood pressure, pulse rate, and respiratory rate are taken every fifteen minutes for the first hour, then every half hour and every hour for several hours or until they become stabilized. They are then taken every four hours. Any changes should be reported to the doctor at once. The patient who has a severe headache may benefit from an ice cap to the head, and he should be given fluids through a straw so that his head is not raised. Acetylsalicylic acid, codeine, meperidine hydrochloride (Demerol) or dextropropoxyphene hydrochloride (Darvon) are given for severe headache. If the patient complains of noises in his head, he should be assured that they are temporary since they are caused by gas in the ventricles and will disappear when the gas is absorbed. If the patient has any history of convulsions or unpredictable behavior, side rails should be placed on the bed and a mouth gag should be at the bedside. Occasionally an emergency tracheotomy set is kept on the unit for forty-eight hours after this procedure has been done.

Occasionally, reactions to pneumoencephalography are severe, including continued vomiting, convulsions, shock, and signs of increased intracranial pressure with respiratory difficulty. Severe prolonged headache

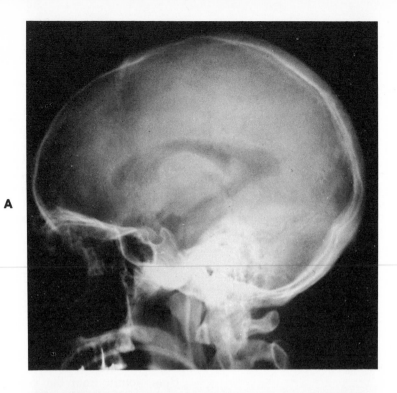

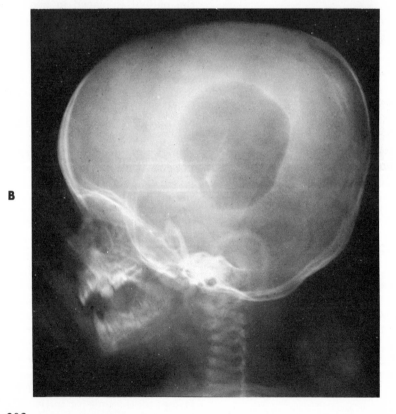

Fig. 203

Pneumoencephalogram. **A,** Lateral view shows the outline of a normal ventricle.
B, Lateral view shows marked distention of the ventricle with cerebrospinal
fluid (due to hydrocephalus).

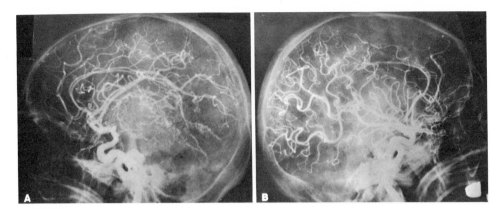

Fig. 204

A, Arteriogram showing elevation of middle cerebral arteries by glioblastoma multiforme containing abnormal vascular network. **B,** Arteriogram showing the opposite normal side for comparison. (From Moseley, H. F., editor: Textbook of surgery, ed. 3, St. Louis, 1959, The C. V. Mosby Co.)

may also follow this diagnostic procedure, although headache usually disappears after twenty-four to thirty-six hours. For the first day or two the patient should be fed and encouraged to be as quiet as possible. He should have assistance even in turning from side to side. Usually after forty-eight hours he can be out of bed gradually. He may find that his headache and nausea increase when he is up, but they will be relieved by lying flat again and will gradually subside.

Ventriculography. Ventriculography is similar to pneumoencephalography except that air is introduced directly into the lateral ventricles through trephine openings (burr holes) in the skull. This procedure is always done in the operating room. It may be used when the suspected diagnosis is such that a spinal puncture is contraindicated because of extreme pressure within the skull or because the spinal canal is blocked. The preparation is similar to that for an encephalogram except that the top or the back of the head must be partially shaved depending on the doctor's orders. An intravenous or general anesthetic is usually used, and the patient may go directly from the x-ray department to the operating room for attempted removal of a tumor or for other necessary brain surgery. If the roentgenogram is normal, the patient is cared for in a manner

similar to that following encephalography. Tissues and skin over the burr holes are sutured and the wounds covered with a collodion dressing.

Arteriography. In this diagnostic procedure a radiopaque substance is injected into the carotid artery. Roentgenograms taken immediately afterward may reveal an intracranial aneurysm, anomaly, or ruptured vessel. The large blood vessels of the circle of Willis at the base of the brain and the larger vessels penetrating the cerebrum can often be seen by this means (Fig. 204). Before the test is performed, a permit is signed by the patient or a responsible relative. Usually a sedative is given the night before if necessary, and scopolamine or atropine sulfate and sodium phenobarbital or Demerol are given a half hour before the procedure is done. Occasionally, when the patient is confused or extremely restless, a general anesthetic may be given If this is necessary, the procedure is usually done in the operating room. If the dye can be injected directly into the carotid vessel without surgical exposure of the artery and if general anesthesia is not necessary, usually the procedure is done in the x-ray department.

Following the test, the patient is watched for changes in the vital signs such as pulse,

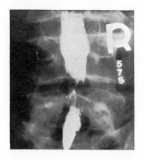

Fig. 205

A myelogram showing an almost complete block of the interspace between the fourth and fifth lumbar vertebrae. (From Moseley, H. F., editor: Textbook of surgery, ed. 3, St. Louis, 1959, The C. V. Mosby Co.)

blood pressure, and respirations. Decreased hand grip upon plantar pressure and facial weakness on the side opposite the injection are significant. Convulsive seizures or aphasia may occur. Occasionally a delayed allergic reaction to the dye occurs, and this reaction may be serious (p. 77). An ice collar applied to the neck helps to prevent bleeding from the vessel and local edema, which might cause respiratory difficulty. Usually, however, the patient experiences little, if any, discomfort and can resume his usual activities within a few hours.

Myelography. In this test either a gas or a radiopaque liquid is injected into the subarachnoid space, usually in the lumbar area, in an attempt to identify a lesion of the spinal cord or in the spinal canal by the distortion it produces (Fig. 205). This test is most often done as part of the diagnosis of cord tumor and occasionally when herniation of an intervertebral disk is suspected. The procedure is similar to that for a spinal puncture except that after the air or the radiopaque substance is injected, the patient's head is elevated on two pillows and he is taken to the x-ray department. After fluoroscopic examination and roentgenograms are completed, the doctor removes the dye, if it is used, by doing another lumbar puncture because it can cause serious irritation to the meninges. If some of it remains, care is taken to keep the patient's head elevated, and repeated attempts to remove the dye are made under fluoroscopy. One disadvantage of this test is the irritating quality of the available dyes. Therefore, the test is not done when relatively certain diagnosis can be made by other means, and air is often used in preference to the dye.

Electroencephalography. The electroencephalogram is a recording of the electrical activity of the brain amplified many times and recorded in a manner similar to that of the electrocardiogram. Certain characteristic patterns in the record are normal, and by study of the recordings of brain action, areas of abnormal action can sometimes be detected. This test is only an adjunct to other diagnostic tests, but it may be helpful in locating the site of a lesion. Before the examination the patient should be quiet, and the procedure should be explained to him so that no undue excitement occurs. The scalp should be clean, but no other local preparation is necessary. Approximately sixteen tiny electrodes are attached to the scalp with collodion, and the patient should be prepared for this procedure. No hair need be cut, which is often reassuring to the patient. (See Fig. 206.) Occasionally the electrodes used are tiny pins that are stuck into the scalp. The patient should know that this procedure will not be really painful because there are very few nerve endings in the scalp. The examination is done in a special room where outside electrical activity is eliminated. The patient usually sits in a comfortable chair or lies on a stretcher or table with his eyes closed. The test may last for an hour or more.

Radioactive iodine–tagged albumin test. Albumin tagged with radioactive iodine has proved useful in locating tumors within the skull cavity; approximately 70% can be localized by this means. Solutions containing the radioactive substance are injected intravenously. Location of a tumor can be determined by using a Geiger-Müller counter since tumor cells tend to hold the radioactive substance. This procedure may be referred to as the scanning test.

Caloric testing. Testing the equilibrium by dropping water into the auditory canal often is done to differentiate neurologic disorders.

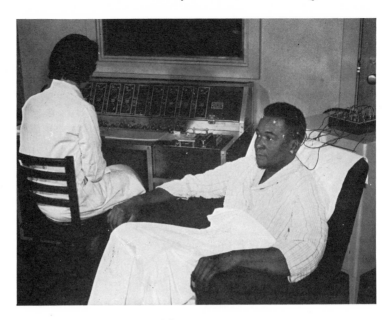

Fig. 206

A patient ready to have an electroencephalo-gram. (From de Gutiérrez-Mahoney, C. G., and Carini, Esta: Neurological and neurosurgical nursing, ed. 4, St. Louis, 1965, The C. V. Mosby Co.)

Degenerative diseases

Multiple sclerosis

Multiple sclerosis is a common neurologic disease in northern climates. The exact prevalence of the disease is not known since in many instances a diagnosis is not made, but probably at least 300,000 persons in the United States are affected. The onset of symptoms usually occurs between 20 and 40 years of age. Symptoms rarely occur before 15 or after 50 years of age. The course of the disease is estimated to be 12 to 27 years. Multiple sclerosis has serious implications for family life since it affects men and women in the active, productive years, when their responsibilities are greatest. Men and women are affected about equally.

The cause of multiple sclerosis is unknown. Mineral deficiency, toxic substances, viruses, and disturbance of blood clotting mechanisms are a few suspected contributory causes, but there is no real evidence that any of them is involved. Patchy, irregular areas of degeneration appear in the white matter of the brain and in the outer part of the spinal cord. The outer myelin sheath of the spinal cord can be compared to the insulation on an electric wire, and its destruction causes interruption of nerve pathways. Because of the wide distribution of areas of degeneration, there is a larger variety of signs and symptoms in multiple sclerosis than in any other neurologic disease.

There is evidence of partial healing of the areas of degeneration, which accounts for the transitory nature of many early symptoms. The scarring that occurs at the site of the degenerative lesion gives the name sclerosis to the disease.

Multiple sclerosis may be acute or chronic. Usually there are acute exacerbations and remissions that may last for a year or more, although eventually exacerbations will recur. There is no record of any patient's having recovered from the disease, although many have lived for twenty or more years and have died from other causes. Exacerbations may be aggravated or precipitated by fatigue, chilling, and emotional disturbances.

Early symptoms are usually transitory and may include double vision (diplopia), spots before the eyes (scotomas), blindness, tremor, weakness or numbness of a part of

865

the body such as the hand, fatigue, susceptibility to upper respiratory infections, and emotional instability. Many patients with early multiple sclerosis are considered neurotic by their associates and sometimes by their physicians because of the wide variety and temporary nature of symptoms and because of their emotional instability. As the disease progresses, symptoms may include nystagmus, disorders of speech, urinary frequency and urgency, constipation, and changes in muscular coordination and gait. Late symptoms may include urinary incontinence, difficulty in swallowing, and severe muscle spasm and contractures. Pain is not a symptom of multiple sclerosis except when there is severe muscle spasm. Death may be caused by pneumonia.

In the hospital, the nurse may care for the patient for short periods when he is admitted for diagnosis or for some other condition. She may also participate in terminal care of patients with advanced disease. Because many patients with multiple sclerosis are not hospitalized, she is likely to encounter them when she cares for patients in their homes as a public health nurse.

Medical treatment and nursing care. There is no specific treatment for multiple sclerosis. Warm baths, physical therapy, psychotherapy, and specific drugs for acquired infections are helpful. Effort is made to keep the patient working for as long as possible, and many men have worked for five to ten years and even longer after the onset of the first symptoms. Women can be helped to plan their shopping, housework, and other duties so that they may continue to function as wives and mothers even when the disease is advanced. The decision as to whether or not the patient is told his diagnosis rests with the doctor, and there is not full agreement among doctors as to the proper course of action. Usually the decision is made on an individual basis and depends on the patient's emotional makeup and upon his family's ability to cope with the economic, social, and emotional problems that a condition of this kind presents.

The patient with multiple sclerosis should have a daily routine for rest and activity, and he should adhere to it strictly. Rest must be balanced with adequate exercise. The patient is usually advised to exercise regularly but never to the point of extreme fatigue. Because he almost always feels tired, he must look for some special sign that tells him he has exercised enough. If he does more, he may suffer ill effects. For example, a tight feeling in the chest may indicate that the patient must rest or else have severe discomfort. After an exacerbation, it may be difficult for the patient to resume exercises, but it is usually best for him to return to an established schedule as soon as possible.

One side of the body is usually affected more than the other, and the patient may learn to stabilize his gait by leaning toward his good side. The annoyance of having the foot slap forward in taking a step may sometimes be overcome by the patient if he puts the heel down in a pronounced fashion and rolls the weight forward on the side of the foot.

The patient with multiple sclerosis needs a peaceful, relaxed environment. He should never be hurried and should not be expected to respond quickly either physically or mentally. He may have slowness in speech and slowness in ability to respond, and this difficulty should be ignored by persons around him. Members of the family and friends need help in understanding this problem and in meeting it calmly. The patient may have sudden explosive emotional outbursts of crying or laughing brought on by such simple acts as putting something hot into the mouth. Close members of the family must protect both the patient and visitors from the embarrassment of prolonged emotional outbursts. Reminding the patient of something sad may stop him from laughing and holding the mouth open will sometimes stop the crying.

A sense of optimism and well-being (euphoria) seems to be characteristic of persons with multiple sclerosis, especially during remissions. It is suspected that this reaction is due largely to the patient's attempts to reassure himself that his condition is not so serious as is supposed. This response is helpful to the patient in many ways, but sometimes it may lead him to overdo and thus increase symptoms.

Good general hygiene is necessary for the patient with multiple sclerosis and includes a well-balanced diet with plenty of high-vitamin foods and fluids. Obesity must be avoided, because it makes it more difficult for the patient to handle himself and detracts from his appearance. The patient should sleep eight hours each night and should have a rest period after lunch. Fresh air and sunshine are good, but chilling and overheating must be avoided because they may aggravate symptoms or bring on exacerbations.

Since association with others is good for physical and mental health, the patient with multiple sclerosis must be encouraged and helped to remain an active, participating member of his family and his community for as long as possible. Personal cleanliness adds to a feeling of acceptance and well-being; consequently these patients should be encouraged to pay careful attention to personal appearance even though they may sometimes feel too tired to put forth the effort. The patient should be encouraged to develop interests and hobbies that will help make up for things he should not do, such as driving a vehicle, and that will help to fill the time when the physical activity becomes more difficult. Music, writing, reading, and question games are good hobbies to develop. Interest in politics and in world affairs, which may be followed on the radio if sight is lost, may stand the patient in good stead. The development of a religious faith should be encouraged.

The National Multiple Sclerosis Society* is a national voluntary organization founded in 1946. Its functions are to encourage the finance research, to gather statistics, and to act as an information center for patients and for the public. Membership is open to doctors nurses, and other health and welfare workers and to patients and their families. Local organizations are located in many of our larger cities.

Paralysis agitans (Parkinson's disease)

Parkinson's disease is a slowly progressive degenerative disease of unknown cause in which there is destruction of nerve cells in the basal ganglia of the brain. It may follow encephalitis and occasionally occurs following carbon monoxide poisoning. The

disease usually affects older persons and is often associated with arteriosclerosis, although this disease is not thought to be a direct cause. Approximately 200,000 persons in the United States have the disease, and its incidence appears to be increasing. Since the disease is more common in persons past their mid-fifties, the increase is probably the result of the increase in the number of persons in this age group.

Parkinson's disease begins with a faint tremor and progresses so slowly that the patient is seldom able to recall its onset. There is no true paralysis and no loss of sensation. Tremor and muscle rigidity are the two outstanding signs of the disease. Muscle rigidity seems to prevent normal response in commonly performed acts and leads to characteristic changes that make the diagnosis almost unmistakable to persons who have observed patients with the disease. There is a masklike appearance to the face and slowed, monotonous speech. Drooling may occur because of the difficulty of swallowing saliva. This may cause skin irritation, which is best prevented or treated by frequent sponging followed by protecting the skin with an emollient such as cold cream. There is a characteristic shuffling gait in which the patient tends to walk on his toes. The trunk is bent forward, and the arms fall rigidly at the sides and do not swing as in a normal rhythmic gait. Neuromuscular control may be altered so that the patient is unable to stop his propulsive gait until he meets an obstruction; finally, he may become unable to walk at all. The patient usually has a moist, oily skin. Judgment defect and emotional instability may occur, but intelligence is not impaired. The appetite may be increased, and there is heat intolerance probably because of the activity of the persistent tremor. All signs and symptoms increase with fatigue, excitement, and frustration.

Medical treatment and nursing care. Treatment for Parkinson's disease is only palliative. Drugs that produce relaxation of the muscles, such as scopolamine hydrobromide and related drugs (hyoscyamus and stramonium), are widely used. These drugs are more effective in lessening muscle rigidity than in controlling the tremor. One of the disadvantages in the use of these drugs is

*Home office: 257 Park Ave. South, New York, N. Y. 10010.

that in order to get the desired effect upon the muscles, the dosage must be such that unpleasant side effects, such as dryness of the mouth, occur. Many other drugs are being used in attempts to find some that are effective yet produce fewer side effects. One synthetic atropine-like preparation, *trihexyphenidyl* (Artane), is used widely. The dosage is usually 2 mg. (1/30 grain) in tablet form given by mouth three or four times a day. Phenobarbital and bromides are used to allay excitement and thereby decrease the tremor and treat the insomnia that is common in this disease. Some of the antihistaminic drugs such as phenindamine tartrate (Thephorin) also seem to be of some benefit.

In recent years a surgical procedure has been used with some success in treatment of selected patients with Parkinson's disease. Descriptions of successful operations in popular magazines have led some patients and their families to believe that a cure for all patients has been found. The nurse should refer those asking her about the operation to a qualified neurologist. Many patients cannot be treated surgically. Results seem to be best in younger patients who have unilateral involvement following other disease and who have marked tremor and rigidity. Treatment consists of destroying portions of the globus pallidus (relieves rigidity) and/or the thalamus (relieves tremor) in the brain by means of cautery, removal, or injection of a chemical (alcohol). More recently, operative techniques involving cooling or freezing with liquid nitrogen (cryogenic surgery) have been attempted with good results in selected cases and with fewer complications than when cautery or alcohol were used.[8] Medications used to control rigidity and tremor are discontinued several days preoperatively so that patients' symptoms will be at their maximum during the operation.[47] Nursing care preoperatively includes seeing that nutrition is adequate as well as other general preoperative care.

Postoperative care includes the most careful attention to the vital signs, use of side rails to prevent accidents in the event of convulsions, disorientation, or temporary hemiplagia, and frequent turning and moving to prevent respiratory and circulatory complications. Excessive salivation and dif-

ficulty in blinking the eye on the operated side may be problems requiring special nursing care.

The progress of Parkinson's disease, a condition that often lasts for years, may be slowed by good nutrition, sufficient rest, moderate exercise in fresh air, and other measures that improve general health. Special attention should be paid to posture. Lying on a firm bed without a pillow during rest periods may help to prevent the spine from bending forward, and lying in the prone position also helps. Holding the hands folded behind the back when walking may help to keep the spine erect and prevent the annoyance of the arms falling stiffly at the sides. The tremor often is less apparent when the patient is sitting in an armchair since he can grip the arms of the chair and partially control the tremor in his hands and arms.

The patient with Parkinson's disease should continue to work as long as possible. Most physicians advise this unless the occupation is such that continued work is dangerous. The patient should reduce his regular work gradually while he builds up hobbies and interests in which he may engage when the disease becomes more advanced. Relatives must have complete understanding of the circumstances so that they may intelligently assist in the adjustments that will eventually be necessary. Such problems as danger of accidents, personality changes, and progressive helplessness must be anticipated. While drooling and difficulty in swallowing often limit the important social outlet of eating at group gatherings, the patient should have his meals at home with the family as long as possible. Feeding the patient becomes a real problem when the disease is far advanced because of the danger of choking in attempts to swallow; eventually, aspiration pneumonia may terminate the patient's life.

Myasthenia gravis

Myasthenia gravis is a relatively rare disease of unknown cause. It usually occurs in young adults. Nerve impulses fail to pass to muscles at the myoneural junction. The outstanding symptom is severe generalized fatigue to the point of exhaustion, which comes on quickly and, in the early stages of the disease, disappears quickly with rest.

Weakness of arms and hands first may be noticed when shaving or combing the hair. Facial muscles innervated by the cranial nerves are often affected, and it may not be possible for the patient to hold his eyelids open, to keep his mouth closed, or to chew and swallow. Occasionally the fatigue becomes so great that the patient cannot breathe, and a respirator must be used.

There is no known cure for myasthenia gravis. There is, however, a very marked improvement following the use of neostigmine (Prostigmin) or pyridostigmine (Mestinon). These drugs block the action of cholinesterase at the myoneural junction and allow action of acetylcholine, a chemical necessary for transmission of impulses to the muscles. Treatment is planned so that the patient may be maintained on the amount of drug that he can tolerate without side effects and yet carry out activities essential for normal living. Usually the patient is permitted to adjust his own dosage. Patients with myasthenia gravis must often change their method of earning a living. The nurse can help the patient and his family plan so that a minimum of energy is used in activities that are essential to his remaining relatively self-sufficient.

The patient with myasthenia gravis should take particular care of his health. Upper respiratory infections may be serious because he may not have the energy to cough effectively and may develop pneumonia or strangle. The patient who is living at home may feel more secure if there is a suction apparatus available and a member of his family knows how to use it if an emergency arises.

During acute episodes of the disease a tracheotomy set is kept in the patient's room ready for immediate use. Often it is necessary to use suction before the patient eats. If swallowing is too dangerous, a nasogastric tube is used, and great care must be taken to be certain that the tube is in the stomach before fluid is introduced, since the patient cannot cough to indicate its presence in the trachea. When caring for the patient with severe symptoms of myasthenia gravis, the nurse should remember that he is too weak to do anything for himself. Therefore, the patient may not take a drink and may not turn over in bed unless the nurse thinks to help him.

Progressive muscular dystrophy

Progressive muscular dystrophy is a relatively rare disease of unknown cause. The characteristic signs are muscle wasting and weakness. The disease develops most often in children, and boys are affected three times as often as girls. In approximately half of all cases there is a history of at least one other family member who has had the disease, and sometimes several siblings are affected.

There are several forms of the disease. One form, *pseudohypertrophic muscular dystrophy,* always develops during childhood and is characterized by enlargement of the muscles of the calf of the leg, accompanied by limitation of muscle function. The child gets from a horizontal to a standing position by turning on his abdomen, getting on his knees and "climbing up his thighs" with the use of his hands.

There is no effective medical treatment known for progressive muscular dystrophy. Physical therapy is sometimes given but its benefit is largely psychologic and to help delay contractures. Progressive muscular dystrophy does not have remissions but becomes very slowly but progressively worse. Few children who develop the disease live to adulthood.

Headache

Headache is the most common of all neurologic conditions. Probably over 98% of all persons suffer from this condition at some time in their lives. Headache is not a disease but a symptom of disease or of bodily reaction to harmful substances such as drugs or to excessive psychic pressure. The conditions that cause headache are almost infinite in number. Headaches may be caused by systemic disease or infection, by hypertension, or by pressure from a lesion such as a tumor. They may be caused by drugs, by foreign substances to which the person is sensitive, and by anoxia or inhalation of poisonous gases. They may be caused by eyestrain, by congestion in the sinuses, and by contraction of neck and scalp muscles due to fatigue or tension. Headaches often occur either before or during the menstrual period.

The nature of headaches varies, depending on their cause. For example, frontal headache may be caused by sinusitis and is characteristically relieved if the patient sits up and if local heat is applied to areas of the face overlying the sinuses. Brain tumors often cause dull, constant headaches. Headaches caused by emotional tension are usually steady and bandlike, usually precede or follow periods of tension, and became worse as the day progresses.

Headaches are probably treated by the laity more often than any other condition, including even the common cold. However, the public should know that persistent headaches are abnormal and need investigation by a physician. Patients have been known to treat a headache for months in the belief that it was due to a sinus infection, only to learn finally that it was due to hypertension or a brain tumor. Persistent headaches, even when physical cause has been ruled out, indicate that the patient should review his mode of living and make some adjustments. The nurse can sometimes help him see the wisdom of this course. She can also advise against the widespread use of the coal-tar analgesics in treatment of headaches. Occasional use of acetylsalicylic acid by the laity for minor indispositions is considered safe by most medical authorities. The use of phenacetin and similar preparations is not advisable unless prescribed by a physician. Prolonged and excessive use of these preparations has caused changes in blood cells.

Migraine syndrome

The layman's term for migraine headache is "sick headache." This condition is now believed to be much more common than was previously supposed. Before the acute onset there may be fatigue, chilliness, and irritability. These symptoms occasionally precede the acute attack by as much as a day or more. The acute symptoms vary in intensity but may be severe. Usually the headache is present upon awakening in the morning, and one side of the head is more affected than the other. Pain is usually keenest in the temporal area but may be anywhere in the head, and sometimes the face is also affected. There may be spots before the eyes, partial blindness, dizziness, nausea, and vomiting. The pain is often so intense that the patient is forced to seek isolation in a dark room. The acute attack usually lasts from a few

hours to a day but occasionally may last for a week or even longer. It concludes with a feeling of relaxation and need for sleep; dull head and neck pain, probably due to tension during the attack, may persist for some time.

The precipitating cause of migraine headache is a constriction and then a dilation of cerebral arteries. The cause of this is unknown, but it has been repeatedly demonstrated that nervous tension contributes to attacks. The person who develops migraine headaches is usually one who works hard and strives for perfection. Migraine headaches often follow a period of overwork and overstrain. After an attack, the patient feels better, probably because he has been forced to rest. Hope for a cure of the condition lies in changing the patient's attitudes toward the world and toward himself, and usually this is not easy.

Acetylsalicylic acid is seldom effective for the true migraine headache. The one drug that is quite effective is ergotamine tartrate. For best results ergotamine tartrate should be given early—before the condition is full-blown. The usual dosage is 2 mg. (1/30 grain) by mouth or 0.25 mg. (1/250 grain) subcutaneously or intramuscularly. Occasionally, it may be given intravenously for quicker action. The disadvantages of the drug are that it can cause nausea and vomiting, tingling sensations, and muscle tightness. Dihydroergotamine is a newer preparation that is being used and is believed to cause fewer toxic reactions.[6] It may be given by any of the parenteral routes.

Convulsive seizures

Convulsions may occur in many illnesses such as uremia, eclampsia, tetanus, and infections accompanied by extremely high temperature. Convulsions may be caused by poisons such as strychnine and may occur with increasing intracranial pressure such as that produced by a brain tumor. Children are more susceptible to convulsive seizures than are adults, presumably because their nervous system is less stable. Children may have generalized convulsions when temperature is elevated in many infectious diseases or with relatively minor conditions such as gastrointestinal upsets. Convulsions may be hysterical in origin rather than due to an organic disease. However, the patient seldom injures himself during a simulated seizure. Actually, simulated seizures are not true convulsions. By far the most common cause of convulsive seizures is epilepsy.

A common name for seizures is "fits." However, the term has an unpleasant connotation. "Attacks" is the best term to use in conversation with the laity. The words seizure and convulsions also describe the condition correctly.

Nursing care during a convulsive seizure

The nurse should observe the patient during a seizure and note the kind of convulsion that is occurring. In a *tonic convulsion* all muscles contract at once, whereas in a *clonic convulsion* opposing muscle groups alternately contract and relax, giving a jerking, convulsive movement of the body. Convulsions may start in one muscle or group of muscles and may spread to parts or all of the body; this type of seizure is known as a *jacksonian seizure*. A brain lesion may be the cause, and the part of the body in which the convulsive movements start may give a clue to its location. A focal attack is one that, by its location, reveals the part of the nervous system involved. The duration of the seizure should be noted. The nurse should observe whether the patient convulses equally in all parts of the body, whether his eyes turn to one side or to the other, and whether his pupils dilate or constrict. She should note how pulse and respirations are affected and whether there are changes in skin color. Grinding or clenching of the teeth, unusual diaphoresis, and urinary or fecal incontinence should be reported.

During a seizure, the nurse should protect the patient from injury. If the patient is in a precarious location where he might fall or otherwise injure himself, he should be lowered to the floor gently and a pillow or soft object placed under his head. Any equipment that might be harmful, such as an electric fan, should be placed out of reach. If the patient has fallen to the floor at the onset of the seizure, no attempt should be made to move him to a bed or sofa during the attack. A hard rubber wedge or two tongue blades fastened together with adhesive should be placed between his back teeth to prevent the tongue from being bitten. In the hospital, a padded tongue blade is kept at the bedside when seizures are anticipated. Care must be taken not to pry open the front or side teeth in an attempt to insert the gag since this may loosen them and cause the patient more inconvenience than a bitten tongue. Tight clothing should be loosened, but no restraint should be used.

Following a seizure, the nurse should question the patient to determine his state of consciousness and to learn if he knows where he is and if he has headache or any other complaints. Convulsions should be described in detail in the nurse's notes or on the special neurologic chart and reported to the physician at once.

Epilepsy

Epilepsy is one of the oldest diseases known to man. It was described in detail by Hippocrates. The term epilepsy means seizure or "state." The disease was at one time thought to be of divine origin and perhaps for this reason has been linked in the public mind with the occult, the strange, and the unmentionable. No disease has been more carefully concealed within families, and many attitudes toward the disease have persisted from early times to the present day. Attitudes may also be affected by the frightening experience of having seen a person during a severe seizure, by the belief that mental deterioration always occurs in epilepsy, and by the belief that epilepsy is inherited.

Because of the emotional overtones associated with convulsive disorders, it is often exceedingly difficult for parents to believe that their child might have such a condition. Sometimes they give an inadequate report to their family physician and receive the sought-for assurance that the child will probably outgrow the disorder. Many children would be spared severely traumatizing experiences at school and elsewhere if parents could only be convinced that the advice of a specialist is needed.

Epilepsy, often called *idiopathic* epilepsy, is a disease of unknown cause. The disease is not directly inherited, although abnormal brain waves, as shown in the electroencephalogram, are found in many relatives of persons having seizures, and it is likely that a predisposition to the disease is inherited. It is believed that some alteration of chemical balance touches off the seizure in susceptible persons. There are over 800,000 persons in the United States with some form of epilepsy, or approximately one out of every 200 of our population. Epilepsy is largely a disease of younger people, approximately three-fourths of sufferers having seizures before the age of 20 years. The life expectancy of persons with epilepsy is less than for the population as a whole, primarily because the person often dies of an accident incurred during a seizure.

Types of seizures. There are several types of epileptic seizures: grand mal seizures, petit mal seizures, and psychic equivalents. Status epilepticus is the term used when the patient goes from one grand mal seizure to another without regaining consciousness.

The term *grand mal seizures* (the big sickness) refers to major convulsions in which the patient may lose consciousness for minutes. This form of epilepsy is by far the most common. Convulsions are preceded by an *aura,* or warning sensation, in about 50% of all patients. This aura may be dizziness, spots before the eyes, numbness, or a wide variety of other sensations that the patient may find difficult to describe but that give him conclusive warning of the impending seizure. It serves a useful purpose in that it enables the patient to seek safety and privacy before the onset of the seizure. Occasionally it occurs as much as a day before the seizure so that the patient who works can remain at home and his fellow workers need not know of his attacks.

The grand mal seizure is usually heralded by a sharp cry as air is rapidly inhaled. Expiration of air does not follow naturally, the muscles are held rigid in a tonic contraction, (tonic phase), and the patient's skin becomes pale and then cyanotic. The eyes are opened widely and the pupils dilate and become fixed. After what seems to the observer to be a long time (usually only a few seconds), jerky (clonic phase) movements and quick irregular respirations begin and continue for as long as a minute or more. Often there is frothing at the mouth; this froth may be streaked with blood if the tongue or lips

have been bitten during the convulsion. During the clonic phase there may be fecal or urinary incontinence. As the convulsion subsides, the patient usually falls asleep, awakening moments of hours later with a dull headache and depression. There is no actual pain from the seizure, and many patients who have seizures during sleep realize that they have had a seizure only when, upon awakening, they find blood on the pillow or soiling of the bed. If convulsions occur often during sleep, it is necessary to protect the bed. However, protection should be given as inconspicuously as possible. Side rails are sometimes necessary, and they are likely to disturb the patient. It is possible that depression following seizures is caused in part by the knowledge that they have occurred.

The *petit mal attack* (the little sickness) is a momentary loss of consciousness. It occurs frequently in children and in adolescents at the onset of puberty. It does not produce the frightening spectacle of the grand mal seizure, but it can be most disconcerting to the patient and is seldom preceded by an aura. Petit mal attacks may be more difficult to control with the drugs available than grand mal seizures. While talking, the patient may stop for a moment and stare into space or drop his head and then go on talking without realizing that his conversation was interrupted. The child may be considered awkward by his parents, since, as he loses consciousness, he may appear to stumble and starts to fall but then regains consciousness before he really falls. He may drop his fork or glass of milk during meals, and again the reason may not be discovered for a time. A serious problem is the momentary loss of consciousness during play, such as when riding a bicycle in traffic, walking on a high fence, or climbing a tree.

Psychic equivalents, or *psychomotor epilepsy,* is a condition in which consciousness is lost or amnesia occurs but in which no convulsion ensues, and activity that in some ways appears normal may be continued during the attack. When the attack is over, the patient has no recollection of what took place. During the attack, he may appear drowsy, intoxicated, or violent, behave normally, or engage in violent antisocial activity. Since serious crimes have been committed by persons with psychic equivalents, diagnosis in such persons is sometimes of great interest to lawyers and judges as well as to medical scientists.

Status epilepticus, or a *continuous major convulsion,* is relatively rare, but it can lead to death from exhaustion. Emergency medical and nursing measures are often needed, and padded side rails must always be used. Inhalation anesthesia or large doses of barbiturates may be given in an effort to halt seizures. Concentrated solutions of glucose may be given intravenously to cause dehydration, and relatively short-acting drugs such as paraldehyde may be given for their sedative effect. Oxygen and cardiac stimulants should be readily available. A suction machine is often needed, and occasionally the head of the bed may be lowered and the patient turned on his side if there is danger of aspiration of mucus. The patient should be kept in a quiet room, and noise and confusion must be reduced to a minimum.

Medical treatment and nursing care. Some authorities believe that the only prevention for epilepsy is applied eugenics since the predisposition to develop the disease appears to be inherited.[5] There is no known cure for idiopathic epilepsy, although seizures can sometimes be controlled by dehydration, quieting the emotional state, increasing the acidity of the body, and using certain drugs. Treatment consists of trying to raise the threshold at which seizures occur. Bromides have long been considered helpful in the treatment of epilepsy, and phenobarbital has been widely used for years. Phenobarbital is usually given in small doses four or more times each day. However, so much of the drug may have to be given in order to control seizures that its sedative effect may give others the impression that the patient is mentally sluggish. One of the most satisfactory drugs is *diphenylhydantoin sodium* (Dilantin sodium). This drug has an anticonvulsive effect with less of a sedative effect than the barbiturates. The dosage is often 0.1 Gm. (1½ grains) three times a day by mouth for adults, but the dosage depends on the reaction of the individual patient to the drug and the severity of symptoms. Tremor, nystagmus, gastric disturbances, rash, and hypertrophy and bleeding of the gums are signs of toxicity from Dilantin sodium. Hypertrophy of the gums may be controlled in most instances by regular, vigorous massage.

Many newer drugs are being used in the treatment of epilepsy. Trimethadione (Tridione) is one that has been particularly useful for petit mal seizures, but it causes a peculiar photophobia (glare phenomenon) in which objects are perceived as if they were reflected from a bright snowy surface. This condition is relieved by wearing dark glasses. *Mephenytoin* (Mesantoin) is particularly helpful for grand mal seizures and for psychic equivalents. Most of the drugs that are helpful in epilepsy produce toxic effects, including severe kidney and liver damage, if given in too large doses and if patients are sensitive to them. The patient must remain under careful medical care, and an important nursing function is to emphasize to the patient that he must take the drug as ordered. He must not take more lest he have ill effects; neither must he decrease his dosage lest he have recurrence of convulsions. Patients with epilepsy tend to indulge in wishful thinking, to hope that they have "outgrown" the disease, and to believe that they can "get by" without taking the drug if they have gone for some time without a seizure.

Special diets in the treatment of epilepsy are prescribed less often than formerly. The *ketogenic diet,* planned to produce a mild ketosis or acidosis, which lessens the predisposition to have seizures, is so high in fat that it is not acceptable to most patients, but it is still ordered occasionally for children. A general well-balanced diet is usually recommended, with avoidance of too much food or fluids. Most patients seem to have fewer seizures when they are mildly dehydrated, presumably because there is less danger of cerebral edema. Alcoholic beverages, particularly beer, are likely to contribute to attacks. The patient should be advised to avoid excesses of any kind, both physical and emotional. This advice may be hard for the young person to follow since the need to participate with those in his age group often makes it difficult for him to avoid physical and emotional stresses.

Home care. Members of the family must learn to care for the person during and following a convulsion. They should have a mouth gag on hand at all times and should know how to insert it correctly, and they should be alert for accident hazards. One of the most important things for the family to learn is the need to be calm and accepting in regard to the patient's seizures. They should attempt to keep him from engaging in activity that may be dangerous and from exposure to curious persons during convulsions, but they should not contribute to the patient's feeling that he is different from others. More widespread general knowledge about the disease would help to prevent friends and neighbors from adding to the problems the patient and his family already have.

Public attitudes. One of the most important aspects in epilepsy is changing the public's attitude toward the disease. The patient and the public must be made to look upon convulsive seizures not as bizarre catastrophes but as relatively normal events that should be dealt with rationally. Many persons with epilepsy lead normal, productive lives. Indeed, many outstanding figures in world history had seizures, including Julius Caesar, Lord Byron, and Napoleon Bonaparte. Recent studies do not bear out the popular assumption that there usually is mental deterioration with epilepsy. Nor is there any evidence that personality changes are the result of pathologic progress. They are probably the result of society's attitude toward the person with epilepsy. For example, most people who are found to have epilepsy are automatically and immediately suspended from their work even when it is such that they are not dangerous to themselves or to others. It is almost impossible for a person with known epilepsy to get new employment, yet at least 80% of all persons with epilepsy are employable. The patient is haunted by fear of being seen during a seizure, fear of being found to have seizures, fear of losing his job, and fear of losing the companionship of others. Children with epilepsy have been segregated in separate schools, and only recently have some major cities passed laws ensuring children with epilepsy the right to attend the public schools if they are under adequate medical care. Children in many schools are barred from the classroom according to the inclina-

tion of the teacher. Limitation of environment and of educational opportunity often limits the patient's knowledge, but this does not mean that his learning capacity is poor.

Interest in epilepsy and in the problems of the epileptic person has been increased by various organizations such as the National Association to Control Epilepsy, Inc.* and the National Epilepsy League, Inc.† Membership in these organizations is open to medical science personnel, to persons with epilepsy, and to other interested citizens. The nurse should encourage public-spirited citizens to support these organizations.

Vascular disease

Cerebrovascular accident is the most common disease of the nervous system and in 1965 was the third highest cause of death in the United States. The condition is often associated with vascular disease of the heart, the kidneys, other organs, and the peripheral blood vessels. Usually the vessel involved in a cerebrovascular accident is a relatively large one and affects one side of the brain, which leads to partial or complete paralysis of the opposite side of the body (hemiplegia). *Shock, hemiplegia,* and *stroke* are other terms used in referring to cerebrovascular accidents. If a small blood vessel is involved there may be symptoms of short duration or that are less severe, as described later in this section.

Vascular lesions of the brain are often categorized as due to embolus, hemorrhage, or thrombosis. Cerebral embolism is usually caused by an embolus breaking away from a thrombosed blood vessel elsewhere in the body. This condition has been less frequent since the treatment of bacterial endocarditis with antibiotic drugs. Anticoagulant drugs given in treatment of coronary artery disease and early ambulation now also prevent much thrombosis of peripheral blood vessels in hospitalized patients.

Cerebral hemorrhage is due either to the rupture of a congenital aneurysm or to the rupture of a sclerosed blood vessel in per-

*Headquarters: 22 East 67th St., New York, N. Y. 10021.
†Headquarters: 130 North Wells St., Chicago 6, Ill. 60606.

sons who have high blood pressure. Although the symptoms of rupture of an aneurysm and of hemorrhage due to arteriosclerosis and high blood pressure may be similar, the treatment is different. Therefore, the nursing care will be considered separately. Cerebral thrombosis is by far the most common cause of hemiplegia and accounts for approximately 90% of all cerebrovascular accidents in persons over 65 years of age. It is caused by the formation of a thrombus, or clot, in a blood vessel of the brain. Because the nursing care of patients with cerebral hemorrhage does not differ very much from that for cerebral thrombosis, it will be considered in one discussion.

Cerebral thrombosis and cerebral hemorrhage

Cerebral thrombosis and cerebral hemorrhage may occur at any time, although thrombosis is more likely to occur when the patient is sleeping, and the hemorrhage is more likely to occur when physical or emotional stress is encountered.

Cerebral hemorrhage may be preceded by headache, vertigo, flushing of the face, momentary loss of consciousness, and foreboding that something is wrong. If a large artery ruptures, a sizable portion of the brain may be deprived of blood supply and the onset may be sudden. If a smaller vessel ruptures, only a small portion of the brain may be affected, and symptoms may become pronounced only when enough blood has flowed into the brain tissue to produce pressure. Symptoms of cerebral thrombosis are most likely to be obvious upon the patient's awakening, but they usually vary in degree. The patient may have only a slight difficulty in speech, in walking, or in recalling events of the day before. The effects of the thrombosis may become progressively worse over a twenty-four-hour period, or the patient may be paralyzed on one side of his body upon awakening. If the thrombosis is massive or develops quickly, the patient may die in his sleep without awakening.

Following a cerebral hemorrhage or a cerebral thrombosis, the patient may fall and lapse into total unconsciousness, and convulsions may occur immediately following the accident. Loss of consciousness may come on slowly or quickly and may last for a few minutes or many days until slow recovery occurs. Or it may continue until death, which usually does not occur for several days. The pulse is rapid and bounding, the respirations are labored or stertorous, and the blood pressure is elevated; vomiting may also occur. The pupils may not react normally to light, and one side of the body may appear limp. If the paralysis is on the right side of the body, the patient may not be able to speak even if consciousness returns, because the speech center in right-handed persons is located on the left side of the brain, along with the sensory and motor areas for the right side of the body. If the patient is hospitalized, a spinal puncture is usually done. It may reveal blood in the spinal fluid if hemorrhage has occurred in an artery that communicates with the spinal fluid system.

Emergency care. A cerebrovascular accident may occur when the patient is at work or elsewhere outside his home and may be confused with convulsive seizures, diabetic coma, or drunkenness. Emergency care at the scene of the episode consists of turning the patient carefully on his affected side (determined by the puffiness of the cheek on this side) and elevating the head without tilting the neck forward, since tilting may constrict blood vessels and in turn cause congestion of blood within the skull. Turning the patient on his affected side permits saliva to drain out of the mouth and lessens the danger of aspiration into the lungs. Elevation of the head may help to prevent edema of the brain. Clothing should be loosened about the throat to further help prevent engorgement of blood vessels in the head, which may lead to cerebral edema. The patient should be kept quiet, moved as little as possible, and protected from chilling. Medical aid should be sought at once.

The prognosis for the patient who has had a cerebrovascular accident is poor, particularly during the first few days. The mortality rate is somewhat higher in cerebral hemorrhage than in cerebral thrombosis. One study showed that of 191 patients sustaining a cerebrovascular accident, 82 survived for two days, 43 for one month, 28 for one year, and only 19 for three years.[14]

General nursing care. Nursing care for the patient who has had a cerebrovascular accident does not differ whether he is in the hospital or in his own home, although oxygen is more likely to be given in the hospital. In an attempt to prevent further thrombosis, bishydroxycoumarin (Dicumarol) and heparin may be given to the patient when he is in the hospital if it is certain that the cause of the trouble is cerebral thrombosis and not cerebral hemorrhage.

If the patient survives the first few days, he may begin to regain consciousness and some of the paralysis may disappear. It is then that the greatest understanding is needed by persons attending him. He may realize that he cannot talk, that he drools, that he cannot move a hand or a leg, or, if he can move the limbs, that the motions are shaky and uncertain. The patient's condition is a terrible shock to him, and it is at this point that the nurse's active part in rehabilitation begins. By her quiet assurance she must make the patient feel that his progress toward recovery and self-sufficiency has begun and will continue. She can help by telling him what she is going to do even though he cannot answer her. If the patient is right-handed and cannot speak, he has the added difficulty of having to learn to write with his left hand in addition to being partially speechless. The nurse should try to anticipate the patient's needs and should make every effort to understand his indistinct speech, since repeated attempts to make himself understood only augment his misery and frustration. Usually, if partial speech is present at the time of return to consciousness, there is likelihood that speech will improve, and the patient is heartened by the knowledge of this fact. Speech may be affected because of involvement of the tongue, mouth, and throat, as well as because of damage to the speech center in the brain. The patient who has sustained a cerebrovascular accident may be overly emotional, and this reaction, combined with his fear and frustration upon becoming aware of his condition, is upsetting to his family. He may cry easily, and sometimes family members believe that they are responsible for his sadness when this is usually not true.

Rest and quiet are important even if the accident has not been serious enough to cause complete loss of consciousness. No attempt should be made to rouse the patient from coma, although respiratory and circulatory stimulants may be prescribed by the physician. The vital signs should be carefully checked, and the nurse should observe for such things as a rise in temperature within the first day or two, slowing of pulse and respirations, and deepening of the coma, all of which indicate pressure on the vital centers and a poor prognosis.

The patient's eye on the affected side should be protected if the lid remains open and there is no blink reflex. Otherwise, damage to the cornea can lead to corneal ulcers and blindness. Irrigations with boric acid solution or physiologic solution of sodium chloride, followed by drops of sterile mineral oil, sterile castor oil, or sterile petroleum jelly, are sometimes used. After the lid is gently closed, an eye pad may be taped over the affected eye. If a pad is used, it must be changed daily and the eye cleansed and carefully examined for signs of inflammation or drying of the cornea. Eye shields are preferable to pads because they lessen the danger of lint entering the eye.

Mouth care is difficult to give since the patient may be unable to retain fluid and is likely to choke if it is introduced into the mouth. (See p. 165 for details of giving mouth care to the unconscious patient.) Mouth care should be given every four hours during the day and night, and special attention must be given to the paralyzed side of the mouth and tongue.

Fluids may be restricted for the first few days after a cerebrovascular accident in an effort to prevent edema of the brain. Then regular diet and fluid intake are desirable. Patience and persistence are necessary in giving food and fluids to the patient. The nurse must make him feel that the problem is not discouraging and that time taken to assist him in eating is well spent. He may encounter so much difficulty in getting food and fluids beyond his partially paralyzed mouth and throat that the effort may not seem worthwhile. Therefore, each small step in improvement should be brought to the attention of the patient. Turning him to his back or to the unaffected side may spare him the annoyance and embarrassment of having food spill from the affected side of the mouth. Foods that may cause choking, such as mashed potatoes, stringy meats, and semicooked vegetables, must be avoided.

Since food may collect in the affected side of the mouth, it must be irrigated after eating to prevent accumulation of food with subsequent poor mouth hygiene. The patient should assist in feeding himself as soon as possible, since the helplessness of having to be fed by others is detrimental to emotional health. Food such as meats must, of course, be cut up. A covered plastic cup is now available with a small center opening through which a straw can be introduced, or one can be improvised by using a straw and a covered plastic food container. This cup is useful for the patient who can draw through a straw but whose hands are unsteady. If the patient can swallow but cannot draw through a straw, an Asepto syringe with a piece of rubber tubing on the end or a pitcher must be used. Turning the patient to his unaffected side before introducing fluids into his mouth often helps him to control the mouthful of fluid and to swallow it successfully. If the patient with dentures can keep them in his mouth, he should have them placed in the mouth as soon as possible since wearing dentures also improves his morale and will increase his interest in eating.

Urinary output should be noted carefully and recorded for several days after a cerebrovascular accident. Retention of urine may occur, but it is more likely that the patient will be incontinent. If urinary incontinence occurs, the patient may be told that his control of excretory function probably will improve day by day. Offering a bedpan or a urinal immediately after meals and at other regular intervals helps to overcome incontinence. A retention catheter may be used for the first few days for women patients.

Fecal incontinence is fairly common following a cerebrovascular accident, and again the patient must be reassured that as general improvement occurs, this condition will be overcome. Some patients develop constipation, and impactions develop readily. Elimination must be noted carefully since diarrhea may develop in the presence of an impaction, thus causing it to go unnoticed for several days. Small daily doses of cathartics may be ordered, and an enema may be given every other day. Massage to the abdomen may be helpful in starting peristalsis, but it is done only when ordered by a physi-

cian. Warm oil-retention enemas are sometimes given regularly in an attempt to prevent impactions and when impactions occur. Mineral oil by mouth is often given, since straining in the act of defecation must be avoided. The patient must be cautioned not to strain and must be assured that the enema can easily be repeated if no results are obtained. He usually needs assistance in getting on and off the bedpan. Side rails which he can hold onto in turning himself or a trapeze that he can reach with his unaffected hand is useful if he is permitted this exertion.

The length of time the patient remains in bed depends entirely on the type of cerebrovascular accident suffered and the judgment of the doctor in regard to early mobilization. Some physicians prescribe fairly long periods of rest following cerebrovascular accidents, whereas others believe that early mobilization is best. However, the trend is toward early mobilization of the patient with cerebral thrombosis, and mobilization sometimes begins a day or two after the accident has occurred.

While the patient is in bed, he must be moved frequently to avoid danger of circulatory stasis and hypostatic pneumonia. Care must be taken to see that body weight is not borne on the paralyzed side or on the back for long intervals because decubitus ulcers occur very easily. Pillows should support the uppermost limbs when the patient lies on his unaffected side to prevent strain on shoulder and hip joints. The patient can suffer complete dislocation of the hip joint from lack of support to the limb when he is placed on his unaffected side and when the flaccid thigh is allowed to fall forward and downward, because the muscles take an active part in holding the head of the femur in its socket. The patient may be turned to a face-lying or partial face-lying position, with pillows again being used to maintain good body alignment. This position is good for the patient who is not fully conscious, since it lessens the danger of aspiration of mucus. There should be a regular schedule for turning the patient, and the sequence of desirable positions should be outlined and recorded on the nursing care plan.

Specific rehabilitative measures. The greatest challenge for the nurse in care of the patient who has had a cerebrovascular accident comes after the patient is past the point of danger, for then he must face the long, slow process of learning to use whatever abilities that remain or can be relearned, and he must adjust to his limitations if he and his family are to be reasonably happy for the remainder of his life. If the patient is hospitalized, the physical therapist may make an evaluation of his functional ability before he goes home. If he is referred to a community nursing agency, a physical therapist who is either on the staff of, or available to, the agency may, with the approval of the physician, assess the patient's limitation in moving about. She may then help the nursing staff in working with the family to set up a regimen of exercises for the patient and to make alterations in and about his home so that the patient can do as much as possible for himself safely and more easily. Simple and relatively inexpensive modifications such as rails on the bathtub and a firm support by the lavatory may make the difference between helplessness and some freedom for the patient. Often, however, no physical therapist is available, and the patient may be cared for at home throughout his illness. If the nurse cares for the patient at home early in his illness, she should take time to teach the family member who is responsible for his care some of the nursing measures already described under general nursing care. The pamphlet *Strike Back at Stroke,** written for patients and their families, should be familiar to all nurses. It is available to any patient who has his doctor's approval for its use. If there is ability to use the arm when consciousness returns, there is reason to believe that the leg function will return sufficiently for the patient to walk. Return of motor impulses and subsequent return of function are evidenced by a tightening and spasticity of the affected part. This may appear from the second day to the second week after the cerebrovascular accident. Return of motor impulses is significant for the future use of the affected part but presents new problems for the patient, the

nurse, and all others who may care for him. Muscles that draw the limbs toward the midline become very active, and the arm may be held tightly adducted against the body. The affected lower limb may be held inward and adducted to, or even beyond, the midline. Muscles that draw the limbs into flexion are also stimulated, with the result that the heel is lifted off the ground, the heel cord shortens, and the knee becomes bent. In the upper limb, flexor muscles draw the elbow into the bent position, and the wrist is flexed and fingers are curled in palmar flexion. This is often seen following a cerebrovascular accident.

Persistent nursing effort must be directed toward keeping any part of the body from remaining in a position of flexion long enough for the occurrence of muscle shortening and of joint changes that might interfere with free joint action. If a physical therapist is not available, the total responsibility for preventive measures may rest with the nurse. Every minute counts in prevention, and the nurse must not miss one opportunity to take a moment from her busy day in the hospital to move the patient's adducted or flexed limbs back to the correct position. In the home she must teach members of the family who are caring for the patient to exert this same careful attention.

If the patient is lying on his back, a pillow can be placed between the upper arm and the body to hold the arm in abduction. A roll made of one or two washcloths serves as a good support to prevent flexion of the fingers, and a splint made from a padded tongue blade may be used to ensure straightening of the thumb or other fingers for periods during the day. A firm box at the foot of the bed holds the foot at right angles and prevents contractures in dropfoot position.

Range of joint motion should be preserved, and passive exercises are often begun early. The nurse needs no order to put the patient's limbs through complete range of joint motion passively once or twice each day. (See Figs. 2 to 4.) But passive exercise in which the limb is to be exercised more than this should be done only when so ordered by the doctor. If the nurse does not have a written order, she should consult the physician as to the amount of

---

*Prepared and published by U. S. Department of Health, Education, and Welfare, Public Health Service, Bureau of State Services, Division of Special Health Services, Chronic Disease Program.

passive exercise he wishes the patient to have. A safe rule to follow in caring for any patient with neuromuscular disease is never to force a muscle or a joint past the point of pain. Passive exercise stimulates circulation and may help to reestablish neuromuscular pathways. No difficulty is encountered with these procedures until tightening of the muscles begins to appear. Then other physical measures are needed, and the patient's treatment should be under the direction of a physical therapist.

Active exercise of the affected side also may be started early. It is ordered by the physician and, in the hospital, may be directed by the physical therapist. Under the guidance of the physical therapist the nurse checks the exercises while the patient is in the hospital, and she or the physical therapist may teach the exercises to the family in preparation for the patient's return home.

Since the patient will depend a good deal on his unaffected arm and leg when he begins to move about, the unaffected part of the body needs attention to prevent contractures and preserve muscle strength. Even while he is in bed, the patient should exercise his good arm and use it in all normal positions. The unaffected leg should be in a position of slight *internal rotation* most of the time while the patient is in bed, and the knee should be bent several times each day. Exercise to strengthen the quadriceps muscle should be done because the quadriceps is the most important muscle, giving stability to the knee joint in walking. Exercises against resistance is obtained by placing two small sandbags that are fastened together saddle fashion over the ankle and having the patient raise his leg. One of the best exercises for strengthening the quadriceps is to have the patient straighten the knee against resistance when he is sitting on the edge of the bed or in a chair; a small bucket of sand hung over the ankle may be used as the resistance, but care should be taken to protect the skin of the ankle from pressure. An ordinary cooking pan with a bucket handle may be used in the home.

When the patient begins to move about and to try to help himself, he may have several problems that can alter his ability to proceed. He may have loss of position sense, so that it is awkward for him to handle his body normally even when he has the muscular coordination to do so. He may have dizziness, diplopia, and altering of skin sensation. He may also have to work harder than other persons to receive a normal amount of air upon inhalation since the involved side of the chest does not expand easily. This difficulty may lead to excessive fatigue unless the nurse and all caring for him plan their work so that the patient's effort is not wasted.

Motivation is considered essential to rehabilitation. Most patients who have suffered a cerebral thrombosis are motivated and desire deeply to help themselves even though some are so overcome with the enormity of their limitations that they are very quiet and are misunderstood by those around them. If there is return of hand function in two to three weeks, fecal incontinence has disappeared, and no contractures, decubiti, or other complications have developed, there is reason to believe that the patient can learn to care for himself.[49]

The patient needs preparation for each new step in learning to move and care for himself. He must be shown each new activity as it will apply to him, and he then needs practice under supervision and recognition of each accomplishment regardless of its size.

Before standing or walking, the patient may practice raising himself up in bed and may sit on the side of the bed while holding firmly to an overbed table or to a strap with his good hand and pressing his feet on a chair or stool. The patient benefits from wearing shoes, since it is good for his morale and keeps his paralyzed foot in good position.

If preparation for walking has been adequate, the patient usually needs only one crutch when he begins to walk, and then he progresses to the use of a cane. When he first begins to walk, the nurse must remain close to him to allay his fear of falling. He may practice balancing himself by standing between parallel bars or by leaning on the backs of two chairs (provided the chairs are heavy enough to support weight safely). Good walking patterns must be established early, because incorrect patterns are difficult, and sometimes impossible, to change. A sideward shuffle should be watched for and avoided. The patient should begin by leaning rather heavily upon his crutch or cane and lifting his body sufficiently to bring the leg and foot forward so that the toes point straight ahead and not inward. The cane or single crutch is held in the hand opposite the damaged side of the body.

The patient may be taught how to help with his own improvement. Careful and detailed instructions on how to hold and support himself will save him much embarrassment and confusion. By using his unaffected hand, he may, for example, straighten out the flexed fingers on the affected side, and can move his affected arm to a position where, with the weight of gravity, the elbow will be straightened.

Long-range plans. General care and the pattern of living that should be followed after a cerebrovascular accident vary for each patient and are determined by his own circumstances, the amount of recovery he has, and the guidance he received in the early stages of his illness. Despite all effort he may, for example, never be able to negotiate stairs. The medical social worker and the public health nurse are indispensable in helping to arrange the patient's home so that he may live with a moderate amount of self-sufficiency and independence. Members of the family often need help in assisting the patient to accept his limitations, both physical and emotional. They must also make adjustments to actual circumstances. Almost all persons who have cerebrovascular accidents need health supervision for the rest of their lives. Whether or not the patient will be able to return to his own home or must go to a nursing home will depend a great deal upon his family's understanding and acceptance of his problems when maximum rehabilitation may have been achieved.

While it is not uncommon for cerebrovascular accidents to recur, the patient may go for years with no further difficulty and eventually die of some other cause. The physician usually explains the prognosis to the patient and to his family. The nurse should know what explanation the physician has given and must sometimes help in interpreting it to the family. Some patients must curtail activity to such a point that

they have little enjoyment in living and still have recurrences, whereas others may be active and escape further accidents for many years.

The patient who has sustained a cerebrovascular accident and who has a high blood pressure is usually advised by his physician to change his mode of life so that more rest is assured and strain and excitement are avoided. If his work is strenuous, he may be urged to take longer and more frequent vacations. He may be advised to lose weight if obesity is putting an extra strain on his circulatory system and to avoid the use of tobacco because of its constricting effect on blood vessels. Activities of daily living may be modified; for example, the patient may be advised to sit while shaving. If the doctor feels that the danger of cerebral hemorrhage is imminent, he may advise against any activities that promote dilation of cerebral blood vessels, such as vigorous exercise, hot or cold baths, violent coughing or laughing, straining at defecation, and sexual activity. Occasionally, retirement at an early age is necessary. Relocation in a warmer climate or in a more rural area is helpful to some people provided they can afford it and it does not upset the living pattern of the patient and his family too much.

The patient who has continued hypertension usually is given drugs such as reserpine or its derivatives. Side effects of these drugs, such as dryness of the nose, depression and mood changes, and tremor, should be explained to the patient if they may possibly occur. Anticoagulant drugs such as bishydroxycoumarin (Dicumarol) or warfarin sodium (coumadin) may be prescribed for an indefinite period following a cerebral thrombosis. The patient and his family should know why blood samples are taken regularly and what signs of overdosage, such as epistaxis, should be reported to the doctor at once.

Cerebral arteriosclerosis and multiple small thrombi

Cerebral arteriosclerosis may lead to deterioration of brain tissue, even though cerebrovascular accidents do not occur. This condition, which usually is associated with high blood pressure, may occur in people in their fifties, though it is usually considered a disease of old age.

Multiple small thrombi may occur in persons whose blood pressure is normal or even below normal if atheromatous changes have occurred in the lining of arteries. This condition causes frequent small and barely perceptible strokes. Both cerebral arteriosclerosis and multiple small strokes from thrombi may produce personality changes. The person who has arteriosclerosis is likely to have a more consistent downward course, whereas the one suffering from multiple small thrombi may have periods of apparently normal physical and mental response between episodes of confusion.

Both cerebral arteriosclerosis and multiple small thrombi cause slowly progressive changes that are particularly distressing to members of the patient's family. Complete brain deterioration may occur. The patient may feel irritable and unhappy with apparently little cause, and no amount of reassurance can make him feel better. The family must be prepared for gradual deterioration in the patient's condition and should make provision for his safety and for the results of the poor judgment he may demonstrate; for example, he may forget to dress appropriately, may give away family possessions, and may enter into unwise business dealings. The family needs help in learning how to treat the patient as an adult and yet deal with his limitations. The doctor, the social case worker, and the nurse can help family members care for the patient in such a way that their own lives are not completely disrupted and yet that they are not plagued by guilt feelings when the patient dies. Institutional care is sometimes necessary, and the family needs encouragement and help in arriving at joint decisions that serve the best interests of all its members.

Cerebral aneurysm

A cerebral aneurysm is a weakening and outpouching of the wall of a cerebral artery and is usually caused by a congenital weakness in the vessel wall. The most common sites are the internal carotid, the posterior communicating, the middle cerebral, and the vertebral and basilar arterial systems.[60] The internal carotid artery comes from the common carotid artery and branches to form the ophthalmic, the anterior, and the middle cerebral arteries. The posterior communicating artery comes from the posterior cerebral artery. The vertebral and basilar arteries come from the subclavin artery; each of these arteries sends communicating branches to the internal carotid branches (anterior and middle cerebral arteries) to form the circle of Willis at the base of the brain. Hemorrhage occurs when the aneurysm ruptures and the blood seeps into the subarachnoid spaces. This condition accounts for the sudden death of young people from "strokes" during strenuous exercise or excitement that causes the blood pressure to rise. The aneurysm commonly ruptures between the ages of 20 and 40 years. Signs and symptoms include sudden explosive headache, neck rigidity, nausea and vomiting, loss of consciousness, shock, convulsions, a full, bounding pulse, and noisy, labored respirations.

The immediate treatment for *subarachnoid hemorrhage* is to keep the patient absolutely quiet. He should be very gently moved to bed, and sometimes it is not advisable to move him to a hospital. He must be kept flat in bed in a darkened room and attended constantly to be sure that he does not raise his head. Blood pressure may be taken as often as every fifteen minutes. This procedure is best accomplished and is less disturbing to the patient if the cuff is left (deflated) about the arm. If he is conscious, he is given small amounts of water by mouth, but water must be given through a straw so that his head is not elevated. Intravenous fluids may be given by slow drip so that blood pressure is not affected, and often an indwelling catheter is inserted to avoid the exertion of voiding. Bowel elimination is usually ignored for several days, and then oil retention enemas or small doses of bulk laxatives may be given. Under no circumstances should the patient be permitted to strain, cough, or otherwise exert himself. Visitors must be carefully prepared so that they will not upset the patient, and no mail should be given to him unless it is certain that no disturbing information is contained therein. Hypothermia may be used to lessen the need of the brain for oxygen and thereby decrease the danger of damage to vital brain tissues (p. 188).

About 50% of patients with rupture of an

aneurysm recover from the initial episode, but at least 50% of these persons will have recurrences of hemorrhage if untreated. Recurrence may occur within two weeks, and the danger of death increases with each recurrence. If the aneurysm is not obliterated by surgery, the patient may die eventually from recurrent hemorrhage.

The only satisfactory treatment for congenital aneurysm is surgery. Before surgery can be done, however, the location of the rupture must be determined. The rupture is found by arteriography (angiography), as described on p. 863. The time after the acute rupture when arteriograms are taken and when surgery is done varies with the patient, his age, the intensity and kind of symptoms he has, and the judgment of the surgeon. Since angiography may increase symptoms, it may be followed by immediate surgery in some instances.

Surgery consists of a craniotomy and location of the aneurysm. If it can be found, the aneurysm may be obliterated by ligation at its neck if this procedure is feasible or by the application of a clamp (Stillman clamp). If the base of the aneurysm is too large for ligation to be practicable, it may be coated with a liquid, adherent, plastic substance that hardens to form a firm support about the weakened vessel wall and thereby prevents rupture. If the aneurysm has not ruptured but has given symptoms, attempts may be made to produce thrombosis within the aneurysm by use of an electric current and other means.[60]

Not all aneurysms can be treated surgically at the site of the lesion. If surgery is not feasible, the proximal arterial vessel may be completely or partially obliterated to lessen the flow of blood to the site of the aneurysm *provided* enough blood can be supplied from collateral vessels to preserve vital brain function. The procedure usually is done in stages of several days. A clamp (Selverstone clamp), which has a detachable screw stem and which can be tightened gradually, is used.[60] Usually the surgeon adjusts it each day, and the nurse who attends the patient watches him closely and is instructed to release the clamp at once if there is evidence of inadequate blood supply. Any signs of muscle weakness in the face or in either extremity on the side opposite the incision,

or any changes in the level of consciousness, in vital signs, or in sensory or muscular coordination or control should be reported to the doctor at once. Immediate removal of the clamps may prevent irreversible complications such as hemiplegia, aphasia, and loss of consciousness. If symptoms of inadequate blood supply appear, further surgical treatment cannot be done safely, although the clamp may be left indefinitely to partially obliterate the vessel. If complete occlusion can be tolerated, the vessel may be permanently ligated. Thrombus formation with resultant cerebral embolism may complicate the patient's postoperative course following any surgery for a cerebral aneurysm. It is a feared and often fatal complication.

Before surgical treatment of an aneurysm is attempted, the surgeon usually explains the hope for cure and the risks involved to the patient's family. The nurse must appreciate how distressing the situation is for the family and should realize that the time spent waiting to know whether or not the outcome will be favorable seems interminable to them. The reasons for details of nursing care should be explained to them if they are with the patient. For example, it is important that both the patient and his family know that blood pressure, pulse rate, respiratory rate, and other pertinent observations will be taken frequently, since these procedures can be most upsetting if they are not explained.

If the surgery is successful, the patient will be cured, although usually he will be advised to avoid strenuous exercise and emotional stress for the rest of his life. Occasionally, he may have a severe physical or mental handicap resulting from damage to brain tissue during surgery.

If the aneurysm cannot be successfully treated, however, the family should be aware that there is always the danger of sudden death. The patient must be protected from strenuous activity and excitement.

Infections

The nervous system may be attacked by a variety of organisms and viruses and may suffer from toxic reactions to bacterial and viral disease. Sometimes the infection becomes walled off and causes an abscess, sometimes the meninges, or coverings of the brain and spinal cord, primarily are involved, and sometimes the brain itself is affected most. Organisms and viruses may reach the nervous system by a variety of routes. Untreated chronic otitis media and mastoiditis, chronic sinusitis, and fracture in any bone adjacent to the meninges may be the source of infection. Some organisms, such as the tubercle bacillus and probably the pneumococcus, reach the nervous system by means of the blood or the lymph system. The exact route by which some infective agents, such as the meningococcus in epidemic meningitis and the viruses that cause encephalitis, reach the central nervous system is not known.

Meningococcal meningitis (epidemic) and poliomyelitis are reportable communicable diseases. Because they are becoming less common and because they are discussed in specialized texts on communicable disease nursing, they will be mentioned only briefly here.

Meningitis

Meningitis is an acute infection of the meninges usually caused by pneumococci, meningococci (epidemic), staphylococci, streptococci, or aseptic agents (usually viral). Any other pathogenic organism, such as the tubercle bacillus, that gains access to the subarachnoid spaces can cause meningitis. Mild forms of the disease do occur and may be referred to as *meningism*. They may be caused by the enteroviruses (the poliovirus, the Coxsackie viruses, and the ECHO visuses) or by the virus that causes herpes simplex. A common form of the disease is lymphocytic meningitis, believed in many instances to be associated with a virus.

The incidence of bacterial meningitis is higher in fall and winter, when upper respiratory infections are common. Children are more often affected than adults because of frequent colds and ear infections. Disease caused by the enteroviruses is more common in the summer and early fall than in other seasons of the year.

The onset of meningitis (except when due to tubercle bacilli) is usually sudden, with severe headache, stiffness of the neck, irritability, malaise, and restlessness. Nausea, vomiting, delirium, and complete disorientation may develop quickly. Temperature, pulse rate, and respirations are increased. The diagnosis is usually confirmed by doing a lumbar puncture. Usually the offending organism can be isolated from the spinal fluid and, if a pyogenic organism is the cause, the fluid is cloudy. Treatment consists of large doses of the antibiotic most specific for the causative organism. This antibiotic may be given directly into the spinal canal as well as administered by other routes.

Nursing care. Isolation is required for the patient with epidemic meningitis until the acute illness is over. Particular care should be taken in handling discharges from the nose, mouth, and throat. Nursing care for the patient with meningitis includes the general care given a critically ill patient, who may be irritable, confused, and unable to take fluids, and yet who is dehydrated because of elevation of temperature. The room should be kept darkened, and noise should be curtailed as much as possible. The patient must be observed very carefully and must be constantly attended if he is disoriented. Side rails should be placed on the bed.

Residual damage from meningitis includes deafness, blindness, paralysis, and mental retardation. However, these complications are now rare, because the infection is effectively treated with antibiotics before permanent damage to the nervous system occurs.

Encephalitis

Encephalitis is inflammation of the brain and its coverings. Occasionally the meninges of the spinal cord are also involved. Encephalitis can have a variety of causes. A generalized inflammation of the brain can be caused by syphilis, and encephalitis can follow exogenous poisoning, such as that which follows the ingestion of lead or arsenic or the inhalation of carbon monoxide. It can be caused by reaction to toxins produced by infections such as typhoid fever, measles, and chickenpox, and occasionally it follows vaccination.

Encephalitis caused by a virus and occurring in epidemic form was first described by von Economo in Austria, and the name von Economo's disease is still used to identify the widespread epidemic in the United States that followed the influenza epidemic in 1918. This form of the disease has not recurred since 1926. Von Economo's disease was also called encephalitis lethargica and sleeping sickness, a term still used by the layman.

The death rate from encephalitis varies with epidemics but is generally fairly high. The most common and most serious sequela for patients who do recover from the acute disease is paralysis agitans, which may come on suddenly or develop slowly. Other residual neurologic symptoms may also occur and occasionally incapacitate the patient completely.

Viral encephalitis. Viral encephalitis appears to be caused by a number of viruses, some of which may be interrelated. Many names are used to identify the kind of virus—for example, St. Louis, western equine, eastern equine, and Japanese B. All are believed to be transmitted by the bite of an insect (arthropod), to have an incubation period of five to fifteen days, not to be transmissible from man to man, and to leave no serious sequelae though the acute illness may be severe enough to cause death. A more complete discussion of this increasingly complex group of pathologic entities can be found in current medical texts.[5,20]

The onset of viral encephalitis may be sudden, with death occurring within twelve to twenty-four hours of the onset of symptoms, although usually the height of symptoms is reached in approximately forty-eight hours. Symptoms vary and include severe headache, malaise, dizziness, nausea and vomiting, restlessness, irritability, lethargy, sleeplessness, vague feelings of fear and misgiving that can be poorly described, difficulty in speech, and twitching and tremor in muscles of the face and hands. Temperature, pulse rate, and respirations may be moderately elevated and, upon neurologic examination, there may be some reflexes absent or otherwise abnormal. The patient's white blood cell count may be normal, and the spinal fluid is usually normal or shows only slight increase in protein and in lymphocytes. If death occurs, a postmortem examination will reveal clouding of the meninges, which can be seen grossly, and small petechiae and degeneration of brain cells can be found upon microscopic examination.

Nursing care consists mainly of symptomatic care and careful observation. Any change in appearance or behavior must be reported at once since the progress in this disease sometimes is extremely rapid. The patient is kept in bed, and side rails are used if disorientation develops. The patient must be constantly attended to prevent injury. If the temperature is high, sponging may be ordered. Frequent changes of linen may be necessary if perspiration is excessive. There is no specific medical treatment for this disease, and the mortality rate ranges from 5 to 60%. No isolation is necessary.

Poliomyelitis

Poliomyelitis is an acute febrile disease caused by three different strains of one of the smallest known viruses. With discovery of the Salk vaccine and its wide use since 1956 and the recent availability of a safe "live virus" vaccine (Sabin vaccine), this disease, which had been a serious crippler of children and young adults, promises to become quite rare. In 1963 there were only 41 deaths in the United States from poliomyelitis.

The incubation period for poliomyelitis is from seven to twenty-one days. The virus attacks the anterior horn cells of the spinal cord where the motor pathways are located and may cause motor paralysis. Sensory perception is not affected since posterior horn cells are not attacked. Poliomyelitis sometimes takes a somewhat different form and attacks primarily the medulla and basal structures of the brain, including the cranial nerves; the term *bulbar* poliomyelitis is used for this form.

An important responsibility of the nurse is to help prevent poliomyelitis by encouraging immunization. Since this dreaded disease is now largely preventable, it is deplorable if all children and young adults do not receive protection. (See p. 299 for recommended immunization schedule.)

Poliomyelitis is probably transmitted by secretions from the nose and throat of infected persons and by means of the gastrointestinal tract. The virus has been found in milk, is known to remain active in sewage for many months, and has been found on insects such as flies. However, none of these has been proved to be a source of epidemic spread. The disease is not easily transmitted, and very few infections have occurred among medical and nursing personnel caring for acutely ill patients. Several members of one family, however, often have the disease in varying degrees of severity. It is believed that, for every person who develops paralysis, there are many who have a milder form of the disease without paralysis and who develop an immunity to subsequent exposure. The incidence of poliomyelitis is highest in the summer and early autumn, and it is higher among rural than urban dwellers. The general health of the person before exposure does not seem to affect his resistance to the disease, although immediate bed rest upon the onset of symptoms may lessen the severity of symptoms.

Medical treatment and nursing care. The treatment of acute poliomyelitis is largely symptomatic. There is no specific drug, and antibiotics are given only to prevent superimposed infection. The patient should be kept warm and quiet, and fluids should be given freely provided there are no signs of bulbar involvement. Narcotics and sedatives are not given because they may mask symptoms of oncoming bulbar involvement. The application of warm, moist packs to tender muscles and warm tub baths often help lessen pain and give comfort if they can be given without causing fatigue and pain from moving. Urinary retention occurs quite often and may require use of an indwelling catheter. This is disturbing to the patient, and he must be assured that the condition is temporary. Bladder function is always regained within a few weeks. A careful record of bowel elimination must be kept since constipation is common.

For the first few days, when pain is severe and the patient is generally quite ill, he should assume any position that is comfortable. After that time attention must be given to good bed posture, keeping weakened muscles in a protected position and being certain that normal range of joint motion is maintained. Ofter the patient is admitted to a bed especially prepared with a fracture board to ensure good alignment of the spine, bath blankets instead of sheets to help prevent chilling, and a board at the foot against which his feet may rest in good alignment. Responsibility for retraining and redeveloping weakened muscles is assumed by the physical therapist, but the nurse must see that postural deformities do not develop, that uninvolved muscles do not undergo unnecessary atrophy, and that range of joint motion is preserved.

Syphilis

In the late, or chronic, stage of syphilis, infection may involve the brain and spinal cord. The oculomotor nerves may be involved, causing inability of the pupil to react to light (Argyll Robertson pupil). *Tabes dorsalis* is the name given to the involvement of the posterior columns of the spinal cord and the posterior nerve roots. Since the sensory nerves are primarily involved, sensory symptoms predominate. The patient may have severe paroxysmal pain anywhere in the body, although perhaps the most common location is in the stomach. This condition, known as gastric crisis, may be confused with ruptured peptic ulcer or other acute conditions of the stomach or gallbladder. There may be areas of severe paresthesia on the skin. A common finding in tabes dorsalis is loss of position sense in the feet and legs. The patient is unable to sense where he places his feet, and his resultant slapping gait is highly characteristic of the disease. He has real difficulty walking at night because he depends on sight in placing his feet normally. Visual loss or even total blindness also occurs. Tabes dorsalis can cause trophic changes in the limbs and changes in the joint so that stability is lost (Charcot's joint).

General paresis is the term used to designate another late manifestation of syphilis in which there is degeneration of the brain with deterioration of mental function and varying evidences of other neurologic disease. Since patients with this condition occupy many beds in mental hospitals, the disease is discussed quite fully in texts dealing with nursing care of the mentally ill.

Head injuries

Since many head injuries are caused by automobile accidents, and deaths from vehicle accidents exceeded 43,000 in 1964, it is likely that almost every nurse will be called upon to care for a patient who has an accidental head injury. Injuries vary from minor scalp wounds to concussions and open fractures of the skull with severe damage to brain tissue. The amount of apparent injury is not necessarily indicative of the seriousness of the trouble. Scalp lacerations, for example, bleed profusely and may be frightening to the patient and to others. Most of them are relatively minor, however, if bleeding is controlled before too much blood is lost.

The brain can be seriously injured even when there is no break in the skin and no evidence of skull fracture when a roentgenogram is taken. When the bony skull strikes a solid object, the soft tissues within the cavity continue to move. This action can be likened to what happens as one stops suddenly when moving quickly with an open dish of fluid—some of the fluid spills. The only difference is that, instead of spilling, the soft contents of the cranial cavity strike the bony covering forcibly and may sustain severe damage. This injury is known as *concussion* and is suspected whenever a patient loses consciousness for even a few moments at the time of or immediately after an accident. *Contusions* and *lacerations* of the brain may occur as the soft brain tissue is forced suddenly against relatively sharp bony protrusions within the skull. They are likely to cause serious damage since, in addition to the brain damage, bleeding almost always occurs, increasing pressure within the enclosed cranial cavity still further.

If lethargy or unconsciousness develops after consciousness has been regained following an accident, an *extradural hemorrhage* should be suspected. It may occur even when consciousness is not lost at the time of injury. Usually one pupil becomes dilated, and the patient may vomit. Bleeding is usually caused by the tearing of the middle meningeal artery. This injury is fairly often sustained in baseball, football, and other vigorous sports.

If the patient has been conscious for several weeks or even months following a head injury and then shows neurologic signs suggestive of a lesion, he may have a *subdural hematoma* caused by slow venous oozing after the accident. This injury may occur following even seemingly inconsequential blows to the head. Careful observation

and recognition of subtle changes may bring patients to medical attention before irreparable brain damage has occurred. Extradural or subdural hemorrhage may, of course, accompany other serious injury, causing unconsciousness.

Fractures *of the base of the skull* usually result in serious damage and cause a high mortality, whereas *linear fractures* of the vault of the skull may be of little significance unless bone fragments are depressed. When a basal fracture has been sustained, the brain tissue and vital nerve pathways may be permanently damaged. Trauma and edema often cause interruption in the flow of cerebrospinal fluid, with resultant increase in intracranial pressure. If the injury has caused a direct communication between the cranial cavity and the middle ear or the sinuses, meningitis or a brain abscess may develop. Bleeding from the nose and ears is highly suggestive of a basal fracture. Occasionally there is serosanguineous drainage that may contain cerebrospinal fluid.

Medical treatment and nursing care

Although the period of unconsciousness usually varies directly with the extent of brain injury, even severely injured patients may regain consciousness, recover almost completely, and return to an active life. Medical and nursing care is directed toward lifesaving measures immediately following the accident and maintaining normal body function until recovery is accomplished.

Care at the scene of the accident

The patient with an obvious head injury should be kept absolutely quiet. The wound should be covered with the cleanest material available, and pressure should be applied to the bleeding scalp *provided* there is no evidence of a depressed fracture. If it is apparent that a sharp instrument has penetrated the bone or if brain tissues is protruding through the wound, the wound must be left strictly alone, and no attempt should be made to remove the instrument of injury. No matter how serious the injury seems to be, no patient should be regarded as hopeless. Some truly remarkable recoveries have followed injuries in which contents of the cranial cavity were exposed. The patient should be kept warm, and a clear airway should be assured. If there is bleeding into the mouth, he should be turned carefully to one side, provided that several persons are available to help. The patient must be turned "in one piece" with the greatest care taken that the cervical spine is kept absolutely straight. A support must be placed under the head when the patient is on his side. No other moving of the patient should be permitted until an ambulance has arrived and experienced help is available.

Any person who has sustained a blow to the head must be watched closely following the accident. Even if consciousness has been regained almost immediately, the patient should sit quietly and not attempt to help others. Pulse and respiratory rate should be noted and cyanosis watched for. Vomiting may be a sign of increased intracranial pressure following injury, although sometimes it is an emotional response to shock.

Care in the hospital

The patient who has a skull fracture or other serious head injury must be attended constantly. Many neurosurgeons feel that alert and intelligent nursing care is often the decisive factor in determining the outcome for the patient. Side rails should always be on the bed, and a mouth gag to protect the tongue should be kept at the bedside since restlessness may come on suddenly and convulsions may occur. Usually the doctor orders that the bed be kept flat, though some doctors believe that the danger of edema to the brain may be reduced by slight elevation of the head of the bed.[10]

Rest. The patient should be kept absolutely quiet. No vigorous effort should be made to "clean the patient up" during the first few hours after an accident. Rest is much more important. Sudden noises, flashes of light, and the clatter of equipment can increase the patient's restlessness and should be avoided. Portable equipment may be used to take roentgenograms. The nurse must remain in the room with the patient to help him move and to protect him from exertion. Restlessness may be due to the need for a slight change of position, the relaxation of a limb, or the need to empty the bladder. If nursing measures fail to allay extreme restlessness, the doctor may order phenobarbital, chloral hydrate, or paraldehyde. Narcotics are avoided because they depress the respiratory center. Sedatives may also be ordered for the patient who is conscious and who complains of severe headache.

Vital signs and respiratory function. Usually the blood pressure, pulse, and respiratory rate are taken and recorded every fifteen minutes until they become stabilized and remain within safe limits. Leaving the deflated blood pressure cuff on the arm helps to prevent disturbing the patient unduly when the pressure must be taken often. Developing the habit of not forcing the mercury column much above the expected reading also sometimes enables the nurse to take the blood pressure and yet barely disturb the patient. The eyes should be observed for inequality of the pupils and the lips and fingernails for cyanosis. A sudden sharp rise in temperature, which may go to 42° C. (106° F.) or higher, and a sudden drop in blood pressure indicates that the regulatory mechanisms have lost control and the prognosis is poor. Deepening of the unconsciousness or coma and any change in depth or rate of respirations are important signs of increase in pressure, which must be reported at once. Twitching or convulsive movement of a body part should be recorded and reported.

The most common complication in severe head injury is lack of proper aeration of the lungs.[10] The nurse must keep the patient on his side. A suction machine should be at the patient's bedside, and suctioning to remove tracheobronchial secretions must be done as often and as deeply as requested by the doctor for the individual patient. A tracheotomy is often done when the patient with a severe head injury experiences any breathing difficulty, and in some medical centers it is done almost routinely. If it has not been done, an emergency tracheotomy set should be on the patient unit and available for immediate use. (See p. 598 for care of the patient who has a tracheostomy.) Oxygen should also be available and is sometimes used, although it is generally considered much less important in treatment than keeping the air passages clear by suctioning and other means.[10]

Drainage from ears and nose. The patient's ears and nose should be observed carefully for signs of blood and for serous drainage, which may indicate that the meninges have been torn (common in basal skull fractures) and that spinal fluid is escaping. No attempt should be made to clean out these orifices. Loose sterile cotton may be placed in the outer openings only. This procedure must be done with caution so that the cotton does not in any way act as a plug to interfere with free flow of fluid. The cotton should be changed as soon as it becomes moistened. Usually the flow of fluid subsides spontaneously. Antibiotics usually are given when a basal fracture has been sustained. Suction is never used to remove nasal secretions on any patient who has a head injury or who has undergone brain surgery because of the danger of causing further damage. Meningitis is a possible complication when communication to the nose and ears occurs. If there is evidence of drainage of spinal fluid from the nose, the patient should not cough, sneeze, or blow his nose. These activities may, in addition to contributing to the development of meningitis, enable air to enter the cranial cavity, where it may increase symptoms of intracranial pressure.[65]

Lumbar puncture. A lumbar puncture is done with caution following a head injury because of the danger of lowering spinal fluid pressure in the spinal canal, which may cause herniation of the brain stem into the foramen magnum, resulting in severe pressure on vital centers. If a spinal puncture is done, the patient must be watched exceedingly carefully during and following the procedure for such signs of pressure on vital centers as changes in respiratory rate and pulse rate.

Dehydration and output. Effort may be made to dehydrate the patient and thereby try to lessen intracranial pressure. Urea in a solution of invert sugar (Urevert) is widely used. Although urea is a normal waste product, giving therapeutic amounts to persons with normal kidney function causes no difficulty and increases the fluid eliminated. It is not given if severe kidney damage is suspected, Sucrose exerts the same effect, but its larger molecule is less readily eliminated by the kidneys. Glucose, 50%, is very seldom used since it has been found that the edema for which it is given recurs very quickly after the height of its effect is reached.[10] Caffeine sodium benzoate or atropine sulfate is given occasionally, although there is not complete medical agree-

ment as to their value as dehydrating agents.[10] Hypertonic mannitol is also given intravenously for its dehydrating effect, and dexamethasone (Decadron) is also prescribed for its effect in reducing edema of the brain.[20]

If at all possible, the patient's urinary output should be recorded, and often an indwelling catheter is inserted following a severe head injury. The urinary output should be approximately 0.6 to 1 ml. per kilogram (2.2 pounds) of body weight per hour. This means that a man weighing 175 pounds should eliminate between 45 and 80 ml. per hour, and if dehydrating drugs have been given, this amount may be greater.

Food and fluids. Following a severe head injury, fluid intake may be limited to 1,500 ml. daily, or fluids up to 2,500 ml. may be permitted. Fluids may be given parenterally, by means of a nasogastric tube or by mouth, depending upon the patient. Food and fluids are not given by mouth if the patient is likely to aspirate or to vomit. A tube in the nose, however, is most annoying to the patient and may interfere seriously with rest.

Bowel function. Bowel function is not encouraged for several days following a head injury. Mild bulk laxatives, bisacodyl (Dulcolax) suppositories, and sometimes oil retention enemas may be prescribed. The patient is cautioned repeatedly not to strain in an effort to defecate since straining increases intracranial pressure.

Metabolic disorder of central origin. If no improvement in level of consciousness and in other vital signs occurs within approximately five days, a metabolic disorder of central nervous system origin may be suspected. This poorly understood syndrome is believed to be caused by too much protein and/or by hypothalamic or frontobasalic brain involvement as a result of the injury.[10] Treatment includes curtailing protein and increasing fluid intake and giving mercurial diuretics. Cortisone and dexamethasone (Decadron) are also often given. If hyperthermia develops, hypothermia may be used (p. 188).

Prolonged unconsciousness. General nursing care as described in Chapter 9 is necessary for the patient with a head injury who remains unconscious for some time. Patients may be unconscious for as long as a month or more and yet finally make a satisfactory recovery provided good supportive care has been given.

Extradural hematoma. Because of the danger of *extradural hematoma,* many doctors believe that any patient who has sustained any injury to the head with loss of consciousness should be hospitalized for at least twenty-four hours. If he is asleep during this time, he should be awakened hourly to determine his state of consciousness. Some doctors believe that fluids should be restricted to 1,000 to 1,500 ml. for the first day or two and that a dehydrating substance should be given. If the patient does remain at home, the family should be told to watch him closely for signs of increased intracranial pressure, to awaken him hourly during the night after injury, and to bring him to a hospital at once if drowsiness, stupor, paralysis, convulsions, or inequality of the pupil size occur. The treatment for extradural hematoma consists of making burr holes through the temporal bone to relieve the pressure caused by the bleeding and to attempt to control the bleeding; sometimes a craniotomy is done. Occasionally the patient has so much damage to the soft tissue of the brain that he dies despite relief of pressure caused by the bleeding. Usually such a patient is unconscious after the accident and is taken to a hospital at once.

Often when a person has sustained a serious head injury, members of his family are in a state of shock and need special attention. Occasionally the doctor orders sedatives for them. If they are not permitted to see the patient because he is in the operating room or undergoing tests, they should be kept informed of his progress. A quiet, pleasant waiting room and a helpful word as to where such facilities as the telephone are located do a great deal to make them more comfortable.

Convalescence

The length of convalescence will depend entirely on how much damage has been done and how rapid recovery has been. Patients are usually urged to resume normal activity as soon as possible, since this seems to decrease the tendency to develop psychoneurotic responses to the injury. Patients may complain of headache and occasional dizziness for some time following a head injury. These difficulties should disappear within three to four months. Loss of memory and loss of initiative may also persist for a time. Occasionally convulsions develop due to the formation of scar tissue in injured brain substance or in its coverings. Such scar tissue may often be surgically removed to effect a complete cure. Loss of hearing and strabismus (cross-eye) sometimes complicate basal skull fractures and require a long period of rehabilitation. Sometimes corrective surgery can be done for the strabismus.

Brain tumors

Every nurse should recognize the early symptoms of brain tumor, since, unless the tumor is diagnosed and treated promptly, death from irreparable brain damage will occur. Although approximately one-half of all brain tumors originating in the brain are benign, they may cause death. As the tumor grows within the cranial cavity, it eventually exerts lethal pressure on vital centers of the brain. Hemorrhage and abscess may cause symptoms similar to those caused by brain tumors.

Early treatment becomes even more important as newer techniques have been developed that improve the operative risks and the postoperative prospects for patients with brain tumors. These techniques include hypothermia, establishment of controlled hypotensive states during operation by means of sympathetic blocking agents such as trimethaphan camphorsulfonate (Arfonad), and dehydration of cerebral tissues by giving urea compounds and/or mannitol before, during, and after surgery. The nurse should be alert so that she is able to detect early signs of brain tumor in patients and urge them to seek medical care at once. The only hope for cure of a brain tumor is early surgical removal. Radiation therapy and craniotomies to lessen pressure are used as palliative measures only when the tumor cannot be removed completely.

Brain tumors cause symptoms by directly affecting portions of the brain, or its related structures and by generally increasing pressure within the cranial cavity as the tumor grows.

In many instances, especially if the tumor is infiltrating brain tissue, an alert observer may recognize subtle changes that suggest

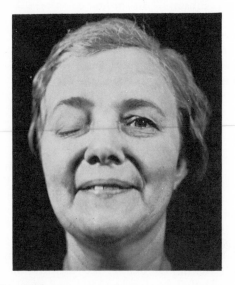

Fig. 207

This patient has a marked ptosis of the right eyelid. (From Davis, Loyal: The principles of neurological surgery, Philadelphia, 1942, Lea & Febiger.)

the need for neurologic examination before symptoms of increased pressure appear. The symptoms depend on the part of the brain affected. They usually are transitory at first but become more frequent as the tumor grows. The first noticeable symptom may be a change in personality or judgment. If motor areas are involved, there may be weakness of a leg, an arm, or any other part of the body (Figs. 207 and 208). Sometimes the patient complains of paresthesia or anesthesia of a part of the body. He may complain of unpleasant odors, a sensation that often accompanies tumors of the frontal lobe. If the speech center is involved, the patient may be unable to use words correctly or he may become unable to understand the written or spoken word. He may complain of loss of visual acuity or of double vision. These signs indicate pressure on the optic nerve or on one or both of the adducens nerves. Unexplained loss of hearing in one ear is suggestive of brain tumor, although there are also many other causes.

The patient may have a change in his gait, perhaps staggering, veering to one side, or walking with an unusually wide base of support. These symptoms often occur with cerebellar tumors. Convulsions

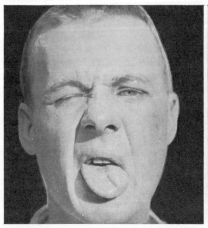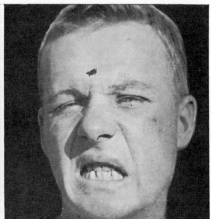

Fig. 208

This patient has weakness of the left facial nerve and hypoglossal palsy. Note the deviation of the tongue and drooping of the mouth on the left side when the patient clenches his teeth. (From Davis, Loyal: The principles of neurological surgery, Philadelphia, 1942, Lea & Febiger.)

occurring for the first time after middle age are suggestive of a brain tumor in the cerebrum or its coverings.

Brain tumors are named for the tissues from which they arise. The more common types are gliomas, arising from the connective tissue, meningiomas, arising from the meningeal coverings, and neuromas, arising from the cranial nerves. Glandular tumors such as pituitary tumors may occur, and tumors that have metastasized from elsewhere in the body are fairly common.

Pituitary tumors may cause a variety of symptoms, depending on their type. *Gigantism* and *acromegaly* (overgrowth of bone) are caused by tumors of the pituitary but are treated medically. (See p. 763.) However, other tumors of the pituitary gland compress the surrounding brain structures and are treated surgically. The most common symptom is a decrease in vision caused by pressure on the optic chiasm, as well as other signs of pituitary anomaly.

Unfortunately, some tumors do not produce any symptoms until they become large enough to displace brain tissue or until they block the flow of cerebrospinal fluid, causing *increased intracranial pressure* and producing the so-called cardinal signs of brain tumor. The patient often complains of slight dimming of vision, which is caused by papilledema, or swelling of the optic nerve head (choked disk). He may have sudden vomiting that is not preceded by nausea. Persistent dull headache that is most severe in the morning often accompanies these signs. Blood pressure progressively rises, and pulse and respirations become slower because of pressure on regulatory centers in the medulla. One of the first signs of increased intracranial pressure may be change in level of consciousness. The patient may first be irritable and restless and then gradually become lethargic and stuporous.

Nursing care of the patient with a brain tumor

When admitting the patient with a brain tumor to the hospital, the nurse should carefully observe his physical and mental status. Limitations of movement, muscle weakness, difficulty in following instructions, speech impairment, loss of vision or hearing, and any symptomatic complaints can easily be noted at this time. Blood pressure, temperature, pulse rate, respirations, and pupillary reaction also should be carefully recorded, since the doctor often needs this information later as a basis for comparison. Even before the doctor examines the patient, necessary plans for nursing care related to his personal needs, such as help in eating, assistance in walking, placement of the bedside stand if he has limitations of movement in the upper extremities, the need for side rails on the bed, a mouth gag at the bedside, and appropriate means of communication, should be made. The patient may be well oriented and very fearful of the probable diagnosis or the anticipated surgery. The nurse should encourage the patient to talk, listen to what he says, and reassure him as to the skill of his surgeon.

The nurse may be able to help the doctor localize a brain lesion by accurately reporting and recording her observations. For example, noting that the patient has less severe headache when his head is in a certain position may be important, because it suggests that this position relieves the pressure. If possible, the exact location of headache should be noted. Careful description of the course of convulsions may help locate a tumor. Any symptoms indicative of increasing intracranial pressure should be reported to the physician at once. These observations, in addition to several of the tests described earlier in this chapter, help the doctor to analyze the patient's trouble and to select the best course of action for the individual patient.

Occasionally a patient enters the hospital with signs of severe intracranial pressure, or signs of increased pressure may appear suddenly while he is undergoing a period of observation and diagnostic study. If the signs appear suddenly, treatment for relief of pressure must be given at once. Urea dissolved in a solution with invert sugar (Urevert) or mannitol, 25%, may be given intravenously to cause dehydration of the brain.

A lumbar puncture may be done to remove cerebrospinal fluid and thereby release pressure, provided it is assured that the lowering of pressure in the spinal canal will not result in an increase of pressure on the vital centers in the medulla. Immediate operation, known as decompression of the skull, may be done to allow for expansion of brain tissue outside the cranial cavity, thus releasing pressure.

Preoperative care. If immediate surgery is not necessary, the patient is given a thorough physical examination and a complete neurologic examination with related investigation, such as endocrine studies, if indicated. Roentgenograms of the skull are always taken, and an electroencephalogram is also ordered routinely when a brain tumor is suspected. A pneumoencephalogram or a ventriculogram may be necessary to establish a diagnosis. Since a ventriculogram requires that the patient have general anesthesia, the operation is usually performed immediately after the test if the results show evidence of a tumor.

Written permission for operations on the brain must be given by the nearest relative unless the patient himself is able to sign a permit. Even then, close relatives are usually consulted, and the doctor obtains their consent before doing surgery. The patient and his family usually feel very much threatened when brain surgery must be done. Thus, every effort should be made to inspire confidence in the surgeon, members of the nursing staff, and the hospital. As before any major surgery, the patient may wish to have his spiritual adviser visit him.

Treatments and procedures should be explained to the patient even though he may not seem to understand clearly. Enemas may not be given because of the danger of increasing intracranial pressure by exertion and by absorption of fluid. Narcotics, except codeine, are rarely ordered preoperatively since they may cause further depression of cerebral function. Any order for their use should be carefully verified by the nurse. If hair is to be shaved the procedure may be delayed until the patient is in the operating room and under anesthesia. Long hair should not be discarded but should be returned to the unit because the patient may wish to have it made into a wig for use until her hair grows again. It is rarely necessary to shave the entire head, and some surgeons have only a small area shaved. Hair along the front hairline can often be left so that after the operation, it can be drawn backward to cover the scar.

Surgery. A surgical opening through the skull is known as a *craniotomy.* The meninges are opened, and the tumor is removed if possible. Brain surgery usually is done under hypothermia to lessen bleeding during the procedure. Drugs for hypotension, such as levarterenol bitartrate (Levophed), may be given also. A dye such as fluorescein sodium may be administered intravenously one hour preoperatively to help localize the tumor. Tumor tissue tends to retain the substance, which can then be seen under ultraviolet light. This dye will cause the skin and the scleras to appear jaundiced for several days. The nursing staff, the patient, and his family should be aware of this.

When the brain lesion is in the *supratentorium* (the cerebrum), the incision is usually made behind the hairline (Fig. 209). When the incision is into the *infratentorium* (the cerebellum and brain stem), it is made slightly above the nape of the neck. Neither of these incisions is apparent when the hair has grown. The scalp is incised, and a piece of the bone over the site of the suspected tumor is removed with a small electric saw. The bone flap is carefully saved, since it usually is replaced following the operation. The bone flap, however, may be left out to prevent pressure from edema postoperatively or to permit expansion of an inoperable tumor. It may be replaced weeks or months later, or a Vitallium plate may be used instead of the preserved bone.

Although a portion of the frontal lobe can be removed with little residual damage, limitation of some functions may necessarily follow complete removal of tumors elsewhere. Tumors located where they are readily accessible to surgery, such as some meningiomas and tumors of the outer cerebrum, have the best prognosis.

Immediate postoperative care. To facilitate change of dressings and other treatment following surgery, the patient may be placed in bed "head to foot." If he returns to the patient unit and not to a recovery room, the nurse should be certain that the following are readily available: side rails for the bed, a suction machine with 14 Fr. and 16 Fr. Robinson catheters, an airway, a mouth gag, a lumbar puncture set, and an emergency medication tray con-

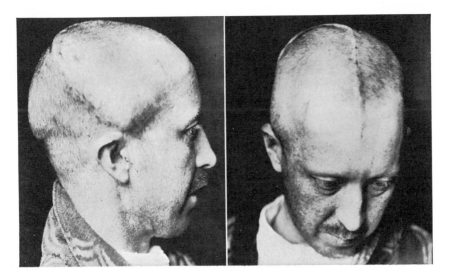

Fig. 209

Subtemporal decompression combined with unilateral frontal flap. These photographs
were taken one week after operation. The only place the scar might show is in
the middle of the forehead. The scar is imperceptible if made accurately in the
median line. Note the slight bulging of the right subtemporal decompression.
(From Sachs, Ernest: Diagnosis and treatment of brain tumors and care of
the neurosurgical patient, ed. 2, St. Louis, 1949, The C. V. Mosby Co.)

taining caffeine sodium benzoate, theobromine, amobarbital sodium (Amytal sodium), syringes, intravenous and hypodermic needles, and a tourniquet. An emergency tracheotomy set should also be readily available on the unit if a tracheotomy has not been done.

Immediately after the patient returns from the operating room, he is placed on his side to allow for an adequate airway. If a large tumor has been removed, he must not be turned onto the affected side since this position may cause displacement of brain structures by gravity. Otherwise, he may be turned to either side. If there has been supratentorial surgery, the head gatch on the bed is elevated 45 degrees and a large pillow is placed under the patient's head and shoulders. This position should lessen the possibility of hemorrhage, provide for better circulation of the cerebrospinal fluid, and decrease cerebral and other tissue edema. If an infratentorial tumor has been removed, the head dressing will extend down to the shoulders, holding the head in slight hyperextension. The bed should be kept flat with only a small pillow under the nape of the neck. (See Fig. 210.)

The head dressing (often a helmet of crinoline and starch) should be inspected to make sure that it is thoroughly dry (Fig. 211). If it is not dry, a hair dryer turned to "cool" should be used. The dryer should never be turned to "hot" because the patient may be burned by the hot air. The face and neck should be covered with a towel since air blowing over them may be very annoying. Serosanguineous drainage on the dressings should be outlined in ink, as is done on other dressings, so that it can be accurately checked for an increase in amount. Yellowish drainage should be reported immediately to the doctor, because it probably indicates loss of spinal fluid. If the head dressing appears to be soaked with any kind of drainage, it should be covered with a sterile towel held in place with adhesive tape. Every half hour the towel should be removed and the dressing checked and reinforced with sterile towels if necessary. An unprotected wet dressing may cause the wound to become infected, which might even lead to meningitis. Sometimes the doctor changes the entire dressing.

The nurse should observe the patient carefully, recording his blood pressure, rectal temperature, pulse rate, respirations, state of consciousness, pupillary responses and inequality of the size of the pupils, muscle strength (hand grip), and ability to move. If he is unconscious or semiconscious, she should note his response to painful stimuli

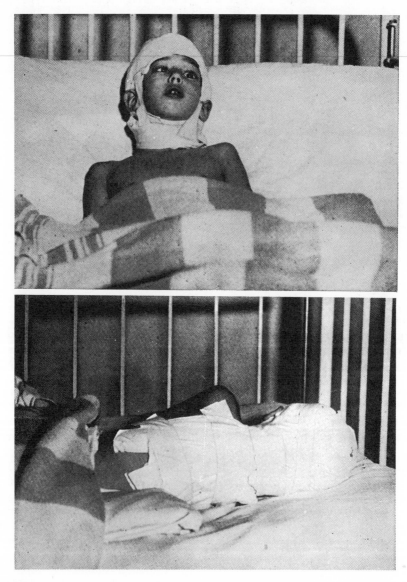

Fig. 210

This patient has had an infratentorial craniotomy. Note that the adhesive straps extend down the back to prevent the patient from flexing his neck. (From Sachs, Ernest: Diagnosis and treatment of brain tumors and care of the neurosurgical patient, ed. 2, St. Louis, 1949, The C. V. Mosby Co.)

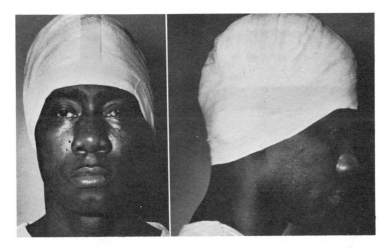

Fig. 211

Typical head dressing for the patient who has had a supratentorial craniotomy.
(From de Gutiérrez-Mahoney, C. G., and Carini, Esta: Neurological and neurosurgical
nursing, ed. 4, St. Louis, 1965, The C. V. Mosby Co.)

such as pinching or pricking. Specific observations are usually made and results recorded every thirty minutes for six hours, every hour for at least a day, and every three to four hours until the third or fourth postoperative day. Frequency of making and recording specific observations depends on the patient's condition. His temperature is usually taken every hour for four hours, and then at least every four hours for twenty-four hours. If the lesion was in the infratentorium, the temperature may be taken every two hours for two or three days, because edema of the brain stem might occur and upset the temperature control center in the medulla. (The treatment for hyperthermia is discussed on p. 66.) Any change in the patient's vital signs, state of consciousness, or ability to use muscles should be reported at once. If he appears to be restless, he should be watched closely for further signs, since restlessness may forewarn of hemorrhage or of irritation to the brain. Irregular or fixed pupils indicate pressure or disturbance that may be due to hemorrhage. In a patient who has intracranial bleeding, the blood pressure rises and the pulse rate drops as the intracranial pressure increases. This process continues until the pressure becomes so great that all regulating control is lost and the

blood pressure drops and the pulse rises just before death.

The family during the postoperative period. The family should be prepared to see the patient. They should know that he will return from the recovery room with a helmetlike head dressing and that edema may distort his features. If he is unconscious or has any noticeable limitation, such as aphasia, they should be so informed before entering his room. If he is alert, members of the family should be advised to sit quietly at the bedside since talking will tire the patient. If a supratentorial incision has been made, the family should be warned that when they see him on the day following surgery he may be unable to open one or both eyes, may have generalized facial edema, and may have discoloration of the skin about the eyes (ecchymosis) (Fig. 212). Periocular edema is caused by postoperative cerebral edema. It usually improves in three or four days. Iced compresses to the eyes may make the patient more comfortable.

Fluids and food. Fluid intake and output should be accurately recorded. If there is no special medical order to the contrary, 2,500 to 3,000 ml. of fluid should be given each day. Some neurosurgeons routinely

895

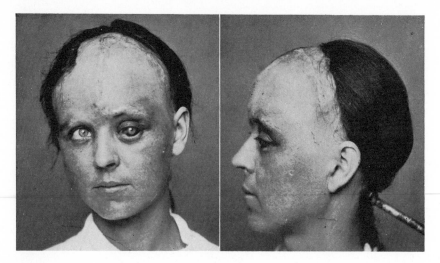

Fig. 212

This patient had surgery for a left-sided brain tumor eight days prior to the taking of these photographs. The conjunctiva of the left eye still shows ecchymosis. Note the area of hair and eyebrow shaved. (From Sachs, Ernest: Diagnosis and treatment of brain tumors and care of the neurosurgical patient, ed. 2, St. Louis, 1949, The C. V. Mosby Co.)

restrict fluids to 1,500 ml. per day for the first three days after a craniotomy.[10]

Since the gag and swallowing reflexes may be depressed or absent after infratentorial brain surgery, fluids by mouth are usually withheld for at least a day and intravenous fluids are substituted. They should be run very slowly to prevent increased intracranial pressure. The doctor tests the patient's reflexes. If they are present, water is carefully given by mouth. A nurse should help the patient until she is sure that there is no danger of his choking or aspirating fluids. The patient should be placed on his side or in a semisitting position. Fluid is most easily given by placing the rubber-protected tip of an Asepto syringe into the patient's mouth and allowing him to suck through it. Fluid should not be injected into his mouth. If he coughs or cannot swallow, the fluid should be discontinued.

A regular diet is usually given as soon as it is tolerated. After supratentorial surgery, the regular diet may be given on the second postoperative day. Any patient who has had a craniotomy, however, should be fed for at least forty-eight hours to prevent undue fa-

tigue. He may need to be fed for a longer time to ensure adequate food and fluid intake. If the patient is unable to take food and fluid by mouth, liquid foods by nasogastric tube are started forty-eight hours postoperatively.

Urinary output. Care must be taken to see that the patient voids. Urinary output must be carefully recorded, and sometimes an indwelling catheter may be used for a few days following surgery. A decrease in output must be reported to the doctor. It may indicate the onset of a metabolic disorder of central nervous system origin. If a pituitary tumor has been removed, special attention must be paid to urinary output because surgery on the pituitary gland may alter the control of water balance. Patients who have had surgery of the pituitary gland usually are given pituitary hormones to control excessive loss of fluid and electrolytes in the urine (p. 763).

Bowel function. Because straining increases intracranial pressure, the patient is urged not to try to have a bowel movement until the third postoperative day. On the second and third postoperative days he may be given a cathartic, and on the fourth postoperative day a small, low enema. He should be instructed not to strain in an attempt to expel the enema. If an impaction develops, it must be removed manually by the doctor.

Headache. Patients who are conscious after intracranial surgery complain of severe headache for twenty-four to forty-eight hours. Codeine sulfate usually is given hypodermically every four hours for this pain, and acetylsalicylic acid may be given by rectum or by mouth if fluids can be swallowed. An ice cap may be placed on the head, and sudden movement and jarring are avoided. He should be protected from loud noises and bright lights. Even if the patient is conscious, he should be turned with a turning sheet for the first forty-eight hours since the effort needed to move himself may cause further headache, increased intracranial pressure, or hemorrhage (Fig. 223). The turning sheet should be placed well above the level of the patient's head. General hygienic care for the patient during the first forty-eight hours is the same whether he is conscious or unconscious.

Ambulation. The patient who has had surgery for a supratentorial lesion usually is allowed out of bed on the third to fifth postoperative day. Activity should be increased gradually and he should be watched carefully for signs of increased intracranial pressure. First, the head of the bed should be elevated to a high Fowler's position, and then the patient should sit on the edge of the bed, with his feet hanging over its side. If he tolerates this position, four to six hours later, with the help of two persons, he may be assisted to a chair and usually may sit up for a half hour. He then progresses to normal activity as quickly as he desires and is able. The patient who has had surgery for an infratentorial lesion usually is not permitted up until the tenth postoperative day. His initial progress may be slower, since patients who have been kept flat in bed for some time may be dizzy upon arising until the circulatory system readjusts to the change in position.

Head dressings. If a drain has been used, the head dressing is changed by the doctor in twenty-four to forty-eight hours. Otherwise it is not disturbed until the sutures can be removed. They are usually removed on the third postoperative day following supratentorial incisions and on the fifth postoperative day following infratentorial incisions. Some neurosurgeons use a protective dressing both in the operating room and after the first dressing is changed. The wound is covered with gauze dressings. Two-inch crinoline bandage or a special head dressing (neurosurgical roll) is then applied in a recurrent fashion from the back to the front of the head. After the dressing has been anchored, a coating of heavy laundry starch is applied. Occasionally a thin plaster-of-Paris cast is used. It must be thoroughly dried with a hair dryer. The crinoline and starch dressing gives an even pressure to the dressings and affords some protection from injury. The dressing, like any encircling dressing, may be too tight when it dries. Signs of tightness such as edema, must be reported to the doctor, who may slit the dressing, taking care to avoid the operative site.

When final dressings are removed, the scalp needs care. It should be gently cleansed with hydrogen peroxide to remove dried blood. Crusts can be loosened with mineral oil. The head may then be shampooed, with care taken not to rub the operative area or put traction on the healed suture line. The patient is often given a head covering, which protects the healed wound from dirt and helps to remind the patient not to scratch. Some doctors prefer that a stockinette cap be worn at first because it readily reveals any bulging of the wound. A cap may be made by tying one end of a 10-inch piece of tubular stockinette. (See Fig. 213.) For women patients, it is psychologically important to cover the operative scar. Many doctors prefer that women patients wear an attractive bandana. The nurse should inspect the wound at least twice a day. The patient who has had a piece of bone left out will eventually have a depression in the scalp, and he should be warned of the danger of bumping his head in this area. Women patients should be encouraged to have the remaining hair restyled. If the hospital has beautician service, restyling may be done, with the doctor's permission, before the patient leaves the hospital.

Protective measures. Sometimes the patient must be protected from self-injury after a brain operation. If he pulls at dressings or

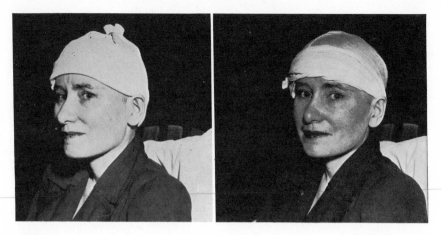

Fig. 213

The patient convalescing after brain surgery. In one picture she wears a stockinette cap; in the other, a turban. Note that she wears makeup. (From Sachs, Ernest: Diagnosis and treatment of brain tumors and care of the neurosurgical patient, ed. 2, St. Louis, 1949, The C. V. Mosby Co.)

a catheter, or if he scratches or hits himself, he should be attended constantly, and occasionally some kind of hand restraint, such as a large mitten made of combination pads, bandages, and stockinette and fastened at the wrist with adhesive tape, may be used. Mittens usually upset the patient less than arm restraints since with mittens he can move his arm freely. The fingers should be separated with gauze to prevent skin irritation and should be curled around a large bandage roll in the palm to prevent hyperextension of the fingers. The hand is then well covered with combination pads held in place with bandage. A piece of stockinette is closed at one end and everted so that the tied end cannot cause injury to the eye. It is then slipped over the bandaged hand and fastened securely at the wrist with adhesive tape. The hair should be shaved from the wrist and the skin protected with tincture of benzoin before adhesive is used. At least every other day the mitten must be removed, the hand washed in warm water, and passive exercise given to the fingers before the mitten is reapplied.

Ventricular drainage. Occasionally a catheter is placed in a ventricle of the brain to drain excess spinal fluid and prevent increased intracranial pressure. The catheter is usually attached to a drainage system on a level with the ventricle. The collection bottle is frequently attached to the head of the bed. The tubing and drainage receptable should be sterile, and care must be taken to prevent kinking of the tubing. If drainage seems to stop, the doctor should be notified. The catheter is usually left in place for twenty-four to forty-eight hours and is then removed by the surgeon.

Complications. Meningitis is a relatively rare complication of brain surgery. It can follow infection during the operation or thereafter. Following supratentorial surgery, the nurse should watch for any clear, watery drainage from the nose. This drainage may be present if there has been a tear in the meninges, which causes subsequent loss of cerebrospinal fluid. The treatment consists of keeping the patient very quiet, avoiding any suctioning or blowing of the nose, and administering antibiotic drugs. The leakage usually subsides spontaneously. Because of the danger of causing damage that might be followed by the drainage of cerebrospinal fluid through the nose, many surgeons request that the nose never be suctioned when supratentorial surgery has been done. A sign with this caution may be placed at the head of the bed.

Respiratory collapse may follow infratentorial surgery. It is caused by edema of the brain stem or edema above the brain stem that causes herniation of the brain stem into the foramen magnum and pressure on the respiratory center. Any irregularity of respirations, dyspnea, or cyanosis should be reported to the surgeon at once. Equipment should be ready for administering oxygen, doing a ventricular tap, and doing a tracheotomy if this procedure has not already been done. (For details of nursing care of the patient with a tracheostomy, see p. 598.) Occasionally a respirator is used (p. 853).

Convulsions are not unusual after a craniotomy, and therefore a mouth gag should be at the bedside and side rails should be used even if the patient is unconscious and it is believed that he cannot move. Diphenylhydantoin sodium (Dilantin sodium) may be ordered prophylactically to prevent convulsions. The drug may be given by rectum until the patient is able to take it by mouth. If the patient has a history of seizures before the operation or if convulsions occurred in the postoperative period, he may be given this drug for several months postoperatively.

Loss of the corneal reflex may follow brain tumors or brain surgery. If the eye appears inflamed or if the patient does not seem to blink when objects approach the open eye, the doctor should be notified. Special eye care, such as that given to patients who have had cerebrovascular accidents or who have surgery for trigeminal neuralgia, may be necessary.

The patient may complain of *double vision* after brain surgery. This condition is often temporary, and the patient should know that it will probably improve. It can be relieved by placing an opaque eye shield over one eye. The eye covered usually is alternated each day to prevent atrophy of eye muscles through disuse.

X-ray therapy is given to many patients following surgery for brain tumors. (See p. 281 for discussion of nursing the patient receiving radiation.)

Long-term care. Some patients who have had cranial surgery will have physical and mental limitations. The patient may have hemiplegia, aphasia, and personality changes, including severe depression. The rehabilitative care and planning both for the patient and for his family are the same as for other patients with chronic and permanent neurologic disease. Specific rehabilitation for patients with hemiplegia and aphasia is similar to that following cerebrovascular accidents. Preventive exercises should be started as soon as possible postoperatively. Regardless of the eventual prognosis, each patient should be helped to be as independent as possible for as long as possible.

The patient who has had brain surgery may need the same protection from injury as do other patients with neurologic disease when judgment defect, disorientation, or locomotor difficulties make it unsafe for him to move above without assistance.

Spinal cord injuries

The spinal cord may be damaged by pressure or erosion from a lesion outside the cord or by a tumor within the cord itself. The more common cause of injury, however, is compression by surrounding structures. Metastatic tumors growing in the vertebral bones may cause injury by direct extension and pressure or by destroying the bony support around the cord. Rupture of an intervertebral disk with protrusion of the nucleus pulposus into the spinal canal is a common cause of cord compression. Accidents involving the spine may cause fractures of the vertebras or laminas, with resultant tearing or compression of the cord and edema, which also causes compression. Since the spinal cord is located within a bony canal, slight edema of the cord, relatively small tumor growths, and minimal protrusions of tissue into the canal may cause symptoms of cord compression. Paralysis may occur in body parts supplied by nerves leaving the cord below the level of injury. (See Fig. 214.)

The symptoms of cord compression depend on the level at which the compression occurs and the degree of compression sustained. Cervical injury may cause paralysis of all four extremities and the trunk. Perspiration may be absent in the paralyzed parts; the patient is unable to void and has fecal incontinence. Since the diaphragm and intercostal muscles are paralyzed, respiratory failure may result, and the patient may die unless he is placed immediately into a respirator. A pulmotor is sometimes used for short

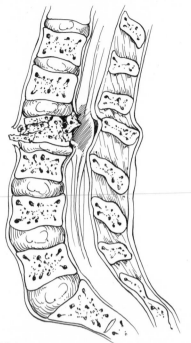

Fig. 214

Damage to the spinal cord and distortion of adjacent structures that may occur in traumatic injuries to the spine.

periods of transportation to a hospital where equipment to aid respirations is available.

Compression of the spinal cord in the thoracic region causes paralysis of the lower extremities, bladder, and rectum. The paralysis is flaccid at first but becomes spastic. Compression of the cord in the lumbar region causes a flaccid paralysis of the lower extremities, bladder, and rectum. This paralysis remains flaccid.

Diagnosis of cord compression can usually be made by the history and the neurologic examination. Roentgenograms of the spine may be taken and lumbar punctures done; myelograms also may be made. Any inability to move an extremity or any loss of sensation should make one suspicious of cord compression, and the patient should be treated accordingly until there is proof to the contrary. This precaution may prevent such a disastrous result as permanent paralysis or death.

900

General principles of care

Position and movement. Before moving a patient with acute spinal cord injury onto a bed from the stretcher on which he is admitted, the doctor should be consulted about the type of bed he wishes used. The selection will depend on the doctor's preference, the type of injury, the size of the patient, and the equipment available. If a regular bed is to be used, a full-length fracture board should be placed on top of the bedspring under the mattress. This board prevents sagging of the bed and motion of the spine. If the bed is to be gatched, the board must be hinged, or two or more boards with correctly placed breaks must be used. Mattresses containing springs should not be used. Instead of springs and one mattress, some doctors prefer two hair mattress placed on top of the fracture board. Some use the knee gatch to provide hyperextension to the spine (Fig. 215); the bed must then be made up "head to foot." Sponge rubber mattresses are widely recommended and, when available, are usually used when there is the possibility that for some time the patient will be moved very little and with extreme difficulty. If available, an alternating air-pressure mattress often is used. It alternates the points of pressure at regular intervals. Since it may be dangerous to move the patient for some time and since he may have loss of sensation and paralysis of part of the body, pressure areas develop easily. The mattress and entire bed foundation must be well protected with plastic sheeting so that incontinence will not cause damage.

Before moving the patient, the bed foundation should be completely adjusted, with gatches raised as ordered, bolsters placed in the desired positions, and a turning sheet available so that a minimum of motion will be necessary. Three to five people are needed to move the patient from the stretcher to the bed, depending upon his size and the location of injury. The doctor should supervise moving the patient. The body should be supported in proper alignment, and, if necessary, a doctor should apply manual hyperextension to the spine as the patient is moved. (See p. 245.)

Observation. The nurse must carefully observe the patient with a spinal fracture, a cord tumor, or a ruptured intervertebral

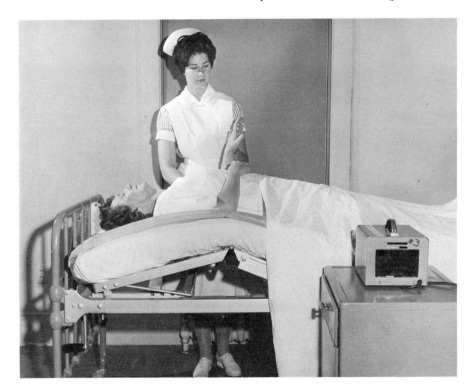

Fig. 215

Hyperextension for spinal fracture can be accomplished by gatching the bed with the patient head to foot in the bed. This patient is placed so that the highest point is directly under the fracture. An alternating air-pressure mattress is often used on the bed to prevent pressure sores. The patient must be observed carefully for changes in sensation or use of the extremities.

disk for signs of cord compression. The motion, strength, and sensation in the extremities should be tested at least four times a day and more frequently if specifically ordered. Any loss of motion or sensation should be reported at once, since immediate surgery may be needed to relieve pressure on the cord. Some of the laminas may be removed to prevent pressure from edema.

General hygiene. If cord damage has occurred, nursing care will depend on the level of the injury. Patients with cervical lesions, for instance, will be unable to do anything for themselves. Meticulous skin care, maintenance of correct body alignment, preservation of range of joint motion, and attempts to preserve muscle tone are imperative nursing measures in the care of any paralyzed patient. No external heat such as a hot-water bottle should be used if the patient has loss of sensation and will not feel a burn. Care should also be taken to be sure that bath water is not too hot, and paralyzed areas should be inspected daily for any signs of skin irritation. There will be no perspiration below the cord injury. At first

this may cause the patient to have an elevated temperature, which may be treated as described on p. 66. Later there may be excessive perspiration of the unaffected areas, which will need to be bathed frequently.

Diet. If the patient's arms are paralyzed or if he is not allowed to move them, he will need to be fed. The diet for any patient who is immobilized because of spinal injuries should be high in protein to increase the resistance to decubiti. Fruit juices and foods high in calcium may be limited since urinary calculi tend to form

901

quite easily in patients who are completely immobilized and in those who have fractures. Unless otherwise ordered, at least 3,000 ml. of fluid should be given daily.

Urinary output. The patient may have urinary retention because of injury to spinal nerves. Since he may have no sensation of needing to void, the nurse should check carefully for voiding and for distention of the bladder. A Foley type of catheter may be inserted into the bladder, or a cystostomy may be done. Later, if the injury is not in the lumbar area, automatic bladder function may be established. (See p. 154.)

Gastrointestinal function. Following an acute injury to the spinal cord, the patient often has abdominal distention. A rectal tube may be used, and neostigmine may be given hypodermically to stimulate peristalsis. A nasogastric tube or a Miller-Abbott or Cantor tube attached to suction equipment may be tried. Cathartics and enemas may be required to maintain normal bowel function. A permanent loss of bowel control may occur. (See p. 157 for care of and rehabilitation measures for patients with fecal incontinence.) If the injury is in the lumbar area, no recovery of automatic control can be hoped for, since the bowel is permanently flaccid, unless partial recovery eventually occurs.

Pain. Patients with spinal injuries often have a great deal of pain at the level of the injury which radiates along the spinal nerves. A thoracic injury causes chest pain, whereas a lumbar injury causes pain in the legs. Analgesics such as acetylsalicylic acid are ordered, and narcotics usually must be given for some time. However, if the patient has a high cervical injury, no narcotics should be given because respirations may be further depressed. Sometimes the paravertebral nerves are injected with 95% alcohol to relieve thoracic pain. This measure may give relief for several weeks or even months.

Prevention of respiratory complications. Respiratory complications are common following injury of the spinal cord. The patient should be encouraged to take frequent deep breaths, fully expanding the lungs. If he cannot be turned, deep-breathing exercises should be supervised, and he should take ten to fifteen deep breaths at least every two hours. Patients who can be turned

should have position changes at least every two hours and should be encouraged to take deep breaths. If coughing is not contraindicated, it should be encouraged also, but the doctor should be consulted before urging the patient to cough. Patients who have injuries of the thoracic spine tend to splint their chests and have shallow breathing. Narcotics may be given to control the pain that causes splinting of the chest and shallow breathing.

Rehabilitation. As the patient recovers, every possible effort should be made to help him do as much as possible for himself. Supplies should be placed within his reach on special trays or on overbed tables, and he must be given time to give what daily personal care he can manage for himself. Diversional activity should be started to keep him constructively occupied. An occupational therapist can help the nurse in selecting appropriate activities. However, if an occupational therapist is not available, the patient may do any light handiwork that he enjoys and that is feasible, provided he can use his arms. A radio, television set, and reading material may help to pass the time. If the patient's neck is hyperextended, books that can be flashed on the ceiling are useful if they do not cause eyestrain. Volunteers are exceedingly helpful in reading to patients. The patient's family and friends should be encouraged to visit often and to keep him up-to-date on activities in his home and community.

Possible rehabilitation depends on the extent of the cord injury, the emotional reactions of the patient, his age, and other factors (Figs. 216 and 217). Muscle exercises often can be started long before the patient is allowed up, and this practice lessens the period of rehabilitation necessary for returning to activity. The patient should be kept in proper body alignment at all times to prevent shortening of muscles and contracture of joints. The patient who must be kept on his back should have a small, round bolster placed under the knees so that the proximal end of the tibia is supported without any popliteal pressure. Bath towels or a small pillow can be used to fashion such a bolster. A firm, flat pillow should be placed under both calves, and the feet should be firmly dorsiflexed against a footboard. Foot drop and contrac-

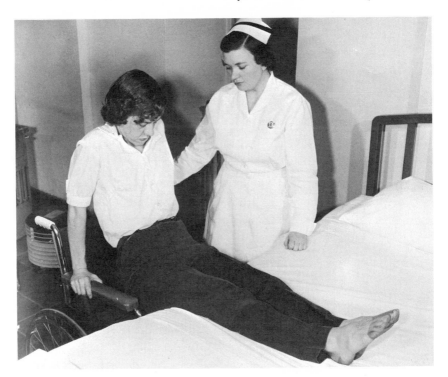

Fig. 216

The paraplegic patient moving from bed to wheelchair. Note placement of the chair. The patient pushes up with her arms when moving the buttocks into the chair seat. The paralyzed legs rest on the bed and must be lifted down. Patients with spinal tumors or injuries are frequently paraplegic.

tures at the hips and knees may take months to overcome, and they may prevent the paralyzed patient from being able to walk even when he uses braces and crutches.

Before the patient is permitted to be up following a spinal injury, a brace may be prescribed. A *Taylor back brace*, made of padded and covered metal bars to support the back, is often used. It has sturdy straps that come forward to be fastened over a muslin "apron." Patients who have ruptured lumbar intervertebral disks may be fitted with a heavy muslin corset with firm stays. All braces and corsets must be custom-made and are quite expensive. The cost usually is at least $75 for a brace and, of course, it cannot be reused by another patient. The brace or corset should be applied before the patient gets out of bed, and he will need help in getting into it. The patient should wear a thin knitted undershirt next to the skin to keep the brace clean and to protect the skin. Correct use so that the brace fits contours of the buttocks and chest as designed makes a great deal of

difference in the patient's comfort. Care should be taken that the apron is smooth and that tapes are not twisted. The patient's emotional reaction to wearing a brace or a corset is important, since it vitally affects ultimate rehabilitation. Attention to small details that help in initial acceptance of this somewhat uncomfortable and unfamiliar piece of "clothing" is important. The patient should practice putting the brace on while he is in the hospital if he must wear it for some time. A close member of his family may visit the hospital and learn to assist him. Patients who live alone and who are unable to care for their braces themselves may need to have a public health nurse help them in the home or teach someone else to assist.

903

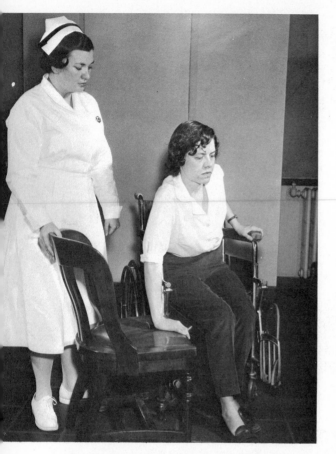

Fig. 217

Teaching the paraplegic patient to move from wheelchair to a straight chair. The same motion is used in moving from a wheelchair to the toilet seat. The patient should push up, turn toward the straight chair, and then swing the buttocks around onto the chair seat.

The patient wearing a brace should be especially careful in crossing streets and in engaging in activities such as walking down stairs, since he is limited in his ability to shift his balance quickly to prevent an accident.

Following fracture of a cervical vertebra, a neck brace may be ordered. This brace fits in such a manner that the chin rests on a cup, and the neck is kept in slight hyperextension. Patients who have a ruptured cervical disk may also need to use a neck brace,

and the *Thomas collar* is often used. (See Fig. 218.) A Thomas collar can be quite cheaply improvised as follows: (1) cut a piece of firm cardboard the depth desired; (2) pad it with cotton or combination pads and secure with bandages; (3) cover the collar with stockinette and carefully stitch at the top and bottom, avoiding bumps or knots that may irritate the skin. The collar is usually anchored at the side with wide adhesive tape and must never be removed without specific orders from the surgeon. The collar extends well up under the chin and prevents flexion of the neck. The patient who wears any brace to hyperextend the neck has difficulty in seeing where he is going and must be cautioned about this problem, because accidents can occur easily during everyday functions, such as crossing streets and going down stairs.

All patients who have had spinal injuries should wear shoes with firm lasts and low heels. If the woman patient has always worn moderately high heels, she should continue to wear them rather than to wear flat-heeled shoes. Shoes that tie are preferable. The patient is usually asked to have his family bring his shoes to the hospital so that they may be examined by the doctor and so that they may be worn when he first walks about in the hospital.

Nursing care of the patient with a fracture of the spine

Fractures of the spine may cause compression of the bodies of the vertebras or smashing of the laminas, with or without dislocation of parts, and compression of the spinal cord may result. (The emergency care of patients suffering fracture of the spine is discussed on p. 245.) Nurses should know and be able to teach others what symptoms indicate spinal fracture and how to care for a patient with a spinal fracture so that cord damage is not caused or increased. Spinal fractures should be suspected after automobile accidents, falls, and diving accidents.

Hyperextension. The patient with a spinal fracture may be placed in hyperextension since this position causes the least pressure on the spinal cord. Hyperextension may be accomplished by various means. Skeletal traction may be used. Small burr holes are drilled in the outer portion of the skull over each parietal region. *Tongs* (usually Crutchfield) are then inserted into the holes, the skin around the tongs is sutured, and a collodion dressing is applied. From ten to twenty pounds of weight are attached to a rope coming from the center of the tongs and extending over a pulley attached to the head of the bed. If Crutchfield tongs are to be used, the bed should be made up "head to foot." The nurse must be sure that the patient does not slip up in the bed enough for the weights to rest on a rung of the bed or on the floor. The rope should be free of the mattress or any other obstruction that might decrease the amount of pull needed and thus harm the patient (Fig. 219). Sandbags are often placed above the patient's shoulders to help prevent his slipping toward the "head" of the bed. Occasionally the "head" of the bed may be elevated by placing the bed on blocks to give countertraction and to prevent the patient from slipping toward the "head" of the bed. Since elevation of the "head" of the bed increases the traction, it must not be done without a specific order from the doctor.

In order to obtain traction and hyperextension, a leather chin strap (Sayre strap) attached to a pulley and weights, as described for use with tongs, may be used. The strap fits snugly under the chin and against the occipital protuberances. Leather straps from front and back meet a metal spreader to which the pulley rope is centrally attached. Skin care of the patient's chin is extremely important when this kind of traction is used. The amount of pressure on the skin and soft tissues depends on the amount of weight used. Traction must not be released without the doctor's order, but the chin may need to be gently massaged as often as every hour. The nurse can exert gentle pressure on one side of the chin as she massages the other side with her other hand. Alcohol and powder should be used, and frequent sponging of the skin is necessary to protect the leather from perspiration and to make the patient more comfortable. A small piece of rubber sponge, sheepswool, or chamois is helpful if signs of skin irritation and pressure occur. When feeding the patient, the nurse should take care not to soil or moisten the leather chin strap.

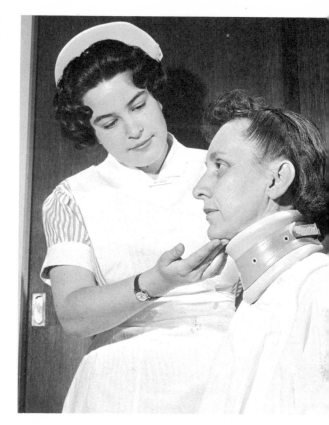

Fig. 218

This patient has been fitted with a neck brace following a cervical fracture. As the patient becomes accustomed to the brace, the nurse checks to see that skin irritation does not occur.

Hyperextension may be accomplished by gatching the bed with the patient head to foot in the bed and placing him so that the high point is directly under the fracture (Fig. 215). If the bed gatch is not at the desired position, a small, firm, round bolster, the width of the mattress, may be placed under the top mattress at the desired level. Several tightly rolled bath blankets may be used to make a bolster of the desired size. Obviously a fracture board must be used to give firm support, and it must be hinged to permit use of the gatches. This method of obtaining hyperextension is commonly used following fracture of a thoracic vertebra.

Members of the family should be prepared for seeing the patient in head or neck trac-

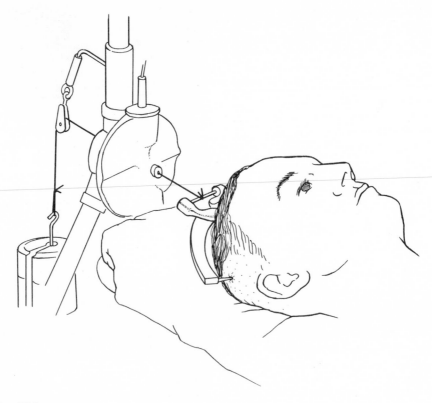

Fig. 219

Patient with Crutchfield tongs inserted into the skull.

tion. Tongs are particularly frightening to them. Both the family and the patient should understand that the tongs do not go through the skull but only into the outer layer of bone. Actually, many patients get so much relief from pain from this type of traction that they accept it surprisingly well. An adjustable mirror attached to the head of the bed enables them to see about the room. Usually they are happier and more content when in a unit with other patients around them.

The patient who is placed in hyperextension cannot be moved about in bed. He must stay flat on his back for as long as six weeks. He must understand why this is necessary, since a sudden movement might cause irreparable cord damage. A drawsheet may be placed over the abdomen and tucked in at the sides of the mattress to remind the restless patient not to move. Occasionally,

sandbags are placed on either side of the body. This is done most often during sleeping hours. If the patient is very restless or unable to cooperate, he must be constantly attended to prevent his moving about in bed.

Patients who are immobilized in head or neck traction or kept in hyperextension develop pneumonia easily. The patient must be instructed to take from ten to fifteen deep breaths regularly each hour when he is awake. The nurse should remain with him to see that it is done at least several times each day. Arms and legs usually may be exercised passively if the patient is paralyzed and unable to move himself, but a doctor should be consulted before this is done.

Care of the skin is a major responsibility of the nurse, and the patient must be given back care at least every two hours. The nurse's work is made much easier if the patient is on a sponge rubber mattress, since two nurses working together can give the patient back care without moving him. Each nurse depresses the mattress with one hand and massages the patient's skin with the palm of the other. No part of the back should be neglected, although not all the surface of the back must be done at once, since this might tire the patient too much. The use of a bedpan presents a problem, but a child's bedpan may be placed under the patient without moving him if two nurses work together. The part of the mattress under the buttocks should be depressed with one hand and the bedpan slipped into place with the other. To maintain correct spinal alignment, one of the the nurses should insert a small towel roll at the small of the patient's back directly above the bedpan.

Extreme care must be taken in feeding any patient who is in hyperextension and lying on his back, since it is difficult to swallow in this position. Obviously if the patient chokes he cannot turn or be raised forward. A suction machine should always be on hand for immediate use in case the patient should aspirate into the trachea. The patient should practice swallowing saliva before he attempts to take fluids or solid foods. Usually he does best when given fairly soft food, such as baked custard, at first, because liquids tend to flow into the nasopharynx quite easily. Feeding the patient, at least until he has become fully accustomed to the awkward position, is a nursing responsibility that should never be delegated to a nonprofessional worker. Since feeding the patient takes time, it must be planned for. He must not be allowed to feel that he is a nursing problem on this account. Adequate food intake is necessary to prevent pressure areas from developing and to preserve general tissue health. Also, since meals are psychologically important to all people, the patient needs the emotional support that attractive meals will give when carefully fed to him.

Stryker frame and Foster bed. If the patient with a spinal injury can be placed flat in bed but cannot be turned in bed, a Stryker frame or a Foster bed may be used (Fig. 184). These beds make it possible to change the patient's position from abdomen to back without altering his alignment. Usu-

ally the patient on one of these beds is turned every two to four hours. The bed cannot be used for very obese patients because space between the frames is inadequate and cannot be adjusted sufficiently. The beds have two metal frames to which canvas covers are attached. The canvas used for the back-lying position has an opening under the buttocks to allow for use of a bedpan, and the canvas used for the prone-lying position can be cut out so that the male patient can void. When the patient is in the prone position, the canvas should extend from below the shoulders to the ankles, and a narrow head strap should be used to support the forehead. In the prone position the patient can eat, read, and do light activities with his hands. The canvasses may be covered with thin sponge rubber mattresses cut the same size as the canvas and covered with bed linen. To turn the patient, the linen, the mattress, and the opposite canvas and frame are placed in that order over the patient. The frame fastens to a metal attachment at head and foot. Straps are placed around both frames, and then two people release pivot pins at either end of the frame and slowly rotate the patient on the frame from his abdomen to his back or vice versa. The pins are reinserted, and the upper frame, canvas, and mattress are removed. The bed has armboard and footboard attachments to use, if desired, for permissible activity or for good alignment. The patient may be quite apprehensive about being placed on this bed, and, if possible, a demonstration of turning should be given to him before he is moved onto it. This type of bed is unsafe for a very restless or disoriented patient, although the straps may be used to give some security and protection. Another advantage of these beds is that they wheel easily, so that the patient may be taken to a sun porch or recreational area for a change of surroundings.

Plaster jacket. A plaster jacket that extends from the shoulders to below the hips is sometimes used to treat the patient with a fractured vertebra below the cervical area. A fracture board and a firm mattress should be used. As soon as the patient returns from the plaster room, the nurse should check the cast at the top and bottom for crumbs of plaster, which can usually be removed at first but later are difficult to remove as they work downward or upward. The cast should be examined to be certain it is cut out enough to permit use of a bedpan. If it is not, the nurse must remind the doctor, since it must be done before the patient has a bowel movement. The patient can usually urinate safely without soiling the cast. Plastic material may be used to cover the cast edges, and the head of the bed may be raised on blocks so that gravity can help to simplify voiding. The gatch must never be raised without the doctor's order, since this may cause the cast to crack. When the cast is dry, its edges should be bound with small pieces of adhesive tape to protect the skin from irritation. This procedure is known as "petaling" the cast.[31] The lower portion should be covered with plastic material fastened on the edge and pushed up under the cast so that it will remain in place when a bedpan is used. This material can easily be removed and changed if it becomes soiled.

If abdominal distention is troublesome, a "window," or opening, may be cut in the cast over the abdomen. The edges of this opening must also be bound. Such a window is useful in checking for distention of the bladder. Skin under the cast should be massaged with alcohol and powder. The nurse should slip her hand palm downward as far as she can reach to feel for crumbs or bits of plaster and any areas of skin tenderness, which may be caused by pressure or irritation. The cast is usually loose enough to permit threading a thin piece of terry cloth toweling from top to bottom under the cast to partially cleanse the patient's skin. This procedure is done by having the patient lie down, which permits the toweling to be pushed along the upper surface of the body, which "falls away" from the cast while he is in this position until it can be reached at the other end of the cast. The patient then turns slowly and supports himself by holding the upper rungs of the bed. Pillows may be needed to support the cast at the hips at this time. The toweling must not be too wet or the lining of the cast will become moist, but soap may be used, and the use of a scented cologne is often gratifying to women patients. (For further details, see orthopedic nursing texts.[31])

Nursing care of a patient with a ruptured intervertebral disk

Although low back pain can be caused by congenital anomalies, poor general use of the back combined with overweight, and changes such as those caused by arthritis, the most common cause with an organic basis is a "slipped disk," or ruptured intervertebral disk. Rupture of an intervertebral disk with protrusion of the nucleus pulposus into the spinal canal is a common spinal injury among middle-aged persons engaged in manual labor (Fig. 220). With age, the anulus fibrosus, or fibrous capsule within which the nucleus pulposus (a soft, cartilaginous pad) is enclosed, becomes less elastic and ruptures easily. Although the disk may rupture at any level in the spine, the most common sites are the last two lumbar interspaces. Rupture of the disk at the fifth and sixth cervical interspaces is seen less frequently.

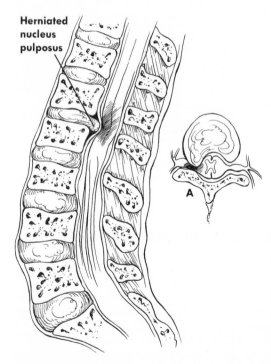

Fig. 220

Note compression of the spinal cord, caused by herniation of nucleus pulposus into the spinal canal and, **A,** pressure on nerves as they leave the spinal cord.

Prevention. Injury to an intervertebral disk usually is caused by stress on the back while it is in acute flexion. Many back injuries of this type could be prevented if persons doing extensive lifting and pulling were taught to observe principles of good body mechanics. When a person is lifting heavy objects, the knees should be flexed and the back kept straight. In this position, the large muscles of the thighs and the buttocks carry the weight—not the back muscles, which give support to the spine. It is always better to pull than to push, and the body should be kept in correct alignment and not twisted to one side whenever one bends, lifts, or carries heavy objects. If one is lifting objects from a high shelf, both hands should be used. This will place the weight of the object on the shoulder muscles rather than on those of the cervical spine.

The nurse must frequently move patients and heavy objects. Therefore, she must learn and practice the principles of good body mechanics. The incidence of back strain and ruptured intervertebral disks is high among nursing personnel. The nurse should be responsible for teaching the principles of good body mechanics to persons who work with her. The industrial nurse may have many opportunities to help workers improve their body mechanics and avoid back injury. (For complete discussion of body mechanics in nursing, see texts on fundamentals of nursing.)

Diagnostic measures. The diagnosis of ruptured intervertebral disk usually is made from the history and neurologic examination. The patient with a ruptured lumbar disk typically has a sciatic pain when the leg on the affected side is raised straight up without bending the knee (Lasègue's sign). The pain is caused by the pressing of the protruding nucleus pulposus against the sciatic nerve. Motor and sensory losses can be traced along the course of the impinged spinal nerves, and manual pressure on the jugular veins will cause increased pain since this measure causes a rise in intracranial pressure. A lumbar puncture is often done to differentiate this condition from an intervertebral tumor. The cerebrospinal protein is elevated in the presence of a tumor. Roentgenograms of the spine are taken, and myelography sometimes is done. The latter procedure is most useful in differentiating a herniated disk from an intervertebral tumor.

The patient with a ruptured intervertebral lumbar disk. The patient with a ruptured intervertebral lumbar disk usually complains of acute pain in the lower back. This pain usually appears suddenly when stress is placed on the back, such as when opening a window, or soon thereafter. Later the pain begins to radiate over one buttock and into the leg, often extending as far as the ankle. It is unilateral since the nucleus pulposus usually presses on nerves arising from one side of the spinal cord. Activities such as sneezing, coughing, bending, or straining to defecate cause increased pain since they temporarily increase intracranial pressure, which puts additional pressure on the pinched spinal nerves. Since motor and sensory nerves to the leg and foot may be impinged upon, the patient may limp and have paresthesia or hyperesthesia in the leg and foot on the affected side. He typically walks on either his toes or his heels because of muscle spasm in the leg. The severity of neurologic damage is indicative of the amount of compression on the cord and may dictate the treatment, since immediate operation may be imperative to prevent permanent cord damage. The nurse should urge anyone who has injured his back to seek immediate medical attention.

Conservative treatment. If possible, the patient with a ruptured intervertebral lumbar disk is treated conservatively. He is placed on bed rest. Sometimes Bucks extension (p. 944) is used, and occasionally head and pelvic traction is tried (see texts on orthopedic nursing). The bed usually is kept flat, and a firm mattress should be used to maintain good body alignment and alleviate pain caused by stress on the affected nerves, and a bed board may be placed under the mattress. If the patient is at home, table leaves or a door may be used. The patient should be taught to turn himself in a log-rolling fashion: to cross his arms over his chest, bend the uppermost knee to the side to which he wishes to turn, and then to roll over (Fig. 221). This position helps him to maintain good spinal alignment. If there is any motor nerve loss, a footboard should be used to prevent foot drop. The patient may complain of a burning sensation in his feet

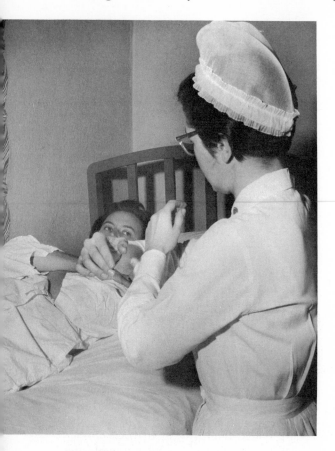

Fig. 221

The nurse is teaching the patient with a ruptured disk how to fold her arms preparatory to "logrolling."

should be taken each day, and a regular time for defecation should be established. A mild laxative such as one of the bulk laxatives may be ordered.

Many patients with a ruptured lumbar intervertebral disk suffer from severe muscle spasm in the lower back. A heating pad may relieve it, although codeine or other analgesic drugs are often necessary. Physical therapy in the form of infrared heat, massage, and active and passive muscle exercise done in warm water may also be ordered to help relieve the muscle spasm. Exercises are more easily performed in water, and the heat helps to relax muscles. The patient should be transferred to the physical therapy department by stretcher, and extra covers, such as a towel to wrap around the head if the hair becomes wet, should be sent with him to avoid chilling after the treatment.

The patient with a ruptured disk may be discouraged by the prospects of a long period of bed rest and possible surgery. If he has motor or sensory losses, he worries lest he become unable to walk. To some people the words spinal surgery are synonymous with paralysis. The patient may worry about his family, his finances, and his job and about collecting compensation if the injury was sustained at work. Doctors, nurses, other professional team members, and the patient's spiritual adviser may need to help alleviate his fears and anxieties. Although the head gatch may not be raised, he may be more content if the head of the bed may be elevated on 6-inch blocks, increasing his range of vision and allowing him to eat more easily. He may also find it easier to use the bedpan in this position. Diversions such as reading, visiting with others, and light handicrafts should be encouraged.

While the patient is still in bed, he should be measured for a corset so that it will be available when he gets up. He should have walking shoes and socks brought to the hospital. The corset should be put on before arising. Since straight leg raising and bending at the waist should be avoided, the patient may need assistance in getting into shoes and stockings. However, it is permissible to bend the knees to bring the foot up, and most patients learn to dress themselves.

The nurse should teach and demonstrate

because of paresthesia, and a footboard helps by keeping the bedclothes off the feet. If the patient has a sensory nerve loss, hot-water bottles or heating pads should not be used on the feet or legs, and other precautions should be taken to prevent further injury. A small bedpan should be used, and a small towel roll should be placed directly behind it to support the arch of the lower back. The patient should roll onto the bedpan instead of lifting his hips. He should be advised not to strain to defecate since straining will increase pain. Constipation is frequent. The patient is urged to increase the amount of roughage eaten, and fresh fruits are helpful. At least 3,000 ml. of fluid

principles of body mechanics to the patient since he will need to be particularly careful in lifting. Some patients may be encouraged by the doctor to change their type of work. Movement and positions that cause poor alignment of the spinal column and put strain on the injured nerves should be avoided until approved by the doctor. Approval usually is given about six weeks after the patient is allowed out of bed. A firm, straight chair should be used instead of an overstuffed one. The knees should not be crossed or the feet or legs elevated on a footstool. It is inadvisable for the patient to drive a car since this activity would necessitate stretching the legs. Stairs should be climbed as infrequently as possible, and great care should be taken in walking over rough ground or in stepping off curbs to avoid sudden twisting of the back. If a tub bath must be taken, the knees should be kept flexed; showers are preferable. The corset should be worn by the patient when he is out of bed except when bathing or taking a shower. In picking things up off the floor, the patient should assume a squatting posture, with the knees bent and the back held straight (Fig. 222). Weights heavier than five pounds should not be carried.

If, when the patient resumes activity, the symptoms recur, surgical excision of the ruptured portion of the nucleus pulposus will usually be necessary. This is done through an opening made by removing part of the bone surrounding the spinal cord. The procedure is called a *laminectomy*. If more than three intervertebral disks are ruptured, a *spinal fusion* usually is done. In a spinal fusion the spinal vertebras in the affected area are ankylosed, permanently preventing movement of this portion of the spine. The bone used is often taken from the iliac crest. The skin incision for both a laminectomy and a spinal fusion is made directly over the spinous processes and is about 10 cm. (4 inches) long.

The postoperative nursing care of the patient having surgery for a ruptured lumbar intervertebral disk is similar to that given the patient being treated more conservatively, with a few additional considerations. The patient should be observed carefully for signs of hemorrhage or leakage of spinal fluid from the wound and for compression

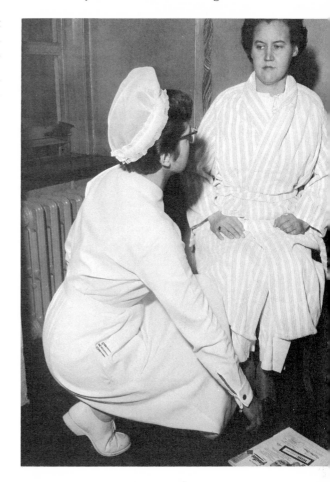

Fig. 222

The nurse is demonstrating to a patient with a ruptured disk how to stoop to pick something up from the floor. Note that her back is held straight and that her knees and hips are flexed sharply.

of the cord caused by edema at the site of operation. Evidence of hemorrhage or a loss of spinal fluid can usually be seen on the dressings. The doctor should be called at once. Usually he changes the dressings, since moisture on the dressings many predispose to infection. The patient who is bleeding from the wound may be placed on his back and the head of the bed elevated on blocks, causing the spinal fluid to put pressure on blood vessels in the area.

Before the operation the patient should

911

be warned that pain will persist for some time postoperatively because of local edema. Time is also needed for the nerve to recover from damage caused by the pressure on it preoperatively. The patient may complain of severe spasm in the back and thigh muscles. It is a result of the nerves being touched during surgery. The spasm may be relieved somewhat by moving the legs in bicycle fashion while the patient is lying on his side. The doctor may wish this exercise to be started on the first postoperative day. The patient may have bladder and bowel dysfunction for several days. These complications are treated in the usual manner—with Foley catheters, rectal tubes, neostigmine (Prostigmin), and carminative enemas.

Some doctors order bed rest for about ten

Fig. 223

The nurse and the aide are turning the patient who has had surgery for the excision of a ruptured disk. Note that the nurse holds the turning sheet taut with one hand at the level of the patient's shoulder and the other below his buttocks.

days after a laminectomy for excision of a protruded lumbar nucleus pulposus. Others have the patient get up on the operative day. If the patient is on bed rest, he should be turned every two hours by two people using a turning sheet (Fig. 223). He should make no attempt to help himself for forty-eight hours to prevent strain on the operative site. It is better if the patient and the nurse practice turning preoperatively, since postoperatively the patient may have a great deal of pain and may be tense and frightened. He should be told not to try to reach for articles on his bedside table but to ask for help. Heat and massage treatments are started the day after sutures have been removed, usually the fifth postoperative day. Hydrotherapy is not resumed until around the tenth day, at which time the patient is usually permitted up wearing a corset and walking shoes.

If the patient is to get up on the operative day, he must be fitted with a corset preoperatively. He should be watched closely for weakness or fainting, and the dressings should be checked for signs of hemorrhage or of leakage of cerebrospinal fluid. The patient may be given special exercises to do to relieve muscle spasm in the back and

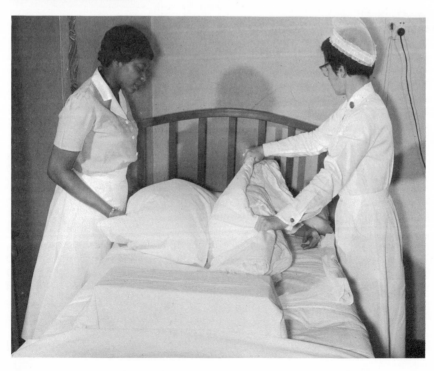

the thighs. The exercises may include the goose step, raising the knees high as he walks, and "woodchopping," which consists of raising both hands over the head and letting them fall to below the knees. The exercise should be done five to ten times three times a day. The patient may be discharged from the hospital by the fifth postoperative day. He should continue to sleep on a firm bed.

Patients who have had a spinal fusion are kept in bed for varying lengths of time (usually a minimum of two weeks) and resume activity slowly. A jacket cast sometimes is applied, and a brace or a corset may be used when it is removed. When such a cast is used, ambulation is possible at an earlier time.

The patient with a ruptured cervical intervertebral disk. The patient with a ruptured cervical intervertebral disk usually complains of pain and muscle weakness in the arms. Immediate operation may be necessary to relieve cord compression, since the compression may cause respiratory failure.

Following surgery for a ruptured cervical disk, the patient should be closely watched for decrease in chest expansion because edema may temporarily paralyze the diaphragm and intercostal muscles. If there is a decrease in chest expansion, the patient may need to be placed in a respirator at once.

The patient who has had surgery for a ruptured cervical disk is placed flat in bed postoperatively with only a small pillow at the nape of the neck. The head should not be flexed, because pressure may then be exerted on the cord and cause respiratory failure. The patient may be turned, but the turning sheet should extend above the head. On the third postoperative day he may be placed in a semi-Fowler's position, and pillows should be placed well down under the shoulders. Arm movements, even to eat, are prohibited until this time. The patient is allowed up on the fifth postoperative day, and a Thomas collar may be used to prevent forward flexion of the head for several weeks.

Nursing care of the patient with an intravertebral tumor

It is unfortunate that intravertebral tumors are infrequent, since they are extremely difficult to remove surgically without causing serious damage to the spinal cord. Tumors of the spinal cord are both intramedullary, involving primarily the substance of the cord, and extramedullary, involving primarily the meninges. Metastatic tumors often involve the vertebrae and may also invade the spinal cord and its coverings. Obviously, tumors involving the meninges are more likely to be removed successfully than the other types. Even when complete removal is not considered possible, surgery is often done to remove part of the tumor and to remove some of the bone surrounding the spinal column and thus reduce the obstruction for a time. This is called a *spinal decompression operation.*

The patient first complains of tenderness over a spinous process that is aggravated by movement and by bed rest. He may also have pain in the areas innervated by the cord at that level. A cervical lesion causes pain in the arms, a thoracic lesion causes pain in the chest, and a lumbar lesion causes pain in the legs. Foot and hand pain are rare, but there may be numbness and tingling. As the lesion grows and further compresses the cord, motor and sensory losses occur until eventually the patient loses all functions below the level of the tumor.

Nursing care for a patient with a tumor of the spinal cord is the same as that given other patients with spinal injury and its resultant neurologic symptoms. The care after a decompression operation is similar to that given the patient who has had excision of a ruptured nucleus pulposus, except that recovery is much slower. The patient often has severe pain and requires narcotics.

Convalescent care and rehabilitation depend entirely on the kind of tumor and whether or not it has been successfully removed. Even if it cannot be removed, the decompression operation may give relief from symptoms for months and sometimes years. X-ray treatment may be given while the patient is recovering in the hospital and continued after his dismissal. The family often needs help in caring for the patient and in meeting the problems that his condition entails. The patient often either knows or guesses if little can be done for him medically because he does not have the mental dulling that often accompanies brain tumors

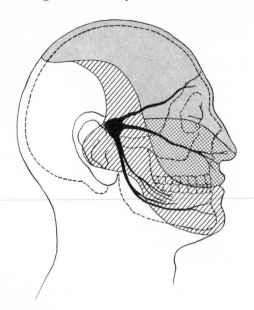

Fig. 224

Pathway of the trigeminal nerve and the facial area innervated by each of the three main branches.

and sometimes accompanies cerebrovascular accidents.

Trigeminal neuralgia

Trigeminal neuralgia, or tic douloureux, is characterized by excruciating, burning pain that radiates along one or more of the three divisions of the fifth cranial nerve (Fig. 224). The pain typically extends only to the midline of the face and head since this is the extent of the tissue supplied by the offending nerve. There are areas along the course of the nerve known as "trigger points," and the slightest stimulation of these areas may cause pain. Patients with trigeminal neuralgia usually are very unhappy individuals who try desperately to avoid "triggering" the pain. It is not unusual to see them lying in bed with the covers over their heads in an effort to avoid drafts. They frequently have been unable to eat properly for some time, since chewing causes pain. They may, therefore, be undernourished and dehydrated. They may have slept poorly and not have washed, shaved, or combed their hair for some time. Oral hygiene must often be neglected because of pain.

In caring for the patient with trigeminal neuralgia preoperatively or in caring for the patient who is being treated medically, it is important that members of the nursing staff be sympathetic toward the patient's behavior. Every effort should be made to avoid placing the patient in a draft and to avoid walking swiftly to his bed, because the slight motion of air created may be enough to cause pain. The bed should not be jarred or the bedclothes fanned. It is unwise to urge the patient to wash or shave the affected area or to comb his hair, since he may either become upset in feeling that it is required or he may comply and set off another seige of pain. He will probably prefer to do things for himself if touching his face is involved. It is sometimes possible for him to give himself mouth care if applicators and a lukewarm mouthwash are provided. Often pureed foods or lukewarm fluids taken through a straw are the only diet that can be tolerated.

Fifth nerve resection is an elective operative procedure. Although surgery relieves pain, some patients find that the side effects due to the numbing are almost unbearable. The patient is usually treated conservatively with such drugs as nicotinic acid, thiamine chloride, potassium chloride, cobra venom, analgesics, and sedatives for a time, and surgery is done only when the condition becomes unbearable. Antiepileptic drugs such as diphenylhydantoin (Dilantin) and carbamazepine (Tegretol) may shorten the duration of attacks. Using chlorpromazine hydrochloride (Thorazine) may permit a spontaneous remission to occur.[20] The peripheral branches of the fifth cranial nerve may also be injected with 95% alcohol, perhaps giving relief for several months. Recently it has been discovered that patients with tic douloureux have a decreased gastric acidity, and it is suspected that the reaction may be one similar to allergy to histamine. Success has been reported from giving hydrochloric acid, desensitizing the patient to histamine, and giving antihistaminic drugs.[19]

Postoperatively it is important to know what branches of the nerve have been cut in order to provide the necessary protection. If the upper branch is completely severed, the patient may lose the corneal reflex on that side. An attempt is made to save a few fibers of the nerve, since even a few seem to preserve this vital reflex. Until the doctor has tested the corneal reflex and verified its presence, an eye shield is used to prevent dust or lint from getting onto the cornea and causing injury.

The patient should be instructed not to touch or rub his eye but to blink it often, since blinking helps to lubricate the eye. Mineral oil or other medications should be used only as ordered by the doctor. If the reflex is completely missing, the eye should be bathed twice a day with normal saline solution or a weak boric acid solution, and a solution of methylcellulose may be prescribed to help keep the cornea moist. The lids should not be dried, since any material such as cotton, gauze, tissue, or toweling may leave lint. The patient should be taught to care for his eye when he returns home. Any contact with the eye should be carefully avoided when washing the face. The eye should be inspected several times a day, and medical attention should be sought if it becomes inflamed. Patients are safer outdoors if they wear glasses, which will protect the eyes from dust and other flying particles.

When the lower branch of the fifth cranial nerve is interrupted, the patient needs to avoid hot foods, since he will not be aware if the mucous membrane is burned. He may have some difficulty chewing and swallowing at first and should be instructed to place the food in the unaffected side of the mouth. Since food may be retained in the mouth on the affected side, mouth care should be given immediately following meals. Dental caries on the affected side will not cause pain. Therefore, the patient should visit the dentist routinely every six months. He should tell the dentist that he has had a fifth nerve resection so that trauma is avoided. Care must be taken in shaving to avoid nicking the insensitive skin.

Within twenty-four hours after a fifth nerve resection, many patients develop herpes simplex (cold sores) about the lips. Campho-Phenique, applied frequently, seems to give more relief than any other treatment. Usually the lesions heal in about a week.

Recently an operation has been devised by which the myelinated sheath of the fifth cranial nerve is partially removed, permitting the nerve to expand. Since the nerve is not resected, there is no sensory loss. However, the operation necessitates an infratentorial craniotomy.

Other cranial nerve surgery

Other cranial nerves may be interrupted if necessary. It is sometimes necessary to resect both the fifth and the ninth nerves to relieve severe pain caused by carcinoma of the sinuses. The nursing problems in each instance are related to the areas that have been desensitized and the resulting handicaps. Often there is temporary and sometimes permanent loss or a change of facial expression after resection of these nerves, which may cause severe psychic problems. When any nerve is resected, whether it be peripheral or cranial, the patient must understand that all sensation in this area is lost and that he will therefore need to avoid injury, especially from heat, cold, and trauma.

Intractable pain

When pain becomes unbearable and cannot be controlled by more conservative means, it is sometimes possible to alleviate it by surgery. Pain may involve the nerve endings in the skin, and scars such as those seen after an attack of herpes zoster may continue to cause severe pain. Such pain usually can be relieved by resecting a piece of the nerve going to the skin and cutting off pathways to the damaged nerve endings.

Neurectomy

When pain is localized in one part of the body, it can be relieved by interruption of the peripheral or cranial nerves supplying the area. The nerve fibers to the affected area are severed from the cord (cell body) in an operation known as a neurectomy. (The nerve may also be effectively destroyed by injecting it with absolute alcohol, but the results are unpredictable.) Not only pain fibers are interrupted by these procedures, but also fibers controlling movement and position sense. Therefore, this type of treatment cannot be used to control pain in the extremities. A neurectomy probably is most often done to relieve the suffering of patients with trigeminal neuralgia, in which case it is referred to as a *fifth nerve resection*. A neurectomy may also be done to control incapacitating dysmenorrhea, and is called a *presacral neurectomy*.

Rhizotomy

Resection of a posterior nerve root just before it enters the spinal cord is known as a rhizotomy. This procedure frequently is useful in controlling severe pain in the upper trunk, such as that caused by carcinoma of the lung. However, it cannot be used to relieve pain in the extremities since position sense is lost. The incision is made high in the thoracic or low in the cervical area and involves a laminectomy. The postoperative observation and care are similar to those necessary for any patient who has had a laminectomy, except that the patient who has had a rhizotomy is usually a poorer operative risk and may be suffering from a severe debilitating disease and therefore develops complications, such as decubiti, more easily. It is important for both the patient and the nurse to realize that this operation will not prevent pain at the level of incision because the resected nerves affect only the area below the incision.

Chordotomy

A chordotomy is an operation done to relieve intractable pain in the lower trunk and legs and is most often done for patients with extensive carcinoma of the pelvis. The incision is made high in the thoracic area, two laminas are removed, and the pain pathways in the spinothalamic tract (anterior and lateral aspect of the cord) on the side opposite the pain are severed (Fig. 225). If the pain is in the midline, the interruption must be made bilaterally. However, the two operations must be done separately to avoid extensive damage to the cord from edema.

Following surgery, nursing care is similar to that given a patient who has had a cervical laminectomy for removal of a protruded nucleus pulposus. Frequently temporary paralysis, or at least leg weakness, and loss of bowel and bladder control follow a chordotomy due to edema of the cord and will gradually disappear in about two weeks. Back care, with special attention given to pressure points, should be given every two or three hours since position sense is lessened and the patient is often debilitated. It is advisable to use an alternating air-pressure mattress until the patient is allowed out of bed. Sometimes a Foster bed or a Stryker frame enables the nurses to give the patient better care. Because of the decreased position sense, special attention needs to be given

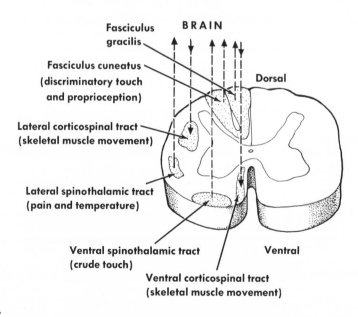

Fig. 225

Nerve pathways to and from the brain.

to placing the patient in proper body alignment by using foot blocks. If quadriceps-setting exercises are begun in the early postoperative period, retraining in walking will be less difficult for the patient. It usually is easier for the patient to use a walker when he first begins to walk, but he should progress to a cane. Many patients will always feel more secure with a cane. Occupational therapy should be designed to strengthen the leg muscles. The use of a treadle sewing machine or a treadle sander will give exercise to the ankle. A bicycle provides for hip and knee flexion and extension. Therapy can be started as soon as the patient can be out of bed comfortably for at least two hours at a time.

Because temperature sensation is permanently lost, the nurse must be careful to avoid burning or otherwise injuring the patient's lower trunk and legs, and she must teach the patient and his family to avoid injury. The lower portion of the body, especially the feet, should be inspected routinely for any breaks in the skin or unnoticed infection.

References and selected readings*

1 Alpers, Bernard J.: Clinical neurology, ed. 5, Philadelphia, 1963, F. A. Davis Co.

2 *Anderson, Eleanor M., and Irving, Jane: Uninterrupted care for long-term patients, Pub. Health Rep. **80:**271-275, March 1965.

3 *Ariagno, Richard P., and Quimby, Margaret Ann: Ultrasonic surgery for Meniere's disease and care of patients with labyrinthine dysfunction, Am. J. Nursing **60:**1778-1781, Dec. 1960.

4 Baker, A. B., editor: Clinical neurology (4 vol.), ed. 2, New York, 1962, Harper & Row, Publishers.

5 Beeson, Paul B., and McDermott, Walsh, editors: Cecil-Loeb textbook of medicine, ed. 11, Philadelphia, 1963, W. B. Saunders Co.

6 Bergersen, Betty S., and Krug, Elsie E.: Pharmacology in nursing, ed. 10, St. Louis, 1966, The C. V. Mosby Co.

7 *Buck, McKenzie: Adjustments during recovery from stroke, Am. J. Nursing **64:**92-95, Oct. 1964.

8 Cooper, Irving S.: Cryogenic surgery, New England J. Med. **268:**743-749, April 4, 1963.

9 Covalt, Donald A., and others: Early management of patients with spinal cord injury, J.A.M.A. **151:**89-94, Jan. 10, 1953.

10 Davis, Loyal, editor: Christopher's textbook of surgery, ed. 8, Philadelphia, 1964, W. B. Saunders Co.

11 *de Brisay, Amy N., and Stuart, C. Keith: Restoration of communication in the elderly, with special reference

to hemiplegic patients, J. Am. Geriatrics Soc. **12:**687-693, July 1964.

12 de Gutiérrez-Mahoney, C. G., and Carini, Esta: Neurological and neurosurgical nursing, ed. 4, St. Louis, 1965, The C. V. Mosby Co.

13 *DeJong, Russell N.: The treatment of migraine, Am. J. Nursing **62:**67-71, July 1962.

14 Eisenberg, Henry, and others: Cerebrovascular accidents, J.A.M.A. **189:**883-888, Sept. 21, 1964.

15 Ford, Frank R.: Diseases of the nervous system in infancy, childhood, and adolescence, ed. 5, New York, 1966, Charles C Thomas, Publisher.

16 Forster, Francis M.: Management of the epileptic patient, M. Clin. North America **47:**1579-1590, Nov. 1963.

17 *Goda, Sidney: Communicating with the aphasic or dysarthric patient, Am. J. Nursing **63:**80-84, July 1963.

18 Gordon, John E., editor: Control of communicable disease in man, ed. 10, New York, 1965, The American Public Health Association.

19 Hanes, William J.: Tic douloureux—a new theory of etiology and treatment, J. Oral Surg., Anaesth. & Hosp. Dent. Serv. **20:**200-205, May 1962.

20 Harrison, T. R., and others, editors: Principles of internal medicine, ed. 5, New York, 1966, McGraw-Hill Book Co.

21 Hawken, Patty: Hypophysectomy with yttrium[90], Am. J. Nursing **65:**122-125, Oct. 1965.

22 Headquarters, Department of the Army: Neuropsychiatric specialist, Technical Manual no. 8-243, Washington, D. C., 1962, U. S. Government Printing Office.

23 *Hodges, Lucien R., and Taufic, Marjorie: Tumors of the brain and rehabilitation after craniotomy, Am. J. Nursing **58:**58-63, Jan. 1958.

24 Holquin, Alfonso H., Reeves, Joan S., and Gelfand, Henry M.: Immunization of infants with the Sabin oral poliovirus vaccine, Am. J. Pub. Health **52:**600-610, April 1962.

25 *Hunkele, Eileen, and Lazier, Rosemary: A patient with fractured cervical vertebrae, Am. J. Nursing **65:**82-84, Sept. 1965.

26 *Hurd, Georgina Greene: Teaching the hemiplegic self-care, Am. J. Nursing **62:**64-68, Sept. 1962.

27 Jeffreys, William H., and Hood, Henry: The supportive management of acute closed head injuries, M. Clin. North America **46:**1599-1604, Nov. 1964.

28 *Jordan, Victoria, and others: Halo body cast and spinal fusion, Am. J. Nursing **63:**77-80, Aug. 1963.

29 *Kottke, Frederic J., and Anderson, Eleanor: Deterioration of the bedfast patient—causes and effects, and nursing care, Pub. Health Rep. **80:**437-451, May 1965.

30 La Roche, Laurent P., and McMechen, Ann: Head injuries at Cape Kennedy, Am. J. Nursing **65:**102-105, June 1965.

31 Larson, Carroll B., and Gould, Marjorie: Calderwood's orthopedic nursing, ed. 6, St. Louis, 1965, The C. V. Mosby Co.

32 *Leavens, Milam E., Hilkemeyer, Renilda, and others: Brain tumors and nursing care of patients with brain tumors, Am. J. Nursing **64:**78-83, March 1964.

33 Lennette, Edwin H., and others: Viral central nervous

*References preceded by an asterisk are particularly well suited for student reading.

system disease, J.A.M.A. 179:687-695, March 3, 1962.

34 *Lennox, W. G.: Epilepsy—a problem in public health, Am. J. Pub. Health 41:533-536, May 1951.

35 Livingston, Samuel: Antiepileptic drugs, Am. J. Nursing 63:103-107, Oct. 1963.

36 *Livingston, Samuel, and others: Petit mal epilepsy, J.A.M.A. 194:227-232, Oct. 18, 1965.

37 *MacKenzie, Marguerite, and Baldwin, Maitland: Cerebral seizures, Am. J. Nursing 57:312-316, March 1957.

38 *Magee, Kenneth R., and Elliott, Alta: Parkinson's disease—neurologic management and nursing care, Am. J. Nursing 55:814-818, July 1955.

39 *Magee, Kenneth R., and Moser, Doris: Myasthenia gravis and nursing care of myasthenic patient, Am. J. Nursing 60:336-343, March 1960.

40 *Martin, John, and Craig, Iris: The early care of patients with injury of the spinal cord, Am. J. Nursing 55:936-939, Aug. 1955.

41 *Martin, M. Arlene: Nursing care in cervical cord injury, Am. J. Nursing 63:60-66, March 1963.

42 McAlpine, Douglas, Lumsden, Charles E., and Acheson, E. D.: Multiple sclerosis, a reappraisal, Baltimore, 1965, The Williams & Wilkins Co.

43 *Mead, Sedwick: The doctor has a stroke, Lancet. 2:574-576, Sept. 14, 1963.

44 *Morrissey, Alice B.: Rehabilitation in hemiplegia—major nursing function, Am. J. Nursing 62:58-61, Sept. 1962.

45 *Moser, Doris: An understanding approach to the aphasic patient, Am. J. Nursing 61:52-55, April 1961.

46 *Mullan, John F., and Van Schoick, Mildred R.: Intractable pain, Am. J. Nursing 58:228-230, Feb. 1958.

47 *Olson, C. Kent, and Tollefsrud, Valborg, E.: Chemosurgery for Parkinsonism and when the patient has chemosurgery, Am. J. Nursing 59:1411-1416, Oct. 1959.

48 *Pasternak, Sophie: The patient with a ruptured disk, Am. J. Nursing 62:77-80, Feb. 1962.

49 *Peszczynski, Mieczyslaw: The rehabilitation potential of the late adult hemiplegic, Am. J. Nursing 63:111-114, April 1963.

50: *Pirnie, Florence A., and Baldwin, Maitland: Observing cerebral seizures, Am. J. Nursing 59:366-369, March 1959.

51 *Potanos, John, Pool, J. Lawrence, and Gleason, Arline M.: Cerebral edema, Am. J. Nursing 61:92-94, March 1961.

52 *Raney, Rupert B.: The minor concussion, Am. J. Nursing 57:1444-1445, Nov. 1957.

53 Reaves, Leonard E., III: Considerations in rehabilitation of patients with cerebrovascular disease, J. Am. Geriatrics Soc. 12:996-1001, Oct. 1964.

54 *Schlesinger, Edward B., and Haber, Martha E.: Trigeminal neuralgia and nursing care of the patient with trigeminal neuralgia, Am. J. Nursing 58:853-858, June 1958.

55 *Schumacher, George A., and Palmer, Mary Ellen: Multiple sclerosis and nursing the patient with multiple sclerosis, Am. J. Nursing 57:751-755, June 1957.

56 Shaternick, Juanita: Living with myasthenia gravis, Am. J. Nursing 63:73-75, Feb. 1963.

57 Silverstein, A.: Arteriography of stroke, Arch. Neurol. 12:387-389, April 1965.

58 Smith, Genevieve Waples: Care of the patient with a stroke, a handbook for the patient's family and the nurse, New York, 1959, Springer Publishing Co., Inc.

59 Steigmann, Frederick: Muscle relaxants, Am. J. Nursing 61:49-51, July 1961.

60 *Taren, James A., and Martin, M. Arlene: Cerebral aneurysm and care of the patient with a cerebral aneurysm, Am. J. Nursing 65:90-95, April 1965.

61 *Turner, Gwendolyn E.: The cerebral vascular accident patient, Nursing Outlook 8:326-330, June 1960.

62 Tweed, G. Gilbert, Coyle, Norma R., and Miller, Barbara: Guillain-Barré syndrome, Am. J. Nursing 66:2222-2226, Oct. 1966.

63 *Ullman, Montague: Disorders of body image after stroke, Am. J. Nursing 64:89-91, Oct. 1964.

64 U. S. Bureau of the Census: Statistical abstract of the United States, 1965, ed. 86, Wasihngton, D. C., 1965, U. S. Government Printing Office.

65 Warren, Richard, and others: Surgery, Philadelphia, 1963, W. B. Saunders Co.

66 *Whitehouse, Frederick A.: Stroke—some psychological problems and causes, Am. J. Nursing 63:81-87, Oct. 1963.

32

The patient with disease
of the joints and
connective tissues

**Study
questions**

1 What part of the joint is the synovial membrane? What tissue constitutes the remainder of the joint?

2 What main types of joints are there in the body? Review the range of motion for the hip, shoulder, knee, elbow, ankle, wrist, and finger joints, and give examples of daily activities for which these joints are used.

3 What are the harmful effects of immobilization of a joint?

4 What is the therapeutic action of acetylsalicylic acid? What are the toxic effects?

5 What are the therapeutic effects of heat? What are some of the measures used to provide heat and the related nursing care?

6 Select a patient from your ward, a member of your family, or an acquaintance who has arthritis. How does this person earn his living? What financial problems has the disease presented? What major modifications in the patient's life have been necessary because of the disease? How has his need for recreation been affected?

7 What substances constitute connective tissue? What is the difference between elastic and fibrous connective tissue?

Rheumatic disease and *rheumatism* are general terms applied to all those conditions in which there are pain and stiffness of some portion of the musculoskeletal system. These conditions include diseases of the connective tissue. Diseases of the joints are commonly designated as *arthritis*. The word arthritis means inflammation of the joint. Not all diseases of the joints, however, are accompanied by inflammation. Hypertrophic arthritis, for instance, is a degenerative process. The term *nonarticular rheumatism* refers to those conditions, such as bursitis, tenosynovitis, and fibromyositis, which affect the soft tissue structures primarily.

Arthritis and the related rheumatic diseases are among the most common chronic illnesses of our times. They are exceeded only by mental illness as a cause of disability. It is estimated that over 10 million people in the United States suffer from forms of rheumatic disease.[8] Of these persons, 4.5 million have arthritis of some kind, 2% or 90,000, are completely disabled, and 11%, or 1,143,000 persons, are partially disabled. Many millions of working days are lost each year because of this disease. In Great Britain, where arthritis is even more common than in the United States, it has been reported that one-sixth of all loss of work in industry due to disability is from this cause.[8]

An inflammatory process in the musculoskeletal system may be caused by pathogenic organisms or their toxins or it may be a reaction to foreign substances, such as urates of sodium or free calcium, which are deposited in the part. Often the cause is unknown.

In a joint the inflammatory process usually begins in the synovial membrane and gradually extends to the outer structure of the joint. The synovial membrane is inflamed, and the joint becomes swollen and painful. Spasm occurs in the muscles attached to the joint. If the process cannot be controlled, the entire joint may be destroyed and replaced by a solid mass of spongy bone, causing immobility of the joint. The attached muscles also may become wasted. The joint appears deformed, and contractures may occur.

If the voluntary muscles or tendons are involved in an inflammatory process, the affected part becomes stiff, exquisitely tender, and painful on movement. If the process is not controlled, muscle fibers or tendons may degenerate and undergo atrophy, causing permanent inability to use the part.

Inflammatory processes involving the collagen substance of connective tissue cause fluid to be exuded from the affected tissues into surrounding spaces such as the joint spaces, the pericardial sac, the pleura, and the peritoneal cavity. This may cause pain, and it hampers function of the organ or part. If the inflammatory process is not controlled, the collagen fibers gradually deteriorate, lessening the elastic quality of the tissues involved.

The normal degenerative processes of aging, trauma, strain, overuse, or disuse, may affect the musculoskeletal system. Inflammation is not involved, and severe crippling seldom occurs. With aging and following trauma, joints may enlarge, their motion may be limited to some degree, and they may be painful. When muscles are strained or overexerted, muscle spasm and pain on motion may occur. The muscle fibers do not degenerate, although if pain is severe, the muscle may atrophy from disuse.

The patient with rheumatic disease needs supportive care during acute episodes of illness in order to control pain and prevent deformity. If the illness is a long-term one such as arthritis, the nurse needs to assist

the patient and his family to adjust to the social, economic, and emotional consequences of the disease. She, in collaboration with the physician and physical therapist, also helps to correct the deformities of patients with long-term illness, including those who have been neglected and those whose disease has progressed despite all medical effort.

The nurse also has a part in the prevention of chronic arthritic diseases and in their detection and treatment in early stages, when hope for arrest is most promising. It can be assumed that poor health habits do play some part in the predisposition to develop arthritis. By teaching the importance of a well-balanced diet, a careful schedule of rest and exercise, avoidance of exposure to infections, and avoidance of severe emotional strain, the nurse may be contributing to prevention. She should help others to understand the warning signs of arthritis. They include frequent morning stiffness, pain and swelling of one or more joints, persistent muscular aches and pains, and unexplained fever or fatigue. If these signs are present, the person should seek medical care as soon as possible to learn if anything is wrong. Early treatment seems to help prevent the progress of crippling by arthritis.

The nurse also may discover sufferers from diseases of the joints and connective tissue who do not know that help is possible. On a home visit, she may find a person with arthritis. In the hospital, while talking to a patient, she may learn of a member of his family who has joint pain and direct him to medical care.

The general aspects of nursing care for patients with rheumatic diseases is included before specific diseases and their medical and nursing treatment. While much of the long-term care refers primarily to the care of patients with atrophic arthritis, care in the acute stage of all diseases affecting the muscles and joints is similar.

Nursing care

To carry out her responsibilities, the nurse must have some understanding of the disease process involved and of what the doctor, the physical therapist, and others are trying to accomplish. The short- and long-term goals for each patient should be determined. These goals and the special nursing care needed by each patient to achieve them should be recorded on the nursing care plan.

Relief of pain

Pain accompanies all musculoskeletal diseases. It may be exquisite in acute stages of diseases such as rheumatic fever, atrophic arthritis, gout, and diseases of the muscles and tendons. The patient requires the greatest care and gentleness when he must be moved. Fear of pain often makes him irritable and can lead to muscular resistance, which makes the pain worse. Care must be taken not to jar the bed. Heavy bedclothes may cause added pain. If cradles are used, the greatest caution must be taken not to accidentally bump an involved part of the body when adjusting or removing the cradle. Footboards help to relieve the pressure of covers, provided the patients can be kept warm during their use. Patients with rheumatic arthritis must be encouraged to change position frequently since their general nutrition is often poor and pressure sores and contractures develop easily. Sometimes a very painful joint such as a wrist, elbow, or ankle can be placed on a pillow, and the pillow and the limb can be moved together when the patient must turn over or otherwise adjust his position (Fig. 226).

Drugs often are used to help control the pain. *Salicylates* such as *acetylsalicylic acid* (aspirin) are widely used for patients with arthritis and have been found to be effective in combating pain and discomfort in almost all types of rheumatic diseases. Sodium bicarbonate is usually given with the salicylates because the large doses that must be used cause gastritis. Sodium bicarbonate also hastens the elimination of salicylates from the body. Fluids are forced for this purpose too. The signs of salicylate poisoning—ringing in the ears, nausea, vomiting, and tachycardia—should be watched for, although aspirin usually can be taken over a long period of time without the occurrence of toxicity or the acquisition of tolerance. Liver damage from salicylates seldom occurs, although massive doses may lower the prothrombin content of the blood.[4] *Methylsalicylate* for local application to inflamed joints is ordered almost universally in the treatment of acute rheumatic fever. It also may help to relieve pain in arthritis and in muscular inflammation and strains. *Phenylbutazone*

Fig. 226

Supporting the painful part on a pillow lessens discomfort when the patient must be moved.

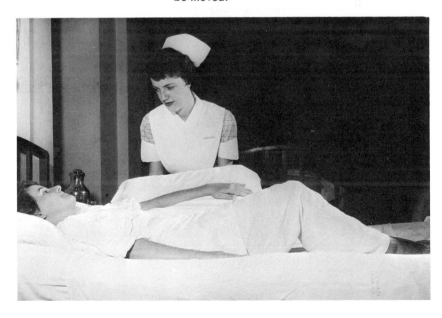

(Butazolidin), has an analgesic effect and may be prescribed for patients with atrophic arthritis and gout. The usual dosage is 100 mg. (1½ grains) four or five times per day for one or two days. The drug is an amino-pyrine derivative and may cause edema, nausea, gastritis, anemia, and serious agranulocytosis. Therefore, it cannot be used for extended periods of time. *Codeine* may be given in acute short-term rheumatic conditions, but it and other habit-forming analgesics are avoided whenever possible in chronic rheumatic diseases because of the danger of addiction.

Corticosteroid preparations frequently are given by mouth or parenterally in inflammatory processes of the musculoskeletal system. They tend to relieve pain, probably by suppressing the inflammation. Hydrocortisone is often given directly into a painful joint and appears to be helpful in controlling local joint inflammation. It is usually injected under sterile precautions after the joint has first been aspirated. Codeine and other narcotics are not given if corticosteroids are used. (The side effects and precautions essential for safe use of these drugs are described on p. 63.)

Maintenance of personal hygiene

Despite acute pain, personal hygiene must not be neglected. The patient with acute rheumatic fever often has profuse, sour-smelling perspiration and needs refreshing warm sponges at least daily, as does the patient with an acute attack of gout. The patient with rheumatoid arthritis is often too tired and discouraged to keep himself as well groomed as he should be, but few things contribute so much to general morale as attention to personal hygiene. The nurse should give time to cutting fingernails and should assist women patients in setting and arranging their hair. The man with rheumatoid arthitis should be encouraged to shave regularly, and nursing personnel can help by having equipment conveniently placed and by providing time for this activity. If the patient is having much pain, the nurse should see that drugs for pain are given about one-half hour before personal hygiene measures are begun.

Every effort should be made to help the patient with a rheumatic disease to become and to remain self-sufficient in caring for his daily needs. Many *self-help devices* for patients with permanent musculoskeletal limitations are now available for purchase, and many others can be improvised by the resourceful person. For example, the patient who has limited shoulder and elbow movements can sometimes comb her hair using a long-handled comb; eating utensils can be equipped with built-up handles that can be grasped more easily by persons who have deformity of the fingers; and special buttons, zippers, and hooks can be used to make dressing easier for the person with limited range of joint motion. The Arthritis and Rheumatism Foundation has a self-help device center from which suggestions can be obtained.

Helping to relieve emotional and socioeconomic difficulties

Patients with chronic rheumatic diseases have many emotional and socioeconomic problems. While care is being given, the nurse should become acquainted with her patient. Nothing is more important in the care of the patient with chronic rheumatic disease, whether he is at home, in a clinic, or in a hospital, than a friendly interest in him and in his particular problems. His relationship to his family should be considered. The family may be overprotecting the patient and thus contributing to his becoming a permanent invalid. On the other hand, they may be tired of the problems the patient is causing, and he, in turn, may be greatly disturbed over the burden he is, or may become, to his family. It is at such times that a well-placed word from the thoughtful nurse may help to direct the patient's thinking along positive lines. New opportunities that are within his physical limitations and that may contribute immeasurably to his rehabilitation may be suggested. The assistance of a social case worker may be needed by the patient in thinking through and talking through his family problems. If the patient is not hospitalized and lives at home, the nurse may refer him to a family service agency for help.

Determining a program of rest and activity

Bed rest is usually ordered for the patient with rheumatic disease who has an elevation of temperature. When the temperature becomes normal, a careful balance of rest and activity should be planned. This balance is especially important for the patient with arthritis.

The nurse should carefully review with the physician the schedule of rest and activity for every patient with arthritis. For the ambulatory patient, this schedule involves consideration of work, recreation patterns, family and community life, and responsibilities. The importance of regular vacations and routine exposure to sunshine is usually stressed. In most instances a change of climate is not advised, since the personal disadvantages for the patient often outweigh the advantages. After the medical limits have been set, each patient must be helped to work out his own schedule.

Maintenance of posture

Although maintenance of good posture is important for all patients, it is especially important for the patient with a chronic arthritic disease. Poor posture exerts further strain on already damaged joints and not only may cause pain and fatigue but predisposes to increased deformity.

The patient's bed. A firm bed lessens pain by preventing motion and consequent pull on painful joints and helps to keep the spine in good alignment. In the home or in the hospital, the bed should have a firm mattress, and often bed boards are needed. Boards should be long enough and wide enough to rest firmly upon the main side and end rails of the bed—not on the bedsprings. The person with arthritis should either use no pillow or should use one small pillow that fits well down under the shoulders so that forward bending of the cervical spine is not encouraged. Knees should not be flexed on pillows, and all patients who must be confined to bed most of the day should lie flat on the abdomen for a part of each day.

Sitting posture. Furniture should be such that good posture can be maintained during working and recreational hours with a minimum of drain on vital energy resources. There are five criteria for a good chair: the seat should be deep enough to support the thighs but not so deep that circulation in the popliteal spaces is hampered; the seat should be high enough so that feet rest firmly on the floor and do not dangle and put strain on knee joints; the seat should be

level or tilted slightly forward so that flexion of the knees and hips is at a minimum and not at less than a right angle; the chair should have arms so that arm and shoulder muscles can provide leverage to help in moving from the chair; the rungs must be such that one foot can be placed partially under the seat in preparation for rising so that the patient is better able to stabilize his center of gravity when he assumes an erect position. Chairs with a seat a little higher than is usually considered comfortable provide better leverage when arising. Sometimes adding an inch of two to the height of the patient's favorite chair will increase his comfort when sitting and upon arising. Occasionally, too, it is necessary to build up the toilet seat. Devices to be placed over the seat to provide height can be improvised. A rail beside the toilet seat is as necessary as arms on any chair the patient uses since he must use his arms to arise from the seat safely.

If the patient with arthritis has been sitting for some time and finds his knees stiff upon attempting to move, he should remember to flex and extend his knees several times before attempting to rise from the chair. By eliminating some of the stiffness before trying to bear weight, he will find that he is much steadier on his feet. Many patients who otherwise find an evening at the movies intolerable are able to enjoy such recreation by remembering this simple practice.

Shoes. The patient with arthritis should always wear properly fitted shoes that give support to the feet. Frequent changes of shoes also are helpful. Sometimes the physician may prescribe corrective shoes or shoes modified to provide special support. For example, a metatarsal bar may be placed on the outside of the sole of the shoe. The patient is usually gratified at the difference such changes make in how he feels after several hours on his feet. Shoes, not soft bedroom slippers, should be worn about the house.

Splints. Splints may be ordered for use during sleeping or waking hours to help prevent deformity caused by muscle spasm. Splints should be well padded and should be removed frequently. The skin should be carefully checked for signs of pressure, particularly over bony prominences. In the home, splints may be made from chicken wire that has been carefully covered and padded.

Exercise

Activities for all patients with arthritic diseases in the chronic stage should be planned to keep joints limber. Most patients with rheumatoid arthritis must do special exercises that are prescribed for them by the physiatrist and taught to them by the physical therapist. The nurse should know what these exercises are. She should not only encourage the patient to do his exercises regularly but also should occasionally watch him do them. Some patients are so eager to get well that they are too vigorous in exercising and may cause aggravation of the disease and damage to the involved joints. Others, who are tired and resigned to their fate, may sit passively, not moving their limbs sufficiently because of slight pain and thus negating the whole purpose of the exercises.

Exercises are often prescribed to be done two or three times a day. To be beneficial, all exercises must involve steady, prolonged contraction before relaxation—not merely "wiggling" the part. Pain experienced during the exercise and disappearing soon afterward is not significant. Pain persisting throughout the rest of the day or into the night probably is an indication that the exercise has been too strenuous and should be decreased. The physician or the physical therapist should be consulted.

The patient and his family need to know why activity is necessary, why exercises are ordered, why it is so important to do them regularly, and what changes take place in muscles and joints when motion is not maintained. They should be told that muscles are very important in holding joints in good position and that without muscle action, joints themselves cannot produce motion. Exercises are necessary to preserve range of joint motion, to strengthen muscles, and to prevent shortening of muscles. If they can understand this explanation, they will know why position in bed is important and what the correct positions are.

The patient needs to understand the normal range of motion for every joint in his body and should be helped to appreciate why the daily efforts demanded to prevent

limitation of any involved joints are so important in his long-term outlook. Drawings and pictures help in this explanation, which is usually given by the doctor and augmented by the nurse and the physical therapist. Members of the patient's family also should be taught the positions and exercises so that they may help the patient as necessary. However, they should encourage the patient to do, without help, the exercises that he is capable of performing alone.

It may be helpful for the patient to take aspirin about one-half hour before doing exercises. Use of heat before beginning the exercises is of great help in making them easier for the patient. The patient may prefer a heating pad, a heat lamp equipped with a 25-watt bulb and placed at least twelve inches from the skin, or warm, moist packs applied for short periods. Bath towels wrung out in hot water and applied directly to the skin are often used, since moist heat seems more effective than dry heat in causing muscle relaxation and alleviating pain. Warm baths rather than moist packs may be preferred by the patient who is caring for himself and who may have difficulty in wringing out the towels. The patient may prefer to do his exercises while lying in a tub of warm water. If bath oils and bath salts can be afforded, their use makes this routine more enjoyable.

Nutrition

There are no special diets that will cure or even materially alter the course of any type of arthritis except possibly gout. Yet thousands of patients follow special and expensive diets in the hope of cure. More patients with arthritis than with any other disease are the victims of advertising and diet fads.

The essentials of good nutrition, which include fruits, vegetables, protein, and vitamins, are recommended for most patients with arthritis. If the arthritis is metabolic in origin, as is gout, or if the patient is overweight, a special diet may be ordered. Otherwise the patient should be permitted to indulge his food likes and dislikes within the range of the essentials of good nutrition.

The patient should be urged to eat regular meals and should be given plenty of time for meals. Even the patient with marked limitation of movement should be urged to feed himself, although food may sometimes have to be cut up or otherwise prepared beforehand. Built-up handles on eating equipment may enable the patient with severe limitations to handle the utensils independently.

Care at home

Many patients with arthritis, unless they are having an acute exacerbation, will be in their own homes and will be treated by their family physicians or at a local hospital clinic. A careful referral to the public health nurse in the patient's local community from the hospital if the patient is hospitalized for diagnosis or intensive treatment will often help the patient to continue a program of regulated rest, exercise, appropriate nutrition, and drug therapy (Fig. 227).

Often the patient needs supportive care at home to prevent severe emotional reaction to stresses as well as assistance in many aspects of particular home schedules. For example, the nurse may help the woman patient with atrophic arthritis to cut down on her work load at home. Sitting down with a piece of paper and plotting the activity for each hour of the day is a good way to help the patient see what changes may be made. It is possible that home arrangements can be altered to save energy. Such simple things as using lightweight aluminum pans, sitting while preparing vegetables and ironing, and using a lightweight iron may be all that are necessary to enable a woman to remain at home and care for her family. If a patient finds that pain and stiffness on awakening prevent him from getting about, the nurse may suggest that he keep aspirin, if it is prescribed, at the bedside and set his alarm clock a little earlier than usual so that he may awaken and take the aspirin. He should then rest for about a half hour before beginning his preparation for the day. The nurse's efforts are directed toward helping the patient to remain at home or at work as long as possible. Planning with other family members and with other agencies may also be necessary.

The Arthritis and Rheumatism Foundation has prepared a pamphlet* that should give the nurse helpful hints in working with persons who have arthritis. Another publication, prepared in both English and Spanish, is available to patients with the approval of their physician and is also helpful to nurses.† The American Rheumatism Asso-

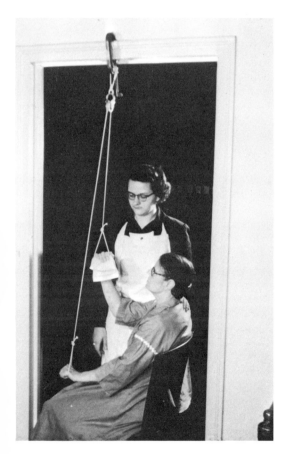

Fig. 227

With the help of the public health nurse this patient who has osteoarthritis is able to improve range of shoulder joint motion by using a pulley attached to a doorway in her home. (Courtesy Visiting Nurse Association of Brooklyn, Inc., Brooklyn, N. Y., and Clay-Adams, Inc., New York, N. Y.)

*Home care in arthritis: The Arthritis and Rheumatism Foundation, National Headquarters, 10 Columbus Circle, New York, N. Y. 10019, 1958.
†U. S. Department of Health, Education, and Welfare in collaboration with the Arthritis and Rheumatism Foundation: Strike back at arthritis, Washington, D. C., 1961, Public Health Service publication no. 747.

ciation suggests a paperback book that is available at bookstores, for use by the patient and his family.*

Providing heat therapy

Many forms of heat are used in the treatment of arthritis to increase circulation to the affected joints and to lessen muscle spasm, thereby decreasing pain. Hot, wet packs applied locally and hot tub baths are often ordered. A cradle with electric light bulbs is sometimes used to supply dry heat. Diathermy also may be used to supply heat, but it sometimes increases joint pain.

Paraffin provides an excellent form of penetrating heat. Sometimes the patient is instructed by his physician to use paraffin at home. Usually he is advised to apply it immediately before doing the prescribed exercises. The nurse may be called upon to help the patient or his family with this procedure in the home. Usually from eight to ten pounds of paraffin are slowly heated in the top of a large double boiler until the paraffin is melted and vaporizes slightly. It is then removed from the stove and cooled until a thin film appears on the surface. At this point it is at the right temperature for use.

The skin should be shaved before paraffin is applied. From eight to ten coats may be applied with a brush, or the part may be immersed in the melted paraffin the same number of times. Waxed paper or Pliofilm is then wrapped about the part, and the part is covered with a bath towel while the patient rests for about a half hour. The paraffin is then peeled off and saved to be reused. During and following this treatment, the patient must be protected from drafts and chilling. If the paraffin is too hot for comfort, soaking the part in hot water preceding the treatment sometimes helps. Another alternative is to use an ounce of mineral oil in the paraffin to lower its melting point and therefore its temperature.

Paraffin can be dangerous unless carefully used. It is flammable, and the greatest care must be taken if gas or other open flame is used for heating it. Pans must be handled carefully, since accidental spilling of hot

---

*Bland, J. H.: Arthritis, medical treatment and home care, a book for family use, rev. ed., New York, 1963, Collier Books.

paraffin can cause serious burns. It goes without saying that this procedure should never be carried out when children are playing nearby. Clothing should be protected from wax by using an apron, and floors can be protected with newspapers. Care must be taken not to clog plumbing with wax.

Care after surgery

There are particular problems in caring for the patient with joint disease following any type of surgery because of the danger of further stiffness and limitation of joint movement throughout the body. Bed posture and bed exercises are important. Muscle-setting exercises, in which a muscle may be consciously contracted, may be ordered if the patient cannot move freely. The patient should be urged to do things for himself to help prevent further stiffness and to improve his morale. In all activities he must be given more time than the average patient.

Mobilization of the patient is difficult following surgery on his joints. Many joints may be involved, and the patient may have been tired and discouraged even before the operation took place. He is cautious and fearful of falling, and rightly so, since he does not have the quickness of action at his command that is necessary for the prevention of many accidents. A walkerette is usually used and is much safer than crutches for the patient who is beginning to walk (Fig. 228). To prevent accidents the greatest care must be taken to see that the floor is dry and not slippery, to provide good supporting shoes, and to see that no bathrobe cords are dangling for the patient to trip over. If the patient's arms are in good condition, the time in bed is well spent in doing resistance exercises to strengthen the triceps muscles of the arms in anticipation of ambulation, first in a walkerette and then perhaps on crutches. (These exercises are described on p. 394.)

Habit-forming drugs are used as little as possible following surgery for arthritis because of the chronic nature of the disease. The nurse can help to make sedatives less necessary by giving attention to simple details of patient comfort. A firm bed, a small, correctly placed pillow, a warm drink, and appropriate lightweight bed coverings all help to induce rest.

The patient with arthritis feels drafts and

changes of temperature more than most patients who move about more readily. If the affected limb is in traction, therefore, it is often a good idea to put a warm sock on the foot or to wrap the whole limb in a light, warm blanket, provided this can be done without interfering with the traction. Sometimes, wrapping an exposed limb in cotton batting and then in a light towel or blanket affords protection from drafts.

The patient with rheumatoid arthritis often expects too much improvement from his operation. He may have been ill a long time and may have made many major adjustments, yet he hopes that an operation will produce a cure. A patient may hope for a cure even when it is obvious to everyone else that, because of the many joints involved, the operation is only one small step toward improving the patient's ability to care for himself. The patient will often need an understanding person to talk with when he begins to accept reality. Morale usually improves visibly when the patient can be up to spend time on a sun porch or recreation room with other patients.

Caution against quick "cures"

An important part of nursing care for the patient with arthritis in the home or elsewhere is to caution him about the danger of seeking quick-cure methods of treatment or miracle drugs that promise cure. Family members as well as the patient may ask the nurse about drug preparations, advertisements, and a host of other related offerings that promise relief in a variety of ways. The nurse should attempt to learn about the product under discussion if it is unknown to her, and if she feels that the patient needs additional counsel from his physician, she should relay this information to him. Each year an enormous amount of money, which most patients can ill afford to spend, is wasted on prepared drugs that are not prescribed by competent physicians. The impatience of the person with a long-term and often discouraging disease such as arthritis is quite understandable. However, his best hope for control of his condition lies in selecting a physician who is qualified and in whom he has confidence and then remaining under his care and following his instructions. Agencies that may be helpful when

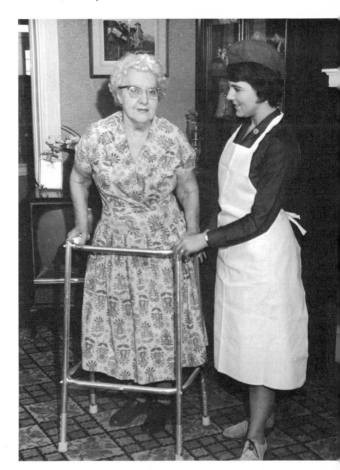

Fig. 228

A walkerette enables the patient to start standing erect, maintaining balance, and walking safely after bone or joint surgery. (Courtesy Hamden Public Health and Visiting Nurse Association, Inc., Hamden, Conn.)

exploitation of the patient by someone who is promoting useless products is suspected are the Better Busines Bureau, the American Medical Association's Bureau of Investigation, and the Arthritis and Rheumatism Foundation and its local chapters throughout the United States.

Specific diseases of the joints

Arthritic disorders

Arthritis is one of the oldest diseases known to man. Although arthritis resulting from bacterial infections, such as those caused by the gonococcus and the tubercle bacillus, respond to drug therapy, other, more common forms of arthritis have not yielded permanently to any of the new drugs of modern times. However, much progress in the diagnosis and treatment of arthritis has been made. Most persons with this disease can benefit substantially from modern physical medicine and rehabilitation provided they have good supportive care physically, socially, and emotionally from the time of the onset of their illness.

The nursing care required by patients with arthritis presents many problems. The patient may have been ill for some time; he may be worried, irritable, pessimistic, or resigned. He may be impatient or discouraged. Indeed, progress is often very slow, and even the nurse may tend to become discouraged. She must have a truly optimistic attitude based on her conviction that arthritis need not be a hopeless disease. She must help the patient set realistic goals. Then, as each small but definite step toward these goals is achieved, she must help him to realize that progress is being made.

Polyarthritis. Because many joints usually are involved, rheumatoid arthritis, Marie-Strümpell disease, and Still's disease are often classified as polyarthritis.

Rheumatoid arthritis (atrophic arthritis, arthritis deformans). Rheumatoid arthritis attacks young adults most often and affects women more often than men. The incidence is higher in persons who are less favored economically. It appears usually during the productive years of life, when family responsibilities are at their height. The cause of rheumatoid arthritis is unknown, though it sometimes appears to be associated in some way with streptococcal infections. There is also some question of its being a disorder of metabolism or an autoimmune reaction. General debility, overfatigue, endocrine imbalance, emotional instability, and psychic trauma all apparently play a part in its development. Thin, asthenic persons seem more susceptible to the disease than others. Because the collagen substance of the connective tissue is involved, rheumatoid arthritis is now considered probably to be a collagen disease (p. 933).

Rheumatoid arthritis is a systemic disease characterized by fatigue, poor appetite, low-grade fever, anemia, mild leukocytosis, and increased blood sedimentation rate. Initially the synovial membrane of a joint becomes involved in a inflammatory and ankylosing process similar to that described on p. 920. Often the proximal interphalangeal joints of the hands are affected early. The fingers develop a characteristic tapering appearance. Several joints may be involved at the same time, and if the disease is not arrested, it may progress steadily to other joints. There is spasm of the muscles attached to the involved joints, and wasting of these muscles is greater than would normally be expected from their lessened activity. Subcutaneous nodules may develop. They are usually near joints, over bony prominences, or along extensor surfaces.

The public should be taught that the outlook for rheumatoid arthritis is not necessarily hopeless. If the disease is intensively treated, some patients recover from the first attack and, with careful attention to their general health, never suffer a recurrence. If not treated early, the disease has a tendency to relapse and to recur in more severe form. The nurse may be helpful in stimulating the patient to seek and continue competent medical care. Approximately 10 to 15% of the patients with rheumatoid arthritis, however, progress to crippling despite any kind of treatment.

Because most patients with arthritis remain ambulatory, a large part of the nurse's work will be in the home and in the clinic. All the nursing measures described previously are usually needed by the patient eventually. Since the patient with rheumatoid arthritis is often underweight, a high-caloric diet with vitamin supplements to stimulate appetite may be needed. Sunshine and fresh air also stimulate appetite.

Unfortunately, the drugs available at present do not cure rheumatoid arthritis, and often symptoms are relieved only as long as the drug is continued. Corticosteroids are given frequently. *Prednisone* and *prednisolone* have now been proved to be superior to hydrocortisone in the treatment of rheumatoid arthritis. Usually treatment starts with 20 to 30 mg. (⅓ to ½ grain) given orally, and the maintenance dose is 5 to 10 mg. (1/12 to ⅙ grain) per day.[4] Steroids given over extended periods of time and in high dosages may cause cataracts or elevate intraocular pressure and cause glaucoma. Any complaints about vision should be reported to the doctor at once. (For general care, see p. 63.)

Gold salts also seem to control the symptoms of rheumatoid arthritis. However, gold salts may cause serious untoward reactions. They have been known to cause severe renal and hepatic damage,[3] and gold may be deposited on the cornea of the eye.[9] Dermatitis and inflammation of the eyelids and the conjunctivas are rather common side effects.[9] If the patient receiving gold has a sore mouth, excessive salivation, nausea, vomiting, diarrhea, or irritated eyes, the drug usually is stopped. Signs of jaundice should be watched for and reported. The urine usually is tested frequently for albumin.

Solganal-B and *Myochrysine* are the two forms of gold most frequently used. The dosage is usually 10 mg. ($\frac{1}{6}$ grain) intramuscularly as a first test dose. If no ill effects are encountered, a second dose of 25 mg. ($\frac{3}{8}$ grain) is given and then 50 mg. ($\frac{3}{4}$ grain) are given at weekly or biweekly intervals until 750 mg. to 1,000 mg. (12 to 15 grains) have been given.[4] A rest period of at least four weeks is usually planned before another series of injections is started, although in some clinics a maintenance dose of 25 to 50 mg. is given every four weeks for months and sometimes years. Dimercaprol (BAL) and vitamin B_{12} may be given with gold preparations to reduce the danger of untoward reactions.

Antimalarial drugs such as chloroquine phosphate (Aralen phosphate) also seem to relieve symptoms of rheumatoid arthritis and are being used by some doctors in the treatment of the disease. However, they have been found to cause changes in the retina, and blindness may result from their use. Early symptoms are blurred vision, halos around lights, difficulty in adjusting to sun or glare, and diplopia. These symptoms should be watched for carefully, and the doctor should be notified at once if they occur.

Several surgical procedures may be performed on selected patients with rheumatoid arthritis to relieve symptoms. Arthrodesis or arthroplasty may be done (p. 934), or nodules may be surgically removed to relieve pain caused by them in areas such as the bottom of the foot or the elbow.

Marie-Strümpell disease (ankylosing, or rheumatoid, spondylitis). Marie-Strümpell disease affects the spine and is seen primarily in young men. The sacroiliac joint usually is involved first. The patient complains of intermittent low back pain that does not radiate into the buttocks or legs, and stiffness. Later the symptoms become constant. The disease progresses upward in the spine and, unless arrested, causes a severe forward-bending deformity. Marie-Strümpell disease sometimes responds to x-ray treatment, and sometimes fusion of the spine is done to prevent further progressive deformity.

Still's disease. Atrophic arthritis that affects children is called Still's disease. It occurs before puberty. There may be slowly progressive joint inflammation, or an acute febrile illness with joint involvement may herald the onset of the disease. The clinical findings and the progress of the disease are almost identical to that in adults except that there may be premature cessation of the growth of bones, and the vertebrae in the cervical spine may become fused. The percentage of patients who develop severe deformities is fairly high. The nursing needs are no different from those of adults except that the technique for accomplishing care must be adapted to the age of the child. (Adaptations needed by children of various ages are described in Chapter 2.)

Hypertrophic arthritis (osteoarthritis, degenerative arthritis). Hypertrophic arthritis is primarily a disease of older people. Almost everyone past 40 years of age has hypertrophic changes in the joints. These changes may become symptomatic, depending on their severity and on such mechanical factors as poor posture, obesity, and occupational strain. Weight-bearing joints such as the knees, hips, and spine are most often affected. The patient with osteoarthritis can be given reassurance that pronounced deformity will not occur. Changes within the joint consist of thinning of the articular cartilages and deposition of calcium on the bone surfaces and in the joint spaces. Some enlargement of the joint occurs, but there is no swelling. There is some discomfort, and motion may be limited. Pain is often intermittent, tending to follow chilling, and is possibly due to muscle tension from the cold. Small fragments of bone or cartilage, known as *joint mice,* occasionally break off, causing severe pain on movement. They may need to be removed surgically. Bony tumors *(exostoses)* may develop. They are benign growths, but if they develop on weight-bearing areas such as the heel, they may need to be removed surgically.

The patient with hypertrophic arthritis often is overweight, and general weight reduction is advised. Pain and discomfort in the joints are usually relieved by aspirin. Activity rarely needs to be limited. In fact, activity alleviates the accompanying stiffness. Care must be taken, however, in placing patients with osteoarthritis in unusual positions such as the lithotomy position, since movement of the hip may be markedly limited. Severe pain and even trauma can be caused by forcing the legs apart or by failure to move both legs in unison.

Although hypertrophic changes in the joints cannot be prevented, their attendant discomforts can be controlled to some extent. This is true particularly if prevention is considered early in life. Obesity should be controlled because it places considerable strain on all weight-bearing joints. Trauma and excessive use of certain joints can lead to hypertrophic arthritis fairly early in life. Examples of professions and occupations that seem to be associated with hypertrophic involvement of the upper spine and shoulder joints are dentistry, barbering, and dishwashing. It seems likely that the position assumed during working hours is a contributing factor. Public education and industrial practices that consider the dangers of prolonged work in a position of strain may help to prevent the development of symptoms in some people. The orthopedic principle of alternate rest and activity to prevent strain on particular joints and muscles has real application in the prevention of hypertrophic arthritis. Poor posture throughout life contributes to hypertrophic arthritis. The child should be taught to stand correctly so that strain due to prolonged hyperextension does not occur in joints such as the knee joints. Holding the pelvis correctly with a forward tilt will prevent increased curvature of the lower back with its resultant strain on mus-

cles and joints. Correct mechanical use of the body, such as stooping with knees and hips flexed rather than bending, prevents strain on muscles, which may pull the joint out of alignment just enough for osteoarthritic changes to develop or to cause symptoms. Holding the head up and back takes a great deal of strain from the joints of the upper spine. It is surprising how many older patients can benefit from posture improvement even though the damage may date from childhood. (For more complete discussion of posture, see specialized texts.[14])

Arthritis associated with metabolic diseases. *Gout,* although it actually is a disease related to faulty metabolism, frequently is classified as an arthritic disease because of the joint symptoms. The Arthritis and Rheumatism Foundation also classifies acromegaly (a disorder arising from excessive secretion of the growth hormone) and the blood disorders, hemophilia and sickle cell anemia, as arthritic diseases. In each of these diseases joint symptoms may be predominant. Only gout, however, is discussed under this form of arthritis in this book.

Gout, or gouty arthritis, is arthritis caused by the deposit of sodium urate crystals in the joints as a result of excessive uric acid in the blood. Eighty-five percent of all patients with gout show a familial tendency to develop the disease, and 95% of all patients with gout are men. Despite the emphasis, in fiction and elsewhere, that has been placed upon overindulgence in food as a cause of gout, the disease occurs most often in the economically less favored.

Gout is a chronic disease, although acute exacerbations occur, causing high temperature, malaise, and headache. Attacks are characterized by acute pain, swelling, and tenderness of joints such as those of the great toe, ankle, instep, knee, and elbow. Renal stones form from the uric acid as it is filtered from the blood. Renal damage may occur when acute attacks are repeated over an extended period of time. Subcutaneous deposits of urates *(tophi)* in locations such as the outer ear occur in about one-third of all patients who have gouty arthritis.

Treatment of gout is directed toward control of acute attacks, since permanent joint damage and deformity as well as renal failure can follow repeated attacks. Prevention of recurrences depends mainly on taking specific prescribed medications to increase the output of urates, on increasing the intake of fluids (particularly those which are alkaline-ash in reaction), and on weight reduction if obesity is present.

The patient with gout often is instructed to avoid foods high in purine, such as brains, kidneys, and sweetbreads, to avoid too much fat, and to avoid alcohol. Meat, fish, and fowl contain less purine, and the patient with gout may be encouraged to follow a diet that is fairly high in proteins in an effort to lose weight. Fruit juices, mineral waters, and alkaline-ash fluids of all kinds are beneficial to the patient with gout, partly because they help supply extra fluid so that any uric acid crystals may be flushed from the kidneys more easily and partly because they inhibit uric acid precipitation. The daily urine output for the patient with gout should be about 2,000 to 3,000 ml. per day, or two or three times that of the average person.

Colchicine is the standard drug used in the treatment of gout. When an acute attack of gout is imminent, the usual treatment is administration of 0.5 mg. (1/120 grain) of the drug each hour by mouth until nausea develops. Camphorated tincture of opium (paregoric) is then sometimes given as treatment for the gastrointestinal irritation. The usual maintenance dose of colchicine (0.5 mg.) is administered daily or two or three times per week. Some patients may require medication two or three times each day. There is no evidence of damage to the body from therapeutic doses of colchicine even when it is taken for years.[4] *Acetylsalicylic acid* also helps to increase the uric acid output and may be regularly prescribed over long periods of time.[4]

Since *probenecid* (Benemid) furthers the excretion of uric acid through the kidneys, it is another drug that is prescribed for the treatment of gout. The usual dosage is 0.5 Gm. (7½ grains) daily by mouth for one week, followed by 1 Gm. daily for months. The drug may cause gastric distress and is best tolerated if taken with meals. Large amounts of fluid must be given to prevent formation of stones in the kidneys. Since the drug works best in an alkaline medium, sodium bicarbonate, 5 to 7.5 Gm. (75 to 110 grains) daily, is often ordered. However, this dosage may disturb the acid-base balance of the body if continued for too long. The nurse may be asked to check the acidity of the patient's urine with litmus paper each time he voids or to teach him to do so and to record the results for the physician. One limitation in the use of Benemid is that salicylates cannot be given at the same time since this combination diminishes the benefit derived from both drugs.[4]

Early treatment of gout prevents serious complications. However, people often fail to recognize the significance of early symptoms. The most prominent early symptom is pain in the foot during the night. The nurse has a responsibility for being aware of the possible cause of this complaint. If it comes to her attention, she should urge the patient to seek medical attention.

Other types of arthritis. Almost any organism can affect the joints. The typhoid bacillus, tubercle bacillus, gonococcus, and staphylococcus were common causes of arthritis before the discovery of the specific antibiotic drugs and the control of communicable diseases. Arthritis can also result from trauma to the joint, or it may be associated with new growths within or about the joint or with neurogenic changes.

Rheumatic fever

Rheumatic fever is a systemic disease causing an elevation of temperature and acute inflammation of the joints with pain and swelling. It occurs most often in children but can occur at any age, and it is particularly important because it is often a precursor of acute rheumatic heart disease (p. 347). The inflammation, a sensitivity response (p. 56), tends to move from joint to joint. Although the pain and swelling may be severe, no permanent joint damage or deformity occurs.

The incidence of rheumatic fever is high in the lower economic groups, and conditions such as poor housing, dampness, lack of sunshine, poor nutrition, and repeated exposure to upper respiratory infections seem to be predisposing factors. Rheumatic fever also seems to be associated with streptococcal infections. Prevention of the disease appears to lie in the improvement of environmental conditions, the early treatment of respiratory infections, and immediate medical care

Table 13

Summary of characteristics of various types of arthritis

Characteristics	Rheumatic fever	Rheumatoid arthritis	Hypertrophic arthritis	Gout
Synonyms	—	Atrophic arthritis Arthritis deformans	Osteoarthritis Degenerative arthritis	—
Average age of onset	5-11 yr.	30-50 yr.	50-70 yr.	20-40 yr.
Sex (ratio)	—	Women 3:1	Women 5:1	Men 19:1
Build and weight	—	Asthenic—underweight	Stocky—overweight	Overweight
Joints involved	Any; moves from joint to joint	Any; often fingers, other joints; progressive	Weight-bearing joints— knees, hips, spine, fingers; localized	Terminal great toe of foot—spreading to any joint, tarsal and metatarsal joints
Subcutaneous lesion	Rheumatic nodules over tendon surfaces; indicate poor prognosis	Nodules over bony prominences; painful on injury; no prognostic significance	Heberden's nodes on fingers; painful at times; no prognostic significance	Tophi; prognostic of difficulty in control of blood urates
X-ray findings	None	Clouding of fluid space, fraying of inner joint margins, lessening of joint space	Lipping of bony margins, lessening of joint space	Clouding of joint spaces
Outward appearance of joints	Swollen, tender, reddened, painful	Swollen, painful, reddened, shiny	Enlarged; no swelling	Swollen, painful, reddened, shiny
Termination	No joint damage or limitation of motion	Ankylosis and deformity	Some limitation of motion, little deformity, no ankylosis	Limitation of motion, deformity; possible renal calculi

if streptococcal infections occur in those who have had previous attacks of rheumatic fever. Prophylactic antibiotic treatment similar to that used following rheumatic heart disease (p. 348) also may be ordered.

Nonarticular rheumatic disease

Bursitis, or inflammation of the connective tissue sac about a joint, may be acute or chronic. It usually is caused by trauma, strain, and overuse of the joint, but pathogenic organisms and toxins may cause it. The shoulder bursa is the one most often affected and may be exceedingly troublesome. Severe pain occurs, especially on movement of the joint.

The main treatment of bursitis consists of controlling the pain and preserving joint motion. Treatment and the response of individual patients vary widely. Treatment includes the local application of heat, diathermy, medications to control pain, and immobilization of the part. X-ray treatment is sometimes given in an attempt to dissolve the calcium deposits that form within the bursa, causing pain. Sometimes the bursa may be aspirated to remove some of the irritating deposits. Sterile normal saline solution or novocaine may be used. Hydrocortisone may be injected into the bursa. If there are large particles of calcium, surgery may be necessary for their removal. In bursitis of the shoulder, attention needs to be given to preserving the range of joint motion in the shoulder. Pendulum exercises are almost always ordered, and the nurse may demonstrate them and stress their importance to the patient.

In some cases recurrence of bursitis may be prevented by avoiding excessive use of the joint. The patient with chronic bursitis should continue physical therapy and exercises as prescribed by the physiatrist.

There are many other forms of nonarticular rheumatism. *Lumbago, stiff neck, fibrositis, tendinitis,* and *tenosynovitis* are examples. These conditions can be very painful and may cause distress out of all proportion to their seriousness. So far, unfortunately, there seems to be no specific cure for any of them, and the greatest comfort comes from the use of local heat and mild analgesic drugs such as acetylsalicylic acid. Constant pain is demoralizing to the patient, and one of his greatest needs is a sympathetic person to listen to his problems and to give encouragement.

Collagen diseases

The collagen, or connective tissue, diseases are a group of not very well understood clinical entities in which there is derangement of collagen substance. It is now thought that it may be an autoimmune reaction.[4] Collagen and elastic substances are the fibrous constituents of connective tissue. Connective tissue makes up the extracellular framework around which cells develop and organs and other essential structures are formed and carry out their function. The collagen substance may respond with inflammation and degeneration. Because of its extremely wide distribution in the body, disease involvement is widespread also. There are several collagen diseases, including polyarteritis, systemic lupus erythematosus, scleroderma, and dermatomyositis. Only two, systemic lupus erythematosus and scleroderma, will be described.

Systemic lupus erythematosus is a serious disease involving the collagen substance of connective tissue in the skin, blood vessels, and serous and synovial membranes. It is now known to be fairly common, and young women are most often affected. The cause of systemic lupus erythematosus is unknown. It may be acute or chronic and usually runs a long course, with exacerbations and remissions. About half the patients have skin lesions, and arthritis is common. There may be cardiac, lymphatic, neurologic, pulmonary, hematologic, renal, hepatic, and gas-trointestinal involvement, causing problems such as pleuritis, pericarditis, peritonitis, neuritis, nephritis, and anemia.

Erythema (redness), usually in a butterfly pattern, appears over the cheeks and bridge of the nose. The margins of the lesions are usually bright red, and the lesions may extend beyond the hairline, with partial alopecia (loss of hair) above the ears. Lesions also occur on the exposed part of the neck. Chronic discoid (round) lesions are also fairly common and may undergo vascularization, degeneration, and subsequent atrophy. Lesions slowly spread to the mucous membranes and other tissues of the body, or they may originate there. The lesions do not ulcerate but cause degeneration and atrophy of tissues.

No specific treatment for lupus is available. Adrenocorticosteroid therapy is used to control active manifestations. With this treatment and supportive treatment of systems involved, many patients live for years. Bed rest and salicylates are used during exacerbations, and antimalarial treatment with chloroquine is sometimes surprisingly helpful. If the patient has skin lesions, rest in a darkened room during the acute stages and permanent avoidance of sunshine are usually prescribed.

Scleroderma (progressive systemic sclerosis) is a generalized systemic disease involving the collagen substance throughout the body. The cause of this relatively rare condition is unknown. Middle-aged persons are most often affected, and women are affected more frequently than men.

The word scleroderma means "hard skin" and accurately describes the skin manifestations that are predominant in this disease. Usually local areas such as the face and fingers are first affected, and sometimes the condition is confused with rheumatoid arthritis and with Raynaud's disease in the early stages. Usually there is pain on joint motion because the skin and muscle contractures produce a deformity of the joint. The skin may first appear slightly edematous, then turn pale, becomes steadily more firm, and finally becomes fixed to underlying tissues and mildly pigmented. The face becomes masklike, and chewing may be impossible. Finally all body motion becomes so restricted that the patient has the appearance of a living mummy. Tissues of essential organs such as the heart, kidneys, and liver may be affected in a similar manner, and fatal impairment of their function may result. Chest expansion may be impaired by firming of the skin so that respiratory failure threatens.

There is no cure and no specific treatment for scleroderma, and the disease is fatal within a period of months or years. Death usually is caused by failure of involved organs or systems such as the liver or the circulatory system. Intensive treatment with cortisone in the early stages has proved helpful in some cases. Salicylates and mild analgesics are used for joint pain, and physical therapy is ordered to slow the development of contractures and deformity.

In advanced stages of the disease, meticulous nursing care is imperative. It includes mouth care, care in eating to prevent choking, skin care and prevention of decubiti, and attention to the emotional problems of the patient, who is becoming more helpless daily.

Operations used for diseases of the musculoskeletal system

Surgery is done to correct deformity and to improve function in diseases of the joints. For example, severe alteration of alignment may prevent the wearing of shoes or may make the wearing of shoes unbearably painful. Contractures at the hip may make it impossible for the patient to use crutches or to be otherwise rehabilitated. The patient with advanced rheumatoid arthritis who has an immobile joint (ankylosis) or a deformed joint may sometimes benefit from surgery.

An *arthrodesis* is a surgical fixation of a joint by fusing the bones in it together so that the joint is immobile. It may be performed to stabilize a joint, such as the knee or ankle, that has become distorted from normal alignment because of muscle spasm, muscle weakness, and joint disease. Vertebrae in the spine may also be fused. As a result of this operation, pain is lessened, and the stabilized joint may make it possible for the patient to walk and move about more easily. Usually a cast is applied following operation, but sometimes bandaging, slings, and traction are used.

Attempts have been made to restore partial function to joints that have become ankylosed. By far the most successful of these operations is an *arthroplasty,* in which a Vitallium cup is inserted into the acetabulum after the head of the femur has been removed from the socket and spongy ankylosed bone has been scooped away. Following this operation, the patient is usually placed on a firm bed in traction. Motion of the hip joint must be started within three or four days if effective use of the joint is to be obtained. A favorite and very satisfactory method used to facilitate this exercise is to place the foot on a roller skate, which in turn is placed on a firm, shellacked board. Using this setup, the patient is able, by an arrangement of pulleys, to exercise the hip joint in adduction and abduction. It is important to prevent external rotation of the hip joint, since this will result in an awkward flat-footed gait, with the entire extremity turning outward. A full-sized bed sheet folded over to form what is usually referred to as a trochanter roll and tucked inward at the crest of the ilium will often suffice to keep the thigh and leg from rolling outward.

Rheumatic nodules may sometimes be removed surgically if they have become irritated by trauma or pressure or if they are particularly unsightly. Hospitalization for this treatment is usually of only one day's duration. In a similar fashion, the *tophi of gout* may be excised, particularly if they have opened and are draining or are causing pain.

Patients with hypertrophic arthritis may be operated upon when bony tumors, or exostoses, develop and cause pain, particularly on weight-bearing areas such as the heel. Calcium deposits within the joint that are causing pain in the patient with hypertrophic arthritis or in the one with bursitis also may be removed surgically. Occasionally the joint is fused when pain is persistent and severe.

References and selected readings*

1 Ansell, Barbara M., and Bywaters, E. G. L.: Rheumatoid arthritis (Still's disease), Pediat. Clin. North America 10:921-939, Nov. 1963.

2 *Barckley, Virginia, and others: Arthritis and a narrow

*References preceded by an asterisk are particularly well suited for student reading.

perspective do not mix, Nursing Outlook 6:638-639, Nov. 1958.

3 Beeson, Paul B., and McDermott, Walsh, editors: Cecil-Loeb textbook of medicine, ed. 11, Philadelphia, 1963, W. B. Saunders Co.

4 Bergersen, Betty S., and Krug, Elsie E.: Pharmacology in nursing, ed. 10, St. Louis, 1966, The C. V. Mosby Co.

5 *Brewer, Earl J., Jr.: Rheumatoid arthritis in childhood, Am. J. Nursing 65:66-71, June 1965.

6 *Campbell, Emily B., Hogsed, Clyde M., and Bogdonoff, Morton: Lupus erythematosus, Am. J. Nursing 62:74-77, June 1962.

7 Committee of the American Rheumatism Association: Primer of the rheumatoid diseases, New York, 1964, The Arthritis Foundation.

8 Harrison, T. R., and others, editors: Principles of internal medicine, ed. 5, New York, 1966, McGraw-Hill Book Co.

9 Henkind, P.: Iatrogenic eye manifestations in rheumatic disease, Geriatrics 20:12-19, Jan. 1965.

10 Hollander, J. L., editor: Arthritis and allied conditions, ed. 7, Philadelphia, 1966, Lea & Febiger.

11 *Jaschik, Eva, and Olsen, Catherine: Nursing care of the arthritic patient at home, Am. J. Nursing 55:429-432, April 1955.

12 *Jessar, Ralph A., and Hollander, Joseph Lee: Types of arthritis and their medical treatment, Am. J. Nursing 55:426-429, April 1955.

13 *Lamont-Havers, Ronald W.: Arthritis quackery, Am. J. Nursing 63:92-95, March 1963.

14 Larson, Carroll B., and Gould, Marjorie: Calderwood's orthopedic nursing, ed. 6, St. Louis, 1965, The C. V. Mosby Co.

15 *Lonergan, Robert C.: Osteoporosis of the spine, Am. J. Nursing 61:79-81, Jan. 1961.

16 Lowman, Edward W.: Rehabilitation of the patient with chronic rheumatoid arthritis, J. Chron. Dis. 1:628-637, June 1955.

17 Marmor, Leonard: Hand surgery in rheumatoid arthritis, Arthritis & Rheumatism 5:419-427, Aug. 1962.

18 *McDermott, Ita K., and Wensley, Edith: We can help arthritic patients, Nursing Outlook 3:582-585, Nov. 1955.

19 Talbott, John H.: Gout, ed. 2, New York, 1964, Grune & Stratton, Inc.

20 *Talbott, John H.: Gout and gouty arthritis, Nursing Outlook 2:540-543, Oct. 1954.

21 Wedgwood, Ralph J., editor: Symposium on collagen diseases, Pediat. Clin. North America 10:855-1093, Nov. 1963.

33

The patient
with
a fracture

Study questions

1 Describe the anatomic structures of bones. What are the functions or purposes of the skeletal system?
2 What are some of the changes that might be observed in the skin if circulation is impaired?
3 Review the methods of assisting a patient in and out of bed and to and from bed to a wheelchair.
4 What are some of the exercises to preserve muscle tone in the legs and arms that you might teach the patient?

The nursing care of patients with fractures is discussed here because fractures are so often encountered by nurses on the medical and surgical units of general hospitals and by nurses who visit patients in their homes. Application of the principles of body mechanics—often referred to as orthopedic principles—is a part of the overall nursing care and has been included in previous chapters. Nursing care of patients with many orthopedic ailments requires specific knowledge beyond the scope of this book. Since there are excellent orthopedic nursing textbooks available, the student nurse should turn to these when she encounters a patient with an orthopedic condition on the medical or surgical floors of the general hospital.

This chapter includes only a few of the more important general principles of care of all patients with fractures and nursing responsibilities when surgical treatment is used. Prevention of fractures and first-aid care are considered on p. 244, amputations and crutch-walking on p. 389, skull fractures and back injuries on pp. 886 and 904, arthritis in the previous chapter, and fracture of the jaw on p. 629.

General statements

Definitions and terminology. A bone is said to be fractured or broken when there is an interruption in its continuity. This is usually caused by a blow or injury sustained in a fall or other accident. A fracture may also occur during normal activity or following a minimal injury when the bone is weakened by disease such as *cancer* or *osteoporosis*. This is called a *pathologic fracture* and causes collapse of the bone. Usually, osteoporosis involves the hip or the lumbar spine and is becoming increasingly common with the increase of aged persons. The real cause of the condition is obscure, but it is thought to be usually related to hormonal activity and is discussed on p. 764. The nurse should bear in mind the possibility of this condition being present whenever she cares for an elderly patient, and she should urge the elderly patient with persistent or recurrent back pain to report it to his doctor so that treatment can be begun before marked collapse of bone occurs.

There are several types of fractures. A fracture is *complete* when there is complete separation of the bone, producing two fragments. It is *incomplete* when only part of the bone is broken. The part of the bone nearest to the body is referred to as a *proximal* fragment, whereas the one most distant from the body is called the *distal* fragment. The proximal is also called the *uncontrollable* fragment since its location and muscle attachments prevent it from being moved or manipulated when attempting to bring the separate fragments into correct alignment. The distal is referred to as the *controllable* fragment since it can usually be moved and manipulated to bring it into the correct relationship to the proximal fragment. Fractures in long bones are designated as being in the proximal, middle, or distal third of the bone.

If the skin is intact, the fracture is classified as *simple* or *closed*. If there is a break in the skin, with or without protrusion of bone, the fracture is called *compound* or *open*. If a bone fragment, such as a rib, has penetrated an internal structure, such as a lung, the fracture is called *complicated.* When the two bone fragments are in good alignment with no change from their normal position despite the break in continuity of bone, the fracture is referred to as a fracture *without displacement*. If the bone frag-

ments have separated at the point of fracture, it is referred to as a fracture *with displacement*. This may be slight, moderate, or marked.

The line of fracture as revealed by x-ray examination or fluoroscopy is usually classified as to type. It may be *greenstick* with splintering on one side of the bone (this occurs most often in young children with soft bones), *transverse* with a break straight across the bone, *oblique* with the line of fracture at an oblique angle to the bone shaft, or *spiral* with the fracture lines partially encircling the bone. The fracture may be referred to as *telescoped* if a bone fragment is forcibly pushed against and into the adjacent fragment. If there are several fragments, the fracture is referred to as a *comminuted* one. (See Fig. 229.)

Symptoms of fracture and related injury. The signs and symptoms of fracture vary according to the location and function of the involved bone, the strength of its muscle attachments, the type of fracture sustained, and the amount of related damage.

Pain is usually immediate and severe following a fracture. It may continue and is aggravated by attempted motion of any kind and by pressure at the site of injury. Loss of function is another characteristic sign. If the patient attempts to use the injured part, he may be unable to do so. If there has been marked displacement of fragments, there will be obvious gross deformity, and there may be motion where motion does not usually occur. Upon moving the fractured limb gently, there may be a characteristic grating sound (crepitus) as the bone fragments come in contact with each other. The nurse should never, under any circumstances, attempt to elicit this sign since it may cause further damage and increase pain. It is possible, though unusual, for a fracture to occur with no displacement of fragments, little or no swelling, and pain only when direct pressure is applied to the site of fracture or upon use of the limb or body part. Fractures of this kind might be missed if x-ray examinations were not routinely ordered when there is any reason to suspect that a fracture may have occurred.

Since the bones are firmer than their surrounding structures, any injury severe enough to cause bone fracture will also cause injury

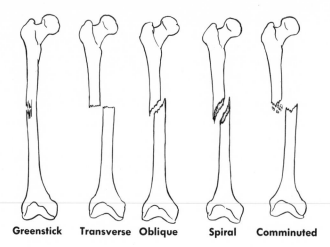

Fig. 229

Types of fractures.

to muscles, nerves, connective tissue, and blood vessels which may be evident by hemorrhage externally or into surrounding tissues. Bleeding may not be fully apparent for several hours, and discoloration of the skin (ecchymosis) may not be apparent until several days after injury. Edema may follow extravasation of blood into the tissues and localization of serous fluid at the site of injury, and paralysis or other evidence of nerve injury may develop. Occasionally a large nerve becomes locked between two bone fragments and causes immediate paralysis. The patient who has a fracture usually has signs and symptoms of injury of both bone and surrounding tissues. He may go quickly into shock if the injury is severe and if he has intense pain.

Immediate care

Perhaps the most important basic principle in the care of a patient with any fracture is to provide some kind of splint before moving him. This is constantly emphasized in the emergency care of patients at the scene of accidents. (See p. 244.) It is equally important for the nurse to remember to preserve body alignment when caring for patients who are in traction or other mechanical apparatus.

When a patient with a known or a suspected fracture is to be admitted to the hospital, his bed should be provided with a fracture board. This is a good practice regardless of the part fractured because the patient with a known fracture of the ankle, for example, may be found, upon further examination, also to have a fracture of the pelvis or of the spine.

Since it can be assumed that edema will occur following a fracture, the injured part usually is elevated routinely. One or more protected pillows should be used, and these can support the extremity if moving must be done. If a temporary splint has been applied, this should not be removed without orders from the doctor no matter how crude or soiled it may be. The limb encased in the splint can be elevated.

The injured part should be observed at frequent intervals for local changes in color, sensation, or temperature. Care should be taken that emergency splinting bandages do not cause constriction as edema develops. Tingling, numbness, or burning pain may indicate nerve injury. Coldness, whiteness, or cyanosis may indicate interference with circulation. Increased warmth and swelling may indicate infection. Gas bacillus infection is a dreaded complication in grossly contaminated compound fractures. Sudden increase in edema and pain associated with darkening of the tissues should be reported to the doctor at once. Tetanus immunization usually is given when a compound fracture has been sustained (p. 299).

General observation is necessary to detect early signs of shock. If the injury has been severe or if there are signs of impending shock, the blood pressure is taken every fifteen minutes for several hours, and the pulse and respiratory rates are noted and recorded frequently.

The nurse should anticipate that the doctor may order cold, local applications during the first twenty-four hours following a fracture, since these help to reduce hemorrhage and edema and contribute to the patient's comfort. Ice bags are often used and must be covered and moved at regular intervals if placed close to the affected area to prevent skin damage.

Pain is usually relieved in the first few hours by giving acetylsalicylic acid or narcotics. Adjustment to sudden immobilization is difficult for the patient, and the nurse must appreciate what it means to him to be unable to move about freely. Even a fracture of an arm bone may make the patient quite helpless at first. He may be unable to move or use the rest of his body without severe pain. Sometimes treatment of the fractured bone makes it physically impossible for him to care for some of his most basic physical needs. The patient usually needs sedation such as phenobarbital to help him sleep the first few nights after he has sustained a fracture.

Occasionally an air or fat embolus may result from compound fractures or from severe comminuted fractures with extensive soft tissue injury. The signs of an embolism of this kind are similar to those of other emboli and consist of sudden severe pain in the chest, pallor, dyspnea, shock, prostration, and collapse. Treatment includes administering oxygen and stimulants and keeping the patient absolutely quiet. (See p. 573.)

Ischemic paralysis (contracture) is a somewhat rare complication of a fracture and develops when an artery is injured by trauma or pressure so that arterial spasm occurs. *Volkmann's contracture* is a complication of fractures about the elbow caused by circulatory impairment due to pressure

from a cast, constricting bandages, or injury to the radial artery. The muscles of the forearm atrophy and the fingers and forearm are permanently flexed (clawhand). Signs of coldness, pallor, cyanosis, pain, and swelling of the part below the cast must be observed and reported promptly so that pressure may be relieved by either loosening the bandage or removing the cast in order that circulation may be restored before this contracture can develop.

Common methods of treatment and related care

Objectives in the treatment and care of fractures include reduction of the fracture, maintenance of the fragments in the correct position while healing takes place, prevention of excessive loss of joint motility and muscle tone, prevention of general complications, and maintenance of good general health so that, with healing of the fractured bone, the patient can continue as before his accident or injury.

Reduction of fractures

Reduction is the term used for the return of bone fragments to their normal position. This may be accomplished by closed manipulation, traction, or operation.

Closed reduction. When closed manipulation is used to reduce a fracture, the patient is usually given a general anesthetic which relieves pain and also causes muscle relaxation. The physician then reduces the fracture by pulling on the distal fragment (manual traction) while he (or someone else) applies countertraction to the proximal fragment until the bone fragments *engage* or fall into their normal alignment. The physician may also apply direct pressure over the site of the fracture to correct angulation or lateral displacement of a fragment. Usually when this type of reduction is used, a cast is applied to hold the fragments in the desired position while healing occurs.

Traction. Continuous traction (pull on the affected extremity) for a period of days or even weeks may be necessary to reduce fractures of the femur, because the large muscles draw the bone fragments out of normal alignment so that immediate reduction by manual traction is impossible. Continuous traction may also be used to reduce fractures when there has been very extensive tissue damage and when the physical condition of the patient is such that anesthetics cannot be given. Traction may therefore be used for immobilizing the limb while soft tissue healing takes place, reducing the fracture and maintaining correct position of fragments during bone healing.

Open reduction. Open reduction may be necessary if closed manipulation or traction fails to reduce a fracture. The operation permits the surgeon to view the bone fragments and adjacent injured structures, to arrange the fragments in their proper positions, and to use, when needed, some internal splinting device such as a metal plate and screws to hold the fragments in position. This may be the procedure of choice in certain fractures such as fracture of the femur, compound fractures, comminuted fractures, fractures involving joints, fractures in which soft tissue is caught between bone fragments, and fractures accompanied by severe blood vessels or nerve injury. The disadvantages of this method of reduction are that it requires anesthesia and imposes surgery upon a patient who has already suffered from the trauma of the original injury. However, since open reduction usually permits excellent approximation of bone fragments, better function and quicker healing usually occur. This is now the treatment of choice for many fractures in adults.

Healing of fractures

When a bone is broken, bleeding occurs and a hematoma forms around the damaged bone ends. The hematoma is not absorbed during healing, as are hematomas that occur elsewhere in the body, but becomes changed into granulation tissue. From the sixth to the tenth day after injury the granulation tissue changes into a tissue called the *callus.* Callus is different from other granulation tissue in that it contains cartilage, calcium and phosphate ions, and osteoblasts. The callus temporarily holds the bone fragments together, but will not support weight or withstand much strain. It eventually is replaced by true bone which grows from beneath the periosteum of each fragment to meet and fuse across the defect. The length of time required for a bone to heal depends on its location, blood circulation to

the part, and age and general physical condition of the patient. Fractures in young children unite much more quickly than do those in older patients. Fractures of the humerus usually heal within ten to twelve weeks; of the forearm, within eight to ten weeks; of the femur, in six months; of the lower leg, in three months; and of the spine, within six to twelve months. The larger the bone, the longer it usually takes to heal.

Delayed healing or *delayed union* is said to occur when the fracture has not healed within the usual time for the particular bone involved. Delayed healing will occur if the space between the two bones is such that neither the callus nor bone cells can bridge the gap, if the callus is broken or torn apart by too much activity, if muscle or fascia is caught between the fragments, if an infection develops, or if there is poor blood supply to the part or marked dietary deficiency. Occasionally delayed union occurs with no obvious cause. Open reduction and more complete immobilization may be necessary.

Nonunion is the term used when healing does not take place even in a much longer time than is usually needed. Congenital conditions and obscure medical disease occasionally account for this, and nonunion may occur in the aged. When this occurs, the patient may have to wear a brace to support the limb. If the fracture is in the lower extremity, crutches may have to be used indefinitely. Surgery may be performed and an attempt made to unite the fragments with a bone graft. Nonunion occurs most often in the middle of the humerus, the neck of the femur in older people, the lower third of the tibia, and the carpal bones.

Treatment by immobilization of the reduced fracture

The purpose of immobilization is to hold the bone fragments in contact with each other until healing takes place. All activity of the part that might cause separation of the fragments is restricted, and the fractured bone is kept in position by immobilizing the entire limb. Usually immobilization includes the joints immediately proximal to and distal to the fractured bone. Bandages, adhesive tape, plaster-of-Paris casts, splints, traction, internal fixation, and bed rest are methods of securing immobilization. Metal pins, screws, plates, and nails, all made of stainless steel or Vitallium, are used to hold the fragments together when an open reduction is done; a plaster-of-Paris cast is often used to provide extra protection when internal fixation is used. This is especially true in treatment of compound fractures of the leg.

Plaster casts

Plaster-of-Paris casts have been used for many years and are still widely used in the treatment of fractures. Unless a cast has been applied to the entire trunk, the patient who is treated with a plaster-of-Paris cast can usually move about and carry on most of the activities of daily living. Often he may, for example, return to school or to work and participate in many activities without damage to the site of injury. Use of casts shortens hospitalization, and many patients with simple fractures can be treated in a doctor's office or the outpatient department of a hospital. After a short period of observation, they can be discharged and treatment continued under close medical supervision.

Plaster-of-Paris casts do, however, restrict activities because of their weight and their inflexibility. A cast can cause complications due to interference with normal physiologic functions and can cause actual physical injury if incorrectly applied and improperly cared for. A cast applied to the arm or shoulder may limit the kind of clothing worn and may interfere with eating, writing, or other uses of the arm. If applied to the leg, a cast may change body alignment, put strain on certain muscle groups, and limit locomotion.

The nurse must not only know how to maintain the effectiveness of the cast, but she must also remember the patient in the cast and understand how he is affected by it. She must help the patient be as independent as possible yet provide assistance as needed. The nurse should help to prevent complications from developing and be alert for early signs of complications which must be reported to the physician promptly.

Application of the cast. Most hospitals have a room set aside for the application of casts which provides the necessary space and contains all the equipment required for this procedure. Some hospitals also have a cart equipped with plaster and other cast materials that can be taken to the bedside for use.

Plaster-of-Paris bandages come in various widths (2 to 8 inches). Each roll is wrapped in waxed paper to prevent sifting of the plaster from the bandage and to prevent deterioration from exposure to moisture. The bandage itself is made of crinoline into which plaster of Paris (gypsum or calcium sulfate dihydrate) has been rubbed. When water is added, the gypsum assumes its crystalline state and the wet plaster bandage can be molded to fit the shape of a body part or wrapped about a limb. When the water evaporates, the cast becomes firm and is able to withstand considerable stress and strain. The number of layers of plaster used determines the strength of the cast.

After reduction has been accomplished and before the cast is applied, the skin is usually protected with sheet wadding (a thick, nonabsorbent cotton web covered with starch to hold it together), and felt or sponge rubber is used over bony prominences to protect them from pressure. Tubular stockinette, from 2 to 18 inches wide, is used as lining for the cast and is applied so that it will extend over the edge to cover the rough edges of the plaster. The excess stockinette and sheet wadding are usually folded back over the cast after it has been applied and bound down with a final roll of plaster.

If the cast is applied elsewhere than in a special plaster room, the floor and table should be protected from wet plaster. When the doctor is ready to apply the cast, the bandage is placed in a bucket of water at 21° to 24° C. (70° to 75° F.) for five seconds. The bandage should be carefully removed from the water so that none of the plaster is lost. It should be held horizontally with an end in the palm of each hand and gently compressed to remove excess water. It should then be quickly handed to the doctor so that it can be used before it begins to set. Only a few bandages should be placed in the water at a time. The bucket containing the water should be lined with a cloth or paper to collect waste plaster. When the procedure has been completed, the cloth or paper containing waste plaster can be removed and discarded into a garbage can and the water emptied into the sink, if there is no loose plaster. Plaster of Paris will clog ordinary plumbing and should never be emptied into ordinary drains.

Care of the cast. Most plaster bandages fall into two categories, fast-setting (five to eight minutes) and extra-fast setting (two to four minutes). Thin casts may dry completely in several hours, but thick casts may require as much as a week or more to dry. The cast can be cracked or broken by inadequate support or by unwise handling before it is dry. A wrinkle in the plaster and indentations caused by the finger tips or from continuous pressure can alter the inner shape of the cast and cause pressure on the body part encased in the plaster.

A fracture board should always be used to provide a firm mattress and prevent uneven weight on the fresh plaster cast. To protect the new cast and ensure its efficiency, the patient should be carefully transferred from the stretcher onto his bed. If he is conscious, he can move onto the bed with the assistance of one nurse while another supports the wet cast with the palms of her hands at the areas of greatest strain—usually at the joints. If the patient is asleep or is in a body cast, three or four people should lift him onto the bed. The entire cast and the patient's head and his free leg below the cast must be fully supported.

The wet cast should not lie unsupported on the hard bed because it may become flattened over bony prominences and weight-bearing areas such as the back of the heel, buttocks, and shoulders, and this can cause pressure. The wet cast should always be fully supported on a pillow or pillows that are protected with waterproof material to prevent their becoming damp. The patient should be in proper body alignment, and there should not be any break in the support provided by the pillows to cause weakening of the cast. If the patient has a cast on the leg, the foot should extend over the edge of the pillow or the bed to avoid pressure upon the heel.

In order for the cast to dry, there must be provision for evaporation by exposure to circulating air. A hair dryer can be used to provide warm moving air; this is particularly helpful when wet, humid weather delays drying. Heat from radiant lamps is not advocated because it can cause severe burns beneath the cast. Cradles equipped with electric bulbs are not recommended unless there is also provision for free circulation of air; moisture-laden air becomes trapped under the cradle and delays the drying process. The cast should not be covered with bed linen until it is dry. Therefore, the bed must be made in such a way that the cast is exposed but the patient kept warm and free from drafts. Blankets should be used to protect body parts not encased in plaster.

The patient in a body cast should be turned to ensure uniform drying of the cast, to prevent continuous pressure on any one area while the cast is drying, and to make him more comfortable. The time of the first turning will depend upon the physician's order, and the nurse should have assistance to give the patient and the cast maximum support. The patient is then usually turned every four hours. He should always be turned toward the uninjured side; the side of the body with the fracture must always be uppermost when the patient is turned. The cast must be very carefully handled and supported until it is completely dry.

To protect body and long leg casts from becoming soiled or wet, waterproof material should be applied around the perineal area. Continuous dampening will soften the cast and impair its effectiveness, and a soiled cast lining will irritate the patient's skin and cause an offensive odor. The area can be covered with plastic material, oiled silk, or waxed paper, which can be anchored with adhesive or cellophane tape and changed as necessary. Shellac and varnish protect the entire cast from staining and soiling but should not be applied until the cast is completely dry. If the cast becomes dirty, it can be cleaned with a damp cloth and an abrasive or scouring powder. Soap and water cannot be used because their continued use may soften the plaster.

Old stockings or stockinette can be used to cover the cast to protect it from soiling and from moisture. Mold may form on a damp cast. When this happens, the cast is usually thoroughly dried, reinforced with fresh plaster, and dried again.

Care of the patient in the cast. After the patient has been carefully transferred into bed and the cast is supported on pillows, the nurse should check the patient's general condition. If he has had an anesthetic, he must be watched carefully until vital signs are normal (p. 193). After reduction and immobilization, he should be observed for signs of *delayed shock* such as sudden faintness, dizziness, pallor, diaphoresis, or change in pulse rate. Medication, if ordered, should be given for *general pain*. Complaints of *pressure* may be relieved by elevating the extremity or changing the patient's position. However, if the patient complains of continuous pressure that is unrelieved by change of position, it should be reported to the physician. It may be possible to relieve pressure by cutting out small edges of the cast, or it may be necessary to bivalve all or part of the cast. Areas of pressure are usually over the instep, the lateral border of the foot, heel, malleoli, iliac crests, and sacrum. Changes in skin color should also be observed carefully since they, too, indicate that pressure may be restricting circulation.

The skin below the cast should be inspected frequently and routinely for signs of *circulatory impairment*. There may be swelling and slow return of color after pressure has been applied to the fingers or the toes below the cast. The skin also may be cold or cyanotic. The patient may complain of tightness of the cast and of numbness or tingling of the fingers or toes. These signs and symptoms should be reported to the doctor immediately so that the cast can be divided to relieve constriction if necessary. Most swelling occurs within the first twenty-four to forty-eight hours. Interference with circulation is usually caused by a tight cast or by edema. Occasionally it is caused by bruising of a blood vessel during manipulation or surgery.

Compression of a nerve can also occur. The nerve most often affected is the peroneal nerve which is located below the head of the fibula on the lateral side of the leg. Continuous pressure on this superficial nerve by a leg cast results in paralysis, with a loss of the ability to dorsiflex the foot or to extend the toes. The patient's complaint of pressure on the lateral side of the leg or of numbness and tingling in the foot must always be reported to the physician at once since pressure must be relieved immediately. This is often done by bivalving the cast.

Plaster on the skin should be removed with plain water. The skin around and directly under the cast edges should be washed and then massaged with alcohol or cream to prevent skin irritation. The skin should also be inspected for pressure areas and signs of irritation from rough plaster edges. As the patient remains in the cast, his elbows may become irritated from bracing himself to move about in bed. Frequent massage and protective pads help, but probably the best thing, if the patient is able to use one, is to provide him with a Balkan frame and crossbar so that he may lift himself.

If the patient is in a body cast or a long leg cast, the head of the bed should be elevated when a bedpan is used. If the cast is new and still damp, it is better to elevate the head of the bed on shock blocks instead of using the gatch, which will put a strain on the cast and may cause it to crack. A pillow should be placed against the small of the back, and a cotton pad protected with plastic material may be tucked under the sacral area to protect the cast from soiling. The leg in the cast should be supported with pillows so that the patient does not feel insecure in this position. An overhanging trapeze will permit him to help lift himself as the nurse places the bedpan under him. Side rails also assist the patient to turn and give him protection from falling out of bed.

Many patients are discharged after the cast is dry if there is no evidence of circulatory or nerve impairment. If a cast is applied to the arm, the patient should wear a sling to support the full weight of the cast, and the hand should be supported to prevent wristdrop from developing. The ends of the sling should be secured with two pins instead of being tied at the back of the neck. If the sling is to be worn for some time, sling ties may be lengthened with bandage or muslin so that they can be crossed in the back and brought around and tied in the front of the body. This helps to prevent forward and downward pull on the neck, which may cause postural defect and fatigue. A member of the patient's family should be taught how to apply the sling correctly.

If a cast is applied to the leg, the patient usually must not bear weight on the cast. If weight-bearing is permitted, the cast is usually fitted with a piece of iron (walking iron), which prevents wear on the plaster. This lengthens the limb and causes the awk-

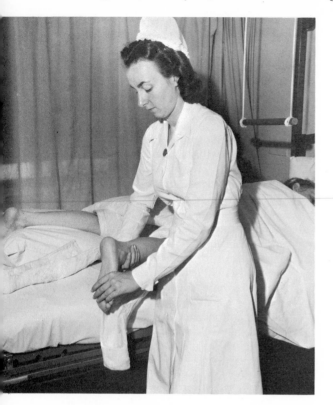

Fig. 230

Use of a bivalved cast permits removal
of the extremity to give care and exercise.
(From Newton, Kathleen, and Anderson, Helen
C.: Geriatric nursing, ed. 4, St. Louis, 1966,
The C. V. Mosby Co.)

ward posture, but its use is usually only
temporary and the patient progresses to the
use of crutches when the cast is removed (p.
394).

Cast removal. The cast is usually removed
when roentgenograms show that union is
sufficient to allow safe removal. This is often
done in the doctor's office or in the hospital
outpatient or emergency departments. The
cast is bivalved with manual or electric plaster cutters. While the procedure is not painful, the patient may feel some pressure or
vibration. The skin is usually dry and scaly
and should be washed with mild soap and
water and lubricated with mineral oil. Since
there is usually some stiffness of the joints,
the limb should be moved very gently. (See

Fig. 230.) The patient is usually encouraged
to move the limb as much as he is able
within limits of pain or stiffness. Exercises
for the stiff joint are usually started. After
a leg cast is removed, swelling and edema
occur for some time when the leg is placed
in a dependent position. The patient is usually advised by his doctor to sleep with the
limb elevated and to elevate it at intervals
during the day. Elastic bandages or stockings
may be prescribed by the physician to help
prevent dependent edema.

Traction

Continuous traction, or pull, is used to
reduce and immobilize fractures, to overcome muscle spasm, and to stretch adhesions
and correct certain deformities.

Skin traction. Skin traction is achieved by
applying wide bands of moleskin or adhesive
directly to the skin and attaching weights
to these. The pull of the weights is transmitted indirectly to the involved bone.
Buck's extension, Bryant's traction, and *Russell traction* are the three most common forms
of skin traction used for injury to the lower
extremities.

Buck's extension is the simplest and provides for straight pull on the affected extremity. It is often used to relieve muscle spasm
and to immobilize a limb temporarily, such
as the leg and thigh when a hip fracture has
been sustained by an elderly person and internal fixation is to be done within a short
time. The nurse usually assists the physician
in applying the traction. The skin of the
thigh and leg is usually shaved, and tincture
of benzoin is applied for protection. As physicians differ about the advantages of shaving and applying tincture of benzoin to the
skin, the nurse should check before proceed-
ing with these measures. Adhesive tape or
moleskin is placed on the lateral and medial
aspects of the thigh and leg and secured with
a circular gauze or elastic bandage. The ends
of the tape extending beyond the ankle are
attached to a foot plate or spreader which
is used to prevent pressure on the toes. Rope
is attached to the spreader, passed through
a pulley on a crossbar at the foot of the
bed, and suspended with weights. (See Fig.
231.) The foot of the bed may be ordered
elevated to provide for countertraction.

Bryant's traction, which is skin traction ap-

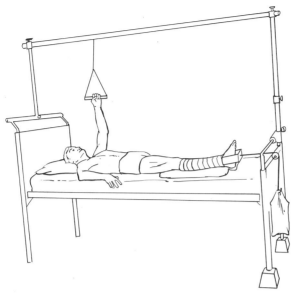

Fig. 231

Buck's extension. Note that the limb is not raised but lies parallel with the bed.
Note also the blocks to raise the foot of the bed to provide countertraction
and to help keep the patient from moving to the foot of the bed.

plied to both lower limbs, can be used to reduce fractures of the femur in children under 6 years of age. Both lower limbs are suspended vertically from a Balkan (overbed) frame. This kind of traction is not used for patients over 6 years of age because the countertraction (weight of the trunk) is not sufficient and because the position hampers arterial circulation to the feet.

Russell traction is widely used because it permits the patient to move about in bed somewhat freely and permits bending of the knee joint. This is skin traction in which four pulleys are used. A Balkan (overbed) frame must be attached to the bed before the procedure is started. Moleskin or adhesive is then applied to the leg as in Buck's extension. The knee is suspended in a hammock or sling to which a rope is attached. This rope is directed upward to a pulley which has been placed on the Balkan frame at a point located over the tubercle of the tibia of the affected extremity. The rope is then passed downward through a pulley on a crossbar at the foot of the bed, back through a pulley on the foot plate, back

again to another pulley on the crossbar, and then suspended with weights. Because there is double pull from the crossbar to the footplate the traction is equal to approximately double the amount of weight used. (See Fig. 232.) Since there is upward pull from the hammock, skin under the popliteal space should be protected with a piece of felt or sponge rubber and should be inspected regularly. The patient's heel should just clear the bed so that there is no weight or pressure on the heel. Usually a pillow is placed lengthwise under the thigh, and a second pillow is placed under the leg. This traction results in slight flexion of the hip. The angle between the thigh and the bed should be approximately 20 degrees. Usually the foot of the bed is elevated on blocks to provide countertraction. Any complaints of pain or discomfort should be reported to the doctor at once. Occasionally thrombophlebitis develops from inactivity and from pressure on the popliteal vessels. Often the patient is permitted to have the head of the bed elevated slightly, but as elevation of the head of the bed does reduce the amount

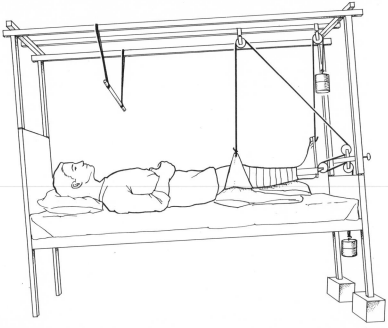

Fig. 232

Russell traction. Note that the Balkan frame is attached to the bed, that the leg is supported on pillows and the heel extends beyond the pillow.

of the traction, the nurse should check with the physician about the amount of elevation permitted. Russell traction is widely used in treatment of aged persons with fractures since it is relatively comfortable for most patients.

Skeletal traction. Skeletal traction is applied directly to the bone. The skin and periosteum are anesthetized with procaine hydrochloride, or general anesthesia may be used. Under the strictest of aseptic precautions, a rustless *Steinmann pin* or *Kirschner wire* is inserted directly through the bone fragment distal to the fracture and out through the skin on the opposite side of the limb. (See Fig. 233.) The ends of the pin or wire are protected with cork, and small sterile dressings are placed around the points of entry and exit. These must be watched for signs of local infection, and care must be taken that they do not become wet or soiled. A metal U-shaped spreader is then attached to the wire or pin, and weights are attached to the spreader. A cast may be applied to

immobilize the extremity when Steinmann pins or Kirschner wires and traction are used to reduce a fracture. Skeletal traction can be used for fractures of the tibia, femur, humerus, and neck or cervical spine. Skeletal traction to the cervical spine is achieved by use of *Crutchfield tongs* applied to the skull. (See p. 905.)

Balanced traction. When a balanced or suspension apparatus is used in conjunction with skin or skeletal traction, the patient is able to move about in bed more freely without disturbing the line of traction. The extremity is balanced with countertraction, and any slack in the traction caused by the patient's movement is taken up by the suspension apparatus. The use of balanced traction also facilitates nursing measures such as bathing the patient, caring for his skin, and placing the bedpan correctly.

A full or half-ring Thomas or Hodgen splint is used for balanced traction. Straps of canvas or muslin are placed over the splint and secured to provide a support for the leg.

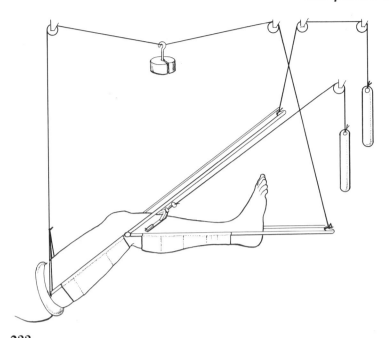

Fig. 233

Balanced traction used in conjunction with skeletal traction.

The areas under the popliteal space and heel are left open to prevent pressure on these parts. If it is desirable to have the knee flexed and to permit movement of the lower leg, a Pearson attachment is clamped or fixed at the level of the knee to the Thomas splint. It is also covered with muslin or canvas to support the lower leg. A Balkan (over-bed) frame is placed on the bed. The leg is put through the ring and placed on the canvas support. The ring is placed firmly against the ischium. When a half-ring is used, the ring is placed on the anterior aspect of the thigh. Rope is attached to the ring or to the frame on either side of the ring and to the end of the Thomas splint, directed upward to pulleys on the frame, and then suspended with weights. Rope is also attached to the end of the Pearson attachment, directed upward to a pulley on the overbed frame, and suspended with weights. (See Fig. 233.) A foot support may be fastened to the Pearson attachment to prevent foot drop, or the foot is left free so that the patient can exercise it more fully. Skin or skeletal traction is applied as described earlier.

The ring is made of smooth, soft plastic material that is moisture resistant. It is not necessary to wrap the ring with padding. The padding cannot be changed after it is applied and inevitably gets damp from perspiration, bedpan accidents, and bathing the skin. The padding holds moisture against the skin and causes skin irritations. When bathing the patient, the skin beneath the ring must be moved back and forth so that all areas are washed and dried thoroughly. The patient may be turned toward the leg in the splint.

Nursing care of the patient in traction. Before the nurse attempts to give care to a patient in traction, she must know the nature of the patient's difficulty and what is to be achieved by the use of traction. Any deviation from the basic rules for care of any patient in traction must be approved by the doctor before it is permitted. For example, the patient with arthritis may be permitted to partially release traction by sitting upright for a few moments whereas the patient with a fresh fracture of the femur might harm himself by doing this.

In order for traction to be effective, the patient must lie on his back. Turning onto the side or sitting up changes body alignment, and the pull (traction) is lost or becomes less effective. The nurse should explain this to the patient and help him to be as comfortable as possible while remaining in the correct position. The patient who must lie flat often feels handicapped and helpless because he cannot readily see what is going on about him; changing the position of the bed sometimes helps.

The nurse must be certain that the *weights hang free* with no obstruction to interfere with straight, even, continuous pull. Traction should be inspected frequently. For example, when traction is being applied to the lower limb, bedclothes must not be pressing on the rope or against the footplate. The footplate must never be pushing against the foot of the bed or the pulley, since this will completely negate traction. There should be no knots in the rope, since these may become caught in the pulley and interfere with traction. The rope should be long enough so that weights will not be hampered by the pulley as the patient pulls himself up in bed, yet not long enough to rest on the floor if he slips to the foot of the bed. The rope must be strong enough so that it will not break if more weights are added. The weights must be securely fastened so that they will not drop off if they are disturbed accidentally, and the equipment should be visible so that it is not jarred or swung inadvertently. Sandbags are often used for weights and are tied to the rope. When regular scale weights are used, they should be fastened with adhesive tape so that they will not slip off. Jarring the bed and swinging the weights may cause pain and are upsetting to the patient.

An important concept in the care of the patient in traction is that the patient should not suffer from lack of any kind of nursing care because of his immobilization. At first glance it might sometimes appear that good back care, for example, is impossible. This is not true. The patient in traction should be on a firm bed and should have a Balkan frame or overhead attachment so that he can help to lift himself and take some weight off his back for short periods. Usually he can be moved enough for good back care to be given and for linen to be changed. This is accomplished by having the patient raise himself straight up in bed with the help of

the trapeze while care is given and the bed linen slid under him. Depending upon the site and the extent of the fracture, the doctor may permit the patient to turn toward the side of the fracture enough for back care to be given. (See Fig. 234.) It is a good practice for a second nurse or an attendant to steady the traction and even increase the pull slightly as the patient carefully and steadily turns or raises himself. The same principles are followed when the patient has the bedpan placed under him. A very small, flat bedpan should be used, and the back above the pan should be supported by a small pillow or a bath blanket folded to the correct height.

The patient who is in traction needs the same attention to nutrition, elimination, exercise of noninvolved extremities, prevention of postural defects, and skin care as any other patient who is immobilized. Particular attention must be given to the skin that comes into contact with any traction apparatus. For example, the skin over bony hip prominences may become reddened and painful if a pelvic band is being used, adhesive tape may work downward and straps may rub against the ankle malleolus when skin traction is used on the lower limb, and a Thomas splint may cause injury to the skin of the groin. Skin irritation of this kind must be reported to the doctor, who may alter the amount of weight used or take other action.

General nursing care of a patient immobilized with a fracture

Nursing care during the time of immobilization includes prevention of complications and maintenance of general health. The patient whose activity is limited by a fracture usually has digestive and elimination problems. Appetite may be poor, yet the body requirements must be met if repair is to progress normally. The diet should be high in protein, iron, calcium, and vitamins. It should also be high in roughage since constipation is often a real problem which causes inconvenience and discomfort and may interfere with appetite. The patient who is ambulatory and being cared for at home should be encouraged to eat plenty of uncooked green vegetables and fresh fruits. The patient in the hospital may be permitted to have relatives bring such foods to him if

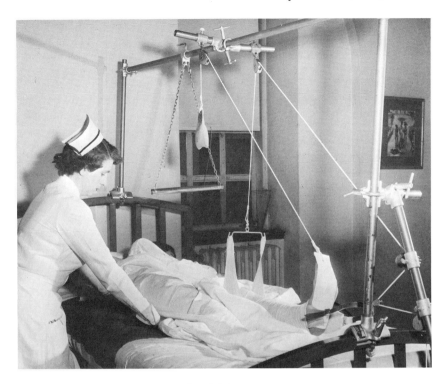

Fig. 234

The patient may turn slightly when Russell traction is used. Note the hammock under the knee, the placement of the four pulleys, and the apparatus used to prevent foot drop.

the hospital menu is somewhat limited in uncooked vegetables and fresh fruits.

Thrombosis and embolism, and muscle and joint changes, with resultant deformity or limitation of function, are possible complications when a patient is immobilized in the treatment of a fracture. It is a nursing responsibility to see that the patient does deep-breathing exercises and exercises his good limbs by means of muscle setting, resistive exercises, or other exercises depending on his particular circumstances. Because of the complex arrangement of muscle attachments and because of muscle action, the nurse needs specific orders from the surgeon before assisting or encouraging the patient to exercise the involved limb. A safe rule is never, under any circumstances, have the patient move or use the joint either immediately distal to or immediately proximal to the fracture unless there is an order permitting this. For example, if the fracture is in the radius, the wrist and elbow joints should not be moved without an order. However, the shoulder can and should be protected from muscle weakness, muscle shortening, and joint changes by regular motion and ex-

ercise. The legs, trunk, and unaffected upper limb should be checked regularly (at least daily) to be certain that the patient is doing some systematic routine exercises.

The patient who must remain in bed for a long period of time in traction or in a cast should be in a bed with a firm mattress, and a fracture board should be placed under the mattress. The patient should, from the beginning of his confinement, pay particular attention to his posture. The lumbar curve in the back can be supported by small pillows or a bath towel or rolled bath blanket. The unaffected foot (or feet) should rest against a footboard at least part of the day. This helps to maintain the foot in the normal walking position, prevents the weight of bedclothes from contributing to foot drop, and provides something firm against which the patient can do resistive foot exercises. The patient should be taught to check the position of his lower limb when at rest. He should "toe in" to prevent external rotation of the hip and pronation of the foot which cause serious difficulty when walking is resumed.

The patient's skin should be inspected for pressure areas or signs of other irritation. In caring for patients who are immobilized for a long time, there should be a regular schedule (such as weekly for cutting the nails) for giving special attention to the skin, for turning and massage, and for cleansing areas such as the perineum. Urinary output should be measured and observed at intervals since the patient who is immobilized for a time may develop urinary retention and renal calculi.

The patient with a fracture who is confined to bed should do full range-of-joint exercises for all unaffected joints daily (Figs. 2 to 4). If he is to eventually use crutches, he should practice push-up exercises or other resistive exercises to strengthen the triceps muscle. These can be done, for example, when the patient in a body cast is turned on his abdomen; the patient in traction and in a back-lying position can straighten his elbows while holding weights on his palms.

Patients who have been on bed rest for some time should be mobilized gradually. The change of position from a flat to an upright one causes weakness and dizziness. The patient should be prepared for this and should be closely supervised until he can be safely left alone. A *tilt table* is useful since it allows the patient to become accustomed to an upright position before actual standing is attempted. The walker is extremely helpful, particularly for elderly patients, since the seat provides a resting place if they become too tired from standing. Often the walker is useful in preparing the patient to use crutches. With increasing frequency, walkerettes, which can be moved by the patient at his own speed, are being used instead of walkers (Fig. 228).

Before leaving the hospital, the patient should be relatively self-sufficient in getting in and out of bed and in and out of a chair. If he lives alone, he must be able to manage stairs. When he practices getting out of bed in the hospital, the casters should be removed from the hospital bed to lower it and to make it more stable. A visiting nurse

can usually help the patient in his home to adjust to his immediate environment and to supervise his progress. A nursing referral should be sent to the public health nursing agency, so that the visiting nurse will know exactly what the patient may or may not do and what his progress was during hospitalization and at discharge.

Treatment by internal fixation

There are several methods that the surgeon may use in the treatment of fractures by operation, depending upon the nature and location of the injury. He may make an incision directly over the fracture site, align the bone fragments, close the incision, and apply a cast. He may, at the time of the operation, also insert steel wires, plates and screws or nails into or along the bone fragments to secure them before he closes the wound. This is called internal fixation. Depending upon the location of the fracture, a cast may also be required. In other cases, such as fractures of the femur, he may reduce the fracture by closed reduction, make an incision at some point distal to the fracture site, and drive a pin or nail through the bone fragments, using guide wires and roentgenograms to assist him in the correct placement of the metal support.

The steel wires, plates and screws, nails, bolts, and intramedullary nails used for internal fixation are made of stainless steel or Vitallium which are nonirritating metals and can be left in place indefinitely or removed after the fracture is healed. The *Smith-Petersen* nail, the *Neufeld* nail, the *Jewett* nail, the *Austin Moore* pins, or other variations may be used to secure fractures of the head and neck of the femur (Fig. 235). This operation is often referred to as *pinning* of the femur. The intramedullary nail and plating with slotted plates and screws are often used for fractures of the shaft of the femur and the tibia (Fig. 236). Securing the bone fragments by internal fixation until union is complete helps prevent deformities that might occur from the strong pull of muscles and permits the patients to get up in a chair or up on crutches without the fear of disturbing the fracture. Early ambulation is desirable because it helps prevent complications such as pneumonia, urinary abnormalities, and gastric disturbances from developing. These are par-ately following the patient's return from the operating room, he should be watched carefully for signs of shock and hemorrhage. If a cast has been applied, it may be impossible to detect external signs of bleeding for some time, and the blood pressure, pulse, and respiratory rate should be taken at frequent intervals until they have become stabilized. Extensive bleeding under a cast will eventually become apparent either as oozing around the edge of the cast or as staining of the cast as blood saturates the damp plaster. Any stain on the cast is marked with pencil, and the time is noted, so that the rate of progress can be noted if bleeding continues. The surgeon usually requests that the extremity

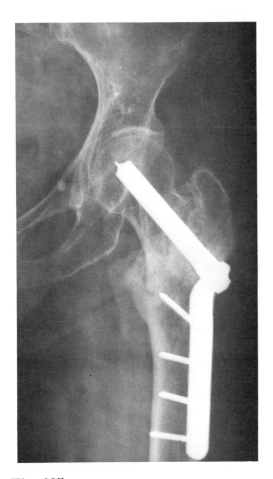

Fig. 235

This roentgenogram shows internal fixation of an intertrochanteric fracture with McLaughlin plate and pins.

ticularly troublesome complications with the older patient.

General nursing care of patients with internal fixation

Preoperative care. When an operation is planned for the treatment of the fracture, the skin is carefully prepared, and the greatest care is taken not to cut the skin or cause even minor abrasions. Bone infection is a serious complication; surgery is delayed and other methods of reduction and immobilization are used if there are lacerations, abrasions, or extensive ecchymosis about the area of the fracture.

Immediate postoperative care. Immedi-

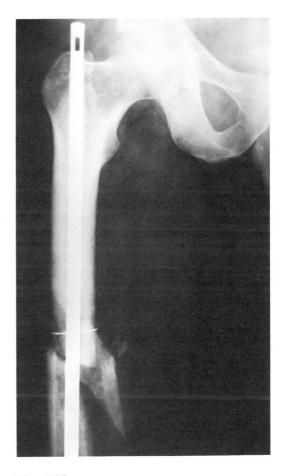

Fig. 236

Internal fixation of fracture of middle third of femur by means of an intramedullary nail (Kirschner nail).

in a cast be elevated on a pillow and that an ice bag be placed on the cast over the fracture site. The nurse should check the circulation of the area below the cast and report any signs of coldness, pallor, cyanosis, or swelling. The other nursing care required is that of any postoperative patient.

Nursing care of patients following operations on the head of the femur. Because the nurse will have many occasions to care for patients who have had a fractured hip pinned, the nursing care of these patients will be discussed in some detail. Casts are not usually applied after the pinning of a hip, and the dressing can be inspected frequently for bleeding. The linen under the patient should also be inspected to be sure that blood has not oozed from under the dressing and down the side of the thigh. Pain usually is severe postoperatively and the patient generally requires narcotics for pain and sedatives for sleep. As these patients are frequently aged women, the nurse needs to give drugs discriminately to prevent too much depression of respirations and activity. The older patient may become confused, particularly when barbiturates have been given. Precautions such as the use of side rails should be taken to prevent falls and further injuries. Side rails also are a help to the patient in moving about in bed.

A patient who has had his hip pinned may be turned for back care the evening of the operation. Although lying on the operative site may be uncomfortable and cause apprehension, the patient can be turned to either side. When turning the patient to the operative side, the nurse should stand on the side of the bed, reach across the patient, place her hands on the opposite hip and shoulder, and gently roll him toward her. When the patient is turned to the unaffected side, the fractured limb should be kept at the same level as the trunk. To prevent the affected hip from rotating externally when the patient is lying on his back, a trochanter roll should be placed gently but firmly against the outer aspect of the hip and upper thigh.

If there are no contraindications, the patient is usually permitted to be up in a chair the morning following surgery. As there can be no weight bearing on the affected extremity for six months, the patient is lifted or assisted to the chair. The extremity is kept elevated to prevent edema and discoloration.

Exercise of the affected extremity should be initiated as early as possible. The nurse should consult with the surgeon regarding the desirable exercises for the affected limb as well as the exercises necessary to prepare the patient for crutch walking. (See p. 392.) Often the physical therapist is needed to help with this. As most of the patients with hip fracture are in the older age group, progress with crutch walking is slow, and the ability to use crutches may be hampered by poor sight and physical limitations. Each patient will need to be observed carefully, and plans for discharge to the family or a nursing home will depend upon the help and facilities needed and available.

References and selected readings*

1 Beeson, Paul B., and McDermott, Walsh: Cecil-Loeb textbook of medicine, ed. 11, Philadelphia, 1963, W. B. Saunders Co.

2 Committee on Trauma of American College of Surgeons: An outline of the treatment of fractures, ed. 8, Philadelphia, 1965, W. B. Saunders Co.

3 Conwell, H. Earle, and Reynolds, Fred C.: Key and Conwell's management of fractures, dislocations, and sprains, St. Louis, 1961, The C. V. Mosby Co.

4 Donaldson, John S., and Williams, Mary Edna: Replacement arthroplasties of the hip and nursing care, Am. J. Nursing 55:566-568, May 1955.

5 Francis, Sister Maria: Nursing the patient with internal hip fixation, Am. J. Nursing 64:111-112, May 1964.

6 Kerr, Avice: Orthodepic nursing procedures, New York, 1959, Springer Publishing Co., Inc.

7 *Larson, Carroll B., and Gould, Marjorie L.: Fractures of the hip and nursing care of the patient with a fractured hip, Am. J. Nursing 58:1558-1563, Nov. 1958.

8 Larson, Carroll B., and Gould, Marjorie L.: Calderwood's orthopedic nursing, ed. 6, St. Louis, 1965, The C. V. Mosby Co.

9 Lonergan, Robert C.: Osteoporosis of the spine, Am. J. Nursing 61:79-81, Jan. 1961.

10 *Mayo, Richard A., and Hughes, Joanne M.: Intramedullary nailing of long bone fractures and nursing care after intramedullary nailing, Am. J. Nursing 59:236-240, Feb. 1959.

11 Neufeld, Alonzo J.: Surgical treatment of hip injuries, Am. J. Nursing 65:80-83, March 1965.

12 Schmeisser, Gerhard, J.: A clinical manual of orthopedic traction techniques, Philadelphia, 1963, W. B. Saunders Co.

13 Wiebe, Anne M.: Orthopedics in nursing, Philadelphia, 1961, W. B. Saunders Co.

14 *Wilde, Delphine: Traction and suspension, Am. J. Nursing 53:1465-1468, Dec. 1953.

*References preceded by an asterisk are particularly well suited for student reading.

Index

Index

Index

Index

Burette test
  biliary system, 724
  ureteral stricture, 455
"Burn bed," 795
"Burn pack," 794
Burns
  accidental, in home, 789
  in atomic bombing, first-aid treatment, 262
  causes and classification, 788
  chemical, of esophagus, 644
  dressings and soaks, 796
  emergency care, 789-790
  emotional aspects, 800-801
  exposure method of treatment, 794-796
  local treatment and general care, 793-797
  long-term problems and rehabilitation, 801
  medical treatment and nursing care, 791-801
  nursing observation of patient, 792-793
  occlusive dressings, 793-794
  prevention of contractures, 798-800
  severe, physiologic changes, 790
  silver nitrate treatment, 796
  skin grafting, 796-797
Bursitis, 932
"Butterfly" adhesive strips for laceration of forearm, 263

C

Caffeine in peripheral vascular disease, 371
Caisson disease, 83
Calcium
  deficit, 100
  excess, 100
  oxalate, urinary calculi due to, 460
  and tooth formation, 617
Calculi
  bladder, 467
  renal, 456-460
Caldwell-Luc operation, 591
Callus in fracture healing, 940
Calluses, 786
Caloric needs
  basic, 87
  variations in, 115
Caloric test for Ménière's syndrome, 610
Caloric testing of equilibrium, 864
Calories, obesity and, 122
Cancer; see also Carcinoma
  alkylating agents for, 288-289
  antimetabolites for, 288
  breast; see Breast carcinoma
  of cervix, 508
    radiation therapy, 512
  of colon, 673-674
  control, 274
  cure
    best hope for, 275
    incidence, 270
  cytologic test for, 484-485
  danger signs, seven, 274
  diagnosis, psychologic reactions to, 277, 278
  drugs for, 288, 289
  of esophagus, 644-647
  facilities for education and care, 275-276
  facts, 269-270
  fracture due to, 937

Cancer—cont'd
  of fundus uteri, 508
    radiation therapy, 512
  hormones for, 288
  incidence, 269, 270
  of larynx, 602-604
  of lips, 624
  of lung, prevention, 273, 274
  in men, common sites, 275
  misconceptions about, 274
  of mouth, 624-629
    prevention, 273
  and the nurse, 267
  nursing care, general, 276-278
  of ovary, 509
  of penis, 523
  plastic surgery following surgical treatment, 212
  possible cause, 272
  prevention, 273-274
  of prostate gland, 521-523
  quack cures, 275
  radiotherapy and, 281-288
  of rectum, 689-691
  research, 272
  of sex organs, increased predisposition with onset of climacteric, 480
  signs and symptoms, 274-275
  skin
    lesions causing, 786-787
    prevention, 273
  status chart, leading sites, table, 268-269
  of stomach, 660-661
  surgical treatment, 278
  term and definition, 271
  terminal, of reproductive system, nursing care, 517
  of testicle, 520-521
  of thyroid gland, 733
  of tongue, 624
  uncontrollable, care of patient with, 290-292
  of vulva, 511
  in women, most common sites, 274
Canker sores, 622, 782
Cantor tube for intestinal decompression, 641
Cap for patients after brain operation, 897, 898
Capacity, lung, tests, 536
Capillary fragility test, 402
  in peripheral vascular disease, 377
Capsule and lens, cataract surgery techniques, 838
Carbohydrate
  metabolism
    insulin and, in diabetes mellitus, 742
    liver function tests based on, 699
  replacement, 105
  refined, and dental caries, 618, 619, 620
Carbon dioxide narcosis, 87, 101, 561
Carbon monoxide poisoning, emergency treatment, 254
Carbon tetrachloride, liver damage from, 712
Carbonate in body fluids, 95
Carbonic acid deficit and excess, 101
Carbuncle of kidney, 455
Carbuncles, 72, 780-781
Carcinoma; see also Cancer
  biliary system, 722
  bladder, 469
  breast; see Breast carcinoma

960

Index

Index

Index

Index

Index

Index

Index

Index